SAUNDERS

Q&A REVIEW *for the*
NCLEX-RN®
EXAMINATION

Linda Anne Silvestri, PhD, RN, FAAN

Nursing Instructor
University of Nevada, Las Vegas
Las Vegas, Nevada

President and Owner
Nursing Reviews, Inc.
Henderson, Nevada

Director and Owner
Professional Nursing Seminars, Inc.
Henderson, Nevada

Elsevier
Next Generation NCLEX® (NGN) Consultant and Subject
Matter Expert

Angela Elizabeth Silvestri, PhD, APRN, FNP-BC, CNE

Associate Professor and *Associate Dean for Entry and Prelicensure Education*
University of Nevada, Las Vegas
Las Vegas, Nevada

President
Nurse Prep, LLC
Henderson, Nevada

Associate Editors

Eileen H. Gray, DNP, RN, CPNP

Nursing Instructor
University of Nevada, Las Vegas
Las Vegas, Nevada

Consultant
Nursing Reviews, Inc.
Henderson, Nevada

Allison E. Bowser, MEd, BSB

Consultant
Nursing Reviews, Inc.
Henderson, Nevada

ELSEVIER

Elsevier
3251 Riverport Lane
St. Louis, Missouri 63043

Notice

Practitioners and researchers must always rely on their own experience and knowledge in evaluating and using any information, methods, compounds or experiments described herein. Because of rapid advances in the medical sciences, in particular, independent verification of diagnoses and drug dosages should be made. To the fullest extent of the law, no responsibility is assumed by Elsevier, authors, editors or contributors for any injury and/or damage to persons or property as a matter of products liability, negligence or otherwise, or from any use or operation of any methods, products, instructions, or ideas contained in the material herein.

Content Strategist: Heather Bays-Petrovic
Director of Content Development: Laurie Gower
Senior Content Development Specialist: Rebecca Leenhouts
Publishing Services Manager: Julie Eddy
Senior Project Manager: Cindy Thoms
Senior Book Designer: Maggie Reid

Printed in India

Last digit is the print number: 9   8   7   6   5   4   3   2   1

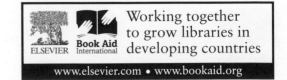

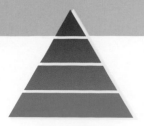

About the Authors

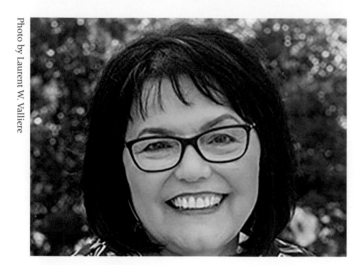

Photo by Laurent W. Valliere

Linda Anne Silvestri

Linda is a well-known author, nurse educator, entrepreneur, and philanthropist whose professional aspirations focus on assisting nursing students to become successful. She has been teaching at all levels of nursing education for many years. Linda is currently a nursing instructor and nursing course developer at the University of Nevada, Las Vegas (UNLV). She earned her PhD in Nursing from UNLV and conducted research on self-efficacy and the predictors of NCLEX® success.

Her research findings are published in the *Journal of Nursing Education and Practice.*

Dr. Silvestri has received several awards and honors. In 2019 she was inducted as a Fellow in the American Academy of Nursing. In 2012 she received the UNLV School of Nursing Alumna of the Year Award. And in 2010 she received the School of Nursing's Certificate of Recognition for Outstanding PhD Student. Linda is a member of several national nursing organizations, including the Honor Society of Nursing, Sigma Theta Tau International, the National League for Nursing, the America Nurses Association, Phi Kappa Phi, the Western Institute of Nursing, and the Golden Key International Honour Society. Additionally, she is a Fellow in the American Academy of Nursing and will be inducted as a Fellow in the National League for Nursing Academy of Nursing Education in the Fall of 2023. Dr. Silvestri is the successful Elsevier author of numerous best-selling national and international NCLEX® preparation resources. She is also co-author of *Strategies for Student Success on the Next Generation NCLEX® (NGN)* and serves as an Elsevier Thought Leader and Subject Matter Expert for the Next Generation NCLEX® (NGN). Linda has presented numerous faculty and student webinars on NCLEX® and NGN preparation and success. She is the President and Owner of Nursing Reviews, Inc., and Director and Owner of Professional Nursing Seminars, Inc. Both companies are dedicated to helping nursing students and graduates achieve their goals of becoming licensed nurses.

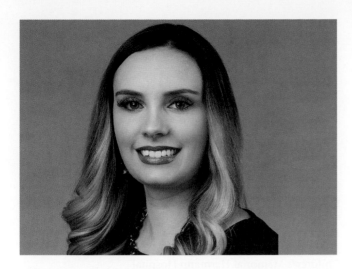

Angela Elizabeth Silvestri

Angela is a well-known nurse educator, researcher, and author. She has been teaching and working in university administrative roles for many years at all levels of nursing education. She has experience teaching in classroom and clinical settings and in working with graduate students on their culminating projects and research dissertations. She currently serves as the Associate Dean for Entry and Prelicensure Education at the University of Nevada, Las Vegas (UNLV). Dr. Silvestri is a successful Elsevier author of numerous best-selling NCLEX® preparation resources on the national and international levels. She also serves as an Elsevier Subject Matter Expert for the Next Generation NCLEX® (NGN).

Angela earned her bachelor's degree in nursing and in sociology from Salve Regina University in Newport, Rhode Island; she earned her master's degree with a focus in nursing education and her PhD from the University of Nevada, Las Vegas. She also has a post-master's graduate certificate in advanced practice and is a board-certified family nurse practitioner. She is a scholar in Sigma Theta Tau's New Academic Leadership Academy. Dr. Silvestri is passionate about college students' success. She works with faculty, staff, and students on managing primary and episodic health care needs at UNLV's Student Wellness Center and Faculty and Staff Treatment Center as a family nurse practitioner. This passion also comes through in her work at the School of Nursing, where she teaches medical-surgical nursing and pharmacology, and in the publication of her research and best-selling licensure exam review resources at the national and international levels.

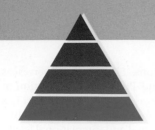

Contributors

CONSULTANTS

Dianne E. Fiorentino
Research Coordinator
Nursing Reviews, Inc.
Henderson, Nevada

Karen Hoem
Editorial and Reviewer Consultant
Nurse Prep, LLC
Henderson, Nevada

Katherine M. Silvestri, MSN, APRN, FNP-BC
Family Nurse Practitioner
Student Health Center, University of Nevada, Las Vegas
Las Vegas, Nevada
Editorial and Reviewer Consultant
Nursing Reviews, Inc.
Henderson, Nevada

CONTRIBUTORS

Natalie Filer, BSN, RN
Level IV Neonatal Intensive Care Unit Nurse
Children's Memorial Hermann Hospital
Houston, Texas

James Guibault Jr., BS, PharmD
Clinical Pharmacist
Orlando, Florida
Pharmacology Consultant
Nursing Reviews, Inc.
Henderson, Nevada

Madison Drew Mahon, BSN, RN
Neonatal ICU Registered Nurse
St. Luke's of Nampa Idaho
Nampa, Idaho

Laurent W. Valliere, BS, DD
Vice President
Nursing Reviews, Inc.,
Henderson, Nevada

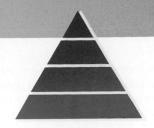

Preface

"Success is climbing a mountain, facing the challenge of obstacles, and reaching the top of the mountain."

Linda Anne Silvestri, PhD, RN, FAAN

"Success is never an accident. To be successful is to have been perseverate, to have sacrificed, and to have loved what you are cultivating to become successful."

Angela Elizabeth Silvestri, PhD, APRN, FNP-BC, CNE

Welcome to *Saunders Pyramid to Success!*

AN ESSENTIAL RESOURCE FOR TEST SUCCESS

Saunders Q&A Review for the NCLEX-RN® Examination is one in a series of products designed to assist you in achieving your goal of becoming a registered nurse. This text and Evolve site package provide you with more than 6000 practice NCLEX-RN test questions based on the current NCLEX-RN test plan.

The current test plan for the NCLEX-RN identifies a framework based on *Client Needs*. The Client Needs categories include Physiological Integrity, Safe and Effective Care Environment, Health Promotion and Maintenance, and Psychosocial Integrity. *Integrated Processes* are also identified as a component of the test plan. These include Caring, Clinical Judgment, Communication and Documentation, Culture and Spirituality, Nursing Process, and Teaching and Learning. This book has been uniquely designed and includes chapters that describe each specific component of the NCLEX-RN test plan framework and five practice tests that contain NCLEX-style questions specific to each component.

NCLEX-RN® TEST PREPARATION

This book begins with information regarding NCLEX-RN preparation. **Chapter 1,** *Clinical Judgment and the NCLEX-RN® Examination,* addresses information about clinical judgment and the related cognitive processes/skills as defined by the National Council of State Boards of Nursing (NCSBN) and all of the information related to the NCLEX-RN test plan and the examination testing procedures. This chapter answers all of the questions that you may have regarding this information.

Chapter 2, *Self-Efficacy and Profiles to Success,* discusses the NCLEX-RN from a nonacademic viewpoint and emphasizes a holistic approach for your individual test preparation. This chapter discusses self-efficacy, the components of a structured study plan, anxiety-reducing techniques, and personal focus

issues. Nursing students also want to hear what other students have to say about their experiences with the NCLEX-RN and what it is really like to take this examination. **Chapter 3,** *The NCLEX-RN® Examination: A Graduate's Perspective,* is a story of success written by a nursing graduate who recently took the NCLEX-RN and addresses the issue of what the examination is all about.

Chapter 4, *Clinical Judgment and Test-Taking Strategies,* includes information about using clinical judgment and the six cognitive processes/skills to answer questions and all of the strategies that will assist in teaching you how to read a question, how not to read into a question, and how to use the process of elimination and various other strategies to select the correct response from the options presented.

CLIENT NEEDS

Chapters 5 through **9** address the NCLEX-RN test plan component, *Client Needs.* **Chapter 5,** *Client Needs and the NCLEX-RN® Test Plan* describes each category of Client Needs as identified by the test plan and lists any subcategories, the percentage of test questions for each category, and some of the content included on the NCLEX-RN. **Chapters 6** through **9** contain practice test questions related specifically to each category of Client Needs. **Chapter 6** comprises questions related to Physiological Integrity; **Chapter 7** contains questions dealing with Safe and Effective Care Environment; **Chapter 8** is made up of questions concerned with Health Promotion and Maintenance; and **Chapter 9** contains Psychosocial Integrity questions.

INTEGRATED PROCESSES

Chapters 10 and **11** address the Integrated Processes as identified in the NCLEX-RN test plan. **Chapter 10,** *Integrated Processes and the NCLEX-RN® Test Plan,* describes each Integrated Process. **Chapter 11** contains practice test questions related specifically to each Integrated Process, including Caring, Communication and Documentation, Culture and Spirituality, Nursing Process, and Teaching and Learning. Clinical Judgment is addressed with practice questions.

SPECIAL FEATURES OF THE BOOK

Book Design

The book is designed with a unique two-column format. The left column presents the practice questions, answer options, and coding areas, while the right column provides the corresponding answers, rationales, priority nursing tips, test-taking strategies, and references. The two-column format makes the review easier because you do not have to flip through pages in search of answers and rationales. A bookmark accompanies this book, and you can use it to hide the right column with the answer section as you are practicing questions.

SPECIAL FEATURES FOUND ON EVOLVE

Pretest and Study Calendar

The accompanying Evolve site contains a pretest that provides you with feedback on your strengths and weaknesses. The results of your pretest will generate an individualized study calendar to guide you in your preparation for the NCLEX examination. A post-test is generated after the pretest is taken and is intended to be completed after using other features of the product.

Heart, Lung, and Bowel Sound Questions

The accompanying Evolve site contains *Audio Questions* representative of content addressed in the current test plan for the NCLEX-RN exam. These questions are in NCLEX-style format, and each question presents an audio sound as a component of the question.

Podcasts

The companion Evolve site includes three *Podcasts*, which cover challenging subject areas under the current NCLEX-RN test plan, including *Pharmacology, Acid-Base Balance,* and *Fluids and Electrolytes.* Information on accessing the podcasts is located in Chapter 4.

NEXT GENERATION NCLEX® (NGN) CASE STUDIES AND NGN TEST QUESTIONS

The accompanying Evolve site contains single-episode case studies and unfolding case studies. These case studies are accompanied by NGN test questions representative of the NGN testing format. The single-episode case studies are accompanied by one NGN test question that measures one of the cognitive processes/skills of the NCSBN Clinical Judgment Measurement Model (NCJMM). The unfolding case studies are accompanied by six NGN test questions, and the questions measure all six cognitive processes/skills of the NCJMM. These cognitive processes/skills include Recognize Cues, Analyze Cues, Prioritize Hypotheses, Generate Solutions, Take Action, and Evaluate Outcomes.

PRACTICE QUESTIONS

Multiple Choice and Alternate Item Format Questions

While preparing for the NCLEX-RN, students need to review practice test questions. This book contains practice questions that are in the multiple choice format or in alternate item test question formats used in the NCLEX-RN examination.

The accompanying Evolve site contains more than 6000 questions: all the questions from the book, plus new questions, including all types of alternate item formats. The alternate item format questions in the book and on the accompanying Evolve site may be presented as one of the following:

- Fill-in-the-blank question
- Multiple response question (select all that apply)
- Prioritizing (ordered response) question
- Figure/illustration question
- Graphic options question, in which each option contains a figure or illustration
- Scenario/exhibit question
- Audio question that includes a heart, lung, or bowel sound
- NGN® Case Studies and NGN test questions

These questions provide you with practice in prioritizing, decision-making and critical thinking, and strengthening your clinical judgment skills. In addition, each practice question provides a review button that links you to common laboratory values for your reference while studying on the Evolve site.

Answer Sections for Practice Questions

Each practice question is accompanied by the correct answer, rationale, priority nursing tip, test-taking strategy, question categories, and reference source. The structure of the answer section is unique and provides the following information for every question:

- **Rationale:** The rationale provides you significant information regarding both correct and incorrect options.
- **Priority Nursing Tip:** The priority nursing tip provides you with an important piece of information that will be helpful to you when answering practice questions and questions on the NCLEX.
- **Test-Taking Strategy:** The test-taking strategy provides a logical path for selecting the correct option and helps you select an answer to a question for which you otherwise might have to guess. In each practice question, the specific strategy that will assist in answering the question correctly is highlighted in bold blue type. The highlighted specific test-taking strategies in the practice questions will guide you on what topics to review for further remediation in *Saunders Clinical Judgment and Test-Taking Strategies: Passing Nursing School and the NCLEX® Exam, Saunders Comprehensive Review for the NCLEX-RN® Exam,* and the *Saunders/HESI Online Review for the NCLEX-RN® Exam.*
- **Question Categories:** Each question on the accompanying Evolve site is identified based on the categories used by the NCLEX-RN test plan. Both Content Area and Health Problem categories are also provided with each question to assist you in identifying areas in need of review. In addition, Priority Concepts codes are included, which provide the specific concept related to nursing practice. This code is especially helpful to students learning in a concept-based curriculum. The categories identified with each question include Level of Cognitive Ability, Client Needs, Clinical Judgment/Cognitive Skill, Integrated Process, Content Area, Health Problem, and Priority Concepts. All categories are identified by their full names so that you do not need to memorize codes or abbreviations.
- **Reference:** The reference source and page number are listed for you so that you can easily find the information you need to review in your undergraduate nursing textbooks.

HOW TO USE THIS BOOK

Saunders Q&A Review for the NCLEX-RN® Examination is specially designed to help you with your successful journey to the peak of the Pyramid to Success: becoming a registered nurse. As you begin your journey through this book, you will be introduced to all of the important points regarding the NCLEX-RN examination, the process of testing, and the unique and special tips regarding how to prepare yourself both academically and nonacademically for this important examination. Read the chapter from the nursing graduate who recently passed the NCLEX-RN and consider what the graduate had to say about the examination. The test-taking strategy chapter will provide you with important strategies that will guide you in applying clinical judgment and selecting the correct option(s). Read this chapter and practice these strategies as you proceed through your journey with this book.

Once you have read the introductory components of this book, it is time to begin the practice questions. As you read through each question and select an answer, be sure to read the rationale, the priority nursing tip, and the test-taking strategy. The rationale provides significant information regarding both the correct and incorrect options. The priority nursing tip provides a piece of important information to remember that will help answer questions on the NCLEX, and the test-taking strategy provides the logic for selecting the correct option. Use the reference source provided so that you can easily find the information you need to review.

CLIMBING THE PYRAMID TO SUCCESS

This step on the *Pyramid to Success* is to get additional practice with a **Q&A review** product. *Saunders Q&A Review for the NCLEX-RN® Examination* offers more than 6000 unique practice questions in the book and on the companion Evolve site. The questions are focused on the Client Needs and Integrated Processes of the NCLEX test plan, making it easy to access your study area of choice.

As you work your way through *Saunders Q&A Review for the NCLEX-RN® Examination* and identify your areas of strength and weakness, you can return to the companion book, *Saunders Comprehensive Review for the NCLEX-RN® Examination,* to focus your study on these areas. The purpose of the *Saunders Comprehensive Review for the NCLEX-RN® Examination* is to provide a **comprehensive review** of the nursing content you will be tested on during the NCLEX-RN examination. However, *Saunders Comprehensive Review for the NCLEX-RN® Examination* is intended to do more than simply prepare you for the rigors of the NCLEX; this book is also meant to serve as a valuable study tool that you can refer to throughout your nursing program, with customizable Evolve site selections to help identify and reinforce key content and health problem areas. Your final step on the Pyramid to Success is to master the **online review.** *HESI/Saunders Online Review for the NCLEX-RN® Examination* provides an interactive and individualized platform to get you ready for your final licensure exam. This online course provides 10 high-level content modules, supplemented with instructional videos and accompanying NGN test items, animations, audio, illustrations, case studies, and several subject matter exams. End-of-module practice tests are provided along with several Crossing the Finish Line: Practice Tests and three Test Yourself Quizzes. In addition, you can assess your strengths and areas in need of improvement with a pretest that generates a study calendar providing guidance on how to proceed through the course and a comprehensive exam in a computerized environment that prepares you for the actual NCLEX-RN exam.

At the base of the Pyramid to Success are our **test-taking strategies,** which provide a foundation for understanding and unpacking the complexities of NCLEX exam questions, including alternate item formats and NGN test items. *Saunders Clinical Judgment and Test-Taking Strategies: Passing Nursing School and the NCLEX® Exam* takes a detailed look at all the test-taking strategies you will need to know to pass any nursing examination, including the NCLEX. Special tips are integrated for nursing students, and there are more than 1200 practice questions included so that you can apply the testing strategies.

To obtain any of these resources that will prepare you for your nursing exams and the NCLEX-RN exam, visit the Elsevier Health Sciences website: www.elsevierhealth.com. You can also visit the Apple App Store and Google Play to locate the app for both this resource and the Saunders Comprehensive Review for the NCLEX-RN® Examination.

Good luck with your journey through the *Saunders Pyramid to Success.* We wish you continued success throughout your new career as a Registered Nurse!

Linda Anne Silvestri, PhD, RN, FAAN
Angela Elizabeth Silvestri, PhD, APRN, FNP-BC, CNE

To All Future Registered Nurses,

Congratulations to you!

You should be very proud of and pleased with yourself for your accomplishments in nursing, as well as for your well-deserved success in completing your nursing program to become a registered nurse. We know you have worked very hard to be successful and that you have proven to yourself that indeed you can achieve your goals.

You are about to enter what is, in our opinion, the most wonderful and rewarding profession. Your willingness, desire, and ability to assist those who need nursing care will bring you great satisfaction. In the profession of nursing, learning is a lifelong process, which makes the profession stimulating and dynamic and ensures that your learning will continue to expand and grow as the profession continues to evolve. Your next very important endeavor will be the learning process needed to achieve success in your examination to become a registered nurse.

We are excited and pleased to be able to provide you with the *Saunders Pyramid to Success* products, which will help you prepare for your next important professional goal: becoming a registered nurse. We want to thank all of our former nursing students whom we have assisted in studying for the NCLEX-RN exam for their willingness to offer ideas for preparing for licensure. Student input certainly is a unique benefit to all of the products available in the *Saunders Pyramid to Success.*

Saunders Pyramid to Success products provide you with everything that you need to ready yourself for the NCLEX-RN exam. These products include material that is required for the NCLEX-RN exam for all nursing students regardless of educational background, specific strengths, areas in need of improvement, or clinical experience during the nursing program.

So let's get started and begin our journey through the *Saunders Pyramid to Success,* and welcome to the wonderful profession of nursing!

Sincerely,

Linda Anne Silvestri, PhD, RN, FAAN

Angela Silvestri, PhD, APRN, FNP-BC, CNE

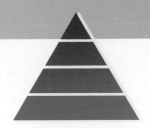

Acknowledgments

A Few Words From Linda

There are many individuals who, in their own ways, have contributed to my success in making my professional dreams become a reality. I extend my sincere appreciation and warmest thanks to all of them.

First, I want to acknowledge my parents, who opened my door of opportunity in education and encouraged and supported me through my profession to work hard to reach my goals. I thank my mother, Frances Mary, for all of her love, support, and assistance as I continuously worked to achieve my professional goals. I thank my father, Arnold Lawrence, who always provided insightful words of encouragement. I miss you both so dearly, and my memories of your love and support will always remain in my heart. I also thank my best friend and the love of my life, my husband, Larry, for always being there for me for whatever I needed; my sister, Dianne Elodia, and her husband, Lawrence, and my brother, Lawrence Peter, and my sister-in-law, Mary Elizabeth, for all their love and continuous support. And I thank all my nieces and nephews, who were continuously supportive, giving, and helpful during my research and preparation of this publication. But I especially want to thank my niece and co-author, Angela, for her love and continuous support and for always being there when I need her.

I want to thank my nursing students at the Community College of Rhode Island who approached me in 1991 and persuaded me to assist them in preparing to take the NCLEX-RN examination. Their enthusiasm and inspiration led to the commencement of my professional endeavors in conducting review courses for the NCLEX-RN exam and writing NCLEX preparation resources for nursing students. I also thank the numerous nursing students who have attended my review courses for their willingness to share their needs and ideas. Their input has certainly added a special uniqueness to this publication.

I wish to acknowledge all of the nursing faculty who taught in my review courses for the NCLEX-RN exam. Their commitment, dedication, and expertise have certainly assisted nursing students in achieving success with the NCLEX-RN exam. Additionally, I want to especially acknowledge my husband, Larry (Laurent W. Valliere), for his contribution to this publication, for teaching in my review courses for the NCLEX-RN exam, and for his commitment and dedication in assisting my nursing students to prepare for the exam from a nonacademic point of view. I also want to extend a very special thank you to my niece, Angela, for joining me in preparing and authoring these NCLEX resources. Angela is so wonderful to work with. Her ideas and her expertise have certainly added to the content of this publication and all of our NCLEX publications. She is dedicated to promoting and ensuring student success. Thank you, Angela! And finally, I again want to thank my husband, Larry, for all of his continuous support as I moved through my personal challenges and professional endeavors; he has been my rock of support!

A Few Words From Angela

There are many people that contributed to my success in my work on this product. I am very grateful for their continued support in all of my endeavors.

First and foremost, I would like to thank my husband, Brent, for his lighthearted and positive attitude. He always knows how to make me laugh, especially when I'm stressed. All of this would not be possible without him!

I would also like to thank my parents, Mary and Larry, for their continued support throughout the years. Their words of encouragement and wisdom have been tremendously important to my success. I also don't know what I would do without their support in caring for my kids!

I would like to thank my sister, Katie, who is a wonderful nurse. Her ambitions as a nursing student are inspiring and remind me every day about why I'm so passionate about being an educator. Thank you to my brother, Nick, who always is positive and encouraging about my work. His wit and sarcasm are always a great way to lift my mood at the end of the day.

I want to extend a special thank you to Linda for her collaboration, guidance, and expertise. Without her, I would not be where I am today. Thank you, Linda!

A Few Words From Both Linda and Angela

We want to thank our Associate Editors, Eileen Gray and Allison Bowser, for all of their dedication and hard work in editing and preparing the entire manuscript for this edition. Their expertise and close attention to detail have certainly added to the quality of this resource. Eileen and Allison, thank you so much!

We also want to acknowledge and thank Laurent W. Valliere for writing a chapter addressing important nonacademic test preparation issues.

In addition, we also sincerely thank Natalie Filer, RN, BSN and Madison Drew Mahon, BSN, RN, for writing a chapter for this book about their experience preparing for and taking the NCLEX-RN examination.

A special thank you and acknowledgment also go to all of the previous contributors who provided contributions to this book. And a very special thank you goes to Katherine Silvestri, MSN, APRN, FNP-BC, CNE, for her work in reviewing, editing, and coding practice questions.

We especially thank Dianne E. Fiorentino for her continuous and endless support and dedication to our work and in her reference support and other secretarial responsibilities for the ninth edition of this book. As well, we thank Karen Hoem for her continuous and endless support and dedication to our work and for all of her expert organizational skills, review, and editing. We thank Jimmy Guibault for reviewing all of the medication questions and providing medication research support.

We sincerely acknowledge and thank some very important and special people from Elsevier. We thank Heather Bays-Petrovic, Content Strategist, for her continuous support, enthusiasm, and expert professional guidance throughout the preparation of this edition. Thank you, Heather—you are the best! We could not have completed this publication without you! A very special thank you goes to Cindy Thoms, Senior Project Manager, for her expert work and for anticipating our needs as we prepared this publication. We worked so closely with Cindy throughout the preparation and publication and could not have done it without her expert help and her support and patience with us. Thank you, Cindy! We also extend a special thank you to Jenny Korte, our copyeditor and proofreader, for her superior work and for paying such close attention to detail in the manuscript. And a very special thank you goes to Rebecca Leenhouts, Senior Content Development Specialist, who provided us with consistent and a tremendous amount of support throughout this publication. Thank you, Rebecca, for maintaining order for all of the work that we submitted for manuscript production.

We want to acknowledge all of the staff at Elsevier for their tremendous help throughout the preparation and production of this publication. A special thanks goes to all of them. We thank Julie Eddy, Publishing Services Manager; Cindy Thoms, Senior Project Manager; and Maggie Reid, Design Direction. You have all played such significant roles in finalizing this publication.

Last, a very special thank you to all our nursing students: past, present, and future. All of you light up our lives! Your love and dedication to the profession of nursing and your commitment to provide health care will bring never-ending rewards!

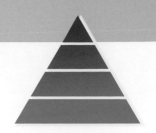

Contents

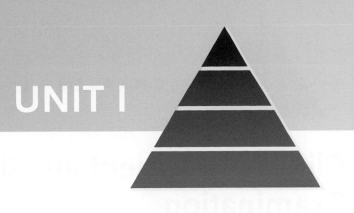

NCLEX-RN® Preparation

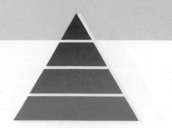

CHAPTER 1

Clinical Judgment and the NCLEX-RN® Examination

The Pyramid to Success

Welcome to *Saunders Q&A Review for the NCLEX-RN® Examination*, the second component of the Pyramid to Success! At this time, you have completed your first path toward the peak of the pyramid with *Saunders Comprehensive Review for the NCLEX-RN® Examination*. Now it is time to continue that journey to become a registered nurse with *Saunders Q&A Review for the NCLEX-RN® Examination*.

As you begin your journey through this book, you will be introduced to all of the important points regarding the NCLEX-RN examination, including the process of testing and unique and special tips for preparing yourself both academically and nonacademically for this important examination. You will read what a nursing graduate who recently passed the NCLEX-RN examination has to say about the test. Important test-taking strategies guide you in selecting the correct option, assist you in making an educated guess if you are not entirely sure about the correct answer, and guide you in ways to answer the Next Generation NCLEX® (NGN) test items. Additionally, the Cognitive Skills presented in the National Council of State Boards of Nursing (NCSBN) Clinical Judgment Measurement Model (NCJMM) are identified in practice questions.

About This Resource

Saunders Q&A Review for the NCLEX-RN® Examination contains more than 6000 NCLEX-style practice questions. Question types include multiple choice; multiple response (select all that apply [SATA]); fill in the blank; prioritizing (ordered response); image ("hot spot") questions; scenario/exhibit questions; graphic options; and audio questions. The Evolve site also includes podcasts for audio review on test-taking strategies for pharmacology, fluids and electrolytes, and acid-base balance. NGN-style questions are also included on the Evolve site. The chapters in the book have been developed to provide a description of the components of the NCLEX-RN test plan, including Client Needs and the Integrated Processes. In addition, chapters have been prepared to contain practice questions specific to each category of Client Needs and the Integrated Processes.

A rationale, priority nursing tip, test-taking strategy, and reference source containing a page number are provided with each question. Each question is coded on the basis of the Level of Cognitive Ability, Client Needs category, Integrated Process, Content Area being tested, Health Problem if applicable, and the Cognitive Skills/Processes of the National Council of State

Boards of Nursing (NCSBN) Clinical Judgment Measurement Model (NCJMM). In addition, two Priority Concepts that relate to the content of the question are identified. This code is helpful specifically for students whose curriculum is concept based. The rationale contains significant information regarding both the correct and incorrect options. The priority nursing tip provides key information to remember about a nursing point. The test-taking strategy maps out a logical path for selecting the correct option, if necessary. The reference source and page number provide easy access to the information that you need to review. The Health Problem code is a unique and helpful feature that allows you to filter and select questions based on a disease process when you are practicing questions on Evolve. For example, if heart failure is your area of interest, you can select "Adult Health, Cardiovascular, Heart Failure" on the Evolve site, and all questions on this content will be generated for practice. Additionally, information about all of the special features of this resource and the question types is located in the preface of this book.

Other Resources in the Saunders Pyramid to Success

There are several other resources in the Saunders Pyramid to Success program. These include the following: The *Saunders Comprehensive Review for the NCLEX-RN® Examination*, *Saunders Clinical Judgment and Test-Taking Strategies: Passing Nursing School and the NCLEX® Exam*, *Strategies for Student Success on the Next Generation NCLEX® (NGN) Test Items*, The HESI/Saunders Online Review for the NCLEX-RN® Examination, *Saunders Q&A Review Cards for the NCLEX-RN® Exam*, and *Saunders RNtertainment for the NCLEX-RN® Examination Review Game*. The HESI® Compass™ Course is also a resource for NCLEX preparation and provides you with an individual coach to guide you in your preparation. Ask your nursing instructors about institutional access to this course.

All of these resources in the Saunders Pyramid to Success are described in the preface of this book and can be obtained online by visiting http://elsevierhealth.com or by calling 1-800-545-2522.

Let's begin our journey through the Pyramid to Success.

Clinical Judgment

⚠ Clinical judgment is the observed outcome of critical thinking and decision-making (Dickison, Haerling, & Lasater, 2019).

In recent years, heightened attention has been paid to clinical judgment as a means of teaching, learning, and assessment and testing. The Next Generation NCLEX-RN examination requires candidates to demonstrate a higher level of ability in applying clinical judgment in the delivery of client care. Clinical judgment can also be used as a test-taking strategy to answer test questions (see Chapter 4). The NCSBN has created a Clinical Judgment Measurement Model (NCJMM) that consists of applying six cognitive skills or processes. These include: (1) recognizing cues; (2) analyzing cues; (3) prioritizing hypotheses; (4) generating solutions; (5) taking actions; and (6) evaluating outcomes (Dickison et al., 2019). Table 1.1 provides a description of these six cognitive skills/processes identified in the NCJMM. The NCJMM also serves as a guide for the NCSBN to create NGN questions. The NGN was launched in April 2023. Scored stand-alone test items (Bowtie and Trend items) and unfolding case studies are presented in the NGN. Some of these NGN item types can be found on the Evolve site accompanying this book, and an example of an NGN item is located in Chapter 4, Box 4.26. We strongly encourage you to frequently access the NCSBN website at https://www.ncsbn.org for updates.

The Examination Process

An important step in the Pyramid to Success is to become as familiar as possible with the examination process. Candidates facing the challenge of this examination can experience significant anxiety. Knowing what the examination is all about and knowing what you will encounter during the process of testing will assist in alleviating fear and anxiety. The information contained in this chapter was obtained from the NCSBN website (http://www.ncsbn.org) and from the NCSBN 2023 test plan for the NCLEX-RN. It includes some procedures related to registering for the examination, testing procedures, and the answers to the questions most commonly asked by nursing students and graduates preparing to take the NCLEX-RN.

TABLE 1.1 Cognitive Skills/Processes and Descriptions

Cognitive Skill/Process	Description
Recognize cues	Identifying significant data; data can be from many sources (assessment)
Analyze cues	Connecting data to the client's clinical presentation—determining if the data is expected? Unexpected? (analysis)
Prioritize hypotheses	Ranking hypotheses; what are the concerns or client needs/problems and their priority? (analysis)
Generate solutions	Using hypotheses or client needs to determine interventions for an expected outcome (planning)
Take actions	Implementing the generated solutions addressing the highest priorities or hypotheses (implementation)
Evaluate outcomes	Comparing observed outcomes with expected ones (evaluation)

From: Dickison, P., Haerling, K.A., & Lasater, K. (2019). Integrating the National Council of State Boards of Nursing Clinical Judgment Model into Nursing Educational Frameworks, *Journal of Nursing Education, 58* (2), 72–78.

You can obtain additional information regarding the test and its development by accessing the NCSBN website and clicking on the NCLEX® & Other Exams tab or by writing to the National Council of State Boards of Nursing, 111 East Wacker Drive, Suite 2900, Chicago, IL 60601. You are encouraged to access the NCSBN website, because this site provides you with valuable information about the NCLEX, the test plan, and other resources available to an NCLEX candidate. You are also encouraged to access the most up-to-date *Candidate Bulletin*. This document provides you with everything you need to know about registration procedures and scheduling a test date.

Computer Adaptive Testing

The acronym *CAT* stands for computerized adaptive test, which means that the examination is created as the test-taker answers each question. All the test questions are categorized on the basis of the test plan structure and the level of difficulty of the question. As you answer a question, the computer determines your competency based on the answer you selected. If you selected a correct answer, the computer scans the question bank and selects a more difficult question. If you selected an incorrect answer, the computer scans the question bank and selects an easier question. This process continues until all test plan requirements are met and a reliable pass-or-fail decision is made.

When you take a CAT, once an answer is recorded, all subsequent questions administered depend, to an extent, on the answer selected for that question. Skipping and returning to earlier questions are not compatible with the logical methodology of a CAT. The inability to skip questions or go back to change previous answers will not be a disadvantage to you; you will not fall into that "trap" of changing a correct answer to an incorrect one with the CAT system.

If you are faced with a question that contains unfamiliar content, you may need to guess at the answer. Although guessing is discouraged when taking any examination, there is no penalty for guessing on the NCLEX. Remember, in almost all of the questions, the answer will be right there in front of you. If you need to guess, use your nursing knowledge, clinical experiences, and clinical judgment skills to their fullest extent and all of the test-taking strategies you have practiced in this review program. Refer to Chapter 4 for information on clinical judgment and test-taking strategies.

You do not need any computer experience to take this examination. A keyboard tutorial is provided and administered to all test-takers at the start of the examination. The tutorial provides instructions for the use of the on-screen optional calculator and the mouse and for recording an answer. The tutorial provides instructions on how to respond to all question types on this examination. This tutorial is on the NCSBN website; you are encouraged to view the tutorial when you are preparing for the NCLEX examination. In addition, at the testing site, a test administrator is present to assist in explaining the use of the computer to ensure your full understanding of how to proceed.

The CAT model will not be used for the NGN items. Instead, the NCSBN will be using selected scoring models that will be applied to your test responses. In addition, you will not be able to skip NGN questions or return to earlier questions. For specific information on the scoring models, refer to the NCSBN website at https://www.ncsbn.org and the National Council of State Boards of Nursing 2021 *Next Generation NCLEX News* at https://www.ncsbn.org/public-files/NGN_Summer21_ENG.pdf.

Development of the Test Plan

The test plan for the NCLEX-RN examination is developed by the NCSBN. The examination is a national examination; the NCSBN considers the legal scope of nursing practice as governed by state laws and regulations, including the Nurse Practice Act, and uses these laws to define the areas on the examination that will assess the competence of the test-taker for licensure.

The NCSBN also conducts an important study every 3 years, known as a *practice analysis study*. The results of this study determine the framework for the test plan for the examination. The participants in this study include newly licensed registered nurses from all types of generalist nursing education programs. Participants of this study provide valuable information about work settings. From a list of nursing care activities (activity statements) provided, the participants are asked about the applicability, frequency, and importance of performing these activities in relation to client safety. A panel of content experts at the NCSBN analyze the results of the study and make decisions regarding the test plan framework. The results of this recently conducted study provided the structure for the test plan implemented in April 2023.

The Test Plan

The content of the NCLEX-RN examination reflects the activities identified in the practice analysis study conducted by the NCSBN. Exam questions are written based on the test plan framework and these activities *rather than* on content areas such as adult health, maternity, pediatrics, and mental health. The questions address Level of Cognitive Ability, Client Needs, and Integrated Processes as identified in the test plan developed by the NCSBN.

Level of Cognitive Ability

Levels of cognitive ability include remembering, understanding, applying, analyzing, evaluating, and creating. The practice of nursing requires complex thought processing and critical thinking in decision-making and in making clinical judgments. Therefore, you will not encounter any remembering or understanding questions on the NCLEX. Table 1.2 provides descriptions and examples of each level of cognitive ability. Box 1.1 presents an example of an applying question.

Client Needs

In the test plan implemented in April 2023, the NCSBN applied a test plan framework based on Client Needs. The NCSBN identifies four major categories of Client Needs, which are Safe and Effective Care Environment, Health Promotion and Maintenance, Psychosocial Integrity, and Physiological Integrity. Some of these categories are further divided into subcategories. Refer to Chapter 5 for a detailed description of the categories of Client Needs and the NCLEX-RN examination, and refer to Table 1.3 for the percentages of questions from each Client Needs category.

TABLE 1.2 Levels of Cognitive Ability: Descriptions and Examples

Level	Description and Example
Remembering	Recalling, retrieving information from memorization, previous learning, or long-term memory Example: A normal blood glucose level is 70–99 mg/dL (3.9–5.5 mmol/L).
Understanding	Determining the meaning of information Example: A blood glucose level of 60 mg/dL (3.34 mmol/L) is lower than the normal reference range.
Applying	Carrying out an appropriate action based on information Example: Administering 10–15 g of carbohydrate such as a ½ glass of fruit juice to treat mild hypoglycemia
Analyzing	Examining concepts or data and interpreting how the concepts or data connect or relate to one another Example: The concept is mild hypoglycemia and the connecting data are the signs and symptoms of mild hypoglycemia, such as hunger, irritability, weakness, headache, blood glucose level lower than 70 mg/dL (3.9 mmol/L).
Evaluating	Making judgments, conclusions, or validations based on evidence Example: Determining that treatment for mild hypoglycemia was effective if the blood glucose level returned to a normal level between 70–99 mg/dL (3.9–5.5 mmol/L)
Creating	Generating or producing a new outcome or plan of care by putting parts of information together Example: Designing a safe and individualized plan of care with the interprofessional health care team for a client with diabetes mellitus that meets the client's physiological, psychosocial, and health maintenance needs

Adapted from: Understanding Bloom's (and Anderson and Krathwohl's) Taxonomy, 2015, ProEdit, Inc. http://www.proedit.com/understanding-blooms-and-anderson-and-krathwohls-taxonomy/

Integrated Processes

The NCSBN identifies six processes in the test plan that are foundational to the practice of nursing. These processes are incorporated throughout the major categories of Client Needs. The Integrated Process subcategories are Caring, Clinical Judgment, Communication and Documentation, Culture and Spirituality, Nursing Process (Assessment, Analysis, Planning, Implementation, and Evaluation), and Teaching and Learning. Refer to Chapter 10 for a detailed description of the Integrated Processes and the NCLEX-RN examination.

Types of Questions on the Examination and Scoring

The types of questions on the current NCLEX include multiple choice; fill-in-the-blank; multiple response; ordered response (prioritizing); image (hot spot) questions; figure, scenario/exhibit, or graphic option items; and audio formats. These question types

---

BOX 1.1   Level of Cognitive Ability: Applying

A client at 32 weeks' gestation is brought into the emergency department after an automobile crash. The client is bleeding vaginally, and fetal assessment indicates moderate fetal distress. Which action would the nurse take **first** in an attempt to reduce the stress on the fetus?

1. Start intravenous (IV) fluids at a keep open rate.
2. Set up for an immediate cesarean section delivery.
3. Elevate the head of the bed to a semi-Fowler's position.
4. Administer oxygen via a face mask at 7 to 10 liters per minute.

Answer: **4**

Note the **strategic word,** *first*. This question requires you to identify the *first* nursing action that you will take. Also use the **ABCs—airway, breathing, and circulation**—to answer correctly. Administering oxygen will increase the amount of oxygen for transport to the fetus, partially compensating for the loss of circulating blood volume. This action is essential regardless of the cause or amount of bleeding. IV fluids will also be initiated. Although a cesarean delivery may be needed, there are no data that indicate it is necessary at this time. The client will be positioned based on the cause of fetal distress and per primary health care provider's prescription.

Level of Cognitive Ability: Applying

TABLE 1.3 Client Needs Categories and Percentage of Questions on the NCLEX-RN Examination

Client Needs Category	Percentage of Questions
Safe and Effective Care Environment	
Management of Care	15-21
Safety and Infection Control	10-16
Health Promotion and Maintenance	6-12
Psychosocial Integrity	6-12
Physiological Integrity	
Basic Care and Comfort	6-12
Pharmacological and Parenteral Therapies	13-19
Reduction of Risk Potential	9-15
Physiological Adaptation	11-17

From: National Council of State Boards of Nursing. (2023). *Next Generation NCLEX®*, *NCLEX-RN test plan*, National Council of State Boards of Nursing.

will continue to be a part of the NCLEX examination, and, except for the multiple response questions, each of these question types will be scored as either correct or incorrect, known as *dichotomous scoring*. No partial credit is given. Thus, the possible points for these question types will be 0 or 1 point. Partial credit will be given for the multiple response questions.

⚠️ The NGN item types use a case study approach as stand-alone cases and unfolding case studies. The stand-alone cases will be accompanied by a question that tests more than one cognitive skill. The unfolding case studies will be accompanied by six NGN item type questions, and each cognitive skill will be tested.

Examples of NGN items can be located on the Evolve site accompanying this book. These are specially designed to simulate the NCLEX experience of testing for these NGN item types. Chapter 4, Box 4.26, provides an example of a Bowtie NGN question. Table 1.4 provides a list of the NGN question types. The NCSBN also identifies three scoring methods for NGN items. These scoring methods are described in Table 1.5.

The NCSBN provides specific directions for you to follow with all question types to guide you through the testing process. Be sure to read these directions as they appear on the computer screen. Examples of some of these types of questions are noted in this chapter. Most question types are also placed in this book, and all types, including the NGN items, are on the accompanying Evolve site.

Multiple Choice Questions

Many of the questions that you will be asked to answer will be in the multiple choice format. These questions provide you with data about a client situation and four answers, or options.

Fill-in-the-Blank Questions

Fill-in-the-blank questions may ask you to perform a medication calculation, determine an intravenous flow rate, or calculate an intake or output record on a client. You will need to type only a number (your answer) in the answer box. If the question requires rounding the answer, this needs to be performed at the end of the calculation. The rules for rounding an answer are described in the tutorial provided by the NCSBN and are also provided in the specific question on the computer screen. In addition, you must type a decimal point if necessary and noted in the question directions. See Box 1.2 for an example of a fill-in-the-blank question.

Multiple Response Questions

For a multiple response question, you will be asked to select or check all of the options, such as nursing interventions, that relate to the information in the question. In this question type, there will be five to ten possible options, and there may be one or more correct answers. Partial credit is given for correct selections. See Box 1.3 for an example.

Ordered Response (Prioritizing) Questions

In ordered response (prioritizing) questions you will be asked to place nursing actions in order of priority. Information will be presented in a question and, based on the data, you need to determine what you will do first, second, third, and so forth. Specific directions for answering are provided with the question. See Fig. 1.1 for an example. Examples of this question type are located on the accompanying Evolve site.

Figure Questions

A question with a picture or graphic will ask you to answer the question based on the picture or graphic. The question could contain a chart, a table, or a figure or illustration. You also may be asked to use the computer mouse to point and click on a

TABLE 1.4 NGN Item Types

Type of Case Scenario	Description	Item Types
Stand-alone	A stand-alone case will include a short scenario about a client and will be accompanied by one question that tests more than one cognitive skill.	Bowtie Trend
Unfolding	An unfolding case study will include phases as the story about the client unfolds and changes. This will be accompanied by six NGN item type questions, and each of the six cognitive skills will be tested.	Highlight in Text Highlight in Table Matrix Multiple Choice Matrix Multiple Response Multiple Response Select N Multiple Response Select All That Apply Multiple Response Grouping Drag and Drop Cloze Drag and Drop Rationale Drop Down Cloze Drop Down Rationale Drop Down in Table

From: Petersen, E., Betts, J., & Muntean, W. (December 2020). *Next Generation NCLEX® (NGN)* Webinar. NCSBN; National Council of State Boards of Nursing. (2021). *Next Generation NCLEX News.* https://www.ncsbn.org/NGN_Summer21_Eng.pdf

TABLE 1.5 NGN Scoring Methods

Method	Description
Plus-Minus (+/−) Scoring	One point is given for each correct response One point is subtracted for each incorrect response If the sum is negative, a zero is assigned Used when the test-taker can select any number of options such as a multiple response, select all that apply, matrix multiple response, highlight in text, highlight in table, multiple response grouping
One-Zero (1/0) Scoring	One point is given for each correct response Points are NOT subtracted for incorrect responses Used for items such as Bowtie, matrix multiple choice, Select N, drop down cloze, drag and drop cloze, or drop down table
Rationale Scoring	One point is given for each correct grouping of response elements Used when elements of a response are linked such as drop down rationale or drag and drop rationale items

From: National Council of State Boards of Nursing. (2021). *Next Generation NCLEX News.* https://www.ncsbn.org/NGN_Summer21_Eng.pdf; National Council of State Boards of Nursing. (2021). *Braving new pathways: Leading the way for regulatory transformation,* 2021 NCSBN Annual Meeting.

specific area in the visual. A figure or illustration may appear in any type of question, including a multiple choice question. See Box 1.4 for an example.

Scenario/Exhibit Questions

In this type of question, you will be presented with a problem and a scenario or exhibit. You will be provided with three or more tabs or buttons that you need to click to obtain the information needed to answer the question. A prompt or message will appear that will indicate the need to click on a tab or button. See Box 1.5 for an example.

BOX 1.2   Fill-in-the-Blank Question

The physician prescribes 12 mEq of liquid potassium chloride. The medication label reads 20 mEq/15 mL. The nurse needs to administer how many milliliters (mL) to the client?

Answer: 9 mL

Focus on the **subject,** the amount of mL to be administered, and on the **data in the question.** For this fill-in-the-blank question, use the formula for calculating medication doses. Once the dose is determined, you will need to type your numeric answer in the answer box. Always follow the specific directions noted on the computer screen when answering a question. Also, remember that there will be an on-screen calculator on the computer for your use to confirm your answer.

Formula:

$$\frac{\text{Desired}}{\text{Available}} \times mL = mL \text{ per dose}$$

$$\frac{12 \text{ mEq}}{20 \text{ mEq}} \times 15 \text{ mL} = 9 \text{ mL}$$

Graphic Option Questions

In graphic option questions the option selections will be pictures rather than text. You will select the option that represents your answer choice. See Box 1.6 for an example.

Audio Questions

Audio questions will require listening to a sound to answer the question. These questions will prompt you to use the headset provided and to click on the sound icon. You will be able to click on the volume button to adjust the volume to your comfort level, and you will be able to listen to the sound as many times as necessary. Content examples include, but are not limited to, various lung sounds, heart sounds, or bowel sounds.

BOX 1.3 Multiple Response Question

The nurse is caring for a client with a terminal condition who is dying. Which respiratory assessment findings would indicate to the nurse that death is imminent? **Select all that apply.**

☑ 1. Dyspnea
☑ 2. Cyanosis
☐ 3. Kussmaul's respiration
☐ 4. Tachypnea without apnea
☑ 5. Irregular respiratory pattern
☑ 6. Adventitious bubbling lung sounds

Answer: 1, 2, 5, 6

Focus on the **subject**, assessment findings in a client who is dying. In a multiple response question, you will be asked to select or check all the options, such as signs and symptoms or interventions that relate to the information in the question. Be sure to follow the specific directions given on the computer screen. Partial credit is given for multiple response questions. To answer this question, think about the respiratory assessment findings that indicate death is imminent. These include altered patterns of respiration, such as slow, labored, irregular, or Cheyne-Stokes pattern (alternating periods of apnea and deep, rapid breathing); increased respiratory secretions and adventitious bubbling lung sounds (death rattle); irritation of the tracheobronchial airway as evidenced by hiccups, chest pain, respiratory fatigue, or exhaustion; and poor gas exchange as evidenced by hypoxia, dyspnea, or cyanosis. Kussmaul's respirations are abnormally deep, very rapid sighing respirations characteristic of diabetic ketoacidosis.

Examples of this question type are located on the accompanying Evolve site (Fig. 1.2).

Case Study Questions

Case study questions are the format for the NGN-style items. These case studies may be stand-alone or unfolding cases. The stand-alone case studies will be accompanied by one NGN-style question, and the unfolding case studies will be accompanied by six questions in NGN style. Each type of case study is aimed at testing one or more of the cognitive skills or processes associated with the NCSBN Clinical Judgment Measurement Model (see Table 1.1). Examples of these NGN item types can be located on the Evolve site accompanying this book.

Registering to Take the Examination

It is important to obtain an NCLEX® Examination Candidate Bulletin from the NCSBN website at https://www.ncsbn.org, because this bulletin provides all of the information you need to register for and schedule your examination. It also provides you with website and telephone information for NCLEX examination contacts. The initial step in the registration process is to submit an application to the state board of nursing in the state in which you intend to obtain licensure. You need to obtain information from the board of nursing regarding the specific registration process because the process may vary from state to state. Then, use the NCLEX® Examination Candidate Bulletin as your guide to complete the registration process.

Following the registration instructions and completing the registration forms precisely and accurately are important.

SAUNDERS Q&A REVIEW *For The* **NCLEX-RN® EXAMINATION 9TH EDITION**   **Silvestri**

| Home | History | **Study Mode** | | | | Calculator | Help |

Question 14 of 20   ‹ [14] Go ›   Bookmark   Stop

A unit of packed red blood cells has been prescribed for a client with low hemoglobin and hematocrit levels. The nurse notifies the blood bank of the prescription, and a blood specimen is drawn from the client for typing and cross-matching. The nurse receives a telephone call from the blood bank and is informed that the unit of blood is ready for administration. In what **priority** order should the nurse perform the actions necessary to administer the blood? **Arrange the actions in the order that they should be performed. All options must be used.**

Drag the text in the left column to the correct order in the right column.

Document that the blood was administered.	1	
Obtain the unit of blood from the blood bank.	2	
Ensure that an informed consent has been signed.	3	
Insert an 18- or 19-gauge intravenous (IV) catheter into the client.	4	
Check the health care provider's prescription for administering blood.	5	
Ask a licensed nurse to assist in confirming blood compatibility and verifying client identity.	6	

| Rationale | Strategy | Nursing Tip | Reference | Submit   **Reset**

FIGURE 1.1 Example of an ordered response question.

BOX 1.4   Figure Question

The nurse performs client rounds and notes that a client with a respiratory disorder is wearing this oxygen device (refer to figure). The nurse would document that the client is receiving oxygen by which type of low-flow oxygen delivery system? **Refer to figure.**

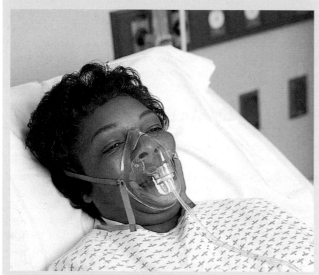

(Figure from Potter, P., Perry, A., Stockert, P. & Hall, A. [2017]. *Fundamentals of nursing.* [9th ed.] Mosby.)

1. Venturi mask
2. Nasal cannula
3. Simple face mask
4. Partial rebreather mask

Answer: 3

Focus on the subject, the type of face mask that the client is wearing. For some of these question types, you need to use the computer mouse and point and click at a designated area to answer the question. For this question, use of the computer mouse is not necessary. A simple face mask is used to deliver low-flow oxygen concentrations of 40% to 60% for short-term oxygen therapy. It also may be used in an emergency. A minimum flow rate of 5 L/min is needed to prevent the rebreathing of exhaled air. The simple face mask fits over the nose and mouth, has exhalation ports, and has a tube that connects to the oxygen source. A Venturi mask is a high-flow oxygen delivery system that delivers an accurate oxygen concentration. An adaptor is located between the bottom of the mask and the oxygen source. The adaptor contains holes of different sizes that allow specific amounts of air to mix with the oxygen. The nasal cannula contains nasal prongs that are used to deliver oxygen flow rates at 1 to 6 L/min. A partial rebreather mask is a mask with a reservoir bag without flaps. It provides oxygen concentrations of 60% to 75% with flow rates of 6 to 11 L/min.

BOX 1.5   Scenario/Exhibit Question

Oral prednisone is prescribed for a hospitalized client. The nurse reviews the client's medical record and is **most** concerned about this prescription because of which documented item? **Refer to chart.**

SCENARIO/EXHIBIT

CLIENT'S CHART

History: Diabetes mellitus
          Hypertension
Medications: Furosemide 40 mg oral daily

Diagnostic Tests: Electrocardiogram: normal

1. Furosemide
2. Hypertension
3. Diabetes mellitus
4. Normal electrocardiogram

Answer: 3

Note the strategic word, *most*. This scenario/exhibit question provides you with data from a client's medical chart, identifies a prescribed medication, and asks about a concern related to this medication. Read all the data in the question and the client's chart. Use nursing knowledge about the interactions and effects of prednisone, and recall that this medication may increase the blood glucose level. This will assist in directing you to option 3. For these question types, be certain to read all of the data in the client's chart before selecting the answer. Remember you will be provided with tabs to click to read information.

Authorization to Test Form and Scheduling an Appointment

Once you are eligible to test, you will receive an Authorization to Test (ATT) form. You cannot make an appointment until you receive an ATT form. Note the validity dates on the ATT form, and schedule a testing date and time before the expiration date on the ATT form. The NCLEX® Examination Candidate Bulletin provides you with the directions for scheduling an appointment, and you do not have to take the examination in the same state in which you are seeking licensure.

The ATT form contains important information, including your test authorization number, candidate identification (ID) number, and validity date. You need to take your ATT form to the testing center on the day of your examination. You will not be admitted to the examination if you do not have this form.

Changing Your Appointment

If for any reason you need to change your appointment to test, you can make the change on the candidate website or by calling candidate services. Refer to the NCLEX® Examination Candidate Bulletin for this contact information and other

---

Registration forms not properly completed or not accompanied by the proper fees in the required method of payment will be returned to you and will delay testing. You must pay a fee for taking the examination; you also may have to pay additional fees to the board of nursing in the state in which you are applying.

BOX 1.6 **Graphic Options Question**

The primary health care provider prescribes a tuberculin skin test to be done on a client. Which syringe would the nurse select to perform the test? **Refer to Figures 1 to 4.**

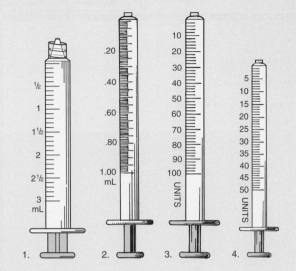

Answer: 2

Focus on the **subject,** the procedure for administering a tuberculin skin test. This question requires you to select the picture that represents your answer choice. To perform a tuberculin skin test, the nurse would use a tuberculin syringe that is marked in 0.01 (hundredths) because the dose for administration is less than 1 mL. Option 1 is a 3-mL syringe and is marked in 0.1 (tenths) and is used for most subcutaneous or intramuscular injections. Insulin syringes are available in 50 and 100 units and are used to administer insulin.

(Figure from Potter, P., Perry, A., Stockert, P., & Hall, A. [2017]. *Fundamentals of nursing.* [9th ed.]. Mosby.)

---

important procedures for canceling and changing an appointment. If you fail to arrive for the examination or fail to cancel your appointment to test without providing appropriate notice, you will forfeit your examination fee, and your ATT form will be invalidated. This information will be reported to the board of nursing in the state in which you have applied for licensure, and you will be required to register and pay the testing fees again.

The Day of the Examination

It is important that you arrive at the testing center at least 30 minutes before the test is scheduled. If you arrive late for the scheduled testing appointment, you may be required to forfeit your examination appointment. If it is necessary to forfeit your appointment, you will need to reregister for the examination and pay an additional fee. The board of nursing will be notified that you did not take the test. A few days before your scheduled date of testing, take the time to drive to the testing center to determine its exact location; the length of time required to arrive at that destination; and any potential obstacles that might delay you, such as road construction, traffic, or parking sites.

In addition to the ATT form, you must have proper identification such as a U.S. driver's license, passport, U.S. state ID, or U.S. military ID to be admitted to take the examination. All acceptable ID must be valid and not expired and contain a photograph and signature (in English). In addition, the first and last names on the ID must match the ATT form. According to the NCSBN guidelines, any name discrepancies require legal documentation, such as a marriage license, divorce decree, or court action legal name change.

Testing Accommodations

If you require testing accommodations, you should contact the board of nursing before submitting a registration form. The board of nursing will provide the procedures for the request. The board of nursing must authorize testing accommodations. After board of nursing approval, the NCSBN reviews the requested accommodations and must approve the request. If the request is approved, the candidate will be notified and provided the procedure for registering for and scheduling the examination.

Testing Center

The testing center is designed to ensure complete security of the testing process. Strict candidate identification requirements have been established. You will be asked to read the rules related to testing. A digital fingerprint and palm vein print will be taken. A digital signature and photograph will also be taken at the testing center. These identity confirmations will accompany the NCLEX exam results. In addition, if you leave the testing room for any reason, you may be required to perform these identity confirmation procedures again to be readmitted to the room.

Personal belongings are not allowed in the testing room; all electronic devices must be placed in a sealable bag provided by the test administrator and kept in a locker. Any evidence of tampering with the bag could result in the need to report the incident and test cancellation. A locker and locker key will be provided for you; however, storage space is limited, so you must plan accordingly. In addition, the testing center will not assume responsibility for your personal belongings. The testing waiting areas are generally small; friends or family members who accompany you are not permitted to wait in the testing center while you are taking the examination.

Once you have completed the admission process, the test administrator will escort you to the assigned computer. You will be seated at an individual workspace area that includes computer equipment, appropriate lighting, an erasable note board, and a marker. No items, including unauthorized scratch paper, are allowed into the testing room. Eating, drinking, and the use of tobacco are not allowed in the testing room. You will be observed at all times by the test administrator while taking the examination. In addition, video and audio recordings of all test sessions are made. The testing center has no control over the sounds made by typing on the computer by others. If these sounds are distracting, raise your hand to summon the test administrator. Earplugs are available on request.

You must follow the directions given by the testing center staff and must remain seated during the test except when authorized to leave. If you think that you have a problem with

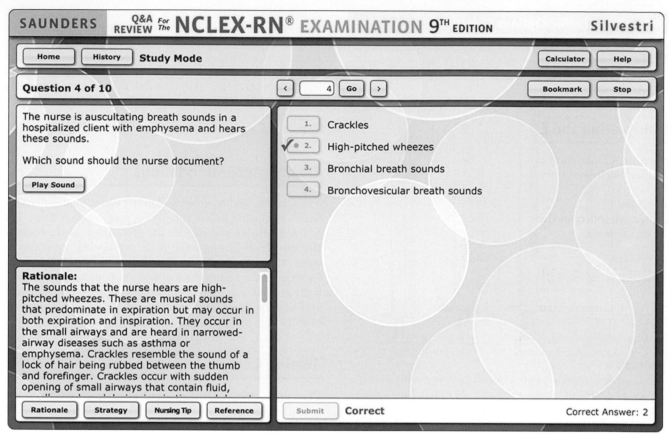

FIGURE 1.2 Example of an audio question.

TABLE 1.6 NGN Test Design

Element	NGN Minimum Length Exam	NGN Maximum Length Exam
Scored Items	85 (70 scored and 15 unscored)	150 (135 scored and 15 unscored)
Unfolding case studies	3 cases (total of 18 items)	3 cases (total of 18 items)
Stand-alone items	Possibly Bowtie or Trend	Possibly Bowtie or Trend
Traditional item types	Approximately 52 (dependent on # of stand-alones)	Approximately 52-117 (dependent on # of stand-alones)
Pretest (Unscored) Items	15	15
Time Allowed	5 hours	5 hours

Adapted from: National Council of State Boards of Nursing. (2021). *Braving new pathways: Leading the way for regulatory transformation*, 2021 NCSBN Annual Meeting.

the computer, need a clean note board, need to take a break, or need the test administrator for any reason, you must raise your hand. You are also encouraged to access the NCSBN candidate website to obtain additional information about acceptable medical devices that can be brought into the testing room and the physical environment of the testing center; you can also view a virtual tour of the testing center.

NGN Test Design

The time allowed for the exam is 5 hours; this period includes the tutorial, the sample items, all breaks, and the examination. All breaks are optional. Remember that all breaks count against

testing time. If you take a break, you must leave the testing room; when you return, you may be required to follow identity confirmation procedures to be readmitted. Pretest items will be a part of the examination. The pretest questions are questions that may be presented as scored questions on future examinations. These pretest questions are not identified as such. In other words, you do not know which questions are the pretest (unscored) questions. Table 1.6 provides information about the test design.

Pass-or-Fail Decisions

All examination questions are categorized by test plan area and level of difficulty. This is an important point to keep in mind when you consider how the computer makes a pass-or-fail decision, because a pass-or-fail decision is not based on a percentage of correctly answered questions. Additional information about pass-or-fail decisions can be found in the NCLEX® Examination Candidate Bulletin located at https://www.ncsbn.org.

Completing the Examination

When the examination has ended, you will complete a brief computer-delivered questionnaire about your testing experience. After you complete this questionnaire, you need to raise your hand to summon the test administrator. The test administrator will collect and inventory all note boards and then permit you to leave.

Processing Results

Every computerized examination is scored twice, once by the computer at the testing center and again after the examination is transmitted to the test scoring center. No results are released at the testing center; testing center staff do not have access to examination results. The board of nursing receives your result, and your result will be mailed to you approximately 6 weeks after you take the examination. In some states, an unofficial result can be obtained via the Quick Results Service 2 business days after taking the examination. There is a fee for this service, and information about obtaining your NCLEX result by this method can be obtained on the NCSBN website by clicking candidate services.

Candidate Performance Report

A candidate performance report is provided to a test-taker who failed the examination. This report provides the test-taker with information about strengths and weaknesses in relation to the test plan framework and provides a guide for studying and retaking the examination. If a retake is necessary, the candidate must wait 45 days between examination administration, depending on state procedures. Test-takers should refer to the state board of nursing in the state in which licensure is sought for procedures regarding when the examination can be taken again.

Interstate Endorsement and Nurse Licensure Compact

Because the NCLEX-RN examination is a national examination, you can apply to take the examination in any state. When licensure is received, you can apply for interstate endorsement, which is obtaining another license in another state to practice nursing in that state. The procedures and requirements for interstate endorsement may vary from state to state, and these procedures can be obtained from the state board of nursing in the state in which endorsement is sought. It may be possible to practice nursing in another state under the mutual recognition model of nursing licensure if the state has enacted a Nurse Licensure Compact. To obtain information about the Nurse Licensure Compact and the states that are part of this interstate compact, access the NCSBN website at https://www.ncsbn.org.

The International-Educated Nurse

An important first step in the process of obtaining information about becoming a registered nurse in the United States is to access the NCSBN website at https://www.ncsbn.org and obtain information provided for international-educated nurses in the NCLEX website link. The NCSBN provides information about some of the documents you need to obtain as an international-educated nurse seeking licensure in the United States and about credentialing agencies. Refer to Box 1.7 for a list of some of these documents. The NCSBN also provides information regarding the requirements for education and English proficiency and immigration requirements such as visas and VisaScreen. You are encouraged to access the NCSBN website to obtain the most current information about seeking licensure as a registered nurse in the United States.

An important factor to consider as you pursue this process is that some requirements may vary from state to state. You need to contact the board of nursing in the state in which you are planning to obtain licensure to determine the specific requirements and documents that you need to submit.

Boards of nursing can decide either to use a credentialing agency to evaluate your documents or to review your documents at the specific state board, known as in-house evaluation. When you contact the board of nursing in the state in which you intend to work as a nurse, inform them that you were educated outside of the United States and ask that they send you an application to apply for licensure by examination.

BOX 1.7   International-Educated Nurse: Some Documents Needed to Obtain Licensure

1. Proof of citizenship or lawful alien status
2. Work visa
3. VisaScreen certificate
4. Commission on Graduates of Foreign Nursing Schools (CGFNS) certificate
5. Criminal background check documents
6. Official transcripts of educational credentials sent directly to credentialing agency or board of nursing from home country school of nursing
7. Validation of a comparable nursing education as that provided in U.S. nursing programs; this may include theoretical instruction and clinical practice in a variety of nursing areas including, but not limited to, medical nursing, surgical nursing, pediatric nursing, maternity and newborn nursing, community and public health nursing, and mental health nursing
8. Validation of safe professional nursing practice in home country
9. Copy of nursing license or diploma or both
10. Proof of proficiency in the English language
11. Photograph(s)
12. Social Security number
13. Application and fees

Be sure to specify that you are applying for RN licensure. You should also ask about the specific documents needed to become eligible to take the NCLEX exam. You can obtain contact information for each state board of nursing through the NCSBN website at https://www.ncsbn.org. In addition, you can write to the NCSBN regarding the NCLEX exam. The address is 111 East Wacker Drive, Suite 2900, Chicago, IL 60601. The telephone number for the NCSBN is 1-866-293-9600; international telephone is 011-1-312-525-3600; the fax number is 1-312-279-1032.

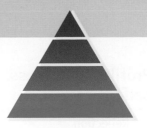

CHAPTER 2

Self-Efficacy and Profiles to Success

Laurent W. Valliere, BS, DD

The Pyramid to Success

Preparing to take the National Council Licensure Examination Next Generation NCLEX® (NGN) can produce a great deal of anxiety in the nursing graduate. You may be thinking that the NCLEX-RN is the most important examination that you will ever have to take and that it reflects the culmination of everything for which you have worked so hard. The NGN is an important examination because achieving that nursing license defines the beginning of your career as a registered nurse. A vital ingredient to your success on the NCLEX is examining your profile to success and avoiding negative thoughts that allow this examination to seem overwhelming and intimidating (Box 2.1). Such thoughts will take full control over your destiny. A strong positive attitude and self-efficacy, a structured plan for preparation, and maintaining control in your pathway to success ensure reaching the peak of the Pyramid to Success (Fig. 2.1). For additional information about study habits and testing and test anxiety, we refer you to *Saunders 2024-2025 Clinical Judgment and Test-Taking Strategies* resource.

Self-Efficacy

The concept of self-efficacy was originally proposed by Albert Bandura in social science research in developing social cognitive theory. According to Bandura (1977), this theory has been used extensively in the field of psychology. Central to Bandura's work are the concepts of self-efficacy and self-efficacy (outcome) expectations. The concept of self-efficacy is described as a type of self-reflection that affects one's behavior (Bandura, 1977). Self-reflection enables an individual to assess their own experiences, develop perceptions about their own capabilities that guide behavior, and determine how much effort will ensure performance. Thus, self-reflection leads to an individual's self-efficacy expectations and confidence in their ability to succeed.

⚠ With regard to NCLEX, a study done by Silvestri, Clark, & Moonie (2013) showed that self-efficacy expectations were an important predictor for NCLEX success.

Self-Efficacy Expectations

Self-efficacy expectations are focused on one's belief in their own capacity to carry out particular behaviors. These expectations determine the behaviors a person chooses to perform, their degree of perseverance, and the quality of the performance. Bandura (1997) describes self-efficacy as an individual's belief regarding their own abilities to successfully perform activities or tasks and indicates that the stronger the sense of self-efficacy, the more confident one is to succeed. In applying Bandura's (1977) theory to NCLEX success, if you have high self-efficacy expectations, you will work hard and persevere and believe that you will achieve NCLEX success. Conversely, if your self-efficacy expectations are low, this could lead to self-doubt about your ability to achieve success on NCLEX.

BOX 2.1 Profiles to Success

- Avoid negative thoughts that allow the examination to seem overwhelming and intimidating.
- Develop a comprehensive plan to prepare for the examination.
- Examine the study methods and strategies that you used in preparing for examinations during nursing school.
- Develop realistic time goals.
- Select a study time period and study place that will be most conducive to your success.
- Commit to your own special study methods and strategies.
- Incorporate a balance of exercise with adequate rest and relaxation time in your preparation schedule.
- Maintain healthy eating habits.
- Learn to control anxiety.
- Remember that discipline and perseverance will automatically bring control.
- Remember that this examination is all about you.
- Remember that your self-confidence and the belief in yourself will lead you to success!

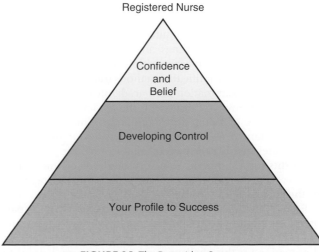

FIGURE 2.1 The Pyramid to Success.

Registered Nurse

Confidence and Belief

Developing Control

Your Profile to Success

Profiles to Success: Increasing Self-Efficacy

Self-Reflection

Self-reflection enables an individual to assess their own experiences, develop perceptions about their own capabilities that guide behavior, and determine how much effort will ensue for performance. Thus, self-reflection leads to an individual's self-efficacy expectations and confidence in their ability to succeed. According to Bandura (1997), individuals possess a self-regulatory function that provides the capability to influence their own cognitive processes and actions and thus alter their environments. Therefore, whatever self-efficacy beliefs an individual holds will help to determine what activities the individual will pursue, the effort that they will expend in pursuing these activities, and how long they will persist in the face of obstacles and hardships.

To start, take some time to self-reflect. Think about the accomplishments you have achieved and how you have achieved these accomplishments. Journal these accomplishments and keep these in mind. Review them whenever you begin to feel any self-doubt about your ability to succeed on the NCLEX. Some self-reflection questions to ask yourself include the following:

1. Am I a goal-setter?
2. Do I develop a plan and determine what activities I need to pursue to achieve my goals?
3. Do I set goals that are unrealistic to achieve in a specific time frame?
4. Do I accomplish the goals that I set?
5. How much time and effort do I put in to accomplish my goals?
6. Do I find ways to achieve my goals when I am faced with life challenges and obstacles?
7. How do I feel when I accomplish a goal?

Developing Your Preparation Plan

The foundation begins with a strong positive attitude and self-efficacy, the belief that you will achieve success, and developing self-control. Nursing graduates preparing for the NCLEX must develop a comprehensive plan to prepare for this examination. The most important component in developing a plan is identifying the study patterns that guided you to your nursing degree. It is important to begin your planning by reflecting on all of the personal and academic challenges you experienced during your nursing education. Take time to focus on the thoughts, feelings, and emotions that you experienced before taking an examination while enrolled in your nursing program. Examine the methods that you used in preparing for that examination both academically and from the standpoint of how you dealt with the anxiety that parallels the experience of facing an examination. These factors are very important considerations in preparing for the NCLEX because they identify the patterns that worked for you. Think about this for a moment. Your own methods of study must have worked, or you would not be at the point of preparing for the NCLEX-RN.

Each individual requires their own methods of preparing for an examination. Graduate nurses who have taken the NCLEX-RN will probably share their experiences and methods of preparing for this challenge with you. It is very helpful to listen to what they tell you. These graduates can provide you with important strategies that they have used. Listen closely to what they have to say, but remember that this examination is all about you. Your identity and what you require in terms of preparation are most important.

Reflect on the methods and strategies that worked for you throughout your nursing program. Do not think that you need to develop new methods and strategies to prepare for the NCLEX. Use what has worked for you. Take some time to reflect on these strategies, write them down on a large blank card, sign your name, and write "RN" after your name. Post this card in a place where you will see it every morning. Commit to your own special strategies. These strategies reflect your profile and identity and will lead you to a successful outcome—registered nurse!

A frequent concern of graduates preparing for the NCLEX relates to deciding whether they should study alone or become a part of a study group. Examining your profile will easily direct you in making this decision. Again, reflect on what has worked for you throughout your nursing program as you prepared for examinations. Remember, your needs are most important. Address your own needs, and do not become pressured by peers who are encouraging you to join a study group if this is not your normal pattern for study. Additional pressure is not what you need at this important time of your life.

You may ask, "What is the best method of preparing?" First, remember that you are prepared. In fact, you began preparing for this examination on the first day that you entered your nursing program. The task you are faced with is to review, in a comprehensive manner, all of the nursing content that you learned in your nursing program. It can become totally overwhelming to look at your bookshelf, which is overflowing with the nursing books you used during nursing school, and your challenge becomes monumental when you look at the boxes of nursing lecture notes that you have accumulated. It is unrealistic to even think that you could read all of those nursing books and lecture notes in preparation for the NCLEX. These books and lecture notes should be used as reference sources, if needed, during your preparation for the NCLEX.

Saunders Comprehensive Review for the NCLEX-RN® Examination has identified for you all of the important nursing content areas relevant to the examination. During the comprehensive review, you should have noted the areas that are unfamiliar or unclear to you. Be sure that you have taken the time to become familiar with these areas. Now, you are progressing through the Pyramid to Success and testing your knowledge in this book, *Saunders Q&A Review for the NCLEX-RN® Examination*. Answer all of the practice questions provided in this book and on the Evolve site: practice question, after question, after question! You may identify nursing content areas that require further review. Take the time to review these nursing content areas, as you are guided to do in this book.

Identifying Your Goals for Success

⚠️ Create a list of your goals related to NCLEX preparation. Open your calendar and start with listing your daily goals and what you want to accomplish each day. Your daily goal could be practicing a specific number of questions or reviewing a specific content area, or it could be a day of rest and relaxation!

Your profile to success requires that you develop realistic time goals to prepare for the NCLEX. It is necessary to take the time to examine your life and all of the commitments you may have. These commitments may include family, work, and friends. As you develop your goals, remember to plan time for fun and exercise. To achieve success, you require a balance of time for both work and enjoyment. If you do not plan for some leisure time, you will become frustrated and perhaps even angry. These sorts of feelings will block your ability to focus and concentrate. Remember that you need time for yourself.

Goal development may be a relatively easy process because you have probably been juggling your life commitments ever since you entered nursing school. Remember that your goal is to identify a daily time frame and time period for you to use in reviewing and preparing for the NCLEX. Open your calendar and identify days on which life commitments will not allow you to spend this time preparing. Block those days off and do not consider them as a part of your review time. Identify the time of day that is best for you in terms of your ability to concentrate and focus so that you can accomplish the most in your identified time frame. Be sure that you consider a time that is quiet and free of distractions. Many individuals find the morning hours most productive, whereas others may find the afternoon and evening hours most productive. Remember that this examination is all about you, so select the time period that will be most conducive to your success.

Selecting Your Study Place

The place of study is very important. Select a place that is quiet and comfortable for study—where you normally do your studying and preparing. If studying at home in your own environment is your normal pattern, be sure to free yourself of distractions during your scheduled preparation time. If you are not able to free yourself of distractions, you may consider spending your preparation time in a library. When selecting your place of study, reflect on what worked best for you during your nursing program.

Deciding on Your Amount of Daily Study Time

Selecting the amount of daily preparation time can be troublesome for many graduates preparing for the NCLEX. It is very important to set a realistic time period that can be adhered to on a daily basis. Set a time frame that will provide you with quality time and a time frame that can be achieved. If you set a time frame that is not realistic and cannot be achieved every day, you will become frustrated. This frustration will block your journey toward the peak of the Pyramid to Success.

The best suggestion is to spend at least 2 hours daily for NCLEX preparation. Two hours is a realistic time period, both in terms of spending quality time and adhering to a time frame. You may find that after 2 hours your ability to focus and concentrate is diminished. You may, however, find that on some days you are able to spend more than the scheduled 2 hours. If you can and feel as though your ability to concentrate and focus is still present, then do so.

Developing Control

Discipline and perseverance will automatically bring control. Control will provide you with the momentum that will sweep you to the peak of the Pyramid to Success.

Discipline yourself to spend time preparing for the NCLEX every day if possible. Daily preparation is very important because it maintains a consistent pattern and keeps you in synchrony with the mind flow needed on the day you are scheduled to take the NCLEX examination. Some days you may think about skipping your scheduled preparation time because you are not in the mood for study or because you just do not feel like studying. On these days, practice discipline and persevere. Stand yourself up, shake off those thoughts of skipping a day of preparation, take a deep breath, and get the oxygen flowing throughout your body. Look in the mirror, smile, and say to yourself, "This time is for me and I can do this!" Look at your card that displays your name with "RN" after it, and get yourself to that special study place. Remember that discipline and perseverance will bring control!

Dealing with Anxiety

In the profile to success, academic preparation directs the path to the peak of the Pyramid to Success. There are, however, additional factors that will influence successful achievement to the peak. These factors include your ability to control anxiety, your physical stamina, the amount of rest and relaxation you get, your self-confidence, and the belief in yourself that you will achieve success on the NCLEX. You need to take time to think about these important factors and incorporate these factors into your daily preparation schedule.

Anxiety is a common concern among students preparing to take the NCLEX. Feeling some anxiety is normal and will keep your senses sharp and alert. A great deal of anxiety, however, can block your process of thinking and hamper your ability to focus and concentrate. You have already practiced the task of controlling anxiety when you took examinations in nursing school. Now you need to continue with this practice and incorporate this control on a daily basis. Each day, before beginning your scheduled preparation time, sit in your quiet special study place, close your eyes, and take a slow, deep breath. Fill your body with oxygen, hold your breath to a count of four, and then exhale slowly through your mouth. Continue with this exercise and repeat it 4–6 times. This exercise helps relieve your mind of any unnecessary chatter and delivers oxygen to all of your body tissues and your brain. On your scheduled day for taking the NCLEX, after the necessary pretesting procedures, you will be escorted to your test computer. Practice this breathing exercise before beginning the examination. Use this exercise during the examination if you feel yourself becoming anxious and distracted and if you are having difficulty focusing or concentrating. Remember that breathing will move that oxygen to your brain!

Ensuring Physical Readiness

Physical stamina is a necessary component of readiness for the NCLEX. Plan to incorporate a balance of exercise with adequate rest and relaxation time in your preparation schedule. It is also important that you maintain healthy eating habits. Begin to practice these healthy habits now, if you have not already done so. There are a few points to keep in mind each day as you plan your daily meals. Three balanced meals are important, with snacks, such as fruits and vegetables, included between meals. Remember that food items that contain fat will slow you down, and food items that contain caffeine could cause increased nervousness. Avoid these items. Healthy foods that are high in complex carbohydrates work best to supply your

---

BOX 2.2 Healthy Eating Habits

Eat three balanced meals each day.
Include snacks, such as fruits and vegetables, between meals.
Avoid food items that contain fat.
Avoid food items that contain caffeine.
Consume healthy foods that are high in complex carbohydrates.

BOX 2.3 Meeting the Challenge

Believe
Believe in your success every day.
Plan
Plan the study strategies that work for you.
Control
Always maintain command of your emotions, and breathe.
Practice
Review, review, review: Practice questions, practice questions, and more practice questions!
Succeed
Believe, plan, control, and practice: "Yes, I can!"

---

energy needs. Remember that your brain works like a muscle. It requires healthy carbohydrates (Box 2.2).

If you are not a breakfast eater, work on changing that habit. Practice the habit of eating breakfast now as you are preparing for the NCLEX. Attempt to provide your brain with energy in the morning with some form of complex carbohydrate food. It will make a difference. On your scheduled day for the NCLEX, feed your brain and eat a healthy breakfast. In addition, on this very important day, bring some form of healthy snack and feed your brain again if you take a break during the exam so that you will have the energy to concentrate, focus, and complete your examination.

Adequate rest, relaxation, and exercise are important in your preparation process. Many graduates preparing for the NCLEX have difficulty sleeping, particularly the night before the examination. Begin now to develop methods that will assist in relaxing your body and mind and allow you to obtain a restful sleep. You may have already developed a particular method to help you sleep. If not, it may be helpful to try the breathing exercise while you lie in bed to assist in eliminating any "mind chatter" that is present. It is also helpful to visualize your favorite and most peaceful place while you do these breathing exercises. Graduates say that listening to quiet music and relaxation tapes assisted in helping them relax and sleep. Begin to practice some of these helpful methods now while you are preparing for the NCLEX. Identify those that work best for you. The night before your scheduled examination is an important one. Spend time having some fun, get to bed early, and incorporate the relaxation method that you have been using to help you sleep.

Confidence and Belief in Yourself

Confidence and belief that you have the ability to achieve success will bring your goals to fruition. Remember, Bandura (1997) describes self-efficacy as an individual's belief regarding their own abilities to successfully perform activities or tasks and indicates that the stronger the sense of self-efficacy, the more confident one is to succeed. Reflect on your profile maintained during your nursing education. Your confidence and belief in yourself, along with your academic achievements, have brought you to the status of graduate nurse. Now you are facing one more important challenge (Box 2.3).

Can you meet this challenge successfully? Yes, you can! There is no reason to think otherwise if you have taken all of the necessary steps to ensure that profile to success. Each morning, place your feet on the floor, stand tall, take a deep breath, and smile. Take both hands and imagine yourself brushing off any negative feelings. Look at your card that bears your name with the letters "RN" after it, and tell yourself, **"Yes, I can!!!!"**

Believe in yourself, and you will reach the peak of the Pyramid to Success!

Congratulations, and I wish you continued success in your career as a registered nurse!

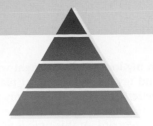

CHAPTER 3

The NCLEX-RN® Examination: A Graduate's Perspective

Natalie Filer, BSN, RN

To be called to serve in the profession of nursing is an honor. We all have our own reasons why we want to become nurses and in what ways we want to impact the world with having a nursing degree and a license to practice nursing. Each individual path to licensure and practice is different but likely with some similarities as well.

I graduated May 14, 2022, with my Bachelor of Science in Nursing (BSN). I was enrolled in a traditional nursing program. I began my program in the fall semester. The pandemic completely shifted what I thought nursing school was going to be like. Looking back now I would not change anything about my nursing school experience because it has made me the person and nurse I am today. Nursing school does not only teach you about how to care and advocate for others but also teaches you valuable lessons you need for yourself. The journey may seem long, the process may seem tedious, but I promise it will all be worth it.

Prior to graduating I accepted a position in a level IV neonatal intensive care unit. I began this position in late July after I graduated. I felt a host of emotions from being excited, to nervous, to anxious. Just like many others I was nervous and anxious because now I would be practicing as a nurse, but to do that I knew I had one task in which I had to be successful: the National Council Licensure Examination for Registered Nurses, commonly known as the NCLEX-RN®. The thought of taking this exam brought so many emotions because it was the determining factor to finally start the career I always wanted. The first thing I must tell you is this: you know yourself best, so please do whatever works for you and do not compare yourself to anyone! Remember this journey is yours! For myself, I knew I wanted to take my NCLEX closer to graduation. I received my Authorization to Test (ATT) from my State Board of Nursing about 2 weeks after graduation, and I scheduled my NCLEX-RN for June 9.

After graduating I took a week-long break just to enjoy, rest, and take in the huge accomplishment of graduating with a BSN. After the break, on the following Monday, I began to study. I studied using question platforms with rationales and test-taking strategies provided as instant feedback. I found practicing questions really helped me to get in testing mode. I first began by going over specific content and systems to get an overall assessment of areas I was comfortable in and others that I was not. After identifying areas that I was not performing strongly in, I reviewed the pathophysiology and interventions and followed this review by doing practice questions. The last 2 weeks of my studying time, I began to take exams without instant feedback to mirror the testing experience. I believe using platforms that had this option was tremendously helpful because it prepared me for what the NCLEX would be like. Taking these exams close to the time I knew I was going to take my NCLEX helped me build a routine.

Throughout nursing school, my school required us to take HESI exams in each of our core classes (Fundamentals, Medical Surgical, Community, Pediatrics, Women's Health, Critical Care, and Mental Health), and our last semester we took the HESI Exit. I strongly believe taking these standardized exams throughout nursing school really helped prepare me for the NCLEX. Taking these exams taught me test-taking strategies that I used while taking the NCLEX. This is a reminder that you have worked hard and studied hard all throughout nursing school, so you can do this. You are more prepared than you think you are.

About a week and a half before my exam, all the emotions started to hit me. The test anxiety started to really impact me, and this is when I was reminded to take breaks. It was not ideal to constantly study and bombard myself with information, and I had to tell myself it is okay to take a break and do things that you love. You must take breaks when studying for anything, whether that be in nursing school or for the NCLEX. Taking breaks to do things you enjoy ultimately helps you in the long run. Having discipline is what is most important. The second thing I realized was to lean on my support system. Reaching out to my close friends, family, and my school faculty and staff really helped me so much because, in that moment, I needed the reassurance and support that they were giving me. This brings me to my last point, repeat to yourself positive affirmations; write them down and say them to yourself! Your mind believes whatever you tell it. Throughout nursing school and while studying for the NCLEX, I would journal and write on sticky notes, "I will be a nurse," "I will achieve this or that," and it worked wonders for me. You must believe in yourself!

I took my NCLEX on a Thursday. That week I did not bombard myself with information or practice questions. I truly did things I enjoyed and engaged in self-care that entire week. That Sunday while I was out, I drove pass the testing center so that I could know where it was and where I would be going. I highly suggest doing this; that alone relieved anxiety. I scheduled my exam for 0800. Again, you know yourself best! Throughout nursing school, I preferred early morning exams and felt this is when I functioned best, so that is why I chose that time. Once I arrived at the PearsonVue Center, I did all the biometric requirements and put my belongings in my locker. All I brought with me was a water, my wallet, and my car keys, which I placed in my locker. The less the better! I was escorted to my testing area and placed at my desk, where I was given noise cancellation headphones and a whiteboard. At this time is when I realized that the moment we all wait for was here. I began my exam. My exam stopped at the minimum number of questions, and after completion of a survey, I raised my hand and was escorted out of the testing area. After leaving the testing center, I engaged in more self-care while I waited for my results. Early Saturday morning I checked my state's board of nursing website, and I saw my license posted. Then I purchased the quick view results and saw I passed. Seeing your license and that you passed the one exam that determines so much brings so much joy. It is a reminder that you can do hard things and, most importantly, that you have a purpose you must fulfill and that no one can stop you from achieving that.

Remember, no matter how long it takes you, how many bumps in the road you may have, or anything else you feel is stopping you from fulfilling your purpose, you have been called to the profession of nursing for a reason, so do not give up on yourself. Be your biggest cheerleader, look at how far you have come, and enjoy the process! You are going to be an amazing nurse!

A Note About The Next Generation NCLEX® (NGN) from Madison Drew Mahon, BSN, RN

During the winter semester of school, I found out that there would be something called next generation, or NGN questions, on the NCLEX. At first, I was terrified because who would try to make the NCLEX harder than it already is? However, after going through many Elsevier case studies as a class and learning new test taking strategies, these turned into my favorite type of question! NGN questions include the Bow-Tie, Trend, dropdown, highlighting, multiple response questions, and some other types. These are included on the NCLEX to test our clinical judgment as well as our critical thinking skills. I like these questions the most because they give more leeway to apply your own decision-making abilities, which to me is simpler than answering multiple choice questions.

The most helpful way to prepare for these questions on the NCLEX is to practice, practice, practice. I suggest going through at least 2-3 NGN case studies a day during your study time leading up to the NCLEX just to get familiar with them. Elsevier has an NGN book with an Evolve site that is all case studies and NGN style questions – that is what I used to prepare. At first it will be hard, and your scores may not be what you hoped for, but with time you will see how much your scores are improving with every case study.

On the NCLEX, you will have a minimum of 85 questions. Among these, you will have at least 3 unfolding case studies and each will contain 6 questions, so that is a total of 18 NGN questions. You may also have single case studies with Bow-Tie or Trend NGN questions. There is no need to be fearful of these questions if you prepare. Critical thinking is crucial in the nursing world, which is why these types of questions are important to practice and be tested on the NCLEX. When you see an NGN case study pop up on your NCLEX, you will have confidence in your critical thinking skills and be able to talk yourself through these questions with ease.

CHAPTER 4

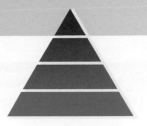

Clinical Judgment and Test-Taking Strategies

If you would like to read more about test-taking strategies after completing this chapter, *Saunders Strategies for Test Success: Passing Nursing School and the NCLEX® Exam* focuses on the test-taking strategies that will help you to pass your nursing examinations while in nursing school and will prepare you for the NCLEX-RN® examination.

I. Clinical Judgment

A. *Clinical judgment* is the observed outcome of critical thinking and decision-making (Dickison, Haerling, & Lasater, 2019). The NCLEX-RN examination requires candidates to demonstrate the ability to use clinical judgment in client care. Thus, clinical judgment skills, along with other traditional test-taking strategies, should be used to answer test questions.

B. The National Council of State Boards of Nursing (NCSBN) has created a Clinical Judgment Measurement Model (NCJMM) that consists of applying six cognitive skills or processes: (1) recognizing cues; (2) analyzing cues; (3) prioritizing hypotheses; (4) generating solutions; (5) taking actions; and (6) evaluating outcomes. See Chapter 1, Table 1.1 for a description of these six cognitive skills/processes. Also, see Box 4.18 for an example of how to apply the six cognitive skills/processes when answering test questions.

II. Key Test-Taking Strategies (Box 4.1)

III. How to Avoid Reading into the Question (Box 4.2)

A. Pyramid Points

1. For traditional NCLEX items, such as multiple choice or multiple response, avoid asking yourself the forbidden words, "Well, what if …?" because this will lead you to the "forbidden" area: Reading into the question.

⚠️ For NGN® items, you will have to ask yourself, "What if…?" because you need to think about and consider all existing and potential concerns, such as complications, that can occur in the clinical scenario.

2. Focus only on the data in the question, read every word, and make a decision about what the question is asking. Reread the question more than one time; ask yourself, "What is this question asking?" and "What content is this question testing?" (see Box 4.2).

3. Recognize cues that determine an abnormality exists. Look at data or information in the question

---

BOX 4.1   Key Test-Taking Strategies

The Question

- Focus on the data, read every word, and make a decision about what the question is asking.
- Note the subject and determine what content is being tested.
- Visualize the event; recognize cues that determine if an abnormality exists in the data provided.
- Consider available resources when reading the question.
- Determine who "the client of the question" is.
- Look for the strategic words; strategic words make a difference regarding what the question is asking about.
- Determine whether the question presents a positive or negative event query.
- For traditional NCLEX items, such as multiple choice or multiple response, avoid asking yourself the forbidden words, "Well, what if …?" because this will lead you to the "forbidden" area: Reading into the question.
- Apply the NCSBN Clinical Judgment Measurement Model (NCJMM) and the six cognitive skills alongside other test-taking strategies.

The Options

- Always use the process of elimination when choices or options are presented and read each option carefully; once you have eliminated options, reread the question before selecting your final choice or choices.
- In multiple-choice questions, look for comparable or alike options and eliminate these.
- Determine whether there is an umbrella or encompassing option; if so, this could be the correct option.
- Identify any closed-ended words; if present, the option is likely incorrect.
- Use the ABCs (airway, breathing, and circulation), Maslow's Hierarchy of Needs, the steps of the nursing process, and the NCJMM to answer questions that require prioritizing; use CAB (compressions, airway, breathing) for cardiopulmonary resuscitation (CPR) questions.
- Use therapeutic communication techniques to answer communication questions and remember to focus on the client's thoughts, feelings, concerns, anxieties, and fears.
- Use delegating and assignment-making guidelines to match the client's needs with the scope of practice of the health care provider.
- Use pharmacology guidelines to select the correct option if the question addresses a medication.

BOX 4.2 Practice Question: Avoiding the "What if ...?" Syndrome and Reading into the Question

The nurse is changing the tapes on a tracheostomy tube. The client coughs and the tube is dislodged. What is the **initial** nursing action?
1. Call the primary health care provider to reinsert the tube.
2. Ventilate the client using a manual resuscitation bag and face mask.
3. Cover the tracheostomy site with a sterile dressing to prevent infection.
4. Call the respiratory therapy department to reinsert the tracheostomy tube.

Answer: 2
Test-Taking Strategy
You may immediately think that because the tube is dislodged, you need to notify the primary health care provider. Read the question carefully and note the strategic word, *initial*. Focus on the subject, the tube is dislodged, and determine if an abnormality exists. The question is asking you for a nursing action, so that is what you need to look for as you eliminate the incorrect options. Eliminate options 1 and 4 because they are comparable or alike and delay the *initial* intervention needed. Eliminate option 3 because this action will block the airway. If the tube is dislodged, the *initial* nursing action is to ventilate the client using a manual resuscitation bag and face mask. Additionally, use of the ABCs—airway, breathing, and circulation—will direct you to the correct option. Remember: Avoid the "What if ...?" syndrome and reading into the question!

BOX 4.3 Ingredients of a Question: Event, Event Query, and Options

Event
The clinic nurse instructs an adolescent with iron deficiency anemia about the administration of oral iron preparations.

Event Query
The nurse would tell the adolescent that it is **best** to take the iron with which item?

Options
1. Cola
2. Soda
3. Water
4. Tomato juice

Answer: 4
Test-Taking Strategy
Note the strategic word, *best*. Remember that vitamin C enhances the absorption of the iron preparation. Tomato juice has a high ascorbic acid (vitamin C) content, whereas cola, soda, and water do not contain vitamin C. Note that options 1 and 2 are comparable or alike, so eliminate these options. Next, recalling that vitamin C increases the absorption of iron will direct you to option 4, tomato juice. As you read a question, remember to note its ingredients: the event, event query, and options!

and in the responses and decide what is abnormal. Pay close attention to this information as you answer the question.
4. Focus on the client in the question. At times, there are other people discussed in the question who also impact how the question should be answered. Remember the concepts of client-centered and family-centered care.
5. Consider available resources as you answer the question. Remember that you will have all the resources you need at the client's bedside to provide quality client care.
6. Look for the strategic words in the question, such as *immediate, initial, first, priority, best, need for follow-up,* and *need for further teaching;* strategic words make a difference regarding what the question is asking (see Box 4.4).

BOX 4.4 Common Strategic Words: Words That Indicate the Need to Prioritize and Words That Reflect Assessment

Words That Indicate the Need to Prioritize
- Best
- Early or late
- Essential
- First
- Highest priority
- Immediate
- Initial
- Most
- Most appropriate
- Most important
- Most likely
- Next
- Priority
- Primary
- Vital

Words That Reflect Assessment
- Ascertain
- Assess
- Check
- Collect
- Determine
- Find out
- Gather
- Identify
- Monitor
- Observe
- Obtain information
- Recognize

Additional Strategic Words
- Need for further teaching or education
- Need for follow-up
- On the day of
- After several days
- Increased, decreased
- Refute, support

7. In multiple-choice questions, multiple-response questions, or questions that require you to arrange nursing interventions or other data in order of priority, read every choice or option presented before answering.

8. *Always* use the process of elimination when choices or options are presented; after you have eliminated options, reread the question before selecting your final choice or choices. Focus on the data in both the question and the options to assist in the process of elimination and directing you to the correct answer (see Box 4.2).

9. With questions that require you to fill in the blank, focus on the information in the question and determine what the question is asking; if the question requires you to calculate a medication dose, an intravenous flow rate, or intake and output amounts, recheck your work in calculating and always use the on-screen calculator to verify the answer.

B. Ingredients of a question (Box 4.3)

1. The ingredients of a question include the cues or event, which is a client or clinical situation; the event query; and the options or answers.

2. The cues or event provides you with the content about the client or clinical situation that you need to think about when answering the question.

3. The event query asks something specific about the content of the event.

4. The options are all of the answers provided with the question.

5. In a multiple-choice question, there will be four options and you must select one; read every option carefully and think about the event and the event query as you use the process of elimination.

6. In a multiple-response question, there will be several options and you must select all options that apply to the event in the question. Each option provided is a true or false statement. Also, visualize the event and use nursing knowledge, clinical judgment, and clinical experiences to answer the question.

7. In an ordered-response (prioritizing)/drag and drop question, you will be required to arrange in order of priority nursing interventions or other data; visualize the event and use nursing knowledge, clinical judgment, and clinical experiences to answer the question. These questions are usually related to nursing procedures.

8. A fill-in-the-blank question does not contain options, and some figure/illustration questions and audio item formats may or may not contain options. A graphic option item will contain options in the form of a picture or graphic.

9. A scenario/exhibit question will most likely contain options; read the question carefully and all of the information in the scenario or exhibit before selecting an answer. In this question type, there will be information in the scenario/exhibit that is significant and/or insignificant. It is necessary to discern what information is significant, what is insignificant, and what the "distractors" are.

10. The NGN item types will use a case study approach. The stand-alone cases will be accompanied by a question that tests more than one cognitive skill. The unfolding case studies will be accompanied by 6 NGN item type questions, and each cognitive skill will be tested. Examples of both stand-alone and unfolding case studies and NGN items can be located on the Evolve site accompanying this book.

IV. **Strategic Words (Boxes 4.4 and 4.5)**

A. Strategic words focus your attention on a critical point to consider when answering the question and will assist you in eliminating the incorrect options. These words can be located in either the event or the query of the question.

B. Some strategic words may indicate that all options are correct and that it will be necessary to prioritize to select the correct option; words that reflect the process of assessment are also important to note (see Box 4.4). Words that reflect assessment usually indicate the need to look for an option that is a first step, because assessment is the first step in the nursing process.

C. As you read the question, look for the strategic words; these words make a difference regarding the focus of the question. Throughout this book, *strategic words* presented in the question, such as those that indicate the need to prioritize, are boldface. If the test-taking strategy is to focus on *strategic words,* then the term *strategic words* is highlighted in blue type where it appears in the test-taking strategy.

V. **Subject of the Question (Box 4.6)**

A. The subject of the question is the specific topic that the question is asking about.

B. Identifying the subject of the question will assist you in eliminating the incorrect options and direct you to select the correct option. Throughout this book, if the *subject*

BOX 4.5 Practice Question: Strategic Words

The home care nurse visits a client with chronic obstructive pulmonary disease (COPD) who is on home oxygen at 2 L per minute. The client's respiratory rate is 22 breaths per minute, and the client is complaining of increased dyspnea. The nurse would take which **initial** action?

1. Determine the need to increase the oxygen.
2. Call emergency services to come to the home.
3. Reassure the client that there is no need to worry.
4. Collect more information about client's respiratory status.

Answer: 4
Test-Taking Strategy
Note the strategic word, *initial*. Completing the assessment and collecting additional information regarding the client's respiratory status is the *initial* nursing action. The oxygen is not increased without validation of the need for further oxygen and the approval of the primary health care provider. Calling emergency services is a premature action. Reassuring the client is appropriate, but it is inappropriate to tell the client not to worry. Use the steps of the nursing process to answer correctly and remember that assessment is the first step. Also, use the ABCs—airway, breathing, and circulation—to direct you to option 4. Remember to look for strategic words!

of the question is a specific strategy to use in answering the question correctly, it is highlighted in blue type in the test-taking strategy.

⚠️ The specific test-taking strategy for every practice question in this book is highlighted in blue type. Highlighting the strategy will provide guidance on what strategies you need to review in *Saunders Clinical Judgment and Test-Taking Strategies: Passing Nursing School and the NCLEX® Exam*. The Health Problem code that accompanies each practice question will provide insight into the content areas in need of further remediation in *Saunders Comprehensive Review for the NCLEX-RN® Examination*.

VI. Positive and Negative Event Queries (Boxes 4.7 and 4.8)

A. A positive event query uses strategic words that ask you to select an option that is correct; for example, the event query may read, "Which statement by a client *indicates*

an understanding of the side effects of the prescribed medication?"

B. A negative event query uses strategic words that ask you to select an option that is an incorrect item or statement; for example, the event query may read, "Which statement by a client *indicates a need for further teaching* about the side effects of the prescribed medication?"

VII. Questions That Require Prioritizing

A. Many questions in the examination will require you to use the skill of prioritizing nursing actions.

B. Look for the strategic words in the question that indicate the need to prioritize (see Box 4.4).

C. Remember that when a question requires prioritization, all options may be correct and you need to determine the correct order of action.

D. Strategies to use to prioritize include the ABCs (airway, breathing, and circulation), Maslow's Hierarchy of Needs theory; the steps of the nursing process; and the cognitive skills in the NCJMM (recognize cues, analyze cues, prioritize hypotheses, generate solutions, take actions, and evaluate outcomes).

⚠️ The cognitive skills in the NCJMM include recognize cues, analyze cues, prioritize hypotheses, generate solutions, take actions, and evaluate outcomes (see Box 4.18).

BOX 4.6　Practice Question: Subject of the Question

The nurse would implement which measures to prevent infection in a hospitalized immunocompromised client? **Select all that apply.**

☐ 1. Use strict aseptic technique for all invasive procedures.
☐ 2. Use good handwashing technique before touching client.
☐ 3. Insert a urinary catheter to eliminate the need to use a bedpan.
☐ 4. Keep fresh flowers and potted plants out of client's room.
☐ 5. Place client in a semiprivate room with another client who is immunocompromised.
☐ 6. Keep frequently used equipment, such as a blood pressure cuff, in client's room for use by client.

Answer: 1, 2, 4, 6
Test-Taking Strategy
Focus on the subject, measures to prevent infection. The nurse needs to use knowledge to generate solutions and the actions to take to prevent infection. An immunocompromised client is at high risk for infection, and specific measures are taken to prevent infection. Strict aseptic technique is necessary for all invasive procedures; however, invasive procedures are avoided as much as possible. Urinary catheters are avoided because of the risk of infection associated with their use. Good handwashing technique is used before touching the client. Fresh fruits, fresh flowers, and potted plants are kept out of the client's room because they harbor organisms, placing the client at risk for infection. The client is placed in a private room. Frequently used equipment, such as a blood pressure cuff, stethoscope, or thermometer, is kept in the client's room for use by the client only. The client is also monitored daily for any signs of infection. Remember to focus on the subject of the question!

BOX 4.7　Practice Question: Positive Event Query

The nurse is teaching a postpartum client to bathe their newborn. The nurse would provide which instructions to the client? **Select all that apply.**

☐ 1. Support the newborn's body during the bath.
☐ 2. Clean any eye discharge using a wet cotton ball.
☐ 3. Fill the bathtub with no more than 10 inches of water.
☐ 4. Clean the eyes, moving from the outer canthus to the inner canthus.
☐ 5. Cover the newborn's body except for the part being washed or rinsed.
☐ 6. Begin the bath with the face, and clean the newborn's diaper area next.

Answer: 1, 2, 5
Test-Taking Strategy
Focus on the subject, instructions for bathing the newborn. Note that the question identifies a positive event query, and you need to select the correct instructions for bathing a newborn. Visualize each option carefully, keeping the principles of safety and infection control in mind. During bathing, the newborn's body is supported at all times by placing a hand under the newborn's head and neck. If the newborn is bathed in a bathtub, the tub should be lined with a towel to provide comfort and traction to prevent slipping, and it is filled with no more than 3 inches of water. The newborn's body is covered except for the part being washed or rinsed. Any eye discharge is cleaned using a wet cotton ball moving from the inner canthus to the outer canthus. The bath is started with the face, then other body areas are washed, and the diaper area is cleaned last. Remember to read the event query and note if it is a positive event type.

E. The ABCs (Box 4.9)
1. Use the ABCs (airway, breathing, and circulation) when selecting an answer or determining the order of priority.
2. Remember the order of priority: airway, breathing, and circulation.
3. Airway is always the first priority. Note that an exception occurs when cardiopulmonary resuscitation (CPR) is performed; in this situation, the nurse follows the CAB (compressions, airway, breathing) guidelines.
F. Maslow's Hierarchy of Needs theory (Box 4.10 and Fig. 4.1)
1. According to Maslow's Hierarchy of Needs theory, physiological needs are the priority, followed by safety and security needs, love and belonging needs, self-esteem needs, and, finally, self-actualization needs; select the option or determine the order of priority by addressing physiological needs first.
2. When a physiological need is not addressed in the question or noted in one of the options, continue to use Maslow's Hierarchy of Needs theory sequentially as a guide and look for the option that addresses safety.

BOX 4.8 Practice Question: Negative Event Query

The nurse provides home care instructions to a client who is taking lithium carbonate. Which statement by the client indicates a **need for further instructions?**
1. "I need to take the medication with meals."
2. "My blood levels must be monitored very closely."
3. "I need to decrease my salt and fluid intake while taking the medication."
4. "I need to call my doctor if I have excessive diarrhea, vomiting, or sweating."

Answer: 3
Test-Taking Strategy
This question identifies an example of a negative event query question. Note the strategic words, *need for further instructions*. These strategic words indicate that you need to select an option that identifies an incorrect client statement. Lithium is irritating to the gastric mucosa; therefore, lithium should be taken with meals. Because therapeutic and toxic dosage ranges are so close, lithium blood levels must be monitored very closely, more frequently at first and then once every several months after that per the primary health care provider's prescription. The client would be instructed to withhold the medication if excessive diarrhea, vomiting, or diaphoresis occurs and to inform the primary health care provider if any of these problems occur. A normal diet with daily recommended sodium (1500 mg) and fluid (3000 mL) intake should be maintained because lithium decreases sodium reabsorption by the renal tubules, which could cause sodium depletion. A low-sodium intake causes a relative increase in lithium retention and could lead to toxicity. Remember that negative event queries ask you to select an option that is an *incorrect* item or statement! Watch for negative event queries!

BOX 4.9 Practice Question: Use of the ABCs

A client is admitted to the emergency department with complaints of severe chest pain. The client is extremely restless, frightened, and dyspneic. Immediate admission orders include oxygen by nasal cannula at 4 L per minute, troponin level, creatinine phosphokinase and isoenzyme blood levels, a chest x-ray, and a 12-lead electrocardiogram (ECG). Which action would the nurse take **first?**
1. Obtain the 12-lead ECG.
2. Draw the blood specimens.
3. Apply the oxygen to the client.
4. Call radiology to obtain the chest x-ray study.

Answer: 3
Test-Taking Strategy
Note the strategic word, *first*. The nurse needs to recognize and analyze cues to determine that the priority hypothesis is oxygenation. The nurse would then generate solutions and take action by applying the oxygen first. Also, use the ABCs—airway, breathing, and circulation. The *first* action would be to apply the oxygen because the client can be experiencing myocardial ischemia. The ECG can provide evidence of cardiac damage and the location of myocardial ischemia. However, oxygen is the priority to prevent further cardiac damage. Drawing the blood specimens would be done after oxygen administration and just before or after the ECG, depending on the situation. Although the chest x-ray can show cardiac enlargement, having the chest x-ray would not influence immediate treatment. Remember to use the ABCs—airway, breathing, and circulation—to prioritize!

BOX 4.10 Practice Question: Maslow's Hierarchy of Needs Theory

A client arrives at the emergency department and states they were just raped. In preparing a plan of care, which is the **priority** intervention?
1. Providing instructions for medical follow-up
2. Obtaining appropriate counseling for the victim
3. Providing anticipatory guidance for police investigations, medical questions, and court proceedings
4. Exploring safety concerns by obtaining permission to notify significant others who can provide shelter

Answer: 4
Test-Taking Strategy
Note the strategic word, *priority*. The nurse needs to have knowledge of the client's priority needs and generate solutions. Use Maslow's Hierarchy of Needs theory. After the provision of medical treatment, the nurse's next *priority* would be obtaining support and planning for safety. Option 1 is concerned with ensuring that the victim understands the importance of and commits to the need for medical follow-up. Options 2 and 3 seek to meet the emotional needs related to the rape and emotional readiness for the process of discovery and legal action. From the options provided, these are not *priority* interventions. Remember that physiological needs are the *priority*, followed by safety needs. Therefore, select option 4 because it addresses the client's safety needs. Remember to use Maslow's Hierarchy of Needs theory to help prioritize and generate solutions!

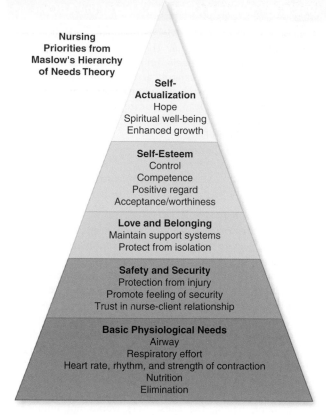

Nursing Priorities from Maslow's Hierarchy of Needs Theory

Self-Actualization
Hope
Spiritual well-being
Enhanced growth

Self-Esteem
Control
Competence
Positive regard
Acceptance/worthiness

Love and Belonging
Maintain support systems
Protect from isolation

Safety and Security
Protection from injury
Promote feeling of security
Trust in nurse-client relationship

Basic Physiological Needs
Airway
Respiratory effort
Heart rate, rhythm, and strength of contraction
Nutrition
Elimination

FIGURE 4.1 Use Maslow's Hierarchy of Needs theory to establish priorities.

G. Steps of the Nursing Process and the NCJMM Cognitive Skills/Processes

1. Assessment/Recognize Cues

   a. The nurse recognizes cues by identifying significant data from many sources.

   b. These questions address the process of gathering subjective and objective data relative to the client, confirming the data, and communicating and documenting the data.

   c. Remember that assessment/recognizing cues is the first step.

   d. When you are asked to select your first, immediate, or initial nursing action, assess/recognize cues first to prioritize when selecting the correct option.

   e. Look for strategic words in the options that reflect assessment (see Box 4.4).

   f. If an option contains the concept of assessment or the collection of client data, the best choice is to select that option (Box 4.11).

   g. Possible exception to the guideline—if the question presents an emergency situation, read carefully; in an emergency situation, an intervention may be the priority rather than taking the time to collect further data.

2. Analysis/Analyze Cues and Prioritize Hypotheses (Box 4.12)

   a. The nurse analyzes cues by connecting significant data to the client's clinical presentation and determining: is the data expected? Unexpected? What are the concerns?

BOX 4.11 Practice Question: Assessment/Recognize Cues

The clinic nurse prepares to develop a diabetic teaching program. To meet the clients' needs, the nurse would consider which of the following **first?**

1. Assess the clients' functional abilities.
2. Ensure that insurance will pay for participation in the program.
3. Discuss the focus of the program with the interprofessional team.
4. Include everyone who comes into the clinic in the teaching sessions.

Answer: 1
Test-Taking Strategy
Note the **strategic word,** *first,* which indicates the need to prioritize. The nurse needs to have knowledge of the teaching/learning process to recognize cues that affect preparation of an individualized teaching program for the clients. Use the **steps of the nursing process** to answer the question, remembering that assessment is the first step. The only option that addresses assessment is option 1. The nurse would focus on individualized disease prevention and health promotion and maintenance. Therefore, the nurse must *first* assess the clients and their needs so as to effectively plan the program. Options 2, 3, and 4 do not directly address the clients' needs.

b. The nurse also prioritizes hypotheses (concerns, client needs) by ranking the hypotheses from highest to lowest priority.

c. These questions are the most difficult questions because they require understanding of the principles of physiologic responses and require interpretation of the data collected.

d. They require critical thinking and decision-making and determining the rationale for therapeutic prescriptions or interventions that may be addressed in the question.

e. These questions may address the formulation of a statement that identifies a client need or problem and may also include the communication and documentation of the results from the process of analyzing cues.

f. Often these types of questions require examining a broad concept and breaking it down into smaller parts and assimilation of the information and application to a client scenario.

3. Planning/Generating Solutions (Box 4.13)

   a. The nurse generates solutions by using hypotheses to determine interventions for an expected outcome.

   b. These questions require prioritizing client problems, determining goals and outcome criteria for goals of care, developing the plan of care, and communicating and documenting the plan of care.

   c. Remember that actual client problems rather than potential client problems will be the priority in most client situations.

4. Implementation/Taking Actions (Box 4.14)

BOX 4.12 Practice Question: Analysis/Analyze Cues

The nurse reviews the arterial blood gas results of a client and notes the following. The nurse analyzes these results as indicating which condition?

Laboratory Results

Test and Results	Reference Range
pH 7.30	pH 7.35–7.45
PO_2 82 mm Hg	80–100 mm Hg
PCO_2 50 mm Hg	35–45 mm Hg
HCO_3 22 mEq/L (22 mmol/L)	21–28 mEq/L (21–28 mmol/L)

1. Metabolic acidosis, compensated
2. Respiratory alkalosis, compensated
3. Metabolic alkalosis, uncompensated
4. Respiratory acidosis, uncompensated

Answer: 4

Test-Taking Strategy

Focus on the **data in the question** and the **subject**, interpreting arterial blood gas results. The nurse needs to analyze the laboratory results and have knowledge of the reference ranges for arterial blood gas results and acid-base disorders to determine the condition the client is experiencing. In a respiratory condition, an opposite effect will be seen between the pH and the PCO_2. In this situation, the pH is below the lower limit of the reference range, and the PCO_2 is elevated. In an acidotic condition, the pH is low. Therefore, the laboratory results indicate respiratory acidosis. Compensation occurs when the pH returns to a value in the reference range. Because the pH is not normal, compensation has not occurred. Remember that in a respiratory imbalance you will find an opposite response between the pH and the PCO_2. Therefore, you can eliminate options 1 and 3. Also, remember that the pH decreases in an acidotic condition and compensation occurs, as evidenced by pH that is in range. Remember, the nurse needs to analyze cues and connect data to the client's presentation.

---

a. The nurse implements the generated solutions addressing the highest priorities or hypotheses.
b. These questions address the process of organizing and managing care, counseling and teaching, providing care to achieve established goals, supervising and coordinating care, and communicating and documenting nursing interventions.
c. Focus on a nursing action rather than on a medical action when you are answering a question, unless the question is asking you what prescribed medical action is anticipated.
d. On the NCLEX-RN examination, the only client whom you need to be concerned about is the client in the question that you are answering; avoid the "What if. . .?" syndrome and remember that the client in the question on the computer screen is your *only* assigned client.
e. Answer the question from a textbook and ideal point of view; remember that the nurse has all of the time and all of the equipment needed to

---

BOX 4.13 Practice Question: Planning/Generating Solutions

A client with active tuberculosis (TB) is to be admitted to a medical-surgical unit. Which action would the nurse take when planning a bed assignment?
1. Tell the admitting office to send the client to the intensive care unit.
2. Place client in a private, airborne infection isolation room (AIIR).
3. Assign client to a room with another client because intravenous antibiotics will be administered.
4. Assign client to a room with another client and place a "strict hand washing" sign outside the door.

Answer: 2

Test-Taking Strategy

Focus on the **subject**, planning nursing care and identifying the safe bed assignment. Note that the question states "active tuberculosis." Tuberculosis is spread via the airborne route. Preventing the spread of infection requires the use of special air handling and ventilation in an AIIR. Therefore, option 2 is the only correct option when planning a bed assignment for this client. Remember, the nurse needs to plan and generate solutions to determine interventions for an expected outcome.

---

care for the client readily available at the bedside; remember that you do not need to run to the supply room to obtain, for example, sterile gloves because the sterile gloves will be at the client's bedside.
5. Evaluation/Evaluate Outcomes (Box 4.15)
   a. The nurse compares observed outcomes with expected ones.
   b. These questions focus on comparing the actual outcomes of care with the expected outcomes and on communicating and documenting findings.
   c. They also focus on assisting in determining the client's response to care, identifying factors that may interfere with achieving expected outcomes.
   d. In these question types, watch for negative event queries because they are frequently used.
H. Determine if an abnormality exists (Box 4.16).
   1. In the question, the client scenario will be described. Use your nursing knowledge to recognize cues and determine whether any of the information presented is indicating an abnormality.
   2. If an abnormality exists, either further nursing assessment or further nursing intervention will be required. Therefore, continuing to monitor or documenting will not likely be a correct answer; do not select these options if they are presented!
I. Focus on the data or information in the question (Box 4.17).
   1. With this strategy, data are provided in either the question or the options (or both) that are important in answering the question correctly.
   2. Data needed to answer the question may be normal or abnormal. If it is normal, there may be another

---

BOX 4.14 Practice Question: Implementation/ Taking Actions

The nurse is performing range-of-motion (ROM) exercises on a client when the client develops spastic muscle contractions. Which actions would the nurse take? **Select all that apply.**

☐ 1. Stop movement of affected part.
☐ 2. Massage the affected part vigorously.
☐ 3. Notify the primary health care provider immediately.
☐ 4. Force movement of the joint supporting the muscle.
☐ 5. Ask the client to stand and walk rapidly around the room.
☐ 6. Place continuous gentle pressure on the muscle group until it relaxes.

Answer: 1, 6
Test-Taking Strategy
Implementation questions address the process of organizing and managing care. Focus on the subject, interventions to relieve spastic muscle contractions. In this question, the hypothesis is spastic muscle contractions. The nurse would use knowledge about the interventions to relieve spasticity, generate solutions, and take actions. ROM exercises should put each joint through as full a range of motion as possible without causing discomfort. An unexpected outcome is the development of spastic muscle contraction during ROM exercises. If this occurs, the nurse would stop movement of the affected part and place continuous gentle pressure on the muscle group until it relaxes. Once the contraction subsides, the exercises are resumed using slower, steady movement. Massaging the affected part vigorously may worsen the contraction. There is no need to notify the primary health care provider unless intervention is ineffective. The nurse would never force movement of a joint. Asking the client to stand and walk rapidly around the room is an inappropriate measure. Additionally, if the client is able to walk, ROM exercises are probably unnecessary. Remember, the nurse needs to generate solutions and then take action.

BOX 4.15 Practice Question: Evaluation/ Evaluate Options

The nurse instructs a client receiving external radiation therapy about skin care. Which statements by the client indicate an understanding of the instructions? **Select all that apply.**

☐ 1. "I can lie in the sun as long as I limit the time to 2 hours daily."
☐ 2. "I should wear snug clothing to support the radiated skin area."
☐ 3. "I should wash the radiated area gently each day with a mild soap and water."
☐ 4. "After bathing I should dry the area with a patting motion using a clean, soft towel."
☐ 5. "I should avoid the use of powders, lotions, or creams on the skin area being radiated."
☐ 6. "I should avoid removing the markings on the skin when bathing until my course of radiation is complete."

Answer: 3, 4, 5, 6
Test-Taking Strategy
Focus on the subject, client's understanding of the instructions. The subject specifies that this is an evaluation-type question. The nurse needs to use knowledge about radiation therapy to evaluate the outcomes of teaching. Recall that external radiation therapy can cause altered skin integrity, and special measures need to be taken to protect the skin. These measures include washing the radiated area gently (using the hand rather than a wash cloth) each day with either water alone or water and a mild soap (rinse soap thoroughly); drying the area with a patting motion (not a rubbing motion) with a clean soft towel; avoiding removing the markings on the skin when bathing until the entire course of radiation is complete because these markings indicate exactly where the beam of radiation is to be focused; avoiding the use of powders, lotions, or creams on the skin area being radiated unless prescribed by the radiologist; avoiding wearing clothing or items that bind or rub the radiated skin area; and avoiding heat exposure or sun exposure to the radiated area. Remember, the nurse needs to evaluate outcomes by comparing observed outcomes with expected ones.

---

event in the question that could cause the data to become abnormal.

J. Choose options that ensure client safety (see Box 4.17).
   1. When choosing an option, think about whether the option could cause a compromise in client safety.
   2. If an option could potentially result in an adverse effect or increase the client's risk for injury, eliminate that option.

VIII. Using the NCJMM to Answer a Test Question (Box 4.18)

IX. Client Needs

A. Physiological Integrity
   1. According to the NCSBN, these questions test the concepts that the nurse provides care as it relates to comfort and assistance in the performance of activities of daily living, as well as care related to the administration of medications and parenteral therapies.
   2. These questions also address the nurse's ability to reduce the client's potential for developing complications or health problems related to treatments,

procedures, or existing conditions and to provide care to clients with acute, chronic, or life-threatening physical health conditions.
   3. Focus on Maslow's Hierarchy of Needs theory in these types of questions and remember that physiological needs are a priority and are addressed first.
   4. Use the ABCs—airway, breathing, and circulation—and the NCJMM when selecting an option addressing Physiological Integrity. Note that when CPR is necessary, follow the CAB guidelines rather than the ABCs.

B. Safe and Effective Care Environment
   1. The NCSBN indicates that these questions test the concepts of providing safe nursing care and collaborating with interprofessional team members to facilitate effective client care; these questions also focus on the protection of clients, significant others, and health care personnel from environmental hazards.

BOX 4.16   Practice Question: Determine if an Abnormality Exists

The nurse is caring for a client who is taking digoxin and is complaining of nausea. The nurse gathers additional assessment data and checks the most recent laboratory results. Which test result requires the **need for follow-up** by the nurse?

Laboratory Results

Test and Results	Reference Range
Sodium 134 mEq/L (134 mmol/L)	135–145 mEq/L (135–145 mmol/L)
Potassium 3.3 mEq/L (3.3 mmol/L)	3.5–5.0 mEq/L (3.5–5.0 mmol/L)
Phosphorus 3.1 mg/dL (1.0 mmol/L)	3.0–4.5 mg/dL (0.97–1.45 mmol/L)
Magnesium 1.8 mg/dL (0.9 mmol/L)	1.8–2.6 mEq/L (0.74–1.07 mmol/L)

1. Sodium
2. Potassium
3. Phosphorus
4. Magnesium

Answer: 2
Test-Taking Strategy
Note the **strategic words**, *need for follow-up*. The first step in approaching the answer to this question is to **determine whether an abnormality exists**. Recognize cues in the question that are significant, and analyze the cues by connecting the data to a possible hypothesis. The client is taking digoxin and is complaining of nausea, and the nurse would suspect toxicity. The sodium result is one point below the reference range, which is insignificant and unrelated to the client scenario. All other laboratory results are within the reference range except for the potassium level. Recall that the potassium level must stay consistent while the client is taking digoxin to prevent adverse effects such as toxicity from occurring. Remember to recognize and analyze cues, and **determine whether an abnormality exists** in the event before choosing the correct option.

BOX 4.17   Practice Question: Focus on the Data in the Question and Ensure Client Safety

The nurse is providing discharge instructions to an adult client with diabetes mellitus and checks the client's glycosylated hemoglobin (HbA1c) level. How would the nurse guide the client?

Laboratory Results

Test and Results	Reference Range
Hemoglobin (HbA1c) 10%	<6% (adult without diabetes)

1. "Increase the amount of vegetables and water intake in your diet regimen."
2. "Change the time of day you exercise because it may cause hypoglycemia."
3. "Continue with the same diet and exercise regimen you are currently using."
4. "Utilize a high-intensity exercise regimen and decrease carbohydrate consumption."

Answer: 1
Test-Taking Strategy
Focus on the **data in the question**, an HbA1c level of 10%. The nurse needs to recognize cues and analyze the cues to determine that the HbA1c level is above the recommended value for an adult client with diabetes mellitus and indicates poor glycemic control. Therefore, an **abnormality exists**. Choose the option that addresses this abnormality and **ensures client safety**. Option 1 is a safe recommendation to make to a diabetic client and will help to reduce the HbA1c level. Changing the time of day for exercise and continuing with the same diet and exercise regimen will not address the client's problem. Note the words *high intensity* in option 4. Using a high-intensity exercise regimen and decreasing carbohydrate consumption could potentially result in a hypoglycemic reaction and does not ensure client safety. Remember to **focus on the data in the question** and recognize and analyze cues to determine if an abnormality is present.

---

2. Focus on safety with these types of questions, and remember the importance of hand washing, call lights or bells, bed positioning, appropriate use of side rails, asepsis, use of standard and other precautions, triage, and emergency response planning.

C. Health Promotion and Maintenance
   1. According to the NCSBN, these questions test the concepts that the nurse provides and assists in directing nursing care to promote and maintain health.
   2. Content addressed in these questions relates to assisting the client and significant others during the normal expected stages of growth and development and providing client care related to the prevention and early detection of health problems.
   3. Use the teaching and learning theory if the question addresses client teaching, remembering that the client's willingness, desire, and readiness to learn is the first priority.

4. Watch for negative event queries because they are frequently used in questions that address Health Promotion and Maintenance and client education.

D. Psychosocial Integrity
   1. The NCSBN notes that these questions test the concepts of nursing care that promote and support the emotional, mental, and social well-being of the client and significant others.
   2. Content addressed in these questions relates to supporting and promoting the client's or significant others' ability to cope, adapt, or problem-solve in situations such as illnesses, disabilities, or stressful events, including abuse, neglect, or violence.
   3. In this Client Needs category, you may be asked communication-type questions that relate to how you would respond to a client, a client's family member or significant other, or other health care team members.

BOX 4.18 Using the NCJMM to Answer Test Questions

A client in the emergency department has anorexia, nausea, vomiting, and visual problems. The nurse asks about medications the client takes at home, and the client provides a list. How would the nurse proceed?

Medication List

- Amiodarone: 400 mg orally daily
- Digoxin: 0.25 mg orally daily
- Lisinopril: 20 mg orally daily
- Furosemide: 40 mg orally daily
- Metformin: 1000 mg orally twice daily
- Tamsulosin: 0.4 mg orally daily

Cognitive Skill: Recognize Cues

- Client observation cues: Anorexia, nausea, vomiting, and visual problems
- Environmental: Emergency department
- Medical record: Medications taken by the client

Cognitive Skill: Analyze Cues

- Need knowledge of the medications and their adverse effects
- The client exhibits signs of digoxin toxicity.

Cognitive Skill: Prioritize Hypotheses

- Check the digoxin level.
- Treat toxicity.
- Treat nausea and vomiting.

Cognitive Skill: Generate Solutions

- Reduce digoxin level—consider an antidote.
- Eliminate nausea and vomiting—consider antiemetics.

Cognitive Skill: Take Actions

- Withhold digoxin.
- Monitor vital signs (VS) and apical heart rate.
- Contact the physician for orders to treat digoxin toxicity and nausea and vomiting.
- Administer antidote and antiemetics.

Cognitive Skill: Evaluate Outcomes

- Digoxin level in therapeutic range
- Clinical symptoms resolved
- VS and apical heart rate stable

BOX 4.19 Practice Question: Communication and the Client of the Question

A client with a diagnosis of depression says to the nurse, "I should have died. I've always been a failure." The nurse would make which therapeutic response to the client?
1. "I see a lot of positive things in you."
2. "You still have a great deal to live for."
3. "Feeling like a failure is part of your illness."
4. "You've been feeling like a failure for some time now?"

Answer: 4
Test-Taking Strategy
Use **therapeutic communication techniques** to answer this question. Recognize cues in the question and analyze them to determine the significance of the client's statement. Remember to address the client's feelings and concerns. Option 4 is the only option that is stated in the form of a question and is open ended, thus encouraging the verbalization of feelings. Remember to recognize and analyze cues, use **therapeutic communication techniques,** and focus on the client.

The nurse is caring for a terminally ill client. The client's spouse, who has served as the caregiver, is at the bedside. The spouse states, "I really hope my partner here can just get better so we can go home." What statement would the nurse make to the client's spouse?
1. "Has the doctor spoken with you about your partner's plan of care?"
2. "It sounds like this is difficult for you. What do you know about your partner's condition?"
3. "I hope your partner gets better too. It would be wonderful for you and your partner to be at home."
4. "I know this is a difficult situation. I've seen this many times before. The spouse always has a hard time."

Answer: 2
Test-Taking Strategy
Focus on the **client of the question,** which in this case is the client's spouse. Recognize cues in the question and analyze them to determine the significance of the client's statement. Also, use **therapeutic communication techniques.** The correct option acknowledges the spouse's feelings and asks for further information to determine understanding of the situation. Option 1 does not acknowledge feelings. Option 3 may offer false reassurance and false hope. Option 4 does not address the spouse's feelings and may cause further emotional distress. Remember to recognize and analyze cues, use **therapeutic communication techniques,** and focus on the client.

4. Use therapeutic communication techniques to answer communication questions because of their effectiveness in the communication process (Box 4.19).
5. Remember to identify the client of the question and select the option that focuses on the thoughts, feelings, concerns, anxieties, or fears of the client, client's family member, or significant other (see Box 4.19).

E. For additional information about Client Needs, refer to Chapter 5 and to the NCLEX-RN test plan at the NCSBN website (http://www.ncsbn.org).

X.   Eliminate Comparable or Alike Options (Box 4.20)

A. When reading the options in multiple-choice or multiple-response questions, look for options that are comparable or alike.

B. Comparable or alike options can be eliminated as possible answers because it is not likely for both options to be correct.

XI. Eliminate Options Containing Closed-Ended Words (Box 4.21)

A. Some closed-ended words are *all, always, every, must, none, never,* and *only.*

BOX 4.20 Practice Question: Eliminate Comparable or Alike Options

The nurse is assessing the leg pain of a client who has just undergone right femoral-popliteal artery bypass grafting. Which question would be **most** useful in determining whether the client is experiencing graft occlusion?

1. "Can you describe what the pain feels like?"
2. "Can you rate the pain on a scale of 1 to 10?"
3. "Did you get any relief from the last dose of pain medication?"
4. "Can you compare this pain to the pain you felt before surgery?"

Answer: 4
Test-Taking Strategy
Note the strategic word, *most,* and focus on recognizing cues related to differentiating expected postoperative pain from pain that indicates graft occlusion. The most frequent indication that a graft is occluding is the return of pain that is similar to that experienced preoperatively. Eliminate options 1, 2, and 3 because they are comparable or alike and are standard pain assessment questions. Remember to eliminate comparable or alike options!

B. Eliminate options that contain closed-ended words because these words imply a fixed or extreme meaning; these types of options are usually incorrect.
C. Options that contain open-ended words, such as *may, usually, normally, commonly,* or *generally,* should be considered as possible correct options.

XII. Look for the Umbrella Option (Box 4.22)

A. When answering a question, look for the umbrella option.
B. The umbrella option is one that is a broad or universal statement and that usually contains the concepts of the other options within it.
C. The umbrella option will be the correct answer.

XIII. Use the Guidelines for Delegating and Assignment-Making (Box 4.23)

A. You may be asked a question that will require you to decide how you will delegate a task or assign clients to other health care providers (HCPs).
B. Focus on the information in the question and what task or assignment is to be delegated and the available HCPs.
C. When you have determined what task or assignment is to be delegated and the available HCPs, consider the client's needs and match the client's needs with the scope of practice of the HCPs identified.
D. The Nurse Practice Act and any practice limitations define which aspects of care can be delegated and which must be performed by a registered nurse. Use nursing scope of practice as a guide to assist in answering questions. Remember that the NCLEX is a national examination, and national standards rather than agency-specific standards must be followed when delegating.
E. In general, noninvasive interventions, such as skin care, range-of-motion exercises, ambulation, grooming, and hygiene measures, can be assigned to an unlicensed

---

BOX 4.21 Practice Question: Eliminate Options That Contain Closed-Ended Words

A client is to undergo an endoscopy, and the nurse provides preprocedure instructions. The nurse would instruct the client to take which action in the preprocedure period?

1. Avoid eating or drinking after midnight before the test.
2. Limit self to only two cigarettes on the morning of the test.
3. Have a clear liquid breakfast only on the morning of the test.
4. Take all routine medications with a glass of water on the morning of the test.

Answer: 1
Test-Taking Strategy
The nurse needs to use knowledge about the preparation for an endoscopy in order to take action with regard to preprocedure instructions. Note the closed-ended words "only" in options 2 and 3 and "all" in option 4. Eliminate options that contain closed-ended words because these options are usually incorrect. Also, note that options 2, 3, and 4 are comparable or alike options in that they all involve taking in something on the morning of the test. Remember to eliminate options that contain closed-ended words.

BOX 4.22 Practice Question: Look for the Umbrella Option

The home care nurse is caring for a client who has just been discharged from the hospital after implantation of a permanent pacemaker. The nurse would assess the client's home for the presence of which high-risk **priority** item?

1. Hair dryer
2. Electric blanket
3. Electric toothbrush with holder
4. Electrical items with strong magnetic fields

Answer: 4
Test-Taking Strategy
The nurse needs to use knowledge about safety measures for a client with a permanent pacemaker to recognize cues indicating risks. Note the strategic word, *priority,* and note the umbrella option. A pacemaker is shielded from interference from most electrical devices. Radios, televisions, electric blankets, toasters, microwave ovens, heating pads, and hair dryers are considered to be safe. Devices to be forewarned about include those with a strong electric current or magnetic field, such as antitheft devices in stores, metal detectors used in airports, and radiation therapy (if applicable and which might require relocation of the pacemaker). Note that option 4 uses the word "strong" and is the umbrella option addressing items with strong electric currents or magnetic fields. Remember that the umbrella option is a broad or universal option that includes the concepts of the other options in it!

---

assistive personnel (UAP), also known as a nursing assistant or certified nursing assistant.
F. A licensed practical nurse (LPN) can perform the tasks that a UAP can perform and can usually perform certain invasive tasks, such as dressings, suctioning, urinary

---

BOX 4.23 Practice Question: Use Guidelines for Delegating and Assignment-Making

The nurse is planning the client assignments for the day and has a licensed practical nurse (LPN) and an unlicensed assistive personnel (UAP) on the nursing team. Which client would the nurse **most appropriately** assign to the LPN?
1. Client with stable heart failure who has early stage Alzheimer's disease
2. Client who is scheduled for an electrocardiogram and a chest radiograph
3. Client who was treated for dehydration and is weak and needs assistance with bathing
4. Client with emphysema who is receiving oxygen at 2 L by nasal cannula and becomes dyspneic on exertion

Answer: 4
Test-Taking Strategy
The nurse needs to have knowledge of the job descriptions and roles of the LPN and UAP in order to generate solutions for planning safe client assignments. Note the **strategic words,** *most appropriately,* and focus on the **subject,** the assignment to be delegated to the LPN. When asked questions related to delegation, think about the role description of the employee and the needs of the client. The nurse would most appropriately assign the client with emphysema to the LPN. This client has an airway problem and has the highest priority needs of the clients presented in the options. The clients described in options 1, 2, and 3 can be cared for appropriately by the UAP. Remember to match the client's needs with the scope of practice of the health care provider!

---

catheterization, and administering medications orally or by the subcutaneous or intramuscular route; some selected piggyback intravenous medications may also be administered.
G. A registered nurse can perform the tasks that an LPN can perform and is responsible for assessment and planning care, analyzing client data, implementing and evaluating client care, supervising care, initiating teaching, and administering medications intravenously.

XIV. Available Resources and Ideal Situations (Box 4.24)

A. When providing care to a client, particularly in emergency situations, keep in mind that all of the resources needed (e.g., blood pressure cuff, dressing supplies) to provide client care will be readily available. Remember, you have everything you need wherever and whenever you need it!

B. Answer traditional NCLEX-style questions as if they were an ideal situation. Remember that traditional questions require that you will answer questions based on textbook information. In contrast, NGN-style questions present authentic clinical scenarios, so you need to consider multiple external factors when answering these question types.

XV. Answering Pharmacology Questions (Box 4.25)

A. If you are familiar with the medication, use nursing knowledge to answer the question.

BOX 4.24 Practice Question: Available Resources

The nurse is called to a client's room to assist the client who has a chest tube. The client states that it felt like the tube pulled out. The nurse assesses the client and finds that the tube has dislodged and is lying on the floor. What action would the nurse take **next?**
1. Obtain a pair of sterile gloves.
2. Contact the charge nurse for help.
3. Cover the insertion site with a sterile dressing.
4. Submerge the dislodged tube into sterile water.

Answer: 3
Test-Taking Strategy
Note the **strategic word,** *next.* Recognize cues in the question and analyze the cues for their significance to identify the action that needs to be taken. When providing care to a client, particularly in emergency situations, keep in mind that all of the **resources** needed to provide client care will be readily available at the client's bedside. Most students would eliminate option 4 first knowing that this action is not necessary in this scenario. From the remaining options, you may think, "I don't have sterile gloves or a sterile dressing with me, so let me call for help first." Remember, you have everything you need wherever and whenever you need it!

BOX 4.25 Practice Question: Answering Pharmacology Questions

The nurse is preparing to administer atenolol. The nurse would check which **priority** item before administering the medication?
1. Temperature
2. Blood pressure
3. Potassium level
4. Blood glucose level

Answer: 2
Test-Taking Strategy
Note the **strategic word,** *priority.* The nurse needs to use knowledge about the medication in order to know the action that would be taken. Focus on the name of the medication. Recall that most beta-blocker medication names end with the letters *-lol* and that these medications are used to treat hypertension. This will direct you to option 2. Remember to use pharmacology guidelines to assist you in answering questions about medications!

B. Remember that the question will identify the generic name of the medication only.
C. If the question identifies a medical diagnosis, try to form a relationship between the medication and the diagnosis; for example, you can determine that cyclophosphamide is an antineoplastic medication if the question refers to a client with breast cancer who is taking this medication. Remember, however, that on the NCLEX, a diagnosis may not be presented in a pharmacology question.

D. Try to determine the classification of the medication being addressed to assist in answering the question. Identifying the classification will assist in determining a medication's action or side/adverse effects or both.

E. Recognize the common side effects and adverse effects associated with each medication classification and relate the appropriate nursing interventions to each effect; for example, if a side effect is hypertension, the associated nursing intervention would be to monitor the blood pressure.

F. Focus on what the question is asking or the subject of the question, for example, intended effect, side effect, adverse effect, or toxic effect.

G. Learn medications that belong to a classification by commonalities in their medication names; for example, medications that act as beta blockers end with *"-lol"* (e.g., ateno*lol*).

H. If the question requires a medication calculation, remember that a calculator is available on the computer; talk yourself through each step to be sure that the answer makes sense, and recheck the calculation before answering the question, particularly if the answer seems like an unusual dosage.

I. Pharmacology: Pyramid Points to remember

1. In general, the client should not take an antacid with medication because the antacid will affect the absorption of the medication.

2. Enteric-coated and sustained-release tablets should not be crushed; also, capsules should not be opened.

3. The client should never adjust or change a medication dose or abruptly stop taking a medication.

4. The nurse never adjusts or changes the client's medication dosage and never discontinues a medication.

5. The client needs to avoid taking any over-the-counter medications or any other medications, such as herbal preparations, unless they are approved for use by the primary health care provider.

6. The client needs to avoid consuming alcohol.

7. Medications are never administered if the prescription is difficult to read, is unclear, or identifies a medication dose that is not a normal one.

8. Additional strategies for answering pharmacology questions are presented in *Saunders Strategies for Test Success: Passing Nursing School and the NCLEX® Exam.*

XVI. Using Enhanced Test-Taking Strategies to Answer Test Questions

A. Using a visual format to answer test questions can be a very helpful way to apply test-taking strategies to answer test questions.

B. Setting up a table to illustrate the thought process is a good way to make sure all information is considered and helps to arrive at the correct answers.

C. Box 4.26 provides an example of a stand-alone bowtie NGN question and an enhanced test-taking strategy.

XVII. Podcasts for Additional Review

For additional review on Acid Base Balance, Fluids and Electrolytes, or Pharmacology Strategies, use this QR code:

BOX 4.26 Practice Question: Stand-Alone Bowtie NGN Question with Enhanced Test-Taking Strategy

Scenario

The nurse is assigned to a newly admitted 49-year-old client and is reviewing the Emergency Department (ED) nurses' notes to prepare the client's plan of care.

Health History	Nurses' Notes	Vital Signs	Lab Results

1530: Client admitted to the ED accompanied by spouse, reporting sharp abdominal pain localized to the right upper quadrant for the last 3 days. Has been experiencing decreased appetite, nausea, and low-grade fever. Past medical history includes cholelithiasis, gastroesophageal reflux disease, pneumonia, and type 1 diabetes mellitus.

*Select one potential condition the client is **most likely** experiencing, two actions the nurse would take to address that condition, and two parameters the nurse would monitor to assess the client's progress.*

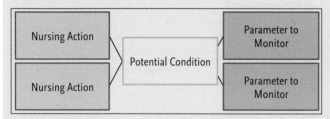

Answer: 2

Actions to Take	Potential Condition	Parameters to Monitor
Insert a urinary catheter	Acute cholecystitis	Temperature hourly
Administer pain medication	Bacterial pneumonia	Hemoglobin level
Give intravenous regular insulin	Diabetic ketoacidosis	Ultrasound results
Start continuous IV fluids	Gastrointestinal bleeding	Liver function tests
Administer oxygen using a simple face mask		Blood glucose level

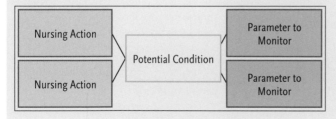

Actions to Take	Potential Condition	Parameters to Monitor
Insert a urinary catheter	Acute cholecystitis	Temperature hourly
Administer pain medication	Bacterial pneumonia	Hemoglobin level
Give intravenous regular insulin	Diabetic ketoacidosis	Ultrasound results
Start continuous IV fluids	Gastrointestinal bleeding	Liver function tests
Administer oxygen using a simple face mask		Blood glucose level

Test-Taking Strategy, Part 1

To begin, a helpful hint with a Bowtie question is to answer the middle section (the middle well) **first**. In this question, you need to first determine the condition.

Since there are three parts that need to be answered, organize your thought process into three parts. It is really important to focus on the **data in the question**. This question is asking you to decide on the potential condition based on the client's assessment findings. Think about each assessment finding presented in the clinical scenario, and decide if it is consistent with the condition listed. The table below provides you with an illustration of how you can organize your thoughts to determine the condition.

The abdominal pain could occur with three potential conditions presented; however, the pain is described as being localized to the right upper quadrant, and this is highly specific to and characteristic of acute cholecystitis. Use knowledge about anatomy, recalling that the gallbladder is located in the right upper quadrant. Decreased appetite and nausea are vague and nonspecific findings and do not help you narrow the list of potential conditions. Low-grade fever can occur with both acute cholecystitis and bacterial pneumonia. The client's past medical history of cholelithiasis places them at higher risk for acute cholecystitis. The past medical history of gastroesophageal reflux disease may elevate their risk for gastrointestinal bleeding. The client may be at higher risk for bacterial pneumonia because of their past medical history of pneumonia. Last, their past medical history of type 2 diabetes mellitus places them at higher risk for diabetic ketoacidosis. Note that acute cholecystitis appears most often in the table below and therefore is the condition the client is most likely experiencing.

BOX 4.26 Practice Question: Stand-Alone Bowtie NGN Question with Enhanced Test-Taking Strategy—cont'd

Assessment Finding	Potential Condition
Sharp abdominal pain	Acute cholecystitis
	Diabetic ketoacidosis
	Gastrointestinal bleeding
Abdominal pain localized to the right upper quadrant	Acute cholecystitis
Decreased appetite	Acute cholecystitis
	Bacterial pneumonia
	Diabetic ketoacidosis
	Gastrointestinal bleeding
Nausea	Acute cholecystitis
	Bacterial pneumonia
	Diabetic ketoacidosis
	Gastrointestinal bleeding
Low-grade fever	Acute cholecystitis
	Bacterial pneumonia
Past medical history of cholelithiasis	Acute cholecystitis
Past medical history of gastroesophageal reflux disease	Gastrointestinal bleeding
Past medical history of pneumonia	Bacterial pneumonia
Past medical history of type 1 diabetes mellitus	Diabetic ketoacidosis

Test-Taking Strategy, Part 2

Now that you've identified the most likely potential condition, the second part of your thought process will be to decide on the most appropriate nursing actions for the care of the client with acute cholecystitis. To decide on the two actions the nurse would take, think about whether there are data to support performing that action, as illustrated in the *Nursing Action and Supporting Data* table.

In acute cholecystitis, pain is often severe. The client is complaining of pain; therefore, administering pain medication will be an important intervention. Even though the client has a history of type 2 diabetes mellitus, there are no data in the clinical scenario to support giving intravenous regular insulin; intravenous insulin is only given in acute management of diabetic ketoacidosis and is not a part of routine treatment. Starting continuous intravenous fluids is an aspect of care for the client with acute cholecystitis to hydrate the client. Often, these clients are placed on nothing by mouth (NPO) status and therefore need supplemental hydration often in the form of intravenous fluids unless contraindicated. Additionally, the client

has nausea. There are no data to support giving supplemental oxygen as the client is not experiencing a problem with oxygenation. There are also no data to support the need to insert a urinary catheter.

Nursing Action	Supporting Data
Administer pain medication	Yes
Give intravenous regular insulin	No
Start continuous intravenous fluids	Yes
Administer oxygen using a simple face mask	No
Insert a urinary catheter	No

Test-Taking Strategy, Part 3

Now that you've decided on the two nursing actions you will take to care for the client with acute cholecystitis, the next step is to decide on the two parameters to monitor for this client. Decide whether each listed parameter is directly related to either the condition or the nursing actions to assist in selecting the correct options as illustrated in the table below.

The hemoglobin level is not specifically related to acute cholecystitis and is probably a distractor because this would be useful in assessing the progress for someone with gastrointestinal bleeding. Although the blood glucose level would be monitored because of the client's history of type 2 diabetes mellitus, it is also not directly related to acute cholecystitis but would be important to monitor for someone with diabetic ketoacidosis. Ultrasound results confirm the diagnosis of acute cholecystitis and therefore are related to the condition. Liver function studies are important because they provide information about any liver involvement related to the gallbladder problem and therefore are also related to the condition. Temperature monitoring hourly is unnecessary, although the temperature would be monitored per protocol probably every 4 hours.

Parameters to Monitor	Related to Condition or Action
Hemoglobin level	No—gastrointestinal bleeding
Ultrasound results	Yes
Liver function tests	Yes
Blood glucose level	No—diabetic ketoacidosis
Temperature hourly	No—hourly is not necessary

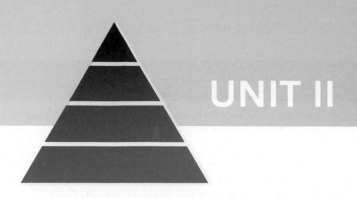

UNIT II

Client Needs

Client Needs

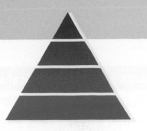

CHAPTER 5

Client Needs and the NCLEX-RN® Test Plan

In the new test plan implemented in April 2023, the National Council of State Boards of Nursing (NCSBN) identified a test plan framework that was based on Client Needs. This framework was selected on the basis of the findings in a practice analysis study of newly licensed registered nurses in the United States. This study identified the nursing activities performed by entry-level nurses. Also, according to the NCSBN, the Client Needs categories provide a structure for defining nursing actions and competencies across all settings for all clients.

⚠ The NCSBN identifies four major categories of Client Needs, Safe and Effective Care Environment, Health Promotion and Maintenance, Psychosocial Integrity, and Physiological Integrity. Some of these categories are further divided into subcategories, and the percentage of test questions in each subcategory is identified in Table 5.1.

The information in this chapter related to the test plan was obtained from the NCSBN website at http://www.ncsbn.org and from the NCSBN *NCLEX-RN® Examination Test Plan*, effective April 2023. Additional information regarding the test

and its development can be obtained by accessing the NCSBN website at http://www.ncsbn.org or by writing to the National Council of State Boards of Nursing, 111 E. Wacker Drive, Suite 2900, Chicago, IL 60601.

Physiological Integrity

The Physiological Integrity category includes four subcategories: Basic Care and Comfort, Pharmacological and Parenteral Therapies, Reduction of Risk Potential, and Physiological Adaptation. The NCSBN describes the content tested in each subcategory. Basic Care and Comfort addresses content that tests the ability of the nurse to make clinical judgments when providing basic care and comfort measures and assisting the client in performing activities of daily living. Pharmacological and Parenteral Therapies addresses content that tests the ability required to administer medications and parenteral therapies and to make clinical judgments about pharmacological therapies. Reduction of Risk Potential addresses content that tests the ability required by the nurse to make clinical judgments in order to prevent complications or health problems related to the client's condition, or any prescribed treatments or procedures. Physiological Adaptation addresses content that tests the nurse's ability to make clinical judgments required to provide care to clients with acute, chronic, or life-threatening conditions.

The NCSBN identifies related content and specific nursing activities for the subcategories of the Physiological Integrity category. For specific content and nursing activities, refer to the NCSBN test plan that can be located at the NCSBN website at http://www.ncsbn.org. See Box 5.1 for examples of questions in this Client Needs category, and refer to Chapter 6 for practice questions reflective of this Client Needs category.

Safe and Effective Care Environment

The Safe and Effective Care Environment category includes two subcategories: (1) Management of Care and (2) Safety and Infection Control. The NCSBN describes the content tested in each subcategory. Management of Care addresses content that tests the clinical judgment skills and ability of the nurse to provide and direct nursing care that will enhance the care delivery setting to protect clients, health care personnel, and others. Safety and Infection Control addresses content that tests the nurse's ability required to protect clients,

TABLE 5.1 Client Needs Categories and Percentage of Questions on the NCLEX-RN® Examination

Client Needs Category	Percentage of Questions
Safe and Effective Care Environment	
Management of Care	15–21
Safety and Infection Control	10–16
Health Promotion and Maintenance	6–12
Psychosocial Integrity	6–12
Physiological Integrity	
Basic Care and Comfort	6–12
Pharmacological and Parenteral Therapies	13–19
Reduction of Risk Potential	9–15
Physiological Adaptation	11–17

From National Council of State Boards of Nursing. (2023). *Next Generation NCLEX®, NCLEX-RN® Test Plan,* Chicago: Author.

BOX 5.1   Physiological Integrity Questions

Basic Care and Comfort

A client with right-sided weakness needs to learn how to use a cane for home maintenance of mobility. The nurse would teach the client to position the cane by holding it in which way?

1. Left hand and 6 inches lateral to the left foot
2. Right hand and 6 inches lateral to the right foot
3. Left hand and placing the cane in front of the left foot
4. Right hand and placing the cane in front of the right foot

Answer: 1

This question addresses content related to the use of an assistive device. Focus on the subject, use of a cane for a client with right-sided weakness. The client is taught to hold the cane on the opposite side of the weakness, because with normal walking the opposite arm and leg move together (called *reciprocal motion*). The cane is placed 6 inches lateral to the fifth toe.

Pharmacological and Parenteral Therapies

A client is receiving furosemide 40 mg orally daily. Which laboratory result would indicate to the nurse that the client is experiencing an adverse effect related to the medication?

Laboratory Results

Test and Results	Reference Range
Chloride 98 mEq/L (98 mmol/L)	98–106 mEq/L (98–106 mmol/L)
Sodium 135 mEq/L (135 mmol/L)	135–145 mEq/L (135–145 mmol/L)
Potassium 3.1 mEq/L (3.1 mmol/L)	3.5–5.0 mEq/L (3.5–5.0 mmol/L)
BUN 15 mg/dL (5.4 mmol/L)	10–20 mg/dL (3.6–7.1 mmol/L)

1. Chloride level
2. Sodium level
3. Potassium level
4. BUN level

Answer: 3

This question addresses content related to a medication. Focus on the subject, an adverse effect. Furosemide is a loop diuretic. The medication can produce acute, profound water loss; volume and electrolyte depletion; dehydration; decreased blood volume; and circulatory collapse. The potassium level is the only result that indicates an electrolyte depletion.

Reduction of Risk Potential

A client is scheduled to undergo a renal biopsy. To minimize the risk of postprocedure complications, the nurse would report which laboratory result to the physician before the procedure?

Laboratory Results

Test and Results	Reference Range
Potassium 3.8 mEq/L (3.8 mmol/L)	3.5–5.0 mEq/L (3.5–5.0 mmol/L)
Prothrombin time: 15 sec (15 sec)	11–12.5 sec (11–12.5 sec)
Creatinine 1.2 mg/dL (106 mcmol/L)	0.5–1.2 mg/dL (44–106 mcmol/L)
BUN 18 mg/dL (6.48 mmol/L)	10–20 mg/dL (3.6–7.1 mmol/L)

1. Potassium level
2. Prothrombin time
3. Creatinine level
4. BUN level

Answer: 2

This question addresses a potential postprocedure complication of a diagnostic test (renal biopsy). Focus on the subject, an abnormal laboratory result. Postprocedure hemorrhage is a complication after renal biopsy. Because of this, prothrombin time is assessed before the procedure. The nurse ensures that these results are available and reports abnormalities promptly.

Physiological Adaptation

A pregnant client tells the nurse about feeling wetness on the peripad and they found some clear fluid. The nurse quickly inspects the perineum and notes the presence of the umbilical cord. The nurse would take which **immediate** action?

1. Monitor the fetal heart rate.
2. Notify the primary health care provider.
3. Transfer the client to the delivery room.
4. Place the client in Trendelenburg position.

Answer: 4

This question addresses an acute and life-threatening physical health condition. Note the strategic word, *immediate*. On inspection of the perineum, if the umbilical cord is noted, the nurse immediately places the client in Trendelenburg position while holding the presenting part upward to relieve the cord compression. This position is maintained while the nurse calls out for assistance with fetal heart rate monitoring and for notification of the primary health care provider. The client is transferred to the delivery room when prescribed by the primary health care provider.

health care personnel, and others from health and environmental hazards.

The NCSBN identifies related content and nursing activities for the subcategories of the Safe and Effective Care Environment category. For specific content and nursing activities, refer to the NCSBN test plan. See Box 5.2 for examples of questions in this Client Needs category, and refer to Chapter 7 for practice questions reflective of this Client Needs category.

Health Promotion and Maintenance

The Health Promotion and Maintenance category addresses the principles related to growth and development. According to the NCSBN, this Client Needs category also addresses content that tests the clinical judgment skills and ability required to assist the client, family members, and/or significant others to prevent health problems, recognize alterations in health to detect health

| BOX 5.2 | Safe and Effective Care Environment Questions |

Management of Care

The registered nurse is planning the client assignments for the day. Which is the appropriate client assignment for the unlicensed assistive personnel (UAP)?

1. Client requiring a colostomy irrigation
2. Client receiving continuous tube feedings
3. Client who requires stool specimen collections
4. Client who has difficulty swallowing food and fluids

Answer: 3

This question addresses content related to assignment-making and delegation. Focus on the subject, the appropriate assignment for the UAP. Work that is delegated to others must be done consistent with the individual's level of expertise and licensure or lack of licensure. In this situation, the most appropriate assignment for the UAP is to care for the client who requires stool specimen collections. Colostomy irrigations and tube feedings are not performed by the UAP. The client with difficulty swallowing food and fluids is at risk for aspiration. Remember, the health care provider needs to be competent and skilled to perform the assigned task or activity.

Safety and Infection Control

A client diagnosed with tuberculosis (TB) is scheduled to go to the radiology department for a chest radiograph. The nurse would take which action when preparing to transport the client?

1. Apply a mask to the client.
2. Apply a mask and gown to the client.
3. Apply a mask, gown, and gloves to the client.
4. Notify the radiology department so that the personnel can be sure to wear masks when the client arrives.

Answer: 1

This question addresses content related to airborne precautions. Focus on the subject, transporting a client with TB. Institution policies and procedures for airborne precautions are always followed; however, clients known or suspected of having TB need to wear a mask when out of the hospital room to prevent the spread of the infection to others. Gown and gloves are not necessary. Although the radiology department may need to be notified, others are not protected unless the infected client wears the mask.

| BOX 5.3 | Health Promotion and Maintenance Questions |

The postpartum nurse has instructed a new birthing parent on how to bathe their newborn. The nurse demonstrates the procedure to the client and on the following day asks the client to perform the procedure. Which observation by the nurse indicates that the client is performing the procedure correctly?

1. Washes the newborn by starting with the eyes and face
2. Washes the entire newborn's body and then washes the eyes, face, and scalp
3. Washes the newborn by starting with the ears and then moves to the eyes and the face
4. Washes the newborn by starting with the arms, chest, and back followed by the neck, arms, and face

Answer: 1

This question addresses the postpartum period. Focus on the subject, that the client can correctly perform the bathing procedure for the newborn. Bathing should start at the eyes and face and with the cleanest area first. Next, the external ears and behind the ears are cleaned. The newborn's neck should be washed because formula, lint, or breast milk often accumulates in the folds of the neck. Hands and arms are then washed. The newborn's legs are washed next, with the diaper area washed last. Remember to always start with the cleanest area of the body first and proceed to the dirtiest area.

A client with atherosclerosis asks the nurse about dietary modifications to lower the risk of heart disease. The nurse would encourage the client to eat which food that will lower this risk?

1. Fresh cantaloupe
2. Broiled cheeseburger
3. Mashed potatoes with gravy
4. Fried chicken without skin

Answer: 1

This question addresses health and wellness. Focus on the subject, the food item that will lower the risk of heart disease. To lower the risk of heart disease, the diet should be low in saturated fat, with the appropriate number of total calories. The diet should include fewer red meats and more white meat, with the skin removed. Both gravy and fried foods are high in fat. Dairy products used should be low in fat, and foods with large amounts of empty calories should be avoided. Fresh fruits and vegetables are naturally low in fat.

problems early, and develop health practices and strategies that promote and support wellness and achieve optimal health.

The NCSBN identifies related content and specific nursing activities for the Health and Promotion and Maintenance category. For specific content and nursing activities, refer to the NCSBN test plan. See Box 5.3 for examples of questions in this Client Needs category, and refer to Chapter 8 for practice questions reflective of this Client Needs category.

Psychosocial Integrity

The Psychosocial Integrity category addresses content that tests the clinical judgment skills required to promote and support the client, family, and/or significant other's ability to cope, adapt, and/or solve problems during stressful events. According to the NCSBN, this Client Needs category also addresses the emotional, mental, and social well-being of the client, family, or significant other, and the clinical judgment skills required to care for the client with an acute or chronic mental illness.

The NCSBN identifies related content and specific nursing activities for the Psychosocial Integrity category. For specific content and nursing activities, refer to the NCSBN test plan. See Box 5.4 for examples of questions in this Client Needs category, and refer to Chapter 9 for practice questions reflective of this Client Needs category.

BOX 5.4   Psychosocial Integrity Questions

The nurse is planning care for a client who is experiencing fear and anxiety following a myocardial infarction. Which nursing intervention would be included in the plan of care?

1. Answer questions with factual information.
2. Provide detailed explanations of all procedures.
3. Limit family involvement during the acute phase.
4. Administer an antianxiety medication to promote relaxation.

Answer: 1

This question addresses content related to fear and anxiety following a myocardial infarction. Focus on the subject, an intervention that will alleviate the client's fear and anxiety. Accurate and factual information reduces fear, strengthens the nurse–client relationship, and assists the client in dealing realistically with the situation. Providing detailed information may increase the client's anxiety. Information should be provided simply and clearly. The client's family may be a source of support for the client. Therefore, limiting family involvement may or may not be helpful. Medication should not be used unless necessary.

The nurse in the mental health clinic is performing an initial assessment of a family with a diagnosis of domestic violence. Which factor would the nurse **initially** include in the assessment?

1. The coping style of each family member
2. The ability of the family to use community resources
3. The family's anger toward the intrusiveness of the nurse
4. The family's denial of the violent nature of their behavior

Answer: 1

This question addresses assessment of a domestic violence situation. Note the strategic word, *initially*. The initial family assessment includes a careful history of each family member. Options 2, 3, and 4 address the family. Option 1 addresses each family member.

CHAPTER 6

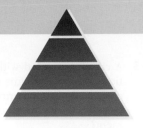

Physiological Integrity Practice Questions

1. The nurse is caring for a client who is receiving blood transfusion therapy. Which clinical manifestations would alert the nurse to a hemolytic transfusion reaction? **Select all that apply.**
- ❑ **1.** Headache
- ❑ **2.** Tachycardia
- ❑ **3.** Hypertension
- ❑ **4.** Apprehension
- ❑ **5.** Distended neck veins
- ❑ **6.** A sense of impending doom

Level of Cognitive Ability: Analyzing
Client Needs: Physiological Integrity
Clinical Judgment/Cognitive Skills: Recognize Cues
Integrated Process: Clinical Judgment; Nursing Process/Assessment
Content Area: Complex Care: Blood Administration
Health Problems: Adult Health: Immune: Hypersensitivity Reactions and Allergy
Priority Concepts: Clinical Judgment; Immunity

Answer: 1, 2, 4, 6
Rationale: Hemolytic transfusion reactions are caused by blood type or Rh incompatibility. When blood containing antigens different from the client's own antigens is infused, antigen-antibody complexes are formed in the client's blood. These complexes destroy the transfused cells and start inflammatory responses in the client's blood vessel walls and organs. The reaction may include fever and chills or may be life-threatening with disseminated intravascular coagulation and circulatory collapse. Other manifestations include headache, tachycardia, apprehension, a sense of impending doom, chest pain, low back pain, tachypnea, hypotension, and hemoglobinuria. The onset may be immediate or may not occur until subsequent units have been transfused. Distended neck veins are characteristics of circulatory overload.
Test-Taking Strategy: Focus on the subject, a hemolytic transfusion reaction. Recall the pathophysiology of this type of reaction to select the correct options. Also think about other types of transfusion reactions that can occur, and recall that distended neck veins are characteristic of circulatory overload.
Priority Nursing Tip: The nurse would suspect a transfusion reaction if the client develops any symptom or complains of anything unusual while receiving the blood transfusion.
Reference: Ignatavicius, D., et al. (2021). *Medical-surgical nursing: Concepts for interprofessional collaborative care* (10th ed., pp. 819–820). Elsevier.

 2. A client has an arteriovenous (AV) fistula in place in the right upper extremity for hemodialysis treatments. When planning care for this client, the nurse would implement which measure to promote client safety?
1. Use the right arm for blood pressure measuremnuent.
2. Use the fistula for all venipunctures and intravenous infusions.
3. Ensure that small clamps are attached to the AV fistula dressing.
4. Assess the fistula for the presence of a bruit and thrill every 4 hours.

Level of Cognitive Ability: Applying
Client Needs: Physiological Integrity
Clinical Judgment/Cognitive Skills: Generate Solutions
Integrated Process: Clinical Judgment; Nursing Process/Planning
Content Area: Adult Health: Renal and Urinary
Health Problems: Adult Health: Renal and Urinary: Acute Kidney Injury/Chronic Kidney Disease
Priority Concepts: Perfusion; Safety

Answer: 4
Rationale: AV fistulas are created by anastomosis of an artery and a vein within the subcutaneous tissues to create access for hemodialysis. Fistulas need to be evaluated for the presence of thrills (palpate over the area) and bruits (auscultate with a stethoscope) as an assessment of patency. Blood pressures or venipunctures are not done on the extremity with the fistula because of the risk of clotting, infection, or damage to the fistula. The fistula is not used for venipunctures or intravenous infusions for the same reason. Clamps may be needed for an external device such as an AV shunt, but the AV fistula is internal.
Test-Taking Strategy: Focus on the subject, an AV fistula and safety. Eliminate option 3 first because this refers to care of an AV shunt, in which there is an external cannula that can become disconnected. If accidental disconnection occurs, the small clamps can be used to occlude the ends of the cannula. Blood pressure measurement, insertion of intravenous access, and venipuncture would never be performed on the affected extremity because of the potential for infection and clotting of the fistula; therefore, eliminate options 1 and 2. The only option that relates to the subject of this question is option 4.
Priority Nursing Tip: For the client receiving hemodialysis, the AV fistula is the client's lifeline, and the client's hemodynamic status needs to be closely monitored. Clients will need teaching on which medications to avoid before dialysis.
Reference: Ignatavicius, D., et al. (2021). *Medical-surgical nursing: Concepts for interprofessional collaborative care* (10th ed., p. 1399). Elsevier.

❖ **3.** A client diagnosed with both a wound infection and osteomyelitis is to receive hyperbaric oxygen therapy. During the therapy, which **priority** intervention would the nurse implement?
1. Maintaining an intravenous access
2. Ensuring that oxygen is being delivered
3. Administering sedation to prevent claustrophobia
4. Providing emotional support to the client's family

Level of Cognitive Ability: Applying
Client Needs: Physiological Integrity
Clinical Judgment/Cognitive Skills: Take Action
Integrated Process: Clinical Judgment; Nursing Process/Implementation
Content Area: Skills: Oxygenation
Health Problems: Adult Health: Integumentary: Wounds
Priority Concepts: Clinical Judgment; Gas Exchange

Answer: 2
Rationale: Hyperbaric oxygen therapy is a process by which oxygen is administered at greater than atmospheric pressure. When oxygen is inhaled under pressure, the level of tissue oxygen is greatly increased. The high levels of oxygen promote the action of phagocytes and promote healing of the wound. Because the client is placed in a closed chamber, the administration of oxygen is of primary importance. Although options 1, 3, and 4 may be appropriate interventions, option 2 is the priority.
Test-Taking Strategy: Note the strategic word, *priority*. Use the ABCs—airway, breathing, and circulation—and Maslow's Hierarchy of Needs theory to direct you to option 2, which addresses oxygen. Also note the relationship of the words hyperbaric oxygen in the question and oxygen in the correct option.
Priority Nursing Tip: Hyperbaric oxygen therapy may be a treatment measure for chronic osteomyelitis to increase tissue perfusion and promote healing.
Reference: Lewis, S., et al. (2020). *Medical-surgical nursing: Assessment and management of clinical problems* (11th ed., p. 167). Elsevier.

❖ **4.** A client is scheduled for hydrotherapy for a burn dressing change. Which action would the nurse take to ensure that the client is comfortable during the procedure?
1. Ensure that client is appropriately dressed.
2. Administer an opioid analgesic 30 to 60 minutes before therapy.
3. Schedule the therapy at a time when client generally takes a nap.
4. Assign an unlicensed assistive personnel (UAP) to stay with client during the procedure.

Level of Cognitive Ability: Applying
Client Needs: Physiological Integrity
Clinical Judgment/Cognitive Skills: Take Action
Integrated Process: Clinical Judgment; Nursing Process/Implementation
Content Area: Pharmacology: Pain: Opioid Analgesics
Health Problems: Adult Health: Integumentary: Burns
Priority Concepts: Pain; Tissue Integrity

Answer: 2
Rationale: The client needs to receive pain medication approximately 30 to 60 minutes before a burn dressing change. This will help the client tolerate an otherwise painful procedure. None of the remaining options addresses the issue of pain effectively.
Test-Taking Strategy: Use Maslow's Hierarchy of Needs theory (physiologic needs are the priority). This will direct you to option 2, which addresses pain management.
Priority Nursing Tip: A burn injury is extremely painful, and the client is adequately medicated before a burn dressing change to reduce pain and prevent fear of future dressing changes. Strict aseptic technique is used for dressing changes because of the risk of infection.
Reference: Lewis, S., et al. (2020). *Medical-surgical nursing: Assessment and management of clinical problems* (11th ed., p. 448). Elsevier.

❖ **5.** The nurse is caring for a client diagnosed with heart failure and is reviewing the client's magnesium level. Based on the laboratory result, which action would the nurse take?

Laboratory Results

Test and Result	Reference Range
Magnesium 0.75 mEq/L (0.3 mmol/L)	1.8–2.6 mEq/L (0.74–1.07 mmol/L)

1. Monitor the client for irregular heart rhythms.
2. Encourage the intake of antacids with phosphate.
3. Teach the client to avoid foods high in magnesium.
4. Provide a diet of ground beef, eggs, and chicken breast.

Level of Cognitive Ability: Applying
Client Needs: Physiological Integrity
Clinical Judgment/Cognitive Skills: Take Action
Integrated Process: Clinical Judgment; Nursing Process/Implementation
Content Area: Foundations of Care: Laboratory Tests
Health Problems: Adult Health: Cardiovascular: Heart Failure
Priority Concepts: Fluids and Electrolytes; Clinical Judgment

Answer: 1
Rationale: The client is experiencing hypomagnesemia. The client needs to be monitored for dysrhythmias because magnesium plays an important role in myocardial nerve cell impulse conduction; thus, hypomagnesemia increases the client's risk of ventricular dysrhythmias. The nurse avoids administering phosphate in the presence of hypomagnesemia because it aggravates the condition. The nurse instructs the client to consume foods high in magnesium; ground beef, eggs, and chicken breast are low in magnesium.
Test-Taking Strategy: Focus on the subject, a client with heart failure who has a magnesium level of 0.75 mEq/L (0.3 mmol/L). Reviewing the reference range for magnesium and noting that the client is experiencing hypomagnesemia will direct you to option 1. Also, the use of the ABCs—airway, breathing, and circulation—will direct you to the correct option.
Priority Nursing Tip: The client with hypomagnesemia is at risk for seizures. Therefore, the nurse needs to initiate seizure precautions if the magnesium level is low.
Reference: Ignatavicius, D., et al. (2021). *Medical-surgical nursing: Concepts for interprofessional collaborative care* (10th ed., pp. 258–259). Elsevier.

6. The nurse is assessing a pregnant client with a diagnosis of abruptio placentae. Which manifestations of this condition would the nurse expect to note? **Select all that apply.**
☐ 1. Uterine irritability
☐ 2. Uterine tenderness
☐ 3. Painless vaginal bleeding
☐ 4. Abdominal and low back pain
☐ 5. Strong and frequent contractions
☐ 6. Nonreassuring fetal heart rate patterns

Level of Cognitive Ability: Analyzing
Client Needs: Physiological Integrity
Clinical Judgment/Cognitive Skills: Recognize Cues
Integrated Process: Nursing Process/Assessment
Content Area: Maternity: Intrapartum
Health Problems: Maternity: Abruptio Placentae
Priority Concepts: Clinical Judgment; Perfusion

Answer: 1, 2, 4, 6
Rationale: Placental abruption, also referred to as abruptio placentae, is the separation of a normally implanted placenta before the fetus is born. It occurs when there is bleeding and formation of a hematoma on the maternal side of the placenta. Manifestations include uterine irritability with frequent low-intensity contractions, uterine tenderness that may be localized to the site of the abruption, aching and dull abdominal and low back pain, painful vaginal bleeding, and a high uterine resting tone identified by the use of an intrauterine pressure catheter. Additional signs include nonreassuring fetal heart rate patterns, signs of hypovolemic shock, and fetal death. Painless vaginal bleeding is a sign of placenta previa.
Test-Taking Strategy: Focus on the subject, manifestations of abruptio placentae. Think about the word *abrupt*. Recalling the pathophysiology associated with this hemorrhagic condition will assist in selecting the correct options. Remember that placental abruption occurs when there is separation of the placenta and bleeding and formation of a hematoma on the maternal side of the placenta.
Priority Nursing Tip: It is important to know the differences between the manifestations of abruptio placentae and placenta previa. In abruptio placentae, dark red vaginal bleeding, uterine pain and/or tenderness, and uterine rigidity are characteristic. In placenta previa, there is painless, bright red vaginal bleeding, and the uterus is soft, relaxed, and nontender.
Reference: McKinney, E. S., et al. (2022). *Maternal child nursing* (6th ed., pp. 537–538). Elsevier.

❖ **7.** The nurse is caring for a client diagnosed with a herniated lumbar intervertebral disk who is experiencing low back pain. Which position would the nurse place the client in to minimize the pain?
1. Supine with the knees slightly raised
2. High-Fowler's position with the foot of the bed flat
3. Semi-Fowler's position with the foot of the bed flat
4. Semi-Fowler's position with the knees slightly raised

Level of Cognitive Ability: Applying
Client Needs: Physiological Integrity
Clinical Judgment/Cognitive Skills: Take Action
Integrated Process: Nursing Process/Implementation
Content Area: Adult Health: Musculoskeletal
Health Problems: Adult Health: Neurologic: Intervertebral Disk
Priority Concepts: Caregiving; Pain

Answer: 4
Rationale: Clients with low back pain are often more comfortable in the semi-Fowler's position with the knees raised sufficiently to flex the knees (William's position). This relaxes the muscles of the lower back and relieves pressure on the spinal nerve root. Keeping the bed flat or lying in a supine position with the knees raised would excessively stretch the lower back. Keeping the foot of the bed flat will enhance extension of the spine and also stretch the lower back.
Test-Taking Strategy: Focus on the **subject**, a client with a herniated lumbar intervertebral disk who is experiencing low back pain. Visualize each of the positions, noting that option 4 places the least amount of pressure on the spine.
Priority Nursing Tip: A physical therapist will work with a client with a herniated lumbar intervertebral disk to develop an individualized exercise program, and the type of exercises prescribed depends on the location and nature of the injury and the type of pain. The client does not begin exercise until acute pain is reduced.
Reference: Ignatavicius, D., et al. (2021). *Medical-surgical nursing: Concepts for interprofessional collaborative care* (10th ed., p. 889). Elsevier.

8. A client admitted to the hospital has been prescribed pyridostigmine as treatment for myasthenia gravis. When assessing the client for side effects of the medication, the nurse would ask the client about the presence of which occurrence?
1. Mouth ulcers
2. Muscle cramps
3. Feelings of depression
4. Unexplained weight gain

Level of Cognitive Ability: Applying
Client Needs: Physiological Integrity
Clinical Judgment/Cognitive Skills: Recognize Cues
Integrated Process: Nursing Process/Assessment
Content Area: Pharmacology: Neurologic: Antimyasthenics
Health Problems: Adult Health: Neurologic: Myasthenia Gravis
Priority Concepts: Clinical Judgment; Safety

Answer: 2
Rationale: Pyridostigmine is an acetylcholinesterase inhibitor used to treat myasthenia gravis, a neuromuscular disorder. Muscle cramps and small muscle contractions are side effects and occur as a result of overstimulation of neuromuscular receptors. Mouth ulcers, depression, and weight gain are not associated with this medication.
Test-Taking Strategy: Focus on the **subject**, the side effects of pyridostigmine. It is necessary to recall that this medication is used to treat myasthenia gravis, a neuromuscular disorder. Select the option that is most closely associated with this disorder. This will direct you to the correct option.
Priority Nursing Tip: Indicators of a therapeutic response to pyridostigmine include increased muscle strength, decreased fatigue, and improved chewing and swallowing functions.
Reference: Lewis, S., et al. (2020). *Medical-surgical nursing: Assessment and management of clinical problems* (11th ed., pp. 1377–1378). Elsevier.

❖ **9.** A client who experienced a fractured right ankle has a short leg cast applied in the emergency department. During discharge teaching, which information would the nurse provide to the client to prevent complications?
1. Trim the rough edges of the cast after it is dry.
2. Weight bearing on the right leg is allowed once the cast feels dry.
3. Expect burning and tingling sensations under the cast for 3 to 4 days.
4. Keep the right ankle elevated above the heart level with pillows for 24 hours.

Level of Cognitive Ability: Applying
Client Needs: Physiological Integrity
Clinical Judgment/Cognitive Skills: Take Action
Integrated Process: Teaching and Learning
Content Area: Adult Health: Musculoskeletal
Health Problems: Adult Health: Musculoskeletal: Skeletal Injury
Priority Concepts: Patient Education; Perfusion

Answer: 4
Rationale: Leg elevation is important to increase venous return and decrease edema. Edema can cause compartment syndrome, a major complication of fractures and casting. The client and/or family may be taught how to "petal" the cast to prevent skin irritation and breakdown, but rough edges, if trimmed, can fall into the cast and cause a break in skin integrity. Weight bearing on a fractured extremity is prescribed by the physician during follow-up examination, after radiographs are obtained. Additionally, a walking heel or cast shoe may be added to the cast if the client is allowed to bear weight and walk on the affected leg. Although the client may feel heat after the cast is applied, burning and/or tingling sensations indicate nerve damage or ischemia and are not expected. These complaints need to be reported immediately.
Test-Taking Strategy: Focus on the subject, measures to prevent complications with a short leg cast. Recall the ABCs—airway, breathing, and circulation. Option 4 is associated with maintenance of circulation.
Priority Nursing Tip: Circulation impairment and peripheral nerve damage can result from tightness of the cast applied to an extremity. The client needs to be taught to assess for adequate circulation, including the ability to move the area distal to the casted extremity.
Reference: Ignatavicius, D., et al. (2021). *Medical-surgical nursing: Concepts for interprofessional collaborative care* (10th ed., p. 1036). Elsevier.

❖ **10.** An adult client who experienced a fractured left tibia has a long leg cast and is using crutches to ambulate. In caring for the client, the nurse assesses for which sign/symptom that indicates a complication associated with crutch walking?
1. Left leg discomfort
2. Weak biceps brachii
3. Triceps muscle spasms
4. Forearm muscle weakness

Level of Cognitive Ability: Analyzing
Client Needs: Physiological Integrity
Clinical Judgment/Cognitive Skills: Recognize Cues
Integrated Process: Clinical Judgment; Nursing Process/Assessment
Content Area: Skills: Activity/Mobility
Health Problems: Adult Health: Musculoskeletal: Skeletal Injury
Priority Concepts: Clinical Judgment; Mobility

Answer: 4
Rationale: Forearm muscle weakness is a sign of radial nerve injury caused by crutch pressure on the axillae. When a client lacks upper body strength, especially in the flexor and extensor muscles of the arms, the client frequently allows weight to rest on the axillae and on the crutch pads instead of using the arms for support while ambulating with crutches. Leg discomfort is expected as a result of the injury. Weak biceps brachii is not a complication of crutch walking but rather is caused by an injury to the brachial plexus itself. Triceps muscle spasms may occur as a result of increased muscle use but is not a complication of crutch walking.
Test-Taking Strategy: Focus on the subject, a complication of crutch walking. When asked about a complication of the use of crutches, think about nerve injury caused by crutch pressure on the axillae. This will direct you to option 4.
Priority Nursing Tip: To prevent pressure on the axillary nerve from the use of crutches, there needs to be two to three fingerbreadths between the axilla and the top of the crutch when the crutch tip is at least 6 inches diagonally in the front of the foot. The crutch is adjusted so that the elbow is flexed no more than 30 degrees when the palm is on the handle.
Reference: Lewis, S., et al. (2020). *Medical-surgical nursing: Assessment and management of clinical problems* (11th ed., p. 1378). Elsevier.

11. A client diagnosed with myasthenia gravis is experiencing prolonged periods of weakness, and the physician prescribes an edrophonium test, also known as a Tensilon test. A test dose is administered and the client becomes weaker. How would the nurse interpret these results?

1. Myasthenic crisis is present.
2. Cholinergic crisis is present.
3. This result is a normal finding.
4. This result is a positive finding.

Level of Cognitive Ability: Analyzing
Client Needs: Physiological Integrity
Clinical Judgment/Cognitive Skills: Analyze Cues
Integrated Process: Clinical Judgment; Nursing Process/Analysis
Content Area: Foundations of Care: Diagnostic Tests
Health Problems: Adult Health: Neurologic: Myasthenia Gravis
Priority Concepts: Clinical Judgment; Functional Ability

Answer: 2
Rationale: An edrophonium test may be performed to determine whether increasing weakness in a client with previously diagnosed myasthenic is a result of cholinergic crisis (overmedication) with anticholinesterase medications or myasthenic crisis (undermedication). Worsening of the symptoms after the test dose of medication is administered indicates a cholinergic crisis.
Test-Taking Strategy: Focus on the subject, a client who becomes weaker after edrophonium is administered. Recalling that edrophonium is a short-acting anticholinesterase and that the treatment for myasthenia gravis includes administration of an anticholinesterase will assist in answering the question. If the client's symptoms worsen after administration of edrophonium, then the client is likely experiencing overmedication.
Priority Nursing Tip: Although rare, the edrophonium test, also known as the Tensilon test, can cause ventricular fibrillation and cardiac arrest. Atropine sulfate is the antidote for edrophonium and needs to be available when the test is performed in case these complications occur.
Reference: Lewis, S., et al. (2020). *Medical-surgical nursing: Assessment and management of clinical problems* (11th ed., pp. 1377–1378). Elsevier.

12. When tranylcypromine is prescribed for a client, which food items would the nurse instruct the client to avoid? **Select all that apply.**
☐ 1. Figs
☐ 2. Apples
☐ 3. Bananas
☐ 4. Broccoli
☐ 5. Sauerkraut
☐ 6. Baked chicken

Level of Cognitive Ability: Applying
Client Needs: Physiological Integrity
Clinical Judgment/Cognitive Skills: Take Action
Integrated Process: Teaching and Learning
Content Area: Pharmacology: Psychotherapeutics: Monoamine Oxidase Inhibitors (MAOIs)
Health Problems: Mental Health: Mood Disorders
Priority Concepts: Patient Education; Safety

Answer: 1, 3, 5
Rationale: Tranylcypromine is a monoamine oxidase inhibitor (MAOI) used to treat depression. Foods that contain tyramine need to be avoided because of the risk of hypertensive crisis associated with use of this medication. Foods to avoid include figs; bananas; sauerkraut; avocados; soybeans; meats or fish that are fermented, smoked, or otherwise aged; some cheeses; yeast extract; and some beers and wine.
Test-Taking Strategy: Focus on the subject, foods to avoid with an MAOI. Focus on the name of the medication and recall that tranylcypromine is an MAOI. Next, recall the foods that contain tyramine to answer the question. Remember that figs, bananas, and sauerkraut are high in tyramine.
Priority Nursing Tip: Hypertensive crisis is characterized by an extreme increase in blood pressure, resulting in an increased risk for stroke, headache, anxiety, and shortness of breath.
Reference: Varcarolis, E., & Fosbre, C. (2021). *Essentials of psychiatric mental health nursing: A communication approach to evidence-based care* (4th ed., pp. 218, 220). Elsevier.

13. The nurse notes an isolated premature ventricular contraction (PVC) on the cardiac monitor of a client recovering from anesthesia. Which action would the nurse take?
   1. Prepare for defibrillation.
   2. Continue to monitor the rhythm.
   3. Prepare to administer a beta blocker.
   4. Notify the physician immediately.

Level of Cognitive Ability: Applying
Client Needs: Physiological Integrity
Clinical Judgment/Cognitive Skills: Take Action
Integrated Process: Clinical Judgment/Nursing Process/Implementation
Content Area: Adult Health: Cardiovascular
Health Problems: Adult Health: Cardiovascular: Dysrhythmias
Priority Concepts: Clinical Judgment; Perfusion

Answer: 2
Rationale: As an isolated occurrence, the PVC is not life threatening. In this situation, the nurse would continue to monitor the client. Frequent PVCs, however, may be precursors of more life-threatening rhythms, such as ventricular tachycardia and ventricular fibrillation. If this occurs, the physician needs to be notified. Defibrillation is done to treat ventricular fibrillation. A beta blocker may be prescribed to treat frequent PVCs but is not prescribed to treat an isolated occurrence.
Test-Taking Strategy: Focus on the **subject**, the action to take for an isolated PVC. Noting the word "isolated" should direct you to the option that addresses continued monitoring.
Priority Nursing Tip: Ventricular tachycardia can progress to ventricular fibrillation, a life-threatening condition.
Reference: Ignatavicius, D., et al. (2021). *Medical-surgical nursing: Concepts for interprofessional collaborative care* (10th ed., p. 763). Elsevier.

14. The clinic nurse prepares to assess a client who is in the second trimester of pregnancy. When measuring the fundal height and comparing it to gestational age, the nurse would expect to note which of the following?
   1. It is less than gestational age.
   2. It correlates with gestational age.
   3. It is greater than gestational age.
   4. It has no correlation with gestational age.

Level of Cognitive Ability: Applying
Client Needs: Physiological Integrity
Clinical Judgment/Cognitive Skills: Recognize Cues
Integrated Process: Nursing Process/Assessment
Content Area: Maternity: Antepartum
Health Problems: N/A
Priority Concepts: Clinical Judgment; Reproduction

Answer: 2
Rationale: Until the third trimester, the measurement of fundal height will, on average, correlate with the gestational age. Therefore, options 1, 3, and 4 are incorrect.
Test-Taking Strategy: Focus on the **subject**, fundal height in the second trimester. Recall the correlation of fundal height and gestational age to direct you to the correct option.
Priority Nursing Tip: Usually a paper tape is used to measure fundal height. Consistency in performing the measurement technique is important to ensure reliability in the findings. If possible, the same care provider should examine the pregnant client at each of the prenatal visits.
Reference: McKinney, E. S., et al. (2022). *Maternal child nursing* (6th ed., p. 234). Elsevier.

15. A pregnant client tells the nurse about feeling wetness on the peripad and found some clear fluid. The nurse inspects the perineum and notes the presence of the umbilical cord. What is the **immediate** nursing action?
   1. Monitor the fetal heart rate.
   2. Notify the primary health care provider.
   3. Transfer client to the delivery room.
   4. Place client in Trendelenburg's position.

Level of Cognitive Ability: Applying
Client Needs: Physiological Integrity
Clinical Judgment/Cognitive Skills: Take Action
Integrated Process: Clinical Judgment; Nursing Process/Implementation
Content Area: Maternity: Intrapartum
Health Problems: Maternity: Prolapsed Umbilical Cord
Priority Concepts: Clinical Judgment; Reproduction

Answer: 4
Rationale: On inspection of the perineum, if the umbilical cord is noted, the nurse immediately places the client in the Trendelenburg's position while gently holding the presenting part upward to relieve the cord compression. This position is maintained and the primary health care provider is notified. The fetal heart rate also needs to be monitored to assess for fetal distress. The client is transferred to the delivery room when prescribed by the primary health care provider.
Test-Taking Strategy: Note the **strategic word**, immediate, which indicates the immediate action on the nurse's part to prevent or relieve cord compression. The only action that will achieve this is option 4.
Priority Nursing Tip: Relieving cord compression is the priority goal if the umbilical cord is protruding from the vagina. The nurse never attempts to push the cord back into the vagina.
Reference: McKinney, E. S., et al. (2022). *Maternal child nursing* (6th ed., p. 599). Elsevier.

Client Needs

❖ **16.** On assessment of a newborn being admitted to the nursery, the nurse palpates the anterior fontanel and notes that it feels soft. The nurse determines that this finding indicates which condition?
1. Dehydration
2. A normal finding
3. Increased intracranial pressure
4. Postterm by at least 2 weeks

Level of Cognitive Ability: Analyzing
Client Needs: Physiological Integrity
Clinical Judgment/Cognitive Skills: Analyze Cues
Integrated Process: Clinical Judgment; Nursing Process/Assessment
Content Area: Maternity: Newborn
Health Problems: N/A
Priority Concepts: Clinical Judgment; Development

Answer: 2
Rationale: The anterior fontanel is normally 2 to 3 cm in width, 3 to 4 cm in length, and diamond-like in shape. It can be described as soft, which is normal, or full and bulging, which could indicate increased intracranial pressure. Conversely a depressed fontanel could mean that the infant is dehydrated. The condition of the anterior fontanel is not generally influenced by a postterm delivery.
Test-Taking Strategy: Focus on the **subject**, an anterior fontanel that is soft. Recalling the normal physiologic findings in the newborn will direct you to the correct option.
Priority Nursing Tip: The anterior fontanel is a diamond-shaped area where the frontal and parietal bones meet. It closes between 12 and 18 months of age. Vigorous crying may cause the fontanel to bulge, which is a normal finding.
Reference: McKinney, E. S., et al. (2022). *Maternal child nursing* (6th ed., p. 449). Elsevier.

17. A client admitted to the hospital with a diagnosis of *Pneumocystis jiroveci* pneumonia is prescribed intravenous (IV) pentamidine. What intervention would the nurse plan to implement to safely administer the medication?
1. Infuse over 1 hour and allow client to ambulate.
2. Infuse over 1 hour with client in a supine position.
3. Administer over 30 minutes with client in a reclining position.
4. Administer by IV push over 15 minutes with client in a supine position.

Level of Cognitive Ability: Applying
Client Needs: Physiological Integrity
Clinical Judgment/Cognitive Skills: Generate Solutions
Integrated Process: Nursing Process/Planning
Content Area: Pharmacology: Immune: Antifungals
Health Problems: Adult Health: Respiratory: Pneumonia
Priority Concepts: Clinical Judgment; Safety

Answer: 2
Rationale: IV pentamidine is an antifungal medication infused over 1 hour with the client supine to minimize severe hypotension and dysrhythmias. Options 1, 3, and 4 are inaccurate in either the length of time that pentamidine is administered or the client's position.
Test-Taking Strategy: Focus on the **subject**, the procedure for administering pentamidine. Eliminate options 3 and 4 first because these time frames are too short for safe administration of this IV medication. From the remaining options, recalling that the medication causes hypotension will direct you to option 2, which addresses both the supine position and the longest time of administration.
Priority Nursing Tip: During the administration of IV pentamidine, the client needs to remain supine, and the nurse would monitor the blood pressure for hypotension and the cardiac pattern for dysrhythmias.
Reference: Gahart, B., Nazareno, A., & Ortega, M. (2021). *Gahart's 2021 Intravenous medications: A handbook for nurses and health professionals* (37th ed., pp. 1080–1081). Elsevier.

❖ **18.** During the postoperative period, the client who underwent a pelvic exenteration reports pain in the calf area. What action would the nurse take?

1. Ask client to walk and observe the gait.
2. Lightly massage calf area to relieve the pain.
3. Check calf area for temperature, color, and size.
4. Administer as needed (PRN) morphine sulfate as prescribed for postoperative pain.

Level of Cognitive Ability: Applying
Client Needs: Physiological Integrity
Clinical Judgment/Cognitive Skills: Take Action
Integrated Process: Clinical Judgment; Nursing Process/Implementation
Content Area: Adult Health: Cardiovascular
Health Problems: Adult Health: Cardiovascular: Deep Vein Thrombosis
Priority Concepts: Clinical Judgment; Perfusion

Answer: 3
Rationale: The nurse monitors the postoperative client for complications such as deep vein thrombosis, pulmonary emboli, and wound infection. Pain in the calf area could indicate a deep vein thrombosis. Change in color, temperature, or size of the client's calf could also indicate this complication. Options 1 and 2 could cause a possible thrombosis to break loose, resulting in an embolus. Administering pain medication for this client is not the appropriate nursing action since further assessment needs to take place.
Test-Taking Strategy: Focus on the information in the question and use the steps of the nursing process. Assessment is the first step. Option 3 is the only option that addresses assessment.
Priority Nursing Tip: The primary signs of deep vein thrombosis are calf or groin tenderness and pain and sudden onset of unilateral swelling of the leg.
Reference: Ignatavicius, D., et al. (2021). *Medical-surgical nursing: Concepts for interprofessional collaborative care* (10th ed., pp. 722–723). Elsevier.

19. A physician prescribes acetaminophen liquid 450 mg orally every 4 hours PRN for a client's report of minor arthritic hand pain. The medication label reads 160 mg/5 mL. The nurse prepares how many milliliters (mL) to administer one dose? Fill in the blank and record your answer to the nearest whole number.

Answer: _____ mL
Level of Cognitive Ability: Applying
Client Needs: Physiological Integrity
Clinical Judgment/Cognitive Skills: Generate Solutions
Integrated Process: Nursing Process/Planning
Content Area: Skills: Dosage Calculations
Health Problems: Adult Health: Musculoskeletal: Rheumatoid Arthritis and Osteoarthritis
Priority Concepts: Clinical Judgment; Safety

Answer: 14
Rationale: Use the formula for calculating medication dosages.

$$\frac{Desired \times Volume}{Available} = mL \text{ per dose}$$

$$\frac{450 \text{ mg} \times 5 \text{ mL}}{160 \text{ mg}} = 14 \text{ mL}$$

Test-Taking Strategy: Focus on the subject, a medication calculation. Identify the components of the question and what the question is asking. In this case, the question asks for milliliters per dose. Set up the formula knowing that the desired dose is 450 mg and that what is available is 160 mg per 5 mL. Verify the answer using a calculator and be sure that the answer makes sense.
Priority Nursing Tip: After performing a medication calculation, ensure that the amount calculated is a reasonable amount.
Reference: Potter, P., et al. (2021). *Fundamentals of nursing* (10th ed., pp. 600–601). Elsevier.

❖ **20.** The client with atrial fibrillation is prescribed sotalol AF. Which assessment finding indicates that the client is experiencing an adverse effect of the medication?

1. Dry mouth
2. Diaphoresis
3. Difficulty swallowing
4. Dizziness and feeling faint

Level of Cognitive Ability: Analyzing
Client Needs: Physiological Integrity
Clinical Judgment/Cognitive Skills: Recognize Cues
Integrated Process: Clinical Judgment; Nursing Process/Assessment
Content Area: Pharmacology: Cardiovascular: Beta Blockers
Health Problems: Adult Health: Cardiovascular: Dysrhythmias
Priority Concepts: Clinical Judgment; Perfusion

Answer: 4
Rationale: Sotalol AF is a beta-adrenergic blocking agent that may be prescribed to treat atrial fibrillation or atrial flutter. Adverse effects include headache with chest pain and severe dizziness, fainting, and fast or pounding heartbeats. Gastrointestinal disturbances, anxiety and nervousness, and unusual tiredness and weakness can also occur. Options 1, 2, and 3 are not adverse effects of this medication.
Test-Taking Strategy: Focus on the subject, adverse effects of sotalol AF. Remember that medication names ending with the letters -*lol* (sotalol AF) are beta blockers, which are commonly used for cardiac disorders. Think about the effects of atrial fibrillation on the body and recall the adverse effects to answer correctly.
Priority Nursing Tip: For the client taking a beta-adrenergic blocking agent, monitor the blood pressure for hypotension and the apical pulse rate for bradycardia. If the client's blood pressure is lower than the client's baseline or the heart rate is below 60 beats/min, notify the physician before administration.
Reference: Ignatavicius, D., et al. (2021). *Medical-surgical nursing: Concepts for interprofessional collaborative care* (10th ed., p. 650). Elsevier.

21. Which action would the nurse take to ensure safety before performing a venipuncture to initiate continuous intravenous (IV) therapy?
1. Apply a cool compress to the affected area.
2. Inspect the IV solution and expiration date.
3. Secure a padded arm board above the IV site.
4. Apply a tourniquet below the venipuncture site.

Level of Cognitive Ability: Applying
Client Needs: Physiological Integrity
Clinical Judgment/Cognitive Skills: Take Action
Integrated Process: Nursing Process/Implementation
Content Area: Foundations of Care: Safety
Health Problems: N/A
Priority Concepts: Clinical Judgment; Safety

Answer: **2**
Rationale: IV solutions need to be free of particles or precipitates to prevent trauma to veins or a thromboembolic event; in addition, the nurse avoids administering IV solutions whose expiration date has passed to prevent infection. Cool compresses cause vasoconstriction, making the vein less visible, smaller, and more difficult to puncture. Arm boards are applied after the IV is started and are used only if necessary. A tourniquet is applied above the chosen vein site to halt venous return and engorge the vein; this makes the vein easier to puncture.
Test-Taking Strategy: Note the word "before" and use the steps of the nursing process. Option 2 is the only option that reflects assessment, the first step of the nursing process.
Priority Nursing Tip: Administration of an IV solution provides immediate access to the vascular system. Check the physician's prescription and ensure that the correct solution and flow rate are administered as prescribed.
Reference: Potter, P., et al. (2021). *Fundamentals of nursing* (10th ed., pp. 1002–1003). Elsevier.

❖ **22.** The nurse is caring for a client who is receiving tacrolimus daily. Which finding indicates to the nurse that the client is experiencing an adverse effect of the medication?
1. Hypotension
2. Photophobia
3. Profuse sweating
4. Decrease in urine output

Level of Cognitive Ability: Analyzing
Client Needs: Physiological Integrity
Clinical Judgment/Cognitive Skills: Recognize Cues
Integrated Process: Nursing Process/Assessment
Content Area: Pharmacology: Immune: Immunosuppressants
Health Problems: Adult Health: Immune: Transplantation
Priority Concepts: Clinical Judgment; Safety

Answer: **4**
Rationale: Tacrolimus is an immunosuppressant medication used in the prophylaxis of organ rejection in clients receiving allogenic liver transplants. Adverse reactions and toxic effects include nephrotoxicity and pleural effusion. Nephrotoxicity is characterized by an increasing serum creatinine level and a decrease in urine output. Frequent side effects include headache, tremor, insomnia, paresthesia, diarrhea, nausea, constipation, vomiting, abdominal pain, and hypertension. None of the other options are associated with an adverse reaction to this medication.
Test-Taking Strategy: Focus on the subject, an adverse effect of tacrolimus. First, determine the medication classification and that it is an immunosuppressant. Next, recalling that nephrotoxicity is an adverse effect of the medication and other immunosuppressant medications will direct you to the correct option.
Priority Nursing Tip: Assess the renal status of the client before administering tacrolimus because the medication is nephrotoxic.
Reference: Lewis, S., et al. (2020). *Medical-surgical nursing: Assessment and management of clinical problems* (11th ed., pp. 206–207). Elsevier.

23. A client was admitted to the hospital 24 hours ago after sustaining blunt chest trauma. Which is the **earliest** clinical manifestation of acute respiratory distress syndrome (ARDS) the nurse would monitor for?
1. Cyanosis with accompanying pallor
2. Diffuse crackles and rhonchi on chest auscultation
3. Increase in respiratory rate from 18 to 30 breaths/min
4. Diffused haziness or "white-out" appearance of lungs on chest radiograph

Level of Cognitive Ability: Analyzing
Client Needs: Physiological Integrity
Clinical Judgment/Cognitive Skills: Recognize Cues
Integrated Process: Clinical Judgment; Nursing Process/Assessment
Content Area: Adult Health: Respiratory
Health Problems: Adult Health: Respiratory: Acute Respiratory Distress Syndrome/Failure
Priority Concepts: Clinical Judgment; Gas Exchange

Answer: 3
Rationale: ARDS usually develops within 24 to 48 hours after an initiating event, such as chest trauma. In most cases, tachypnea and dyspnea are the earliest clinical manifestations as the body compensates for mild hypoxemia through hyperventilation. Cyanosis and pallor are late findings and are the result of severe hypoxemia. Breath sounds in the early stages of ARDS are usually clear but then progress to diffuse crackles and rhonchi as pulmonary edema occurs. Chest radiographic findings may be normal during the early stages but will show diffuse haziness or "white-out" appearance in the later stages.
Test-Taking Strategy: Note the strategic word, *earliest*. Remember that with ARDS initial presenting symptoms are tachypnea, dyspnea, and restlessness as hypoxia develops. Knowing the definition of tachypnea and possible etiologies will direct you to the correct option.
Priority Nursing Tip: If the client sustains a chest injury, assess the respiratory status of the client. This quick assessment is followed by the treatment of life-threatening conditions.
Reference: Lewis, S., et al. (2020). *Medical-surgical nursing: Assessment and management of clinical problems* (11th ed., pp. 1598–1599). Elsevier.

24. The nurse, caring for a client with Buck's traction, is monitoring the client for complications of the traction. Which assessment finding indicates a complication of this form of traction?
1. Weak pedal pulses
2. Drainage at the pin sites
3. Complaints of leg discomfort
4. Toes are warm and demonstrate a brisk capillary refill

Level of Cognitive Ability: Analyzing
Client Needs: Physiological Integrity
Clinical Judgment/Cognitive Skills: Recognize Cues
Integrated Process: Clinical Judgment; Nursing Process/Assessment
Content Area: Adult Health: Musculoskeletal
Health Problems: Adult Health: Musculoskeletal: Skeletal Injury
Priority Concepts: Mobility; Perfusion

Answer: 1
Rationale: Buck's traction is skin traction. Weak pedal pulses are a sign of vascular compromise, which can be caused by pressure on the tissues of the leg by the elastic bandage or prefabricated boot used to secure this type of traction. Skeletal (not skin) traction uses pins. Discomfort is expected. Warm toes with brisk capillary refill is a normal finding.
Test-Taking Strategy: Use the ABCs—airway, breathing, and circulation—to direct you to option 1, indicative of vascular compromise. Also eliminate option 2 because Buck's traction does not use pins. Options 3 and 4 can be eliminated because they are comparable and alike and are both expected and normal findings.
Priority Nursing Tip: If the client in traction exhibits signs of neurovascular compromise such as changes in temperature, sensation, or the ability to move digits of the affected extremity, the physician is notified immediately.
Reference: Ignatavicius, D., et al. (2021). *Medical-surgical nursing: Concepts for interprofessional collaborative care* (10th ed., p. 1040). Elsevier.

25. A prenatal client has been diagnosed with a vaginal infection from the organism *Candida albicans*. What would the nurse expect to note on assessment of the client?
1. Costovertebral angle pain
2. Absence of any observable signs
3. Pain, itching, and vaginal discharge
4. Proteinuria, hematuria, and hypertension

Level of Cognitive Ability: Analyzing
Client Needs: Physiological Integrity
Clinical Judgment/Cognitive Skills: Recognize Cues
Integrated Process: Nursing Process/Assessment
Content Area: Maternity: Antepartum
Health Problems: Maternity: Infections/Inflammations
Priority Concepts: Infection; Sexuality

Answer: 3
Rationale: Clinical manifestations of a *Candida* infection include pain; itching; and a thick, white vaginal discharge. Proteinuria and hypertension are signs of preeclampsia. Costovertebral angle pain, proteinuria, and hematuria are clinical manifestations associated with urinary tract infections.
Test-Taking Strategy: Focus on the subject, a vaginal infection. Note the relationship between the subject and option 3.
Priority Nursing Tip: *Candida albicans* is a fungal infection of the skin and mucous membranes. Common areas of occurrence include the mucous membranes of the mouth, perineum, vagina, axilla, and under the breasts.
Reference: McKinney, E. S., et al. (2022). *Maternal child nursing* (6th ed., pp. 221, 570). Elsevier.

❖ **26.** A prenatal client has a suspected diagnosis of iron deficiency anemia. On assessment, which finding would the nurse expect to note as a result of this condition?
1. Dehydration
2. Fluid overload
3. A high hematocrit level
4. A low hemoglobin level

Level of Cognitive Ability: Analyzing
Client Needs: Physiological Integrity
Clinical Judgment/Cognitive Skills: Recognize Cues
Integrated Process: Nursing Process/Assessment
Content Area: Maternity: Antepartum
Health Problems: Adult Health: Hematologic: Anemias
Priority Concepts: Cellular Regulation; Reproduction

Answer: 4
Rationale: Pathologic anemia of pregnancy is caused primarily by iron deficiency. When the hemoglobin level is below 11 g/dL (110 g/L), iron deficiency is suspected; reference range for hemoglobin is 12–16 g/dL (120–160 g/L). An indirect index of the oxygen-carrying capacity is determined via a packed red blood cell volume or hematocrit level. Dehydration and overhydration are not specifically associated with iron deficiency anemia.
Test-Taking Strategy: Focus on the subject, manifestations of iron deficiency anemia. Note the relationship between the words "deficiency" in the diagnosis and "low" in the correct option.
Priority Nursing Tip: The ferritin level is a laboratory test that is used to diagnose iron deficiency anemia. A ferritin level of less than 10 ng/mL (10 mcg/L) confirms the diagnosis. Reference range for ferritin for a biologically born male is 12–300 ng/mL (12–300 mcg/L); for a biologically born female is 10–150 ng/mL (10–150 mcg/L).
Reference: McKinney, E. S., et al. (2022). *Maternal child nursing* (6th ed., p. 567). Elsevier.

27. The nurse caring for a postpartum client would suspect that the client is experiencing endometritis if what is noted during an assessment?
1. Breast engorgement
2. Elevated white blood cell count
3. Lochia rubra on the second day postpartum
4. Fever over 38° C (100.4° F), beginning 2 days postpartum

Level of Cognitive Ability: Analyzing
Client Needs: Physiological Integrity
Clinical Judgment/Cognitive Skills: Recognize Cues
Integrated Process: Clinical Judgment; Nursing Process/Assessment
Content Area: Maternity: Postpartum
Health Problems: Maternity: Infections/Inflammations
Priority Concepts: Infection; Reproduction

Answer: 4
Rationale: Endometritis is a common cause of postpartum infection. The presence of fever of 38° C (100.4° F) or more on 2 successive days of the first 10 postpartum days (not counting the first 24 hours after birth) is indicative of a postpartum infection. Breast engorgement is a normal response in the postpartum period and is not associated with endometritis. The white blood cell count of a postpartum client is normally elevated; thus, this method of detecting infection is not of great value in the puerperium. Lochia rubra on the second day postpartum is a normal finding.
Test-Taking Strategy: Focus on the subject, endometritis. Recalling the normal findings in the postpartum period will assist in eliminating options 1, 2, and 3.
Priority Nursing Tip: A postpartum infection may also be termed "a puerperal infection" and is described as an infection of the genital canal that occurs within 28 days after a miscarriage, induced abortion, or childbirth.
Reference: McKinney, E. S., et al. (2022). *Maternal child nursing* (6th ed., pp. 615–616). Elsevier.

❖ **28.** The nurse is performing an assessment on a postterm infant. Which physical characteristic would the nurse expect to observe in this infant?
1. Peeling of the skin
2. Smooth soles without creases
3. Lanugo covering the entire body
4. Vernix that covers the body in a thick layer

Level of Cognitive Ability: Analyzing
Client Needs: Physiological Integrity
Clinical Judgment/Cognitive Skills: Recognize Cues
Integrated Process: Clinical Judgment; Nursing Process/Assessment
Content Area: Maternity: Newborn
Health Problems: Newborn: Preterm and Postterm Newborn
Priority Concepts: Development; Health Promotion

Answer: 1
Rationale: The postterm infant (born after the 42nd week of gestation) exhibits dry, peeling, cracked, almost leather-like skin over the body, which is called desquamation. The preterm infant (born between 24 and 37 weeks of gestation) exhibits smooth soles without creases, lanugo covering the entire body, and thick vernix covering the body.
Test-Taking Strategy: Focus on the **subject**, the postterm infant. Think about the physiology associated with the postterm infant. Recalling that the postterm infant is born after the 42nd week of gestation will assist in directing you to the correct option.
Priority Nursing Tip: The postterm infant may exhibit meconium staining on the fingernails, long nails and hair, and the absence of vernix.
Reference: McKinney, E. S., et al. (2022). *Maternal child nursing* (6th ed., pp. 641–642). Elsevier.

29. A postterm infant, delivered vaginally, is exhibiting tachypnea, grunting, retractions, and nasal flaring. The nurse interprets that these assessment findings are indicative of which condition?
1. Hypoglycemia
2. Respiratory distress syndrome
3. Meconium aspiration syndrome
4. Transient tachypnea of the newborn

Level of Cognitive Ability: Analyzing
Client Needs: Physiological Integrity
Clinical Judgment/Cognitive Skills: Analyze Cues
Integrated Process: Clinical Judgment; Nursing Process/Analysis
Content Area: Maternity: Newborn
Health Problems: Newborn: Respiratory Problems
Priority Concepts: Development; Gas Exchange

Answer: 3
Rationale: Tachypnea, grunting, retractions, and nasal flaring are symptoms of respiratory distress related to meconium aspiration syndrome (MAS). MAS occurs often in postterm infants and develops when meconium in the amniotic fluid enters the lungs during fetal life or at birth. The symptoms noted in the question are unrelated to hypoglycemia; in hypoglycemia, the infant is more likely to present with low body temperature (hypothermia), floppy muscles (poor muscle tone), and a lack of interest in feeding. Respiratory distress syndrome is a complication of preterm infants. Transient tachypnea of the newborn is primarily found in infants delivered via cesarean section.
Test-Taking Strategy: Focus on the **subject**, a postterm infant, and note the symptoms identified in the question. Option 1 is eliminated first because hypoglycemia is not a respiratory condition. Eliminate option 2 because this is a complication in preterm infants. From the remaining options, think about a postterm infant and recall the complications that can occur. This will direct you to the correct option.
Priority Nursing Tip: The primary health care provider is notified if meconium is noted in the amniotic fluid during labor. Although meconium is sterile, aspiration can lead to lung damage, which promotes the growth of bacteria; thus, the newborn needs to be closely monitored for infection.
Reference: McKinney, E. S., et al. (2022). *Maternal child nursing* (6th ed., p. 642). Elsevier.

❖ **30.** The nurse is caring for a client who had an orthopedic injury of the leg that required surgery and the application of a cast. Postoperatively, which nursing assessment is of **highest priority** to ensure client safety?
1. Monitoring for heel breakdown
2. Monitoring for bladder distention
3. Monitoring for extremity shortening
4. Monitoring for blanching ability of toenail beds

Level of Cognitive Ability: Analyzing
Client Needs: Physiological Integrity
Clinical Judgment/Cognitive Skills: Prioritize Hypotheses
Integrated Process: Clinical Judgment; Nursing Process/Assessment
Content Area: Adult Health: Musculoskeletal
Health Problems: Adult Health: Musculoskeletal: Skeletal Injury
Priority Concepts: Mobility; Perfusion

Answer: 4
Rationale: With cast application, concern for compartment syndrome development is of the highest priority. If postsurgical edema compromises circulation, the client will experience numbness, tingling, loss of blanching of toenail beds, and pain that will not be relieved by opioids. Although heel breakdown, bladder distention, or extremity lengthening or shortening can occur, these complications are not potentially life-threatening complications.
Test-Taking Strategy: Note the strategic words, *highest priority.* Use the ABCs—airway, breathing, and circulation—to answer the question. Assessment for circulation to the foot, including observations for numbness and tingling and the ability of the nail beds to blanch, will direct you to the correct option.
Priority Nursing Tip: Monitor the client with a cast for early signs of compartment syndrome. Assess the client for the "six Ps," which include pain, pressure, paralysis, paresthesia, pallor, and pulselessness.
Reference: Ignatavicius, D., et al. (2021). *Medical-surgical nursing: Concepts for interprofessional collaborative care* (10th ed., pp. 1031, 1040). Elsevier.

31. A client experiencing an exacerbation of their asthma symptoms requires mechanical ventilation. An arterial blood gas (ABG) specimen is to be sent to the laboratory for analysis. What information would the nurse include on the laboratory requisition? **Select all that apply.**
❏ 1. Ventilator settings
❏ 2. List of client allergies
❏ 3. Client's temperature
❏ 4. Date and time the specimen was drawn
❏ 5. Any supplemental oxygen client is receiving
❏ 6. Extremity from which the specimen was obtained

Level of Cognitive Ability: Applying
Client Needs: Physiological Integrity
Clinical Judgment/Cognitive Skills: Take Action
Integrated Process: Clinical Judgment; Nursing Process/Implementation
Content Area: Foundations of Care: Laboratory Tests
Health Problems: Adult Health: Respiratory: Asthma
Priority Concepts: Clinical Judgment; Communication

Answer: 1, 3, 4, 5
Rationale: An ABG requisition usually contains information about the date and time the specimen was drawn, the client's temperature, whether the specimen was drawn on room air or using supplemental oxygen, and the ventilator settings if the client is on a mechanical ventilator. The client's allergies and the extremity from which the specimen was drawn do not have a direct bearing on the laboratory results.
Test-Taking Strategy: Focus on the subject, procedures for preparing an ABG draw. Review the pieces of information from the viewpoint of the relevance of the item to the client's airway status or oxygen use. The only pieces of information that do not relate to airway status or oxygen use are the client's allergies and the extremity from which the specimen was drawn.
Priority Nursing Tip: An ABG specimen must be transported to the laboratory for processing within 15 minutes from the time that it was obtained.
References: Lewis, S., et al. (2020). *Medical-surgical nursing: Assessment and management of clinical problems* (11th ed., p. 470). Elsevier; Pagana, K., Pagana, T., & Pagana, T. N. (2021). *Mosby's Diagnostic and laboratory test reference* (15th ed., pp. 108–109). Elsevier.

❖ **32.** The nurse is reviewing the laboratory results for a client diagnosed with chronic heart failure (HF) who is receiving torsemide 5 mg orally daily. Which result would indicate to the nurse that the client might be experiencing an adverse effect of the medication?

Laboratory Results

Test and Result	Reference Range
Chloride 98 mEq/L (98 mmol/L)	98–106 mEq/L (98–106 mmol/L)
Sodium 146 mEq/L (146 mmol/L)	135–145 mEq/L (135–145 mmol/L)
Potassium 3.1 mEq/L (3.1 mmol/L)	3.5–5.0 mEq/L (3.5–5.0 mmol/L)
BUN 15 mg/dL (5.4 mmol/L)	10–20 mg/dL (3.6–7.1 mmol/L)

1. Chloride level
2. Sodium level
3. Potassium level
4. BUN level

Level of Cognitive Ability: Analyzing
Client Needs: Physiological Integrity
Clinical Judgment/Cognitive Skills: Analyze Cues
Integrated Process: Clinical Judgment; Nursing Process/Analysis
Content Area: Pharmacology: Cardiovascular: Diuretics
Health Problems: Adult Health: Cardiovascular: Heart Failure
Priority Concepts: Fluids and Electrolytes; Clinical Judgment

Answer: 3
Rationale: Torsemide is a loop diuretic. The medication can produce acute, profound water loss; volume and electrolyte depletion; dehydration; decreased blood volume; and circulatory collapse. Option 3 indicates electrolyte depletion. The sodium level is only elevated by 1 mEq/L (1 mmol/L), and this elevation is not significant.
Test-Taking Strategy: Focus on the subject, adverse effects of torsemide. Recall knowledge of normal laboratory values to assist in selecting option 3, which is the only abnormal laboratory value presented.
Priority Nursing Tip: Nursing interventions for a client taking a loop diuretic include monitoring the blood pressure, weight, intake and output, and serum electrolytes (especially potassium), and assessing the client for any hearing abnormality.
Reference: Lewis, S., et al. (2020). *Medical-surgical nursing: Assessment and management of clinical problems* (11th ed., pp. 278–279, 689). Elsevier.

33. During history taking of a client admitted with newly diagnosed Hodgkin's disease, the nurse would ask the client about which expected symptom?
1. Weight gain
2. Night sweats
3. Severe lymph node pain
4. Headache with minor visual changes

Level of Cognitive Ability: Applying
Client Needs: Physiological Integrity
Clinical Judgment/Cognitive Skills: Recognize Cues
Integrated Process: Nursing Process/Assessment
Content Area: Adult Health: Oncology
Health Problems: Adult Health: Cancer: Lymphoma, Hodgkin's and Non-Hodgkin's
Priority Concepts: Cellular Regulation; Clinical Judgment

Answer: 2
Rationale: Assessment of a client with Hodgkin's disease most often reveals night sweats; enlarged, painless lymph nodes; fever; and malaise. Weight loss may be present if metastatic disease occurs. Headache and visual changes may occur if brain metastasis is present.
Test-Taking Strategy: Focus on the subject, symptoms associated with Hodgkin's disease. Eliminate options 3 and 4 first because they are comparable or alike in that they relate to discomfort. Weight gain is rarely the symptom of a cancer diagnosis, so eliminate option 1.
Priority Nursing Tip: The most common assessment finding in Hodgkin's disease is the presence of a large and painless lymph node(s), often located in the neck. Biopsy of the node reveals the presence of Reed-Sternberg cells.
Reference: Lewis, S., et al. (2020). *Medical-surgical nursing: Assessment and management of clinical problems* (11th ed., p. 643). Elsevier.

34. The nurse is assessing a 3-day-old preterm neonate being treated for a diagnosis of respiratory distress syndrome (RDS). Which assessment finding indicates that the neonate's respiratory condition is improving?
1. Edema of the hands and feet
2. Urine output of 3 mL/kg/hr
3. Presence of a systolic murmur
4. Respiratory rate between 60 and 70 breaths/min

Level of Cognitive Ability: Evaluating
Client Needs: Physiological Integrity
Clinical Judgment/Cognitive Skills: Evaluate Outcomes
Integrated Process: Clinical Judgment; Nursing Process/Evaluation
Content Area: Maternity: Newborn
Health Problems: Newborn: Respiratory Problems
Priority Concepts: Clinical Judgment; Gas Exchange

Answer: 2
Rationale: RDS is a serious lung disorder caused by immaturity and the inability to produce surfactant, resulting in hypoxia and acidosis. Lung fluid, which occurs in RDS, moves from the lungs into the bloodstream as the condition improves and the alveoli open. This extra fluid circulates to the kidneys, which results in increased voiding. Therefore, normal urination is an early sign that the neonate's respiratory condition is improving (normal urinary output is 2 to 5 mL/kg/hr). Edema of the hands and feet occurs within the first 24 hours after the development of RDS as a result of low protein concentrations, a decrease in colloidal osmotic pressure, and transudation of fluid from the vascular system to the tissues. Systolic murmurs usually indicate the presence of a patent ductus arteriosus, which is a common complication of RDS. Respiratory rates above 60 breaths/min are indicative of tachypnea, which is a sign of respiratory distress.
Test-Taking Strategy: Note the **subject**, sign of improvement of a preterm neonate with a diagnosis of RDS. Option 2 is the only normal finding and indicates a normal urine output, which would indicate resolution of excess lung fluid.
Priority Nursing Tip: Surfactant replacement therapy is used for the rescue treatment of RDS in premature infants. The surfactant is instilled into the endotracheal tube.
Reference: McKinney, E. S., et al. (2022). *Maternal child nursing* (6th ed., p. 628). Elsevier.

35. The nurse is caring for a term newborn. Which assessment finding would predispose the newborn to the occurrence of jaundice?
1. Presence of a cephalhematoma
2. Infant blood type of O negative
3. Birth weight of 8 pounds 6 ounces
4. A negative direct Coombs' test result

Level of Cognitive Ability: Analyzing
Client Needs: Physiological Integrity
Clinical Judgment/Cognitive Skills: Analyze Cues
Integrated Process: Clinical Judgment; Nursing Process/Assessment
Content Area: Maternity: Newborn
Health Problems: Newborn: Cephalohematoma
Priority Concepts: Cellular Regulation; Development

Answer: 1
Rationale: A cephalhematoma is swelling caused by bleeding into an area between the bone and its periosteum of the skull (does not cross over the suture line). Enclosed hemorrhage, such as with cephalhematoma, predisposes the newborn to jaundice by producing an increased bilirubin load as the cephalhematoma resolves (usually within 6 weeks) and is absorbed into the circulatory system. The classic Rh incompatibility situation involves an Rh-negative birthing parent with an Rh-positive fetus/newborn. The birth weight in option 3 is within the acceptable range for a term newborn and therefore does not contribute to an increased bilirubin level. A negative direct Coombs' test result indicates that there are no maternal antibodies on fetal erythrocytes.
Test-Taking Strategy: Focus on the **subject**, a term newborn's predisposition to jaundice. Recalling the risk factors associated with jaundice and the association between hemorrhage and jaundice will direct you to the correct option.
Priority Nursing Tip: Normal or physiologic jaundice appears after the first 24 hours in a full-term newborn. Jaundice occurring before this time is known as pathologic jaundice and warrants primary health care provider notification.
Reference: McKinney, E. S., et al. (2022). *Maternal child nursing* (6th ed., p. 449). Elsevier.

36. To ensure client safety, which assessment is **most important** for the nurse to make before advancing a client recovering from an appendectomy from liquid to solid food?
1. Bowel sounds
2. Chewing ability
3. Current appetite
4. Food preferences

Level of Cognitive Ability: Analyzing
Client Needs: Physiological Integrity
Clinical Judgment/Cognitive Skills: Prioritize Hypotheses
Integrated Process: Clinical Judgment; Nursing Process/Assessment
Content Area: Foundations of Care: Therapeutic Diets
Health Problems: Adult Health: Gastrointestinal: Appendicitis
Priority Concepts: Nutrition; Safety

Answer: 2
Rationale: The nurse needs to assess the client's chewing ability before advancing a client from liquid to solid food. It may be necessary to modify a client's diet to a soft or mechanical chopped diet if the client has difficulty chewing because of the risk of aspiration. Bowel sounds need to be present before introducing any diet, including liquids. Appetite will affect the amount of food eaten, but not the type of diet prescribed. Food preferences should be ascertained on admission assessment.
Test-Taking Strategy: Note the strategic words, *most important.* Also, focusing on the subject, advancing a diet from liquid to solid, will direct you to the correct option because the primary difference between a liquid and a solid diet is that the food needs mechanical processing (chewing) before it can be safely swallowed.
Priority Nursing Tip: The consistency of food may need to be altered based on the client's ability to chew or swallow. Liquid can be added to food to alter its consistency, but the liquid used should complement the food and its original flavor.
References: Lewis, S., et al. (2020). *Medical-surgical nursing: Assessment and management of clinical problems* (11th ed., p. 938). Elsevier; Potter, P., et al. (2021). *Fundamentals of nursing* (10th ed., p. 1122). Elsevier.

37. The nurse, caring for a client in the active stage of labor, is monitoring the fetal status and notes that the monitor strip shows a late deceleration. Based on this observation, which action would the nurse take **immediately**?
1. Document the findings.
2. Prepare for immediate birth.
3. Increase the rate of an oxytocin infusion.
4. Administer oxygen to client via face mask.

Level of Cognitive Ability: Analyzing
Client Needs: Physiological Integrity
Clinical Judgment/Cognitive Skills: Take Action
Integrated Process: Clinical Judgment; Nursing Process/Implementation
Content Area: Maternity: Intrapartum
Health Problems: Maternity: Fetal Distress/Demise
Priority Concepts: Perfusion; Reproduction

Answer: 4
Rationale: Late decelerations are caused by uteroplacental insufficiency as the result of decreased blood flow and oxygen transfer to the fetus through the intervillous space during the uterine contractions. This causes hypoxemia; therefore, oxygen is necessary. Although the finding needs to be documented, documentation is not the priority action in this situation. Late decelerations are considered an ominous sign but do not necessarily require immediate birth of the baby. The oxytocin infusion needs to be discontinued when a late deceleration is noted. The oxytocin would cause further hypoxemia because the medication stimulates contractions and leads to increased uteroplacental insufficiency.
Test-Taking Strategy: Note the strategic word, *immediately.* Recall that late decelerations are an indication of decreased oxygenation. Use the ABCs—airway, breathing, and circulation—to direct you to option 4.
Priority Nursing Tip: Late decelerations are nonreassuring patterns that reflect impaired placental exchange or uteroplacental insufficiency. The patterns look similar to early decelerations, but they begin well after the contraction begins and return to baseline after the contraction ends.
Reference: McKinney, E. S., et al. (2022). *Maternal child nursing* (6th ed., pp. 345–346). Elsevier.

38. The nurse is caring for an obese client on a weight loss program. Which method would the nurse use to **most** accurately assess the program's **effectiveness**?
1. Monitor client's weight.
2. Monitor client's intake and output.
3. Calculate client's daily caloric intake.
4. Frequently check client's serum protein levels.

Level of Cognitive Ability: Evaluating
Client Needs: Physiological Integrity
Clinical Judgment/Cognitive Skills: Evaluate Outcomes
Integrated Process: Clinical Judgment; Nursing Process/Evaluation
Content Area: Health Assessment/Physical Exam: General Assessment Techniques
Health Problems: Adult Health: Gastrointestinal: Nutrition Problems
Priority Concepts: Evidence; Nutrition

Answer: 1
Rationale: The most accurate measurement of weight loss is weighing of the client. This needs to be done at the same time of the day, in the same clothes, and using the same scale. Options 2, 3, and 4 measure nutrition and hydration status but are not associated with effectiveness of the weight loss program.
Test-Taking Strategy: Focus on the subject, weight loss, and note the strategic words, *most* and *effectiveness.* Assessing weight will most accurately identify weight changes. Also note that options 2, 3, and 4 are comparable or alike and measure nutrition and hydration status.
Priority Nursing Tip: Clothing and shoes affect the obtained weight measurement. It is important to make a notation about any clothing, shoes, accessories (heavy jewelry), or other items such as casts or braces worn by the client while obtaining the weight.
Reference: Lewis, S., et al. (2020). *Medical-surgical nursing: Assessment and management of clinical problems* (11th ed., p. 275). Elsevier.

39. A client has fallen and sustained a leg injury. Which question would the nurse ask to help determine if the client sustained a fracture?
1. "Is the pain a dull ache?"
2. "Is the pain sharp and continuous?"
3. "Does the discomfort feel like a cramp?"
4. "Does the pain feel like the muscle was stretched?"

Level of Cognitive Ability: Applying
Client Needs: Physiological Integrity
Clinical Judgment/Cognitive Skills: Recognize Cues
Integrated Process: Nursing Process/Assessment
Content Area: Health Assessment/Physical Exam: Musculoskeletal
Health Problems: Adult Health: Musculoskeletal: Skeletal Injury
Priority Concepts: Mobility; Pain

Answer: 2
Rationale: Fracture pain is generally described as sharp, continuous, and increasing in frequency. Bone pain is often described as a dull, deep ache. Muscle injury is often described as an aching or cramping pain, or soreness. Strains result from trauma to a muscle body or the attachment of a tendon from overstretching or overextension.
Test-Taking Strategy: Focus on the subject, manifestations of a fracture. Recalling that pain from a new injury such as a fracture is more likely to be described as sharp will direct you to the correct option.
Priority Nursing Tip: Some fractures can be identified on inspection and exhibit manifestations such as an obvious deformity, edema, and bruising; others are detected only on x-ray examination.
Reference: Ignatavicius, D., et al. (2021). *Medical-surgical nursing: Concepts for interprofessional collaborative care* (10th ed., pp. 1033, 1035). Elsevier.

❖ **40.** The nurse reviews the arterial blood gas (ABG) results of a client with a bowel obstruction who has a nasogastric tube attached to continuous suction. The nurse determines that the client is experiencing which acid–base imbalance?

Laboratory Results

Test and Result	Reference Range
pH 7.49	7.35–7.45
Po_2 80 mm Hg	80–100 mm Hg
Pco_2 38 mm Hg	35–45 mm Hg
HCO_3 30 mEq/L	21–28 mEq/L
(30 mmol/L)	(21–28 mmol/L)

1. Respiratory acidosis
2. Metabolic acidosis
3. Respiratory alkalosis
4. Metabolic alkalosis

Level of Cognitive Ability: Analyzing
Client Needs: Physiological Integrity
Clinical Judgment/Cognitive Skills: Analyze Cues
Integrated Process: Clinical Judgment; Nursing Process/Analysis
Content Area: Foundations of Care: Acid–Base
Health Problems: Adult Health: Gastrointestinal: Bowel Obstruction
Priority Concepts: Acid–Base Balance; Clinical Judgment

Answer: 4
Rationale: The anticipated ABG finding in the client with a nasogastric tube to continuous suction is metabolic alkalosis resulting from loss of acid. In uncompensated metabolic alkalosis, the pH will be elevated (greater than 7.45), bicarbonate will be elevated (greater than 28 mEq/mL), Po_2 and the Pco_2 will most likely be in range. Therefore, options 1, 2, and 3 are incorrect.
Test-Taking Strategy: Focus on the subject, the acid–base imbalance that occurs in a client with continuous nasogastric suctioning. Note that the question addresses a gastrointestinal situation. Eliminate options 1 and 3 because they both identify a respiratory imbalance (opposite effects between the pH and the Pco_2). From the remaining options, remember that acid will be removed with nasogastric suctioning, so an alkalotic condition will result. This will direct you to the correct option.
Priority Nursing Tip: The reference range for pH is 7.35 to 7.45. A pH level lower than 7.35 indicates an acidotic condition. A pH greater than 7.45 indicates an alkalotic condition.
Reference: Ignatavicius, D., et al. (2021). *Medical-surgical nursing: Concepts for interprofessional collaborative care* (10th ed., p. 272). Elsevier.

41. The nurse is monitoring a client with malnutrition who was started on total parenteral nutrition (TPN) and obtains a finger-stick glucose reading. Based on the result, which action would the nurse take?

Laboratory Results

Test and Result	Reference Range
Glucose 425 mg/dL (23.7 mmol/L)	70–99 mg/dL (3.9–5.5 mmol/L)—fasting

1. Stop the TPN.
2. Decrease oral intake.
3. Notify the physician.
4. Decrease the flow rate of the TPN.

Level of Cognitive Ability: Applying
Client Needs: Physiological Integrity
Clinical Judgment/Cognitive Skills: Take Action
Integrated Process: Clinical Judgment; Nursing Process/Implementation
Content Area: Skills: Nutrition
Health Problems: Adult Health: Gastrointestinal: Nutrition/Malabsorption Problems
Priority Concepts: Glucose Regulation; Clinical Judgment

Answer: 3
Rationale: Hyperglycemia is a complication of TPN, and the nurse would report abnormalities to the physician so that specific parameters for insulin administration can be prescribed. Options 1, 2, and 4 are not done without a physician's order. Additionally, depending on the client situation, it may be harmful to decrease oral intake.
Test-Taking Strategy: Focus on the subject, a finger-stick glucose reading of 425 mg/dL (23.7 mmol/L). Note that options 1, 2, and 4 are comparable or alike and are not within the scope of nursing practice and require a physician's order. A blood glucose of 425 mg/dL (23.7 mmol/L) requires notification of the physician.
Priority Nursing Tip: When a client is receiving TPN, the risk of hyperglycemia exists because of the high concentration of dextrose (glucose) in the solution.
References: Ignatavicius, D., et al. (2021). *Medical-surgical nursing: Concepts for interprofessional collaborative care* (10th ed., p. 1208). Elsevier; Pagana, K., Pagana, T., & Pagana, T. N. (2021). *Mosby's Diagnostic and laboratory test reference* (15th ed., p. 464). Elsevier.

42. The nurse provides information to a preoperative client who will be receiving relaxation therapy. What effects would the nurse teach the client to expect regarding this type of therapy? **Select all that apply.**
☐ 1. Increased heart rate
☐ 2. Improved well-being
☐ 3. Lowered blood pressure
☐ 4. Increased respiratory rate
☐ 5. Decreased muscle tension
☐ 6. Increased neural impulses to the brain

Level of Cognitive Ability: Applying
Client Needs: Physiological Integrity
Clinical Judgment/Cognitive Skills: Take Action
Integrated Process: Teaching and Learning
Content Area: Skills: Perioperative Care
Health Problems: Mental Health: Coping
Priority Concepts: Health Promotion; Patient Education

Answer: 2, 3, 5
Rationale: Relaxation is the state of generalized decreased cognitive, physiologic, and/or behavioral arousal. Relaxation elongates the muscle fibers, reduces the neural impulses to the brain, and thus decreases the activity of the brain and other systems. The effects of relaxation therapy include improved well-being; lowered blood pressure, heart rate, and respiratory rate; decreased muscle tension; and reduced symptoms of distress in persons who need to undergo treatments, those experiencing complications from medical treatment or disease, or those grieving the loss of a significant other. This therapy does not cause an increased heart rate, increased respiratory rate, or increased neural impulses to the brain.
Test-Taking Strategy: Focus on the subject, the effects of relaxation therapy. Thinking about the definition of relaxation and recalling that it is the state of generalized decreased cognitive, physiologic, and/or behavioral arousal will assist in directing you to the correct options.
Priority Nursing Tip: A simple relaxation exercise should be incorporated into an individual's daily routine to decrease stress levels; stress can be a significant factor in the development of disease.
Reference: Lewis, S., et al. (2020). *Medical-surgical nursing: Assessment and management of clinical problems* (11th ed., pp. 81–83). Elsevier.

43. A client has developed atrial fibrillation resulting in a ventricular rate of 150 beats/min. The nurse would assess the client for which effects of this cardiac occurrence? **Select all that apply.**
- ❏ **1.** Dyspnea
- ❏ **2.** Flat neck veins
- ❏ **3.** Nausea and vomiting
- ❏ **4.** Chest pain or discomfort
- ❏ **5.** Hypotension and dizziness
- ❏ **6.** Hypertension and headache

Level of Cognitive Ability: Analyzing
Client Needs: Physiological Integrity
Clinical Judgment/Cognitive Skills: Recognize Cues
Integrated Process: Clinical Judgment; Nursing Process/Assessment
Content Area: Adult Health: Cardiovascular
Health Problems: Adult Health: Cardiovascular: Dysrhythmias
Priority Concepts: Clinical Judgment; Perfusion

Answer: 1, 4, 5
Rationale: The client with uncontrolled atrial fibrillation with a ventricular rate over 100 beats/min is at risk for low cardiac output caused by loss of atrial kick. The nurse would assess the client for palpitations, chest pain or discomfort, hypotension, pulse deficit, fatigue, weakness, dizziness, syncope, shortness of breath, and distended neck veins. Neither headache nor nausea and vomiting are directly associated with the effects of uncontrolled atrial fibrillation.
Test-Taking Strategy: Focus on the subject, the effects of uncontrolled atrial fibrillation. Recalling that flat neck veins are normal or indicate hypovolemia will assist you in eliminating option 2. Remembering that nausea and vomiting are associated with vagus nerve activity, not a tachycardic state, will assist you in eliminating option 3. In addition, the vagus nerve is associated with lowering the heart rate. From the remaining options, thinking of the effects of a falling cardiac output will direct you to the correct option.
Priority Nursing Tip: Clients with atrial fibrillation are at risk for thromboembolism. Monitor the client closely for signs of this life-threatening situation.
Reference: Ignatavicius, D., et al. (2021). *Medical-surgical nursing: Concepts for interprofessional collaborative care* (10th ed., p. 652). Elsevier.

❖ **44.** A preschooler with a history of cleft palate repair comes to the clinic for a routine well-child checkup. To determine whether this child is experiencing a long-term effect of cleft palate, which question would the nurse ask the parent?
- **1.** "Does the child play with an imaginary friend?"
- **2.** "Was the child recently treated for pneumonia?"
- **3.** "Does the child respond when called by name?"
- **4.** "Has the child had any difficulty swallowing food?"

Level of Cognitive Ability: Applying
Client Needs: Physiological Integrity
Clinical Judgment/Cognitive Skills: Recognize Cues
Integrated Process: Nursing Process/Assessment
Content Area: Pediatrics: Gastrointestinal
Health Problems: Pediatric-Specific: Disorders of Prenatal Development
Priority Concepts: Development; Sensory Perception

Answer: 3
Rationale: A child with cleft palate is at risk for developing frequent otitis media, which can result in hearing loss. Unresponsiveness may be an indication that the child is experiencing hearing loss. Option 1 is normal behavior for a preschool child. Many preschoolers with vivid imaginations have imaginary friends. Options 2 and 4 are unrelated to cleft palate after repair.
Test-Taking Strategy: Focus on the subject, a long-term effect of cleft palate. Think about the anatomy of this disorder and the pathophysiology associated with it. Recalling that hearing loss can occur in a child with cleft palate will direct you to the correct option.
Priority Nursing Tip: After a cleft palate repair, avoid the use of oral suction or placing objects in the child's mouth such as a tongue depressor, thermometer, straws, spoons, forks, or pacifiers because of the risk of disrupting the surgical site.
Reference: McKinney, E. S., et al. (2022). *Maternal child nursing* (6th ed., p. 967). Elsevier.

45. The nurse is performing a respiratory assessment on a client being treated for an asthma attack. The nurse determines that the client's respiratory status is worsening based upon which finding?
1. Loud wheezing
2. Wheezing on expiration
3. Noticeably diminished breath sounds
4. Increased displays of emotional apprehension

Level of Cognitive Ability: Evaluating
Client Needs: Physiological Integrity
Clinical Judgment/Cognitive Skills: Evaluate Outcomes
Integrated Process: Clinical Judgment; Nursing Process/Evaluation
Content Area: Adult Health: Respiratory
Health Problems: Adult Health: Respiratory: Asthma
Priority Concepts: Clinical Judgment; Gas Exchange

Answer: 3
Rationale: Noticeably diminished breath sounds are an indication of severe obstruction and impending respiratory failure. Wheezing is not a reliable manifestation to determine the severity of an asthma attack. Clients with minor attacks may experience loud wheezes, whereas others with severe attacks may not wheeze. Also, the client with severe asthma attacks may have no audible wheezing because of the decrease of airflow. For wheezing to occur, the client must be able to move sufficient air to produce breath sounds. Emotional apprehension is likely whatever the degree of respiratory distress is being experienced.
Test-Taking Strategy: Note the **subject**, evidence of worsening respiratory status in a client being treated for an asthma attack. Use **Maslow's Hierarchy of Needs theory** to eliminate option 4. Next, use the **ABCs—airway, breathing, and circulation.** Remember that diminished breath sounds indicate obstruction and impending respiratory failure; this will direct you to the correct option. Also note that options 1 and 2 are **comparable or alike** and address wheezing.
Priority Nursing Tip: During an acute asthma attack, position the client in a high-Fowler's or sitting position to aid in breathing.
Reference: Lewis, S., et al. (2020). *Medical-surgical nursing: Assessment and management of clinical problems* (11th ed., p. 545). Elsevier.

 46. The nurse is assessing the casted extremity of a client for signs of infection. Which finding is indicative of the presence of an infection?
1. Dependent edema
2. Diminished distal pulse
3. Coolness and pallor of the skin
4. Presence of warm areas on the cast

Level of Cognitive Ability: Analyzing
Client Needs: Physiological Integrity
Clinical Judgment/Cognitive Skills: Analyze Cues
Integrated Process: Clinical Judgment; Nursing Process/Analysis
Content Area: Adult Health: Musculoskeletal
Health Problems: Adult Health: Musculoskeletal: Skeletal Injury
Priority Concepts: Infection; Mobility

Answer: 4
Rationale: Manifestations of infection under a casted area include a musty odor or purulent drainage from the cast or the presence of areas on the cast that are warmer than others. The physician needs to be notified if any of these occur. Dependent edema, diminished arterial pulse, and coolness and pallor of the skin all signify impaired circulation in the distal extremity.
Test-Taking Strategy: Focus on the **subject**, manifestations of infection under the cast. Eliminate options 1, 2, and 3 because edema, diminished distal pulse, and coolness and pallor of the skin are **comparable or alike,** and all signify impaired circulation in the distal extremity. Also thinking about the signs of infection (i.e., redness, swelling, heat, and drainage) will direct you to option 4.
Priority Nursing Tip: Teach the client and family to monitor for signs of infection under a casted area. Teach them to monitor for warm areas on the cast and to smell the area for a musty or unpleasant odor, which would indicate the presence of infected material.
Reference: Ignatavicius, D., et al. (2021). *Medical-surgical nursing: Concepts for interprofessional collaborative care* (10th ed., p. 1037). Elsevier.

47. The home care nurse assesses a client diagnosed with chronic obstructive pulmonary disease (COPD) who is reporting increased dyspnea. The client is on home oxygen via a concentrator at 2 L/min and has a respiratory rate of 22 breaths/min. Which action would the nurse take?
1. Determine the need to increase the oxygen.
2. Reassure client that there is no need to worry.
3. Conduct further assessment of client's respiratory status.
4. Call emergency services to take client to the emergency department.

Level of Cognitive Ability: Applying
Client Needs: Physiological Integrity
Clinical Judgment/Cognitive Skills: Take Action
Integrated Process: Clinical Judgment; Nursing Process/Implementation
Content Area: Adult Health: Respiratory
Health Problems: Adult Health: Respiratory: Chronic Obstructive Pulmonary Disease
Priority Concepts: Clinical Judgment; Gas Exchange

Answer: **3**
Rationale: With the client's respiratory rate at 22 breaths/min, the nurse needs to obtain further assessment. Oxygen is not increased without the approval of the physician, especially because the client with COPD can retain carbon dioxide. Reassuring the client that there is "no need to worry" is inappropriate. Calling emergency services is a premature action.
Test-Taking Strategy: Focus on the subject, the action to take for a client with COPD experiencing increased dyspnea. Eliminate option 2 first because it is an inappropriate communication technique and dismisses the client's complaint of dyspnea. Option 4 can be eliminated because calling emergency services is a premature action and there are no data to support the notion that an emergency exists. Remember that oxygen is not increased without physician approval, and there is no evidence to support that the client is exhibiting tissue hypoxia. Also, use of the steps of the nursing process will direct you to the correct option.
Priority Nursing Tip: For some clients with COPD, a low concentration of oxygen may be prescribed (1 to 2 L/min) by the physician because the stimulus to breathe is a low arterial Pao_2 instead of an increased $Paco_2$.
Reference: Ignatavicius, D., et al. (2021). *Medical-surgical nursing: Concepts for interprofessional collaborative care* (10th ed., pp. 484, 548). Elsevier.

❖ **48.** The nurse reviews the chart of a client with hypertension to note the client's vital signs. Based on these data findings, what is the client's pulse pressure? **Refer to chart. Fill in the blank.**
Answer: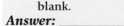

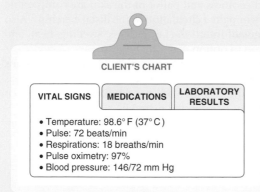

CLIENT'S CHART

| VITAL SIGNS | MEDICATIONS | LABORATORY RESULTS |

- Temperature: 98.6° F (37° C)
- Pulse: 72 beats/min
- Respirations: 18 breaths/min
- Pulse oximetry: 97%
- Blood pressure: 146/72 mm Hg

Level of Cognitive Ability: Applying
Client Needs: Physiological Integrity
Clinical Judgment/Cognitive Skills: Recognize Cues
Integrated Process: Nursing Process/Assessment
Content Area: Skills: Vital Signs
Health Problems: Adult Health: Cardiovascular: Hypertension
Priority Concepts: Clinical Judgment; Perfusion

Answer: **74**
Rationale: The difference between the systolic and diastolic blood pressure is the pulse pressure. Therefore, if the client has a blood pressure of 146/72 mm Hg, then the pulse pressure is 74.
Test-Taking Strategy: Focus on the subject, determining the pulse pressure. Recall that the pulse pressure is the difference between the systolic and diastolic blood pressure, and then use simple mathematics to subtract 72 from 146 to yield 74.
Priority Nursing Tip: The pulse pressure value is an indirect measure of cardiac output. A narrow pulse pressure is seen in clients with heart failure, hypovolemia, or shock. An increased pulse pressure is noted in clients with hypertension, increased intracranial pressure, slow heart rate, aortic regurgitation, atherosclerosis, and aging.
References: Lewis, S., et al. (2020). *Medical-surgical nursing: Assessment and management of clinical problems* (11th ed., p. 660). Elsevier; Potter, P., et al. (2021). *Fundamentals of nursing.* (10th ed., p. 484). Elsevier.

49. The home care nurse is making a follow-up visit to a client after receiving a renal transplant. Which assessment data support the possible existence of acute graft rejection? **Select all that apply.**

❑ **1.** Pale skin color
❑ **2.** Urine output of 45 mL/hr
❑ **3.** Blood pressure of 164/98 mm Hg
❑ **4.** Temperature of 102.4° F (39.1° C)
❑ **5.** Client reporting "feeling so very tired"
❑ **6.** Client reporting that graft site is tender when touched

Level of Cognitive Ability: Analyzing
Client Needs: Physiological Integrity
Clinical Judgment/Cognitive Skills: Analyze Cues
Integrated Process: Clinical Judgment; Nursing Process/Analysis
Content Area: Adult Health: Immune
Health Problems: Adult Health: Immune: Transplantation
Priority Concepts: Cellular Regulation; Immunity

Answer: 3, 4, 5, 6
Rationale: Acute rejection usually occurs within the first 3 months after transplant, although it can occur for up to 2 years after transplant. The client exhibits fever, hypertension, malaise, and graft tenderness. Treatment is immediately begun with corticosteroids and possibly also with monoclonal antibodies and antilymphocyte agents. None of the other options present symptomology associated with acute graft rejection.
Test-Taking Strategy: Focus on the subject, the manifestations of acute graft rejection. Think about the pathophysiology that occurs with acute graft rejection. Eliminate option 1 because pale skin color is related to low hemoglobin and hematocrit status or vascular status rather than acute rejection. Option 2 can be eliminated because an output of 45 mL/hr is adequate (output should be at least 30 mL/hr).
Priority Nursing Tip: The priority focus of care for the renal transplant recipient is the prevention and early recognition of graft rejection. Goals of care include preventing infection and rejection, maintaining hydration, promoting diuresis, and avoiding fluid overload.
Reference: Ignatavicius, D., et al. (2021). *Medical-surgical nursing: Concepts for interprofessional collaborative care* (10th ed., p. 1407). Elsevier.

❖ **50.** The nurse is caring for a client who is receiving tobramycin sulfate intravenously every 8 hours for a lower urinary tract infection. Which laboratory result would indicate to the nurse that the client is experiencing an adverse effect of the medication?

Laboratory Results

Test and Result	Reference Range
Total bilirubin 0.5 mg/dL (8.5 mcmol/L)	0.3–1.0 mg/dL (5.1–17 mcmol/L)
ESR 15 mm/hr (15 mm/hr)	≤15–20 mm/hr (≤15–20 mm/hr)
BUN 30 mg/dL (10.8 mmol/L)	10–20 mg/dL (3.6–7.1 mmol/L)
WBC count 6000/mm³ (6 × 10⁹/L)	5000–10,000/mm³ (5–10 × 10⁹/L

1. Total bilirubin
2. ESR level
3. BUN level
4. WBC count

Level of Cognitive Ability: Analyzing
Client Needs: Physiological Integrity
Clinical Judgment/Cognitive Skills: Analyze Cues
Integrated Process: Clinical Judgment; Nursing Process/Analysis
Content Area: Pharmacology: Immune: Aminoglycosides
Health Problems: Adult Health: Renal and Urinary: Urinary Tract Inflammation/Infection/Trauma
Priority Concepts: Clinical Judgment; Safety

Answer: 3
Rationale: Tobramycin sulfate is an aminoglycoside antibiotic. Adverse effects or toxic effects of tobramycin sulfate include nephrotoxicity, as evidenced by an increased BUN and serum creatinine; irreversible ototoxicity as evidenced by tinnitus, dizziness, ringing, or roaring in the ears, and reduced hearing; and neurotoxicity as evidenced by headaches, dizziness, lethargy, tremors, and visual disturbances.
Test-Taking Strategy: Focus on the subject, an adverse effect of tobramycin sulfate. Think about these adverse effects and review the laboratory results to assist in directing you to the correct option, which is the only abnormal laboratory value presented in the laboratory results table.
Priority Nursing Tip: Aminoglycoside antibiotics are potentially nephrotoxic substances.
References: Gahart, B., Nazareno, A., & Ortega, M. (2021). *Gahart's 2021 Intravenous medications: A handbook for nurses and health professionals* (37th ed., pp. 1287, 1289). Elsevier; Pagana, K., Pagana, T., & Pagana, T. N. (2021). *Mosby's Diagnostic and laboratory test reference* (15th ed., p. 157). Elsevier.

51. A client's telemetry monitor displays ventricular tachycardia. Upon reaching the client's bedside, which action would the nurse take **first**?
1. Call a code.
2. Prepare for cardioversion.
3. Prepare to defibrillate the client.
4. Check the client's level of consciousness.

Level of Cognitive Ability: Applying
Client Needs: Physiological Integrity
Clinical Judgment/Cognitive Skills: Take Action
Integrated Process: Nursing Process/Implementation
Content Area: Complex Care: Emergency Situations/Management
Health Problems: Adult Health: Cardiovascular: Dysrhythmias
Priority Concepts: Clinical Judgment; Perfusion

Answer: 4
Rationale: Determining unresponsiveness is the first assessment action to take. When a client is in ventricular tachycardia, there is a significant decrease in cardiac output. However, assessing for unresponsiveness helps determine whether the client is affected by the decreased cardiac output. If the client is unconscious, then cardiopulmonary resuscitation is initiated.
Test-Taking Strategy: Note the strategic word, *first*. Use the steps of the nursing process, remembering that assessment is the first action.
Priority Nursing Tip: For the client with stable ventricular tachycardia (with a pulse and no signs or symptoms of decreased cardiac output), oxygen and antidysrhythmics may be prescribed.
Reference: Ignatavicius, D., et al. (2021). *Medical-surgical nursing: Concepts for interprofessional collaborative care* (10th ed., pp. 657–658). Elsevier.

❖ **52.** Which nursing assessment question would be asked to help determine the client's risk for developing malignant hyperthermia in the perioperative period?
1. "Have you ever had heat exhaustion or heat stroke?"
2. "What is the normal range for your body temperature?"
3. "Do you or any of your family members have frequent infections?"
4. "Do you or any of your family members have problems with general anesthesia?"

Level of Cognitive Ability: Applying
Client Needs: Physiological Integrity
Clinical Judgment/Cognitive Skills: Recognize Cues
Integrated Process: Clinical Judgment; Nursing Process/Assessment
Content Area: Skills: Perioperative Care
Health Problems: Adult Health: Neurologic: Thermoregulation
Priority Concepts: Clinical Judgment; Thermoregulation

Answer: 4
Rationale: Malignant hyperthermia is a dominantly inherited disorder in which a combination of anesthetic agents (the muscle relaxant succinylcholine and inhalation agents such as halothanes) triggers uncontrolled skeletal muscle contractions that can quickly lead to a potentially fatal hyperthermia. Questioning the client about the family history of general anesthesia problems may reveal this as a risk for the client. Options 1, 2, and 3 are unrelated to this surgical complication.
Test-Taking Strategy: Focus on the subject, malignant hyperthermia. Think about the pathophysiology associated with this disorder. Recalling that this disorder is inherited will direct you to the correct option.
Priority Nursing Tip: Early indicators of malignant hyperthermia include masseter muscle contractions and tachycardia. An elevated temperature is a late sign.
Reference: Ignatavicius, D., et al. (2021). *Medical-surgical nursing: Concepts for interprofessional collaborative care* (10th ed., pp. 155–156). Elsevier.

53. A client has developed oral mucositis as a result of radiation to the head and neck. Which measure would the nurse teach the client to incorporate in a daily home care routine to help manage this condition?

1. A glass of wine per day will introduce useful bacteria to the oral cavity.
2. High-protein foods such as peanut butter needs to be incorporated in the diet.
3. Clean teeth and rinse mouth with a weak saline and water solution before and after each meal.
4. Oral hygiene, including brushing and flossing, needs to be performed in the morning and evening.

Level of Cognitive Ability: Applying
Client Needs: Physiological Integrity
Clinical Judgment/Cognitive Skills: Generate Solutions
Integrated Process: Teaching and Learning
Content Area: Adult Health: Oncology
Health Problems: Adult Health: Integumentary: Inflammations/Infections
Priority Concepts: Patient Education; Inflammation

Answer: 3
Rationale: Oral mucositis (irritation, inflammation, and/or ulceration of the mucosa), also known as stomatitis, commonly occurs in clients receiving radiation to the head and neck. Measures need to be taken to soothe the mucosa and provide effective cleansing of the oral cavity. A combination of a weak saline and water solution is an effective cleansing agent. Oral hygiene needs to be performed more frequently than in the morning and evening. Alcohol would dry and irritate the mucosa and not affect the oral bacteria. Peanut butter has a thick consistency and will stick to the irritated mucosa.
Test-Taking Strategy: Focus on the subject, oral mucositis. Knowing the definition of mucositis will help you eliminate the incorrect options. First, eliminate option 1, knowing that alcohol will have a further drying and irritating effect on the mucosa. Next, eliminate option 2, knowing that although high-protein foods are necessary, peanut butter would not be a good choice because of its consistency. From the remaining options, choose option 3 over option 4 because of the frequency noted in option 4.
Priority Nursing Tip: Special "swish and spit" mixtures are available to treat mucositis (stomatitis), and many contain a local anesthetic combined with anti-inflammatory agents. The client needs to be taught not to swallow these mixtures.
Reference: Lewis, S., et al. (2020). *Medical-surgical nursing: Assessment and management of clinical problems* (11th ed., pp. 250, 893). Elsevier.

 54. A client who is being treated for acute heart failure has the following vital signs: blood pressure (BP), 85/50 mm Hg; pulse, 96 beats/min; respirations, 26 breaths/min. The physician prescribes digoxin. To evaluate a therapeutic response to this medication, which changes in the client's vital signs would the nurse expect?

1. BP 85/50 mm Hg, pulse 60 beats/min, respirations 26 breaths/min
2. BP 98/60 mm Hg, pulse 80 beats/min, respirations 24 breaths/min
3. BP 130/70 mm Hg, pulse 104 beats/min, respirations 20 breaths/min
4. BP 110/40 mm Hg, pulse 110 beats/min, respirations 20 breaths/min

Level of Cognitive Ability: Evaluating
Client Needs: Physiological Integrity
Clinical Judgment/Cognitive Skills: Evaluate Outcomes
Integrated Process: Clinical Judgment; Nursing Process/Evaluation
Content Area: Pharmacology: Cardiovascular: Cardiac Glycosides
Health Problems: Adult Health: Cardiovascular: Heart Failure
Priority Concepts: Perfusion; Safety

Answer: 2
Rationale: The main function of digoxin is inotropic. It produces increased myocardial contractility that is associated with an increased cardiac output. This causes a rise in the BP in a client with heart failure. Digoxin also has a negative chronotropic effect (decreases heart rate) and will therefore cause a slowing of the heart rate. As cardiac output improves, there should be an improvement in respirations as well. Options 1, 3, and 4 do not reflect the physiologic changes attributed to this medication.
Test-Taking Strategy: Focus on the subject, the physiologic changes that occur with digoxin administration. Recalling that digoxin slows the heart rate will assist in eliminating options 3 and 4, which show an increase in the heart rate. Next recalling that digoxin improves cardiac output will assist in eliminating option 1, which does not show improvement in blood pressure.
Priority Nursing Tip: The nurse needs to monitor the client taking digoxin for digoxin toxicity. A normal serum digoxin level is 0.5 to 2.0 ng/mL (0.64 to 2.56 nmol/L).
References: Ignatavicius, D., et al. (2021). *Medical-surgical nursing: Concepts for interprofessional collaborative care* (10th ed., pp. 650, 675). Elsevier; Potter, P., et al. (2021). *Fundamentals of nursing* (10th ed., p. 468). Elsevier.

55. A client diagnosed with hypertension has been taking a prescribed calcium channel blocker for approximately 2 months. The home care nurse monitoring the effects of therapy would determine that drug tolerance has developed if which is noted in the client?
1. Decrease in weight
2. Increased joint pain
3. Output greater than intake
4. Gradual rise in blood pressure

Level of Cognitive Ability: Analyzing
Client Needs: Physiological Integrity
Clinical Judgment/Cognitive Skills: Recognize Cues
Integrated Process: Clinical Judgment; Nursing Process/Assessment
Content Area: Pharmacology: Cardiovascular: Calcium Channel Blockers
Health Problems: Adult Health: Cardiovascular: Hypertension
Priority Concepts: Perfusion; Clinical Judgment

Answer: 4
Rationale: Drug tolerance can develop in a client taking an antihypertensive such as a calcium channel blocker, which is evident by rising blood pressure levels. The physician needs to be notified, who may then increase the medication dosage, change medication, or add a diuretic to the medication regimen. The client is also at risk of developing fluid retention, which would be manifested as dependent edema, intake greater than output, and an increase in weight. This would also warrant adding a diuretic to the course of therapy. Joint pain is not associated with this form of tolerance.
Test-Taking Strategy: Focus on the subject, drug tolerance with antihypertensives such as calcium channel blockers. Recall the definition of drug tolerance; that is, as one adjusts to a medication, the therapeutic effect diminishes. These concepts will direct you to the correct option.
Priority Nursing Tip: Hypertension is a major risk factor for coronary, cerebral, renal, and peripheral vascular disease.
Reference: Lewis, S., et al. (2020). *Medical-surgical nursing: Assessment and management of clinical problems* (11th ed., p. 687). Elsevier.

❖ **56.** A client with a known history of panic disorder comes to the emergency department and states to the nurse, "Please help me. I think I'm having a heart attack." What is the **priority** nursing action?
1. Assess the client's vital signs.
2. Encourage the client to use relaxation techniques.
3. Identify the manifestations related to the panic disorder.
4. Determine what the client's activity involved when the pain started.

Level of Cognitive Ability: Analyzing
Client Needs: Physiological Integrity
Clinical Judgment/Cognitive Skills: Take Action
Integrated Process: Clinical Judgment; Nursing Process/Implementation
Content Area: Mental Health
Health Problems: Mental Health: Anxiety Disorder
Priority Concepts: Anxiety; Clinical Judgment

Answer: 1
Rationale: Clients with a panic disorder can experience acute physical symptoms, such as chest pain and palpitations. The priority is to assess the client's physical condition to rule out a physiologic disorder for these signs and symptoms. Although options 2, 3, and 4 may be appropriate at some point in the care of the client, they are not the priority.
Test-Taking Strategy: Note the strategic word, *priority*. Focus on Maslow's Hierarchy of Needs theory, recalling that physiologic needs are the priority. Also, use of the ABCs—airway, breathing, and circulation—as well as the steps of the nursing process—will direct you to the correct option.
Priority Nursing Tip: A client complaint of chest pain is always a priority. Immediate assessment and treatment is needed.
References: Potter, P., et al. (2021). *Fundamentals of nursing* (10th ed., p. 468). Elsevier; Varcarolis, E., & Fosbre, C. (2021). *Essentials of psychiatric mental health nursing: A communication approach to evidence-based care* (4th ed., p. 142). Elsevier.

57. A client experiencing trigeminal neuralgia (tic douloureux) asks the nurse for a snack and something to drink. Which is the **best** selection the nurse would provide for the client?
1. Hot cocoa with honey and toast
2. Vanilla pudding and lukewarm milk
3. Hot herbal tea with graham crackers
4. Iced coffee and peanut butter and crackers

Level of Cognitive Ability: Applying
Client Needs: Physiological Integrity
Clinical Judgment/Cognitive Skills: Generate Solutions
Integrated Process: Nursing Process/Implementation
Content Area: Adult Health: Neurologic
Health Problems: Adult Health: Neurologic: Trigeminal Neuralgia
Priority Concepts: Clinical Judgment; Pain

Answer: 2
Rationale: Because mild tactile stimulation of the face of clients with trigeminal neuralgia can trigger pain, the client needs to eat or drink lukewarm, nutritious foods that are soft and easy to chew. Extremes of temperature will cause trigeminal pain.
Test-Taking Strategy: Focus on the strategic word, *best*. Note that options 1, 3, and 4 are comparable or alike because these options contain hot or iced items and foods that are mechanically difficult to chew and swallow.
Priority Nursing Tip: Monitor the nutritional status of the client with trigeminal neuralgia closely. Because of the facial pain associated with the disorder, the client may not eat enough to meet their daily nutritional needs.
Reference: Lewis, S., et al. (2020). *Medical-surgical nursing: Assessment and management of clinical problems* (11th ed., pp. 1422–1423). Elsevier.

❖ **58.** An adolescent is admitted to the orthopedic nursing unit after spinal rod insertion for the treatment of scoliosis. Which assessments are **most important** in the immediate postoperative period when considering the client's neurovascular status? **Select all that apply.**
- ❏ 1. Pain level
- ❏ 2. Urinary output
- ❏ 3. Ability to move all extremities
- ❏ 4. Capillary refill in all extremities
- ❏ 5. Ability to flex and extend the feet
- ❏ 6. Ability to detect sensations in all extremities

Level of Cognitive Ability: Analyzing
Client Needs: Physiological Integrity
Clinical Judgment/Cognitive Skills: Take Action
Integrated Process: Clinical Judgment; Nursing Process/Assessment
Content Area: Pediatrics: Neurologic
Health Problems: Pediatric-Specific: Scoliosis
Priority Concepts: Mobility; Perfusion

Answer: 3, 4, 5, 6
Rationale: When the spinal column is manipulated during surgery, altered neurovascular status is a possible complication; therefore, neurovascular checks, including circulation, sensation, and motion, needs to be done at least every 2 hours. Level of pain and urinary output are important postoperative assessments, but are not specific to neurovascular status.
Test-Taking Strategy: Note the strategic words, *most important.* Focus on the subject, neurovascular status. Note that the correct options relate to the client's extremities and address circulatory status.
Priority Nursing Tip: Contact the physician immediately if signs of neurovascular impairment are noted in a postoperative client or a client with a cast, traction, or brace.
Reference: McKinney, E. S., et al. (2022). *Maternal child nursing* (6th ed., pp. 1221, 1231, 1234). Elsevier.

59. The nurse has just finished assisting the physician in placing a central intravenous (IV) line in a client with gastric cancer. Which is a **priority** intervention to ensure the client's safety?
1. Assessing the client's pain level
2. Assessing the client's temperature
3. Preparing the client for a chest x-ray
4. Monitoring the client's blood pressure (BP)

Level of Cognitive Ability: Analyzing
Client Needs: Physiological Integrity
Clinical Judgment/Cognitive Skills: Take Action
Integrated Process: Clinical Judgment; Nursing Process/Implementation
Content Area: Complex Care: Invasive Devices
Health Problems: Adult Health: Cancer: Esophageal/Gastric/Intestinal
Priority Concepts: Clinical Judgment; Safety

Answer: 3
Rationale: A major risk associated with central line placement is the possibility of a pneumothorax developing from an accidental puncture of the lung. Assessing the results of a chest radiograph is one of the best methods to determine if this complication has occurred and verify catheter tip placement before initiating IV therapy. A temperature elevation related to central line insertion would not likely occur immediately after placement. Pain management is important but is not the priority at this point. Although BP assessment is always important in assessing a client's status after an invasive procedure, fluid volume overload is not a concern until IV fluids are started.
Test-Taking Strategy: Note the strategic word, *priority.* Think about the complications associated with central IV line placement. Recall that assessment of accurate placement is essential before initiating IV therapy.
Priority Nursing Tip: A chest x-ray is needed to ensure that the tip of a newly inserted central IV catheter resides in the superior vena cava. IV solutions would not be infused into the catheter until this is verified.
Reference: Ignatavicius, D., et al. (2021). *Medical-surgical nursing: Concepts for interprofessional collaborative care* (10th ed., p. 281). Elsevier.

❖ **60.** A child sustains a greenstick fracture of the humerus from a fall out of a tree house. The nurse describes this type of fracture to the parents and would provide them with which picture? **Refer to figure.**

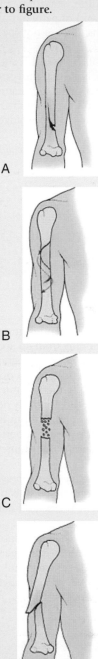

A

B

C

D

(In part from Ignatavicius, D., Workman, M. L., & Rebar, C. R. [2018]. *Medical-surgical nursing concepts for interprofessional collaborative care* [9th ed.]. Saunders.)

☐ 1. A
☐ 2. B
☐ 3. C
☐ 4. D

Level of Cognitive Ability: Applying
Client Needs: Physiological Integrity
Clinical Judgment/Cognitive Skills: Take Action
Integrated Process: Teaching and Learning
Content Area: Pediatrics: Musculoskeletal
Health Problems: Pediatric-Specific: Fractures
Priority Concepts: Patient Education; Mobility

Answer: 1
Rationale: A greenstick fracture is a break that occurs through the periosteum on one side of the bone with only bowing or buckling on the other side. A spiral fracture (option 2) is characterized by a twisted or circular break that affects the length rather than the width. In a comminuted fracture (option 3), the bone is splintered into pieces. In an open (compound) fracture (option 4), the skin surface over the fracture is disrupted causing an external wound.

Test-Taking Strategy: Focus on the subject, greenstick fracture. Recalling that the definition of a greenstick fracture is a break that occurs through the periosteum on one side of the bone, and use of the process of elimination will assist in directing you to the correct option.

Priority Nursing Tip: The nurse would closely monitor the affected extremity of a client who sustained a fracture. Of particular importance are color, sensation, and motion of the affected limb. Compartment syndrome, which occurs when pressure builds within the muscle causing decreased blood flow and oxygen delivery, is a common complication associated with breaks and fractures.

Reference: McKinney, E. S., et al. (2022). *Maternal child nursing* (6th ed., p. 1227). Elsevier.

Client Needs

61. A 2-year-old toddler has just returned from surgery where a hip spica cast was applied. Which nursing action will **best** maintain the child's skin integrity?
1. Changing the toddler's diapers every 2 hours
2. Keeping the toddler's genital area open to the air
3. Implementing a 3-hour turning schedule for the toddler
4. Assessing the toddler's perineal area for redness regularly

Level of Cognitive Ability: Applying
Client Needs: Physiological Integrity
Clinical Judgment/Cognitive Skills: Take Action
Integrated Process: Nursing Process/Implementation
Content Area: Pediatrics: Integumentary
Health Problems: Pediatric-Specific: Developmental Dysplasia of Hip
Priority Concepts: Safety; Tissue Integrity

Answer: 1
Rationale: The spica cast is often needed to treat developmental hip dysplasia (DDH) or after hip/pelvis surgery. The cast encases the child's trunk and one or both legs while leaving access to the genital area. Considering the age of the child, diapers will be in use and will need to be changed at least every 2 hours during the day and 3 to 4 hours during the night to help minimize the effect of urine and feces on the child's diaper area. Exposing the genital and perineal area to the air is an intervention that is implemented to assist in healing damaged skin tissue. Turning the child regularly is appropriate care but has no impact on the major issue of incontinence. Assessment of the skin is necessary but identifies skin breakdown once it has begun.
Test-Taking Strategy: Focus on the subject, maintaining skin integrity for the client in a hip spica cast. Note the strategic word, *best*. Eliminate option 4 that is an intervention that is directed toward addressing skin breakdown once it occurs. Next eliminate options 2 and 3 because they are not the best interventions to maintain skin integrity.
Priority Nursing Tip: If a hip spica cast is placed, the cast edges around the perineum and buttocks may need to be taped with waterproof tape to prevent the cast from becoming wet or soiled during elimination.
Reference: McKinney, E. S., et al. (2022). *Maternal child nursing* (6th ed., p. 1240). Elsevier.

62. The nurse uses the Glasgow Coma Scale while assessing a client with a brainstem injury. Which additional interventions would the nurse be prepared to implement? **Select all that apply.**
1. Assisting with arterial blood gases
2. Assisting with a lumbar puncture
3. Assessing cranial nerve functioning
4. Assessing respiratory rate and rhythm
5. Assessing pulmonary wedge pressure
6. Assessing cognitive abilities, including memory

Level of Cognitive Ability: Applying
Client Needs: Physiological Integrity
Clinical Judgment/Cognitive Skills: Take Action
Integrated Process: Nursing Process/Implementation
Content Area: Adult Health: Neurologic
Health Problems: Adult Health: Neurologic: Head Injury/Trauma
Priority Concepts: Clinical Judgment; Intracranial Regulation

Answer: 3, 4
Rationale: Assessment needs to be specific to the area of the brain involved. Assessing the respiratory status and cranial nerve function is a critical component of the assessment process in a client with a brainstem injury because the respiratory center is located in the brainstem. Options 1, 2, 5, and 6 are not necessary based on the data in the question.
Test-Taking Strategy: Noting that the client sustained a cranial injury will assist in selecting option 3. Next, focus on the ABCs—airway, breathing, and circulation. Recall the anatomic location of the respiratory center to direct you to option 4. Remember that the respiratory center is located in the brainstem.
Priority Nursing Tip: For a client with a head injury, priority is given to maintaining a patent airway, breathing, and circulation.
Reference: Ignatavicius, D., et al. (2021). *Medical-surgical nursing: Concepts for interprofessional collaborative care* (10th ed., pp. 835, 879). Elsevier.

63. A client with a bowel obstruction has had a nasointestinal (NI) tube in place for 24 hours. Which assessment finding indicates that the tube is properly located in the intestine?
1. Bowel sounds are absent.
2. Client denies being nauseous.
3. Aspirate from the tube has a pH of 7.
4. The abdominal x-ray indicates that the end of the tube is above the pylorus.

Level of Cognitive Ability: Analyzing
Client Needs: Physiological Integrity
Clinical Judgment/Cognitive Skills: Recognize Cues
Integrated Process: Clinical Judgment; Nursing Process/Assessment
Content Area: Skills: Tube Care
Health Problems: Adult Health: Gastrointestinal: Bowel Obstruction
Priority Concepts: Clinical Judgment; Safety

Answer: 3
Rationale: The NI tube is used to decompress the intestine and correct a bowel obstruction. Nausea should subside as decompression is accomplished, but this does not indicate proper tube placement. The pH of the gastric fluid is acidic, and the pH of the intestinal fluid is alkaline (7 or higher). Although bowel sounds will be abnormal in the presence of obstruction, the presence or absence of bowel sounds is not associated with the location of the tube. The end of the tube needs to be located in the intestine (below the pylorus). Location of the tube can also be determined by radiographs.
Test-Taking Strategy: Focus on the subject, an NI tube and determining its intestinal location. Recalling that intestinal fluid is alkaline will direct you to the correct option.
Priority Nursing Tip: The client who has had an intestinal tube inserted needs to be positioned on the right side to facilitate passage of the weighted bag in the tube through the pylorus of the stomach and into the small intestine.
Reference: Potter, P., et al. (2021). *Fundamentals of nursing* (10th ed., p. 1226). Elsevier.

64. A client diagnosed with myxedema reports having experienced a lack of energy, cold intolerance, and puffiness around the eyes and face. The nurse plans care knowing that these clinical manifestations are caused by a lack of production of which hormones? **Select all that apply.**
☐ 1. Thyroxine (T_4)
☐ 2. Prolactin (PRL)
☐ 3. Triiodothyronine (T_3)
☐ 4. Growth hormone (GH)
☐ 5. Luteinizing hormone (LH)
☐ 6. Adrenocorticotropic hormone (ACTH)

Level of Cognitive Ability: Applying
Client Needs: Physiological Integrity
Clinical Judgment/Cognitive Skills: Generate Solutions
Integrated Process: Clinical Judgment; Nursing Process/Planning
Content Area: Adult Health: Endocrine
Health Problems: Adult Health: Endocrine: Thyroid Disorders
Priority Concepts: Hormonal Regulation; Clinical Judgment

Answer: 1, 3
Rationale: Although all of these hormones originate from the anterior pituitary, only T_3 and T_4 are associated with the client's symptoms. Myxedema results from inadequate thyroid hormone levels (T_3 and T_4). Low levels of thyroid hormone result in an overall decrease in the basal metabolic rate, affecting virtually every body system and leading to weakness, fatigue, and a decrease in heat production. A decrease in LH results in the loss of secondary sex characteristics. A decrease in ACTH is seen in Addison's disease. PRL stimulates breast milk production by the mammary glands, and GH affects bone and soft tissue by promoting growth through protein anabolism and lipolysis.
Test-Taking Strategy: Focus on the subject, myxedema. Recalling that myxedema is associated with the thyroid gland (hypothyroidism) will assist in connecting the subject of the question and the client's symptoms to the correct options.
Priority Nursing Tip: Myxedema is a rare but serious disorder that results from severe or prolonged thyroid deficiency.
Reference: Ignatavicius, D., et al. (2021). *Medical-surgical nursing: Concepts for interprofessional collaborative care* (10th ed., pp. 1250, 1252–1253). Elsevier.

65. A client is admitted to the hospital with a suspected diagnosis of Graves' disease. On assessment, which manifestation related to the client's menstrual cycle would the nurse expect the client to report?
1. Amenorrhea
2. Menorrhagia
3. Metrorrhagia
4. Dysmenorrhea

Level of Cognitive Ability: Applying
Client Needs: Physiological Integrity
Clinical Judgment/Cognitive Skills: Recognize Cues
Integrated Process: Nursing Process/Assessment
Content Area: Adult Health: Endocrine
Health Problems: Adult Health: Endocrine: Thyroid Disorders
Priority Concepts: Hormonal Regulation; Clinical Judgment

Answer: 1
Rationale: Amenorrhea or a decreased menstrual flow is common in the client with Graves' disease. Menorrhagia, metrorrhagia, and dysmenorrhea are also disorders related to the reproductive system; however, they do not manifest in the presence of Graves' disease. Menorrhagia refers to menstrual periods with abnormally heavy or prolonged bleeding. Metrorrhagia refers to uterine bleeding at irregular intervals, particularly between the expected menstrual periods. Dysmenorrhea refers to pain during menstrual periods.
Test-Taking Strategy: Focus on the subject, Graves' disease. Thinking about the pathophysiology associated with Graves' disease will direct you to the correct option.
Priority Nursing Tip: Graves' disease is also known as toxic diffuse goiter and results in a hyperthyroid state from the hypersecretion of thyroid hormones.
Reference: Ignatavicius, D., et al. (2021). *Medical-surgical nursing: Concepts for interprofessional collaborative care* (10th ed., p. 1255). Elsevier.

66. A client diagnosed with gestational hypertension has just been admitted and is in early active labor. Which assessment finding would the nurse **most likely** expect to note?
1. Increased urine output
2. Increased blood pressure
3. Decreased fetal heart rate
4. Decreased brachial reflexes

Level of Cognitive Ability: Analyzing
Client Needs: Physiological Integrity
Clinical Judgment/Cognitive Skills: Recognize Cues
Integrated Process: Clinical Judgment; Nursing Process/Assessment
Content Area: Maternity: Intrapartum
Health Problems: Maternity: Gestational Hypertension/Preeclampsia and Eclampsia
Priority Concepts: Perfusion; Reproduction

Answer: 2
Rationale: The major manifestation of gestational hypertension is increased blood pressure. As the condition progresses, it is possible that increased brachial reflexes, decreased fetal heart rate and variability, and decreased urine output will occur, particularly during labor.
Test-Taking Strategy: Note the strategic words, *most likely*, and focus on the subject of gestational hypertension. Noting the name of the disorder will easily direct you to the correct option.
Priority Nursing Tip: Gestational hypertension can lead to preeclampsia. Manifestations of preeclampsia are hypertension and proteinuria.
Reference: McKinney, E. S., et al. (2022). *Maternal child nursing* (6th ed., pp. 541–542.) Elsevier.

67. The nurse has just administered a purified protein derivative (PPD) tuberculin skin test (Mantoux test) to a client who is at low risk for developing tuberculosis. The nurse determines that the test is positive if which occurs?
1. An induration of 15 mm
2. The presence of a wheal
3. A large area of erythema
4. Itching at the injection site

Level of Cognitive Ability: Analyzing
Client Needs: Physiological Integrity
Clinical Judgment/Cognitive Skills: Recognize Cues
Integrated Process: Clinical Judgment; Nursing Process/Assessment
Content Area: Foundations of Care: Diagnostic Tests
Health Problems: Adult Health: Respiratory: Tuberculosis
Priority Concepts: Clinical Judgment; Infection

Answer: 1
Rationale: An induration of 10 mm or more is considered positive for clients in low-risk groups. The presence of a wheal would indicate that the skin test was administered appropriately. Erythema or itching at the site is not indicative of a positive reaction.
Test-Taking Strategy: Focus on the subject, a positive Mantoux test, and note that the client is at low risk for developing tuberculosis. This will direct you to the correct option.
Priority Nursing Tip: A positive Mantoux test does not mean that active tuberculosis is present, but rather indicates previous exposure to tuberculosis or the presence of inactive (dormant) disease.
Reference: Ignatavicius, D., et al. (2021). *Medical-surgical nursing: Concepts for interprofessional collaborative care* (10th ed., p. 577). Elsevier.

❖ **68.** The nurse is performing an otoscopic examination on a client with a suspected diagnosis of mastoiditis. Which finding would the nurse expect to note if this disorder was present?
1. A dull red tympanic membrane
2. A mobile tympanic membrane
3. A transparent tympanic membrane
4. A pearly colored tympanic membrane

Level of Cognitive Ability: Analyzing
Client Needs: Physiological Integrity
Clinical Judgment/Cognitive Skills: Recognize Cues
Integrated Process: Clinical Judgment; Nursing Process/Assessment
Content Area: Adult Health: Ear
Health Problems: Adult Health: Ear: Inflammation/Infections/Structural Problems
Priority Concepts: Infection; Sensory Perception

Answer: 1
Rationale: Mastoiditis is an infection of the mastoid air cells surrounding the middle and inner ear. Otoscopic examination of a client with mastoiditis reveals a red, dull, thick, and immobile tympanic membrane with or without perforation. Options 2, 3, and 4 indicate normal findings in an otoscopic examination.
Test-Taking Strategy: Focus on the subject, manifestations of mastoiditis. Recall knowledge of normal assessment findings on an ear examination to direct you to the correct option, the only abnormal finding.
Priority Nursing Tip: Mastoiditis may be acute or chronic and results from untreated or inadequately treated chronic or acute otitis media. Interventions focus on stopping the infection before it spreads to other structures.
Reference: Ignatavicius, D., et al. (2021). *Medical-surgical nursing: Concepts for interprofessional collaborative care* (10th ed., p. 967). Elsevier.

69. The nurse is reviewing the record of a client with a disorder involving the inner ear. Which finding would the nurse **most likely** note as an assessment finding in this client?
1. Tinnitus
2. Burning in the ear
3. Itching in the affected ear
4. Severe pain in the affected ear

Level of Cognitive Ability: Applying
Client Needs: Physiological Integrity
Clinical Judgment/Cognitive Skills: Recognize Cues
Integrated Process: Nursing Process/Assessment
Content Area: Adult Health: Ear
Health Problems: Adult Health: Ear: Inflammatory/Infections/Structural Problems
Priority Concepts: Inflammation; Sensory Perception

Answer: 1
Rationale: Tinnitus is the most common complaint of clients with ear disorders, especially disorders involving the inner ear. Manifestations of tinnitus can range from mild ringing in the ear that can go unnoticed during the day to a loud roaring in the ear that can interfere with the client's thinking process and attention span. The assessment findings noted in options 2, 3, and 4 are not specifically noted in the client with an inner ear disorder.
Test-Taking Strategy: Note the strategic words, *most likely.* Focus on the subject, inner ear disorder. Recalling the function of the inner ear will direct you to the correct option.
Priority Nursing Tip: The inner ear contains the semicircular canals, cochlea, and the distal end of the eight cranial nerves, and maintains a sense of balance or equilibrium.
Reference: Ignatavicius, D., et al. (2021). *Medical-surgical nursing: Concepts for interprofessional collaborative care* (10th ed., pp. 958, 967–968). Elsevier.

70. The nurse has a prescription to administer hydroxyzine in conjunction with an opioid analgesic for severe pain to a client by the intramuscular route. Before administering the medication, what information would the nurse share with the client?
1. Excessive salivation is a side effect.
2. There will be some pain at the injection site.
3. There should be relief from nausea within 5 minutes.
4. Client may experience increased agitation for about 2 hours.

Level of Cognitive Ability: Applying
Client Needs: Physiological Integrity
Clinical Judgment/Cognitive Skills: Take Action
Integrated Process: Nursing Process/Implementation
Content Area: Pharmacology: Pain Medications: Opioid Analgesics
Health Problems: Adult Health: Neurologic: Pain
Priority Concepts: Pain; Clinical Judgment

Answer: 2
Rationale: Hydroxyzine is an antiemetic and sedative/hypnotic that may be used in conjunction with opioid analgesics for added effect. The injection can be painful. Hydroxyzine causes dry mouth and drowsiness as side effects. Agitation is not a usual side effect. Medications administered by the intramuscular route generally take 20 to 30 minutes to become effective.
Test-Taking Strategy: Focus on the subject, intramuscular injection of hydroxyzine. Read each option carefully. Recall that the medication is an antiemetic and sedative/hypnotic. Eliminate options 1 and 4 first because they are the least likely effects. From the remaining options, noting that the medication is administered by the intramuscular route will direct you to the correct option.
Priority Nursing Tip: In an adult, a maximum of 3 mL of solution should be administered by the intramuscular route. Larger volumes are difficult for the injection site to absorb and, if prescribed, need to be verified.
Reference: Kizior, R., & Hodgson, B. (2022). *Saunders Nursing drug handbook 2022* (p. 588). Elsevier.

71. The nurse reviews the results of a blood glucose test done on a client with a diagnosis of diabetes mellitus. Based on the result, the nurse interprets that this client is at risk of developing which type of acid–base imbalance?

Laboratory Results

Test and Result	Reference Range
Blood glucose 644 mg/dL (35.8 mmol/L)	70–99 mg/dL (3.9–5.5 mmol/L)—fasting

1. Metabolic acidosis
2. Metabolic alkalosis
3. Respiratory acidosis
4. Respiratory alkalosis

Level of Cognitive Ability: Analyzing
Client Needs: Physiological Integrity
Clinical Judgment/Cognitive Skills: Analyze Cues
Integrated Process: Clinical Judgment; Nursing Process/Analysis
Content Area: Adult Health: Endocrine
Health Problems: Adult Health: Endocrine: Diabetes Mellitus
Priority Concepts: Acid–Base Balance; Glucose Regulation

Answer: 1
Rationale: Diabetes mellitus can lead to metabolic acidosis. When the body does not have sufficient circulating insulin, the blood glucose level rises. At the same time, the cells of the body use all available glucose. The body then breaks down glycogen and fat for fuel. The by-products of fat metabolism are acidotic and can lead to the condition known as diabetic ketoacidosis. Options 2, 3, and 4 are incorrect.
Test-Taking Strategy: Focus on the subject, diabetes mellitus. Noting the client's diagnosis will assist in eliminating options 3 and 4. From the remaining options, remember that the client with diabetes mellitus is at risk for developing acidosis.
Priority Nursing Tip: In metabolic acidosis, to compensate for the acidosis, hyperpnea with Kussmaul's respiration occurs as the lungs attempt to exhale excess carbon dioxide (CO_2), an acidotic by-product of respiration.
Reference: Ignatavicius, D., et al. (2021). *Medical-surgical nursing: Concepts for interprofessional collaborative care* (10th ed., pp. 267–268, 1268). Elsevier.

❖ **72.** The nurse reviews the most recent blood gas results of a client diagnosed with asthma. Based on these results, the nurse determines that which acid–base imbalance is present?

Laboratory Results

Test and Result	Reference Range
pH 7.43	7.35–7.45
Po_2 84 mmHg	80–100 mm Hg
Pco_2 31 mm Hg	35–45 mm Hg
HCO_3 21 mEq/L (21 mmol/L)	21–28 mEq/L (21–28 mmol/L)

1. Compensated metabolic acidosis
2. Compensated respiratory alkalosis
3. Uncompensated respiratory acidosis
4. Uncompensated metabolic alkalosis

Level of Cognitive Ability: Analyzing
Client Needs: Physiological Integrity
Clinical Judgment/Cognitive Skills: Analyze Cues
Integrated Process: Clinical Judgment; Nursing Process/Analysis
Content Area: Foundations of Care: Acid–Base
Health Problems: Adult Health: Respiratory: Asthma
Priority Concepts: Acid–Base Balance; Clinical Judgment

Answer: 2
Rationale: The pH is elevated in alkalosis and low in acidosis. In a respiratory condition, the pH and the Pco_2 move in opposite directions; that is, the pH rises and the Pco_2 drops (alkalosis) or vice versa (acidosis). In a metabolic condition, the pH and the bicarbonate move in the same direction; if the pH is low, the bicarbonate level will be low also. In this client, the pH is at the high end of normal, indicating compensation and alkalosis. The Pco_2 is low, indicating a respiratory condition (opposite direction of the pH).
Test-Taking Strategy: Focus on the subject, an acid–base imbalance. Remember that in a respiratory imbalance you will find that the pH and Pco_2 move in opposite directions. Therefore, options 1 and 4 are eliminated first. Next, remember that the pH is elevated with alkalosis, but compensation has occurred if the pH is within normal range. Option 2 reflects a respiratory alkalotic condition and compensation because the Pco_2 is below normal, but the pH is at the high end of normal.
Priority Nursing Tip: If the client has a condition that causes overstimulation of the respiratory system, monitor the client for respiratory alkalosis.
Reference: Ignatavicius, D., et al. (2021). *Medical-surgical nursing: Concepts for interprofessional collaborative care* (10th ed., pp. 272–273, 536). Elsevier.

73. The nurse is caring for a client with a possible bowel obstruction who has been prescribed a nasogastric tube that is attached to low suction. Arterial blood gases are prescribed and the nurse reviews the results. Based on the results, the nurse determines that the client is experiencing which acid–base imbalance?

Laboratory Results

Test and Result	Reference Range
pH 7.52	7.35–7.45
Po_2 90 mm Hg	80–100 mm Hg
Pco_2 40 mm Hg	35–45 mm Hg
HCO_3 30 mEq/L (30 mmol/L)	21–28 mEq/L (21–28 mmol/L)

1. Metabolic acidosis
2. Metabolic alkalosis
3. Respiratory acidosis
4. Respiratory alkalosis

Level of Cognitive Ability: Analyzing
Client Needs: Physiological Integrity
Clinical Judgment/Cognitive Skills: Analyze Cues
Integrated Process: Clinical Judgment; Nursing Process/Analysis
Content Area: Foundations of Care: Acid–Base
Health Problems: Adult Health: Gastrointestinal: Bowel Obstruction
Priority Concepts: Acid–Base Balance; Clinical Judgment

Answer: 2
Rationale: Loss of gastric fluid via nasogastric suction or vomiting causes metabolic alkalosis because of the loss of hydrochloric acid (HCl), an acid secreted in the stomach. This occurs as HCO_3 rises above normal. Thus, the loss of hydrogen ions in the HCl acid results in alkalosis. A pH above the reference range would be noted.
Test-Taking Strategy: Focus on the subject, complications of gastrointestinal suctioning and acid–base disorders. Eliminate options 1 and 3 first because the loss of HCl acid would cause an alkalotic condition. Next, noting that the client is experiencing a gastrointestinal problem will direct you to the correct option.
Priority Nursing Tip: Monitor the client experiencing excessive vomiting or the client with gastrointestinal suctioning for manifestations of metabolic alkalosis.
Reference: Ignatavicius, D., et al. (2021). *Medical-surgical nursing: Concepts for interprofessional collaborative care* (10th ed., pp. 271–272, 1111). Elsevier.

❖ **74.** The nurse reviews the results of a blood chemistry profile for a client who is experiencing late-stage salicylate poisoning and metabolic acidosis. Which serum study would the nurse review for data about the client's acid–base balance?
   1. Sodium
   2. Potassium
   3. Magnesium
   4. Phosphorus

Level of Cognitive Ability: Analyzing
Client Needs: Physiological Integrity
Clinical Judgment/Cognitive Skills: Take Action
Integrated Process: Clinical Judgment; Nursing Process/Assessment
Content Area: Complex Care: Poisoning
Health Problems: N/A
Priority Concepts: Acid–Base Balance; Clinical Judgment

Answer: 2
Rationale: A client with late-stage salicylate poisoning is at risk for metabolic acidosis because acetylsalicylic acid increases the client's hydrogen ion (H^+) concentration, decreases the pH, and creates a bicarbonate deficit. Hyperkalemia develops as the body attempts to compensate for the influx of H^+ by moving H^+ into the cell and potassium out of the cell; thus, potassium accumulates in the extracellular space. Clinical manifestations of metabolic acidosis include the clinical indicators of hyperkalemia, including hyperpnea, central nervous system depression, twitching, and seizures. Options 1, 3, and 4 are not primary concerns.
Test-Taking Strategy: Focus on the subject, an acid–base imbalance and salicylate poisoning. Specific knowledge about the effect of an influx of H+ in an acid–base disorder and the potassium shifts that occur will direct you to the correct option.
Priority Nursing Tip: In acidosis, the potassium moves out of the cell to make room for the hydrogen ions; thus, the potassium level increases. In alkalosis, the potassium moves into the cell and the potassium level decreases.
Reference: Ignatavicius, D., et al. (2021). *Medical-surgical nursing: Concepts for interprofessional collaborative care* (10th ed., p. 267). Elsevier.

75. An emergency department nurse is planning care for a child diagnosed with acetaminophen overdose. The nurse reviews the physician's prescriptions and prepares to administer which medication?
   1. Succimer
   2. Vitamin K
   3. N-acetylcysteine
   4. Protamine sulfate

Level of Cognitive Ability: Analyzing
Client Needs: Physiological Integrity
Clinical Judgment/Cognitive Skills: Generate Solutions
Integrated Process: Clinical Judgment; Nursing Process/Planning
Content Area: Complex Care: Poisoning
Health Problems: Pediatric-Specific: Poisoning
Priority Concepts: Clinical Judgment; Safety

Answer: 3
Rationale: N-acetylcysteine is the antidote for acetaminophen overdose. It is administered orally or via nasogastric tube in a diluted form with water, juice, or soda. It can also be administered intravenously. Protamine sulfate is the antidote for heparin. Succimer is used in the treatment of lead poisoning. Vitamin K is the antidote for warfarin.
Test-Taking Strategy: Focus on the subject, acetaminophen overdose management. Specific knowledge regarding the antidote for acetaminophen overdose is required to answer this question. Remember that N-acetylcysteine is the antidote for acetaminophen overdose.
Priority Nursing Tip: When it is used as an antidote via oral administration, dilute N-acetylcysteine in juice or soda because of its offensive odor.
Reference: McKinney, E. S., et al. (2022). *Maternal child nursing* (6th ed., p. 774). Elsevier.

❖ **76.** What would the nurse consider when determining whether a client diagnosed with chronic obstructive pulmonary disease (COPD) could tolerate and benefit from active progressive relaxation? **Select all that apply.**
❑ **1.** Social status
❑ **2.** Financial status
❑ **3.** Functional status
❑ **4.** Medical diagnosis
❑ **5.** Ability to expend energy
❑ **6.** Motivation of the individual

Level of Cognitive Ability: Analyzing
Client Needs: Physiological Integrity
Clinical Judgment/Cognitive Skills: Analyze Cues
Integrated Process: Clinical Judgment; Nursing Process/Analysis
Content Area: Adult Health: Respiratory
Health Problems: Adult Health: Respiratory: Chronic Obstructive Pulmonary Disease
Priority Concepts: Clinical Judgment; Gas Exchange

Answer: 3, 4, 5, 6
Rationale: Active progressive relaxation training teaches the client how to effectively rest and reduce tension in the body. Some important considerations when choosing the type of relaxation technique are the client's physiologic and psychological status. Because active progressive relaxation training requires a moderate expenditure of energy, the nurse needs to consider the client's functional status, medical diagnosis, and ability to expend energy. For example, a client with an advanced respiratory disease like COPD may not have sufficient energy reserves to participate in active progressive relaxation techniques. The client needs to be motivated to participate in this form of alternative therapy to obtain beneficial results. The client's social or financial status has no relationship with their ability to tolerate and benefit from active progressive relaxation.
Test-Taking Strategy: Focus on the subject, determining whether a client could tolerate and benefit from active progressive relaxation. Use teaching and learning principles, recalling that motivation is a key factor. From the remaining options, noting the word "active" will assist in determining that options 3, 4, and 5 are correct.
Priority Nursing Tip: Relaxation techniques are important to learn and integrate into daily activities to aid in the prevention of potential stress-related disease processes.
Reference: Ignatavicius, D., et al. (2021). *Medical-surgical nursing: Concepts for interprofessional collaborative care* (10th ed., pp. 549–550). Elsevier.

❖ **77.** An adult client suspected of having developed encephalitis has undergone a lumbar puncture to obtain cerebrospinal fluid (CSF) for analysis. After reviewing the results of the analysis, the nurse recognizes that the CSF is suggestive of the infection when which element is noted?
1. Protein
2. Glucose
3. Lymphocytes
4. Red blood cells

Level of Cognitive Ability: Analyzing
Client Needs: Physiological Integrity
Clinical Judgment/Cognitive Skills: Analyze Cues
Integrated Process: Clinical Judgment; Nursing Process/Analysis
Content Area: Foundations of Care: Diagnostic Tests
Health Problems: Adult Health: Neurologic: Inflammation/Infections
Priority Concepts: Clinical Judgment; Intracranial Regulation

Answer: 3
Rationale: Lymphocytes are generally rare in CSF. Therefore, lymphocytes in the CSF can indicate an infection. Protein (reference range of 15 to 45 mg/dL [0.15 to 0.45 g/L]) and glucose (reference range of 50 to 75 mg/dL [2.8 to 4.2 mmol/L]) are normally present in CSF. Normally there are no red blood cells in CSF.
Test-Taking Strategy: Focus on the subject, the finding that is suggestive of an infection in CSF. Recall that protein and glucose are normally present in CSF. Next recall that the presence of red blood cells is abnormal and would indicate blood vessel rupture or meningeal irritation. This will direct you to the correct option.
Priority Nursing Tip: Cerebrospinal fluid is normally clear. A pink or red specimen may be caused by the presence of red blood cells.
Reference: Lewis, S., et al. (2020). *Medical-surgical nursing: Assessment and management of clinical problems* (11th ed., pp. 190, 1295). Elsevier.

78. A client who has sustained a burn injury receives a prescription for a regular diet. Which is the **best** meal for the nurse to provide to the client to promote wound healing?
1. Peanut butter and jelly sandwich, apple, tea
2. Chicken breast, broccoli, strawberries, milk
3. Veal chop, boiled potatoes, Jell-O, orange juice
4. Pasta with tomato sauce, garlic bread, ginger ale

Level of Cognitive Ability: Applying
Client Needs: Physiological Integrity
Clinical Judgment/Cognitive Skills: Take Action
Integrated Process: Nursing Process/Implementation
Content Area: Foundations of Care: Therapeutic Diets
Health Problems: Adult Health: Integumentary: Burns
Priority Concepts: Health Promotion; Nutrition

Answer: 2
Rationale: The meal with the best potential to promote wound healing includes nutrient-rich food choices, including protein, such as chicken and milk, and vitamin C, such as broccoli and strawberries. The remaining options include one or more items with a low nutritional value, especially the tea, jelly, Jell-O, and ginger ale.
Test-Taking Strategy: Note the strategic word, *best*. Focus on the subject, nutrition for a client with a burn injury. Knowledge that protein and vitamin C are necessary for wound healing assists in selecting the option that contains those nutrients, and the option with the most nutrients is the best choice. Eliminate options 1 and 3 first because jelly, tea, and Jell-O have no nutritional value related to healing. From the remaining options, select option 2 over option 4 because option 2 contains foods with greater nutritional value.
Priority Nursing Tip: Depending on the extent of the injury, the basal metabolic rate is 40 to 100 times higher than normal in a client with a burn injury.
Reference: Ignatavicius, D., et al. (2021). *Medical-surgical nursing: Concepts for interprofessional collaborative care* (10th ed., pp. 129, 580). Elsevier.

79. The nurse is developing a care plan for a client experiencing urge urinary incontinence. Which interventions would be helpful for this type of incontinence? **Select all that apply.**
☐ 1. Surgery
☐ 2. Bladder retraining
☐ 3. Scheduled toileting
☐ 4. Dietary modifications
☐ 5. Pelvic muscle exercises
☐ 6. Intermittent catheterization

Level of Cognitive Ability: Applying
Client Needs: Physiological Integrity
Clinical Judgment/Cognitive Skills: Generate Solutions
Integrated Process: Nursing Process/Planning
Content Area: Skills: Elimination
Health Problems: Adult Health: Renal and Urinary: Urinary Incontinence
Priority Concepts: Clinical Judgment; Elimination

Answer: 2, 3, 4, 5
Rationale: Urge incontinence is the involuntary passage of urine after a strong sense of the urgency to void. It is characterized by urinary urgency, often with frequency (more often than every 2 hours); bladder spasm or contraction; and voiding in either small amounts (less than 100 mL) or large amounts (greater than 500 mL). It can be caused by decreased bladder capacity, irritation of the bladder stretch receptors, infection, and alcohol or caffeine ingestion. Interventions to assist the client with urge incontinence include bladder retraining, scheduled toileting, dietary modifications such as eliminating alcohol and caffeine intake, and pelvic muscle exercises to strengthen the muscles. Surgery and urinary catheterization are invasive measures and will not assist in the treatment of urge incontinence.
Test-Taking Strategy: Focus on the subject, urge urinary incontinence and recall the definition of this type of incontinence. Also note that options 1 and 6 are invasive measures, and these types of measures are avoided.
Priority Nursing Tip: During bladder retraining, to aid in ensuring complete bladder emptying, teach the client to urinate as much as possible, relax for a few moments, then attempt to urinate again. This is known as "double-voiding."
Reference: Ignatavicius, D., et al. (2021). *Medical-surgical nursing: Concepts for interprofessional collaborative care* (10th ed., pp. 1332–1333, 1335). Elsevier.

❖ **80.** The nurse caring for a client diagnosed with a stroke is planning care to maintain nutritional status. The nurse is concerned about the client's swallowing ability. Which food item would the nurse eliminate from this client's diet?
  1. Spinach
  2. Custard
  3. Scrambled eggs
  4. Mashed potatoes

Level of Cognitive Ability: Applying
Client Needs: Physiological Integrity
Clinical Judgment/Cognitive Skills: Take Action
Integrated Process: Nursing Process/Implementation
Content Area: Foundations of Care: Therapeutic Diets
Health Problems: Adult Health: Neurologic: Stroke
Priority Concepts: Nutrition; Safety

Answer: 1
Rationale: Raw vegetables; chunky vegetables such as diced beets; and stringy vegetables such as spinach, corn, and peas are foods commonly excluded from the diet of a client with a poor swallowing reflex. In general, flavorful, warm, or well-chilled foods with texture stimulate the swallowing reflex. Soft and semisoft foods such as custards or puddings, egg dishes, and potatoes are usually effective.
Test-Taking Strategy: Focus on the subject, concern about a client's swallowing ability. Select option 1 as the food that is stringy and with the least amount of substance or consistency.
Priority Nursing Tip: Pureed foods may be necessary as a means of providing nutritional intake to a client with an altered swallowing ability. Molding the pureed food into the shape of the original food can enhance the appeal of the food item and thus enhance the client's appetite.
Reference: Nix, S. (2022). *Williams' Basic nutrition and diet therapy* (16th ed., pp. 319–320). Elsevier.

81. An adult client arrives in the emergency department with burns to both entire legs and the perineal area. Using the rule of nines, the nurse would determine that approximately what percentage of the client's body surface has been burned? **Fill in the blank.**

Answer: _____ %
Level of Cognitive Ability: Analyzing
Client Needs: Physiological Integrity
Clinical Judgment/Cognitive Skills: Analyze Cues
Integrated Process: Clinical Judgment; Nursing Process/Assessment
Content Area: Adult Health: Integumentary
Health Problems: Adult Health: Integumentary: Burns
Priority Concepts: Clinical Judgment; Tissue Integrity

Answer: 37
Rationale: The most rapid method used to calculate the size of a burn injury in adult clients whose weights are in normal proportion to their heights is the rule of nines. This method divides the body into areas that are multiples of 9%, except for the perineum. Each entire leg is 18%, each arm is 9%, and the head is 9%. The trunk is 36%, and the perineal area is 1%. Both legs and perineal area equal 37%.
Test-Taking Strategy: Focus on the subject, rule of nines. Knowledge regarding the percentages associated with this method of calculating burn injuries is required to answer this question. Remember that each leg is 18%, each arm is 9%, the head is 9%, the trunk is 36%, and the perineal area is 1%.
Priority Nursing Tip: The rule of nines gives an inaccurate estimate of the extent of the burn injury in a child because of the difference in body proportion between children and adults. Instead, in children, the extent of the burn is expressed as a percentage of the total body surface area using age-related charts.
Reference: Ignatavicius, D., et al. (2021). *Medical-surgical nursing: Concepts for interprofessional collaborative care* (10th ed., pp. 460–461). Elsevier.

Client Needs

❖ **82.** A client is resuming a diet after a Billroth II procedure performed because of a gastric carcinoma tumor. To minimize complications associated with eating, which actions would the nurse teach the client? **Select all that apply.**
- ❑ 1. Lying down after eating
- ❑ 2. Eating a diet high in protein
- ❑ 3. Drinking liquids with meals
- ❑ 4. Eating six small meals per day
- ❑ 5. Eating concentrated sweets only between meals

Level of Cognitive Ability: Applying
Client Needs: Physiological Integrity
Clinical Judgment/Cognitive Skills: Take Action
Integrated Process: Clinical Judgment; Nursing Process/Implementation
Content Area: Foundations of Care: Therapeutic Diets
Health Problems: Adult Health: Cancer: Esophageal/ Gastric/Intestinal
Priority Concepts: Patient Education; Elimination

Answer: 1, 2, 4
Rationale: The client who has had a Billroth II procedure is at risk for dumping syndrome. The client should lie down after eating and avoid drinking liquids with meals to prevent this syndrome. The client should be placed on a dry diet that is high in protein, moderate in fat, and low in carbohydrates. Frequent small meals are encouraged, and the client needs to avoid concentrated sweets.
Test-Taking Strategy: Focusing on the subject, Billroth II procedure, and recalling that dumping syndrome is a complication of this surgical procedure will direct you to the correct options. Eliminate option 5 because of the closed-ended word "only." Also thinking about the pathophysiology associated with dumping syndrome will assist in eliminating option 3.
Priority Nursing Tip: Dumping syndrome is a complication of gastric resection and results from the rapid emptying of the gastric contents into the small intestine after eating.
Reference: Ignatavicius, D., et al. (2021). *Medical-surgical nursing: Concepts for interprofessional collaborative care* (10th ed., pp. 1106–1107). Elsevier.

83. The nurse is ambulating a client for the first time after having abdominal surgery. What clinical manifestations would indicate to the nurse that the client may be experiencing orthostatic hypotension? **Select all that apply.**
- ❑ 1. Nausea
- ❑ 2. Dizziness
- ❑ 3. Bradycardia
- ❑ 4. Lightheadedness
- ❑ 5. Flushing of the face
- ❑ 6. Reports of seeing spots

Level of Cognitive Ability: Analyzing
Client Needs: Physiological Integrity
Clinical Judgment/Cognitive Skills: Recognize Cues
Integrated Process: Clinical Judgment; Nursing Process/Assessment
Content Area: Adult Health: Cardiovascular
Health Problems: Adult Health: Cardiovascular: Vascular Disorders
Priority Concepts: Clinical Judgment; Perfusion

Answer: 1, 2, 4, 6
Rationale: Orthostatic hypotension occurs when a normotensive person develops symptoms of low blood pressure when rising to an upright position. Whenever the nurse gets a client up and out of a bed or chair, there is a risk for orthostatic hypotension. Symptoms of nausea, dizziness, lightheadedness, tachycardia, pallor, and reports of seeing spots are characteristic of orthostatic hypotension. A drop of approximately 15 mm Hg in the systolic blood pressure and 10 mm Hg in the diastolic blood pressure also occurs. Fainting can result without intervention, which includes immediately assisting the client to a lying position.
Test-Taking Strategy: Focus on the subject, the manifestations of orthostatic hypotension. As you read each option, think about the physiologic changes that occur when the blood pressure drops. This will assist in answering the question.
Priority Nursing Tip: Baroreceptors (located in the walls of the aortic arch and carotid sinuses) are specialized nerve endings affected by changes in the blood pressure. Increases in the arterial pressure stimulate baroreceptors to decrease the pressure. Conversely, decreases in arterial pressure reduce stimulation and the blood pressure increases.
Reference: Ignatavicius, D., et al. (2021). *Medical-surgical nursing: Concepts for interprofessional collaborative care* (10th ed., p. 247). Elsevier.

❖ **84.** The nurse who has been closely monitoring a child who has been exhibiting decorticate (flexor) posturing after sustaining severe head trauma notes that the child suddenly exhibits decerebrate (extensor) posturing. The nurse interprets that this change in the child's posturing indicates what?
1. An insignificant finding
2. An improvement in condition
3. Decreasing intracranial pressure
4. Deteriorating neurologic function

Level of Cognitive Ability: Analyzing
Client Needs: Physiological Integrity
Clinical Judgment/Cognitive Skills: Analyze Cues
Integrated Process: Clinical Judgment; Nursing Process/Analysis
Content Area: Pediatrics: Neurologic
Health Problems: Pediatric-Specific: Head Injury
Priority Concepts: Clinical Judgment; Intracranial Regulation

Answer: 4
Rationale: The progression from decorticate to decerebrate posturing usually indicates deteriorating neurologic function and warrants physician notification. Options 1, 2, and 3 are inaccurate interpretations.
Test-Taking Strategy: Focus on the subject, decorticate and decerebrate posturing. Eliminate options 2 and 3 first because they are comparable or alike. From the remaining options, recalling the significance of decerebrate posturing will assist in eliminating option 1.
Priority Nursing Tip: Posturing indicates deterioration in the client's neurologic status.
Reference: McKinney, E. S., et al. (2022). *Maternal child nursing* (6th ed., p. 1293). Elsevier.

85. The nurse, while caring for a hospitalized infant being monitored for hydrocephalus, notes that the anterior fontanel bulges when the infant cries. Based on this assessment finding, which conclusion would the nurse draw?
1. No action is required.
2. The head of the bed needs to be lowered.
3. The infant needs to be placed on nothing by mouth (NPO) status.
4. The physician needs to be notified immediately.

Level of Cognitive Ability: Analyzing
Client Needs: Physiological Integrity
Clinical Judgment/Cognitive Skills: Analyze Cues
Integrated Process: Nursing Process/Analysis
Content Area: Maternity: Newborn
Health Problems: Pediatric-Specific: Hydrocephalus
Priority Concepts: Clinical Judgment; Development

Answer: 1
Rationale: The anterior fontanel is diamond shaped and located on the top of the head. It should be soft and flat in a normal infant, and it normally closes by 12 to 18 months of age. The posterior fontanel closes by 2 to 3 months of age. A bulging or tense fontanel may result from crying or increased intracranial pressure (ICP). Noting a bulging fontanel when the infant cries is a normal finding that requires no action. It is not necessary to notify the physician. Options 2 and 3 are inappropriate actions.
Test-Taking Strategy: Focus on the subject, bulging anterior fontanel. Note that the question states that the anterior fontanel bulges when the infant cries. Remember that a bulging or tense fontanel may result from crying; therefore, it is a normal finding.
Priority Nursing Tip: A full or bulging anterior fontanel in a quiet infant may indicate increased ICP.
Reference: Hockenberry, M., Wilson, D., & Rodgers, C. (2019). *Wong's Nursing care of infants and children* (11th ed., pp. 211, 1159–1160). Elsevier.

❖ **86.** The nurse assessing the vital signs of a 3-year-old child hospitalized with a diagnosis of croup notes that the respiratory rate is 28 breaths/min. Based on this finding, which nursing action is appropriate?
   1. Begin administering supplemental oxygen.
   2. Document the findings according to facility policies.
   3. Notify the child's physician immediately.
   4. Reassess the respiratory rate, rhythm, and depth in 15 minutes.

Level of Cognitive Ability: Applying
Client Needs: Physiological Integrity
Clinical Judgment/Cognitive Skills: Take Action
Integrated Process: Nursing Process/Implementation
Content Area: Pediatrics: Throat/Respiratory
Health Problems: Pediatric-Specific: Croup
Priority Concepts: Development; Gas Exchange

Answer: 2
Rationale: The normal respiratory rate for a 3-year-old child is approximately 20 to 30 breaths/min. Because the respiratory rate is normal, options 1, 3, and 4 are unnecessary actions. The nurse would document the findings.
Test-Taking Strategy: Focus on the subject, pediatric vital signs. Recalling that the normal respiratory rate for a 3-year-old child is approximately 20 to 30 breaths per minute will direct you to the correct option.
Priority Nursing Tip: Nasal flaring, sternal retractions, and inspiratory stridor are signs of a compromised airway and respiratory distress.
References: McKinney, E. S., et al. (2022). *Maternal child nursing* (6th ed., pp. 1048–1049). Elsevier; Potter, P., et al. (2021). *Fundamentals of nursing* (10th ed., p. 482). Elsevier.

87. The nurse is performing an assessment on a client who is suspected of having mittelschmerz. Which subjective finding supports the possibility of this condition?
   1. Experiences pain during intercourse
   2. Has pain at the onset of menstruation
   3. Experiences profuse vaginal bleeding
   4. Has sharp pelvic pain during ovulation

Level of Cognitive Ability: Applying
Client Needs: Physiological Integrity
Clinical Judgment/Cognitive Skills: Recognize Cues
Integrated Process: Nursing Process/Assessment
Content Area: Adult Health: Reproductive
Health Problems: Adult Health: Reproductive: Menstruation Problems/Fertility/Infertility
Priority Concepts: Pain; Reproduction

Answer: 4
Rationale: Mittelschmerz (middle pain) refers to pelvic pain that occurs midway between menstrual periods or at the time of ovulation. The pain is caused by a growth follicle within the ovary, or rupture of the follicle and subsequent spillage of follicular fluid and blood into the peritoneal space. The pain is fairly sharp and is felt on the right or left side of the pelvis. It generally lasts 1 to 3 days, and slight vaginal bleeding may accompany the discomfort.
Test-Taking Strategy: Focus on the subject, mittelschmerz. Recalling that mittelschmerz is "middle pain" will direct you to the correct option.
Priority Nursing Tip: The discomfort that occurs with mittelschmerz is usually relieved with a mild analgesic.
Reference: Dorlands's Illustrated medical dictionary (2020). (33rd ed., p. 1154). Elsevier.

❖ **88.** During a health assessment, the client tells the nurse about being diagnosed with endometriosis. Which explanation presented by the client demonstrates an understanding of the description of the condition?
  1. "Endometriosis is known as primary dysmenorrhea."
  2. "Endometriosis is what causes me the pain that occurs when I ovulate."
  3. "Endometriosis is the condition that has caused me to stop menstruating."
  4. "Endometriosis means that I have uterine tissue growing outside my uterus."

Level of Cognitive Ability: Evaluating
Client Needs: Physiological Integrity
Clinical Judgment/Cognitive Skills: Evaluate Outcomes
Integrated Process: Clinical Judgment; Nursing Process/Evaluation
Content Area: Adult Health: Reproductive
Health Problems: Adult Health: Reproductive: Inflammatory/Infectious Problems
Priority Concepts: Patient Education; Reproduction

Answer: 4
Rationale: *Endometriosis* is the presence of tissue outside the uterus that resembles the endometrium in structure, function, and response to estrogen and progesterone during the menstrual cycle. Primary dysmenorrhea refers to menstrual pain without identified pathology. *Mittelschmerz* refers to pelvic pain that occurs midway between menstrual periods coinciding with ovulation. *Amenorrhea,* the cessation of menstruation for a period of at least three cycles or 6 months in a client who has established a pattern of menstruation, can result from a variety of causes.
Test-Taking Strategy: Focus on the **subject**, endometriosis. Note the relationship between "endometriosis" in the question and "uterus" in the correct option.
Priority Nursing Tip: Nonpharmacologic measures such as rest and the application of heat to the lower abdomen will assist in relieving the discomfort associated with menstrual discomfort.
Reference: Lewis, S., et al. (2020). *Medical-surgical nursing: Assessment and management of clinical problems* (11th ed., pp. 1238–1239). Elsevier.

89. A client has developed an infection after sustaining second-degree burns. The physician prescribes 250 mg of amikacin sulfate every 12 hours. How many milliliters (mL) would the nurse prepare to administer one dose? **Refer to the figure. Fill in the blank.**

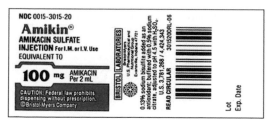

(From Kee, J., & Marshall, S. (2012). *Clinical calculations* (7th ed.). Saunders.)

Answer: _____ mL
Level of Cognitive Ability: Applying
Client Needs: Physiological Integrity
Clinical Judgment/Cognitive Skills: Generate Solutions
Integrated Process: Nursing Process/Planning
Content Area: Skills: Dosage Calculations
Health Problems: Adult Health: Integumentary: Burns
Priority Concepts: Infection; Safety

Answer: 5
Rationale: Use the medication calculation formula.

$$\frac{Desired \times mL}{Available} = mL \text{ per dose}$$

$$\frac{250\,mg \times 2\,mL}{100\,mg} = 5\,mL \text{ per dose}$$

Test-Taking Strategy: Focus on the **subject**, amikacin sulfate and note the data on the medication label. Follow the formula for calculating the correct dose. Once you have performed the calculation, recheck your work with a calculator and ensure that the answer makes sense.
Priority Nursing Tip: Amikacin sulfate is an aminoglycoside that can cause ototoxicity and renal toxicity as adverse effects.
Reference: Potter, P., et al. (2021). *Fundamentals of nursing* (10th ed., pp. 600–601). Elsevier.

90. A hepatitis B screen is performed on a postpartum client, and the results indicate the presence of antigens in the birthing parent's blood. Which intervention would the nurse anticipate will be prescribed to protect the neonate? **Select all that apply.**
- ❏ 1. Obtaining serum liver enzymes
- ❏ 2. Administering hepatitis vaccine
- ❏ 3. Supporting breast-/chest-feeding every 5 hours
- ❏ 4. Repeating hepatitis B screen in 1 week
- ❏ 5. Administering hepatitis B immune globulin
- ❏ 6. Administering antibiotics while hospitalized

Level of Cognitive Ability: Applying
Client Needs: Physiological Integrity
Clinical Judgment/Cognitive Skills: Generate Solutions
Integrated Process: Nursing Process/Planning
Content Area: Maternity: Newborn
Health Problems: Newborn: Infections
Priority Concepts: Infection; Safety

Answer: 2, 5
Rationale: A hepatitis B screen is performed to detect the presence of antigens in birthing parent's blood. If antigens are present, the neonate would receive the hepatitis vaccine and hepatitis B immune globulin within 12 hours after birth. Obtaining serum liver enzymes, retesting the birthing parent's blood in a week, breast-/chest-feeding every 5 hours, and administering antibiotics would not decrease the chance of the neonate contracting the hepatitis B virus.
Test-Taking Strategy: Focus on the subject, hepatitis B in pregnancy. Think about the concerns for the neonate. Eliminate options 1, 3, 4, and 6 because they are actions that would not decrease the chance of the neonate contracting the hepatitis B virus. Recall that the hepatitis B vaccine and the hepatitis B immune globulin will protect the neonate.
Priority Nursing Tip: The risks of prematurity, low birth weight, and neonatal death increase if the birthing parent has hepatitis B infection.
Reference: McKinney, E. S., et al. (2022). *Maternal child nursing* (6th ed., p. 573). Elsevier.

91. The nurse is counseling the family of a terminally ill client about palliative care. When planning care, the nurse identifies which goals as being those of palliative care? **Select all that apply.**
- ❏ 1. The delay of the impending death
- ❏ 2. Offering a caring support system
- ❏ 3. Providing measures focused on pain management
- ❏ 4. Introduction of interventions that enhance the quality of life
- ❏ 5. Expanding the focus of care to both client and family
- ❏ 6. Addressing the expressed spiritual needs of client and family

Level of Cognitive Ability: Applying
Client Needs: Physiological Integrity
Clinical Judgment/Cognitive Skills: Generate Solutions
Integrated Process: Caring
Content Area: Developmental Stages: End-of-Life
Health Problems: Mental Health: Grief/Loss
Priority Concepts: Caregiving; Palliative Care

Answer: 2, 3, 4, 5, 6
Rationale: Palliative care is a philosophy of total care. Palliative care goals include the following: offering a support system to help the client live as actively as possible until death; providing relief from pain and other distressing symptoms; enhancing the quality of life; offering a support system to help families cope during the client's illness and their own bereavement; affirming life and regarding dying as a normal process, neither hastening nor postponing death; and integrating psychological and spiritual aspects of client care.
Test-Taking Strategy: Focus on the subject, goals of palliative care. Recall that palliative care interventions are designed to relieve or reduce the intensity of uncomfortable symptoms but not to produce a cure, and that palliative care is a philosophy of total care. With this in mind, read each option and determine if it meets this description.
Priority Nursing Tip: Palliative care is designed to assist the client and family in achieving the best quality of life during the entire course of an illness.
Reference: Ignatavicius, D., et al. (2021). *Medical-surgical nursing: Concepts for interprofessional collaborative care* (10th ed., pp. 137, 139). Elsevier.

❖ **92.** A pregnant client reports that the last menstrual period (LMP) was February 9, 2025. Using Näegele's rule, what will the nurse determine as the estimated date of birth?
1. October 7, 2025
2. October 16, 2025
3. November 7, 2025
4. November 16, 2025

Level of Cognitive Ability: Applying
Client Needs: Physiological Integrity
Clinical Judgment/Cognitive Skills: Recognize Cues
Integrated Process: Nursing Process/Assessment
Content Area: Maternity: Antepartum
Health Problems: N/A
Priority Concepts: Reproduction; Development

Answer: 4
Rationale: Accurate use of Näegele's rule requires that the client has a regular 28-day menstrual cycle. The Naegele's formula is a simple arithmetic method for calculating the EDD (estimated date of delivery) based on the LMP. To the date of the first day of the LMP (February 9, 2025): subtract 3 months (November 9, 2024), then add 7 days (November 16, 2024) and 1 year as appropriate; or Due Date = LMP + 9 months + 7 days
Test-Taking Strategy: Focus on the subject, Näegele's rule, to answer this question. Be careful when following the steps to determine the estimated date of birth using this rule. Read all of the options carefully, noting the dates and years before selecting an option.
Priority Nursing Tip: There are several formulas that can be used by the primary health care provider to determine the estimated date of birth. Näegele's rule is one method that is used.
Reference: McKinney, E. S., et al. (2022). *Maternal child nursing* (6th ed., p. 231). Elsevier.

93. The nurse is creating a plan of care for a client who suffered a pelvic fracture following a motor vehicle crash (MVC). Which interventions would be included in the nursing care plan to prevent skin breakdown? **Select all that apply.**
❑ 1. Minimize the force and friction applied to the skin.
❑ 2. Massage vigorously over bony prominences twice daily.
❑ 3. Perform a systematic skin inspection at least once a day.
❑ 4. Cleanse the skin at the time of soiling and at routine intervals.
❑ 5. Use pillows to keep the knees and other bony prominences from direct contact with one another.
❑ 6. Use hot water and a mild cleansing agent that minimizes irritation and dryness of the skin when bathing the client.

Level of Cognitive Ability: Creating
Client Needs: Physiological Integrity
Clinical Judgment/Cognitive Skills: Generate Solutions
Integrated Process: Clinical Judgment; Nursing Process/Planning
Content Area: Adult Health: Integumentary
Health Problems: Adult Health: Musculoskeletal: Skeletal Injury
Priority Concepts: Clinical Judgment; Tissue Integrity

Answer: 1, 3, 4, 5
Rationale: The client in this question is at high risk for pressure injury. Interventions for prevention of pressure injuries include minimizing the force and friction applied to the skin; performing a systematic skin inspection at least once a day, giving particular attention to the bony prominences; cleansing the skin at the time of soiling and at routine intervals; avoiding the use of hot water; and using a mild cleansing agent that minimizes irritation and dryness of the skin. Pillows should be used to keep the knees and other bony prominences from direct contact with one another, because skin contact can promote breakdown. Massaging over bony prominences (especially vigorous) can be harmful to at-risk skin surfaces.
Test-Taking Strategy: Focus on the subject, preventing skin breakdown. Visualize each of the options in terms of how it will prevent or promote skin breakdown. Eliminate option 2 because of the word, *vigorously,* and option 6 because of the word, *hot.*
Priority Nursing Tip: The skin is the first line of defense against infection; therefore, a major role of the nurse is to prevent skin breakdown.
Reference: Ignatavicius, D., et al. (2021). *Medical-surgical nursing: Concepts for interprofessional collaborative care* (10th ed., pp. 1036–1037). Elsevier.

❖ **94.** The nurse is preparing to measure the fundal height of a client whose fetus is 28 weeks of gestation. In what position would the nurse place the client to perform the procedure?
1. In a standing position
2. In Trendelenburg's position
3. Supine with the head of the bed elevated to 45 degrees
4. Supine with the head on a pillow and knees slightly flexed

Level of Cognitive Ability: Applying
Client Needs: Physiological Integrity
Clinical Judgment/Cognitive Skills: Take Action
Integrated Process: Nursing Process/Implementation
Content Area: Maternity: Antepartum
Health Problems: N/A
Priority Concepts: Reproduction; Development

Answer: 4
Rationale: When fundal height is measured, the client lies in a supine (back) position with their head on a pillow and knees slightly flexed. The standing position, Trendelenburg's (head lowered), or supine with the head of the bed elevated to 45 degrees would prevent the nurse from getting an accurate measurement.
Test-Taking Strategy: Focus on the subject, measuring fundal height. Visualize this assessment technique to direct you to the correct option. Options 1, 2, or 3 would not give an accurate measurement.
Priority Nursing Tip: During the second and third trimesters of pregnancy (weeks 18 to 30), fundal height in centimeters (cm) approximately equals fetal age in weeks plus 2 cm.
Reference: McKinney, E. S., et al. (2022). *Maternal child nursing* (6th ed., pp. 234–235). Elsevier.

95. The nurse is measuring the fundal height on a client who is 36 weeks of gestation when the client reports feeling lightheaded. What finding would the nurse expect to note when assessing the client?
1. Fear
2. Anemia
3. A full bladder
4. Pallor and hypotension

Level of Cognitive Ability: Analyzing
Client Needs: Physiological Integrity
Clinical Judgment/Cognitive Skills: Recognize Cues
Integrated Process: Clinical Judgment; Nursing Process/Assessment
Content Area: Maternity: Antepartum
Health Problems: Maternity: Supine Hypotension
Priority Concepts: Perfusion; Reproduction

Answer: 4
Rationale: Compression of the inferior vena cava and aorta by the uterus may cause supine hypotension syndrome (vena cava syndrome) late in pregnancy. Pallor and hypotension would be noted. Having the client turn onto the left side or elevating the left buttock during fundal height measurement will prevent the problem. Options 1, 2, and 3 are unrelated to this syndrome.
Test-Taking Strategy: Focus on the subject, vena cava syndrome. Recalling that compression of the inferior vena cava and aorta by the uterus may cause supine hypotension syndrome will direct you to the correct option.
Priority Nursing Tip: Signs of supine hypotension (vena cava syndrome) in a pregnant client include pallor, lightheadedness, breathlessness, tachycardia, hypotension, sweating, cool and damp skin, and fetal distress.
Reference: McKinney, E. S., et al. (2022). *Maternal child nursing* (6th ed., pp. 222–223). Elsevier.

❖ **96.** The nurse in the prenatal clinic is monitoring a client who is pregnant with twins. The nurse monitors the client closely for which **priority** complication that is associated with a twin pregnancy?
1. Hemorrhoids
2. Postterm labor
3. Birthing parent anemia
4. Costovertebral angle tenderness

Level of Cognitive Ability: Analysis
Client Needs: Physiological Integrity
Clinical Judgment/Cognitive Skills: Analyze Cues
Integrated Process: Clinical Judgment; Nursing Process/Analysis
Content Area: Maternity: Antepartum
Health Problems: Maternity: Multiple Gestation
Priority Concepts: Clinical Judgment; Reproduction

Answer: 3
Rationale: Birthing parent anemia often occurs in twin pregnancies because of a greater demand for iron by the fetuses. Options 1 and 4 occur in a twin pregnancy but would not be as high a priority as anemia. Option 2 is incorrect because twin pregnancies often end in prematurity.
Test-Taking Strategy: Focus on the subject, twin pregnancy, and note the strategic word, *priority*. Thinking about the physiologic occurrences of a twin pregnancy will direct you to the correct option.
Priority Nursing Tip: The pregnant client with a multifetal pregnancy needs to be monitored closely for signs of anemia. Adequate nutrition is critical, and supplemental vitamins are prescribed to meet the needs of each fetus without depleting birthing parent stores.
Reference: McKinney, E. S., et al. (2022). *Maternal child nursing* (6th ed., p. 567). Elsevier.

97. A clinic nurse is assessing a prenatal client who has been diagnosed with heart disease. The nurse carefully assesses the client's vital signs, weight, and fluid and nutritional status to detect complications caused by which pregnancy-related concern?
1. Rh incompatibility
2. Fetal cardiomegaly
3. The increase in circulating blood volume
4. Hypertrophy and increased contractility of the heart

Level of Cognitive Ability: Analyzing
Client Needs: Physiological Integrity
Clinical Judgment/Cognitive Skills: Analyze Cues
Integrated Process: Clinical Judgment; Nursing Process/Analysis
Content Area: Maternity: Antepartum
Health Problems: Maternity: Cardiac Disease
Priority Concepts: Perfusion; Reproduction

Answer: 3
Rationale: Pregnancy taxes the circulating system of every client because the blood volume increases, which causes the cardiac output to increase. Stroke volume × heart rate = cardiac output (SV × HR = CO). Options 1, 2, and 4 are not directly associated with pregnancy in a client with a cardiac condition.
Test-Taking Strategy: Focus on the subject, a prenatal client with heart disease. Eliminate options 1 and 2 first because they address the fetus, not the prenatal client. From the remaining options, recalling the changes that take place in the client during pregnancy will direct you to the correct option. Also, remember that hypertrophy of the heart may occur in cardiac disease, but the outcome would be a decrease in contractility, not an increase.
Priority Nursing Tip: A pregnant client with cardiac disease may be unable to physiologically cope with the added blood volume that occurs during pregnancy.
Reference: McKinney, E. S., et al. (2022). *Maternal child nursing* (6th ed., pp. 565, 567). Elsevier.

98. The nurse is providing care for a client with a history of nonalcoholic fatty liver disease (hepatic steatosis) who has just experienced a liver biopsy performed at the bedside. Which position would the nurse place the client in after the biopsy?
1. Supine with the head elevated on one pillow
2. Semi-Fowler's with two pillows under the legs
3. Left side-lying with a small pillow under the puncture site
4. Right side-lying with a folded towel under the puncture site

Level of Cognitive Ability: Applying
Client Needs: Physiological Integrity
Clinical Judgment/Cognitive Skills: Take Action
Integrated Process: Nursing Process/Implementation
Content Area: Foundations of Care: Diagnostic Tests
Health Problems: Adult Health: Gastrointestinal: Fatty Liver Disease
Priority Concepts: Clinical Judgment; Clotting

Answer: 4
Rationale: The liver is located on the right side of the body. After a liver biopsy, the nurse positions the client on the right side with a small pillow or folded towel under the puncture site for 2 hours. This position compresses the liver against the abdominal wall at the biopsy site to tamponade bleeding from the puncture site.
Test-Taking Strategy: Focus on the subject, liver biopsy. Use knowledge regarding the anatomy of the body and principles of hemostasis to answer this question. Remember that the liver is on the right side of the body, and by applying pressure at the puncture site, the nurse helps prevent the escape of blood or bile.
Priority Nursing Tip: Because of the concern for bleeding after a liver biopsy, coagulation blood studies (prothrombin time, partial thromboplastin time, platelet count) are performed before the procedure is done.
References: Lewis, S., et al. (2020). *Medical-surgical nursing: Assessment and management of clinical problems* (11th ed., pp. 846–847). Elsevier; Pagana, K., Pagana, T., & Pagana, T. N. (2021). *Mosby's Diagnostic and laboratory test reference* (15th ed., pp. 576–578). Elsevier.

Client Needs

99. A client has a prescription to receive an enema before a surgical procedure to remove a bowel tumor. The nurse assists the client into which **best** position to administer the enema? **Refer to figure.**

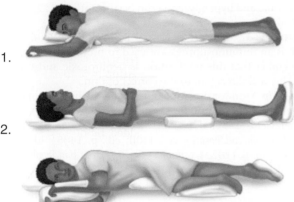

1.

2.

3.

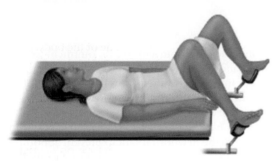

4.

Level of Cognitive Ability: Applying
Client Needs: Physiological Integrity
Clinical Judgment/Cognitive Skills: Take Action
Integrated Process: Nursing Process/Implementation
Content Area: Skills: Elimination
Health Problems: Adult Health: Cancer: Esophageal/Gastric/Intestinal
Priority Concepts: Clinical Judgment; Elimination

Answer: 3
Rationale: When administering an enema, the nurse places the client in a modified lateral position (option 3) exposing the rectal area and allowing the enema solution to flow by gravity in the natural direction of the colon. In the prone position (option 1), the client is lying on the stomach. In the supine position (option 2), the client is lying on the back. The dorsal recumbent position (option 4) is used for abdominal assessment because it promotes relaxation of abdominal muscles.
Test-Taking Strategy: Note the strategic word, *best*. Focus on the subject, enema administration. Use knowledge regarding the anatomy of the bowel to answer the question. This will assist in eliminating options 2 and 4. From the remaining options, visualize the procedure for administering an enema and eliminate option 1 because, in the prone position, the client is lying on the stomach.
Priority Nursing Tip: Administering an enema with the client sitting on the toilet can cause injury to the rectal mucosa because the rectal tubing is curved and could scratch the tissue.
Reference: Potter, P., et al. (2021). *Fundamentals of nursing* (10th ed., pp. 1220–1221). Elsevier.

❖ **100.** The nurse is caring for a client who is receiving cyclosporine following a kidney transplant. Which condition indicates to the nurse that the client is experiencing an adverse effect of the medication?
1. Acne
2. Sweating
3. Joint pain
4. Hyperkalemia

Level of Cognitive Ability: Analyzing
Client Needs: Physiological Integrity
Clinical Judgment/Cognitive Skills: Analyze Cues
Integrated Process: Clinical Judgment; Nursing Process/Assessment
Content Area: Pharmacology: Immune: Immunosuppressants
Health Problems: Adult Health: Immune: Transplantation
Priority Concepts: Immunity; Clinical Judgment

Answer: 4
Rationale: Cyclosporine is an immunosuppressant medication used in the prophylaxis of organ rejection. Adverse effects include nephrotoxicity, infection, hepatotoxicity, hypomagnesemia, coma, hypertension, tremor, and hirsutism. Additionally, neurotoxicity, gastrointestinal effects, hyperkalemia, and hyperglycemia can occur. Options 1, 2, and 3 are not associated with this medication.
Test-Taking Strategy: Focus on the **subject**, cyclosporine. Recall that this medication is an immunosuppressant used to prevent organ rejection. Next, remember that this medication is nephrotoxic and causes hyperkalemia. This will direct you to the correct option.
Priority Nursing Tip: Monitor the urine output and the potassium level if a client is receiving a medication that is nephrotoxic.
References: Ignatavicius, D., et al. (2021). *Medical-surgical nursing: Concepts for interprofessional collaborative care* (10th ed., p. 1408). Elsevier; Kizior, R., & Hodgson, B. (2022). *Saunders Nursing drug handbook 2022* (pp. 286, 288). Elsevier.

101. A nursing childbirth educator tells a class of expectant parents that it is standard routine to instill the ophthalmic ointment form of which medication into the eyes of a newborn infant as a preventive measure against ophthalmia neonatorum?
1. Penicillin
2. Neomycin
3. Vitamin K
4. Erythromycin

Level of Cognitive Ability: Applying
Client Needs: Physiological Integrity
Clinical Judgment/Cognitive Skills: Generate Solutions
Integrated Process: Teaching and Learning
Content Area: Maternity: Newborn
Health Problems: Newborn: Infections
Priority Concepts: Infection; Safety

Answer: 4
Rationale: Ophthalmic erythromycin 0.5% ointment is a broad-spectrum antibiotic and is used prophylactically to prevent ophthalmia neonatorum, an eye infection acquired from the newborn infant's passage through the birth canal. Infection from these organisms can cause blindness or serious eye damage. Erythromycin is effective against *Neisseria gonorrhoeae* and *Chlamydia trachomatis*. Vitamin K is administered in an injectable form to the newborn infant to prevent abnormal bleeding, and it promotes liver formation of the clotting factors II, VII, IX, and X. Options 1 and 2 are incorrect and are not medications routinely used in the newborn.
Test-Taking Strategy: Focus on the **subject**, eye medication used for the prophylaxis of ophthalmia neonatorum. This will assist in eliminating option 3, an injection. From the remaining options, recalling that erythromycin is a broad-spectrum antibiotic will direct you to the correct option.
Priority Nursing Tip: Administer prophylactic eye medication to a newborn within 1 hour after birth.
Reference: McKinney, E. S., et al. (2022). *Maternal child nursing* (6th ed., pp. 469–470). Elsevier.

❖ **102.** The nurse is reviewing the records of recently admitted clients to the postpartum unit. The nurse determines which clients would have an increased risk for developing a puerperal infection? **Select all that apply.**
- ❏ **1.** A client who has given birth to a set of twins
- ❏ **2.** A client with a history of previous infections
- ❏ **3.** A client who had numerous vaginal examinations
- ❏ **4.** A client who has experienced three previous miscarriages
- ❏ **5.** A client who underwent a vaginal delivery of the newborn
- ❏ **6.** A client who experienced prolonged rupture of the membranes

Level of Cognitive Ability: Analyzing
Client Needs: Physiological Integrity
Clinical Judgment/Cognitive Skills: Analyze Cues
Integrated Process: Clinical Judgment; Nursing Process/Assessment
Content Area: Maternity: Postpartum
Health Problems: Maternity: Infections/Inflammations
Priority Concepts: Infection; Reproduction

Answer: 2, 3, 6
Rationale: Risk factors associated with puerperal infection include a history of previous infections, excessive number of vaginal examinations, cesarean births, prolonged rupture of the membranes, prolonged labor, trauma, and retained placental fragments. A vaginal delivery, a history of miscarriages, and the delivery of twins are not considered as risk factors for developing a puerperal infection.
Test-Taking Strategy: Focus on the subject, risks for developing a puerperal infection. Think about the causes of infection and select the options that present a pathway for bacteria to enter into the client's body.
Priority Nursing Tip: The temperature may be elevated during the first 24 hours postpartum because of the dehydrating effects of labor. However, a temperature higher than 100.4° F needs to be reported to the primary health care provider because it is an indication of infection.
Reference: McKinney, E. S., et al. (2022). *Maternal child nursing* (6th ed., pp. 614–615). Elsevier.

103. After assisting with a vaginal delivery, what would the nurse do to prevent heat loss via conduction in the newborn?
1. Wrap the newborn in a blanket.
2. Close the doors to the delivery room.
3. Dry the newborn with a warm blanket.
4. Place the newborn on a warm crib pad.

Level of Cognitive Ability: Applying
Client Needs: Physiological Integrity
Clinical Judgment/Cognitive Skills: Take Action
Integrated Process: Nursing Process/Implementation
Content Area: Maternity: Newborn
Health Problems: Newborn: Thermoregulation
Priority Concepts: Development; Thermoregulation

Answer: 4
Rationale: Hypothermia caused by conduction occurs when the newborn is on a cold surface, such as a cold pad or mattress. Warming the crib pad will assist in preventing hypothermia by conduction. Radiation occurs when heat from the newborn radiates to a colder surface. Convection occurs as air moves across the newborn's skin from an open door and heat is transferred to the air. Evaporation of moisture from a wet body dissipates heat along with the moisture. Keeping the newborn dry by drying the wet newborn at birth will prevent hypothermia via evaporation.
Test-Taking Strategy: Focus on the subject, preventing heat loss in the newborn. Note the word "conduction" in the question to assist in selecting the correct option. Recalling that conduction occurs when a baby is on a cold surface will assist in directing you to the correct option.
Priority Nursing Tip: Newborns do not shiver to produce heat. Instead, they have brown fat deposits, which produce heat.
Reference: McKinney, E. S., et al. (2022). *Maternal child nursing* (6th ed., pp. 432–433). Elsevier.

❖ **104.** After assessment and diagnostic evaluation, it has been determined that the client has a diagnosis of Lyme disease, stage II. The nurse assesses the client for which manifestation that is **most** indicative of this stage?
1. Lethargy
2. Headache
3. Erythematous rash
4. Cardiac dysrhythmias

Level of Cognitive Ability: Analyzing
Client Needs: Physiological Integrity
Clinical Judgment/Cognitive Skills: Recognize Cues
Integrated Process: Clinical Judgment; Nursing Process/Assessment
Content Area: Adult Health: Immune
Health Problems: Adult Health: Immune: Lyme Disease
Priority Concepts: Clinical Judgment; Immunity

Answer: 4
Rationale: Stage II of Lyme disease develops within 1 to 3 months in most untreated individuals. The most serious problems in this stage include cardiac dysrhythmias, dyspnea, dizziness, and neurologic disorders such as Bell's palsy and paralysis. These problems are not usually permanent. Flulike symptoms (headache and lethargy), muscle pain and stiffness, and a rash appear in stage I.
Test-Taking Strategy: Note the strategic word, *most.* Focus on the subject, Lyme disease. Recalling that a rash and flulike symptoms occur in stage I will assist you in eliminating options 1, 2, and 3 and direct you to the correct option.
Priority Nursing Tip: The typical ring-shaped rash of Lyme disease does not occur in all clients. Additionally, if a rash does occur, it can occur anywhere on the body, not only at the site of the tick bite.
Reference: Ignatavicius, D., et al. (2021). *Medical-surgical nursing: Concepts for interprofessional collaborative care* (10th ed., pp. 359–360). Elsevier.

105. The nurse is caring for a client with a diagnosis of pemphigus vulgaris. On assessment of the client, the nurse would look for which sign characteristic of this condition?
1. Turner's sign
2. Chvostek's sign
3. Nikolsky's sign
4. Trousseau's sign

Level of Cognitive Ability: Applying
Client Needs: Physiological Integrity
Clinical Judgment/Cognitive Skills: Recognize Cues
Integrated Process: Nursing Process/Assessment
Content Area: Adult Health: Immune
Health Problems: Adult Health: Immune: Autoimmune Disease
Priority Concepts: Clinical Judgment; Tissue Integrity

Answer: 3
Rationale: A hallmark sign of pemphigus vulgaris is Nikolsky's sign, which occurs when the epidermis can be rubbed off by slight friction or injury. Other characteristics include flaccid bullae that rupture easily and emit a foul-smelling drainage, leaving crusted, denuded skin. The lesions are common on the face, back, chest, and umbilicus. Even slight pressure on an intact blister may cause spread to adjacent skin. *Turner's sign* refers to a grayish discoloration of the flanks and is seen in clients with acute pancreatitis. *Chvostek's sign,* seen in tetany, is a spasm of the facial muscles elicited by tapping the facial nerve in the region of the parotid gland. *Trousseau's sign* is a sign for tetany, in which carpal spasm can be elicited by compressing the upper arm with a blood pressure cuff inflated above the systolic pressure and causing ischemia to the nerves distally.
Test-Taking Strategy: Focus on the subject, pemphigus vulgaris. Eliminate options 2 and 4 first because they are comparable or alike and both relate to tetany. From the remaining options, recalling that Turner's sign is related to pancreatitis will direct you to the correct option.
Priority Nursing Tip: Pemphigus vulgaris is a rare autoimmune disease that causes blister (bullae) formation. The nurse needs to provide gentle care to prevent disruption of the skin lesions.
Reference: Heuther, S., McCance, K., & Brashers, V. (2020). *Understanding pathophysiology* (7th ed., p. 1026). Elsevier.

❖ **106.** The nurse is caring for a child recovering from a tonsillectomy. Which fluid or food item would be offered to the child?
1. Green Jell-O
2. Cold soda pop
3. Butterscotch pudding
4. Cool cherry-flavored Kool-Aid

Level of Cognitive Ability: Applying
Client Needs: Physiological Integrity
Clinical Judgment/Cognitive Skills: Take Action
Integrated Process: Nursing Process/Implementation
Content Area: Pediatrics: Throat/Respiratory
Health Problems: Pediatric-Specific: Tonsillitis and Adenoiditis
Priority Concepts: Nutrition; Safety

Answer: 1
Rationale: After tonsillectomy, clear, cool liquids should be administered. Citrus, carbonated, and extremely hot or cold liquids need to be avoided because they may irritate the throat. Milk and milk products (pudding) are avoided because they coat the throat and cause the child to clear the throat, thus increasing the risk of bleeding. Red liquids need to be avoided because they give the appearance of blood if the child vomits.
Test-Taking Strategy: Focus on the subject, care after tonsillectomy. Avoiding foods and fluids that may irritate or cause bleeding is the concern. This will assist in eliminating options 2 and 3. The words "cherry-flavored" in option 4 is the clue that this is not an appropriate food item.
Priority Nursing Tip: After tonsillectomy, position the client prone or side-lying to facilitate mouth drainage.
Reference: McKinney, E. S., et al. (2022). *Maternal child nursing* (6th ed., pp. 1046–1048). Elsevier.

107. The nurse provides a class to new parents on newborn care. When teaching cord care, the nurse would instruct the parents to take which action?
   1. If antibiotic ointment has been applied to the cord, it is not necessary to do anything else to it.
   2. All that is necessary is to wash the cord with antibacterial soap and allow it to air-dry once a day.
   3. Apply alcohol thoroughly to the cord, being careful not to move the cord because it will cause pain to the newborn infant.
   4. Apply the prescribed cleansing agent to the cord, ensuring that all areas around the cord are cleaned two to three times a day.

Level of Cognitive Ability: Applying
Client Needs: Physiological Integrity
Clinical Judgment/Cognitive Skills: Generate Solutions
Integrated Process: Teaching and Learning
Content Area: Maternity: Newborn
Health Problems: N/A
Priority Concepts: Patient Education; Infection

Answer: 4
Rationale: The cord and base need to be cleansed with an agent as prescribed (some agencies use alcohol) thoroughly, two to three times per day. The steps are (1) lift the cord; (2) wipe around the cord, starting at the top; (3) clean the base of the cord; and (4) fold the diaper below the umbilical cord to allow the cord to air-dry and prevent contamination from urine. Antibiotic ointment is not normally prescribed. Continuation of cord care is necessary until the cord falls off within 7 to 14 days. Water and antibacterial soap are not necessary; in fact, the cord needs to be kept from getting wet. The infant does not feel pain in this area.
Test-Taking Strategy: Focus on the **subject**, umbilical cord care. Simply recalling that the cord needs to be cleansed two to three times a day will direct you to the correct option. Also, note the words "prescribed cleansing agent" in the correct option.
Priority Nursing Tip: The nurse needs to teach the parents of a newborn about the importance of providing cord care because the umbilical cord stump provides a medium for bacterial growth and can easily become infected.
Reference: McKinney, E. S., et al. (2022). *Maternal child nursing* (6th ed., pp. 475, 481). Elsevier.

❖ **108.** The nurse monitoring a preterm newborn infant for manifestations of respiratory distress syndrome (RDS) would assess the infant for which manifestations? **Select all that apply.**
   ☐ 1. Cyanosis
   ☐ 2. Tachypnea
   ☐ 3. Retractions
   ☐ 4. Nasal flaring
   ☐ 5. Acrocyanosis
   ☐ 6. Grunting respirations

Level of Cognitive Ability: Analyzing
Client Needs: Physiological Integrity
Clinical Judgment/Cognitive Skills: Recognize Cues
Integrated Process: Clinical Judgment; Nursing Process/Assessment
Content Area: Maternity: Newborn
Health Problems: Newborn: Respiratory Problems
Priority Concepts: Clinical Judgment; Gas Exchange

Answer: 1, 2, 3, 4, 6
Rationale: The newborn infant with RDS may present with clinical manifestation of cyanosis, tachypnea or apnea, chest wall retractions, audible grunts, or nasal flaring. Acrocyanosis, the bluish discoloration of the hands and feet, is associated with immature peripheral circulation and is not uncommon in the first few hours of life.
Test-Taking Strategy: Focus on the **subject**, manifestations of respiratory distress syndrome. Think about the pathophysiology associated with this disorder. Also, recalling that acrocyanosis may be a normal sign in a newborn infant will assist in eliminating it as an option.
Priority Nursing Tip: The presence of retractions indicates respiratory distress and possible hypoxemia.
Reference: McKinney, E. S., et al. (2022). *Maternal child nursing* (6th ed., p. 640). Elsevier.

109. The nurse assessing the apical heart rates of several different newborn infants notes that which heart rate is normal for this newborn population?
   1. 90 beats/min
   2. 140 beats/min
   3. 180 beats/min
   4. 190 beats/min

Level of Cognitive Ability: Applying
Client Needs: Physiological Integrity
Clinical Judgment/Cognitive Skills: Recognize Cues
Integrated Process: Nursing Process/Assessment
Content Area: Maternity: Newborn
Health Problems: N/A
Priority Concepts: Development; Perfusion

Answer: 2
Rationale: The normal heart rate in a newborn infant is approximately 120 to 160 beats/min. Options 1, 3, and 4 are incorrect. Option 1 indicates bradycardia, and options 3 and 4 indicate tachycardia.
Test-Taking Strategy: Focus on the **subject**, a newborn infant heart rate. Recalling the normal heart rate for a newborn infant will direct you to the correct option.
Priority Nursing Tip: To measure the apical heart rate of a newborn infant, the nurse would place the stethoscope at the fourth intercostal space and auscultate for 1 full minute.
Reference: McKinney, E. S., et al. (2022). *Maternal child nursing* (6th ed., p. 448). Elsevier.

❖ **110.** The physician prescribes a dose of intravenous (IV) potassium chloride for a client diagnosed with a cardiac dysrhythmia. When administering the IV potassium chloride, which action would the nurse take?
   1. Inject it as a bolus.
   2. Use a filter in the IV line.
   3. Dilute it per medication instructions.
   4. Apply cool compresses to the IV site.

Level of Cognitive Ability: Applying
Client Needs: Physiological Integrity
Clinical Judgment/Cognitive Skills: Take Action
Integrated Process: Nursing Process/Implementation
Content Area: Pharmacology: Fluid and Electrolyte Balance: Intravenous Fluids
Health Problems: Adult Health: Cardiovascular: Dysrhythmias
Priority Concepts: Clinical Judgment; Fluids and Electrolytes

Answer: 3
Rationale: Potassium chloride is very irritating to the vein, must be diluted to prevent phlebitis, and is administered using an IV pump. Potassium chloride is never administered as a bolus injection because it can cause cardiac arrest. A filter is not necessary for potassium solutions. Cool compresses would constrict the blood vessel, which could possibly be more irritating to the vein.
Test-Taking Strategy: Focus on the **subject**, intravenous potassium administration. Recalling that potassium chloride is always diluted before administration will eliminate option 1. From the remaining options, noting the words "per medication instructions" in option 3 will direct you to the correct option.
Priority Nursing Tip: After adding potassium to an intravenous (IV) solution, rotate and invert the solution bag to ensure that the potassium is distributed evenly throughout the IV solution. It is also important to rotate and invert the solution bag frequently during the infusion.
Reference: Gahart, B., Nazareno, A., & Ortega, M. (2021). *Gahart's 2021 Intravenous medications: A handbook for nurses and health professionals* (37th ed., pp. 1124–1125). Elsevier.

111. The nurse managing a child's post-supratentorial craniotomy care would ensure that the client is maintained in which position?
   1. Prone
   2. Supine
   3. Semi-Fowler's
   4. Dorsal recumbent

Level of Cognitive Ability: Applying
Client Needs: Physiological Integrity
Clinical Judgment/Cognitive Skills: Take Action
Integrated Process: Nursing Process/Implementation
Content Area: Pediatrics: Neurologic
Health Problems: Pediatric-Specific: Cancers
Priority Concepts: Intracranial Regulation; Clinical Judgment

Answer: 3
Rationale: After supratentorial surgery (surgery above the brain's tentorium sometimes preformed for glioma tumor removal), the child's head is usually elevated 30 degrees to promote venous outflow through the jugular veins and modulate intracranial pressure (ICP). Options 1, 2, and 4 are incorrect positions after this surgery because they are likely to increase ICP.
Test-Taking Strategy: Focus on the **subject**, supratentorial craniotomy. A helpful strategy is to remember the following: supra, above the brain's tentorium, head up. Also note that options 1 and 2 are **comparable or alike** in that they are flat positions; option 4 is eliminated because the increased intraabdominal pressure from this position is more likely to inhibit venous return from the brain.
Priority Nursing Tip: To prevent increased ICP, position the client to avoid extreme hip or neck flexion and maintain the head in a midline, neutral position.
Reference: Hockenberry, M., Wilson, D., & Rodgers, C. (2019). *Wong's Nursing care of infants and children* (11th ed., pp. 1094–1095). Elsevier.

❖ **112.** An infant has been found to be human immunodeficiency virus (HIV) positive. When teaching condition-specific care, which action would the nurse instruct the birthing parent to take to minimize the infant's risk for condition-related injury?
1. Check the anterior fontanel for bulging and the sutures for widening each day.
2. Feed the infant in an upright position with the head and chest tilted slightly back to avoid aspiration.
3. Feed the infant with a special nipple and burp the infant frequently to decrease the tendency to swallow air.
4. Provide meticulous skin care to the infant and change the infant's diaper after each voiding or stool.

Level of Cognitive Ability: Applying
Client Needs: Physiological Integrity
Clinical Judgment/Cognitive Skills: Generate Solutions
Integrated Process: Teaching and Learning
Content Area: Pediatrics: Immune
Health Problems: Pediatric-Specific: Immunodeficiency Disease
Priority Concepts: Patient Education; Immunity

Answer: 4
Rationale: Meticulous skin care helps protect the HIV-infected infant from secondary infections. Bulging fontanels, feeding the infant in an upright position, and using a special nipple are unrelated to the pathology associated with HIV.
Test-Taking Strategy: Focus on the **subject,** a newborn with HIV. Read the question carefully. The question specifically asks for instructions to be given to the birthing parent regarding HIV. Although options 1, 2, and 3 may be correct or partially correct, the content does not specifically relate to care of the infant infected with HIV.
Priority Nursing Tip: Newborns born to HIV-positive clients may test positive because the birthing parent's antibodies may persist in the newborn for 18 months after birth.
Reference: McKinney, E. S., et al. (2022). *Maternal child nursing* (6th ed., pp. 949–950). Elsevier.

113. The nurse is checking postoperative prescriptions and planning care for a 110-pound adolescent after spinal fusion. Morphine sulfate, 8 mg subcutaneously every 4 hours PRN for pain, is prescribed. The pediatric medication reference states that the safe dose is 0.1 to 0.2 mg/kg/dose every 3 to 4 hours. From this information, the nurse determines what about the prescription?
1. The dose is too low.
2. There is no safe range for children
3. The dose is within the safe dosage range.
4. There is not enough information to determine the safe dose.

Level of Cognitive Ability: Analyzing
Client Needs: Physiological Integrity
Clinical Judgment/Cognitive Skills: Analyze Cues
Integrated Process: Clinical Judgment; Nursing Process/Analysis
Content Area: Skills: Dosage Calculations
Health Problems: Pediatric-Specific: Pain
Priority Concepts: Clinical Judgment; Safety

Answer: 3
Rationale: Use the formula to determine the dosage parameters. Convert pounds to kilograms by dividing the weight by 2.2. Therefore, 110 lb ÷ 2.2 = 50 kg.
Dosage parameters:

$$0.1\,mg/kg/dose \times 50\,kg = 5\,mg$$

$$0.2\,mg/kg/dose \times 50\,kg = 10\,mg$$

Dosage is within the safe dosage range.
Test-Taking Strategy: Focus on the **subject,** a medication calculation. Identify the important components of the question and what the question is asking. In this case, the question asks for the safe dosage range for medication for a child. Change pounds to kilograms. Calculate the dosage parameters using the safe dose range identified in the question and the child's weight in kilograms. Use a calculator to verify the answer.
Priority Nursing Tip: Conversion is the first step in the calculation of medication doses.
Reference: Potter, P., et al. (2021). *Fundamentals of nursing* (10th ed., pp. 601–602). Elsevier.

❖ **114.** What action would the nurse take to assess the pharyngeal reflex on a child prescribed liquids post-appendectomy?
1. Ask client to swallow.
2. Pull down on the lower eyelid.
3. Shine a light toward the bridge of the nose.
4. Stimulate the back of the throat with a tongue depressor.

Level of Cognitive Ability: Applying
Client Needs: Physiological Integrity
Clinical Judgment/Cognitive Skills: Take Action
Integrated Process: Nursing Process/Assessment
Content Area: Health Assessment/Physical Exam: Neurologic
Health Problems: Pediatric-Specific: Appendicitis
Priority Concepts: Clinical Judgment; Health Promotion

Answer: 4
Rationale: The pharyngeal (gag) reflex is tested by touching the back of the throat with an object, such as a tongue depressor. A positive response to this reflex is considered normal. Asking the client to swallow assesses the swallowing reflex. To assess the palpebral conjunctiva, the nurse would pull down and evert the lower eyelid. The corneal light reflex is tested by shining a penlight toward the bridge of the nose at a distance of 12 to 15 inches (light reflection should be symmetric in both corneas).
Test-Taking Strategy: Focus on the subject, pharyngeal reflex. Recalling that "pharyngeal" refers to the pharynx, or back of the throat, will assist in determining how this reflex is tested and direct you to the correct option.
Priority Nursing Tip: If a client receives a local throat anesthetic for a diagnostic or other procedure, the client must remain nothing by mouth (NPO) until the gag reflex returns.
Reference: Jarvis, C. (2020). *Physical examination and health assessment* (8th ed., p. 376). Elsevier.

115. The nurse is monitoring a child with mumps for complications. Which manifestation is a sign of the **most** common complication of this disease?
1. Pain
2. Nuchal rigidity
3. Impaired hearing
4. A red, swollen testicle

Level of Cognitive Ability: Analyzing
Client Needs: Physiological Integrity
Clinical Judgment/Cognitive Skills: Recognize cues
Integrated Process: Nursing Process/Assessment
Content Area: Pediatrics: Infectious and Communicable Diseases
Health Problems: Pediatric-Specific: Communicable Diseases
Priority Concepts: Clinical Judgment; Infection

Answer: 2
Rationale: The most common complication of mumps is aseptic meningitis, with the virus being identified in the cerebrospinal fluid. Common signs include nuchal rigidity, lethargy, and vomiting. Muscular pain, parotid pain, or testicular pain may occur, but pain does not indicate a sign of a common complication. Although mumps is one of the primary causes of unilateral nerve deafness, it does not occur frequently. A red, swollen testicle may be indicative of orchitis. Although this complication appears to cause most concern among parents, it is not the most common complication.
Test-Taking Strategy: Focus on the subject, the most common complication of mumps, and the strategic word, *most*. Recalling that aseptic meningitis is the most common complication of mumps will direct you to the correct option.
Priority Nursing Tip: Transmission of mumps is via direct contact or droplet spread from an infected person.
Reference: McKinney, E. S., et al. (2022). *Maternal child nursing* (6th ed., p. 918). Elsevier.

❖ **116.** An adolescent is hospitalized with a diagnosis of Rocky Mountain spotted fever (RMSF). The nurse anticipates which medication will be prescribed?
1. Ganciclovir
2. Amantadine
3. Doxycycline
4. Amphotericin B

Level of Cognitive Ability: Applying
Client Needs: Physiological Integrity
Clinical Judgment/Cognitive Skills: Generate Solutions
Integrated Process: Nursing Process/Planning
Content Area: Pediatrics: Infectious and Communicable Diseases
Health Problems: Pediatric-Specific: Communicable Diseases
Priority Concepts: Clinical Judgment; Immunity

Answer: 3
Rationale: The nursing care of an adolescent with RMSF includes the administration of doxycycline. An alternative medication is chloramphenicol. Ganciclovir is used to treat cytomegalovirus. Amantadine is used to treat Parkinson's disease. Amphotericin B is used for fungal infections.
Test-Taking Strategy: Focus on the subject, Rocky Mountain spotted fever (RMSF). Knowledge regarding the treatment plan associated with RMSF is required to answer this question. Remember that RMSF is treated with doxycycline.
Priority Nursing Tip: The agent that causes RMSF is *Rickettsia rickettsii*; transmission is via the bite of an infected tick.
Reference: McKinney, E. S., et al. (2022). *Maternal child nursing* (6th ed., pp. 925–926). Elsevier.

117. A clinical nurse specialist is asked to present a clinical conference to the student group about brain tumors in children younger than 3 years. The nurse would include which information in the presentation?
   1. Radiation is the treatment of choice.
   2. The most significant symptoms are headache and vomiting.
   3. Head shaving is not required before removal of the brain tumor.
   4. Surgery is not normally performed because of the increased risk of functional deficits.

Level of Cognitive Ability: Applying
Client Needs: Physiological Integrity
Clinical Judgment/Cognitive Skills: Generate Solutions
Integrated Process: Teaching and Learning
Content Area: Pediatrics: Oncologic
Health Problems: Pediatric-Specific: Cancers
Priority Concepts: Cellular Regulation; Development

Answer: 2
Rationale: The classic symptoms of children with brain tumors are headaches and vomiting. The treatment of choice is total surgical removal of the tumor. Before surgery, the child's head will be shaved, although every effort is made to shave only as much hair as is necessary. Radiation therapy is avoided in children younger than 3 years because of the toxic side effects on the developing brain, particularly in very young children.
Test-Taking Strategy: Focus on the subject, brain tumors in children. Eliminate options 3 and 4 first because of the closed-ended word "not." From the remaining options, recalling that radiation therapy is avoided in children younger than 3 years because of the toxic side effects on the developing brain will lead you to the correct option.
Priority Nursing Tip: The headache associated with a brain tumor in a child is worse on awakening and improves during the day.
Reference: McKinney, E. S., et al. (2022). *Maternal child nursing* (6th ed., pp. 1164–1166). Elsevier.

❖ **118.** The nurse caring for a child admitted to the hospital with a diagnosis of viral pneumonia describes the treatment plan to the parents. The nurse determines the **need for further teaching** when the parents make which statement regarding the treatment?
   1. "We need to be very careful since oxygen is extremely flammable."
   2. "It's important that the child isn't allergic to the antibiotic that is prescribed."
   3. "It's difficult to watch the needle be inserted when intravenous fluids are needed."
   4. "Chest physiotherapy will loosen the congestion, so coughing will clear the lungs."

Level of Cognitive Ability: Evaluating
Client Needs: Physiological Integrity
Clinical Judgment/Cognitive Skills: Evaluate Outcomes
Integrated Process: Teaching and Learning
Content Area: Pediatrics: Throat/Respiratory
Health Problems: Pediatric-Specific: Pneumonia
Priority Concepts: Patient Education; Gas Exchange

Answer: 2
Rationale: The therapeutic management for viral pneumonia is supportive. Antibiotics are not given unless the pneumonia is bacterial. More severely ill children may be hospitalized and given oxygen, chest physiotherapy, and intravenous fluids.
Test-Taking Strategy: Note the strategic words, *need for further teaching.* These words indicate a negative event query and ask you to select an option that is an incorrect statement. Also note the word "viral" in the question. Recalling that viral infections are not treated with antibiotics will direct you to option 2. Oxygen, intravenous fluids, and chest physiotherapy are all appropriate interventions for this child.
Priority Nursing Tip: If a specimen culture is prescribed, the culture is obtained before prescribed antibiotics are initiated.
Reference: McKinney, E. S., et al. (2022). *Maternal child nursing* (6th ed., p. 1057). Elsevier.

119. Tretinoin gel has been prescribed for a client with acne. What is the nurse's response when the client calls and reports that, "My skin has become very red and is beginning to peel"?
1. "Discontinue the medication immediately."
2. "Come to the clinic immediately for an assessment."
3. "I'll notify your physician of these results."
4. "This is a normal occurrence with the use of this medication."

Level of Cognitive Ability: Applying
Client Needs: Physiological Integrity
Clinical Judgment/Cognitive Skills: Take Action
Integrated Process: Teaching and Learning
Content Area: Pharmacology: Integumentary: Acne Products
Health Problems: Adult Health: Integumentary: Inflammations/Infections
Priority Concepts: Patient Education; Safety

Answer: 4
Rationale: Tretinoin decreases cohesiveness of the epithelial cells, increasing cell mitosis and turnover. It is potentially irritating, particularly when used correctly. Within 48 hours of use, the skin generally becomes red and begins to peel. Options 1, 2, and 3 are incorrect statements to the client.
Test-Taking Strategy: Focus on the subject, tretinoin. Options 2 and 3 can be eliminated first because they are comparable or alike. Eliminate option 1 next because it is not within the scope of nursing practice to advise a client to discontinue a medication.
Priority Nursing Tip: Tretinoin is a derivative of vitamin A; therefore, vitamin A supplements need to be discontinued during therapy with tretinoin.
Reference: Skidmore-Roth, L. (2021). *2021 Mosby's Nursing drug reference* (34th ed., pp. 1265–1266). Elsevier.

❖ **120.** A child hospitalized with a diagnosis of lead poisoning is prescribed chelation therapy. The nurse caring for the child would prepare to administer which medication?
1. Ipecac syrup
2. Activated charcoal
3. Sodium bicarbonate
4. Sodium calcium edetate (sodium calcium EDTA)

Level of Cognitive Ability: Applying
Client Needs: Physiological Integrity
Clinical Judgment/Cognitive Skills: Generate Solutions
Integrated Process: Clinical Judgment; Nursing Process/Planning
Content Area: Complex Care: Poisoning
Health Problems: Pediatric-Specific: Poisoning
Priority Concepts: Clinical Judgment; Safety

Answer: 4
Rationale: EDTA is a chelating agent that is used to treat lead poisoning. Ipecac syrup may be prescribed by the physician for use in the hospital setting but would not be used to treat lead poisoning. Activated charcoal is used to decrease absorption in certain poisoning situations. Sodium bicarbonate may be used in salicylate poisoning.
Test-Taking Strategy: Focus on the subject, treatment related to lead poisoning. Think about the classifications of the medications in the options. Recalling that EDTA is a chelating agent will direct you to the correct option.
Priority Nursing Tip: During chelation therapy, provide adequate hydration and monitor kidney function for nephrotoxicity because the medication is excreted via the kidneys.
Reference: Hockenberry, M., Wilson, D., & Rodgers, C. (2019). *Wong's Nursing care of infants and children* (11th ed., pp. 449–450). Elsevier.

---

121. The nurse is performing pin-site care on a client in skeletal traction. Which normal finding would the nurse expect to note when assessing the pin sites?
1. Numbness at the pin sites
2. Warm skin around the pin sites
3. Clear drainage from the pin sites
4. Redness and swelling around the pin sites

Level of Cognitive Ability: Applying
Client Needs: Physiological Integrity
Clinical Judgment/Cognitive Skills: Recognize Cues
Integrated Process: Nursing Process/Assessment
Content Area: Adult Health: Musculoskeletal
Health Problems: Adult Health: Musculoskeletal: Skeletal Injury
Priority Concepts: Clinical Judgment; Mobility

Answer: 3
Rationale: A small amount of clear drainage ("weeping") may be expected after cleaning and removing crusting around the pin sites of skeletal traction. Warmth, numbness, redness and swelling around the pin sites may be indicative of an infection.
Test-Taking Strategy: Focus on the subject, pin-site care. Option 1 is not an expected finding and can be eliminated first because it could indicate a neurovascular problem. Eliminate options 2 and 4 next because they are comparable or alike and indicate signs of infection.
Priority Nursing Tip: Skeletal traction is applied mechanically to the bone with pins, wires, or tongs. Because skin integrity is disrupted, the client is at risk for infection.
Reference: Ignatavicius, D., et al. (2021). *Medical-surgical nursing: Concepts for interprofessional collaborative care* (10th ed., p. 1039). Elsevier.

❖ **122.** The nurse, caring for a client who has been placed in Buck's extension traction while awaiting surgical repair of a fractured femur, would perform a complete neurovascular assessment of the affected extremity that includes which assessments? **Select all that apply.**
   - ❑ 1. Vital signs
   - ❑ 2. Bilateral lung sounds
   - ❑ 3. Pulse in the affected extremity
   - ❑ 4. Level of pain in the affected leg
   - ❑ 5. Skin color of the affected extremity
   - ❑ 6. Capillary refill of the affected toes

Level of Cognitive Ability: Applying
Client Needs: Physiological Integrity
Clinical Judgment/Cognitive Skills: Take Action
Integrated Process: Clinical Judgment; Nursing Process/Assessment
Content Area: Adult Health: Musculoskeletal
Health Problems: Adult Health: Musculoskeletal: Skeletal Injury
Priority Concepts: Mobility; Perfusion

Answer: 3, 4, 5, 6
Rationale: A complete neurovascular assessment of an extremity includes color, sensation, movement, capillary refill, and pulse of the affected extremity. Options 1 and 2 are not related to neurovascular assessment.
Test-Taking Strategy: Focus on the subject, complete neurovascular assessment. Eliminate options that are not considered components of a neurovascular assessment. Also, use the ABCs—airway, breathing, and circulation—to direct you to the correct option.
Priority Nursing Tip: Buck's extension traction is a type of skin traction used to alleviate muscle spasms and immobilize a lower limb. It is applied by using elastic bandages or adhesive, a foam boot, or a sling, and counterweights, and the foot of the bed is elevated to provide the traction.
Reference: Ignatavicius, D., et al. (2021). *Medical-surgical nursing: Concepts for interprofessional collaborative care* (10th ed., pp. 1033, 1040). Elsevier.

123. The nurse prepares to transfer the client with a newly applied arm cast into the bed using which method?
   1. Placing ice on top of the cast
   2. Supporting the cast with the fingertips only
   3. Asking client to support the cast during transfer
   4. Using the palms of the hands and soft pillows to support the cast

Level of Cognitive Ability: Applying
Client Needs: Physiological Integrity
Clinical Judgment/Cognitive Skills: Generate Solutions
Integrated Process: Nursing Process/Planning
Content Area: Adult Health: Musculoskeletal
Health Problems: Adult Health: Musculoskeletal: Skeletal Injury
Priority Concepts: Mobility; Tissue Integrity

Answer: 4
Rationale: The palms or the flat surface of the extended fingers should be used when moving a wet cast to prevent indentations. Pillows are used to support the curves of the cast to prevent cracking or flattening of the cast from the weight of the body. Half-full bags of ice may be placed next to the cast to prevent swelling, but this would be done after the client is placed in bed. Asking the client to support the cast during transfer is inappropriate.
Test-Taking Strategy: Focus on the subject, cast care. Eliminate option 1 because ice can be used for swelling after the client is placed in bed. Eliminate option 2 because of the closed-ended word "only" in this option. Eliminate option 3 because it is inappropriate to ask the client to support the cast.
Priority Nursing Tip: Instruct the client with a cast not to stick objects inside the cast because the object can disrupt skin integrity and result in infection. If the skin under the cast is itchy, instruct the client to direct cool air from a hair dryer inside the cast.
Reference: Ignatavicius, D., et al. (2021). *Medical-surgical nursing: Concepts for interprofessional collaborative care* (10th ed., pp. 1036–1037). Elsevier.

❖ **124.** A magnetic resonance imaging (MRI) scan is prescribed for a client with a suspected brain tumor. Which prescription would the nurse expect to be prescribed for the client before the procedure?
1. An opioid
2. A mild sedative
3. A corticosteroid
4. An antihistamine

Level of Cognitive Ability: Applying
Client Needs: Physiological Integrity
Clinical Judgment/Cognitive Skills: Generate Solutions
Integrated Process: Nursing Process/Planning
Content Area: Foundations of Care: Diagnostic Tests
Health Problems: Adult Health: Cancer: Brain Tumors
Priority Concepts: Clinical Judgment; Safety

Answer: **2**
Rationale: An MRI scan is a noninvasive diagnostic test that visualizes the body's tissues, structure, and blood flow. For an MRI, the client is positioned on a padded table and moved into a cylinder-shaped scanner. Relaxation techniques, an eye mask, and sedation are used before the procedure to reduce claustrophobic effects; however, because the client must remain very still during the scan, the nurse avoids oversedating the client to ensure client cooperation. There is no useful purpose for administering an opioid, corticosteroid, or antihistamine. Open MRI systems are available in some diagnostic facilities and this method of testing can be used for clients with claustrophobia.
Test-Taking Strategy: Focus on the **subject,** magnetic resonance imaging (MRI) scan. Recalling that claustrophobia is a concern will direct you to the correct option.
Priority Nursing Tip: In an MRI scan, magnetic fields are used to produce an image. Therefore, all metallic objects such as a watch, other jewelry, clothing with metal fasteners, and metal hair fasteners must be removed.
Reference: Pagana, K., Pagana, T., & Pagana, T. N. (2021). *Mosby's Diagnostic and laboratory test reference* (15th ed., p. 606). Elsevier.

125. A dose of ondansetron is prescribed for a client receiving chemotherapy for a brain tumor. The nurse anticipates that the physician will prescribe the medication by which route during the chemotherapy infusion?
1. Oral
2. Intranasal
3. Intravenous
4. Subcutaneous

Level of Cognitive Ability: Applying
Client Needs: Physiological Integrity
Clinical Judgment/Cognitive Skills: Generate Solutions
Integrated Process: Clinical Judgment; Nursing Process/Planning
Content Area: Pharmacology: Gastrointestinal: Antiemetics
Health Problems: Adult Health: Cancer: Brain Tumors
Priority Concepts: Cellular Regulation; Safety

Answer: **3**
Rationale: Ondansetron is an antiemetic used to control nausea, vomiting, and motion sickness. It is available for administration by the oral, intramuscular (IM), or intravenous (IV) routes. The IV route is the route used when relief of nausea is needed in the client receiving chemotherapy. The IM route may be used when the medication is used as an adjunct to anesthesia. Option 1 should not be used in clients who are nauseated. Options 2 and 4 are not routes of administration of this medication.
Test-Taking Strategy: Focus on the **subject,** ondansetron administration to a client receiving chemotherapy. Noting that the client is receiving chemotherapy will direct you to the correct option.
Priority Nursing Tip: Antiemetics can cause drowsiness and hypotension; therefore, a priority intervention is to protect the client from injury.
Reference: Gahart, B., Nazareno, A., & Ortega, M. (2021). *Gahart's 2021 Intravenous medications: A handbook for nurses and health professionals* (37th ed., p. 1011). Elsevier.

❖ **126.** The nurse is teaching the parents of a child diagnosed with celiac disease about dietary measures. The nurse would instruct the parents to take which measure?
1. Restrict corn and rice in the diet.
2. Restrict fresh vegetables in the diet.
3. Substitute grain cereals with pasta products.
4. Avoid foods that contain hidden sources of gluten.

Level of Cognitive Ability: Applying
Client Needs: Physiological Integrity
Clinical Judgment/Cognitive Skills: Take Action
Integrated Process: Teaching and Learning
Content Area: Foundations of Care: Therapeutic Diets
Health Problems: Pediatric-Specific: Nutrition Problems
Priority Concepts: Patient Education; Nutrition

Answer: **4**
Rationale: Gluten is found primarily in the grains of wheat, rye, barley, and oats. Gluten is added to many foods as hydrolyzed vegetable protein that is derived from cereal grains; therefore, labels need to be read. Corn and rice, as well as vegetables, are acceptable in a gluten-free diet, and corn and rice become substitute foods. Many pasta products contain gluten. Grains are frequently added to processed foods for thickness or fillers.
Test-Taking Strategy: Focus on the **subject,** celiac diet. Recall that a gluten-free diet is required in celiac disease. Select option 4 because it is the **umbrella option.**
Priority Nursing Tip: Celiac crisis is precipitated by fasting, infection, or the ingestion of gluten. It causes profuse watery diarrhea and vomiting, leading to rapid dehydration, electrolyte imbalance, and severe acidosis.
Reference: McKinney, E. S., et al. (2022). *Maternal child nursing* (6th ed., pp. 996–997). Elsevier.

127. A client, admitted to the hospital for evaluation of recurrent runs of ventricular tachycardia, is scheduled for electrophysiology studies (EPS). Which statement would the nurse include in a teaching plan for this client?
1. "You will continue to take your medications until the morning of the test."
2. "You will be sedated during the procedure and will not remember what has happened."
3. "This test is a noninvasive method of determining the effectiveness of your medication regimen."
4. "The test uses a special wire to increase the heart rate and produce the irregular beats that cause your signs and symptoms."

Level of Cognitive Ability: Applying
Client Needs: Physiological Integrity
Clinical Judgment/Cognitive Skills: Take Action
Integrated Process: Teaching and Learning
Content Area: Foundations of Care: Diagnostic Tests
Health Problems: Adult Health: Cardiovascular: Dysrhythmias
Priority Concepts: Patient Education; Perfusion

Answer: 4
Rationale: The purpose of EPS is to study the heart's electrical system. During this invasive procedure, a special wire is introduced into the heart to produce dysrhythmias. To prepare for this procedure, the client needs to be nothing by mouth (NPO) for 6 to 8 hours before the test, and all antidysrhythmics are held for at least 24 hours before the test to study the dysrhythmias without the influence of medications. Because the client's verbal responses to the rhythm changes are extremely important, sedation is avoided if possible.
Test-Taking Strategy: Focus on the **subject,** electrophysiology studies (EPS). Note the relationship between the words "recurrent runs of ventricular tachycardia" in the question and "produce the irregular beats" in option 4.
Priority Nursing Tip: Inducing a dysrhythmia during electrophysiology studies assists the physician in making a diagnosis and determining the appropriate treatment.
Reference: Lewis, S., et al. (2020). *Medical-surgical nursing: Assessment and management of clinical problems* (11th ed., pp. 672, 676). Elsevier.

❖ **128.** The nurse providing diet teaching to a client experiencing heart failure instructs the client to avoid which food item?
1. Sherbet
2. Steak sauce
3. Apple juice
4. Leafy green vegetables

Level of Cognitive Ability: Applying
Client Needs: Physiological Integrity
Clinical Judgment/Cognitive Skills: Take Action
Integrated Process: Teaching and Learning
Content Area: Foundations of Care: Therapeutic Diets
Health Problems: Adult Health: Cardiovascular: Heart Failure
Priority Concepts: Patient Education; Nutrition

Answer: 2
Rationale: Steak sauce is high in sodium. Leafy green vegetables, any juice (except tomato or V8 brand vegetable), and sherbet are all low in sodium. Clients with heart failure need to monitor sodium intake.
Test-Taking Strategy: Focus on the **subject,** a client with heart failure. Note the word "avoid." This word asks you to select an inappropriate food choice. Note that options 1, 3, and 4 are **comparable or alike** in that they are low-sodium foods. Recalling that the client with heart failure needs to limit sodium intake will direct you to the correct option.
Priority Nursing Tip: Clients with heart failure need to monitor sodium intake because sodium causes the retention of fluid.
References: Ignatavicius, D., et al. (2021). *Medical-surgical nursing: Concepts for interprofessional collaborative care* (10th ed., pp. 674, 681). Elsevier; Nix, S. (2022). *Williams' Basic nutrition and diet therapy* (16th ed., p. 532). Elsevier.

129. The nurse is creating a plan of care for a client diagnosed with type 1 diabetes mellitus who is also experiencing acute gastroenteritis. To maintain food and fluid intake in order to prevent dehydration, which action would the nurse plan to include?
1. Offering only water until client is able to tolerate solid foods
2. Withholding all fluids until vomiting has ceased entirely for at least 4 hours
3. Encouraging client to take 8 to 12 ounces of fluid every hour while awake
4. Maintaining a clear liquid diet for at least 5 days before advancing to solid foods

Level of Cognitive Ability: Creating
Client Needs: Physiological Integrity
Clinical Judgment/Cognitive Skills: Generate Solutions
Integrated Process: Clinical Judgment; Nursing Process/Planning
Content Area: Foundations of Care: Fluids and Electrolytes
Health Problems: Adult Health: Endocrine: Diabetes Mellitus
Priority Concepts: Fluids and Electrolytes; Glucose Regulation

Answer: 3
Rationale: Dehydration needs to be prevented in the client with type 1 diabetes mellitus because of the risk of diabetic ketoacidosis (DKA). Small amounts of fluid may be tolerated, even when vomiting is present. The client needs to be offered liquids containing both glucose and electrolytes. The diet should be advanced as tolerated and include a minimum of 100 to 150 g of carbohydrates daily. Offering water only and maintaining liquids for 5 days will not prevent dehydration but may promote it in this client.
Test-Taking Strategy: Focus on the subject, type 1 diabetes mellitus. Eliminate options 1 and 2 because of the closed-ended words "only" and "all" in these options, respectively. From the remaining options, note the words "for at least 5 days" in option 4. Thinking about the subject, a client with diabetes mellitus and preventing dehydration, will assist in eliminating this option.
Priority Nursing Tip: Diabetic ketoacidosis is a life-threatening complication of type 1 diabetes mellitus that develops when a severe insulin deficiency occurs.
Reference: Ignatavicius, D., et al. (2021). *Medical-surgical nursing: Concepts for interprofessional collaborative care* (10th ed., p. 1294). Elsevier.

❖ **130.** The nurse in the postpartum unit is assessing for signs of breast-feeding problems demonstrated by either the newborn or the birthing parent. Which findings indicate a problem? **Select all that apply.**
❑ 1. The infant exhibits dimpling of the cheeks.
❑ 2. The infant makes smacking or clicking sounds.
❑ 3. The breast gets softer during a feeding.
❑ 4. Milk drips from the breast occasionally.
❑ 5. The infant falls asleep after feeding less than 5 minutes.
❑ 6. The infant can be heard swallowing frequently during a feeding.

Level of Cognitive Ability: Analyzing
Client Needs: Physiological Integrity
Clinical Judgment/Cognitive Skills: Recognize Cues
Integrated Process: Nursing Process/Assessment
Content Area: Maternity: Postpartum
Health Problems: Newborn: Newborn Feeding
Priority Concepts: Nutrition; Reproduction

Answer: 1, 2, 5
Rationale: It is important for the nurse to identify breast-feeding problems while the birthing parent is hospitalized so that the nurse can teach the client how to prevent and treat any problems. Infant signs of breast-feeding problems include dimpling of the cheeks; making smacking or clicking sounds; falling asleep after feeding less than 5 minutes; refusing to breast-feed; tongue thrusting; failing to open the mouth at latch-on; turning the lower lip in; making short, choppy motions of the jaw; and not swallowing audibly. Softening of the breast during feeding, noting milk in the infant's mouth or dripping from the breast occasionally, and hearing the infant swallow are signs that the infant is receiving adequate nutrition.
Test-Taking Strategy: Focus on the subject, signs of breast-feeding problems. Think about the process of feeding and visualize the effect of each observation identified in the options. This will direct you to the correct options.
Priority Nursing Tip: If the birthing parent is breast-feeding, calorie needs increase by 200 to 500 calories per day; increased fluids and the continuance of prenatal vitamins and minerals are important.
Reference: McKinney, E. S., et al. (2022). *Maternal child nursing* (6th ed., pp. 496, 498). Elsevier.

131. The nurse has completed tracheostomy care for a client whose tracheostomy tube has a non-disposable inner cannula. Which intervention will the nurse implement **immediately** before reinserting the inner cannula?
1. Rinsing it in sterile water
2. Suctioning the client's airway
3. Tapping it gently against a sterile basin
4. Drying it with the sterile gauze or specialized pipe cleaner

Level of Cognitive Ability: Applying
Client Needs: Physiological Integrity
Clinical Judgment/Cognitive Skills: Take Action
Integrated Process: Nursing Process/Implementation
Content Area: Skills: Tube Care
Health Problems: Adult Health: Respiratory: Artificial Airways
Priority Concepts: Clinical Judgment; Safety

Answer: 4
Rationale: After washing and rinsing the inner cannula, the nurse taps it dry to remove large water droplets and then uses sterile gauze or pipe cleaners specifically for use with a tracheostomy to dry it; then the nurse inserts the cannula into the tracheostomy and turns it clockwise to lock it into place. The nurse would avoid shaking or tapping the inner cannula to prevent contamination. A wet cannula would not be inserted into a tracheostomy because water is a lung irritant. Suctioning is not performed without an inner cannula in place.
Test-Taking Strategy: Note the strategic word, *immediately*. Also note the word "nondisposable" and visualize the procedure. Eliminate option 1 because a wet cannula would not be inserted and option 2 because you would not suction a client without the inner cannula in place. Eliminate option 3 because tapping could contaminate the inner cannula.
Priority Nursing Tip: Keep a tracheostomy obturator and a tracheostomy tube of the same size by the bedside for emergency replacement if the tracheostomy is dislodged.
Reference: Lewis, S., et al. (2020). *Medical-surgical nursing: Assessment and management of clinical problems* (11th ed., p. 491). Elsevier.

❖ **132.** The nurse suspects that an air embolism has occurred when the client's central venous catheter disconnects from the intravenous (IV) tubing. The nurse **immediately** places the client on the left side in which position?
1. Fetal
2. High-Fowler's
3. Trendelenburg's
4. Lateral recumbent

Level of Cognitive Ability: Applying
Client Needs: Physiological Integrity
Clinical Judgment/Cognitive Skills: Take Action
Integrated Process: Clinical Judgment; Nursing Process/Implementation
Content Area: Complex Care: Emergency Situations/Management
Health Problems: Adult Health: Respiratory: Pulmonary Embolism
Priority Concepts: Clinical Judgment; Gas Exchange

Answer: 3
Rationale: If the client develops an air embolism, the immediate action is to place the client in Trendelenburg's position on the left side. This position raises the client's feet higher than the head and traps any air in the right atrium. If necessary, the air can then be directly removed by intracardiac aspiration. Option 2 is incorrect because that position elevates the head, putting the air in a dependent position, and increasing the risk of a cerebral embolism; lying flat in either the lateral or fetal position does not help trap the air in the right atrium.
Test-Taking Strategy: Focus on the subject, air embolism. Note the strategic word, *immediately*. Visualize each position in the options and recall cardiac anatomy. Recalling that the goal of action is to trap air in the right atrium will direct you to the correct option.
Priority Nursing Tip: If an air embolism is suspected, the intravenous tubing is clamped off immediately.
Reference: Ignatavicius, D., et al. (2021). *Medical-surgical nursing: Concepts for interprofessional collaborative care* (10th ed., p. 291). Elsevier.

133. An anxious client enters the emergency department, seeking treatment for a laceration of the finger. The client's vital signs are pulse 106 beats/min, blood pressure (BP) 158/88 mm Hg, and respirations 28 breaths/min. After cleansing the injury and reassuring the client, the nurse rechecks the vital signs and notes a pulse of 82 beats/min, BP 130/80 mm Hg, and respirations 20 breaths/min. Which factor likely accounts for the change in vital signs?
1. Cooling effects of the cleansing agent
2. Client's adaptation to the air conditioning
3. Early clinical indicators of cardiogenic shock
4. Decline in sympathetic nervous system discharge

Level of Cognitive Ability: Analyzing
Client Needs: Physiological Integrity
Clinical Judgment/Cognitive Skills: Analyze Cues
Integrated Process: Clinical Judgment; Nursing Process/Analysis
Content Area: Adult Health: Integumentary
Health Problems: Adult Health: Integumentary: Wounds
Priority Concepts: Perfusion; Stress

Answer: 4
Rationale: Physical or emotional stress triggers sympathetic nervous system stimulation. Increased epinephrine and norepinephrine cause tachycardia, high blood pressure, and tachypnea. Stress reduction then returns these parameters to baseline as the sympathetic discharge falls. Options 1 and 2 are unrelated to the changes in vital signs. Based on the vital signs and injury type, the client exhibits no indication of cardiogenic shock.
Test-Taking Strategy: Focus on the subject, stress effects on vital signs. Eliminate options 1 and 2 first because they are comparable or alike in that they are not related to factors that could notably change the vital signs. Next, note that the client is anxious and has an injury. These two pieces of information guide you to think about the body's response to stress. Recalling the relationship of stress to the sympathetic nervous system will direct you to the correct option.
Priority Nursing Tip: Anxiety can cause an increase in the pulse rate, respiratory rate, and blood pressure.
Reference: Ignatavicius, D., et al. (2021). *Medical-surgical nursing: Concepts for interprofessional collaborative care* (10th ed., p. 829). Elsevier.

❖ **134.** An echocardiogram, chest x-ray (CXR), and computed axial tomography (CAT) scan are prescribed for a client being evaluated for possible coronary artery disease who has been demonstrating activity intolerance. In which order would the nurse plan to schedule the procedures to meet the needs of this client safely and **effectively**?
1. CAT scan and CXR in the morning and echocardiogram on the following morning
2. CXR and echocardiogram together in the morning and CAT scan in the afternoon of the same day
3. Echocardiogram in the morning and CXR and CAT scans together in the afternoon of the same day
4. CXR in the morning, echocardiogram in the afternoon, and CAT scan in the morning of the following day

Level of Cognitive Ability: Analyzing
Client Needs: Physiological Integrity
Clinical Judgment/Cognitive Skills: Generate Solutions
Integrated Process: Clinical Judgment; Nursing Process/Planning
Content Area: Foundations of Care: Diagnostic Tests
Health Problems: Adult Health: Cardiovascular: Coronary Artery Disease
Priority Concepts: Functional Ability; Perfusion

Answer: 4
Rationale: CAT scans are always performed in radiology, and CXR and echocardiograms can be done at the bedside; however, the best results usually occur when the test is performed in the related department. As long as the client is stable and transportation is provided, the nurse can schedule each procedure in its department with two procedures on the first day separated by a rest period, and the remaining procedure the next day. The nurse would plan the CXR and echocardiogram on the same day because if the client's condition deteriorates after the first procedure, the nurse can obtain a portable CXR or echocardiogram.
Test-Taking Strategy: Focus on the subject, scheduling multiple diagnostic procedures for the client with heart failure who has activity intolerance. Note the strategic word, *effectively*. Recalling that the client will do best if activities are spaced will direct you to the correct option.
Priority Nursing Tip: The nurse would instruct the client with heart failure to balance periods of rest and activity and avoid performing isometric activities because they increase pressure in the heart.
Reference: Lewis, S., et al. (2020). *Medical-surgical nursing: Assessment and management of clinical problems* (11th ed., pp. 472, 669–670). Elsevier.

135. The nurse is preparing to initiate an intravenous nitroglycerin drip on a client who has experienced an acute myocardial infarction. In the absence of an arterial monitoring line, the nurse prepares to have which piece of equipment for use at the bedside to help ensure the client's safety?
1. Defibrillator
2. Pulse oximeter
3. Central venous pressure (CVP) tray
4. Noninvasive blood pressure monitor

Level of Cognitive Ability: Applying
Client Needs: Physiological Integrity
Clinical Judgment/Cognitive Skills: Generate Solutions
Integrated Process: Clinical Judgment; Nursing Process/Planning
Content Area: Complex Care: Emergency Situations/Management
Health Problems: Adult Health: Cardiovascular: Myocardial Infarction
Priority Concepts: Perfusion; Safety

Answer: 4
Rationale: Nitroglycerin dilates arteries and veins (vasodilator), causing peripheral blood pooling, thus reducing preload, afterload, and myocardial workload. This action accounts for the primary side effect of nitroglycerin, which is hypotension. In the absence of an arterial monitoring line, the nurse needs to have a noninvasive blood pressure monitor for use at the bedside. None of the other options would monitor blood pressure. Additionally, the client needs to be on a cardiac monitor.
Test-Taking Strategy: Focus on the **subject**, initiating an intravenous nitroglycerin drip on a client with acute myocardial infarction. Note the words "arterial monitoring line." Recalling the purpose of this type of monitoring device and the action of nitroglycerin will direct you to the correct option.
Priority Nursing Tip: An intravenous infusion device such as a pump or controller must be used when administering nitroglycerin via the intravenous route.
Reference: Gahart, B., Nazareno, A., & Ortega, M. (2021). *Gahart's 2021 Intravenous medications: A handbook for nurses and health professionals* (37th ed., p. 973). Elsevier.

❖ **136.** A client in labor has a diagnosis of sickle cell anemia. Which action would the nurse take to assist in preventing the client from experiencing a sickling crisis during labor?
1. Being reassuring
2. Administering oxygen
3. Preventing bearing down
4. Maintaining strict asepsis

Level of Cognitive Ability: Applying
Client Needs: Physiological Integrity
Clinical Judgment/Cognitive Skills: Take Action
Integrated Process: Clinical Judgment; Nursing Process/Implementation
Content Area: Maternity: Intrapartum
Health Problems: Adult Health: Hematologic: Anemias
Priority Concepts: Clinical Judgment; Gas Exchange

Answer: 2
Rationale: During the labor process, the client with sickle cell anemia is at high risk for being unable to meet the oxygen demands of labor. Administering oxygen will prevent sickle cell crisis during labor. Intravenous (IV) fluid therapy will also reduce the risk of a sickle cell crisis. Options 1 and 4 are appropriate actions but are unrelated to sickle cell crisis. Option 3 is inappropriate.
Test-Taking Strategy: Focus on the client's diagnosis and use the ABCs—airway, breathing, and circulation—to direct you to the correct option.
Priority Nursing Tip: During labor, the client with sickle cell anemia needs to receive oxygen and fluids to prevent hypoxemia and dehydration because these conditions stimulate the sickling process.
Reference: McKinney, E. S., et al. (2022). *Maternal child nursing* (6th ed., p. 568). Elsevier.

137. A client is scheduled for computed tomography (CT) of the kidneys to rule out renal cancer. Which would the nurse assess the client for before the procedure to **best** ensure the client's safety?
1. Allergies
2. Familial renal disease
3. Frequent antibiotic use
4. Long-term diuretic therapy

Level of Cognitive Ability: Applying
Client Needs: Physiological Integrity
Clinical Judgment/Cognitive Skills: Recognize Cues
Integrated Process: Nursing Process/Assessment
Content Area: Foundations of Care: Diagnostic Tests
Health Problems: Adult Health: Cancer: Bladder and Kidney
Priority Concepts: Clinical Judgment; Safety

Answer: 1
Rationale: The client undergoing any type of diagnostic testing involving possible dye administration needs to be questioned about allergies, specifically an allergy to shellfish or iodine. This is essential to identify the risk for potential allergic reaction to contrast dye, which may be used. The other items are also useful as part of the assessment but are not as critical as the allergy determination in the preprocedure period in the attempt to maximize client safety.
Test-Taking Strategy: Note the strategic word, *best,* and focus on the subject, preprocedural CT scan. Because the question indicates that CT of the kidneys is planned, the items in the options are evaluated against their potential connection to this aspect of care. Recalling that contrast dye may be used during CT to enhance visualization of the kidneys will direct you to the correct option.
Priority Nursing Tip: The nurse needs to ask the client if they ever had an allergic reaction to contrast media used for diagnostic testing. If so, the client is at high risk for experiencing another reaction if contrast media is administered.
Reference: Pagana, K., Pagana, T., & Pagana, T. N. (2021). *Mosby's Diagnostic and laboratory test reference* (15th ed., p. 276). Elsevier.

❖ **138.** The nurse assists a client diagnosed with pyelonephritis in collecting a 24-hour urine specimen. Which instruction does the nurse provide to the client to ensure proper collection of the 24-hour urine specimen?
1. Void at the start time and discard the specimen.
2. Strain the specimen before pouring the urine into the container.
3. Save all urine, beginning with the urine voided at the start time.
4. Once completed, refrigerate the urine collection until you can bring it to the laboratory.

Level of Cognitive Ability: Applying
Client Needs: Physiological Integrity
Clinical Judgment/Cognitive Skills: Take Action
Integrated Process: Nursing Process/Implementation
Content Area: Skills: Specimen Collection
Health Problems: Adult Health: Renal and Urinary: Urinary Tract Inflammation/Infection/Trauma
Priority Concepts: Elimination; Patient Education

Answer: 1
Rationale: The nurse instructs the client to void at the beginning of the collection period and discard this urine sample because this urine has been stored in the bladder for an undetermined length of time. All urine thereafter is saved in an iced or refrigerated container. The client is asked to void at the finish time, and this sample is the last specimen added to the collection. Straining the urine is not done for timed urine collections. The container is labeled, placed on fresh ice, and brought to the laboratory immediately after the 24-hour urine collection has ended.
Test-Taking Strategy: Focusing on the subject, a 24-hour urine collection, will assist in eliminating options 2 and 4. Straining the urine is not done, and the urine must be sent to the laboratory immediately after the collection time has ended. For the remaining options, think about the procedure. Remember that it is best to discard the first specimen.
Priority Nursing Tip: If the client is collecting a 24-hour urine specimen, check with the laboratory about the need to restrict certain foods or avoid taking certain medications before and during the collection. Some foods and medications affect test results.
Reference: Ignatavicius, D., et al. (2021). *Medical-surgical nursing: Concepts for interprofessional collaborative care* (10th ed., pp. 1315–1316). Elsevier.

139. The nurse is caring for a client in active labor. Which intervention would the nurse implement to prevent fetal heart rate decelerations?
1. Discourage client from walking.
2. Increase the rate of the oxytocin infusion.
3. Monitor the fetal heart rate every 30 minutes.
4. Encourage upright or side-lying positions.

Level of Cognitive Ability: Applying
Client Needs: Physiological Integrity
Clinical Judgment/Cognitive Skills: Take Action
Integrated Process: Nursing Process/Implementation
Content Area: Maternity: Intrapartum
Health Problems: Maternity: Fetal Distress/Demise
Priority Concepts: Perfusion; Reproduction

Answer: 4
Rationale: Side-lying and upright positions such as walking, standing, and squatting can improve venous return and encourage effective uterine activity. There are many nursing actions to prevent fetal heart rate decelerations without necessitating surgical intervention. Monitoring the fetal heart rate every 30 minutes will not prevent fetal heart rate decelerations. The nurse needs to discontinue an oxytocin infusion in the presence of fetal heart rate decelerations, thereby reducing uterine activity and increasing uteroplacental perfusion.
Test-Taking Strategy: Focus on the subject, preventing fetal heart rate decelerations. Options 1, 2, and 3 will not prevent fetal heart rate decelerations. Side-lying and upright positions will improve venous return and encourage effective uterine activity.
Priority Nursing Tip: Early fetal heart rate decelerations are not associated with fetal compromise and require no intervention. Late decelerations indicate impaired placental exchange or uteroplacental insufficiency.
Reference: McKinney, E. S., et al. (2022). *Maternal child nursing* (6th ed., pp. 345–346). Elsevier.

140. A client diagnosed with gestational diabetes is at 36 weeks of gestation. The client has had weekly reactive nonstress tests for the last 3 weeks. This week, the nonstress test was nonreactive after 40 minutes. Based on these results, the nurse would prepare the client for which intervention?
1. A contraction stress test
2. Immediate induction of labor
3. Hospitalization with continuous fetal monitoring
4. A return appointment in 2 days to repeat the nonstress test

Level of Cognitive Ability: Analyzing
Client Needs: Physiological Integrity
Clinical Judgment/Cognitive Skills: Generate Solutions
Integrated Process: Clinical Judgment; Nursing Process/Planning
Content Area: Maternity: Antepartum
Health Problems: Maternity: Gestational Diabetes Mellitus
Priority Concepts: Clinical Judgment; Reproduction

Answer: 1
Rationale: A nonreactive nonstress test needs further assessment. A contraction stress test is the next test needed to further assess the fetal status. There are not enough data in the question to indicate that the procedures in options 2 and 3 are necessary at this time. To send the client home for 2 days may place the fetus in jeopardy.
Test-Taking Strategy: Focus on the subject, a change in nonstress test results from reactive to nonreactive. Options 2 and 3 can be eliminated first because they are unnecessary at this time. Option 4 can be eliminated next because repeating the test at a later time is not a safe intervention, especially considering the fact that previous test results were reactive.
Priority Nursing Tip: A nonstress test is performed to assess placental function and oxygenation and evaluate the fetal heart rate response to fetal movement.
Reference: McKinney, E. S., et al. (2022). *Maternal child nursing* (6th ed., pp. 287–288). Elsevier.

Client Needs

141. The nurse is administering magnesium sulfate to a client experiencing severe preeclampsia. What intervention would the nurse implement during the administration of magnesium sulfate for this client?
1. Schedule a daily ultrasound to assess fetal movement.
2. Schedule a nonstress test every 4 hours to assess fetal well-being.
3. Assess client's temperature every 2 hours because client is at high risk for infection.
4. Assess for signs and symptoms of labor since client's level of consciousness may be altered.

Level of Cognitive Ability: Applying
Client Needs: Physiological Integrity
Clinical Judgment/Cognitive Skills: Take Action
Integrated Process: Clinical Judgment; Nursing Process/Implementation
Content Area: Pharmacology: Maternity/Newborn: Magnesium Sulfate
Health Problems: Maternity: Gestational Hypertension/Preeclampsia and Eclampsia
Priority Concepts: Reproduction; Safety

Answer: 4
Rationale: Magnesium sulfate is a central nervous system depressant and anticonvulsant. Because of the sedative effect of the magnesium sulfate, the client may not perceive labor. Daily ultrasounds are not necessary for this client. A nonstress test may be done, but not every 4 hours. This client is not at high risk for infection.
Test-Taking Strategy: Focus on the subject, magnesium sulfate administration. Use the steps of the nursing process to answer the question. Assessment is the first step; therefore, eliminate options 1 and 2. From the remaining options, knowledge that the client is not at high risk for infection will assist in directing you to the correct option.
Priority Nursing Tip: Calcium gluconate is the antidote to magnesium sulfate.
Reference: McKinney, E. S., et al. (2022). *Maternal child nursing* (6th ed., pp. 545–546). Elsevier.

❖ **142.** When the nasogastric (NG) tube of a client diagnosed with acute pancreatitis stops draining, which intervention would the nurse implement to maintain client safety?
1. Remove and replace the tube.
2. Verify the tube placement according to agency procedure.
3. Clamp the tube for 2 hours to allow the drainage to accumulate.
4. Retract the tube by 2 inches so that it is above a possible obstruction.

Level of Cognitive Ability: Applying
Client Needs: Physiological Integrity
Clinical Judgment/Cognitive Skills: Take Action
Integrated Process: Clinical Judgment; Nursing Process/Implementation
Content Area: Skills: Tube Care
Health Problems: Adult Health: Gastrointestinal: Pancreatitis
Priority Concepts: Clinical Judgment; Safety

Answer: 2
Rationale: If a client's nasogastric tube stops draining, the nurse verifies placement first to ensure that the tube remains in the stomach. After checking placement and verifying a prescription for tube irrigation, the nurse irrigates the tube with 30 to 60 mL of the fluid per agency procedure. Clamping the tube increases the risk of aspiration and is contraindicated; besides, this intervention cannot unclog a tube. Retracting the tube may displace the tube and place the client at risk for aspiration. Replacement of the tube is the last step if other actions are unsuccessful.
Test-Taking Strategy: Focus on the subject, the NG tube stopped draining. Eliminate option 1 because this would be done only if other interventions are unsuccessful. Next, eliminate options 3 and 4 because these interventions increase client risk of aspiration. Also use the steps of the nursing process; option 2 is the only assessment action.
Priority Nursing Tip: Accurate placement of a gastrointestinal tube is always checked before instilling feeding solutions, medications, or any other solution.
Reference: Ignatavicius, D., et al. (2021). *Medical-surgical nursing: Concepts for interprofessional collaborative care* (10th ed., pp. 1113–1114). Elsevier.

143. The nurse is planning to give a tepid tub bath to a child experiencing hyperthermia. Which action would the nurse plan to perform?
1. Obtain isopropyl alcohol to add to the bath water.
2. Allow 5 minutes for the child to soak in the bath water.
3. Have cool water available to add to the warm bath water.
4. Warm the water to the same body temperature as the child's.

Level of Cognitive Ability: Applying
Client Needs: Physiological Integrity
Clinical Judgment/Cognitive Skills: Generate Solutions
Integrated Process: Clinical Judgment; Nursing Process/Planning
Content Area: Pediatrics: Metabolic/Endocrine
Health Problems: Pediatric-Specific: Fever
Priority Concepts: Clinical Judgment; Thermoregulation

Answer: 3
Rationale: Adding cool water to an already warm bath allows the water temperature to slowly drop. The child is able to gradually adjust to the changing water temperature and will not experience chilling. Alcohol is toxic, can cause peripheral vasoconstriction, and is contraindicated for tepid sponge or tub baths. The child needs to be in a tepid tub bath for 20 to 30 minutes to achieve maximum results. To achieve the best cooling results, the water temperature needs to be at least 2 degrees lower than the child's body temperature.
Test-Taking Strategy: Focus on the **subject**, tepid water bath. Eliminate option 1, recalling that alcohol is toxic, as well as irritating, to the skin. Eliminate option 4 because water that is the same as body temperature will not reduce hyperthermia. Eliminate option 2 because of the 5-minute time frame.
Priority Nursing Tip: Perform a complete assessment on a child with a fever. Assessment findings associated with the fever provide important indications of the seriousness of the fever.
Reference: Hockenberry, M., Wilson, D., & Rodgers, C. (2019). *Wong's Nursing care of infants and children* (11th ed., pp. 693–694). Elsevier.

❖ **144.** The nurse is assigned to care for an infant on the first postoperative day after a surgical repair of a cleft lip. Which nursing intervention is appropriate when caring for this child's surgical incision?
1. Rinsing the incision with sterile water after feeding
2. Cleaning the incision only when serous exudate forms
3. Rubbing the incision gently with a sterile cotton-tipped swab
4. Replacing the Logan bar carefully after cleaning the incision

Level of Cognitive Ability: Applying
Client Needs: Physiological Integrity
Clinical Judgment/Cognitive Skills: Take Action
Integrated Process: Clinical Judgment; Nursing Process/Implementation
Content Area: Pediatrics: Gastrointestinal
Health Problems: Pediatric-Specific: Disorders of Prenatal Development
Priority Concepts: Clinical Judgment; Tissue Integrity

Answer: 1
Rationale: The incision needs to be rinsed with sterile water after every feeding. Rubbing alters the integrity of the suture line. Rather, the incision needs to be patted or dabbed. The purpose of the Logan bar is to maintain the integrity of the suture line. Removing the Logan bar on the first postoperative day would increase tension on the surgical incision.
Test-Taking Strategy: Focus on the **subject**, cleft lip repair. Eliminate options 2 and 3 first because of the word "only" in option 2 and "rubbing" in option 3. Focus on the words "first postoperative day." This will assist in eliminating option 4.
Priority Nursing Tip: After cleft lip repair, avoid positioning the infant on the side of the repair or in the prone position because these positions can cause rubbing of the surgical site on the mattress. Additionally, the lip repair site is cleaned per surgeon's prescription.
Reference: McKinney, E. S., et al. (2022). *Maternal child nursing* (6th ed., p. 968). Elsevier.

145. A client is in ventricular tachycardia and the physician prescribes intravenous (IV) lidocaine. The nurse would dilute the concentrated solution of lidocaine with which solution?
1. Lactated Ringer's
2. Normal saline 0.9%
3. 5% Dextrose in water
4. Normal saline 0.45%

Level of Cognitive Ability: Applying
Client Needs: Physiological Integrity
Clinical Judgment/Cognitive Skills: Take Action
Integrated Process: Clinical Judgment; Nursing Process/Implementation
Content Area: Pharmacology: Cardiovascular: Antidysrhythmics
Health Problems: Adult Health: Cardiovascular: Dysrhythmias
Priority Concepts: Clinical Judgment; Safety

Answer: 3
Rationale: Lidocaine for IV administration is dispensed in concentrated and dilute formulations. The concentrated formulation must be diluted with 5% dextrose in water. Therefore, options 1, 2, and 4 are incorrect.
Test-Taking Strategy: Focus on the **subject**, IV lidocaine. Eliminate options 2 and 4 first because they are **comparable or alike** since they are similar solutions. From the remaining options, it is necessary to know that the concentrated formulation must be diluted with 5% dextrose in water.
Priority Nursing Tip: When administering IV lidocaine, be sure that the medication label reads "for IV use" and is preservative free; additionally, resuscitative equipment needs to be readily available.
References: Gahart, B., Nazareno, A., & Ortega, M. (2021). *Gahart's 2021 Intravenous medications: A handbook for nurses and health professionals* (37th ed., p. 843). Elsevier; Kizior, R., & Hodgson, B. (2022). *Saunders Nursing drug handbook 2022* (p. 701). Elsevier.

❖ **146.** A client being treated for a bowel obstruction is receiving total parenteral nutrition (TPN) via a central venous catheter (CVC) and is scheduled to receive an intravenous (IV) antibiotic. Which intervention would the nurse implement before administering the antibiotic?
1. Turn off the TPN for 30 minutes.
2. Ensure a separate IV access route.
3. Flush the CVC with normal saline.
4. Check for compatibility with TPN.

Level of Cognitive Ability: Applying
Client Needs: Physiological Integrity
Clinical Judgment/Cognitive Skills: Take Action
Integrated Process: Clinical Judgment; Nursing Process/Implementation
Content Area: Skills: Medication Administration
Health Problems: Adult Health: Gastrointestinal: Bowel Obstruction
Priority Concepts: Clinical Judgment; Safety

Answer: 2
Rationale: The TPN line is used only for the administration of the TPN solution to prevent crystallization in the CVC tubing and disruption of the TPN infusion. Any other IV medication must be administered through a separate IV access site, including a separate infusion port of the CVC catheter. Therefore, options 1, 3, and 4 are incorrect actions.
Test-Taking Strategy: Focus on the **subject**, total parenteral nutrition. Eliminate options 1, 3, and 4 because they are **comparable or alike** in that they involve using the TPN line for the administration of the antibiotic.
Priority Nursing Tip: Parenteral nutrition solutions that are cloudy or darkened would not be used for administration and need to be returned to the pharmacy.
References: Lewis, S., et al. (2020). *Medical-surgical nursing: Assessment and management of clinical problems* (11th ed., p. 862). Elsevier; Potter, P., et al. (2021). *Fundamentals of nursing* (10th ed., pp. 618–619). Elsevier.

147. The nurse monitoring a postoperative client would recognize which behaviors as indicators that the client is in pain? **Select all that apply.**
❑ 1. Gasping
❑ 2. Lip biting
❑ 3. Muscle tension
❑ 4. Pacing activities
❑ 5. Staring out the window
❑ 6. Asking for the television to be turned off

Level of Cognitive Ability: Analyzing
Client Needs: Physiological Integrity
Clinical Judgment/Cognitive Skills: Recognize Cues
Integrated Process: Clinical Judgment; Nursing Process/Assessment
Content Area: Skills: Vital Signs
Health Problems: Adult Health: Neurologic: Pain
Priority Concepts: Clinical Judgment; Pain

Answer: 1, 2, 3, 4
Rationale: The nurse would assess verbalization, vocal response, facial and body movements, and social interaction as indicators of pain. Behavioral indicators of pain include gasping, lip biting (facial expressions), muscle tension, pacing activities, moaning, crying, grunting (vocalizations), grimacing, clenching teeth, wrinkling the forehead, tightly closing or widely opening the eyes or mouth, restlessness, immobilization, increased hand and finger movements, rhythmic or rubbing motions, protective movements of body parts (body movement), avoidance of conversation, focusing only on activities for pain relief, avoiding social contacts and interactions, and reduced attention span. Options 5 and 6 are not to be assumed as pain-related behaviors because there can be a variety of reasons for such actions.
Test-Taking Strategy: Focus on the subject, behavioral indicators of pain. Think about the physiologic and psychosocial responses that occur during the pain experience as you read each option. This will assist in answering correctly.
Priority Nursing Tip: It is important for the nurse to monitor for behavioral indicators of pain, particularly if the client is unable to verbalize the presence of pain.
Reference: Potter, P., et al. (2021). *Fundamentals of nursing* (10th ed., pp. 1063, 1073–1074). Elsevier.

❖ **148.** A client who experienced a stroke and has dysphagia is receiving enteral nutrition. The nurse plans care considering which conditions that place the client receiving enteral nutrition at increased risk for aspiration? **Select all that apply.**
❑ 1. Sedation
❑ 2. Coughing
❑ 3. An artificial airway
❑ 4. Head-elevated position
❑ 5. Nasotracheal suctioning
❑ 6. Decreased level of consciousness

Level of Cognitive Ability: Analyzing
Client Needs: Physiological Integrity
Clinical Judgment/Cognitive Skills: Recognize Cues
Integrated Process: Clinical Judgment; Nursing Process/Assessment
Content Area: Foundations of Care: Safety
Health Problems: Adult Health: Neurologic: Stroke
Priority Concepts: Gas Exchange; Safety

Answer: 1, 2, 3, 5, 6
Rationale: A serious complication associated with enteral feedings is aspiration of formula into the tracheobronchial tree. Some common conditions that increase the risk of aspiration include sedation, coughing, an artificial airway, nasotracheal suctioning, decreased level of consciousness, and lying flat. A head-elevated position does not increase the risk of aspiration.
Test-Taking Strategy: Focus on the subject, the risks associated with aspiration. Recall that aspiration is the inhalation of foreign material into the tracheobronchial tree. Next read each option and think about the effect it produces with regard to aspiration. This will direct you to the correct options.
Priority Nursing Tip: The nurse must assess the client for conditions that place the client at risk of aspiration. Aspiration can result in airway obstruction.
Reference: Potter, P., et al. (2021). *Fundamentals of nursing* (10th ed., pp. 1132–1133). Elsevier.

149. A client, experiencing a sudden onset of chest pain and dyspnea, is diagnosed with a pulmonary embolus. The nurse **immediately** implements which expected prescriptions for this client? **Select all that apply.**
- ❑ 1. Supplemental oxygen
- ❑ 2. High-Fowler's position
- ❑ 3. Semi-Fowler's position
- ❑ 4. Morphine sulfate intravenously
- ❑ 5. Meperidine hydrochloride intravenously
- ❑ 6. Two tablets of acetaminophen with codeine

Level of Cognitive Ability: Applying
Client Needs: Physiological Integrity
Clinical Judgment/Cognitive Skills: Take Action
Integrated Process: Clinical Judgment; Nursing Process/Implementation
Content Area: Complex Care: Emergency Situations/Management
Health Problems: Adult Health: Respiratory: Pulmonary Embolism
Priority Concepts: Gas Exchange; Perfusion

Answer: 1, 3, 4
Rationale: Standard therapeutic intervention for the client with pulmonary embolus includes proper positioning, oxygen, and intravenous analgesics. The head of the bed is placed in semi-Fowler's position. High-Fowler's is avoided because extreme hip flexure slows venous return from the legs and increases the risk of new thrombi. The usual analgesic of choice is morphine sulfate administered intravenously. This medication reduces pain, alleviates anxiety, and can diminish congestion of blood in the pulmonary vessels because it causes peripheral venous dilation.
Test-Taking Strategy: Note the strategic word, *immediately*. Eliminate option 2 first because a high-Fowler's position could place the client at risk for development of new thrombi. From the remaining options, recall that morphine is used for its vasodilating effects as well as its opioid effects for a client experiencing chest pain.
Priority Nursing Tip: Clients prone to pulmonary embolism are those at risk for deep vein thrombosis.
Reference: Ignatavicius, D., et al. (2021). *Medical-surgical nursing: Concepts for interprofessional collaborative care* (10th ed., pp. 589–591, 674). Elsevier.

❖ **150.** A client is scheduled to have a percutaneous transluminal coronary angioplasty (PTCA) to treat coronary artery disease. What information about the balloon-tipped catheter would the nurse plan to include when providing client education concerning the procedure?
1. A mesh-like device within the catheter will be inflated, causing it to spring open.
2. The catheter will be used to compress the plaque against the coronary blood vessel wall.
3. The catheter will cut away the plaque from the coronary vessel wall using an embedded blade.
4. The catheter will be positioned in a coronary artery to take pressure measurements in the vessel.

Level of Cognitive Ability: Applying
Client Needs: Physiological Integrity
Clinical Judgment/Cognitive Skills: Generate Solutions
Integrated Process: Teaching and Learning
Content Area: Adult Health: Cardiovascular
Health Problems: Adult Health: Cardiovascular: Coronary Artery Disease
Priority Concepts: Patient Education; Perfusion

Answer: 2
Rationale: In PTCA, a balloon-tipped catheter is used to compress the plaque against the coronary blood vessel wall. Option 1 describes placement of a coronary stent, option 3 describes coronary atherectomy, and option 4 describes part of the process used in cardiac catheterization.
Test-Taking Strategy: Focus on the subject, percutaneous transluminal coronary angioplasty (PTCA). Look at the name of the procedure. "Angioplasty" refers to repair of a blood vessel; this will assist in eliminating options 1 and 4. From the remaining options, recalling that a procedure that cuts something away would have the suffix *-ectomy* will assist in eliminating option 3.
Priority Nursing Tip: Complications of PTCA include arterial dissection or rupture, embolization of plaque fragments, spasm, and acute myocardial infarction.
Reference: Ignatavicius, D., et al. (2021). *Medical-surgical nursing: Concepts for interprofessional collaborative care* (10th ed., pp. 628, 761–762). Elsevier.

151. The nurse is caring for a client who has been placed in skin traction to treat a femur fracture. Which action by the nurse provides for countertraction to reduce shear and friction?
1. Using a footboard
2. Providing an overhead trapeze
3. Slightly elevating the foot of the bed
4. Slightly elevating the head of the bed

Level of Cognitive Ability: Applying
Client Needs: Physiological Integrity
Clinical Judgment/Cognitive Skills: Take Action
Integrated Process: Nursing Process/Implementation
Content Area: Adult Health: Musculoskeletal
Health Problems: Adult Health: Musculoskeletal: Skeletal Injury
Priority Concepts: Clinical Judgment; Mobility

Answer: 3
Rationale: The part of the bed under an area in traction is usually elevated to aid in countertraction. For the client in skin traction to treat a femur fracture (which is applied to a leg), the foot of the bed is elevated. Option 3 provides a force that opposes the traction force effectively without harming the client. A footboard, an overhead trapeze, or elevating the head of the bed is not used to provide countertraction.
Test-Taking Strategy: Focus on the subject, countertraction for skin traction. Eliminate option 4, noting that the skin extension traction is applied to the leg. From the remaining options, focus on the subject to eliminate options 1 and 2.
Priority Nursing Tip: The physician's prescription is always followed regarding the amount of weight applied to the traction device. For Buck's extension, weight of usually not more than 8 to 10 pounds is prescribed.
Reference: Lewis, S., et al. (2020). *Medical-surgical nursing: Assessment and management of clinical problems* (11th ed., p. 1453). Elsevier.

❖ 152. The nurse is preparing to initiate a bolus enteral feedings via nasogastric (NG) tube to a client. Which action represents safe practice by the nurse?
1. Checking the volume of the residual after administering the bolus feeding
2. Aspirating gastric contents before initiating the feeding to ensure that pH is greater than 9
3. Elevating the head of the bed to 15 degrees and maintaining that position for 30 minutes after feeding
4. Verifying correct nasogastric tube position with aspiration and administration of air bolus with auscultation

Level of Cognitive Ability: Applying
Client Needs: Physiological Integrity
Clinical Judgment/Cognitive Skills: Take Action
Integrated Process: Nursing Process/Implementation
Content Area: Skills: Tube Care
Health Problems: Adult Health: Gastrointestinal: Nutrition/Malabsorption Problems
Priority Concepts: Nutrition; Safety

Answer: 4
Rationale: After initial radiographic confirmation of NG tube placement, methods used to verify nasogastric tube placement include measuring the length of the tube from the point it protrudes from the nose to the end, injecting 10 to 30 mL of air into the tube and auscultating over the left upper quadrant of the abdomen, and aspirating the secretions and checking to see if the pH is less than 3.5 (safest method). Residual needs to be assessed before administration of the next feeding. Fowler's position is recommended for bolus feedings, if permitted, and needs to be maintained for 1 hour after instillation.
Test-Taking Strategy: Focus on the subject, bolus enteral feedings via nasogastric (NG) tube. Note the words "safe practice." Knowing that the pH of gastric contents should be between 1 and 5 will assist you in eliminating option 2. Option 3 can be eliminated because the head of the bed elevation needs to be at a minimum of 30 degrees for all types of enteral feedings to prevent aspiration. From the remaining two options, use knowledge of when to check residuals to assist you in eliminating option 1.
Priority Nursing Tip: Residual volumes are checked every 4 hours, before each feeding or the instillation of any solution, and before giving medications.
References: Lewis, S., et al. (2020). *Medical-surgical nursing: Assessment and management of clinical problems* (11th ed., pp. 862–863). Elsevier; Potter, P., et al. (2021). *Fundamentals of nursing* (10th ed., p. 1138). Elsevier.

153. The nurse is learning the procedure for inserting a nasogastric (NG) tube and is being supervised while inserting the tube into a client with a bowel obstruction. The nurse inserts the tube to the level of the oropharynx and has repositioned the client's head in a flexed-forward position. The client has been asked to begin swallowing, but as the nurse starts to slowly advance the NG tube with each swallow, the client begins to gag. Which action if taken by the nurse at this point would indicate a **need for further instruction** regarding the insertion of an NG tube?
1. Pulling the tube back slightly
2. Instructing the client to breathe slowly
3. Continuing to advance the tube to the desired distance
4. Checking the back of the pharynx using a tongue blade and flashlight

Level of Cognitive Ability: Analyzing
Client Needs: Physiological Integrity
Clinical Judgment/Cognitive Skills: Analyze Cues
Integrated Process: Clinical Judgment; Teaching and Learning
Content Area: Skills: Tube Care
Health Problems: Adult Health: Gastrointestinal: Bowel Obstruction
Priority Concepts: Clinical Judgment; Safety

Answer: 3
Rationale: As the NG tube is passed through the oropharynx, the gag reflex is stimulated, which may cause gagging. Instead of passing through to the esophagus, the NG tube may coil around itself in the oropharynx, or it may enter the larynx and obstruct the airway. Because the tube may enter the larynx, advancing the tube may position it in the trachea. The nurse would check the back of the pharynx using a tongue blade and flashlight to check for coiling and then pull the tube back slightly to prevent entrance into the larynx. Slow breathing helps the client relax to reduce the gag response. The tube may be advanced after the client relaxes.
Test-Taking Strategy: Note the strategic words, *need for further instruction.* These words indicate a negative event query and the need to select the incorrect nursing action. Focusing on these words and noting that the client is gagging will direct you to the correct option.
Priority Nursing Tip: To determine the insertion length of a nasogastric tube, measure the length of the tube from the bridge of the nose to the earlobe to the xiphoid process and indicate this length with a piece of tape.
Reference: Potter, P., et al. (2021). *Fundamentals of nursing* (10th ed., p. 1226). Elsevier.

❖ 154. The nurse is caring for a client with a terminal condition who is dying. Which respiratory assessment findings would indicate to the nurse that death is imminent? **Select all that apply.**
☐ 1. Dyspnea
☐ 2. Cyanosis
☐ 3. Tachypnea
☐ 4. Kussmaul's respiration
☐ 5. Irregular respiratory pattern
☐ 6. Adventitious bubbling lung sounds

Level of Cognitive Ability: Analyzing
Client Needs: Physiological Integrity
Clinical Judgment/Cognitive Skills: Recognize Cues
Integrated Process: Clinical Judgment; Nursing Process/Assessment
Content Area: Developmental Stages: End-of-Life
Health Problems: N/A
Priority Concepts: Gas Exchange; Perfusion

Answer: 1, 2, 5, 6
Rationale: Respiratory assessment findings that indicate death is imminent include poor gas exchange as evidenced by hypoxia, dyspnea, or cyanosis; altered patterns of respiration, such as slow, labored, irregular, or Cheyne-Stokes pattern (alternating periods of apnea and deep, rapid breathing); increased respiratory secretions and adventitious bubbling lung sounds (death rattle); and irritation of the tracheobronchial airway as evidenced by hiccups, chest pain, fatigue, or exhaustion. Kussmaul's respirations are abnormally deep, very rapid sighing respirations characteristic of diabetic ketoacidosis. Tachypnea is defined as rapid breathing. In an adult, it would indicate a respiratory rate of over 20 breaths/min.
Test-Taking Strategy: Focus on the subject, respiratory assessment findings near death. Think about the physiologic processes that occur in the dying person as you read each option. This will assist in answering the question correctly.
Priority Nursing Tip: As death approaches, metabolism is reduced, and the body gradually slows down until all function ends.
References: Lewis, S., et al. (2020). *Medical-surgical nursing: Assessment and management of clinical problems* (11th ed., p. 130). Elsevier; Potter, P., et al. (2021). *Fundamentals of nursing* (10th ed., p. 753). Elsevier.

155. An infant diagnosed with spina bifida cystica (meningomyelocele type) has had the sac surgically removed. The nurse plans which intervention in the postoperative period to maintain the infant's safety?
1. Covering the back dressing with a binder
2. Placing the infant in a head-down position
3. Strapping the infant in a baby seat sitting up
4. Elevating the head with the infant in the prone position

Level of Cognitive Ability: Applying
Client Needs: Physiological Integrity
Clinical Judgment/Cognitive Skills: Generate Solutions
Integrated Process: Clinical Judgment; Nursing Process/Planning
Content Area: Pediatrics: Neurologic
Health Problems: Pediatric-Specific: Neural Tube Defects
Priority Concepts: Intracranial Regulation; Safety

Answer: 4
Rationale: Spina bifida is a central nervous system defect that results from failure of the neural tube to close during embryonic development. Care of the operative site is carried out under the direction of the surgeon and includes close observation for signs of leakage of cerebrospinal fluid. The prone position is maintained after surgical closure to decrease the pressure on the surgical site on the back; however, many neurosurgeons allow the side-lying or partial side-lying position, unless it aggravates a coexisting hip dysplasia or permits undesirable hip flexion. This offers an opportunity for position changes, which reduces the risk of pressure sores and facilitates feeding. Elevating the head will decrease the chance of cerebrospinal fluid collecting in the cranial cavity. If permitted, the infant can be held upright against the body with care taken to avoid pressure on the operative site. Binders and a baby seat should not be used because of the pressure they would exert on the surgical site.
Test-Taking Strategy: Focus on the subject, postoperative care for an infant with spina bifida who had the sac removed. Recall that preventing pressure on the surgical site and preventing intracranial cerebrospinal fluid collection are goals for the postoperative period. Options 1 and 3 would increase pressure on the surgical site, and option 2 would not promote drainage of cerebrospinal fluid from the cranial cavity.
Priority Nursing Tip: In the preoperative period, the myelomeningocele sac is protected by covering with a sterile, moist (normal saline), nonadherent dressing to maintain the moisture of the sac and contents.
Reference: McKinney, E. S., et al. (2022). *Maternal child nursing* (6th ed., pp 1295–1296). Elsevier.

❖ **156.** The nurse is assessing a client with a history of angina who is being treated with a beta-adrenergic blocker. Which assessment findings would indicate that the client may be experiencing dose-related side effects of the medication? **Select all that apply.**
❏ 1. Dizziness
❏ 2. Bradycardia
❏ 3. Chest pain
❏ 4. Reflex tachycardia
❏ 5. Sexual dysfunction
❏ 6. Cardiac dysrhythmias

Level of Cognitive Ability: Analyzing
Client Needs: Physiological Integrity
Clinical Judgment/Cognitive Skills: Recognize Cues
Integrated Process: Clinical Judgment; Nursing Process/Assessment
Content Area: Pharmacology: Cardiovascular: Beta Blockers
Health Problems: Adult Health: Cardiovascular: Coronary Artery Disease
Priority Concepts: Clinical Judgment; Safety

Answer: 1, 2, 5
Rationale: Beta-adrenergic blockers, commonly called beta blockers, are useful in treating cardiac dysrhythmias, mild hypertension, mild tachycardia, and angina pectoris. Side effects commonly associated with beta blockers are usually dose related and include dizziness (hypotensive effect), bradycardia, hypotension, and sexual dysfunction (impotence). Options 3, 4, and 6 are reasons for prescribing a beta blocker; however, these are general side effects of alpha-adrenergic blockers.
Test-Taking Strategy: Focus on the subject, beta blockers. Specific knowledge regarding the side effects of beta blockers is needed to select the correct options. However, if you can remember that beta blockers are useful in treating cardiac dysrhythmias, mild hypertension, mild tachycardia, and angina pectoris, you will be able to eliminate the incorrect options.
Priority Nursing Tip: Advise the client with diabetes mellitus who is taking beta-adrenergic blockers that the medication can mask the early signs of hypoglycemia such as nervousness and tachycardia.
Reference: Ignatavicius, D., et al. (2021). *Medical-surgical nursing: Concepts for interprofessional collaborative care* (10th ed., pp. 703, 758). Elsevier.

157. A client at risk for respiratory failure is receiving oxygen via nasal cannula at 6 L/min. The nurse reviews the arterial blood gas (ABG) results. What intervention would the nurse anticipate that the physician will order for respiratory support for this client?

Laboratory Results

Test and Result	Reference Range
pH 7.29	7.35–7.45
Pco_2 49 mm Hg	35–45 mm Hg
Po_2 58 mm Hg	80–100 mm Hg
HCO_3 18 mEq/L	21–28 mEq/L
(18 mmol/L)	(21–28 mmol/L)

1. Intubating for mechanical ventilation
2. Keeping the oxygen at 6 L/min via nasal cannula
3. Lowering the oxygen to 4 L/min via nasal cannula
4. Adding a partial rebreather mask to the current prescription

Level of Cognitive Ability: Analyzing
Client Needs: Physiological Integrity
Clinical Judgment/Cognitive Skills: Analyze Cues
Integrated Process: Clinical Judgment; Nursing Process/Analysis
Content Area: Complex Care: Emergency Situations/Management
Health Problems: Adult Health: Respiratory: Acute Respiratory Distress Syndrome/Failure
Priority Concepts: Clinical Judgment; Gas Exchange

Answer: 1
Rationale: If respiratory failure occurs and supplemental oxygen cannot maintain acceptable Po_2 and Pco_2 levels, endotracheal intubation and mechanical ventilation are necessary. The client is exhibiting respiratory acidosis, metabolic acidosis, and hypoxemia. Lowering or keeping the oxygen at the same liter flow will not improve the client's condition. A partial rebreather mask will raise Co_2 levels even further.
Test-Taking Strategy: Focus on the subject, ABG analysis in a client at risk for respiratory failure. Note the ABG values. Noting that the oxygen level is low will eliminate options 2 and 3. Knowing that the Pco_2 is high will eliminate option 4 because a partial rebreather mask will raise Co_2 levels even further.
Priority Nursing Tip: The manifestations of respiratory failure are related to the extent and rapidity of change in the Pao_2 and $Paco_2$.
Reference: Lewis, S., et al. (2020). *Medical-surgical nursing: Assessment and management of clinical problems* (11th ed., pp. 1591–1592). Elsevier.

❖ **158.** The nurse is preparing to assess the respirations of several newborns in the nursery. The nurse performs the procedure and determines that the respiratory rate is normal if which finding is noted?
   ❑ 1. A respiratory rate of 28 breaths/min in a crying newborn
   ❑ 2. A respiratory rate of 46 breaths/min in an awake newborn
   ❑ 3. A respiratory rate of 65 breaths/min in a sleeping newborn
   ❑ 4. A respiratory rate of 76 breaths/min in a newly delivered newborn

Level of Cognitive Ability: Analysis
Client Needs: Physiological Integrity
Clinical Judgment/Cognitive Skills: Recognize Cues
Integrated Process: Clinical Judgment; Nursing Process/Assessment
Content Area: Maternity: Newborn
Health Problems: N/A
Priority Concepts: Development; Gas Exchange

Answer: 2
Rationale: Normal respiratory rate varies from 30 to 60 breaths/min when the infant is not crying. Respirations need to be counted for 1 full minute to ensure an accurate measurement because the newborn infant may be a periodic breather. Observing and palpating respirations while the infant is quiet promotes accurate assessment. Palpation aids observation in determining the respiratory rate. Option 1 indicates bradypnea, and options 3 and 4 indicate tachypnea.
Test-Taking Strategy: Focus on the subject, newborn respiratory rate. Recall knowledge regarding the normal respiratory rate for a newborn infant to answer this question. Remember that the normal respiratory rate varies from 30 to 60 breaths/min.
Priority Nursing Tip: The newborn infant's respiratory rate and apical heart rate are counted for 1 full minute to detect irregularities in rate or rhythm.
Reference: McKinney, E. S., et al. (2022). *Maternal child nursing* (6th ed., p. 442). Elsevier.

159. During a routine prenatal visit, a client in the third trimester of pregnancy reports having frequent calf pain when walking. The nurse suspects superficial thrombophlebitis and checks for which sign associated with this condition?
1. Severe chills
2. Kernig's sign
3. Brudzinski's sign
4. Palpable, hard thrombus

Level of Cognitive Ability: Applying
Client Needs: Physiological Integrity
Clinical Judgment/Cognitive Skills: Recognize Cues
Integrated Process: Nursing Process/Assessment
Content Area: Maternity: Antepartum
Health Problems: Adult Health: Cardiovascular: Vascular Disorders
Priority Concepts: Clinical Judgment; Clotting

Answer: 4
Rationale: Pain in the calf during walking could indicate venous thrombosis or peripheral arterial disease. The manifestations of superficial thrombophlebitis include a palpable thrombus that feels bumpy and hard, tenderness and pain in the affected lower extremity, and a warm and pinkish red color over the thrombus area. Severe chills can occur in a variety of inflammatory or infectious conditions and are also a manifestation of pelvic thrombophlebitis. Brudzinski's sign and Kernig's sign test for meningeal irritability.
Test-Taking Strategy: Focus on the subject, thrombophlebitis. Eliminate options 2 and 3 first because they are comparable or alike options since both test for meningeal irritation. From the remaining options, focus on the words "frequent calf pain when walking" and "thrombophlebitis" to assist in directing you to the correct option.
Priority Nursing Tip: If a thrombus is suspected, never massage the site because of the risk of dislodging it and causing it to travel to the pulmonary system.
Reference: McKinney, E. S., et al. (2022). *Maternal child nursing* (6th ed., pp. 239, 612–613). Elsevier.

160. The nurse evaluates the patency of a peripheral intravenous (IV) site and suspects an infiltration. Which action would the nurse take to determine if the IV has infiltrated?
1. Strip the tubing and assess for a blood return.
2. Check the regional tissue for redness and warmth.
3. Increase the infusion rate and observe for swelling.
4. Gently palpate regional tissue for edema and coolness.

Level of Cognitive Ability: Applying
Client Needs: Physiological Integrity
Clinical Judgment/Cognitive Skills: Take Action
Integrated Process: Nursing Process/Implementation
Content Area: Foundations of Care: Safety
Health Problems: N/A
Priority Concepts: Clinical Judgment; Safety

Answer: 4
Rationale: When assessing an IV for clinical indicators of infiltration, the nurse would assess the site for edema and coolness, which signifies leakage of the IV fluid into the surrounding tissues. Stripping the tubing will not cause a blood return but will force IV fluid into the surrounding tissues, which can increase the risk of tissue damage. Redness and warmth are more likely to indicate infection or phlebitis. Increasing the IV flow rate can further damage the tissues if the IV has infiltrated. Additionally, a physician's prescription is needed to increase an IV flow rate.
Test-Taking Strategy: Focus on the subject, IV infiltration. Recalling that the site will feel cool will direct you to the correct option. Also note the word "gently" in the correct option.
Priority Nursing Tip: If an IV infiltration occurs, the IV device is removed from the client's vein; if IV therapy is still needed, a new IV device is inserted into a vein in a different extremity.
Reference: Ignatavicius, D., et al. (2021). *Medical-surgical nursing: Concepts for interprofessional collaborative care* (10th ed., p. 294). Elsevier.

161. A client who has sustained a neck injury is unresponsive and pulseless. What would the emergency department nurse do to open the client's airway?
1. Insert an oropharyngeal airway.
2. Tilt the head and lift the chin.
3. Place in the recovery position.
4. Stabilize the skull and push up the jaw.

Level of Cognitive Ability: Applying
Client Needs: Physiological Integrity
Clinical Judgment/Cognitive Skills: Take Action
Integrated Process: Clinical Judgment; Nursing Process/Implementation
Content Area: Complex Care: Emergency Situations/Management
Health Problems: Adult Health: Musculoskeletal: Skeletal Injury
Priority Concepts: Gas Exchange; Safety

Answer: 4
Rationale: The health care team uses the jaw-thrust maneuver to open the airway until a radiograph confirms that the client's cervical spine is stable to avoid potential aggravation of a cervical spine injury. Options 1 and 2 require manipulation of the spine to open the airway, and option 3 can be ineffective for opening the airway.
Test-Taking Strategy: Focus on the ABCs—airway, breathing, and circulation. Recalling the principles related to airway management will assist in eliminating options 1 and 2. From the remaining options, visualize each and eliminate option 3 because this action can be ineffective if the client is unable to maintain the airway.
Priority Nursing Tip: If a neck injury is suspected in a victim who sustained an injury, the jaw-thrust maneuver (rather than the head-tilt chin-lift) is used to open the airway to prevent further spine damage.
Reference: Lewis, S., et al. (2020). *Medical-surgical nursing: Assessment and management of clinical problems* (11th ed., pp. 1607, 1609). Elsevier.

❖ **162.** The nurse is caring for a child diagnosed with Reye's syndrome. The nurse monitors for manifestations of which condition associated with this syndrome?
1. Protein in the urine
2. Symptoms of hyperglycemia
3. Increased intracranial pressure
4. A history of a *Staphylococcus* infection

Level of Cognitive Ability: Analyzing
Client Needs: Physiological Integrity
Clinical Judgment/Cognitive Skills: Recognize Cues
Integrated Process: Clinical Judgment; Nursing Process/Assessment
Content Area: Pediatrics: Neurologic
Health Problems: Pediatric-Specific: Reye's Syndrome
Priority Concepts: Clinical Judgment; Intracranial Regulation

Answer: 3
Rationale: Reye's syndrome is an acute encephalopathy that follows a viral illness and is characterized pathologically by cerebral edema and fatty changes in the liver. Intracranial pressure and encephalopathy are major problems associated with Reye's syndrome. Protein is not present in the urine. Reye's syndrome is related to a history of viral infections, and hypoglycemia is a symptom of this disease.
Test-Taking Strategy: Focus on the subject, Reye's syndrome. Recalling that Reye's syndrome is an acute encephalopathy will assist in directing you to the correct option.
Priority Nursing Tip: The administration of aspirin and non-aspirin-containing salicylates is not recommended for a child with a febrile illness or a child with varicella or influenza because of its association with Reye's syndrome.
Reference: McKinney, E. S., et al. (2022). *Maternal child nursing* (6th ed., p. 1317). Elsevier.

163. The nurse analyzed an electrocardiogram (ECG) strip **(refer to figure)** for a client demonstrating left-sided heart failure and interprets the ECG strip as which rhythm?

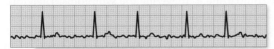

1. Atrial fibrillation
2. Sinus dysrhythmia
3. Ventricular fibrillation
4. Third-degree heart block

Level of Cognitive Ability: Analyzing
Client Needs: Physiological Integrity
Clinical Judgment/Cognitive Skills: Analyze Cues
Integrated Process: Clinical Judgment; Nursing Process/Analysis
Content Area: Adult Health: Cardiovascular
Health Problems: Adult Health: Cardiovascular: Dysrhythmias
Priority Concepts: Clinical Judgment; Perfusion

Answer: 1
Rationale: Atrial fibrillation is characterized by rapid, chaotic atrial depolarization. Ventricular rates may be less than 100 beats/min (controlled) or greater than 100 beats/min (uncontrolled). The ECG reveals chaotic or no identifiable P waves and an irregular ventricular rhythm. A sinus dysrhythmia has a normal P wave and PR interval and QRS complex. In ventricular fibrillation, there are no identifiable P waves, QRS complexes, or T waves. In third-degree heart block, the atria and ventricles beat independently, and the PR interval varies in length.
Test-Taking Strategy: Focus on the **subject**, ECG interpretation. Look at the rhythm and compare it to what a normal rhythm would look like. Recall that in atrial fibrillation the P wave is usually absent or chaotic and the ventricular rhythm is irregular. This will direct you to the correct option.
Priority Nursing Tip: The client with atrial fibrillation is at risk for pulmonary embolism because thrombi can form in the right atrium as a result of atrial quivering and travel to the right atrium to the lungs.
Reference: Ignatavicius, D., et al. (2021). *Medical-surgical nursing: Concepts for interprofessional collaborative care* (10th ed., pp. 652–653). Elsevier.

❖ **164.** The nurse admits a client with a suspected diagnosis of bulimia nervosa. While performing the admission assessment, the nurse expects to elicit which data about the client's beliefs?
1. Is accepting of body size
2. Views purging as an accepted behavior
3. Overeats for the enjoyment of eating food
4. Gorges in response to losing control of diet

Level of Cognitive Ability: Applying
Client Needs: Physiological Integrity
Clinical Judgment/Cognitive Skills: Recognize Cues
Integrated Process: Nursing Process/Assessment
Content Area: Mental Health
Health Problems: Mental Health: Eating Disorders
Priority Concepts: Clinical Judgment; Nutrition

Answer: 2
Rationale: Individuals with bulimia nervosa develop cycles of binge eating, followed by purging. They seldom attempt to diet and have no sense of loss of control. Options 1, 3, and 4 are true of the obese person who may binge eat (not purge).
Test-Taking Strategy: Focus on the **subject**, bulimia nervosa. Eliminate options 3 and 4 because they are **comparable or alike** since both involve overconsumption of food. From the remaining options, recalling the definition of bulimia will direct you to the correct option.
Priority Nursing Tip: The client with an eating disorder experiences an altered body image.
Reference: Varcarolis, E., & Fosbre, C. (2021). *Essentials of psychiatric mental health nursing: A communication approach to evidence-based care* (4th ed., pp. 186–187). Elsevier.

165. The nurse is caring for a client who develops compartment syndrome as a result of a severely fractured arm. When the client asks why this happens, how would the nurse respond?
1. A bone fragment has injured the nerve supply in the area.
2. An injured artery causes impaired arterial perfusion through the compartment.
3. Bleeding and swelling cause increased pressure in an area that cannot expand.
4. The fascia expands with injury, causing pressure on underlying nerves and muscles.

Level of Cognitive Ability: Applying
Client Needs: Physiological Integrity
Clinical Judgment/Cognitive Skills: Generate Solutions
Integrated Process: Teaching and Learning
Content Area: Adult Health: Musculoskeletal
Health Problems: Adult Health: Musculoskeletal: Skeletal Injury
Priority Concepts: Mobility; Perfusion

Answer: 3
Rationale: Compartment syndrome is caused by bleeding and swelling within a compartment, which is lined by fascia that does not expand. The bleeding and swelling place pressure on the nerves, muscles, and blood vessels in the compartment, triggering the symptoms. Therefore, options 1, 2, and 4 are incorrect statements.
Test-Taking Strategy: Focus on the subject, compartment syndrome. Option 2 is eliminated first because this syndrome is not caused by an arterial injury. Knowing that the fascia cannot expand eliminates option 4. From the remaining options, it is necessary to know that bleeding and swelling (not a nerve injury) cause the symptoms.
Priority Nursing Tip: Within 4 to 6 hours after the onset of compartment syndrome, neurovascular damage is irreversible if not treated.
Reference: Ignatavicius, D., et al. (2021). *Medical-surgical nursing: Concepts for interprofessional collaborative care* (10th ed., pp. 1031, 1033–1034). Elsevier.

❖ **166.** A client with an extremity burn injury has undergone a fasciotomy. The nurse prepares to provide which type of wound care to the fasciotomy site?
1. Dry sterile dressings
2. Hydrocolloid dressings
3. Wet, sterile saline dressings
4. One-half-strength povidone-iodine dressings

Level of Cognitive Ability: Applying
Client Needs: Physiological Integrity
Clinical Judgment/Cognitive Skills: Generate Solutions
Integrated Process: Nursing Process/Planning
Content Area: Skills: Wound Care
Health Problems: Adult Health: Integumentary: Burns
Priority Concepts: Clinical Judgment; Tissue Integrity

Answer: 3
Rationale: A fasciotomy is an incision made extending through the subcutaneous tissue and fascia. The fasciotomy site is not sutured but is left open to relieve pressure and edema. The site is covered with wet sterile saline dressings. After 3 to 5 days, when perfusion is adequate and edema subsides, the wound is debrided and closed. A hydrocolloid dressing is not indicated for use with clean, open incisions. The incision is clean, not dirty, so there should be no reason to require povidone-iodine. Additionally, povidone-iodine can be irritating to normal tissues.
Test-Taking Strategy: Focus on the subject, fasciotomy. Recall knowledge of what a fasciotomy involves and the basics of wound care. Recall that the skin is not sutured closed but left open for pressure relief. Remembering that moist tissue needs to remain moist will direct you to the correct option.
Priority Nursing Tip: After fasciotomy, assess pulses, color, movement, and sensation of the affected extremity, and control any bleeding with pressure.
Reference: Ignatavicius, D., et al. (2021). *Medical-surgical nursing: Concepts for interprofessional collaborative care* (10th ed., pp. 447, 1031). Elsevier.

167. The nurse is caring for a client who was recently admitted with a diagnosis of anorexia nervosa. When the nurse enters the room, the client is engaged in rigorous push-ups. Which action would the nurse implement?
1. Allowing client to complete the exercise program
2. Stopping the exercising and weigh client immediately
3. Interrupting client and offer to take the client for a walk
4. Telling client that they are not allowed to exercise rigorously

Level of Cognitive Ability: Applying
Client Needs: Physiological Integrity
Clinical Judgment/Cognitive Skills: Take Action
Integrated Process: Nursing Process/Implementation
Content Area: Mental Health
Health Problems: Mental Health: Eating Disorders
Priority Concepts: Anxiety; Nutrition

Answer: 3
Rationale: Clients with anorexia nervosa are frequently preoccupied with rigorous exercise and push themselves beyond normal limits to work off caloric intake. The nurse must provide for appropriate exercise, as well as place limits on rigorous activities. Allowing the client to complete the exercise program could be harmful. Weighing the client reinforces the altered self-concept that the client experiences and the client's need to control weight. Telling the client that they are not allowed to exercise rigorously will increase their anxiety.
Test-Taking Strategy: Focus on the subject, a client with anorexia nervosa. Focus on the need for the nurse to set limits with clients who have this disorder. Also, recalling that the nurse needs to provide and guide the client to perform appropriate exercise will direct you to the correct option.
Priority Nursing Tip: The client with an eating disorder experiences an altered body image.
Reference: Varcarolis, E., & Fosbre, C. (2021). *Essentials of psychiatric mental health nursing: A communication approach to evidence-based care* (4th ed., pp. 187, 189–190). Elsevier.

❖ **168.** The nurse assesses a peripheral intravenous (IV) dressing and notes that it is damp and the tape is loose. What action would the nurse take **initially?**
1. Stop the infusion immediately.
2. Apply a sterile, occlusive dressing.
3. Ensure all IV tubing connections are tight.
4. Gather the supplies needed to insert a new IV.

Level of Cognitive Ability: Applying
Client Needs: Physiological Integrity
Clinical Judgment/Cognitive Skills: Take Action
Integrated Process: Nursing Process/Implementation
Content Area: Foundations of Care: Safety
Health Problems: N/A
Priority Concepts: Clinical Judgment; Safety

Answer: 3
Rationale: To determine subsequent nursing interventions, the nurse checks all connections to ensure tight seals while the IV infuses to help locate the source of the leak. If the leak is at the insertion site, the nurse stops the infusion, removes the IV, and inserts a new IV catheter. The nurse applies a new sterile occlusive dressing after resolving the source of the leak.
Test-Taking Strategy: Note the strategic word, *initially*, and recall that the nurse needs to determine the cause of the leaking. Use the steps of the nursing process and remember that assessment is the first step. Read each option carefully to determine which option indicates assessment to direct you to the correct option.
Priority Nursing Tip: Administration of an IV solution provides immediate access to the vascular system. Always ensure that the correct solution is administered as prescribed.
Reference: Potter, P., et al. (2021). *Fundamentals of nursing* (10th ed., pp. 1027, 1031). Elsevier.

169. The nurse assists the physician with the removal of a chest tube inserted to treat a client who experienced a pneumothorax. During the procedure, the nurse instructs the client to perform which action?
1. Inhale deeply.
2. Breathe normally.
3. Breathe out forcefully.
4. Take a deep breath and hold it.

Level of Cognitive Ability: Applying
Client Needs: Physiological Integrity
Clinical Judgment/Cognitive Skills: Take Action
Integrated Process: Nursing Process/Implementation
Content Area: Skills: Tube Care
Health Problems: Adult Health: Respiratory: Pneumothorax
Priority Concepts: Clinical Judgment; Gas Exchange

Answer: 4
Rationale: The client is instructed to take a deep breath and hold it for chest tube removal. This maneuver will increase intrathoracic pressure, thereby lessening the potential for air to enter the pleural space. Therefore, options 1, 2, and 3 are incorrect.
Test-Taking Strategy: Focus on the subject, chest tube removal. Eliminate options 1 and 2 because they are comparable or alike in that breathing will cause air to enter the pleural space. From the remaining options, eliminate option 3 because of the word "forcefully."
Priority Nursing Tip: Never clamp a chest tube without a written prescription from the physician. Additionally, agency policy regarding clamping a chest tube needs to be followed.
Reference: Lewis, S., et al. (2020). *Medical-surgical nursing: Assessment and management of clinical problems* (11th ed., pp. 528–529). Elsevier.

❖ **170.** The nurse assesses the water seal chamber of a closed chest drainage system and notes fluctuations in the chamber. What action would the nurse implement?
1. Unkinking the tubing
2. Assessing for an air leak
3. Documenting that the lung has reexpanded
4. Documenting that the lung has not yet reexpanded

Level of Cognitive Ability: Applying
Client Needs: Physiological Integrity
Clinical Judgment/Cognitive Skills: Take Action
Integrated Process: Nursing Process/Implementation
Content Area: Skills: Tube Care
Health Problems: Adult Health: Respiratory: Pneumothorax
Priority Concepts: Clinical Judgment; Gas Exchange

Answer: 4
Rationale: Fluctuations (tidaling) in the water seal chamber are normal during inhalation and exhalation until the lung reexpands and the client no longer requires chest drainage. If fluctuations are absent, it could indicate occlusion of the tubing or that the lung has reexpanded. Excessive bubbling in the water seal chamber indicates that an air leak is present.
Test-Taking Strategy: Focus on the subject, chest tube system. Recalling the normal expectations related to the functioning of chest tube drainage systems will direct you to the correct option.
Priority Nursing Tip: In the water seal chamber, the tip of the tube is underwater, allowing fluid and air to drain from the pleural space and preventing air from entering the pleural space.
Reference: Potter, P., et al. (2021). *Fundamentals of nursing* (10th ed., p. 970). Elsevier.

171. The nurse is creating a care plan for an older client being admitted to a long-term care facility. Which information would the nurse use to plan interventions for this client? **Select all that apply.**
- ❑ **1.** Older clients tend to be incontinent.
- ❑ **2.** Older clients are at risk for dehydration.
- ❑ **3.** Depression is a normal part of the aging process.
- ❑ **4.** Age-related skin changes require special monitoring.
- ❑ **5.** Older clients are at risk for complications of immobility.
- ❑ **6.** Confusion and cognitive changes are common findings in the older population.

Level of Cognitive Ability: Creating
Client Needs: Physiological Integrity
Clinical Judgment/Cognitive Skills: Generate Solutions
Integrated Process: Clinical Judgment; Nursing Process/Planning
Content Area: Developmental Stages: Later Adulthood
Health Problems: N/A
Priority Concepts: Development; Health Promotion

Answer: 2, 4, 5
Rationale: Older clients are at risk for dehydration and complications related to immobility. Another normal physiologic change that occurs during the aging process is loss of skin integrity. Incontinence, depression, confusion, and cognitive changes are not normal parts of the aging process.
Test-Taking Strategy: Focus on the subject, an older client being admitted to a long-term care facility. Read each option carefully and recall normal manifestations of the aging process to lead you to the correct options.
Priority Nursing Tip: During the aging process, normal physiologic body changes occur.
Reference: Potter, P., et al. (2021). *Fundamentals of nursing* (10th ed., pp. 179–181). Elsevier.

❖ **172.** The nurse plans care for a client with dehydration requiring intravenous (IV) fluids and electrolytes, understanding that which are findings that correlate with the need for this type of therapy? **Select all that apply.**
- ❑ **1.** Hyponatremia
- ❑ **2.** Bounding pulse rate
- ❑ **3.** Chronic kidney disease
- ❑ **4.** Isolated syncope episodes
- ❑ **5.** Rapid, weak, and thready pulse
- ❑ **6.** Abnormal serum and urine osmolality levels

Level of Cognitive Ability: Analyzing
Client Needs: Physiological Integrity
Clinical Judgment/Cognitive Skills: Recognize Cues
Integrated Process: Clinical Judgment; Nursing Process/Assessment
Content Area: Foundations of Care: Fluids and Electrolytes
Health Problems: Adult Health: Gastrointestinal: Dehydration
Priority Concepts: Fluids and Electrolytes; Clinical Judgment

Answer: 1, 5, 6
Rationale: Abnormal assessment findings of major body systems offer clues to fluid and electrolyte imbalances. Rapid, weak, and thready pulse is an assessment abnormality found with fluid and electrolyte imbalances, such as hyponatremia. Abnormal serum and urine osmolality are laboratory tests that are helpful in identifying the presence of or risk of fluid imbalances. Isolated episodes of syncope are not indicators for intravenous therapy unless fluid and electrolyte imbalances are identified. A bounding pulse rate is a manifestation of fluid volume excess; therefore, IV fluids are not indicated. Clients with chronic kidney disease experience the inability of the kidneys to regulate the body's water balance; fluid restrictions may be used.
Test-Taking Strategy: Focus on the subject, clinical indicators of intravenous fluid and electrolyte therapy. Think about the purpose of IV therapy and circumstances in which it is prescribed to lead you to the correct options.
Priority Nursing Tip: The assessment process will provide cues that are necessary to consider before intravenous therapy is initiated. The nurse needs to recognize these cues and analyze them to make a clinical judgment about the client's needs.
Reference: Potter, P., et al. (2021). *Fundamentals of nursing* (10th ed., pp. 984, 1201). Elsevier.

173. A child is admitted to the hospital with a diagnosis of rheumatic fever. The nurse reviews the blood laboratory findings, knowing that which finding will confirm the likelihood of this disorder?
1. Increased leukocyte count
2. Decreased hemoglobin count
3. Increased antistreptolysin-O (ASO titer)
4. Decreased erythrocyte sedimentation rate

Level of Cognitive Ability: Analyzing
Client Needs: Physiological Integrity
Clinical Judgment/Cognitive Skills: Recognize Cues
Integrated Process: Clinical Judgment; Nursing Process/Assessment
Content Area: Pediatrics: Cardiovascular
Health Problems: Pediatric-Specific: Rheumatic Fever
Priority Concepts: Clinical Judgment; Inflammation

Answer: 3
Rationale: Children suspected of having rheumatic fever are tested for streptococcal antibodies. The most reliable and best standardized test to confirm the diagnosis is the ASO titer. An elevated level indicates the presence of rheumatic fever. The remaining options are unrelated to diagnosing rheumatic fever. Additionally, an increased leukocyte count indicates the presence of infection but is not specific in confirming a particular diagnosis.
Test-Taking Strategy: Note the word "confirm." Focusing on the **subject** of rheumatic fever will assist in eliminating options 2 and 4. From the remaining options, recall that an increased leukocyte count indicates the presence of infection but is not specific in confirming a particular diagnosis.
Priority Nursing Tip: Rheumatic fever manifests 2 to 6 weeks after a group A beta-hemolytic streptococcal infection of the upper respiratory tract.
Reference: McKinney, E. S., et al. (2022). *Maternal child nursing* (6th ed., p. 1117). Elsevier.

❖ **174.** The nurse caring for a 5-year-old with a history of tetralogy of Fallot notes that the child has clubbed fingers. This finding is indicative of which associated condition?
1. Tissue hypoxia
2. Chronic hypertension
3. Delayed physical growth
4. Destruction of bone marrow

Level of Cognitive Ability: Analyzing
Client Needs: Physiological Integrity
Clinical Judgment/Cognitive Skills: Analyze Cues
Integrated Process: Clinical Judgment; Nursing Process/Analysis
Content Area: Pediatrics: Cardiovascular
Health Problems: Pediatric-Specific: Congenital Cardiac Defects
Priority Concepts: Gas Exchange; Perfusion

Answer: 1
Rationale: Clubbing, a thickening and flattening of the tips of the fingers and toes, is thought to occur because of chronic tissue hypoxia and polycythemia. Options 2, 3, and 4 do not cause clubbing.
Test-Taking Strategy: Focus on the **subject**, tetralogy of Fallot. Use the ABCs—**airway, breathing, and circulation.** Hypoxia relates to oxygenation, which is a concern with this disorder.
Priority Nursing Tip: Hypercyanotic spells (acute episodes of cyanosis and hypoxia) are also called *blue spells* or *tet spells* and occur when the child's oxygen requirements exceed the blood supply, such as during feeding, crying, or defecating.
Reference: McKinney, E. S., et al. (2022). *Maternal child nursing* (6th ed., p.1103) Elsevier.

175. The nurse plans care for a client diagnosed with end-stage renal disease (ESRD). Which assessment findings does the nurse expect to note documented in the client's medical record? **Select all that apply.**
❑ 1. Edema
❑ 2. Anemia
❑ 3. Polyuria
❑ 4. Bradycardia
❑ 5. Hypotension
❑ 6. Osteoporosis

Level of Cognitive Ability: Applying
Client Needs: Physiological Integrity
Clinical Judgment/Cognitive Skills: Recognize Cues
Integrated Process: Nursing Process/Assessment
Content Area: Adult Health: Renal and Urinary
Health Problems: Adult Health: Renal and Urinary: Acute Kidney Injury and Chronic Kidney Disease
Priority Concepts: Elimination; Fluids and Electrolytes

Answer: 1, 2
Rationale: The manifestations of ESRD are the result of impaired kidney function. Two functions of the kidney are maintenance of water balance in the body and the secretion of erythropoietin, which stimulates red blood cell formation in bone marrow. Impairment of these functions results in edema and anemia. Kidney failure results in decreased urine production and increased blood pressure. Tachycardia is a result of increased fluid load on the heart. Osteoporosis is not a common finding with ESRD.
Test-Taking Strategy: Focus on the **subject**, ESRD. Recalling the anatomy and physiology of the renal system and focusing on how the kidney functions and pathophysiology of ESRD will lead you to the correct options.
Priority Nursing Tip: The manifestations of kidney failure are primarily caused by the retention of nitrogenous wastes, the retention of fluids, and the inability of the kidneys to regulate electrolytes.
Reference: Ignatavicius, D., et al. (2021). *Medical-surgical nursing: Concepts for interprofessional collaborative care* (10th ed., p. 1388). Elsevier.

❖ **176.** The nurse is performing range-of-motion (ROM) exercises on a client when the client unexpectedly develops spastic muscle contractions. Which interventions would the nurse implement? **Select all that apply.**
- ❑ 1. Stop movement of the affected part.
- ❑ 2. Massage the affected part vigorously.
- ❑ 3. Notify the physician immediately.
- ❑ 4. Force movement of the joint supporting the muscle.
- ❑ 5. Ask client to stand and walk rapidly around the room.
- ❑ 6. Place continuous gentle pressure on the muscle group until it relaxes.

Level of Cognitive Ability: Applying
Client Needs: Physiological Integrity
Clinical Judgment/Cognitive Skills: Take Action
Integrated Process: Clinical Judgment; Nursing Process/Implementation
Content Area: Skills: Activity/Mobility
Health Problems: N/A
Priority Concepts: Mobility; Pain

Answer: 1, 6
Rationale: ROM exercises should put each joint through as full a range of motion as possible without causing discomfort. An unexpected outcome is the development of spastic muscle contraction during ROM exercises. If this occurs, the nurse would stop movement of the affected part and place continuous gentle pressure on the muscle group until it relaxes. Once the contraction subsides, the exercises are resumed, using slower, steady movement. Massaging the affected part vigorously may worsen the contraction. There is no need to notify the physician unless intervention is ineffective. The nurse would never force movement of a joint. Asking the client to stand and walk rapidly around the room is an inappropriate measure. Additionally, if the client is able to walk, ROM exercises are probably unnecessary.
Test-Taking Strategy: Focus on the subject, interventions to relieve spastic muscle contractions. Eliminate option 2 because of the word *vigorously*, option 3 because of the word *immediately*, and option 4 because of the word *force*. Next eliminate option 5 because if the client is able to walk, ROM exercises are probably unnecessary.
Priority Nursing Tip: ROM exercises provide adequate muscle use and maintain strength and flexibility of the muscles and joints.
Reference: Lewis, S., et al. (2020). *Medical-surgical nursing: Assessment and management of clinical problems* (11th ed., p. 1432). Elsevier.

177. A client has been admitted with a diagnosis of acute glomerulonephritis. During history taking, the nurse would ask the client about a recent history of which event?
1. Bleeding ulcer
2. Myocardial infarction
3. Deep vein thrombosis
4. Streptococcal infection

Level of Cognitive Ability: Applying
Client Needs: Physiological Integrity
Clinical Judgment/Cognitive Skills: Recognize Cues
Integrated Process: Nursing Process/Assessment
Content Area: Adult Health: Renal and Urinary
Health Problems: Adult Health: Renal and Urinary: Urinary Tract Inflammation/Infection/Trauma
Priority Concepts: Fluids and Electrolytes; Infection

Answer: 4
Rationale: The predominant cause of acute glomerulonephritis is infection with beta-hemolytic *Streptococcus* 3 weeks before the onset of symptoms. In addition to bacteria, other infectious agents that could trigger the disorder include viruses, fungi, and parasites. Bleeding ulcer, myocardial infarction, and deep vein thrombosis are not precipitating causes.
Test-Taking Strategy: Focus on the subject, glomerulonephritis. Recalling that infection is a common trigger for glomerulonephritis assists in eliminating options 1, 2, and 3. It is also necessary to know that streptococcal infections are a common cause of this problem.
Priority Nursing Tip: Edema, hematuria, and proteinuria are manifestations of glomerulonephritis.
Reference: Ignatavicius, D., et al. (2021). *Medical-surgical nursing: Concepts for interprofessional collaborative care* (10th ed., p. 1360). Elsevier.

❖ **178.** A client has just been admitted to the emergency department with reports of chest pain. Serum cardiac enzyme levels are drawn, and the results indicate an elevated serum creatine kinase (CK)-MB isoenzyme, troponin T, and troponin I. The nurse concludes that these results are compatible with what diagnosis?
1. Valve disease
2. Unstable angina
3. Coronary artery disease
4. New-onset myocardial infarction (MI)

Level of Cognitive Ability: Analyzing
Client Needs: Physiological Integrity
Clinical Judgment/Cognitive Skills: Analyze Cues
Integrated Process: Clinical Judgment; Nursing Process/Analysis
Content Area: Foundations of Care: Laboratory Tests
Health Problems: Adult Health: Cardiovascular: Myocardial Infarction
Priority Concepts: Clinical Judgment; Perfusion

Answer: 4
Rationale: Creatine kinase (CK)-MB isoenzyme is a sensitive indicator of myocardial damage. Levels begin to rise 3 to 6 hours after the onset of chest pain, peak at approximately 24 hours, and return to normal in about 3 days. Troponin is a regulatory protein found in striated muscle (skeletal and myocardial). Increased amounts of troponins are released into the bloodstream when an infarction causes damage to the myocardium. Troponin I is particularly sensitive to myocardial muscle injury; therefore, the client's results are compatible with new-onset MI. Options 1, 2, and 3 all result in chest pain, these levels would not be elevated in these options.
Test-Taking Strategy: Focus on the subject, cardiac enzymes. Eliminate options 1, 2, and 3 because they are not likely to elevate cardiac enzymes as stated.
Priority Nursing Tip: Troponin I has a high affinity for myocardial injury. The level rises within 3 hours after injury and persists up to 7 to 10 days.
Reference: Ignatavicius, D., et al. (2021). *Medical-surgical nursing: Concepts for interprofessional collaborative care* (10th ed., pp. 626–627). Elsevier.

179. As part of cardiac assessment, to palpate the apical pulse, the nurse places the fingertips at which location?
1. At the left midclavicular line at the fifth intercostal space
2. At the left midclavicular line at the third intercostal space
3. To the right of the left midclavicular line at the fifth intercostal space
4. To the right of the left midclavicular line at the third intercostal space

Level of Cognitive Ability: Applying
Client Needs: Physiological Integrity
Clinical Judgment/Cognitive Skills: Take Action
Integrated Process: Nursing Process/Assessment
Content Area: Health Assessment/Physical Exam: Heart and Peripheral Vascular
Health Problems: N/A
Priority Concepts: Clinical Judgment; Perfusion

Answer: 1
Rationale: The point of maximal impulse (PMI), where the apical pulse is palpated, is normally located in the fourth or fifth intercostal space, at the left midclavicular line. Options 2, 3, and 4 are not descriptions of the location for palpation of the apical pulse.
Test-Taking Strategy: Focus on the subject, point of maximal impulse (PMI). Recalling that the PMI corresponds to the left ventricular apex and visualizing each position in the options will direct you to the correct option.
Priority Nursing Tip: The apical impulse may not be palpable in obese clients or clients with thick chest walls.
Reference: Potter, P., et al. (2021). *Fundamentals of nursing* (10th ed., p. 478). Elsevier.

❖ **180.** The nurse is caring for a client receiving bolus feedings via a nasogastric (NG) tube after surgery for stomach cancer. The nurse would place the client in which position to administer the feeding?
1. Supine
2. Semi-Fowler's
3. Trendelenburg's
4. Lateral recumbent

Level of Cognitive Ability: Applying
Client Needs: Physiological Integrity
Clinical Judgment/Cognitive Skills: Take Action
Integrated Process: Nursing Process/Implementation
Content Area: Skills: Nutrition
Health Problems: Adult Health: Cancer: Esophageal/Gastric/Intestinal
Priority Concepts: Nutrition; Safety

Answer: 2
Rationale: Clients are at high risk for aspiration during an NG tube feeding because the tube bypasses a protective mechanism, the gag reflex. The head of the bed is elevated 35 to 40 degrees (semi-Fowler's) to prevent this complication by facilitating gastric emptying. The remaining options increase the risk of aspiration by blunting the effect of gravity on gastric emptying.
Test-Taking Strategy: Focus on the subject, nasogastric (NG) tube feeding. Eliminate options 1, 3, and 4 because they are comparable or alike and increase the risk of aspiration.
Priority Nursing Tip: Check the expiration date on the formula before administering the nasogastric tube feeding.
Reference: Potter, P., et al. (2021). *Fundamentals of nursing* (10th ed., pp. 1131, 1134). Elsevier.

181. The nurse monitors a client diagnosed with acute pancreatitis. Which assessment finding indicates that paralytic ileus has developed?
1. Inability to pass flatus
2. Loss of anal sphincter control
3. Severe, constant pain with rapid onset
4. Firm, nontender mass palpable at the lower right costal margin

Level of Cognitive Ability: Analyzing
Client Needs: Physiological Integrity
Clinical Judgment/Cognitive Skills: Recognize Cues
Integrated Process: Clinical Judgment; Nursing Process/Assessment
Content Area: Adult Health: Gastrointestinal
Health Problems: Adult Health: Gastrointestinal: Pancreatitis
Priority Concepts: Clinical Judgment; Elimination

Answer: 1
Rationale: An inflammatory reaction such as acute pancreatitis can cause paralytic ileus, the common form of nonmechanical obstruction. Inability to pass flatus is a clinical manifestation of paralytic ileus. Loss of sphincter control is not a sign of paralytic ileus. Pain is associated with paralytic ileus, but the pain usually presents as a more constant generalized discomfort. Pain that is severe, constant, and rapid in onset is more likely caused by strangulation of the bowel. Option 4 is the description of the physical finding of liver enlargement. The liver is usually enlarged in the client with cirrhosis or hepatitis. An enlarged liver is not a sign of paralytic ileus.
Test-Taking Strategy: Focus on the subject, a sign of paralytic ileus. Recalling the definition of this complication and noting the word "paralytic" will direct you to the correct option.
Priority Nursing Tip: Cullen's sign (discoloration of the abdomen and periumbilical area) and Turner's sign (bluish discoloration of the flanks) are indicative of pancreatitis.
Reference: Lewis, S., et al. (2020). *Medical-surgical nursing: Assessment and management of clinical problems* (11th ed., pp. 945, 993). Elsevier.

❖ **182.** After performing an initial abdominal assessment on a client with a diagnosis of cholelithiasis, the nurse documents that the bowel sounds are normal. How would the nurse describe this finding?

1. Waves of loud gurgles auscultated in all four quadrants
2. Soft gurgling or clicking sounds auscultated in all four quadrants
3. Low-pitched swishing sounds auscultated in one or two quadrants
4. Very high-pitched loud rushes auscultated, especially in one or two quadrants

Level of Cognitive Ability: Applying
Client Needs: Physiological Integrity
Clinical Judgment/Cognitive Skills: Recognize Cues
Integrated Process: Nursing Process/Assessment
Content Area: Health Assessment/Physical Exam: Abdomen
Health Problems: Adult Health: Gastrointestinal: Gallbladder Disease
Priority Concepts: Clinical Judgment; Health Promotion

Answer: 2
Rationale: Although frequency and intensity of bowel sounds will vary depending on the phase of digestion, normal bowel sounds are relatively soft gurgling or clicking sounds that occur irregularly 5 to 35 times per minute. Loud gurgles (borborygmi) indicate hyperperistalsis. A swishing or buzzing sound represents turbulent blood flow associated with a bruit. No aortic bruits should be heard. Bowel sounds will be higher pitched and loud (hyperresonance) when the intestines are under tension, such as in intestinal obstruction.
Test-Taking Strategy: Focus on the subject, normal bowel sounds. Normally, bowel sounds would be audible in all four quadrants; therefore, options 3 and 4 can be eliminated. From the remaining options, select option 2 because of the word "soft" in this option.
Priority Nursing Tip: Murphy's sign (the client cannot take a deep breath when the examiner's fingers are passed below the hepatic margin because of pain) is a characteristic of cholecystitis.
Reference: Lewis, S., et al. (2020). *Medical-surgical nursing: Assessment and management of clinical problems* (11th ed., pp. 841, 998–999). Elsevier.

183. Which important parameter would the nurse assess daily for a child diagnosed with nephrotic syndrome?

1. Weight
2. Albumin levels
3. Activity tolerance
4. BUN level

Level of Cognitive Ability: Applying
Client Needs: Physiological Integrity
Clinical Judgment/Cognitive Skills: Take Action
Integrated Process: Nursing Process/Assessment
Content Area: Pediatrics: Renal and Urinary
Health Problems: Pediatric-Specific: Nephrotic Syndrome
Priority Concepts: Clinical Judgment; Fluids and Electrolytes

Answer: 1
Rationale: The child with nephrotic syndrome typically presents with edema, hypoalbuminemia, and proteinuria. The nurse carefully assesses the fluid balance of the child, which includes daily monitoring of weight, intake and output, edema, and girth measurements. Albumin levels are monitored as they are prescribed, as are the BUN and creatinine levels. The child's activity level is adjusted according to the amount of edema and water retention. As edema increases, the child's activity level should be restricted.
Test-Taking Strategy: Focus on the subject, a child with nephrotic syndrome. Note the word "daily." Recalling that the typical signs of nephrotic syndrome are edema, hypoalbuminemia, and proteinuria will direct you to the correct option.
Priority Nursing Tip: In nephrotic syndrome, the blood pressure may be normal or slightly decreased from normal.
Reference: McKinney, E. S., et al. (2022). *Maternal child nursing* (6th ed., pp. 1025–1026). Elsevier.

❖ **184.** A client is being admitted with a diagnosis of urolithiasis and ureteral colic. The nurse expects to note which finding on pain assessment?
1. Dull and aching pain in the costovertebral area
2. Aching and cramplike pain throughout the abdomen
3. Pain that is sharp and radiating posteriorly to the spinal column
4. Pain that is excruciating, wavelike, and radiating toward the genitalia

Level of Cognitive Ability: Analyzing
Client Needs: Physiological Integrity
Clinical Judgment/Cognitive Skills: Recognize Cues
Integrated Process: Clinical Judgment; Nursing Process/Assessment
Content Area: Adult Health: Renal and Urinary
Health Problems: Adult Health: Renal and Urinary: Calculi
Priority Concepts: Clinical Judgment; Pain

Answer: 4
Rationale: The pain of ureteral colic is caused by movement of a stone through the ureter and is sharp, excruciating, and wavelike, radiating to the genitalia and thigh. The stone causes reduced flow of urine, and the urine also contains blood because of the stone's abrasive action on urinary tract mucosa. Stones in the renal pelvis cause pain that is a dull ache in the costovertebral area. Renal colic is characterized by pain that is acute, with tenderness over the costovertebral area. Options 1, 2, and 3 are not characteristics of urolithiasis and ureteral colic.
Test-Taking Strategy: Focus on the subject, urolithiasis and ureteral colic. Recall the anatomic location of the kidneys and the ureters. Because the kidneys are located in the posterior abdomen near the ribcage, pain in the costovertebral area is more likely to be associated with stones in the renal pelvis. On the other hand, sharp wavelike pain that radiates toward the genitalia is more consistent with the location of the ureters in the abdomen.
Priority Nursing Tip: For the client with renal calculi, strain all urine for the presence of stones and send the stones to the laboratory for analysis.
Reference: Ignatavicius, D., et al. (2021). *Medical-surgical nursing: Concepts for interprofessional collaborative care* (10th ed., pp. 1344, 1346). Elsevier.

185. The client with heart failure states the need to use three pillows under the head and upper torso at night to be able to breathe comfortably while sleeping. The nurse documents that the client is experiencing which clinical finding?
1. Orthopnea
2. Dyspnea at rest
3. Dyspnea on exertion
4. Paroxysmal nocturnal dyspnea

Level of Cognitive Ability: Applying
Client Needs: Physiological Integrity
Clinical Judgment/Cognitive Skills: Analyze Cues
Integrated Process: Communication and Documentation
Content Area: Foundations of Care: Sleep and Rest
Health Problems: Adult Health: Cardiovascular: Heart Failure
Priority Concepts: Functional Ability; Gas Exchange

Answer: 1
Rationale: Dyspnea is a subjective complaint that can range from an awareness of breathing to physical distress and does not necessarily correlate with the degree of heart failure. Dyspnea can be exertional or at rest. Orthopnea is a more severe form of dyspnea, requiring the client to assume a "three-point" position while upright and use pillows to support the head and upper torso at night. Paroxysmal nocturnal dyspnea is a severe form of dyspnea, occurring suddenly at night because of rapid fluid reentry into the vasculature from the interstitium during sleep.
Test-Taking Strategy: Focus on the subject, a client with heart failure who has trouble breathing while sleeping. Recall knowledge of the different degrees of dyspnea. Eliminate options 3 and 4 because the question mentions nothing about exertion or a sudden (paroxysmal) event. From the remaining options, select option 1 because the client is breathing "comfortably" with the use of pillows.
Priority Nursing Tip: Signs of left-sided heart failure are evident in the pulmonary system. Signs of right-sided heart failure are evident in the systemic circulation.
Reference: Ignatavicius, D., et al. (2021). *Medical-surgical nursing: Concepts for interprofessional collaborative care* (10th ed., p. 594). Elsevier.

❖ **186.** The nurse admits a client who is in sickle cell crisis. The nurse would prepare for which intervention as a **priority** in the management of the client?
1. Blood transfusion
2. Intravenous fluid therapy
3. Oxygen administration
4. Pain management with an opioid

Level of Cognitive Ability: Applying
Client Needs: Physiological Integrity
Clinical Judgment/Cognitive Skills: Prioritize Hypotheses
Integrated Process: Nursing Process/Planning
Content Area: Adult Health: Hematologic
Health Problems: Adult Health: Hematologic: Anemias
Priority Concepts: Caregiving; Gas Exchange

Answer: 3
Rationale: The priority nursing intervention for a client in sickle cell crisis is to administer supplemental oxygen because the client is hypoxemic, and as a result, the red blood cells change to the sickle shape. In addition, oxygen is the priority because airway and breathing are more important than circulatory needs. The nurse also plans for fluid therapy to promote hydration and reverse the agglutination of sickled cells, opioid analgesics for relief from severe pain, and blood transfusions (rather than iron administration) to increase the blood's oxygen-carrying capacity.
Test-Taking Strategy: Focus on the subject, sickle cell crisis, and focus on the strategic word, *priority*. Recalling the ABCs—airway, breathing, and circulation—will assist in answering correctly. Recalling that clumping of sickled cells occurs when the sickle cell client is hypoxemic will direct you to the correct option.
Priority Nursing Tip: In sickle cell anemia, situations that precipitate sickling include fever, dehydration, and emotional and physical stress.
Reference: Ignatavicius, D., et al. (2021). *Medical-surgical nursing: Concepts for interprofessional collaborative care* (10th ed., p. 796). Elsevier.

187. The nurse suspecting that a client is developing cardiogenic shock would assess for which peripheral vascular manifestation of this complication? **Select all that apply.**
☐ 1. Flushed, dry skin
☐ 2. Warm, moist skin
☐ 3. Cool, clammy skin
☐ 4. Irregular pedal pulses
☐ 5. Bounding pedal pulses
☐ 6. Weak or thready pedal pulses

Level of Cognitive Ability: Analyzing
Client Needs: Physiological Integrity
Clinical Judgment/Cognitive Skills: Recognize Cues
Integrated Process: Clinical Judgment; Nursing Process/Assessment
Content Area: Complex Care: Shock
Health Problems: Adult Health: Cardiovascular: Cardiogenic Shock
Priority Concepts: Gas Exchange; Perfusion

Answer: 3, 6
Rationale: Some of the manifestations of cardiogenic shock include increased pulse (weak and thready); decreased blood pressure; decreasing urinary output; signs of cerebral ischemia (confusion, agitation); and cool, clammy skin. None of the remaining options are associated with the peripheral vascular aspects of cardiogenic shock.
Test-Taking Strategy: Focus on the subject, cardiogenic shock. Recall the signs and symptoms of shock. The words "clammy" and "weak or thready" will direct you to the correct option.
Priority Nursing Tip: The goals of treatment for cardiogenic shock are to maintain tissue oxygenation and perfusion and improve the pumping ability of the heart.
Reference: Ignatavicius, D., et al. (2021). *Medical-surgical nursing: Concepts for interprofessional collaborative care* (10th ed., pp. 733–734). Elsevier.

188. The nurse teaching an older client about general hygienic measures for foot and nail care would include which instructions? **Select all that apply.**

- ❑ 1. Wear knee-high hose to prevent edema.
- ❑ 2. Soak and wash the feet daily using cool water.
- ❑ 3. Use commercial removers for corns or calluses.
- ❑ 4. Use over-the-counter preparations to treat ingrown nails.
- ❑ 5. Apply lanolin or baby oil if dryness is noted along the feet.
- ❑ 6. Pat the feet dry thoroughly after washing and dry well between toes.

Level of Cognitive Ability: Applying
Client Needs: Physiological Integrity
Clinical Judgment/Cognitive Skills: Take Action
Integrated Process: Teaching and Learning
Content Area: Skills: Hygiene
Health Problems: N/A
Priority Concepts: Patient Education; Health Promotion

Answer: 5, 6
Rationale: The nurse would offer the following guidelines in a general hygienic foot and nail care program: Inspect the feet daily, including the tops and soles of the feet, the heels, and the areas between the toes; wash the feet daily using lukewarm water, and avoid soaks to the feet, thoroughly patting the feet dry and drying well between toes; and avoid cutting corns or calluses or using commercial removers. Additional general hygienic measures include gently rubbing lanolin, baby oil, or corn oil into the skin if dryness is noted along the feet; filing the toenails straight across and square (do not use scissors or clippers); avoiding the use of over-the-counter preparations to treat ingrown toenails and consulting a physician for these problems; and avoiding wearing elastic stockings (unless prescribed by a health care professional), knee-high hose, or constricting garters.
Test-Taking Strategy: Focus on the subject, general hygienic measures for foot and nail care. Eliminate option 1, recalling that constricting items need to be avoided. Eliminate option 2 because of the words "soak" and "cool." Eliminate options 3 and 4 because of the words "commercial removers" and "over-the-counter," respectively.
Priority Nursing Tip: A complication of diabetes mellitus is peripheral neuropathy, which results in decreased sensation, particularly in the feet. A client with diabetes mellitus needs to be cautious about temperature exposure and injuries to the feet as they may not be felt because of the decreased sensation.
Reference: Potter, P., et al. (2021). *Fundamentals of nursing* (10th ed., pp. 902–904). Elsevier.

189. A client diagnosed with renal cancer is being treated preoperatively with radiation therapy. The nurse evaluates that the client has an understanding of proper care of the skin over the treatment field when the client makes which statement?

1. "I'll be able to wash the ink marks off my skin after the initial treatment."
2. "Direct sunlight is something I'll have to really avoid exposing my skin to."
3. "I'll have my family bring me some unscented lotion to keep my skin soft."
4. "Wearing snug fitting clothing over the skin site will help provide good support."

Level of Cognitive Ability: Evaluating
Client Needs: Physiological Integrity
Clinical Judgment/Cognitive Skills: Evaluate Outcomes
Integrated Process: Clinical Judgment; Nursing Process/Evaluation
Content Area: Adult Health: Oncology
Health Problems: Adult Health: Cancer: Bladder and Kidney
Priority Concepts: Cellular Regulation; Tissue Integrity

Answer: 2
Rationale: The client undergoing radiation therapy must keep the affected skin protected from temperature extremes, direct sunlight, and chlorinated water (as from swimming pools). The client needs to wash the site using mild soap and warm or cool water and pat the area dry. Lines or ink marks that are placed on the skin to guide the radiation therapy need to be left in place. No lotions, creams, alcohol, perfumes, or deodorants should be placed on the skin over the treatment site. The client needs to wear cotton clothing over the skin site and guard against irritation from tight or rough clothing such as belts or bras.
Test-Taking Strategy: Focus on the subject, care of the skin over the treatment field after radiation therapy. Note the words "understanding of proper care." Recalling that the goal of care is to prevent skin irritation will direct you to the correct option.
Priority Nursing Tip: Radiation therapy is effective on tissues directly within the path of the radiation beam.
Reference: Ignatavicius, D., et al. (2021). *Medical-surgical nursing: Concepts for interprofessional collaborative care* (10th ed., p. 382). Elsevier.

❖ **190.** A client diagnosed with chronic kidney disease is prescribed epoetin alfa. When discussing measures needed to support this medication therapy, the nurse would include information regarding which supplement?
1. Iron
2. Zinc
3. Calcium
4. Magnesium

Level of Cognitive Ability: Applying
Client Needs: Physiological Integrity
Clinical Judgment/Cognitive Skills: Take Action
Integrated Process: Teaching and Learning
Content Area: Pharmacology: Hematologic Medications: Hematopoietic Agents
Health Problems: Adult Health: Renal and Urinary: Acute Kidney Injury and Chronic Kidney Disease
Priority Concepts: Cellular Regulation; Adherence

Answer: 1
Rationale: Iron is needed for red blood cell (RBC) production; otherwise, the body cannot produce sufficient erythrocytes. In either case the client is not receiving the full benefit of epoetin alfa therapy if iron is not taken. Options 2, 3, or 4 are not prescribed for RBC production.
Test-Taking Strategy: Focus on the subject, measures needed to support therapy with epoetin alfa. Focus on this medication classification. Recalling that it is a hematologic medication will direct you to the correct option.
Priority Nursing Tip: A side effect of epoetin alfa is hypertension.
Reference: Kizior, R., & Hodgson, B. (2022). *Saunders Nursing drug handbook 2022* (p. 442). Elsevier.

191. The home health nurse is performing an initial assessment on a client who has been discharged after an insertion of a permanent pacemaker for a bradydysrhythmia. Which client statement indicates that an understanding of self-care is evident?
1. "I will never be able to operate a microwave oven again."
2. "I should expect occasional feelings of dizziness and fatigue."
3. "I will take my pulse in the wrist or neck daily and record it in a log."
4. "Moving my arms and shoulders vigorously helps check pacemaker functioning."

Level of Cognitive Ability: Evaluating
Client Needs: Physiological Integrity
Clinical Judgment/Cognitive Skills: Evaluate Outcomes
Integrated Process: Clinical Judgment; Nursing Process/Evaluation
Content Area: Adult Health: Cardiovascular
Health Problems: Adult Health: Cardiovascular: Dysrhythmias
Priority Concepts: Patient Education; Perfusion

Answer: 3
Rationale: Clients with permanent pacemakers must be able to take their pulse in the wrist and/or neck accurately so as to note any variation in the pulse rate or rhythm that may need to be reported to the physician. Clients can safely operate most appliances and tools, such as microwave ovens, video recorders, AM-FM radios, electric blankets, lawn mowers, and leaf blowers, as long as the devices are grounded and in good repair. If the client experiences any feelings of dizziness, fatigue, or an irregular heartbeat, the physician is notified. The arms and shoulders should not be moved vigorously for 6 weeks after insertion.
Test-Taking Strategy: Focus on the subject, client understanding about care to a pacemaker. Recalling that a pacemaker assists in controlling cardiac rate and rhythm will direct you to the correct option.
Priority Nursing Tip: A responsibility of the nurse is to teach a client with a pacemaker how to measure the pulse rate for 1 full minute at the same time each day.
Reference: Ignatavicius, D., et al. (2021). *Medical-surgical nursing: Concepts for interprofessional collaborative care* (10th ed., p. 649). Elsevier.

❖ **192.** A client experiencing a major depressive episode is unable to address activities of daily living (ADLs). Which nursing intervention **best** meets the client's current needs therapeutically?
1. Have the client's peers approach the client about how noncompliance in addressing ADLs affects the milieu.
2. Structure the client's day so that adequate time can be devoted to client's assuming responsibility for ADLs.
3. Offer the client choices and describe the consequences for the failure to comply with the expectation of maintaining one's own ADLs.
4. Feed, bathe, and dress the client as needed until the client's condition improves so that these activities can be performed independently.

Level of Cognitive Ability: Applying
Client Needs: Physiological Integrity
Clinical Judgment/Cognitive Skills: Take Action
Integrated Process: Nursing Process/Implementation
Content Area: Mental Health
Health Problems: Mental Health: Mood Disorders
Priority Concepts: Caregiving; Functional Ability

Answer: 4
Rationale: The symptoms of major depression include depressed mood, loss of interest or pleasure, changes in appetite and sleep patterns, psychomotor agitation or retardation, fatigue, feelings of worthlessness or guilt, diminished ability to think or concentrate, and recurrent thoughts of death. Often, the client does not have the energy or interest to complete activities of daily living. Option 1 will increase the client's feelings of poor self-esteem and of unworthiness. Option 2 is incorrect because the client still lacks the energy and motivation to do these independently. Option 3 may lead to increased feelings of worthlessness as the client fails to meet expectations.
Test-Taking Strategy: Focus on the subject, major depression. Note the strategic word, *best.* Use Maslow's Hierarchy of Needs theory and remember that physiologic needs are the priority. This will direct you to the correct option.
Priority Nursing Tip: For the client with depression, the nurse needs to avoid pushing the client to make decisions that the client is not ready to make.
Reference: Varcarolis, E., & Fosbre, C. (2021). *Essentials of psychiatric mental health nursing: A communication approach to evidence-based care* (4th ed., p. 211). Elsevier.

193. A pregnant client at 32 weeks of gestation is admitted to the obstetric unit for observation after a motor vehicle crash. When the client begins experiencing slight vaginal bleeding and mild cramps, which action would the nurse take to determine the viability of the fetus?
1. Insert an intravenous line and begin an infusion at 125 mL/hr.
2. Administer oxygen to the client via a face mask at 7 to 10 L/min.
3. Position and connect the ultrasound transducer to the external fetal monitor.
4. Position and connect a spiral electrode to the fetal monitor for internal fetal monitoring.

Level of Cognitive Ability: Applying
Client Needs: Physiological Integrity
Clinical Judgment/Cognitive Skills: Take Action
Integrated Process: Clinical Judgment; Nursing Process/Implementation
Content Area: Maternity: Antepartum
Health Problems: Maternity: Fetal Distress/Demise
Priority Concepts: Perfusion; Reproduction

Answer: 3
Rationale: External fetal monitoring will allow the nurse to determine any change in the fetal heart rate and rhythm that would indicate that the fetus is in jeopardy. The amount of bleeding described is insufficient to require intravenous fluid replacement. Because fetal distress has not been determined at this time, oxygen administration is premature. Internal monitoring is contraindicated when there is vaginal bleeding, especially in preterm labor.
Test-Taking Strategy: Focus on the subject, to determine viability of the fetus. Next use the steps of the nursing process, and note that option 3 is an assessment and a noninvasive measure.
Priority Nursing Tip: Internal fetal monitoring is invasive and requires rupturing of the membranes and attaching an electrode to the presenting part of the fetus.
Reference: McKinney, E. S., et al. (2022). *Maternal child nursing* (6th ed., pp. 601–602). Elsevier.

❖ **194.** The nurse is reviewing the results of a sweat test performed on a child with a suspected diagnosis of cystic fibrosis (CF). The nurse interprets the result as indicating which of the following?

Laboratory Results

Test and Result	Reference Range
Sweat chloride concentration 80 mEq/L (80 mmol/L)	<40 mEq/L (<40 mmol/L)

1. Normal finding
2. Equivocal finding
3. Indeterminate finding
4. Supportive finding

Level of Cognitive Ability: Analyzing
Client Needs: Physiological Integrity
Clinical Judgment/Cognitive Skills: Recognize Cues
Integrated Process: Clinical Judgment; Nursing Process/Assessment
Content Area: Foundations of Care: Diagnostic Tests
Health Problems: Pediatric-Specific: Cystic Fibrosis
Priority Concepts: Hormonal Regulation; Clinical Judgment

Answer: 4
Rationale: Cystic fibrosis is a chronic multisystem disorder characterized by exocrine gland dysfunction. A consistent finding of abnormally high chloride concentrations in the sweat is a unique characteristic of CF. Normally the sweat chloride concentration is less than 40 mEq/L (40 mmol/L). A sweat chloride concentration greater than 60 mEq/L (60 mmol/L) is diagnostic of CF.
Test-Taking Strategy: Focus on the subject, sweat test results supporting the diagnosis of cystic fibrosis. Noting that the test result is high will assist in determining that the finding is supportive.
Priority Nursing Tip: Usually more than 75 mg of sweat is needed to perform the sweat test. This amount is difficult to obtain from an infant; therefore, an immunoreactive trypsinogen analysis and direct deoxyribonucleic acid (DNA) analysis for mutant genes may be done to test for cystic fibrosis.
Reference: McKinney, E. S., et al. (2022). *Maternal child nursing* (6th ed., p. 1076). Elsevier.

195. The emergency department nurse is assessing a client who abruptly discontinued benzodiazepine therapy and is experiencing withdrawal. Which manifestations of withdrawal would the nurse expect to note? **Select all that apply.**
❏ 1. Tremors
❏ 2. Sweating
❏ 3. Lethargy
❏ 4. Agitation
❏ 5. Nervousness
❏ 6. Muscle weakness

Level of Cognitive Ability: Analyzing
Client Needs: Physiological Integrity
Clinical Judgment/Cognitive Skills: Recognize Cues
Integrated Process: Clinical Judgment; Nursing Process/Assessment
Content Area: Pharmacology: Psychotherapeutics: Antianxiety/Anxiolytics
Health Problems: Mental Health: Addictions
Priority Concepts: Clinical Judgment; Safety

Answer: 1, 2, 4, 5
Rationale: Benzodiazepines should not be abruptly discontinued because withdrawal symptoms are likely to occur. Withdrawal symptoms include tremor, sweating, agitation, nervousness, insomnia, anorexia, and muscular cramps. Withdrawal symptoms from long-term, high-dose benzodiazepine therapy include paranoia, delirium, panic, hypertension, and status epilepticus. Lethargy is not associated with benzodiazepine withdrawal.
Test-Taking Strategy: Focus on the subject, benzodiazepines. Specific knowledge regarding the withdrawal symptoms of benzodiazepines is needed to select the correct options. However, if you can remember that the therapeutic effect of benzodiazepines is anxiolytic, you will be able to eliminate the incorrect options because abrupt withdrawal will produce the opposite effect of an anxiolytic.
Priority Nursing Tip: Abrupt withdrawal of benzodiazepines can be potentially life threatening.
Reference: Varcarolis, E., & Fosbre, C. (2021). *Essentials of psychiatric mental health nursing: A communication approach to evidence-based care* (4th ed., p. 311). Elsevier.

❖ **196.** The nurse performs a neurovascular assessment on a client with a newly applied cast. The nurse would determine that there is a need for close observation and a **need for follow-up** if which is noted?
1. Palpable pulses distal to the cast
2. Capillary refill greater than 6 seconds
3. Blanching of the nail bed when it is depressed
4. Sensation when the area distal to the cast is pinched

Level of Cognitive Ability: Evaluating
Client Needs: Physiological Integrity
Clinical Judgment/Cognitive Skills: Evaluate Outcomes
Integrated Process: Clinical Judgment; Nursing Process/Evaluation
Content Area: Adult Health: Musculoskeletal
Health Problems: Adult Health: Musculoskeletal: Skeletal Injury
Priority Concepts: Clinical Judgment; Perfusion

Answer: 2
Rationale: To assess for adequate circulation, the nail bed of each finger or toe is depressed until it blanches and then the pressure is released. This is known as capillary refill time. Optimally, the color will change from white to pink rapidly (less than 3 seconds). If this does not occur, the toes or fingers will require close observation and follow-up. Palpable pulses and sensations distal to the cast are expected. However, if pulses could not be palpated or if the client complained of numbness or tingling, the physician needs to be notified.
Test-Taking Strategy: Focus on the subject, client assessment after cast application. Note the strategic words, *need for follow-up*. This creates a negative event query and requires you to select a finding that is not normal. Eliminate options 1, 3, and 4 because these options identify normal expected findings. Option 2 identifies an abnormal or unexpected finding.
Priority Nursing Tip: For the client with a cast applied to an extremity, if pulses could not be palpated or the client complains of numbness or tingling, the physician needs to be notified.
Reference: Ignatavicius, D., et al. (2021). *Medical-surgical nursing: Concepts for interprofessional collaborative care* (10th ed., p. 1033). Elsevier.

197. The nurse is monitoring an unconscious client who sustained a head injury. Which observed posturing supports the suspicion that the client sustained an upper brainstem injury?
1. Abnormal involuntary flexion of the extremities
2. Abnormal involuntary extension of the extremities
3. Upper extremity extension with lower extremity flexion
4. Upper extremity flexion with lower extremity extension

Level of Cognitive Ability: Analyzing
Client Needs: Physiological Integrity
Clinical Judgment/Cognitive Skills: Analyze Cues
Integrated Process: Clinical Judgment; Nursing Process/Analysis
Content Area: Adult Health: Neurologic
Health Problems: Adult Health: Neurologic: Head Injury/Trauma
Priority Concepts: Clinical Judgment; Intracranial Regulation

Answer: 2
Rationale: Decerebrate posturing, which can occur with upper brainstem injury, is characterized by abnormal involuntary extension of the extremities. Options 1, 3, and 4 are incorrect descriptions of this type of posturing.
Test-Taking Strategy: Focus on the subject, decerebrate posturing. Remember that decerebrate may also be known as extension. Recalling this concept will direct you to the correct option.
Priority Nursing Tip: Decerebrate or decorticate posturing is an indication of neurologic deterioration, warranting immediate notification of the physician.
Reference: Ignatavicius, D., et al. (2021). *Medical-surgical nursing: Concepts for interprofessional collaborative care* (10th ed., pp. 833–834). Elsevier.

❖ **198.** The nurse caring for a client returning to the unit after right radical mastectomy to treat breast cancer includes which intervention in the nursing plan of care for this client?
1. Takes blood pressures in the right arm only
2. Draws serum laboratory samples from the right arm only
3. Positions client supine and flat with the right arm elevated on a pillow
4. Checks the right posterior axilla area when assessing the surgical dressing

Level of Cognitive Ability: Applying
Client Needs: Physiological Integrity
Clinical Judgment/Cognitive Skills: Generate Solutions
Integrated Process: Clinical Judgment; Nursing Process/Planning
Content Area: Adult Health: Oncology
Health Problems: Adult Health: Cancer: Breast
Priority Concepts: Clotting; Safety

Answer: 4
Rationale: If there is drainage or bleeding from the surgical site after mastectomy, gravity will cause the drainage to seep down and soak the posterior axillary portion of the dressing first. The nurse checks this area to detect early bleeding. Blood pressure measurement, venipuncture, and intravenous sites should not involve use of the operative arm. The client needs to be positioned with the head in semi-Fowler's position and the arm on the operative side elevated on pillows to decrease edema. Edema is likely to occur because lymph drainage channels have been resected during the surgical procedure.
Test-Taking Strategy: Focus on the subject, postmastectomy care. Eliminate options 1 and 2 first because of the words "right arm only." From the remaining options, use knowledge of the effects of gravity to direct you to the correct option.
Priority Nursing Tip: Breast self-examination (BSE) should be done monthly, 7 to 10 days after menses. Postmenopausal clients need to select a specific day of the month and perform BSE monthly on that day.
Reference: Ignatavicius, D., et al. (2021). *Medical-surgical nursing: Concepts for interprofessional collaborative care* (10th ed., p. 1443). Elsevier.

199. The nurse is assisting a client diagnosed with hepatic encephalopathy to fill out the dietary menu. The nurse advises the client to avoid which entree item?
1. Tomato soup
2. Fresh fruit plate
3. Vegetable lasagna
4. Ground beef patty

Level of Cognitive Ability: Applying
Client Needs: Physiological Integrity
Clinical Judgment/Cognitive Skills: Take Action
Integrated Process: Nursing Process/Implementation
Content Area: Foundations of Care: Therapeutic Diets
Health Problems: Adult Health: Gastrointestinal: Cirrhosis
Priority Concepts: Nutrition; Safety

Answer: 4
Rationale: Clients with hepatic encephalopathy have impaired ability to convert ammonia to urea and must limit intake of protein and ammonia-containing foods in the diet. The client needs to avoid foods such as chicken, beef, ham, cheese, milk, peanut butter, and gelatin. The food items in options 1, 2, and 3 are acceptable to eat.
Test-Taking Strategy: Focus on the subject, hepatic encephalopathy, and note the word "avoid." Note that options 1, 2, and 3 are comparable or alike in that they address food items that include fruits and vegetables.
Priority Nursing Tip: Some food sources of protein include bread and cereal products, dairy products, beans, eggs, meats, fish, and poultry.
Reference: Ignatavicius, D., et al. (2021). *Medical-surgical nursing: Concepts for interprofessional collaborative care* (10th ed., p. 1164). Elsevier.

❖ **200.** A client with a colostomy reports gas buildup in the colostomy bag. The nurse instructs the client that consuming which food items would help prevent this problem? **Select all that apply.**
- ❑ 1. Yogurt
- ❑ 2. Broccoli
- ❑ 3. Cabbage
- ❑ 4. Crackers
- ❑ 5. Cauliflower
- ❑ 6. Toasted bread

Level of Cognitive Ability: Applying
Client Needs: Physiological Integrity
Clinical Judgment/Cognitive Skills: Generate Solutions
Integrated Process: Teaching and Learning
Content Area: Foundations of Care: Therapeutic Diets
Health Problems: Adult Health: Gastrointestinal: Nutrition/Malabsorption Problems
Priority Concepts: Elimination; Nutrition

Answer: 1, 4, 6
Rationale: Consumption of yogurt, crackers, and toasted bread can help prevent gas. Gas-forming foods include broccoli, mushrooms, cauliflower, onions, peas, and cabbage. These foods should be avoided by the client with a colostomy until tolerance to them is determined.
Test-Taking Strategy: Focus on the **subject**, prevention of gas buildup in the colostomy bag. Note the similarity between options 2, 3, and 5 in terms of their food substance to assist you in eliminating these options.
Priority Nursing Tip: The best way for a client with a colostomy to control flatus is through diet. Every client is different, and the client needs to learn which foods will be problematic. Also available are ostomy bags with a vent that allow the release of flatus through a deodorizing filter.
Reference: Ignatavicius, D., et al. (2021). *Medical-surgical nursing: Concepts for interprofessional collaborative care* (10th ed., p. 1123). Elsevier.

201. A client receiving total parenteral nutrition (TPN) reports nausea, polydipsia, and polyuria. To determine the cause of the client's report, the nurse would assess which client data?
1. Rectal temperature
2. Last serum potassium
3. Capillary blood glucose
4. Serum blood urea nitrogen and creatinine

Level of Cognitive Ability: Analyzing
Client Needs: Physiological Integrity
Clinical Judgment/Cognitive Skills: Analyze Cues
Integrated Process: Clinical Judgment; Nursing Process/Analysis
Content Area: Skills: Nutrition
Health Problems: Adult Health: Gastrointestinal: Nutrition/Malabsorption Problems
Priority Concepts: Glucose Regulation; Nutrition

Answer: 3
Rationale: Clients receiving TPN are at risk for hyperglycemia related to the increased glucose load of the solution. The symptoms exhibited by the client are consistent with hyperglycemia. The nurse would need to assess the client's blood glucose level to verify these data. The other food options would not provide any information that would correlate with the client's symptoms.
Test-Taking Strategy: Focus on the **subject**, total parenteral nutrition (TPN) therapy. Review the client's symptoms and think about the complications of TPN. Recalling that hyperglycemia is a complication will direct you to the correct option.
Priority Nursing Tip: Hyperglycemia occurs in the client receiving total parenteral nutrition because of the high concentration of dextrose (glucose) in the solution.
Reference: Lewis, S., et al. (2020). *Medical-surgical nursing: Assessment and management of clinical problems* (11th ed., p. 865). Elsevier.

❖ **202.** A client admitted to the hospital with a diagnosis of cirrhosis demonstrates massive ascites causing dyspnea. The nurse performs which intervention as a **priority** measure to assist the client with this complication?
1. Repositions side to side every 2 hours
2. Elevates the head of the bed 60 degrees
3. Auscultates the lung fields every 4 hours
4. Encourages deep breathing exercises every 2 hours

Level of Cognitive Ability: Applying
Client Needs: Physiological Integrity
Clinical Judgment/Cognitive Skills: Take Action
Integrated Process: Clinical Judgment; Nursing Process/Implementation
Content Area: Adult Health: Gastrointestinal
Health Problems: Adult Health: Gastrointestinal: Cirrhosis
Priority Concepts: Caregiving; Gas Exchange

Answer: 2
Rationale: The client is having difficulty breathing because of upward pressure on the diaphragm from the ascitic fluid in the abdomen. Elevating the head of the bed enlists the aid of gravity in relieving pressure on the diaphragm. Although assessment is the first step of the nursing process, the stem of the question identifies the assessment findings ascites and difficulty breathing, so the best answer is to intervene based on the assessment data, by elevating the head of the bed to make the client's breathing easier. The other options are general measures in the care of a client with ascites, but the priority measure is the one that relieves diaphragmatic pressure thus assisting effective respirations.
Test-Taking Strategy: Note the strategic word, *priority*, and the subject, to assist with breathing in a client with massive ascites. Recalling that elevating the head will provide immediate relief of symptoms associated with difficulty breathing will direct you to the correct option.
Priority Nursing Tip: A paracentesis may be performed to remove abdominal fluid in a client with cirrhosis and ascites.
Reference: Ignatavicius, D., et al. (2021). *Medical-surgical nursing: Concepts for interprofessional collaborative care* (10th ed., pp. 1162–1163). Elsevier.

203. The nurse who practices culturally sensitive nursing care incorporates which concepts into client care when addressing issues related to pain? **Select all that apply.**
❑ 1. The expression of pain is affected by learned behaviors.
❑ 2. Physiologically, all individuals experience pain in a similar manner.
❑ 3. Ethnic culture has an effect on the physiologic response to pain medications.
❑ 4. Clients need to be assessed for pain regardless of a lack of overt symptomatology.
❑ 5. The use of a standardized pain assessment tool ensures unbiased pain assessment.

Level of Cognitive Ability: Applying
Client Needs: Physiological Integrity
Clinical Judgment/Cognitive Skills: Take Action
Integrated Process: Culture/Spirituality
Content Area: Foundations of Care: Spirituality, Culture, and Ethnicity
Health Problems: Adult Health: Neurologic: Pain
Priority Concepts: Culture; Pain

Answer: 1, 3, 4
Rationale: Pain and its expression are often affected by an individual's ethnic culture in ways that include learned means of pain expression, the physiologic response to pain medications, and attitudes regarding acceptable ways of dealing with pain. Physiologically not all individuals, even those of the same ethnic culture, will respond to pain in a similar manner, and so a standardized pain assessment tool is not effective in measuring pain in all clients.
Test-Taking Strategy: Focus on the subject, pain and cultural awareness. Considering the effects of culture on pain will direct you to the correct options. Also note the closed-ended word "all" in option 2 and the words "ensures unbiased" in option 5.
Priority Nursing Tip: Pain and the expression of pain are individual specific responses that are greatly influenced by an individual's ethnic culture.
Reference: Potter, P., et al. (2021). *Fundamentals of nursing* (10th ed., pp. 1068–1069). Elsevier.

❖ **204.** While gathering data, the nurse notes that the client has been prescribed tolterodine tartrate. The nurse would determine that the client is taking the medication to treat which disorder?
  1. Glaucoma
  2. Pyloric stenosis
  3. Renal insufficiency
  4. Urinary frequency and urgency

Level of Cognitive Ability: Analyzing
Client Needs: Physiological Integrity
Clinical Judgment/Cognitive Skills: Analyze Cues
Integrated Process: Clinical Judgment; Nursing Process/Analysis
Content Area: Pharmacology: Renal and Urinary: Anticholinergics/Antispasmodics
Health Problems: N/A
Priority Concepts: Elimination; Clinical Judgment

Answer: 4
Rationale: Tolterodine tartrate is an antispasmodic used to treat overactive bladder and symptoms of urinary frequency, urgency, or urge incontinence. It is contraindicated in urinary retention and uncontrolled narrow-angle glaucoma. It is used with caution in renal function impairment, bladder outflow obstruction, and gastrointestinal obstructive disease such as pyloric stenosis.
Test-Taking Strategy: Focus on the subject, the action and use of tolterodine tartrate. Recalling that tolterodine tartrate is an antispasmodic will direct you to the correct option.
Priority Nursing Tip: Extended-release capsules of tolterodine tartrate should not be split, chewed, or crushed.
Reference: Ignatavicius, D., et al. (2021). *Medical-surgical nursing: Concepts for interprofessional collaborative care* (10th ed., p. 1331). Elsevier.

205. The nurse provides discharge instructions to a client with diabetes mellitus beginning oral hypoglycemic therapy. Which statements if made by the client indicate a **need for further teaching? Select all that apply.**
  ❑ 1. "If I am ill, I should skip my daily dose."
  ❑ 2. "If I overeat, I will double my dosage of medication."
  ❑ 3. "Oral agents are effective in managing type 2 diabetes."
  ❑ 4. "If I become pregnant, I will discontinue my medication."
  ❑ 5. "Oral hypoglycemic medications will cause my urine to turn orange."
  ❑ 6. "My medications are used to manage my diabetes along with diet and exercise."

Level of Cognitive Ability: Evaluating
Client Needs: Physiological Integrity
Clinical Judgment/Cognitive Skills: Evaluate Outcomes
Integrated Process: Teaching and Learning
Content Area: Pharmacology: Endocrine: Oral Hypoglycemics
Health Problems: Adult Health: Endocrine: Diabetes Mellitus
Priority Concepts: Patient Education; Glucose Regulation

Answer: 1, 2, 4, 5
Rationale: Clients are instructed that oral agents are used in addition to diet and exercise as therapy for diabetes mellitus. During illness or periods of intense stress, the client would be instructed to monitor their blood glucose level frequently and to contact the physician if the blood glucose is elevated because insulin may be needed to prevent symptoms of acute hyperglycemia. The medication should not be skipped, and the dosage should not be doubled. Taking extra medication is avoided unless specifically prescribed by the physician. Medication would never be discontinued unless instructed to do so by the physician. However, the client with diabetes who becomes pregnant will need to contact the physician because the oral diabetic medication may have to be changed to insulin therapy because some oral hypoglycemics can be harmful to the fetus. These medications do not change the color of the urine.
Test-Taking Strategy: Focus on the subject, oral hypoglycemic therapy. Note the strategic words, *need for further teaching*. These words indicate a negative event query and the need to select the incorrect options. Think about the pathophysiology of diabetes mellitus and its treatment, and use general medication guidelines to select the correct options.
Priority Nursing Tip: Any changes to prescribed medication usage or amounts should not be made by clients without prior physician approval.
Reference: Burchum, J., & Rosenthal, L. (2019). *Lehne's Pharmacology for nursing care* (10th ed., pp. 876–877, 879). Elsevier.

❖ **206.** The nurse evaluates a client after treatment for carbon monoxide poisoning following a burn injury. The nurse would document that the treatment was **effective** if which finding was present? **Select all that apply.**
- ❑ 1. Client is sleeping soundly.
- ❑ 2. Client is difficult to arouse.
- ❑ 3. Respiratory rate is 26 breaths/min.
- ❑ 4. Client's heart rate is 84 beats/min.
- ❑ 5. Carboxyhemoglobin levels are less than 5%.
- ❑ 6. The heart monitor shows normal sinus rhythm.

Level of Cognitive Ability: Evaluating
Client Needs: Physiological Integrity
Clinical Judgment/Cognitive Skills: Evaluate Outcomes
Integrated Process: Clinical Judgment; Nursing Process/Evaluation
Content Area: Complex Care: Poisoning
Health Problems: Adult Health: Integumentary: Burns
Priority Concepts: Gas Exchange; Perfusion

Answer: 4, 5, 6
Rationale: Normal carboxyhemoglobin levels are less than 5% for a nonsmoking adult. The symptoms of carbon monoxide poisoning are tachycardia, tachypnea, and central nervous system depression.
Test-Taking Strategy: Focus on the **subject**, carbon monoxide poisoning. Note the **strategic word**, *effective*. Think about the effects of carbon monoxide on the body and what manifestations occur. Recalling that tachycardia, tachypnea, and central nervous system depression can occur will assist in eliminating options 1, 2, and 3. Also note that the correct options are normal findings.
Priority Nursing Tip: A carbon monoxide level of 61% or above is fatal poisoning.
Reference: Ignatavicius, D., et al. (2021). *Medical-surgical nursing: Concepts for interprofessional collaborative care* (10th ed., p. 466). Elsevier.

207. The nurse instructs a preoperative client about the proper use of an incentive spirometer to minimize the risk of postoperative complications. What result would the nurse use to determine that the client is using the incentive spirometer **effectively?**
1. Cloudy sputum
2. Shallow breathing
3. Unilateral wheezing
4. Productive coughing

Level of Cognitive Ability: Evaluating
Client Needs: Physiological Integrity
Clinical Judgment/Cognitive Skills: Evaluate Outcomes
Integrated Process: Clinical Judgment; Nursing Process/Evaluation
Content Area: Skills: Oxygenation
Health Problems: N/A
Priority Concepts: Patient Education; Gas Exchange

Answer: 4
Rationale: Incentive spirometry helps reduce atelectasis and pneumonia, open airways, stimulate coughing, and help mobilize secretions for expectoration, via vital client participation in recovery. Cloudy sputum, shallow breathing, and wheezing indicate that the incentive spirometry is not effective because they point to infection, counterproductive depth of breathing, and bronchoconstriction, respectively.
Test-Taking Strategy: Focus on the **subject**, incentive spirometer. Note the **strategic word**, *effectively*. Think about the purpose of an incentive spirometer. Eliminate options 1, 2, and 3, which indicate abnormal findings.
Priority Nursing Tip: The client needs to assume a sitting or upright position when using an incentive spirometer.
Reference: Potter, P., et al. (2021). *Fundamentals of nursing* (10th ed., pp. 935–936). Elsevier.

❖ **208.** A client prescribed prazosin hydrochloride asks the nurse why the first dose must be taken at bedtime. Which response by the nurse is based on the understanding of the first dose use of prazosin hydrochloride?
  1. Treatment with prazosin hydrochloride results in drowsiness.
  2. Prazosin hydrochloride needs to be taken when the stomach is empty.
  3. Treatment with prazosin hydrochloride can cause dependent edema.
  4. Treatment with prazosin hydrochloride can cause dizziness or possible syncope.

Level of Cognitive Ability: Applying
Client Needs: Physiological Integrity
Clinical Judgment/Cognitive Skills: Take Action
Integrated Process: Teaching and Learning
Content Area: Pharmacology: Cardiovascular: Antihypertensives
Health Problems: Adult Health: Cardiovascular: Hypertension
Priority Concepts: Patient Education; Safety

Answer: 4
Rationale: Prazosin is an alpha-adrenergic blocking agent that reduces peripheral resistance and relaxes vascular smooth muscles. "First-dose hypotensive reaction" may occur during early therapy, which is characterized by dizziness, lightheadedness, and possible loss of consciousness. The occurrence of these effects is better tolerated if the client is in bed. This also can occur when the dosage is increased. This effect usually disappears with continued use or the dosage is decreased. Options 1, 2, and 3 are not characteristics of the medication.
Test-Taking Strategy: Focus on the subject, prazosin hydrochloride. Note the name of the medication. This will assist in determining that the medication is an antihypertensive agent. Recalling that orthostatic hypotension occurs with the use of antihypertensives will direct you to the correct option.
Priority Nursing Tip: When prescribed, it is best to administer the first dose of prazosin hydrochloride at bedtime. If the first dose needs to be given during the daytime, the client must remain supine for 3 to 4 hours.
Reference: Lilley, L., Rainforth Collins, S., & Snyder, J. (2020). *Pharmacology and the nursing process* (9th ed., p. 304). Elsevier.

209. The nurse has applied the prescribed dressing to the leg of a client with an ischemic arterial leg ulcer. Which method would the nurse use to cover the dressing?
  1. Apply a Kerlix roll and tape it to the skin.
  2. Apply a large, soft pad and tape it to the skin.
  3. Apply small Montgomery straps and tie the edges together.
  4. Apply a Kling roll and tape the edge of the roll onto the bandage.

Level of Cognitive Ability: Applying
Client Needs: Physiological Integrity
Clinical Judgment/Cognitive Skills: Take Action
Integrated Process: Nursing Process/Implementation
Content Area: Skills: Wound Care
Health Problems: Adult Health: Cardiovascular: Vascular Disorders
Priority Concepts: Perfusion; Tissue Integrity

Answer: 4
Rationale: Standard dressing technique includes the use of Kling rolls on circumferential dressings. With an arterial leg ulcer, the nurse applies tape only to the bandage. Tape is never used directly on the skin because it could cause further tissue damage. For the same reason, Montgomery straps should not be applied to the skin (although these are generally intended for use on abdominal wounds, anyway).
Test-Taking Strategy: Focus on the subject, care of ischemic arterial leg ulcers. Note that options 1, 2, and 3 are comparable or alike. In options 1 and 2, tape is applied to the skin. For the same reason, eliminate option 3, because the Montgomery straps would need to be adhered to the skin as well.
Priority Nursing Tip: Because swelling in the extremities prevents arterial blood flow, the client with peripheral arterial disease is instructed to elevate the feet at rest but to avoid elevating them above the level of the heart because extreme elevation slows arterial blood flow to the feet.
References: Ignatavicius, D., et al. (2021). *Medical-surgical nursing: Concepts for interprofessional collaborative care* (10th ed., pp. 444–445). Elsevier; Potter, P., et al. (2021). *Fundamentals of nursing* (10th ed., pp. 1258, 1262–1263). Elsevier.

210. A child is admitted to the pediatric unit with a diagnosis of celiac disease. Based on this diagnosis, the nurse expects that the child's stools will have which characteristic?
1. Malodorous
2. Dark in color
3. Unusually hard
4. Abnormally small in amount

Level of Cognitive Ability: Analyzing
Client Needs: Physiological Integrity
Clinical Judgment/Cognitive Skills: Recognize Cues
Integrated Process: Clinical Judgment; Nursing Process/Assessment
Content Area: Pediatrics: Gastrointestinal
Health Problems: Pediatric-Specific: Nutrition Problems
Priority Concepts: Elimination; Nutrition

Answer: 1
Rationale: Celiac disease is a disorder in which the child has intolerance to gluten, the protein component of wheat, barley, rye, and oats. The stools of a child with celiac disease are characteristically malodorous, pale, large (bulky), and soft (loose). Excessive flatus is common, and bouts of diarrhea may occur.
Test-Taking Strategy: Focus on the **subject**, celiac disease. Thinking about the pathophysiology that occurs in celiac disease and the manifestations will direct you to the correct option.
Priority Nursing Tip: Teach the parents of a child with celiac disease to read all food labels for the presence of gluten; if the food contains gluten, it needs to be avoided.
References: Hockenberry, M., Wilson, D., & Rodgers, C. (2019). *Wong's Nursing care of infants and children* (11th ed., pp. 862–863). Elsevier; Potter, P., et al. (2021). *Fundamentals of nursing* (10th ed., p. 522). Elsevier.

❖ **211.** A clinic nurse is caring for a client with a suspected diagnosis of gestational hypertension. The nurse assesses the client, expecting to note which set of findings if gestational hypertension is present?
1. Edema, ketonuria, and obesity
2. Edema, tachycardia, and ketonuria
3. Glycosuria, hypertension, and obesity
4. Sudden weight gain and proteinuria

Level of Cognitive Ability: Analyzing
Client Needs: Physiological Integrity
Clinical Judgment/Cognitive Skills: Recognize Cues
Integrated Process: Clinical Judgment; Nursing Process/Assessment
Content Area: Maternity: Antepartum
Health Problems: Maternity: Gestational Hypertension/Preeclampsia and Eclampsia
Priority Concepts: Perfusion; Reproduction

Answer: 4
Rationale: Gestational hypertension is the most common hypertensive disorder in pregnancy. It is characterized by the development of hypertension, fluid retention, sudden weight gain, and proteinuria. Glycosuria and ketonuria occur in diabetes mellitus. Tachycardia and obesity are not specifically related to diagnosing gestational hypertension.
Test-Taking Strategy: Focus on the **subject**, gestational hypertension. Eliminate options 1 and 2 because they do not address hypertension. From the remaining options, recalling that glycosuria is an indication of diabetes mellitus will assist in directing you to the correct option.
Priority Nursing Tip: Gestational hypertension can be mild or severe and can lead to preeclampsia and then eclampsia (seizures).
Reference: McKinney, E. S., et al. (2022). *Maternal child nursing* (6th ed. pp. 541–542). Elsevier.

212. A client who undergoes a gastric resection is at risk for developing dumping syndrome. Which manifestation would the nurse monitor the client for in association with eating? **Select all that apply.**
❑ 1. Pallor
❑ 2. Dizziness
❑ 3. Diaphoresis
❑ 4. Bradycardia
❑ 5. Constipation
❑ 6. Extreme thirst

Level of Cognitive Ability: Applying
Client Needs: Physiological Integrity
Clinical Judgment/Cognitive Skills: Recognize Cues
Integrated Process: Nursing Process/Assessment
Content Area: Adult Health: Gastrointestinal
Health Problems: Adult Health: Gastrointestinal: Nutrition/Malabsorption Problems
Priority Concepts: Clinical Judgment; Elimination

Answer: 1, 2, 3
Rationale: Dumping syndrome is the rapid emptying of the gastric contents into the small intestine that occurs after gastric resection resulting in diarrhea. Early manifestations of dumping syndrome occur 5 to 30 minutes after eating. Manifestations also include vasomotor disturbances such as dizziness, tachycardia, syncope, sweating, pallor, palpitations, and the desire to lie down.
Test-Taking Strategy: Focus on the **subject**, dumping syndrome. Recalling that the symptoms of this disorder are vasomotor in nature will direct you to the correct option.
Priority Nursing Tip: The client with dumping syndrome should eat small meals and avoid consuming fluids with meals.
Reference: Ignatavicius, D., et al. (2021). *Medical-surgical nursing: Concepts for interprofessional collaborative care* (10th ed., pp. 1106–1107). Elsevier.

❖ **213.** The nurse is monitoring a client in the telemetry unit who has recently been admitted with the diagnosis of chest pain and notes this heart rate pattern on the monitoring strip **(refer to figure)**. What is the **initial** action to be taken by the nurse?

1. Notify the physician.
2. Initiate cardiopulmonary resuscitation (CPR).
3. Continue to monitor the client and the heart rate patterns.
4. Administer oxygen with a face mask at 8 to 10 L/min.

Level of Cognitive Ability: Applying
Client Needs: Physiological Integrity
Clinical Judgment/Cognitive Skills: Take Action
Integrated Process: Clinical Judgment; Nursing Process/Implementation
Content Area: Complex Care: Emergency Situations/Management
Health Problems: Adult Health: Cardiovascular: Dysrhythmias
Priority Concepts: Gas Exchange; Perfusion

Answer: 2
Rationale: The monitor is showing ventricular fibrillation, a life-threatening dysrhythmia that requires CPR and defibrillation to maintain life. Although the physician must be notified, CPR is the initial action. Oxygen is necessary, but again the initiation of CPR is the priority because it will provide more than just oxygen to the client. Monitoring the client is necessary, but not as an initial action; emergency resuscitative treatment must be provided to the client immediately.
Test-Taking Strategy: Knowledge regarding emergency care is essential. Note the strategic word, *initial.* Recalling that ventricular fibrillation is a life-threatening dysrhythmia that requires CPR and defibrillation to maintain life will direct you to the correct option.
Priority Nursing Tip: There is no cardiac output with ventricular fibrillation, and it must be treated immediately to save the client's life.
Reference: Ignatavicius, D., et al. (2021). *Medical-surgical nursing: Concepts for interprofessional collaborative care* (10th ed., pp. 658–660). Elsevier.

214. Which nursing assessment finding indicates the presence of an inguinal hernia on a child?
1. Reports of difficulty defecating
2. Reports of a dribbling urinary stream
3. Absence of the testes within the scrotum
4. Painless groin swelling noticed when the child cries

Level of Cognitive Ability: Applying
Client Needs: Physiological Integrity
Clinical Judgment/Cognitive Skills: Recognize Cues
Integrated Process: Clinical Judgment; Nursing Process/Assessment
Content Area: Pediatrics: Gastrointestinal
Health Problems: Pediatric-Specific: Developmental GI Defects
Priority Concepts: Clinical Judgment; Tissue Integrity

Answer: 4
Rationale: Inguinal hernia is a common defect that may appear as a painless inguinal (groin) swelling when the child cries or strains. Option 1 is a symptom indicating a partial obstruction of the herniated loop of intestine. Option 2 describes a sign of phimosis, a narrowing or stenosis of the preputial opening of the foreskin. Option 3 describes cryptorchidism.
Test-Taking Strategy: Focus on the subject, assessment of an inguinal hernia. Note the relationship between the child's diagnosis, inguinal hernia, and the words "groin swelling" in option 4.
Priority Nursing Tip: An inguinal hernia is characterized by painless inguinal swelling that is reducible. Swelling may disappear during periods of rest and is most noticeable when the infant cries or coughs.
Reference: Hockenberry, M., Wilson, D., & Rodgers, C. (2019). *Wong's Nursing care of infants and children* (11th ed., pp. 127, 877–878). Elsevier.

❖ **215.** At 0900 a client experiencing difficulty breathing and increased pulmonary congestion as a result of heart failure was prescribed furosemide 40 mg to be given intravenously. After an hour which assessment finding indicates that the therapy has been **effective**?

Laboratory Results

Test and Result 0900	Test and Result 1000	Reference Range
Potassium 4.7 mEq (4.7 mmol/L)	Potassium 4.1 mEq (4.1 mmol/L)	3.5–5.0 mEq/L (3.5–5.0 mmol/L)

1. The lungs are now clear upon auscultation.
2. The urine output has increased by 400 mL.
3. The blood pressure has decreased from 118/64 to 106/62 mm Hg.
4. The potassium has decreased from 4.7 to 4.1 mEq (4.7 to 4.1 mmol/L).

Level of Cognitive Ability: Evaluating
Client Needs: Physiological Integrity
Clinical Judgment/Cognitive Skills: Evaluate Outcomes
Integrated Process: Clinical Judgment; Nursing Process/Evaluation
Content Area: Pharmacology: Cardiovascular: Diuretics
Health Problems: Adult Health: Cardiovascular: Heart Failure
Priority Concepts: Perfusion; Clinical Judgment

Answer: 1
Rationale: Furosemide is a diuretic. In this situation, it was given to decrease preload and reduce the pulmonary congestion and associated difficulty in breathing. Although all options may occur, the difficulty breathing and increased pulmonary congestion are the reasons that the furosemide was administered.
Test-Taking Strategy: Focus on the subject, furosemide administration in a client with heart failure who was experiencing difficulty breathing and increased pulmonary congestion. Note the strategic word, *effective*. Specific knowledge of the use of furosemide in heart failure and its side effects is essential. Note the relationship between the words "pulmonary congestion" in the question and option 1.
Priority Nursing Tip: When administering a medication, knowing its purpose will assist in evaluating its effectiveness.
Reference: Gahart, B., Nazareno, A., & Ortega, M. (2021). *Gahart's 2021 Intravenous medications: A handbook for nurses and health professionals* (37th ed., pp. 664–665). Elsevier.

❖ **216.** Skin closure with heterograft will be performed on a client with a burn injury. When the client asks the nurse where the heterograft comes from, the nurse would explain it is from which source?

1. A cadaver
2. Another animal species
3. The burned client themselves
4. A human-made synthetic source

Level of Cognitive Ability: Applying
Client Needs: Physiological Integrity
Clinical Judgment/Cognitive Skills: Take Action
Integrated Process: Clinical Judgment; Nursing Process/Implementation
Content Area: Adult Health: Integumentary
Health Problems: Adult Health: Integumentary: Burns
Priority Concepts: Patient Education; Tissue Integrity

Answer: 2
Rationale: Biologic dressings are usually heterograft or homograft material. Heterograft is skin from another species. The most commonly used type of heterograft is pig skin because of its availability and its relative compatibility with human skin. Homograft is skin from another human, which is usually obtained from a cadaver and is provided through a skin bank. Autograft is skin from the client. Synthetic dressings are also available for covering burn wounds.
Test-Taking Strategy: Focus on the subject, a heterograft. Also, note that options 1 and 3 are comparable or alike and relate to grafts from human skin. Next it is necessary to know that heterograft is skin from another species.
Priority Nursing Tip: Autografting provides permanent wound coverage.
Reference: Urden, L., Stacy, K., & Lough, M. (2022). *Critical care nursing: Diagnosis and management* (9th ed., pp. 882–883). Elsevier.

217. The nurse would place a client who sustained a head injury in which position to prevent increased intracranial pressure (ICP)?
1. In reverse Trendelenburg's position
2. In modified left lateral position
3. With the head elevated on a small, flat pillow
4. With the head of the bed elevated at least 30 degrees

Level of Cognitive Ability: Applying
Client Needs: Physiological Integrity
Clinical Judgment/Cognitive Skills: Take Action
Integrated Process: Nursing Process/Implementation
Content Area: Adult Health: Neurologic
Health Problems: Adult Health: Neurologic: Head Injury/Trauma
Priority Concepts: Clinical Judgment; Intracranial Regulation

Answer: 4
Rationale: The client with a head injury is positioned to avoid extreme flexion or extension of the neck and to maintain the head in the midline, neutral position. The head of the bed is elevated to at least 30 degrees or as recommended by the physician. Therefore, options 1, 2, and 3 are incorrect since they contradict appropriate care.
Test-Taking Strategy: Focus on the **subject**, preventing an increase in ICP. Recall that the client with a head injury is at risk for increased ICP. Bearing this in mind and considering the principles of gravity will direct you to the correct option.
Priority Nursing Tip: Altered level of consciousness is the most sensitive and earliest indication of increased ICP.
Reference: Ignatavicius, D., et al. (2021). *Medical-surgical nursing: Concepts for interprofessional collaborative care* (10th ed., p. 919). Elsevier.

❖ 218. A newborn infant is diagnosed with esophageal atresia. Which assessment finding supports this diagnosis?
1. Slowed reflexes
2. Continuous drooling
3. Diaphragmatic breathing
4. Passage of large amounts of frothy stool

Level of Cognitive Ability: Analyzing
Client Needs: Physiological Integrity
Clinical Judgment/Cognitive Skills: Recognize Cues
Integrated Process: Clinical Judgment; Nursing Process/Assessment
Content Area: Pediatrics: Gastrointestinal
Health Problems: Pediatric-Specific: Disorders of Prenatal Development
Priority Concepts: Development; Safety

Answer: 2
Rationale: In esophageal atresia, the esophagus terminates before it reaches the stomach, ending in a blind pouch. This condition prevents the passage of swallowed mucus and saliva into the stomach. After fluid has accumulated in the pouch, it flows from the mouth and the infant then drools continuously. Responsiveness of the infant to stimulus would depend on the overall condition of the infant and is not considered a classic sign of esophageal atresia. Diaphragmatic breathing is not associated with this disorder. The inability to swallow amniotic fluid in utero prevents the accumulation of normal meconium, and lack of stools results.
Test-Taking Strategy: Focus on the **subject**, esophageal atresia. Review the anatomic location of the disorder to eliminate options 1 and 4 first. From the remaining options, recalling the pathophysiology associated with esophageal atresia and recalling that the word "atresia" indicates narrowing will direct you to the correct option.
Priority Nursing Tip: Tracheoesophageal fistula should be suspected if the child exhibits the "3 Cs"—coughing, choking with feedings, and cyanosis.
Reference: McKinney, E. S., et al. (2022). *Maternal child nursing* (6th ed., p. 967). Elsevier.

219. Which observation by the nurse indicates a need to suction a client with an endotracheal (ET) tube attached to a mechanical ventilator to help manage a pneumothorax? **Select all that apply.**
- ❏ **1.** Audible crackles
- ❏ **2.** Client notably restless
- ❏ **3.** Visible mucus bubbling in the ET tube
- ❏ **4.** Apical pulse rate of 72 beats/min
- ❏ **5.** Low peak inspiratory pressure on the ventilator
- ❏ **6.** High alarm pressures identified by the ventilator

Level of Cognitive Ability: Analyzing
Client Needs: Physiological Integrity
Clinical Judgment/Cognitive Skills: Recognize Cues
Integrated Process: Clinical Judgment; Nursing Process/Assessment
Content Area: Skills: Oxygenation
Health Problems: Adult Health: Respiratory: Pneumothorax
Priority Concepts: Clinical Judgment; Gas Exchange

Answer: 1, 2, 3, 6
Rationale: Indications for suctioning include visible mucus bubbling in the ET tube, wet respirations, restlessness, rhonchi or crackles on auscultation of the lungs, increased pulse and respiratory rates, and increased peak inspiratory pressures on the ventilator and high-pressure alarms on the ventilator. A low peak inspiratory pressure indicates a leak in the mechanical ventilation system.
Test-Taking Strategy: Focus on the **subject**, the need for suctioning in a client with an ET tube attached to a mechanical ventilator. Eliminate option 4 first because it is normal findings. From the remaining options, note that a low-pressure alarm is sounded if there is an air leak.
Priority Nursing Tip: The nurse needs to hyperoxygenate the client before and after performing respiratory suctioning.
Reference: Lewis, S., et al. (2020). *Medical-surgical nursing: Assessment and management of clinical problems* (11th ed., pp. 1550–1552). Elsevier.

❖ **220.** A client is intubated and receiving mechanical ventilation after experiencing lung aspiration. The physician has added 7 cm of positive end-expiratory pressure (PEEP) to the client's ventilator settings. The nurse would assess for which expected but adverse effect of PEEP?
1. Decreased peak pressure on the ventilator
2. Increased rectal temperature from 98° F (36.6° C) to 100° F (37.7° C)
3. Decreased heart rate from 78 to 64 beats/min
4. Systolic blood pressure decrease from 122 to 98 mm Hg

Level of Cognitive Ability: Analyzing
Client Needs: Physiological Integrity
Clinical Judgment/Cognitive Skills: Analyze Cues
Integrated Process: Clinical Judgment; Nursing Process/Analysis
Content Area: Skills: Oxygenation
Health Problems: Adult Health: Respiratory: Foreign Body Airway Obstruction
Priority Concepts: Gas Exchange; Perfusion

Answer: 4
Rationale: PEEP improves oxygenation by enhancing gas exchange and preventing atelectasis. PEEP leads to increased intrathoracic pressure, which in turn leads to decreased cardiac output. This is manifested in the client by decreased systolic blood pressure and increased pulse (compensatory). Peak pressures on the ventilator should not be affected, although the pressure at the end of expiration remains positive at the level set for the PEEP. Fever indicates respiratory infection or infection from another source.
Test-Taking Strategy: Focus on the **subject**, expected but adverse effect of PEEP. Knowing that PEEP increases intrathoracic pressure leads you to look for the option that reflects a consequence of this event. Fever is irrelevant, and option 2 is eliminated first. From the remaining options, think about the effects of PEEP to direct you to the correct option.
Priority Nursing Tip: The need for PEEP indicates a severe gas exchange disturbance.
Reference: Lewis, S., et al. (2020). *Medical-surgical nursing: Assessment and management of clinical problems* (11th ed., p. 1554). Elsevier.

221. The nurse is assessing the respiratory status of a client with pleural effusion after a thoracentesis has been performed. The nurse would become concerned with which assessment finding?
1. Equal bilateral chest expansion
2. Respiratory rate of 22 breaths/min
3. Diminished breath sounds on the affected side
4. Few scattered wheezes, unchanged from baseline

Level of Cognitive Ability: Analyzing
Client Needs: Physiological Integrity
Clinical Judgment/Cognitive Skills: Take Action
Integrated Process: Clinical Judgment; Nursing Process/Analysis
Content Area: Adult Health: Respiratory
Health Problems: Adult Health: Respiratory: Pleural Effusion
Priority Concepts: Clinical Judgment; Gas Exchange

Answer: 3
Rationale: After thoracentesis, the nurse assesses vital signs and breath sounds. The nurse especially notes increased respiratory rates, dyspnea, retractions, diminished breath sounds, or cyanosis, which could indicate pneumothorax. Any of these manifestations need to be reported to the physician. Options 1 and 2 are normal findings. Option 4 indicates a finding that is unchanged from the baseline.
Test-Taking Strategy: Focus on the subject, respiratory status. Eliminate options 1 and 2 first because they are normal findings. Option 4 is an abnormality, but note that the wheezes are unchanged from the client's baseline. Option 3 is the abnormal finding.
Priority Nursing Tip: For a thoracentesis, the client is positioned sitting upright, with the arms and shoulders supported by a bedside table. If the client cannot sit up, the client is placed lying in bed on the unaffected side, with the head of the bed elevated.
Reference: Lewis, S., et al. (2020). *Medical-surgical nursing: Assessment and management of clinical problems* (11th ed., p. 531). Elsevier.

❖ 222. The nurse is preparing to administer a tuberculin skin test to a client. The nurse determines which area is to be used for injection of the medication?
1. Dorsal aspect of the upper arm near a mole
2. Inner aspect of the forearm that is close to a burn scar
3. Inner aspect of the forearm that is not heavily pigmented
4. Dorsal aspect of the upper arm that has a small amount of hair

Level of Cognitive Ability: Applying
Client Needs: Physiological Integrity
Clinical Judgment/Cognitive Skills: Take Action
Integrated Process: Nursing Process/Implementation
Content Area: Foundations of Care: Diagnostic Tests
Health Problems: Adult Health: Respiratory: Tuberculosis
Priority Concepts: Clinical Judgment; Safety

Answer: 3
Rationale: Intradermal injections are most commonly given in the inner surface of the forearm. Other sites include the dorsal area of the upper arm or the upper back beneath the scapulae. The nurse finds an area that is not heavily pigmented and is clear of hairy areas or lesions that could interfere with reading the results.
Test-Taking Strategy: Focus on the subject, tuberculin skin test. Note that options 1, 2, and 4 are comparable or alike in that they indicate areas that are not clear of lesions or hair.
Priority Nursing Tip: After administering a skin test, document the date and time of administration and the test site. Interpret the reaction at the injection site 48 to 72 hours after administration of the test antigen.
Reference: Pagana, K., Pagana, T., & Pagana, T. N. (2021). *Mosby's Diagnostic and laboratory test reference* (15th ed., pp. 904–905). Elsevier.

223. Which questions would the nurse ask when assessing a client for possible manifestations of Meniere's disease? **Select all that apply.**
- ❑ 1. "Do you experience ringing in your ears?"
- ❑ 2. "Are you prone to vertigo that can last for days?"
- ❑ 3. "Can you hear better out of one ear than the other?"
- ❑ 4. "Is there a history of Meniere's disease in your family?"
- ❑ 5. "Have you ever experienced a head injury in the area of your ears?"

Level of Cognitive Ability: Analyzing
Client Needs: Physiological Integrity
Clinical Judgment/Cognitive Skills: Take Action
Integrated Process: Clinical Judgment; Nursing Process/Assessment
Content Area: Adult Health: Ear
Health Problems: Adult Health: Ear: Meniere's Disease
Priority Concepts: Clinical Judgment; Sensory Perception

Answer: 1, 2, 3
Rationale: Meniere's disease is characterized by dilation of the endolymphatic system by overproduction or decreased reabsorption of endolymphatic fluid. Manifestations include tinnitus, vertigo that can last for days, and one-sided sensorineural hearing loss. Although the exact cause of the disease is unknown, there does not seem to be a connection with either genetics or head trauma.
Test-Taking Strategy: Focus on the subject, Meniere's disease. Specific knowledge regarding the manifestations of Meniere's disease will direct you to the correct options 1, 2, and 3. Remember that tinnitus, hearing loss, and vertigo are characteristic of this disease.
Priority Nursing Tip: Meniere's disease has characteristic manifestations that include tinnitus, unilateral hearing impairment, and severe episodes of vertigo.
Reference: Ignatavicius, D., et al. (2021). *Medical-surgical nursing: Concepts for interprofessional collaborative care* (10th ed., p. 968). Elsevier.

❖ 224. A client has been diagnosed with left tension pneumothorax. Which finding observed by the nurse indicates that the pneumothorax is rapidly worsening? **Select all that apply.**
- ❑ 1. Hypertension
- ❑ 2. Flat neck veins
- ❑ 3. Increased cyanosis
- ❑ 4. Tracheal deviation to the right
- ❑ 5. Observable asymmetry of the thorax
- ❑ 6. Diminished breath sounds on the left

Level of Cognitive Ability: Analyzing
Client Needs: Physiological Integrity
Clinical Judgment/Cognitive Skills: Recognize Cues
Integrated Process: Clinical Judgment; Nursing Process/Assessment
Content Area: Complex Care: Emergency Situations/Management
Health Problems: Adult Health: Respiratory: Pneumothorax
Priority Concepts: Gas Exchange; Perfusion

Answer: 3, 4, 5, 6
Rationale: A tension pneumothorax is characterized by distended neck veins, displaced point of maximal impulse (PMI), tracheal deviation to the unaffected side, asymmetry of the thorax, decreased to absent breath sounds on the affected side, worsening cyanosis, and worsening dyspnea. The increased intrathoracic pressure causes the blood pressure to fall, not rise.
Test-Taking Strategy: Focus on the subject, tension pneumothorax, and note the words "rapidly worsening." Pain and hypertension are the least specific indicators and are eliminated first. From the remaining options, remember that a tension pneumothorax causes the trachea to be pushed in the opposite direction, to the unaffected side.
Priority Nursing Tip: After insertion of a central venous catheter, catheter placement must be confirmed by radiography before infusing fluids into it.
Reference: Lewis, S., et al. (2020). *Medical-surgical nursing: Assessment and management of clinical problems* (11th ed., pp. 524–525). Elsevier.

225. A client is admitted to the hospital with a diagnosis of right lower lobe pneumonia. The nurse auscultates the affected lung area, expecting to note which type of breath sounds?
1. Absent
2. Vesicular
3. Bronchial
4. Bronchovesicular

Level of Cognitive Ability: Analyzing
Client Needs: Physiological Integrity
Clinical Judgment/Cognitive Skills: Recognize Cues
Integrated Process: Clinical Judgment; Nursing Process/Assessment
Content Area: Health Assessment/Physical Exam: Thorax and Lungs
Health Problems: Adult Health: Respiratory: Pneumonia
Priority Concepts: Clinical Judgment; Gas Exchange

Answer: 3
Rationale: Bronchial sounds are normally heard over the trachea. The client with pneumonia will have bronchial breath sounds over area(s) of consolidation because the consolidated tissue carries bronchial sounds to the peripheral lung fields. The client may also have crackles in the affected area resulting from fluid in the interstitium and alveoli. Absent breath sounds are not likely to occur unless a serious complication of the pneumonia occurs. Vesicular sounds are normally heard over the lesser bronchi, bronchioles, and lobes. Bronchovesicular sounds are normally heard over the main bronchi.
Test-Taking Strategy: Focus on the subject, breath sounds in a client with lower lobe pneumonia. Recalling that vesicular breath sounds are normal in the lung periphery and bronchovesicular sounds are normally heard over the main bronchi helps eliminate options 2 and 4. From the remaining options, recall that pneumonia transmits bronchial breath sounds, so they are heard over the area of consolidation.
Priority Nursing Tip: Pneumonia can be community acquired or hospital acquired. The sputum culture identifies organisms that may be present and assists in determining appropriate treatment.
Reference: Ignatavicius, D., et al. (2021). *Medical-surgical nursing: Concepts for interprofessional collaborative care* (10th ed., p. 572). Elsevier.

226. The nurse assesses the client diagnosed with acquired immunodeficiency syndrome (AIDS) for **early** signs of Kaposi's sarcoma. What characteristics would be consistent with that lesion? **Select all that apply.**
1. Flat
2. Raised
3. Light blue in color
4. Resembling a blister
5. Brownish and scaly in appearance
6. Color varies from pink to dark violet or black

Level of Cognitive Ability: Analyzing
Client Needs: Physiological Integrity
Clinical Judgment/Cognitive Skills: Recognize Cues
Integrated Process: Clinical Judgment; Nursing Process/Assessment
Content Area: Adult Health: Immune
Health Problems: Adult Health: Immune: Immunodeficiency Syndrome
Priority Concepts: Clinical Judgment; Tissue Integrity

Answer: 1, 6
Rationale: Kaposi's sarcoma generally starts with an area that is flat and pink that changes to dark violet or black. The lesions are usually present bilaterally. They may appear in many areas of the body and are treated with radiation, chemotherapy, and cryotherapy. None of the other options are associated with this type of lesion.
Test-Taking Strategy: Note the strategic word, *early*. Focus on the subject, Kaposi's sarcoma. Recalling that Kaposi's sarcoma lesions are flat and have a variety of colors from pink to dark violet or black eliminates the remaining options.
Priority Nursing Tip: Kaposi's sarcoma is characterized by skin lesions that occur in individuals with a compromised immune system.
Reference: Lewis, S., et al. (2020). *Medical-surgical nursing: Assessment and management of clinical problems* (11th ed., p. 219). Elsevier.

227. When a client who sustained a chest injury is suspected of experiencing a pleural effusion, the nurse would assess for which typical manifestations of this respiratory problem? **Select all that apply.**
- ❑ 1. Dry cough
- ❑ 2. Moist cough
- ❑ 3. Dyspnea at rest
- ❑ 4. Productive cough
- ❑ 5. Dyspnea on exertion
- ❑ 6. Nonproductive cough

Level of Cognitive Ability: Analyzing
Client Needs: Physiological Integrity
Clinical Judgment/Cognitive Skills: Recognize Cues
Integrated Process: Clinical Judgment; Nursing Process/Assessment
Content Area: Adult Health: Respiratory
Health Problems: Adult Health: Respiratory: Pleural Effusion
Priority Concepts: Clinical Judgment; Gas Exchange

Answer: 1, 5, 6
Rationale: A pleural effusion is the collection of fluid in the pleural space. Typical assessment findings in the client with a pleural effusion include dyspnea, which usually occurs with exertion, and a dry, nonproductive cough. The cough is caused by bronchial irritation and possible mediastinal shift.
Test-Taking Strategy: Focus on the subject, pleural effusion. Specific knowledge that pleural effusion is in the pleural space and not the airway helps eliminate options 2 and 4 (moist productive cough does not occur). Remembering that dyspnea occurs on exertion before it occurs at rest will direct you to the correct option from the remaining options.
Priority Nursing Tip: Any condition that interferes with the secretion or drainage of pleural fluid will lead to pleural effusion.
Reference: Lewis, S., et al. (2020). *Medical-surgical nursing: Assessment and management of clinical problems* (11th ed., p. 531). Elsevier.

❖ **228.** After a client diagnosed with pleural effusion had a thoracentesis, a sample of fluid was sent to the laboratory. Analysis of the fluid reveals a high red blood cell count. Based on this test result, what was the cause of this client's pleural effusion?
1. Trauma
2. Infection
3. Liver failure
4. Heart failure

Level of Cognitive Ability: Analyzing
Client Needs: Physiological Integrity
Clinical Judgment/Cognitive Skills: Analyze Cues
Integrated Process: Clinical Judgment; Nursing Process/Analysis
Content Area: Foundations of Care: Diagnostic Tests
Health Problems: Adult Health: Respiratory: Pleural Effusion
Priority Concepts: Clinical Judgment; Gas Exchange

Answer: 1
Rationale: Pleural fluid from an effusion that has a high red blood cell count may result from trauma and may be treated with placement of a chest tube for drainage. Other causes of pleural effusion include infection, heart failure, liver or renal failure, malignancy, or inflammatory processes. Infection would be accompanied by white blood cells. The fluid portion of the serum would accumulate with liver failure and heart failure.
Test-Taking Strategy: Focus on the subject, pleural effusion with a high red blood cell count. Recall that infection would be accompanied by white blood cells, not red, to eliminate option 2. Remember that in liver and heart failure, the fluid portion of the serum would accumulate to direct you to eliminate options 3 and 4.
Priority Nursing Tip: With a pleural effusion, the client experiences pleuritic pain that is sharp and increases with inspiration.
Reference: Heuther, S., McCance, K., & Brashers, V. (2020). *Understanding pathophysiology* (7th ed., pp. 675–676). Elsevier.

229. The nurse is scheduling a client diagnosed with possible diverticulosis for a series of diagnostic studies of the gastrointestinal (GI) system. Which of these studies would the nurse schedule last to avoid altering the results of the remaining tests?
1. Ultrasound
2. Colonoscopy
3. Barium enema
4. Computed tomography

Level of Cognitive Ability: Analyzing
Client Needs: Physiological Integrity
Clinical Judgment/Cognitive Skills: Generate Solutions
Integrated Process: Clinical Judgment; Nursing Process/Planning
Content Area: Foundations of Care: Diagnostic Tests
Health Problems: Adult Health: Gastrointestinal: Diverticulosis/Diverticulitis
Priority Concepts: Care Coordination; Elimination

Answer: 3
Rationale: When barium is instilled into the lower GI tract, it may take up to 72 hours to clear the GI tract. The presence of barium could cause interference with obtaining clear visualization and accurate results of the other tests listed if performed before the client has fully excreted the barium. For this reason, diagnostic studies that involve barium contrast are scheduled at the conclusion of other medical imaging studies.
Test-Taking Strategy: Focus on the subject, diagnostic studies of the GI system. Note the word "last." Recall that barium shows up on x-ray as opaque and that this substance would impair visualization during other tests.
Priority Nursing Tip: After a barium enema, the client is instructed to increase oral fluid intake to help pass the barium.
Reference: Lewis, S., et al. (2020). *Medical-surgical nursing: Assessment and management of clinical problems* (11th ed., p. 844). Elsevier.

❖ **230.** The nurse is caring for a client who is scheduled to have a liver biopsy to rule out liver cancer. Before the procedure, it is important for the nurse to assess which parameter to ensure client safety?
1. Tolerance for pain
2. Allergy to iodine or shellfish
3. History of nausea and vomiting
4. Ability to lie still and hold the breath

Level of Cognitive Ability: Analyzing
Client Needs: Physiological Integrity
Clinical Judgment/Cognitive Skills: Take Action
Integrated Process: Clinical Judgment; Nursing Process/Assessment
Content Area: Foundations of Care: Diagnostic Tests
Health Problems: Adult Health: Cancer: Liver
Priority Concepts: Clinical Judgment; Safety

Answer: 4
Rationale: It is most important for the nurse to assess the client's ability to lie still and hold the breath for the procedure. This helps the physician avoid complications, such as puncturing the lung or other organs. The client's tolerance for pain is a useful item to know. However, the area will receive a local anesthetic. Assessment of allergy to iodine or shellfish is unnecessary for this procedure because no contrast dye is used. Knowledge of the history related to nausea and vomiting is generally a part of assessment of the gastrointestinal system but has no relationship to the procedure.
Test-Taking Strategy: Focus on the subject, a liver biopsy. Visualizing this procedure and thinking about its complications will direct you to the correct option.
Priority Nursing Tip: Bleeding is a concern after a liver biopsy. Assess the results of coagulation tests (prothrombin time, partial thromboplastin time, platelet count) before a liver biopsy is performed and report abnormal results to the physician.
Reference: Lewis, S., et al. (2020). *Medical-surgical nursing: Assessment and management of clinical problems* (11th ed., pp. 846–847). Elsevier.

231. The nurse is caring for a client diagnosed with pneumonia. To ensure tolerance of activities, the nurse would plan to take the client for a short walk after which of the following?
1. Eating lunch
2. Taking a brief nap
3. Using the metered-dose inhaler
4. Assessing client's oxygen saturation

Level of Cognitive Ability: Analyzing
Client Needs: Physiological Integrity
Clinical Judgment/Cognitive Skills: Generate Solutions
Integrated Process: Clinical Judgment; Nursing Process/Planning
Content Area: Adult Health: Respiratory
Health Problems: Adult Health: Respiratory: Pneumonia
Priority Concepts: Gas Exchange; Mobility

Answer: 3
Rationale: The nurse should schedule activities for the client with pneumonia after the client has received respiratory treatments or medications. After the administration of bronchodilators (often administered by metered-dose inhaler), the client has the best oxygen exchange possible and would tolerate the activity best. Still, the nurse implements activity cautiously, so as not to increase the client's dyspnea. The client would become fatigued after eating; therefore, this is not a good time to ambulate the client. Although the client may be rested somewhat after a nap, the respiratory status of the client may not be at its best. Although monitoring oxygen saturation is appropriate, the intervention itself does not affect the client's respiratory function.
Test-Taking Strategy: Focus on the subject, ambulation of the respiratory client. Use the ABCs—airway, breathing, and circulation. The use of bronchodilator medication would widen the air passages, allowing for more air to enter the client's lungs.
Priority Nursing Tip: Clients with a respiratory disorder need to be positioned with the head of the bed elevated.
Reference: Lewis, S., et al. (2020). *Medical-surgical nursing: Assessment and management of clinical problems* (11th ed., pp. 509, 553–554). Elsevier.

❖ 232. The nurse inserts an indwelling urinary catheter into the distended bladder of a postoperative client who has not voided for 8 hours. After the tubing is secured and the collection bag is hung on the bed frame, the nurse notices that 900 mL of urine has drained into the collection bag. What is the appropriate nursing action for the safety of this client?
1. Check the specific gravity of the urine.
2. Clamp the tubing for 30 minutes and then release.
3. Provide suprapubic pressure to maintain a steady flow of urine.
4. Raise the collection bag high enough to slow the rate of drainage.

Level of Cognitive Ability: Applying
Client Needs: Physiological Integrity
Clinical Judgment/Cognitive Skills: Take Action
Integrated Process: Clinical Judgment; Nursing Process/Implementation
Content Area: Skills: Elimination
Health Problems: N/A
Priority Concepts: Elimination; Safety

Answer: 2
Rationale: Rapid emptying of a large volume of urine may cause engorgement of pelvic blood vessels and hypovolemic shock, prolapse of the bladder, or bladder spasms. Clamping the tubing for 30 minutes allows for equilibration to prevent complications. Specific gravity is an assessment and would not affect the flow of urine or prevent possible hypovolemic shock. Applying suprapubic pressure would increase the flow of urine, which could lead to hypovolemic shock. Raising the collection bag could cause backflow of urine. Infection is likely to develop if urine is allowed to flow back into the bladder.
Test-Taking Strategy: Focus on the subject, slowing the urine drainage in a postoperative client with an indwelling urinary catheter. Note the amount: "900 mL." Recall the physiology of the hemodynamic changes after the rapid collapse of an overdistended bladder. Eliminate options 3 and 4; these actions will increase flow rate. Note that option 1 is an assessment action rather than an action that affects the amount of urine drainage.
Priority Nursing Tip: The total bladder capacity is approximately 1 L, and normal adult urine output is 1500 mL/day.
Reference: Potter, P., et al. (2021). *Fundamentals of nursing* (10th ed., p. 1187). Elsevier.

233. The nurse has a prescription to administer amphotericin B intravenously to the client diagnosed with histoplasmosis. Which would the nurse specifically plan to implement during administration of the medication to minimize the client's risk for injury? **Select all that apply.**
- ❑ **1.** Monitoring for hyperthermia
- ❑ **2.** Monitoring for an excessive urine output
- ❑ **3.** Administering a concurrent fluid challenge
- ❑ **4.** Assessing the intravenous (IV) infusion site
- ❑ **5.** Assessing for back, leg, or neck pain
- ❑ **6.** Monitoring client's orientation to time, place, and person

Level of Cognitive Ability: Applying
Client Needs: Physiological Integrity
Clinical Judgment/Cognitive Skills: Generate Solutions
Integrated Process: Clinical Judgment; Nursing Process/Planning
Content Area: Pharmacology: Immune: Antifungals
Health Problems: Adult Health: Respiratory: Infections of the Lower Airway
Priority Concepts: Clinical Judgment; Safety

Answer: 1, 4
Rationale: Amphotericin B is an antifungal medication and is a toxic medication, which can produce symptoms during administration such as chills, fever (hyperthermia), headache, vomiting, and impaired renal function (decreased urine output). The medication is also very irritating to the IV site, commonly causing thrombophlebitis. The nurse administering this medication monitors for these complications. Administering a concurrent fluid challenge is not necessary. Back, leg, or neck pain may be associated with spinal injection of the medication. Disorientation is not specific to this medication.
Test-Taking Strategy: Focus on the **subject**, amphotericin B administration. Recalling the toxic effects of this medication will help direct you to the correct options.
Priority Nursing Tip: If a medication is nephrotoxic, assess kidney function before, during, and after administration. The physician may prescribe blood urea nitrogen (BUN) and creatinine studies. Urine output is also monitored closely.
Reference: Gahart, B., Nazareno, A., & Ortega, M. (2021). *Gahart's 2021 Intravenous medications: A handbook for nurses and health professionals* (37th ed., pp. 78, 81–82). Elsevier.

234. A client who experienced repeated pleural effusions from inoperable lung cancer is to undergo pleurodesis. What intervention would the nurse plan to implement after the physician injects the sclerosing agent through the chest tube?
1. Ambulate client.
2. Clamp the chest tube.
3. Ask client to cough and deep breathe.
4. Ask client to remain in a side-lying position.

Level of Cognitive Ability: Applying
Client Needs: Physiological Integrity
Clinical Judgment/Cognitive Skills: Generate Solutions
Integrated Process: Clinical Judgment; Nursing Process/Planning
Content Area: Adult Health: Respiratory
Health Problems: Adult Health: Cancer: Laryngeal and Lung
Priority Concepts: Collaboration; Gas Exchange

Answer: 2
Rationale: After injection of the sclerosing agent, the chest tube is clamped to prevent the agent from draining back out of the pleural space. Depending on physician preference, a repositioning schedule is used to disperse the substance. Ambulation, coughing, and deep breathing have no specific purpose in the immediate period after injection.
Test-Taking Strategy: Focus on the **subject**, pleurodesis. Recalling the purpose of the procedure will help direct you to the correct option. It is most reasonable to clamp the chest tube so that the sclerosing agent cannot flow back out of the tube. Coughing and deep breathing have no specific purpose in this situation. Ambulation is not advised.
Priority Nursing Tip: The agent injected during pleurodesis creates an inflammatory response that scleroses pleural tissue together.
Reference: Lewis, S., et al. (2020). *Medical-surgical nursing: Assessment and management of clinical problems* (11th ed., p. 531). Elsevier.

235. A client with a posterior wall bladder injury has had surgical repair and placement of a suprapubic catheter. What intervention would the nurse plan to implement to prevent complications associated with the use of this catheter?
1. Monitor urine output every shift.
2. Measure specific gravity once a shift.
3. Encourage a high intake of oral fluids.
4. Avoid kinking of the catheter tubing.

Level of Cognitive Ability: Applying
Client Needs: Physiological Integrity
Clinical Judgment/Cognitive Skills: Generate Solutions
Integrated Process: Clinical Judgment; Nursing Process/Planning
Content Area: Skills: Elimination
Health Problems: Adult Health: Renal and Urinary: Urinary Tract Inflammation/Infection/Trauma
Priority Concepts: Clinical Judgment; Elimination

Answer: 4
Rationale: A complication after surgical repair of the bladder is disruption of sutures caused by tension on them from urine buildup. The nurse prevents this from happening by ensuring that the catheter is able to drain freely. This involves basic catheter care, including keeping the tubing free from kinks, keeping the tubing below the level of the bladder, and monitoring the flow of urine frequently. Monitoring urine output every shift is insufficient to detect decreased flow from catheter kinking. Measurement of urine specific gravity and a high oral fluid intake do not prevent complications of bladder surgery.
Test-Taking Strategy: Focus on the subject, suprapubic catheter. Eliminate option 1 first, because once-a-shift measurement is not a preventive action and is also insufficient in frequency. Eliminate option 2 next because specific gravity measurement is not a preventive action. From the remaining options, knowing that a high oral fluid intake will not prevent complications with the catheter directs you to the correct option.
Priority Nursing Tip: A blunt or penetrating injury to the lower abdomen can cause bladder trauma. Monitor the client for hematuria and pain below the level of the umbilicus, which can radiate to the shoulders.
Reference: Potter, P., et al. (2021). *Fundamentals of nursing* (10th ed., p. 1171). Elsevier.

❖ 236. A client undergoes transurethral resection of the prostate (TURP). Which solution would the nurse infuse postoperatively for continuous bladder irrigation (CBI)?
1. Sterile water
2. Sterile normal saline
3. Sterile Dakin's solution
4. Sterile water with 5% dextrose

Level of Cognitive Ability: Applying
Client Needs: Physiological Integrity
Clinical Judgment/Cognitive Skills: Take Action
Integrated Process: Nursing Process/Implementation
Content Area: Foundations of Care: Fluids and Electrolytes
Health Problems: Adult Health: Renal and Urinary: Obstructive Problems
Priority Concepts: Clinical Judgment; Elimination

Answer: 2
Rationale: Continuous bladder irrigation is done after TURP using sterile normal saline, which is isotonic. Sterile water is not used because the solution could be absorbed systemically, precipitating hemolysis and possibly kidney failure. Dakin's solution contains hypochlorite and is used only for wound irrigation in selected circumstances. Solutions containing dextrose are not introduced into the bladder.
Test-Taking Strategy: Note the subject, continuous bladder irrigation. Recalling that normal saline is isotonic will direct you to the correct option.
Priority Nursing Tip: Bleeding is common after TURP, and the surgeon usually prescribes continuous or intermittent bladder irrigation. An isotonic solution is used for irrigation. Hypotonic solutions absorb into the bloodstream and place the client at risk for transurethral resection syndrome; therefore, they are not used.
Reference: Potter, P., et al. (2021). *Fundamentals of nursing* (10th ed., p. 1193). Elsevier.

237. A client diagnosed with acquired immunodeficiency syndrome (AIDS) is being admitted to the hospital for treatment of a *Pneumocystis jiroveci* respiratory infection. Which intervention would the nurse include when creating the plan of care to assist in maintaining the comfort of this client?
1. Monitoring for bloody sputum
2. Evaluating arterial blood gas results
3. Keeping the head of the bed elevated
4. Assessing respiratory rate, rhythm, depth, and breath sounds

Level of Cognitive Ability: Creating
Client Needs: Physiological Integrity
Clinical Judgment/Cognitive Skills: Generate Solutions
Integrated Process: Clinical Judgment; Nursing Process/Planning
Content Area: Adult Health: Respiratory
Health Problems: Adult Health: Immune: Immunodeficiency Syndrome
Priority Concepts: Caregiving; Gas Exchange

Answer: 3
Rationale: Clients with respiratory difficulties are often more comfortable with the head of the bed elevated. Options 1, 2, and 4 are appropriate measures to evaluate respiratory function and avoid complications. Option 3 is the only choice that addresses planning for client comfort.
Test-Taking Strategy: Focusing on the subject, maintaining comfort, will direct you to the correct option. Also, note that options 1, 2, and 4 are comparable or alike and are all measures to evaluate respiratory function.
Priority Nursing Tip: *Pneumocystis jiroveci* infection is a major source of mortality in the client with AIDS. The client must be monitored closely for manifestations of this respiratory infection.
Reference: Ignatavicius, D., et al. (2021). *Medical-surgical nursing: Concepts for interprofessional collaborative care* (10th ed., p. 339). Elsevier.

❖ **238.** A client with significant flail chest has arterial blood gases (ABGs) drawn at 1200 and again at 1400. Based on the results noted at 1400, which item would the nurse ensure easy access to in order to help ensure client safety?

Laboratory Results

Test and Result 1200	Test and Result 1400	Reference Range
Po$_2$ 82 mm Hg	Po$_2$ 68 mm Hg	80–100 mm Hg
Pco$_2$ 44 mm Hg	Pco$_2$ 51 mm Hg	35–45 mm Hg

1. Intubation tray
2. Injectable lidocaine
3. Chest tube insertion set
4. Portable chest x-ray machine

Level of Cognitive Ability: Analyzing
Client Needs: Physiological Integrity
Clinical Judgment/Cognitive Skills: Analyze Cues
Integrated Process: Clinical Judgment; Nursing Process/Planning
Content Area: Complex Care: Emergency Situations/Management
Health Problems: Adult Health: Respiratory: Chest Injuries
Priority Concepts: Clinical Judgment; Gas Exchange

Answer: 1
Rationale: Flail chest occurs from a blunt trauma to the chest. The loose segment from the chest wall becomes paradoxical to the expansion and contraction of the rest of the chest wall. The client with flail chest has painful, rapid, shallow respirations while experiencing severe dyspnea. The laboratory results indicate worsening oxygenation status. The effort of breathing and the paradoxical chest movement have the net effect of producing hypoxia and hypercapnia. The client develops respiratory failure and requires intubation and mechanical ventilation, usually with positive end-expiratory pressure (PEEP); therefore, an intubation tray is necessary. None of the other options have a direct purpose with the client's current respiratory status.
Test-Taking Strategy: Focus on the subject, flail chest. Review the changes in the ABG values. Recall that a falling arterial oxygen level and a rising carbon dioxide level indicate respiratory failure. The usual treatment for respiratory failure is intubation, which will lead you to the correct option.
Priority Nursing Tip: The client with a flail chest experiences paradoxical respirations (inward movement of a segment of the thorax during inspiration with outward movement during expiration).
Reference: Ignatavicius, D., et al. (2021). *Medical-surgical nursing: Concepts for interprofessional collaborative care* (10th ed., pp. 607–608). Elsevier.

239. A client experiencing empyema is to have a bedside thoracentesis performed. The nurse plans to have which equipment available in the event that the procedure itself is not **effective**?

1. Code cart
2. A small-bore needle
3. Extra-large drainage bottle
4. Chest tube and drainage system

Level of Cognitive Ability: Applying
Client Needs: Physiological Integrity
Clinical Judgment/Cognitive Skills: Generate Solutions
Integrated Process: Nursing Process/Planning
Content Area: Adult Health: Respiratory
Health Problems: Adult Health: Respiratory: Pleural Effusion
Priority Concepts: Gas Exchange; Safety

Answer: 4

Rationale: Empyema is the collection of pus within the pleural cavity. If the exudate is too thick for drainage via thoracentesis, the client may require placement of a chest tube to adequately drain the purulent effusion. A small-bore needle would not effectively allow exudate to drain. Options 1 and 3 are also unnecessary.

Test-Taking Strategy: Note the strategic word, *effective*. Focus on the subject, empyema and thoracentesis. A client with empyema will have exudate that is often very thick. Recalling that the purpose of thoracentesis is to provide drainage of the pleura will direct you to the correct option.

Priority Nursing Tip: Empyema is usually caused by pulmonary infection and lung abscess after thoracic surgery or chest trauma in which bacteria is introduced directly into the pleural space.

Reference: Ignatavicius, D., et al. (2021). *Medical-surgical nursing: Concepts for interprofessional collaborative care* (10th ed., pp. 562, 574). Elsevier.

❖ **240.** The nurse caring for a client being treated for severe back pain is preparing to administer an opioid via an epidural catheter. Before administering the medication, the nurse aspirates and obtains 5 mL of clear fluid. Based on this finding, which action would the nurse take?

1. Inject the opioid with force that is steady but slow.
2. Hold the medication and notify the anesthesiologist.
3. Inject the aspirate back into the catheter and administer the opioid.
4. Flush the catheter with 6 mL of sterile water before injecting the opioid.

Level of Cognitive Ability: Applying
Client Needs: Physiological Integrity
Clinical Judgment/Cognitive Skills: Take Action
Integrated Process: Clinical Judgment; Nursing Process/Implementation
Content Area: Complex Care: Emergency Situations/Management
Health Problems: Adult Health: Musculoskeletal: Skeletal Injury
Priority Concepts: Collaboration; Safety

Answer: 2

Rationale: Aspiration of clear fluid of less than 1 mL is indicative of epidural catheter placement. More than 1 mL of clear fluid or bloody return means that the catheter may be in the subarachnoid space or a vessel. Therefore, the nurse would not inject the medication and would notify the anesthesiologist. Options 1, 3, and 4 are incorrect actions.

Test-Taking Strategy: Focus on the subject, epidural catheter. Eliminate options 1, 3, and 4 because they are comparable or alike and indicate administering the opioid.

Priority Nursing Tip: The use of strict aseptic technique is required when caring for an epidural catheter to prevent the introduction of bacteria into the epidural space.

Reference: Ignatavicius, D., et al. (2021). *Medical-surgical nursing: Concepts for interprofessional collaborative care* (10th ed., pp. 83, 88). Elsevier.

241. The nurse is planning care for a client with a chest tube attached to a Pleur-Evac drainage system for the management of pleural effusion. The nurse would include which interventions in the plan? **Select all that apply.**
- ❏ 1. Changing the client's position often
- ❏ 2. Clamping the chest tube intermittently
- ❏ 3. Maintaining the collection chamber below client's waist
- ❏ 4. Adding water to the suction control chamber as it evaporates
- ❏ 5. Taping the connection between the chest tube and the drainage system

Level of Cognitive Ability: Analyzing
Client Needs: Physiological Integrity
Clinical Judgment/Cognitive Skills: Generate Solutions
Integrated Process: Clinical Judgment; Nursing Process/Planning
Content Area: Skills: Tube Care
Health Problems: Adult Health: Respiratory: Pleural Effusion
Priority Concepts: Clinical Judgment; Gas Exchange

Answer: 1, 3, 4, 5
Rationale: Changing the client's position frequently is necessary to promote drainage and ventilation. Maintaining the system below waist level is indicated to prevent fluid from reentering the pleural space. Adding water to the suction control chamber is an appropriate nursing action and is done as needed to maintain the full suction level prescribed. Taping the connection between the chest tube and system is also indicated to prevent accidental disconnection. To prevent a tension pneumothorax, the nurse avoids clamping the chest tube, unless specifically prescribed. In many facilities, clamping of the chest tube is contraindicated by agency policy.
Test-Taking Strategy: Focus on the **subject**, interventions in the care of the client with a chest tube. Recall that tension pneumothorax occurs when air is trapped in the pleural space and has no exit. Therefore, it is necessary to evaluate each of the options in terms of relative risk for air trapping in the pleural space. Clamping the chest tube could trap air in the pleural space.
Priority Nursing Tip: Confirmation of pneumothorax is made by chest radiography.
Reference: Ignatavicius, D., et al. (2021). *Medical-surgical nursing: Concepts for interprofessional collaborative care* (10th ed., p. 561). Elsevier.

❖ **242.** The nurse is assisting a client with a chest tube, who is recovering from pneumothorax, to get out of bed, when the chest tubing accidentally gets caught in the bed rail and disconnects. While trying to reestablish the connection, the Pleur-Evac drainage system falls over and cracks. The nurse would take which action to minimize the client's risk for injury?
1. Clamp the chest tube.
2. Call the physician.
3. Apply a petroleum gauze over the end of the chest tube.
4. Immerse the chest tube in a bottle of sterile water or normal saline.

Level of Cognitive Ability: Analyzing
Client Needs: Physiological Integrity
Clinical Judgment/Cognitive Skills: Take Action
Integrated Process: Clinical Judgment; Nursing Process/Implementation
Content Area: Complex Care: Emergency Situations/ Management
Health Problems: Adult Health: Respiratory: Pneumothorax
Priority Concepts: Clinical Judgment; Gas Exchange

Answer: 4
Rationale: If a chest tube accidentally disconnects from the tubing of the drainage apparatus, the nurse would first reestablish an underwater seal to prevent tension pneumothorax and mediastinal shift. This can be accomplished by reconnecting the chest tube or, in this case, immersing the end of the chest tube 1 to 2 inches below the surface of a 250-mL bottle of sterile water or normal saline until a new chest tube can be set up. The physician would be notified but only after taking corrective action. If the physician is called first, tension pneumothorax has time to develop. Clamping the chest tube could also cause tension pneumothorax. A petroleum gauze would be applied to the skin over the chest tube insertion site if the entire chest tube was accidentally removed from the chest.
Test-Taking Strategy: Focus on the **subject**, care of a chest tube. Option 1 would create a tension pneumothorax because this action does not reestablish an underwater seal. Eliminate option 2 because it is too time consuming to be the immediate action. From the remaining options, noting that an underwater seal must be established will direct you to the correct option.
Priority Nursing Tip: If a closed chest tube drainage system cracks or breaks, insert the chest tube into a bottle of sterile water, remove the cracked or broken system, and replace it with a new system.
Reference: Ignatavicius, D., et al. (2021). *Medical-surgical nursing: Concepts for interprofessional collaborative care* (10th ed., p. 561). Elsevier.

243. When planning care for a client diagnosed with Cushing's syndrome, the nurse would plan to include which intervention to prevent a common complication of this disorder?
1. Monitoring glucose levels
2. Encouraging rigorous exercise
3. Monitoring epinephrine levels
4. Encouraging visits from friends

Level of Cognitive Ability: Analyzing
Client Needs: Physiological Integrity
Clinical Judgment/Cognitive Skills: Generate Solutions
Integrated Process: Clinical Judgment; Nursing Process/Planning
Content Area: Adult Health: Endocrine
Health Problems: Adult Health: Endocrine: Adrenal Disorders
Priority Concepts: Clinical Judgment; Glucose Regulation

Answer: 1
Rationale: Cushing's syndrome is a metabolic disorder resulting from the chronic and excessive production of cortisol by the adrenal cortex or the administration of glucocorticoids in large doses for several weeks or longer. In the client with Cushing's syndrome, increased levels of glucocorticoids can result in hyperglycemia and signs and symptoms of diabetes mellitus. Clients experience activity intolerance related to muscle weakness and fatigue; therefore, option 2 is incorrect. Epinephrine levels are not affected. Visitors need to be limited because of the client's impaired immune response.
Test-Taking Strategy: Focus on the subject, complications of Cushing's syndrome. Recalling that increased levels of glucocorticoids can result in hyperglycemia will direct you to the correct option.
Priority Nursing Tip: Hyperglycemia, hypernatremia, hypokalemia, and hypocalcemia occur in Cushing's syndrome. The opposite effects occur in Addison's disease.
Reference: Ignatavicius, D., et al. (2021). *Medical-surgical nursing: Concepts for interprofessional collaborative care* (10th ed., p. 1242). Elsevier.

❖ **244.** A client with a central venous catheter who is receiving total parenteral nutrition (TPN) suddenly experiences signs/symptoms associated with an air embolism. The nurse would implement which interventions to minimize the client's risk for injury? **Select all that apply.**
☐ 1. Clamps the catheter
☐ 2. Checks the line for air
☐ 3. Notifies the physician
☐ 4. Boluses the client with 500 mL normal saline
☐ 5. Places the client in Trendelenburg's position on the left side

Level of Cognitive Ability: Analyzing
Client Needs: Physiological Integrity
Clinical Judgment/Cognitive Skills: Take Action
Integrated Process: Clinical Judgment; Nursing Process/Implementation
Content Area: Complex Care: Emergency Situations/Management
Health Problems: Adult Health: Respiratory: Pulmonary Embolism
Priority Concepts: Gas Exchange; Perfusion

Answer: 1, 3, 5
Rationale: If the client experiences air embolus, the client is placed in the lateral Trendelenburg's position on the left side to trap the air in the right atrium. The nurse would also clamp the catheter and notify the physician for emergency prescriptions. Checking the line for air would not help the client or minimize the client's risk for injury. A fluid bolus would cause the air embolus to travel.
Test-Taking Strategy: Focus on the subject, suspected air embolism. Recall that air embolism is a life-threatening condition requiring immediate nursing intervention to prevent the air embolus from traveling. Since this is a life-threatening emergency, the physician is notified.
Priority Nursing Tip: Air embolism can be caused by an inadequately primed intravenous (IV) line or a loose connection. Air embolism may occur during tubing change or during removal of the IV.
Reference: Urden, L., Stacy, K., & Lough, M. (2022). *Critical care nursing: Diagnosis and management* (9th ed., p. 101). Elsevier.

245. The nurse is caring for client who is 33 weeks pregnant and has experienced a premature rupture of the membranes (PROM). Which interventions would the nurse expect to be part of the plan of care? **Select all that apply.**
- ❏ **1.** Perform frequent biophysical profiles.
- ❏ **2.** Monitor for elevated serum creatinine.
- ❏ **3.** Monitor for manifestations of infection.
- ❏ **4.** Teach the client how to count fetal movements.
- ❏ **5.** Use strict sterile technique for vaginal examinations.
- ❏ **6.** Inform the client about the need for tocolytic therapy.

Level of Cognitive Ability: Analyzing
Client Needs: Physiological Integrity
Clinical Judgment/Cognitive Skills: Generate Solutions
Integrated Process: Clinical Judgment; Nursing Process/Planning
Content Area: Maternity: Antepartum
Health Problems: Maternity: Premature Rupture of the Membranes
Priority Concepts: Caregiving; Reproduction

Answer: 1, 3, 4, 5
Rationale: PROM is membrane rupture before 37 weeks of gestation. Frequent biophysical profiles are performed to determine fetal health status and estimate amniotic fluid volume. Monitoring for signs of infection is a major part of the nursing care. The client needs to also be taught how to count fetal movements, because slowing of fetal movement has been shown to be a precursor to severe fetal compromise. Whenever PROM is suspected, strict sterile technique should be used in any vaginal examination to prevent infection. Elevated serum creatinine does not occur in PROM but may be noted in severe preeclampsia. Tocolytic therapy is used for women in preterm labor (not for PROM).
Test-Taking Strategy: Focus on the subject, premature rupture of the membranes (PROM). Think about the pathophysiology of this condition. Select options 3 and 5 because they relate to preventing infection. Next select options 1 and 4 because they relate to determining fetal health status. Recalling the causes of an elevated serum creatinine and the purpose of tocolytic therapy will assist in eliminating these options.
Priority Nursing Tip: An assessment finding in PROM is the evidence of fluid pooling in the vaginal vault. The fluid tests positive with the Nitrazine test.
Reference: McKinney, E. S., et al. (2022). *Maternal child nursing* (6th ed., pp. 289, 586–587). Elsevier.

❖ **246.** A client who has been diagnosed with carbon monoxide poisoning is asking that the oxygen mask be removed. The nurse shares with the client that the oxygen may be safely removed once the carboxyhemoglobin level decreases to less than which level?
1. 5%
2. 10%
3. 15%
4. 25%

Level of Cognitive Ability: Applying
Client Needs: Physiological Integrity
Clinical Judgment/Cognitive Skills: Generate Solutions
Integrated Process: Clinical Judgment; Nursing Process/Planning
Content Area: Complex Care: Poisoning
Health Problems: Adult Health: Respiratory: Environmental
Priority Concepts: Clinical Judgment; Gas Exchange

Answer: 1
Rationale: Oxygen may be removed safely from the client with carbon monoxide poisoning once carboxyhemoglobin levels are less than 5%. Normal carboxyhemoglobin (HbCO) levels are 0% to 3% for nonsmokers and 3% to 8% for smokers. Levels of 10% to 20% cause headaches, nausea, vomiting, and dyspnea. Levels of 30% to 40% cause severe headaches, syncope, and tachydysrhythmias. Levels greater than 40% cause Cheyne-Stokes respiration or respiratory failure, seizures, unconsciousness, permanent brain damage, cardiac arrest, and even death. Options 2, 3, and 4 are elevated levels.
Test-Taking Strategy: Focus on the subject, safely removing the oxygen in CO poisoning. If you are unsure, it would be best to select the lowest level as identified in the correct option.
Priority Nursing Tip: Carbon monoxide is a colorless, odorless, and tasteless gas.
Reference: Ignatavicius, D., et al. (2021). *Medical-surgical nursing: Concepts for interprofessional collaborative care* (10th ed., p. 466). Elsevier.

247. The nurse is teaching a pregnant client about prenatal nutritional needs. The nurse would include which information in the client's teaching plan?

1. All pregnant clients are at high risk for nutritional deficiencies.
2. Calcium intake is not necessary until the third trimester.
3. Iron supplements are not necessary unless the pregnant client has iron deficiency anemia.
4. The nutritional status of the pregnant client significantly influences fetal growth and development.

Level of Cognitive Ability: Applying
Client Needs: Physiological Integrity
Clinical Judgment/Cognitive Skills: Generate Solutions
Integrated Process: Teaching and Learning
Content Area: Maternity: Antepartum
Health Problems: N/A
Priority Concepts: Patient Education; Nutrition

Answer: 4
Rationale: Poor nutrition during pregnancy can negatively influence fetal growth and development. Although pregnancy poses some nutritional risk for the pregnant client, not all clients are at high risk. Calcium intake is critical during the third trimester but must be increased from the onset of pregnancy. Intake of dietary iron is insufficient for the majority of pregnant clients, and iron supplements are routinely prescribed.
Test-Taking Strategy: Focus on the subject, nutrition during pregnancy. Option 1 uses the closed-ended word "all"; therefore, eliminate this option. Options 2 and 3 offer specific time frames or conditions for interventions; therefore, eliminate these options. Option 4 is also a general statement that is true for any stage of pregnancy.
Priority Nursing Tip: An increase of about 300 calories/day is needed during the last 6 months of pregnancy.
Reference: McKinney, E. S., et al. (2022). *Maternal child nursing* (6th ed., p. 260). Elsevier.

❖ **248.** A client is admitted to the hospital with a diagnosis of acute bacterial pericarditis. Which assessment findings are associated with this form of heart disease? **Select all that apply.**

❑ 1. Fever
❑ 2. Leukopenia
❑ 3. Bradycardia
❑ 4. Pericardial friction rub
❑ 5. Decreased erythrocyte sedimentation rate
❑ 6. Precordial chest pain that is intensified by the supine position

Level of Cognitive Ability: Analyzing
Client Needs: Physiological Integrity
Clinical Judgment/Cognitive Skills: Recognize Cues
Integrated Process: Clinical Judgment; Nursing Process/Assessment
Content Area: Adult Health: Cardiovascular
Health Problems: Adult Health: Cardiovascular: Inflammatory and Structural Heart Disorders
Priority Concepts: Infection; Inflammation

Answer: 1, 4, 6
Rationale: In acute bacterial pericarditis, the membranes surrounding the heart become inflamed and rub against each other, producing the classic pericardial friction rub. Fever typically occurs and is accompanied by leukocytosis and an elevated erythrocyte sedimentation rate. The client reports severe precordial chest pain that intensifies when lying supine and decreases in a sitting position. The pain also intensifies when the client breathes deeply. Malaise, myalgia, and tachycardia are common.
Test-Taking Strategy: Focus on the subject, bacterial pericarditis. The diagnosis will assist in determining that the client has a fever (option 1); the compensatory response to fever is an increased metabolic rate and tachycardia. Also remember that when the client has an inflammatory disease, the erythrocyte sedimentation rate will increase, as will the white blood cell count (leukocytosis, not leukopenia). Last, focusing on the diagnosis will assist in determining that a pericardial friction rub and severe precordial chest pain are present (options 4 and 6).
Priority Nursing Tip: Monitor the client with pericarditis for signs of heart failure or cardiac tamponade as complications.
Reference: Ignatavicius, D., et al. (2021). *Medical-surgical nursing: Concepts for interprofessional collaborative care* (10th ed., p. 690). Elsevier.

249. A client is admitted to the hospital with a diagnosis of Cushing's syndrome. The nurse monitors the client for which problem that is likely to occur with this diagnosis?
1. Hypovolemia
2. Hypoglycemia
3. Mood disturbances
4. Deficient fluid volume

Level of Cognitive Ability: Analyzing
Client Needs: Physiological Integrity
Clinical Judgment/Cognitive Skills: Analyze Cues
Integrated Process: Clinical Judgment; Nursing Process/Analysis
Content Area: Adult Health: Endocrine
Health Problems: Adult Health: Endocrine: Adrenal Disorders
Priority Concepts: Clinical Judgment; Mood and Affect

Answer: 3
Rationale: Cushing's syndrome is a metabolic disorder resulting from the chronic and excessive production of cortisol. When Cushing's syndrome develops, the normal function of the glucocorticoids becomes exaggerated and the classic picture of the syndrome emerges. This exaggerated physiologic action can cause mood disturbances, including memory loss, poor concentration and cognition, euphoria, and depression. It can also cause persistent hyperglycemia along with sodium and water retention (hypernatremia), producing edema (hypervolemia; fluid volume excess), and hypertension.
Test-Taking Strategy: Focus on the **subject**, Cushing's syndrome. Eliminate options 1 and 4 first because they are **comparable or alike** since both involve a deficiency in blood volume. Recalling that hyperglycemia rather than hypoglycemia occurs in this condition will direct you to the correct option.
Priority Nursing Tip: Cushing's syndrome is characterized by an excessive amount of cortisol, whereas Addison's disease is characterized by a hyposecretion of adrenal cortex hormones (glucocorticoids and mineralocorticoids).
Reference: Ignatavicius, D., et al. (2021). *Medical-surgical nursing: Concepts for interprofessional collaborative care* (10th ed., p. 1242). Elsevier.

250. An assessment of a client's vocal cords with suspected malignancy requires indirect visualization of the larynx. Which instruction would the nurse give the client to facilitate this procedure?
1. Try to swallow.
2. Hold your breath.
3. Breathe normally.
4. Roll the tongue to the back of the mouth.

Level of Cognitive Ability: Applying
Client Needs: Physiological Integrity
Clinical Judgment/Cognitive Skills: Take Action
Integrated Process: Nursing Process/Implementation
Content Area: Foundations of Care: Diagnostic Tests
Health Problems: Adult Health: Cancer: Laryngeal and Lung
Priority Concepts: Clinical Judgment; Gas Exchange

Answer: 3
Rationale: Indirect laryngoscopy is done to assess the function of the vocal cords or to obtain tissue for biopsy. Observations are made during rest and phonation by using a laryngeal mirror, head mirror, and light source. The client is placed in an upright position to facilitate passage of the laryngeal mirror into the mouth and is instructed to breathe normally. Swallowing cannot be done with the mirror in place. The procedure takes longer than the time the client would be able to hold the breath, and this action is ineffective anyway. The tongue cannot be moved back because it would occlude the airway.
Test-Taking Strategy: Focus on the **subject**, indirect laryngoscopy. Option 4 is eliminated first because it is not possible to move the tongue back with the mirror in place. It would also cause the airway to become occluded. Given the length of time needed to do the procedure, the client could not realistically hold their breath, so option 2 is eliminated next. Trying to swallow would actually cause the larynx to move against the mirror and could cause gagging; therefore, eliminate option 1.
Priority Nursing Tip: After laryngoscopy, maintain an NPO status until the gag reflex returns.
Reference: Lewis, S., et al. (2020). *Medical-surgical nursing: Assessment and management of clinical problems* (11th ed., pp. 494–495). Elsevier.

251. The nurse is caring for a client scheduled for a bilateral adrenalectomy for treatment of an adrenal tumor. What information would the nurse give the client about the postsurgical needs?
1. "You will need to undergo chemotherapy after surgery."
2. "You will need to wear an abdominal binder after surgery."
3. "You will not need any special long-term treatment after surgery."
4. "You will need to take daily hormone replacements beginning after the surgery."

Level of Cognitive Ability: Applying
Client Needs: Physiological Integrity
Clinical Judgment/Cognitive Skills: Take Action
Integrated Process: Teaching and Learning
Content Area: Adult Health: Endocrine
Health Problems: Adult Health: Endocrine: Adrenal Disorders
Priority Concepts: Patient Education; Cellular Regulation

Answer: 4
Rationale: The major cause of primary hyperaldosteronism is an aldosterone-secreting tumor called an aldosteronoma. Surgery is the treatment of choice. Clients undergoing a bilateral adrenalectomy require permanent replacement of adrenal hormones. Options 1, 2, and 3 are inaccurate statements regarding this surgery.
Test-Taking Strategy: Focus on the subject, bilateral adrenalectomy. Recalling the function of the adrenal glands and that glucocorticoids and mineralocorticoids are essential to sustain life will direct you to the correct option.
Priority Nursing Tip: After adrenalectomy, monitor for signs of acute adrenal insufficiency, which is also known as Addisonian crisis.
Reference: Ignatavicius, D., et al. (2021). *Medical-surgical nursing: Concepts for interprofessional collaborative care* (10th ed., p. 1245). Elsevier.

❖ **252.** The nurse is caring for a client who is scheduled for an adrenalectomy. The nurse plans to administer which medication in the preoperative period to prevent Addisonian crisis?
1. Prednisone orally
2. Fludrocortisone orally
3. Spironolactone intramuscularly
4. Methylprednisolone sodium succinate intravenously

Level of Cognitive Ability: Analyzing
Client Needs: Physiological Integrity
Clinical Judgment/Cognitive Skills: Generate Solutions
Integrated Process: Clinical Judgment; Nursing Process/Planning
Content Area: Pharmacology: Endocrine: Corticosteroids
Health Problems: Adult Health: Endocrine: Adrenal Disorders
Priority Concepts: Clinical Judgment; Fluids and Electrolytes

Answer: 4
Rationale: A glucocorticoid preparation will be administered intravenously or intramuscularly in the immediate preoperative period to a client scheduled for an adrenalectomy. Methylprednisolone sodium succinate protects the client from developing acute adrenal insufficiency (Addisonian crisis) that can occur as a result of the adrenalectomy. Prednisone is an oral corticosteroid. Fludrocortisone is a mineralocorticoid. Spironolactone is a potassium-sparing diuretic.
Test-Taking Strategy: Focus on the subject, preventing Addisonian crisis in a client scheduled for adrenalectomy. Recalling the function of the adrenals will assist in eliminating options 2 and 3. From the remaining options, select option 4 because the client is preoperative and should receive medications via routes other than orally.
Priority Nursing Tip: Emergency care of the client with Addisonian crisis includes hormone replacement and hyperkalemia and hypoglycemia management.
References: Gahart, B., Nazareno, A., & Ortega, M. (2021). *Gahart's 2021 Intravenous medications: A handbook for nurses and health professionals* (37th ed., p. 892). Elsevier; Ignatavicius, D., et al. (2021). *Medical-surgical nursing: Concepts for interprofessional collaborative care* (10th ed., p. 1244). Elsevier.

253. The nurse is preparing a client diagnosed with Graves' disease to receive radioactive iodine therapy. What information would the nurse share with the client about the therapy?
1. After the initial dose, subsequent treatments must continue lifelong.
2. The radioactive iodine is designed to destroy the entire thyroid gland with just one dose.
3. High radioactivity levels prohibit contact with family for 4 weeks after the initial treatment.
4. It takes 6 to 8 weeks after treatment to experience relief from the symptoms of the disease.

Level of Cognitive Ability: Applying
Client Needs: Physiological Integrity
Clinical Judgment/Cognitive Skills: Generate Solutions
Integrated Process: Teaching and Learning
Content Area: Adult Health: Endocrine
Health Problems: Adult Health: Endocrine: Thyroid Disorders
Priority Concepts: Cellular Regulation; Patient Education

Answer: 4
Rationale: Graves' disease is also known as toxic diffuse goiter and is characterized by a hyperthyroid state resulting from hypersecretion of thyroid hormones. After treatment with radioactive iodine therapy, a decrease in the thyroid hormone level should be noted, which helps alleviate symptoms. Relief of symptoms does not occur until 6 to 8 weeks after initial treatment. Occasionally, a client may require a second or third dose, but treatments are not lifelong. This form of therapy is not designed to destroy the entire gland; rather, some of the cells that synthesize thyroid hormone will be destroyed by the local radiation. The nurse must reassure the client and family that, unless the dosage is extremely high, clients are not required to observe radiation precautions. The rationale for this is that the radioactivity quickly dissipates.
Test-Taking Strategy: Focus on the subject, Graves' disease. Recall knowledge regarding this treatment. Note the closed-ended words "must," "entire," and "prohibit" in the incorrect options.
Priority Nursing Tip: The consumption or administration of any substance that contains a stimulant needs to be avoided in the client with hyperthyroidism.
Reference: Ignatavicius, D., et al. (2021). *Medical-surgical nursing: Concepts for interprofessional collaborative care* (10th ed., p. 1257). Elsevier.

❖ **254.** A client arrives at the emergency department with upper gastrointestinal (GI) bleeding that began 3 hours ago. What is the **priority** action?
1. Obtaining vital signs
2. Inserting a nasogastric (NG) tube
3. Completing an abdominal physical assessment
4. Asking the client about the precipitating events

Level of Cognitive Ability: Analyzing
Client Needs: Physiological Integrity
Clinical Judgment/Cognitive Skills: Take Action
Integrated Process: Clinical Judgment; Nursing Process/Implementation
Content Area: Complex Care: Emergency Situations/Management
Health Problems: Adult Health: Gastrointestinal: Gastrointestinal Hemorrhage
Priority Concepts: Clotting; Perfusion

Answer: 1
Rationale: The priority action for the client with GI bleeding is to obtain vital signs to determine whether the client is in shock from blood loss and obtain a baseline by which to monitor the progress of treatment. The client may not be able to provide subjective data until the immediate physical needs are met. A complete abdominal physical assessment must be performed but is not the priority. Insertion of an NG tube may be prescribed but is not the priority action.
Test-Taking Strategy: Note the strategic word, *priority*. Recall that the client with a GI bleed is at risk for shock. Also, the correct option addresses the ABCs—airway, breathing, and circulation.
Priority Nursing Tip: For the client experiencing active gastrointestinal bleeding, assess for signs of dehydration and hypovolemic shock.
Reference: Lewis, S., et al. (2020). *Medical-surgical nursing: Assessment and management of clinical problems* (11th ed., p. 918). Elsevier.

255. A client who has chronic kidney disease is prescribed a fluid restriction of 1500 mL per day. Which interventions would the nurse implement to assist the client in maintaining this restriction? **Select all that apply.**
- ❑ 1. Removing the water pitcher from the bedside
- ❑ 2. Using mouthwash with alcohol for mouth care
- ❑ 3. Prohibiting beverages with sugar to minimize thirst
- ❑ 4. Providing client with lip balm to keep lips moist
- ❑ 5. Offering client ice chips at intervals during the day

Level of Cognitive Ability: Applying
Client Needs: Physiological Integrity
Clinical Judgment/Cognitive Skills: Take Action
Integrated Process: Nursing Process/Implementation
Content Area: Foundations of Care: Fluids and Electrolytes
Health Problems: Adult Health: Renal and Urinary: Acute Kidney Injury and Chronic Kidney Disease
Priority Concepts: Clinical Judgment; Fluids and Electrolytes

Answer: 1, 4, 5
Rationale: The nurse can help the client maintain fluid restriction through a variety of means. The water pitcher needs to be removed from the bedside to aid in compliance. The use of ice chips and lip ointments is another intervention that may be helpful to the client on fluid restriction. Frequent mouth care is important; however, alcohol-based products need to be avoided because they are drying to mucous membranes. Beverages that the client enjoys are provided and are not restricted based on sugar content.
Test-Taking Strategy: Focus on the subject, a client with chronic kidney disease who is on fluid restriction. Eliminate options 2 and 3 because they are ineffective or unnecessary.
Priority Nursing Tip: As long as the beverage is not contraindicated, allow the client on fluid restriction to select preferred beverages.
References: Ignatavicius, D., et al. (2021). *Medical-surgical nursing: Concepts for interprofessional collaborative care* (10th ed., p. 1390). Elsevier; Potter, P., et al. (2021). *Fundamentals of nursing* (10th ed., p. 999). Elsevier.

❖ **256.** The nurse has administered approximately half of a high-cleansing enema when the client reports pain and cramping. Which nursing action is appropriate?
1. Reassuring client that those sensations will subside
2. Raising the enema bag so that the solution can be introduced quickly
3. Discontinuing the enema and notifying the physician
4. Clamping the tubing for 30 seconds and restarting the flow at a slower rate

Level of Cognitive Ability: Applying
Client Needs: Physiological Integrity
Clinical Judgment/Cognitive Skills: Take Action
Integrated Process: Nursing Process/Implementation
Content Area: Skills: Elimination
Health Problems: N/A
Priority Concepts: Clinical Judgment; Elimination

Answer: 4
Rationale: The enema fluid should be administered slowly. If the client complains of pain or cramping, the flow is stopped for 30 seconds and restarted at a slower rate. Slow enema administration and stopping the flow temporarily, if necessary, will decrease the likelihood of intestinal spasm and premature ejection of the solution. The client's report of pain and cramping should not be ignored. The higher the solution container is held above the rectum, the faster the flow and the greater the force in the rectum. There is no need to discontinue the enema and notify the physician at this time.
Test-Taking Strategy: Focus on the subject, alleviating pain and cramping with enema instillation. Noting that there is no need to notify the primary health care provider will allow you to eliminate that option.
Priority Nursing Tip: During enema administration, ask the client to breathe slowly in through the nose and out through the mouth. This will assist the client in tolerating the instillation of the solution.
Reference: Potter, P., et al. (2021). *Fundamentals of nursing* (10th ed., p. 1222). Elsevier.

257. The client diagnosed with chronic kidney disease is scheduled for hemodialysis. When would the nurse plan to administer the client's daily dose of enalapril to ensure its **effectiveness?**

1. During dialysis
2. Just before dialysis
3. The day after dialysis
4. Upon return from dialysis

Level of Cognitive Ability: Applying
Client Needs: Physiological Integrity
Clinical Judgment/Cognitive Skills: Generate Solutions
Integrated Process: Nursing Process/Planning
Content Area: Pharmacology: Cardiovascular: Angiotensin-Converting Enzyme (ACE) Inhibitors
Health Problems: Adult Health: Renal and Urinary: Acute Kidney Injury and Chronic Kidney Disease
Priority Concepts: Clinical Judgment; Fluids and Electrolytes

Answer: 4
Rationale: Antihypertensive medications, such as enalapril, are administered to the client after hemodialysis. This prevents the client from becoming hypotensive during dialysis and also from having the medication removed from the bloodstream by dialysis. There is no rationale for waiting a full day to resume the medication. This would lead to ineffective control of the blood pressure.
Test-Taking Strategy: Note the strategic word, *effectiveness.* Focus on the subject, medication administration with hemodialysis. Think about the effects of an antihypertensive medication on the blood pressure when fluid is being removed from the body. Because hypotension is much more likely to occur in this circumstance, eliminate options 1 and 2. Most clients are hemodialyzed three times a week, so if the medication were held for dialysis until the following day, the client would miss three of the seven doses that would usually be given in a week. This would lead to ineffective blood pressure control; therefore, eliminate option 3.
Priority Nursing Tip: In addition to antihypertensive medications, water-soluble vitamins, certain antibiotics, and digoxin are withheld before a hemodialysis treatment because they can be removed by dialysis.
Reference: Ignatavicius, D., et al. (2021). *Medical-surgical nursing: Concepts for interprofessional collaborative care* (10th ed., p. 1400). Elsevier.

❖ 258. The client reports smoking three-fourths of a pack per day over the last 10 years. The nurse calculates that the client has a smoking history of how many pack-years? **Fill in the blank and record your answer using one decimal place.**
Answer: _____ pack-years
Level of Cognitive Ability: Applying
Client Needs: Physiological Integrity
Clinical Judgment/Cognitive Skills: Recognize Cues
Integrated Process: Nursing Process/Assessment
Content Area: Adult Health: Respiratory
Health Problems: Adult Health: Respiratory: Environmental
Priority Concepts: Clinical Judgment; Health Promotion

Answer: 7.5
Rationale: The standard method for quantifying smoking history is to multiply the number of packs smoked per day by the number of years of smoking. The number is recorded as the number of pack-years. The calculation for the number of pack-years for the client who has smoked three-fourths of a pack per day for 10 years is 0.75 pack × 10 years = 7.5 pack-years.
Test-Taking Strategy: Focus on the subject, number of pack-years. Review the information in the question and multiply the number of packs of cigarettes smoked per day by the number of years of smoking.
Priority Nursing Tip: When obtaining a smoking history, ask the client about possible exposure to passive smoke.
Reference: Ignatavicius, D., et al. (2021). *Medical-surgical nursing: Concepts for interprofessional collaborative care* (10th ed., pp. 478–479). Elsevier.

259. The nurse is preparing to provide postsurgical care for a client after a subtotal thyroidectomy. The nurse anticipates the need for which item to be placed at the bedside to minimize the client's risk for injury?
1. Hypothermia blanket
2. Emergency tracheostomy kit
3. Magnesium sulfate in a ready-to-inject vial
4. Ampule of saturated solution of potassium iodide

Level of Cognitive Ability: Applying
Client Needs: Physiological Integrity
Clinical Judgment/Cognitive Skills: Generate Solutions
Integrated Process: Clinical Judgment; Nursing Process/Planning
Content Area: Adult Health: Endocrine
Health Problems: Adult Health: Endocrine: Thyroid Disorders
Priority Concepts: Caregiving; Safety

Answer: **2**
Rationale: Respiratory distress can occur after thyroidectomy as a result of swelling in the tracheal area. The nurse would ensure that an emergency tracheostomy kit is available. Surgery on the thyroid does not alter the heat control mechanism of the body. Magnesium sulfate would not be indicated because the incidence of hypomagnesemia is not a common problem after thyroidectomy. Saturated solution of potassium iodide is typically administered preoperatively to block thyroid hormone synthesis and release and to place the client in a euthyroid state.
Test-Taking Strategy: Focus on the **subject**, postoperative thyroidectomy. Recall the anatomic location of the thyroid gland to direct you to the correct option. Also, use the ABCs—**airway, breathing, and circulation.** Maintaining a patent airway is critical.
Priority Nursing Tip: After thyroidectomy, maintain the client in a semi-Fowler's position to assist in preventing edema at the operative site.
Reference: Ignatavicius, D., et al. (2021). *Medical-surgical nursing: Concepts for interprofessional collaborative care* (10th ed., p. 1259). Elsevier.

❖ **260.** When caring for a client diagnosed with myasthenia gravis, the nurse would be alert for which manifestations of myasthenic crisis? **Select all that apply.**
☐ 1. Bradycardia
☐ 2. Increased diaphoresis
☐ 3. Decreased lacrimation
☐ 4. Bowel and bladder incontinence
☐ 5. Absent cough and swallow reflex
☐ 6. Sudden marked rise in blood pressure

Level of Cognitive Ability: Analyzing
Client Needs: Physiological Integrity
Clinical Judgment/Cognitive Skills: Recognize Cues
Integrated Process: Clinical Judgment; Nursing Process/Assessment
Content Area: Adult Health: Neurologic
Health Problems: Adult Health: Neurologic: Myasthenia Gravis
Priority Concepts: Clinical Judgment; Safety

Answer: **2, 4, 5, 6**
Rationale: Myasthenic crisis is caused by undermedication or can be precipitated by an infection or sudden withdrawal of anticholinesterase medications. It may also occur spontaneously. Clinical manifestations include increased diaphoresis, bowel and bladder incontinence, absent cough and swallow reflex, sudden marked rise in blood pressure because of hypoxia, increased heart rate, severe respiratory distress and cyanosis, increased secretions, increased lacrimation, restlessness, and dysarthria.
Test-Taking Strategy: Focus on the **subject**, myasthenia gravis. Specific knowledge regarding the manifestations of myasthenic crisis is needed to answer this question. Recall that myasthenic crisis is caused by undermedication. With this in mind, think about the manifestations of myasthenia gravis to assist in selecting the correct options.
Priority Nursing Tip: Myasthenic crisis is an acute exacerbation of myasthenia gravis; one cause is undermedication. Cholinergic crisis is caused by overmedication with an anticholinesterase. It is imperative that the nurse documents the time of medication administration, as well as the time of any change in client condition.
Reference: Lewis, S., et al. (2020). *Medical-surgical nursing: Assessment and management of clinical problems* (11th ed., pp. 1377–1378). Elsevier.

261. The nurse is encouraging the client to cough and deep breathe after cardiac surgery to avoid developing pneumonia. The nurse ensures that which item is available to maximize the **effectiveness** of this procedure?
1. Nebulizer
2. Ambu bag
3. Suction equipment
4. Incisional splinting pillow

Level of Cognitive Ability: Applying
Client Needs: Physiological Integrity
Clinical Judgment/Cognitive Skills: Generate Solutions
Integrated Process: Nursing Process/Planning
Content Area: Adult Health: Cardiovascular
Health Problems: Adult Health: Respiratory: Pneumonia
Priority Concepts: Gas Exchange; Health Promotion

Answer: 4
Rationale: The use of an incisional splint such as a "cough pillow" can ease discomfort during coughing and deep breathing. The client who is comfortable will do more effective deep breathing and coughing exercises. Use of an incentive spirometer is also indicated. Options 1, 2, and 3 will not encourage the client to cough and deep breathe.
Test-Taking Strategy: Focus on the subject, coughing and deep breathing after cardiac surgery. Note the strategic word, *effectiveness*. The cough pillow is an item that will maximize effectiveness. Eliminate Ambu bag and suction equipment, which are items used by the nurse. A nebulizer is used to deliver medication.
Priority Nursing Tip: If a surgical incision is located in the abdominal or thoracic area, instruct the client to place a folded towel or pillow, or one hand with the other on top, over the incisional area to splint it during coughing and deep breathing.
Reference: Ignatavicius, D., et al. (2021). *Medical-surgical nursing: Concepts for interprofessional collaborative care* (10th ed., p. 166). Elsevier.

❖ **262.** The nurse caring for a client being treated for a bowel obstruction is preparing to administer an intermittent tube feeding through a nasogastric (NG) tube and assesses for residual volume. How do the resulting data assist in ensuring the client's safety?
1. Confirm proper NG tube placement.
2. Determine client's nutritional status.
3. Evaluate the adequacy of gastric emptying.
4. Assess client's fluid and electrolyte status.

Level of Cognitive Ability: Analyzing
Client Needs: Physiological Integrity
Clinical Judgment/Cognitive Skills: Analyze Cues
Integrated Process: Clinical Judgment; Nursing Process/Analysis
Content Area: Skills: Tube Care
Health Problems: Adult Health: Gastrointestinal: Bowel Obstruction
Priority Concepts: Nutrition; Safety

Answer: 3
Rationale: All stomach contents are aspirated and measured before administering a tube feeding to determine the gastric residual volume. If the stomach fails to empty and propel its contents forward, the tube feeding accumulates in the stomach and increases the client's risk of aspiration. If the aspirated gastric contents exceed the predetermined limit, the nurse withholds the tube feeding and collaborates with the physician on a plan of care. Assessing gastric residual volume does not confirm placement or assess fluid and electrolyte status. The nurse uses clinical indicators, including serum albumin levels, to determine the client's nutritional status.
Test-Taking Strategy: Focus on the subject, the purpose for assessing the gastric residual volume. Eliminate options 1 and 4 because assessing gastric residual volume does not confirm proper tube placement or assess fluid and electrolyte status. Other clinical indicators will determine client nutritional status, so eliminate option 2. Note the relationship between the subject and option 3 to direct you to this option.
Priority Nursing Tip: When administering a nasogastric tube feeding, warm the feeding to room temperature to prevent stomach cramps and diarrhea.
Reference: Potter, P., et al. (2021). *Fundamentals of nursing* (10th ed., pp. 1140, 1143). Elsevier.

263. The nurse is caring for a client scheduled to undergo a renal biopsy to confirm suspected malignancy. To minimize the risk of postprocedure complications, the nurse reports which laboratory result to the physician before the procedure?

Laboratory Results

Test and Result	Reference Range
PT 15 seconds (15 seconds)	11–12.5 seconds (11–12.5 seconds)
Potassium 3.8 mEq/L (3.8 mmol/L)	3.5–5.0 mEq/L (3.5–5.0 mmol/L)
Creatinine 1.2 mg/dL (106 mcmol/L)	0.5–1.2 mg/dL (44–106 mcmol/L)
BUN 22 mg/dL (7.92 mmol/L)	10–20 mg/dL (3.6–7.1 mmol/L)

1. Prothrombin time
2. Potassium
3. Creatinine
4. BUN

Level of Cognitive Ability: Applying
Client Needs: Physiological Integrity
Clinical Judgment/Cognitive Skills: Take Action
Integrated Process: Clinical Judgment; Nursing Process/Implementation
Content Area: Foundations of Care: Diagnostic Tests
Health Problems: Adult Health: Cancer: Bladder and Kidney
Priority Concepts: Collaboration; Safety

Answer: 1
Rationale: Postprocedure hemorrhage is a complication after renal biopsy. Because of this, prothrombin time is assessed before the procedure. The client's PT is prolonged, placing the client at risk for bleeding. Although the BUN is slightly elevated, this is unrelated to hemorrhage and could possibly be due to slight dehydration. The remaining test results are within the reference range.
Test-Taking Strategy: Focus on the subject, renal biopsy. When a client is to have a biopsy, remember that bleeding is a concern. This will direct you to the correct option.
Priority Nursing Tip: After renal biopsy, monitor for bleeding. Provide pressure to the site and check the biopsy site and under the client for bleeding.
Reference: Lewis, S., et al. (2020). *Medical-surgical nursing: Assessment and management of clinical problems* (11th ed., pp. 847, 1020). Elsevier.

❖ **264.** A client who survived a house fire is experiencing respiratory distress, and an inhalation injury is suspected. What would the nurse monitor to determine the presence of carbon monoxide poisoning?
1. Pulse oximetry
2. Urine myoglobin
3. Sputum carbon levels
4. Serum carboxyhemoglobin levels

Level of Cognitive Ability: Analyzing
Client Needs: Physiological Integrity
Clinical Judgment/Cognitive Skills: Recognize Cues
Integrated Process: Clinical Judgment; Nursing Process/Assessment
Content Area: Complex Care: Poisoning
Health Problems: Adult Health: Integumentary: Burns
Priority Concepts: Gas Exchange; Perfusion

Answer: 4
Rationale: Serum carboxyhemoglobin levels are the most direct measure of carbon monoxide poisoning, provide the level of poisoning, and thus determine the appropriate treatment measures. The carbon monoxide molecule has a 200 times greater affinity for binding with hemoglobin than an oxygen molecule, causing decreased availability of oxygen to the cells. Clients are treated with 100% oxygen under pressure (hyperbaric oxygen therapy). Options 1, 2, and 3 would not identify carbon monoxide poisoning.
Test-Taking Strategy: Focus on the subject, carbon monoxide poisoning. Note the relationship between "carbon monoxide" and the correct option.
Priority Nursing Tip: The reference range for carboxyhemoglobin in nonsmokers is up to 3% and up to 10% to 15% in smokers.
Reference: Lewis, S., et al. (2020). *Medical-surgical nursing: Assessment and management of clinical problems* (11th ed., pp. 433, 1619). Elsevier.

265. The nurse is assigned to care for a client experiencing hypertonic labor contractions. The nurse plans to conserve the client's energy and promote rest by performing which intervention?

1. Keeping the TV or radio on to provide distraction
2. Assisting client with breathing and relaxation techniques
3. Keeping the room brightly lit so that the client can watch the monitor
4. Avoiding uncomfortable procedures such as intravenous infusions or epidural anesthesia

Level of Cognitive Ability: Applying
Client Needs: Physiological Integrity
Clinical Judgment/Cognitive Skills: Generate Solutions
Integrated Process: Nursing Process/Planning
Content Area: Maternity: Intrapartum
Health Problems: Maternity: Dystocia
Priority Concepts: Health Promotion; Reproduction

Answer: 2
Rationale: Breathing and relaxation techniques aid the client in coping with the discomfort of labor and conserving energy. Noise from a TV or radio and light stimulation do not promote rest. A quiet, dim environment would be more advantageous. Intravenous or epidural pain relief can be useful. Intravenous hydration can increase perfusion and oxygenation of birthing parent and fetal tissues and provide glucose for energy needs.
Test-Taking Strategy: Focus on the subject, hypertonic labor contractions. Review conserving energy and promoting rest for the client. Noting the word "assisting" in option 2 will direct you to the correct option.
Priority Nursing Tip: In hypertonic labor contractions, the uterine resting tone between contractions is high, reducing uterine blood flow and decreasing fetal oxygen supply.
Reference: McKinney, E. S., et al. (2022). *Maternal child nursing* (6th ed., pp. 580–581, 586). Elsevier.

❖ **266.** A client diagnosed with acute pyelonephritis is scheduled for an intravenous pyelogram this morning. During report the nurse learns that the client vomited several times during the night and continues to report being nauseated. What intervention would the nurse implement to ensure the client's safety regarding the scheduled procedure?

1. Cancels the pyelogram
2. Monitors the client closely for any additional vomiting
3. Medicates the client with a standing order for metoclopramide
4. Requests a prescription for a 0.9% saline intravenous infusion

Level of Cognitive Ability: Applying
Client Needs: Physiological Integrity
Clinical Judgment/Cognitive Skills: Take Action
Integrated Process: Clinical Judgment; Nursing Process/Implementation
Content Area: Foundations of Care: Diagnostic Tests
Health Problems: Adult Health: Renal and Urinary: Urinary Tract Inflammation/Infection/Trauma
Priority Concepts: Fluids and Electrolytes; Safety

Answer: 4
Rationale: The highest priority of the nurse would be to request a prescription for an intravenous infusion. This is needed to replace fluid lost with vomiting, will provide an access site for dye injection for the procedure, and will assist with the elimination of the dye after the procedure. The cancellation of the procedure is premature. Neither monitoring nor medicating the client with an antiemetic will address the fluid loss problem.
Test-Taking Strategy: Focus on the subject, the effect of vomiting on an intravenous pyelogram. Using Maslow's Hierarchy of Needs theory will assist in directing you to the correct option.
Priority Nursing Tip: Inform the client who will undergo an intravenous pyelogram (IVP) about the possibility of experiencing throat irritation, flushing of the face, warmth, or a salty or metallic taste during the test.
References: Lewis, S., et al. (2020). *Medical-surgical nursing: Assessment and management of clinical problems* (11th ed., p. 1019). Elsevier; Pagana, K., Pagana, T., & Pagana, T. N. (2021). *Mosby's Diagnostic and laboratory test reference* (15th ed., p. 761). Elsevier.

267. The nurse is planning care for a client who has experienced a T3 spinal cord injury. The nurse would include which intervention in the plan to prevent autonomic dysreflexia (hyperreflexia)?

1. Assist client to develop a daily bowel routine to prevent constipation.
2. Teach client to manage emotional stressors by using mental imaging.
3. Assess vital signs and observe for hypotension, tachycardia, and tachypnea.
4. Administer dexamethasone orally per the physician's prescription.

Level of Cognitive Ability: Applying
Client Needs: Physiological Integrity
Clinical Judgment/Cognitive Skills: Generate Solutions
Integrated Process: Clinical Judgment; Nursing Process/Planning
Content Area: Adult Health: Neurologic
Health Problems: Adult Health: Neurologic: Spinal Cord Injury
Priority Concepts: Caregiving; Intracranial Regulation

Answer: 1
Rationale: Autonomic dysreflexia is a potentially life-threatening condition and may be triggered by bladder distention, bowel distention, visceral distention, or stimulation of pain receptors in the skin. A daily bowel program eliminates this trigger. Options 3 and 4 are unrelated to this specific condition. A client with autonomic hyperreflexia would be severely hypertensive and bradycardic. Removal of the stimuli results in prompt resolution of the signs and symptoms.
Test-Taking Strategy: Focus on the subject, autonomic dysreflexia. Focus on the word "prevent" to eliminate options 2 and 3. From the remaining options, remembering that this condition may be triggered by bowel distention will direct you to the correct option.
Priority Nursing Tip: Autonomic dysreflexia is a neurologic emergency and must be treated immediately to prevent a hypertensive stroke.
Reference: Ignatavicius, D., et al. (2021). *Medical-surgical nursing: Concepts for interprofessional collaborative care* (10th ed., pp. 880, 882). Elsevier.

268. The nurse monitors a client prescribed a thiazide diuretic as part of treatment from hypertension for which clinical manifestations of hypokalemia? **Select all that apply.**

1. Muscle twitches
2. Deep tendon hyporeflexia
3. Prominent U wave on ECG
4. General skeletal muscle weakness
5. Hypoactive to absent bowel sounds
6. Tall T waves on electrocardiogram (ECG)

Level of Cognitive Ability: Applying
Client Needs: Physiological Integrity
Clinical Judgment/Cognitive Skills: Recognize Cues
Integrated Process: Clinical Judgment; Nursing Process/Assessment
Content Area: Pharmacology: Fluids and Electrolyte Balance: Diuretics
Health Problems: Adult Health: Cardiovascular: Hypertension
Priority Concepts: Clinical Judgment; Fluids and Electrolytes

Answer: 2, 3, 4, 5
Rationale: The reference range for potassium is 3.5–5.0 mEq/L (3.5–5.0 mmol/L). Hypokalemia is a serum potassium level less than 3.5 mEq/L (3.5 mmol/L). Clinical manifestations include ECG abnormalities such as ST depression, inverted T wave, prominent U wave, and heart block. Other manifestations include deep tendon hyporeflexia, general skeletal muscle weakness, decreased bowel motility, hypoactive to absent bowel sounds, shallow ineffective respirations and diminished breath sounds, polyuria, decreased ability to concentrate urine, and decreased urine specific gravity. Tall T waves and muscle twitches are manifestations of hyperkalemia.
Test-Taking Strategy: Focus on the subject, the manifestations of hypokalemia. Note that options 3, 4, and 5 are comparable or alike in that they identify a decreased, or hypo-, response; these are manifestations of hypokalemia. Next remember that an inverted T wave and a prominent U wave on ECG are manifestations of hypokalemia.
Priority Nursing Tip: A potassium deficit is potentially life threatening because every body system is affected.
Reference: Lewis, S., et al. (2020). *Medical-surgical nursing: Assessment and management of clinical problems* (11th ed., pp. 280–281). Elsevier.

269. A client diagnosed with left pleural effusion has just been admitted for treatment. The nurse would plan to have which procedure tray available for use at the bedside?

1. Intubation
2. Paracentesis
3. Thoracentesis
4. Central venous line insertion

Level of Cognitive Ability: Applying
Client Needs: Physiological Integrity
Clinical Judgment/Cognitive Skills: Generate Solutions
Integrated Process: Nursing Process/Planning
Content Area: Foundations of Care: Diagnostic Tests
Health Problems: Adult Health: Respiratory: Pleural Effusion
Priority Concepts: Clinical Judgment; Gas Exchange

Answer: 3
Rationale: The client with a significant pleural effusion is usually treated by thoracentesis. This procedure allows drainage of the fluid from the pleural space, which may then be analyzed to determine the precise cause of the effusion. The nurse ensures that a thoracentesis tray is readily available in case the client's symptoms should rapidly become more severe. A paracentesis tray is needed for the removal of abdominal effusion. Options 1 and 4 are not specifically indicated for this procedure.
Test-Taking Strategy: Focus on the subject, pleural effusion and thoracentesis. Recall knowledge regarding the usual treatment for pleural effusion. Note the relationship between the words "pleural" in the question and "thoracentesis" in the correct option.
Priority Nursing Tip: Instruct the client undergoing thoracentesis not to cough, breathe deeply, or move during the procedure.
Reference: Lewis, S., et al. (2020). *Medical-surgical nursing: Assessment and management of clinical problems* (11th ed., pp. 473, 530–531). Elsevier.

❖ 270. A client has been prescribed procainamide. The nurse implements which intervention before administering the medication to minimize the client's risk for injury?

1. Obtaining a chest x-ray
2. Assessing blood pressure and pulse
3. Obtaining a complete blood cell count and liver function studies
4. Scheduling a drug level to be drawn 1 hour after the dose is administered

Level of Cognitive Ability: Applying
Client Needs: Physiological Integrity
Clinical Judgment/Cognitive Skills: Take Action
Integrated Process: Clinical Judgment; Nursing Process/Implementation
Content Area: Pharmacology: Cardiovascular: Antidysrhythmics
Health Problems: Adult Health: Cardiovascular: Dysrhythmias
Priority Concepts: Clinical Judgment; Safety

Answer: 2
Rationale: Procainamide is an antidysrhythmic medication. Before the medication is administered, the client's blood pressure and pulse are checked. This medication can cause toxic effects, and serum blood levels would be checked before administering the medication (therapeutic serum reference range is 4 to 8 mcg/mL [17.00 to 34 mcmol/L]). A chest x-ray, a complete blood cell count, and liver function studies are unnecessary. The medication is administered via an infusion controller device.
Test-Taking Strategy: Focus on the subject, the medication procainamide. Use the steps of the nursing process. This will direct you to option 2 because it is the only assessment action. Also recalling that this medication is an antidysrhythmic will direct you to the correct option.
Priority Nursing Tip: Antidysrhythmic medications suppress dysrhythmias by inhibiting abnormal pathways of electrical conduction through the heart.
Reference: Lilley, L., Rainforth Collins, S., & Snyder, J. (2020). *Pharmacology and the nursing process* (9th ed., pp. 391, 396). Elsevier.

271. A client diagnosed with urolithiasis is being evaluated to determine the type of calculi that are present. The nurse would plan to keep which item available in the client's room to assist in this process?

1. A urine strainer
2. A calorie count sheet
3. A vital signs graphic sheet
4. An intake and output record

Level of Cognitive Ability: Applying
Client Needs: Physiological Integrity
Clinical Judgment/Cognitive Skills: Generate Solutions
Integrated Process: Nursing Process/Planning
Content Area: Adult Health: Renal and Urinary
Health Problems: Adult Health: Renal and Urinary: Calculi
Priority Concepts: Caregiving; Elimination

Answer: 1
Rationale: The urine is strained until the stone is passed, obtained, and analyzed. Straining the urine will catch small stones that should be sent to the laboratory for analysis. Once the type of stone is determined, an individualized plan of care for prevention and treatment is developed. Options 2, 3, and 4 are unrelated to determining the type of existing calculi.
Test-Taking Strategy: Focus on the subject, urolithiasis. You will need an item that will help determine the type of stone. Eliminate options 2, 3, and 4 because these items give information about food intake, vital signs, and fluid balance, but they will not provide data that will help determine the type of stone.
Priority Nursing Tip: Urolithiasis refers to the formation of urinary calculi and these calculi form in the ureters.
Reference: Lewis, S., et al. (2020). *Medical-surgical nursing: Assessment and management of clinical problems* (11th ed., p. 1040). Elsevier.

❖ **272.** The nurse provides dietary instructions to a client with heart failure who needs to limit intake of sodium. The nurse instructs the client that which food items must be avoided because of their high sodium content? **Select all that apply.**
- ❑ 1. Ham
- ❑ 2. Apples
- ❑ 3. Broccoli
- ❑ 4. Soy sauce
- ❑ 5. Asparagus
- ❑ 6. Cantaloupe

Level of Cognitive Ability: Applying
Client Needs: Physiological Integrity
Clinical Judgment/Cognitive Skills: Generate Solutions
Integrated Process: Teaching and Learning
Content Area: Foundations of Care: Therapeutic Diets
Health Problems: Adult Health: Cardiovascular: Heart Failure
Priority Concepts: Patient Education; Nutrition

Answer: 1, 4
Rationale: Foods highest in sodium include table salt, some cheeses, soy sauce, cured pork, canned foods because of the preservatives, and foods such as cold cuts. Fruits and vegetables contain minimal amounts of sodium.
Test-Taking Strategy: Focus on the subject, foods high in sodium. Eliminate options 2, 3, 5, and 6 because they are comparable or alike in that they are fruits and vegetables and are low in sodium.
Priority Nursing Tip: Sodium causes the retention of fluid, and the physician may prescribe limited sodium intake for clients with hypertension, heart disease, respiratory disease, and certain gastrointestinal and neurologic disorders.
References: Ignatavicius, D., et al. (2021). *Medical-surgical nursing: Concepts for interprofessional collaborative care* (10th ed., pp. 674, 681). Elsevier; Nix, S. (2022). *Williams' Basic nutrition and diet therapy* (16th ed., pp. 124, 353). Elsevier.

273. The nurse is preparing to care for a client post ureterolithotomy who has a ureteral catheter in place. The nurse would plan to implement which action in the management of this catheter when the client arrives from the recovery room?
1. Clamp the catheter.
2. Place tension on the catheter.
3. Check the drainage from the catheter.
4. Irrigate the catheter using 10 mL sterile normal saline.

Level of Cognitive Ability: Applying
Client Needs: Physiological Integrity
Clinical Judgment/Cognitive Skills: Generate Solutions
Integrated Process: Nursing Process/Planning
Content Area: Skills: Elimination
Health Problems: Adult Health: Renal and Urinary: Calculi
Priority Concepts: Caregiving; Elimination

Answer: 3
Rationale: Drainage from the ureteral catheter needs to be checked when the client returns from the recovery room and at least every 1 to 2 hours thereafter. The catheter drains urine from the renal pelvis, which has a capacity of 3 to 5 mL. If the volume of urine or fluid in the renal pelvis increases, tissue damage to the pelvis will result from pressure. Therefore, the ureteral tube is never clamped. Additionally, irrigation is not performed unless there is a specific physician's prescription to do so.
Test-Taking Strategy: Focus on the subject, a ureteral catheter, and think about the anatomy of the kidney. Recalling both that the ureteral catheter is placed in the renal pelvis and the anatomy of this anatomic location will assist in eliminating options 1, 2, and 4.
Priority Nursing Tip: If the client has a ureteral catheter, monitor urine output closely. If the urine output is less than 30 mL/hr or there is a lack of urine output for more than 15 minutes, the physician needs to be notified immediately.
References: Lewis, S., et al. (2020). *Medical-surgical nursing: Assessment and management of clinical problems* (11th ed., p. 1052). Elsevier; Potter, P., et al. (2021). *Fundamentals of nursing* (10th ed., pp. 1169–1170). Elsevier.

❖ **274.** In preparation to administer an intermittent tube feeding, the nurse aspirates 40 mL of undigested formula from the client's nasogastric tube. Which intervention would the nurse implement as a result of this finding?
1. Discard the aspirate and record as client output.
2. Mix with new formula to administer the feeding.
3. Dilute with water and inject into the nasogastric tube.
4. Reinstill the aspirate through the nasogastric tube via gravity and syringe.

Level of Cognitive Ability: Applying
Client Needs: Physiological Integrity
Clinical Judgment/Cognitive Skills: Take Action
Integrated Process: Nursing Process/Implementation
Content Area: Skills: Tube Care
Health Problems: N/A
Priority Concepts: Clinical Judgment; Fluids and Electrolytes

Answer: 4
Rationale: After checking residual feeding contents, the nurse reinstills the gastric contents into the stomach by removing the syringe bulb or plunger and pouring the gastric contents via the syringe into the nasogastric tube. Gastric contents should be reinstilled (unless they exceed an amount of 100 mL or as defined by agency policy) to maintain the client's fluid and electrolyte balance. The nurse avoids mixing gastric aspirate with fresh formula to prevent contamination. Because the gastric aspirate is a small volume, it should be reinstilled; however, mixing the formula with water can also disrupt the client's fluid and electrolyte balance unless the client is dehydrated.
Test-Taking Strategy: Focus on the **subject,** residual tube feeding. Eliminate option 1 because it increases the risk of dehydration and disrupts the client's fluid and electrolyte balance. Also, recalling that aspirated gastric contents are not mixed with formula will assist in directing you to the correct option.
Priority Nursing Tip: If the client is receiving nasogastric tube feedings, check the gastric residual volume before each feeding if the client is receiving intermittent feedings, and every 4 to 6 hours if the client is receiving continuous feedings.
Reference: Potter, P., et al. (2021). *Fundamentals of nursing* (10th ed., pp. 1140–1142). Elsevier.

275. To ensure the desired results, how would the nurse instruct the client who is prescribed oral bisacodyl to take the medication?
1. At bedtime
2. With a large meal
3. With a glass of milk
4. On an empty stomach

Level of Cognitive Ability: Applying
Client Needs: Physiological Integrity
Clinical Judgment/Cognitive Skills: Take Action
Integrated Process: Nursing Process/Implementation
Content Area: Pharmacology: Gastrointestinal: Laxatives
Health Problems: N/A
Priority Concepts: Clinical Judgment; Elimination

Answer: 4
Rationale: Bisacodyl is a laxative. The most rapid effect from bisacodyl occurs when it is taken on an empty stomach. If it is taken at bedtime, the client will have a bowel movement in the morning. It will not have a rapid effect if taken with a large meal. Taking the medication with a glass of milk will not speed up its effect.
Test-Taking Strategy: Focus on the **subject,** bisacodyl. Recalling that medications generally are more effective if taken on an empty stomach will direct you to the correct option.
Priority Nursing Tip: The client taking a laxative needs to increase fluid intake to prevent dehydration.
Reference: Burchum, J., & Rosenthal, L. (2022). *Lehne's Pharmacology for nursing care* (11th ed., p. 968). Elsevier.

❖ **276.** A client diagnosed with acute respiratory distress syndrome has a prescription to be placed on a continuous positive airway pressure (CPAP) face mask. What intervention would the nurse implement for this procedure to be beneficial?
1. Obtain baseline arterial blood gases.
2. Obtain baseline pulse oximetry levels.
3. Apply the mask to the face with a snug fit.
4. Remove the mask for deep-breathing exercises.

Level of Cognitive Ability: Applying
Client Needs: Physiological Integrity
Clinical Judgment/Cognitive Skills: Take Action
Integrated Process: Clinical Judgment; Nursing Process/Implementation
Content Area: Complex Care: Acute Respiratory Failure
Health Problems: Adult Health: Respiratory: Acute Respiratory Distress Syndrome/Failure
Priority Concepts: Caregiving; Gas Exchange

Answer: 3
Rationale: The CPAP face mask must be applied over the nose and mouth with a snug fit, which is necessary to maintain positive pressure in the client's airways. The nurse obtains baseline respiratory assessments and arterial blood gases to evaluate the effectiveness of therapy, but these are not done to increase the effectiveness of the procedure. A disadvantage of the CPAP face mask is that the client must remove it for coughing, eating, or drinking. This removes the benefit of positive pressure in the airway each time it is removed.
Test-Taking Strategy: Focus on the subject, continuous positive airway pressure (CPAP). Options 1 and 2 do not make the therapy more beneficial and are eliminated. From the remaining options, knowing that positive pressure must be maintained to be effective will direct you to the correct option.
Priority Nursing Tip: In acute respiratory distress syndrome, the major site of injury is the alveolar capillary membrane.
Reference: Potter, P., et al. (2021). *Fundamentals of nursing* (10th ed., pp. 938–939). Elsevier.

277. The nurse is caring for a client scheduled to undergo a cardiac catheterization for the first time. Which information would the nurse share with the client regarding the procedure?
1. "The procedure is performed in the operating room."
2. "The initial catheter insertion is quite painful; after that, there is little or no pain."
3. "You may feel fatigue and have various aches because it is necessary to lie quietly on a stationary x-ray table for about 4 hours."
4. "You may feel certain sensations at various points during the procedure, such as a fluttery feeling, flushed warm feeling, desire to cough, or palpitations."

Level of Cognitive Ability: Applying
Client Needs: Physiological Integrity
Clinical Judgment/Cognitive Skills: Take Action
Integrated Process: Nursing Process/Implementation
Content Area: Foundations of Care: Diagnostic Tests
Health Problems: Adult Health: Cardiovascular: Coronary Artery Disease
Priority Concepts: Patient Education; Perfusion

Answer: 4
Rationale: Cardiac catheterization is an invasive test that involves the insertion of a catheter and the injection of dye into the heart and surrounding vessels to obtain information about the structure and function of the heart chambers and valves and the coronary circulation. Access is made by the insertion of a needle in either side of the groin into an artery or vein and the catheter is advanced up to the heart through the abdomen and chest. Preprocedure teaching points include that the procedure is done in a darkened cardiac catheterization room and that ECG leads are attached to the client. A local anesthetic is used so that there is little to no pain with catheter insertion. The x-ray table is hard but can be tilted periodically. The procedure may take up to 2 hours, and the client may feel various sensations with catheter passage and dye injection.
Test-Taking Strategy: Focus on the subject, cardiac catheterization. The location (operating room) eliminates option 1. The duration of the procedure, 4 hours, eliminates option 3. From the remaining options, noting the words "quite painful" in option 2 will assist in eliminating this option.
Priority Nursing Tip: Monitor the postcardiac catheterization client closely. Notify the physician immediately if the client complains of numbness or tingling of the affected extremity; the extremity becomes cool, pale, or cyanotic; or loss of peripheral pulses occurs.
Reference: Ignatavicius, D., et al. (2021). *Medical-surgical nursing: Concepts for interprofessional collaborative care* (10th ed., pp. 628–630). Elsevier.

❖ **278.** The nurse hangs an intravenous (IV) bag of 1000 mL of 5% dextrose in water (D_5W) at 1500 and sets the flow rate to infuse at 75 mL/hr. At 2300, the nurse would expect the fluid remaining in the IV bag to be at approximately which level? **Fill in the blank.**

Answer: _____ mL
Level of Cognitive Ability: Evaluating
Client Needs: Physiological Integrity
Clinical Judgment/Cognitive Skills: Evaluate Outcomes
Integrated Process: Nursing Process/Evaluation
Content Area: Skills: Dosage Calculations
Health Problems: N/A
Priority Concepts: Clinical Judgment; Safety

Answer: 400
Rationale: In an 8-hour period, 600 mL would infuse if an IV is set to infuse at 75 mL/hr. Therefore, 400 mL would remain in the IV bag.
Test-Taking Strategy: Focus on the **subject**, IV calculations. Review the data in the question and use simple math to determine that in an 8-hour period (1500 to 2300), 600 mL would infuse (8 hours × 75 mL/hr = 600 mL). This means that 400 mL would remain. Perform the calculation and then verify your answer using a calculator.
Priority Nursing Tip: If a solution of 5% dextrose in water (D_5W) is prescribed for a client with diabetes mellitus, confirm the prescription because the solution can increase the client's blood glucose level.
Reference: Potter, P., et al. (2021). *Fundamentals of nursing* (10th ed., pp. 1022–1023). Elsevier.

279. The nurse admitting a client diagnosed with myocardial infarction (MI) to the coronary care unit (CCU) would plan care by implementing which intervention?
1. Beginning thrombolytic therapy
2. Placing client on continuous cardiac monitoring
3. Infusing intravenous (IV) fluid at a rate of 150 mL per hour
4. Administering oxygen at a rate of 6 L per minute by nasal cannula

Level of Cognitive Ability: Applying
Client Needs: Physiological Integrity
Clinical Judgment/Cognitive Skills: Generate Solutions
Integrated Process: Clinical Judgment; Nursing Process/Planning
Content Area: Complex Care: Emergency Situations/Management
Health Problems: Adult Health: Cardiovascular: Myocardial Infarction
Priority Concepts: Perfusion; Safety

Answer: 2
Rationale: Standard interventions upon admittance to the CCU as they relate to this question include continuous cardiac monitoring. Thrombolytic therapy may or may not be prescribed by the physician. Thrombolytic agents are most effective if administered within the first 6 hours of the coronary event. The nurse needs to ensure that there is an adequate IV line insertion of an intermittent lock. If an IV infusion is administered, it is maintained at a keep-vein-open rate to prevent fluid overload and heart failure. Oxygen should be administered at a rate of 2 to 4 L/min unless otherwise prescribed.
Test-Taking Strategy: Focus on the **subject**, myocardial infarction care. Eliminate options 3 and 4 because the values related to the rates of IV fluid and oxygen are high. From the remaining options, note the relationship between the client's diagnosis and option 2.
Priority Nursing Tip: Not all clients experience the classic symptoms of myocardial infarction. Some individuals may experience atypical discomfort, shortness of breath, or fatigue, and often present with NSTEMI (non-ST elevation myocardial infarction) or T-wave inversion.
Reference: Lewis, S., et al. (2020). *Medical-surgical nursing: Assessment and management of clinical problems* (11th ed., p. 723). Elsevier.

❖ **280.** The nurse is analyzing an electrocardiogram (ECG) rhythm strip on an assigned client with a suspected myocardial infarction (**refer to figure**). What would the nurse record as the client's PR interval?

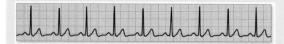

1. 0.12 second
2. 0.20 second
3. 0.24 second
4. 0.40 second

Level of Cognitive Ability: Applying
Client Needs: Physiological Integrity
Clinical Judgment/Cognitive Skills: Take Action
Integrated Process: Clinical Judgment; Nursing Process/Implementation
Content Area: Adult Health: Cardiovascular
Health Problems: Adult Health: Cardiovascular: Myocardial Infarction
Priority Concepts: Clinical Judgment; Perfusion

Answer: 1
Rationale: Standard ECG graph paper measurements are 0.04 seconds for each small box on the horizontal axis (measuring time) and 1 mm (measuring voltage) for each small box on the vertical axis. The PR interval is the period of time from the onset of the P wave to the beginning of the QRS complex. It normally ranges from 0.12 to 0.20 seconds in duration.
Test-Taking Strategy: Focus on the subject, electrocardiogram (ECG). Knowledge regarding ECG basics is necessary to answer this question. Knowing that each small box is equal to 0.04 seconds and that there are three small boxes will direct you to the correct option.
Priority Nursing Tip: Inform the client that an electrical shock will not occur when performing an electrocardiogram test.
Reference: Ignatavicius, D., et al. (2021). *Medical-surgical nursing: Concepts for interprofessional collaborative care* (10th ed., p. 641). Elsevier.

281. The nurse is applying electrocardiogram (ECG) electrodes to a diaphoretic client experiencing tachycardia. Which intervention would the nurse take to facilitate adherence of the electrodes to the skin?
1. Secure the electrodes with adhesive tape.
2. Place clear, transparent dressings over the electrodes.
3. Apply lanolin to the skin before applying the electrodes.
4. Cleanse the skin with alcohol before applying the electrodes.

Level of Cognitive Ability: Applying
Client Needs: Physiological Integrity
Clinical Judgment/Cognitive Skills: Take Action
Integrated Process: Nursing Process/Implementation
Content Area: Adult Health: Cardiovascular
Health Problems: Adult Health: Cardiovascular: Dysrhythmias
Priority Concepts: Clinical Judgment; Perfusion

Answer: 4
Rationale: Alcohol defats the skin and helps the electrodes adhere to the skin. Placing adhesive tape or a clear dressing over the electrodes will not help the adhesive gel of the actual electrode make better contact with the diaphoretic skin. Lanolin or any other lotion makes the skin slippery and prevents good initial adherence.
Test-Taking Strategy: Focus on the subject, electrocardiogram (ECG). Note that options 1 and 2 are comparable or alike in that they both provide an external form of providing security of the electrodes. From the remaining options, note that option 4 addresses cleansing the skin.
Priority Nursing Tip: To obtain an accurate reading when performing an electrocardiogram, instruct the client to lie still, breathe normally, and refrain from talking during the test.
Reference: Pagana, K., Pagana, T., & Pagana, T. N. (2021). *Mosby's Diagnostic and laboratory test reference* (15th ed., p. 352). Elsevier.

❖ **282.** The nurse has created a plan of care for a client with a diagnosis of anterior cord syndrome. Which intervention would the nurse include in the plan of care to minimize the client's long-term risk for injury?
1. Change the client's positions slowly.
2. Assess the client for decreased sensation to touch.
3. Assess the client for decreased sensation to vibration.
4. Teach the client about loss of motor function and decreased pain sensation.

Level of Cognitive Ability: Creating
Client Needs: Physiological Integrity
Clinical Judgment/Cognitive Skills: Generate Solutions
Integrated Process: Clinical Judgment; Nursing Process/Planning
Content Area: Adult Health: Neurologic
Health Problems: Adult Health: Neurologic: Spinal Cord Injury
Priority Concepts: Mobility; Intracranial Regulation

Answer: 4
Rationale: Anterior cord syndrome is caused by damage to the anterior portion of the gray and white matter associated with the spinal cord. Clinical findings related to anterior cord syndrome include loss of motor function, temperature sensation, and pain sensation below the level of injury. The syndrome does not affect sensations of fine touch, position, and vibration.
Test-Taking Strategy: Focus on the subject, anterior cord syndrome. Specific knowledge of anterior cord syndrome is necessary to answer this question. Eliminate option 1 first, knowing that position is not affected below the level of injury. Eliminate options 2 and 3, knowing that in anterior cord syndrome, sensations of touch and vibration remain intact. Remember that this type of injury involves complete motor function loss and decreased temperature and pain sensation, directing you to the correct option.
Priority Nursing Tip: The level of the spinal cord injury is determined by assessing for the lowest spinal cord segment with intact motor and sensory function.
Reference: Lewis, S., et al. (2020). *Medical-surgical nursing: Assessment and management of clinical problems* (11th ed., p. 1406). Elsevier.

283. The nurse is caring for a client who has experienced a thoracic spinal cord injury. In the event that spinal shock occurs, which intravenous (IV) fluid would the nurse anticipate being prescribed?
1. Dextran
2. 0.9% Normal saline
3. 5% Dextrose in water
4. 5% Dextrose in 0.9% normal saline

Level of Cognitive Ability: Understanding
Client Needs: Physiological Integrity
Clinical Judgment/Cognitive Skills: Generate Solutions
Integrated Process: Nursing Process/Planning
Content Area: Complex Care: Shock
Health Problems: Adult Health: Neurologic: Spinal Cord Injury
Priority Concepts: Intracranial Regulation; Perfusion

Answer: 2
Rationale: Normal saline 0.9% is an isotonic solution that primarily remains in the intravascular space, increasing intravascular volume. This IV fluid would increase the client's blood pressure. Dextran is rarely used in spinal shock because isotonic fluid administration is usually sufficient. Additionally, Dextran has potential adverse effects. Dextrose 5% in water is a hypotonic solution that pulls fluid out of the intravascular space and is not indicated for shock. Dextrose 5% in normal saline 0.9% is hypertonic and may be indicated for shock resulting from hemorrhage or burns.
Test-Taking Strategy: Focus on the subject, spinal shock. Thinking about the manifestations of shock and using knowledge of the treatment for spinal shock and the purpose of the various IV fluids will direct you to the correct option. Also, remember that normal saline 0.9% is an isotonic solution that primarily remains in the intravascular space, increasing intravascular volume.
Priority Nursing Tip: Spinal shock occurs within the first hour of spinal cord injury and can last days to months.
Reference: Ignatavicius, D., et al. (2021). *Medical-surgical nursing: Concepts for interprofessional collaborative care* (10th ed., p. 881). Elsevier.

Client Needs

❖ **284.** The nurse is caring for a client experiencing severe macular degeneration who will be taught to ambulate with a cane. Before cane-assisted ambulation instructions begin, what would the nurse check for as the **priority** to ensure client safety?
1. A high level of stamina and energy
2. Self-consciousness about using a cane
3. Full range of motion in lower extremities
4. Balance, muscle strength, and confidence

Level of Cognitive Ability: Applying
Client Needs: Physiological Integrity
Clinical Judgment/Cognitive Skills: Prioritize Hypotheses
Integrated Process: Clinical Judgment; Nursing Process/Planning
Content Area: Skills: Activity/Mobility
Health Problems: Adult Health: Eye: Macular Degeneration
Priority Concepts: Functional Ability; Mobility

Answer: 4
Rationale: Assessing the client's balance, strength, and confidence helps determine if the cane is a suitable assistive device for the client. A high level of stamina and full range of motion are not needed for walking with a cane. Although body image (self-consciousness) is a component of the assessment, it is not the priority.
Test-Taking Strategy: Note the strategic word, *priority,* and focus on the subject, cane-assisting ambulation. Eliminate options 1 and 2 first because they are not required for the use of a cane. Use Maslow's Hierarchy of Needs theory to assist in directing you to the correct option.
Priority Nursing Tip: Safety is a priority concern when the client uses an assistive device such as a cane.
Reference: Potter, P., et al. (2021). *Fundamentals of nursing* (10th ed., pp. 797–798). Elsevier.

285. A physician prescribes 1000 mL of normal saline to infuse at 100 mL/hr for a client experiencing clinical dehydration. The drop factor is 10 drops/mL. The nurse would set the flow rate at how many drops per minute? **Fill in the blank and round your answer to the nearest whole number.**

Answer: _____ drops per minute
Level of Cognitive Ability: Applying
Client Needs: Physiological Integrity
Clinical Judgment/Cognitive Skills: Generate Solutions
Integrated Process: Nursing Process/Planning
Content Area: Skills: Dosage Calculations
Health Problems: Adult Health: Gastrointestinal: Dehydration
Priority Concepts: Clinical Judgment; Safety

Answer: 17
Rationale: It will take 10 hours for 1000 mL to infuse at 100 mL/hr (1000 mL ÷ 100 mL = 10 hour × 60 min = 600 min). Next, use the intravenous (IV) flow rate formula.

$$\frac{\text{Total volume} \times \text{Drop factor}}{\text{Time in minutes}} = \text{drops/minutes}$$

$$\frac{1000\ \text{mL} \times 10\ \text{drops / mL}}{600\ \text{min}} = \frac{10,000}{600} = 16.6, \text{or } 17\ \text{drops/minute}$$

Test-Taking Strategy: Focus on the subject, IV calculations. First, determine how many hours that it will take for 1000 mL to infuse at 100 mL/hr. Next use the formula for calculating IV flow rates and verify the answer using a calculator. Remember to round the answer to the nearest whole number.
Priority Nursing Tip: The nurse would never increase the rate of an IV solution to catch up if the infusion is running behind schedule.
Reference: Potter, P., et al. (2021). *Fundamentals of nursing* (10th ed., pp. 1022–1023). Elsevier.

❖ **286.** The nurse is assessing a client diagnosed with cardiac disease at the 30 weeks of gestation antenatal visit. The nurse assesses lung sounds in the lower lobes after a routine blood pressure screening. The nurse performs this assessment to elicit what information?
  1. Identify mitral valve prolapse.
  2. Identify cardiac dysrhythmias.
  3. Rule out the possibility of pneumonia.
  4. Assess for early signs of heart failure (HF).

Level of Cognitive Ability: Analyzing
Client Needs: Physiological Integrity
Clinical Judgment/Cognitive Skills: Analyze Cues
Integrated Process: Clinical Judgment; Nursing Process/Analysis
Content Area: Maternity: Antepartum
Health Problems: Maternity: Cardiac Disease
Priority Concepts: Perfusion; Reproduction

Answer: 4
Rationale: Fluid volume during pregnancy peaks between 18 and 32 weeks of gestation. During this period, it is essential to observe and record client data that would indicate further signs of cardiac decompensation or HF in the pregnant client with cardiac disease. By assessing lung sounds, the nurse may identify early symptoms of diminished oxygen exchange and potential HF. Options 1, 2, and 3 are not related to the data in the question.
Test-Taking Strategy: Focus on the subject, a pregnant client with cardiac disease. Note the relationship between cardiac disease and lung sounds in the question and the words "heart failure" in the correct option.
Priority Nursing Tip: Monitor the client with cardiac disease for manifestations of cardiac stress and decompensation, such as cough, fatigue, dyspnea, chest pain, and tachycardia.
Reference: Lowdermilk, D., et al. (2020). *Maternity & women's health care* (12th ed.). Elsevier. pp. 640–641, 643.

287. A digoxin level is ordered for a client prescribed digoxin to help manage heart failure. Based on the result, which manifestations would the nurse expect to note in the client? **Select all that apply.**

Laboratory Results

Test and Result	Reference Range
Digoxin 2.3 ng/dL (2.93 nmol/L)	0.5–2.0 ng/mL (0.63–2.56 nmol/L)

  ❑ 1. Nausea
  ❑ 2. Drowsiness
  ❑ 3. Photophobia
  ❑ 4. Increased appetite
  ❑ 5. Increased energy level
  ❑ 6. Seeing halos around bright objects

Level of Cognitive Ability: Analyzing
Client Needs: Physiological Integrity
Clinical Judgment/Cognitive Skills: Analyze Cues
Integrated Process: Clinical Judgment; Nursing Process/Analysis
Content Area: Pharmacology: Cardiovascular: Antidysrhythmics
Health Problems: Adult Health: Cardiovascular: Heart Failure
Priority Concepts: Clinical Judgment; Safety

Answer: 1, 2, 3, 6
Rationale: Digoxin is a cardiac glycoside used to manage and treat heart failure, control ventricular rate in clients with atrial fibrillation, and treat and prevent recurrent paroxysmal atrial tachycardia. Signs of toxicity include gastrointestinal disturbances, including anorexia, nausea, and vomiting; neurologic abnormalities such as fatigue, headache, depression, weakness, drowsiness, confusion, and nightmares; facial pain; personality changes; and ocular disturbances such as photophobia, halos around bright lights, and yellow or green color perception.
Test-Taking Strategy: Focus on the subject, a digoxin level of 2.3 ng/dL (2.93 nmol/L). Recalling that signs of digoxin toxicity include gastrointestinal disturbances, neurologic abnormalities, and ocular disturbances will assist in answering the question correctly.
Priority Nursing Tip: The nurse needs to check the client's apical pulse rate for 1 full minute before administering digoxin. If it is lower than 60 beats/min, the medication is withheld and the physician is notified. A toxic blood level may be lowered with repeated doses of charcoal given orally or via nasogastric (NG) tube.
Reference: Ignatavicius, D., et al. (2021). *Medical-surgical nursing: Concepts for interprofessional collaborative care* (10th ed., pp. 651, 675). Elsevier.

❖ **288.** Which interventions would the emergency department nurse prepare for in the care of a child diagnosed with croup and epiglottitis? **Select all that apply.**
- ❑ 1. Obtaining a chest x-ray
- ❑ 2. Obtaining a throat culture
- ❑ 3. Monitoring pulse oximetry
- ❑ 4. Maintaining a patent airway
- ❑ 5. Providing humidified oxygen
- ❑ 6. Administering antipyretics and antibiotics

Level of Cognitive Ability: Analyzing
Client Needs: Physiological Integrity
Clinical Judgment/Cognitive Skills: Generate Solutions
Integrated Process: Clinical Judgment; Nursing Process/Planning
Content Area: Complex Care: Emergency Situations/Management
Health Problems: Pediatric-Specific: Epiglottitis
Priority Concepts: Clinical Judgment; Inflammation

Answer: 1, 3, 4, 5, 6
Rationale: Epiglottitis is an acute inflammation and swelling of the epiglottis and surrounding tissue. It is a life-threatening, rapidly progressive condition that may cause complete airway obstruction within a few hours of onset. The most reliable diagnostic sign is an edematous, cherry-red epiglottis. Some interventions include obtaining a chest x-ray film, monitoring pulse oximetry, maintaining a patent airway, providing humidified oxygen, and administering antipyretics and antibiotics. The child may also require intubation and mechanical ventilation. The primary concern in a child with epiglottitis is the development of complete airway obstruction. Therefore, the child's throat is not examined or cultured because any stimulation with a tongue depressor or culture swab could trigger complete airway obstruction.
Test-Taking Strategy: Focus on the subject, epiglottitis. Focus on ABCs—airway, breathing, and circulation. Remember that the primary concern is the development of complete airway obstruction and that any stimulation with a tongue depressor or culture swab could trigger complete airway obstruction. This will assist in eliminating the only incorrect option, option 2.
Priority Nursing Tip: Epiglottitis is considered an emergency situation because it can progress rapidly to severe respiratory distress.
Reference: McKinney, E. S., et al. (2022). *Maternal child nursing* (6th ed., pp. 1037, 1052–1053). Elsevier.

289. A child diagnosed with rheumatic fever is admitted to the hospital. The nurse prepares to manage which clinical manifestations of this disorder? **Select all that apply.**
- ❑ 1. Cardiac murmur
- ❑ 2. Cardiac enlargement
- ❑ 3. Cool, pale skin over the joints
- ❑ 4. White, painful skin lesions on the trunk
- ❑ 5. Small, nontender lumps on bony prominences
- ❑ 6. Purposeless, jerky movements of the extremities and face

Level of Cognitive Ability: Analyzing
Client Needs: Physiological Integrity
Clinical Judgment/Cognitive Skills: Recognize Cues
Integrated Process: Clinical Judgment; Nursing Process/Assessment
Content Area: Pediatrics: Cardiovascular
Health Problems: Pediatric-Specific: Rheumatic Fever
Priority Concepts: Clinical Judgment; Inflammation

Answer: 1, 2, 5, 6
Rationale: Rheumatic fever is a systemic inflammatory disease that may develop as a delayed reaction to an inadequately treated infection of the upper respiratory tract by group A beta-hemolytic streptococci. Clinical manifestations of rheumatic fever are related to the inflammatory response. Major manifestations include carditis manifested as inflammation of the endocardium, including the valves, myocardium, and pericardium; cardiac murmur and cardiac enlargement; subcutaneous nodules, manifested as small nontender lumps on joints and bony prominences; chorea, manifested as involuntary, purposeless jerky movements of the legs, arms, and face with speech impairment; arthritis manifested as tender, warm erythematous skin over the joints; and erythema marginatum, manifested as red, painless skin lesions usually over the trunk.
Test-Taking Strategy: Focus on the subject, rheumatic fever. Recalling that rheumatic fever is a systemic inflammatory disease and noting the words "cool" in option 3 and "white" in option 4 will assist in answering this question. Remember that the client will exhibit tender, warm, erythematous skin over the joints and red, painless skin lesions usually over the trunk.
Priority Nursing Tip: Initiate seizure precautions if the child with rheumatic fever exhibits manifestations of chorea (involuntary, purposeless jerky movements of the legs, arms, and face with speech impairment).
Reference: McKinney, E. S., et al. (2022). *Maternal child nursing* (6th ed., pp. 1116–1117). Elsevier.

❖ **290.** A client hospitalized with a diagnosis of thrombophlebitis is being treated with heparin infusion therapy. About 24 hours after the infusion has begun, a partial thromboplastin time (PTT) is drawn and the nurse reviews the result. Based on the result, what action would the nurse take?

Laboratory Results

Test and Result	Reference Range
aPTT 65 seconds, control 30 seconds	30–40 seconds

1. Discontinue the heparin infusion.
2. Prepare to administer protamine sulfate.
3. Notify the physician of the laboratory results.
4. Include in report that client is adequately anticoagulated.

Level of Cognitive Ability: Applying
Client Needs: Physiological Integrity
Clinical Judgment/Cognitive Skills: Take Action
Integrated Process: Nursing Process/Implementation
Content Area: Pharmacology: Cardiovascular: Anticoagulants
Health Problems: Adult Health: Cardiovascular: Deep Vein Thrombosis
Priority Concepts: Clotting; Safety

Answer: 4
Rationale: The effectiveness of heparin therapy is monitored by the results of the PTT. Desired range for therapeutic anticoagulation is 1.5 to 2.5 times the control. A PTT of 65 seconds is within the therapeutic range. Therefore, options 1, 2, and 3 are incorrect actions.
Test-Taking Strategy: Focus on the subject, heparin infusion therapy. Remember that the desired range for therapeutic anticoagulation is 1.5 to 2.5 times the control. Noting that the control is 30 and that 1.5 to 2.5 times the control is a range of 45 to 75 will direct you to the correct option.
Priority Nursing Tip: Heparin is an anticoagulant and the priority concern when a client is receiving an anticoagulant is bleeding.
Reference: Gahart, B., Nazareno, A., & Ortega, M. (2021). *Gahart's 2021 Intravenous medications: A handbook for nurses and health professionals* (37th ed., pp. 703, 706). Elsevier.

291. A client is brought to the emergency department reporting chest pain. Assessment shows vital signs that include a blood pressure (BP) of 150/90 mm Hg, pulse (P) 88 beats/min, and respirations (R) 20 breaths/min. The nurse administers nitroglycerin 0.4 mg sublingually. In addition to pain relief, the treatment is found to be **effective** when the reassessment of vital signs shows which data?
1. BP 150/90 mm Hg, P 70 beats/min, R 24 breaths/min
2. BP 100/60 mm Hg, P 96 beats/min, R 20 breaths/min
3. BP 100/60 mm Hg, P 70 beats/min, R 24 breaths/min
4. BP 160/100 mm Hg, P 120 beats/min, R 16 breaths/min

Level of Cognitive Ability: Evaluating
Client Needs: Physiological Integrity
Clinical Judgment/Cognitive Skills: Evaluate Outcomes
Integrated Process: Clinical Judgment; Nursing Process/Evaluation
Content Area: Pharmacology: Cardiovascular: Vasodilators
Health Problems: Adult Health: Cardiovascular: Coronary Artery Disease
Priority Concepts: Clinical Judgment; Perfusion

Answer: 2
Rationale: Nitroglycerin dilates both arteries and veins, causing blood to pool in the periphery. This causes a reduced preload and therefore a drop in cardiac output. This vasodilation causes the BP to fall. The drop in cardiac output causes the sympathetic nervous system to respond and attempt to maintain cardiac output by increasing the pulse. Beta blockers, such as propranolol, are often used in conjunction with nitroglycerin to prevent this rise in heart rate. If chest pain is reduced and cardiac workload is reduced, the client will be more comfortable; therefore, a rise in respirations should not be seen.
Test-Taking Strategy: Focus on the subject, nitroglycerin administration. Note the strategic word, *effective*. Knowing that nitroglycerin is a vasodilator and that it causes the BP to drop will assist in eliminating options 1 and 4. Next recall that if chest pain is reduced and cardiac workload is reduced, the client will be more comfortable; therefore, a rise in respirations should not be seen. This assists in eliminating option 3.
Priority Nursing Tip: Check the client's blood pressure before administering each dose of nitroglycerin. Nitroglycerin dilates the blood vessels and causes a drop in BP.
Reference: Ignatavicius, D., et al. (2021). *Medical-surgical nursing: Concepts for interprofessional collaborative care* (10th ed., pp. 758, 766). Elsevier.

❖ **292.** A client who underwent surgical repair of an abdominal aortic aneurysm is 1 day postoperative. The nurse performs an abdominal assessment and notes the absence of bowel sounds. What action would the nurse take?
1. Start client on sips of water.
2. Remove the nasogastric (NG) tube.
3. Call the surgeon immediately.
4. Document the finding and continue to assess for bowel sounds.

Level of Cognitive Ability: Applying
Client Needs: Physiological Integrity
Clinical Judgment/Cognitive Skills: Take Action
Integrated Process: Clinical Judgment; Nursing Process/Implementation
Content Area: Adult Health: Cardiovascular
Health Problems: Adult Health: Cardiovascular: Vascular Disorders
Priority Concepts: Clinical Judgment; Perfusion

Answer: 4
Rationale: Bowel sounds may be absent for 3 to 4 postoperative days because of bowel manipulation during surgery. The nurse would document the finding and continue to monitor the client. The NG tube should stay in place if present, and the client is kept nothing by mouth (NPO) until after the onset of bowel sounds. Additionally, the nurse does not remove the tube without a prescription to do so. There is no need to call the surgeon immediately at this time.
Test-Taking Strategy: Focus on the subject, postoperative care. Note the words "1 day postoperative." Eliminate option 2 because there are no data in the question regarding the presence of an NG tube. Additionally, an NG tube would not be removed and the client would not be fed either liquids or solids if bowel sounds were absent. Recalling that bowel sounds may not return for 3 to 4 postoperative days will direct you to the correct option from the remaining options.
Priority Nursing Tip: In the postoperative period, ask the client about the passage of flatus. This is the best initial indicator of the return of intestinal activity.
Reference: Ignatavicius, D., et al. (2021). *Medical-surgical nursing: Concepts for interprofessional collaborative care* (10th ed., pp. 176, 717). Elsevier.

293. The nurse has admitted a client diagnosed with gestational hypertension who is in labor. The nurse monitors the client closely for which complication of gestational hypertension?
1. Seizures
2. Hallucinations
3. Placenta previa
4. Altered respiratory status

Level of Cognitive Ability: Applying
Client Needs: Physiological Integrity
Clinical Judgment/Cognitive Skills: Take Action
Integrated Process: Clinical Judgment; Nursing Process/Assessment
Content Area: Maternity: Intrapartum
Health Problems: Maternity: Gestational Hypertension/Preeclampsia and Eclampsia
Priority Concepts: Perfusion; Reproduction

Answer: 1
Rationale: Gestational hypertension can lead to preeclampsia and eclampsia; therefore, a major complication of gestational hypertension is seizures. Hallucinations, placenta previa, and altered respiratory status are not directly associated with gestational hypertension.
Test-Taking Strategy: Focus on the subject, complications of gestational hypertension. Remember that seizures are a concern with gestational hypertension to direct you to the correct option.
Priority Nursing Tip: Gestational hypertension refers to a condition in which blood pressure elevation is first detected after mid-pregnancy. Proteinuria is absent.
Reference: McKinney, E. S., et al. (2022). *Maternal child nursing* (6th ed., p. 542). Elsevier.

❖ **294.** Which medication instructions would the nurse provide to a client who has been prescribed levothyroxine? **Select all that apply.**
- ❑ 1. Monitor your own pulse rate.
- ❑ 2. Take the medication in the morning.
- ❑ 3. Take the medication at the same time each day.
- ❑ 4. Notify the physician if chest pain occurs.
- ❑ 5. Expect the pulse rate to be greater than 100 beats/min.
- ❑ 6. It may take 1 to 3 weeks for a full therapeutic effect to occur.

Level of Cognitive Ability: Applying
Client Needs: Physiological Integrity
Clinical Judgment/Cognitive Skills: Take Action
Integrated Process: Teaching and Learning
Content Area: Pharmacology: Endocrine: Thyroid Hormones
Health Problems: Adult Health: Endocrine: Thyroid Disorders
Priority Concepts: Patient Education; Safety

Answer: 1, 2, 3, 4, 6
Rationale: Levothyroxine is a thyroid hormone. The client is instructed to monitor their own pulse rate. The client is also instructed to take the medication in the morning before breakfast to prevent insomnia and to take the medication at the same time each day to maintain hormone levels. The client is told not to discontinue the medication and that thyroid replacement is lifelong. Additional instructions include contacting the physician if the heart rate is greater than 100 beats/min and notifying the physician if chest pain occurs, or if weight loss, nervousness and tremors, or insomnia develops. The client is also told that full therapeutic effect may take 1 to 3 weeks and that they need to have follow-up thyroid blood studies to monitor therapy.
Test-Taking Strategy: Focus on the subject, levothyroxine. Think about the effects of the medication as you read each option. Noting the words "greater than 100 beats/min" in option 5 will assist in eliminating this option.
Priority Nursing Tip: Foods that can inhibit thyroid hormone secretion include strawberries, peaches, pears, cabbage, turnips, spinach, kale, Brussels sprouts, cauliflower, radishes, and peas.
Reference: Burchum, J., & Rosenthal, L. (2022). *Lehne's Pharmacology for nursing care* (11th ed., pp. 698–699, 703). Elsevier.

295. The hemoglobin levels of a client in the first trimester of pregnancy are indicative of iron deficiency anemia. Which assessment findings support the diagnosis of this type of anemia? **Select all that apply.**
- ❑ 1. Yellowish sclera
- ❑ 2. Reports of severe fatigue
- ❑ 3. Pink mucous membranes
- ❑ 4. Increased vaginal secretions
- ❑ 5. Reports of frequent headaches
- ❑ 6. Reports of increased frequency of voiding

Level of Cognitive Ability: Analyzing
Client Needs: Physiological Integrity
Clinical Judgment/Cognitive Skills: Recognize Cues
Integrated Process: Clinical Judgment; Nursing Process/Assessment
Content Area: Maternity: Antepartum
Health Problems: Adult Health: Hematologic: Anemias
Priority Concepts: Gas Exchange; Reproduction

Answer: 2, 5
Rationale: Iron deficiency anemia is described as a hemoglobin blood concentration of less than 11.0 g/dL (110 g/L); the reference range for hemoglobin is 12–16 g/dL (120–160 g/L). Complaints of headaches and severe fatigue are abnormal findings and may reflect complications of this type of anemia caused by the decreased oxygen supply to vital organs. Options 3, 4, and 6 are normal findings in the first trimester of pregnancy. Yellow sclera (whites of the eyes) is associated with jaundice.
Test-Taking Strategy: Focus on the subject, iron deficiency anemia, and note that the client is in the first trimester of pregnancy. Options 2 and 5 are abnormal and may reflect complications caused by the decreased oxygen supply to vital organs. The remaining options are normal occurrences of pregnancy, whereas yellow sclera are not associated with either pregnancy or iron deficiency anemia.
Priority Nursing Tip: The hemoglobin and hematocrit levels decline during pregnancy as a result of increased plasma volume.
Reference: McKinney, E. S., et al. (2022). *Maternal child nursing* (6th ed., p. 567). Elsevier.

❖ **296.** A client diagnosed with multiple myeloma is receiving intravenous hydration at 100 mL per hour. Which finding indicates to the nurse that the client is experiencing a positive response to the treatment plan?

Laboratory Results

Test and Result	Reference Range
Creatinine 1.0 mg/dL (88 mcmol/L)	0.5–1.2 mg/dL (44–106 mcmol/L)
WBC count 6000/mm³ (6 × 10⁹/L)	5000–10,000/mm³ (5–10 × 10⁹/L)

1. Weight increase of 1 kilogram
2. Respirations of 18 breaths per minute
3. Creatinine level
4. WBC count

Level of Cognitive Ability: Evaluating
Client Needs: Physiological Integrity
Clinical Judgment/Cognitive Skills: Evaluate Outcomes
Integrated Process: Clinical Judgment; Nursing Process/Evaluation
Content Area: Adult Health: Oncology
Health Problems: Adult Health: Cancer: Multiple Myeloma
Priority Concepts: Cellular Regulation; Fluids and Electrolytes

Answer: 3
Rationale: Multiple myeloma is a malignant proliferation of plasma cells within the bone. Renal failure is a concern in the client with multiple myeloma. In multiple myeloma, hydration is essential to prevent renal damage resulting from precipitation of protein in the renal tubules and excessive calcium and uric acid in the blood. Creatinine is the most accurate measure of renal function. Options 2 and 4 are unrelated to the subject of hydration. Weight gain is not a positive sign when concerned with renal status.
Test-Taking Strategy: Focus on the subject, hydration and multiple myeloma. Recalling that kidney failure is a concern in multiple myeloma will direct you to the correct option. Additionally, option 3 is the only choice that is related to hydration status.
Priority Nursing Tip: The client with multiple myeloma is at risk for pathologic fractures.
Reference: Ignatavicius, D., et al. (2021). *Medical-surgical nursing: Concepts for interprofessional collaborative care* (10th ed., pp. 814, 1313). Elsevier.

297. The nurse provides discharge instructions to a client who is recovering from testicular cancer surgery. Which instruction would the nurse include?
1. To avoid driving a car for at least 2 weeks
2. To avoid sitting for long periods for at least 2 weeks
3. Not to be fitted for a prosthesis for at least 3 months
4. To report any fever to the surgeon immediately

Level of Cognitive Ability: Applying
Client Needs: Physiological Integrity
Clinical Judgment/Cognitive Skills: Generate Solutions
Integrated Process: Teaching and Learning
Content Area: Adult Health: Oncology
Health Problems: Adult Health: Cancer: Testicular
Priority Concepts: Cellular Regulation; Patient Education

Answer: 4
Rationale: For the client who has had testicular surgery, the nurse would emphasize the importance of notifying the surgeon if chills, fever, drainage, redness, or discharge occurs. These symptoms may indicate the presence of an infection. One week after testicular surgery, the client may drive. Often, a prosthesis is inserted during surgery. Sitting needs to be avoided with prostate surgery because of the risk of hemorrhage, but this risk is not as high with testicular surgery.
Test-Taking Strategy: Focus on the subject, post-testicular surgery care. Use Maslow's Hierarchy of Needs theory and principles related to prioritizing. Infection is a priority. After any surgical procedure, elevation of temperature could signal an infection and needs to be reported immediately. Also note the lengthy time periods in options 1, 2, and 3. These will assist in eliminating these options.
Priority Nursing Tip: Testicular self-examination needs to be performed monthly. A day of the month is selected, and the examination is performed on the same day each month.
Reference: Ignatavicius, D., et al. (2021). *Medical-surgical nursing: Concepts for interprofessional collaborative care* (10th ed., p. 1488). Elsevier.

❖ **298.** A multidisciplinary team working with the spouse of a home care client diagnosed with end-stage liver failure is teaching the spouse about pain management. Which statement by the spouse indicates the **need for further teaching?**

1. "I will help prevent constipation with increased fluids."
2. "My partner can use breathing exercises to control pain."
3. "If the pain increases, I will report it to the nurse promptly."
4. "The medication causes very deep sleep that my partner needs."

Level of Cognitive Ability: Evaluating
Client Needs: Physiological Integrity
Clinical Judgment/Cognitive Skills: Evaluate Outcomes
Integrated Process: Clinical Judgment; Nursing Process/Evaluation
Content Area: Skills: Client Teaching
Health Problems: Adult Health: Neurologic: Pain
Priority Concepts: Pain; Safety

Answer: 4
Rationale: In the client with liver disease, the ability to metabolize medication is affected. A decreased level of consciousness is a potential clinical indicator of medication overdose, as well as fluid, electrolyte, and oxygenation deficiencies; thus, the nurse teaches the client's spouse about the differences between sleep related to pain relief and a deteriorating change in neurologic status. Options 1, 2, and 3 all indicate an understanding of suitable steps to be taken in pain management.
Test-Taking Strategy: Note the strategic words, *need for further teaching.* These words indicate a negative event query and the need to select the option that is an incorrect statement. Note that the client has end-stage liver disease, meaning that analgesics take longer to metabolize, so the dosage is likely to have a greater and longer effect than in a client without liver disease. Focusing on the subject, pain management in a client who has end-stage liver failure, will direct you to the correct option.
Priority Nursing Tip: The administration of opioids, sedatives, barbiturates, and any hepatotoxic medications is avoided in the client with liver disease.
Reference: Lewis, S., et al. (2020). *Medical-surgical nursing: Assessment and management of clinical problems* (11th ed., pp. 989–990). Elsevier.

299. The nurse is reviewing the antenatal history of a several clients in early labor. The nurse recognizes which factor documented in the history as having the potential for causing neonatal sepsis after delivery? **Select all that apply.**

❑ 1. Of Asian heritage
❑ 2. Two previous miscarriages
❑ 3. Prenatal care began during the third trimester
❑ 4. History of substance abuse during pregnancy
❑ 5. Dietary assessment identified poor eating habits
❑ 6. Spontaneous rupture of membranes 24 hours ago

Level of Cognitive Ability: Analyzing
Client Needs: Physiological Integrity
Clinical Judgment/Cognitive Skills: Recognize Cues
Integrated Process: Clinical Judgment; Nursing Process/Assessment
Content Area: Maternity: Intrapartum
Health Problems: Maternity: Infections/ Inflammations
Priority Concepts: Clinical Judgment; Infection

Answer: 3, 4, 5, 6
Rationale: Risk factors for neonatal sepsis can arise from maternal, intrapartal, or neonatal conditions. Maternal risk factors before delivery include a history of substance abuse during pregnancy, low socioeconomic status, and poor prenatal care and nutrition. Premature rupture of the membranes or prolonged rupture of membranes greater than 18 hours before birth is also a risk factor for neonatal acquisition of infection. There is no research to associate heritage or previous miscarriages to the development of neonatal sepsis.
Test-Taking Strategy: Focus on the subject, risk factor for neonatal sepsis. Eliminate options that have no connection to the risk of infection.
Priority Nursing Tip: If antibiotics are prescribed for a newborn, monitor the newborn carefully for toxicity because a newborn's liver and kidneys are immature.
Reference: Lowdermilk, D., et al. (2020). *Maternity & women's health care* (12th ed., pp. 768–769). Elsevier.

❖ **300.** The nurse performing a prenatal assessment on a client in the first trimester of pregnancy discovers that the client frequently consumes beverages containing alcohol. Why would the nurse initiate interventions **immediately** to assist the client in avoiding alcohol consumption?

1. To reduce the potential for fetal growth restriction in utero
2. To promote the normal psychosocial adaptation of the client to pregnancy
3. To minimize the potential for placental abruptions during the intrapartum period
4. To reduce the risk of teratogenic effects to embryo's developing fetal organs and tissue

Level of Cognitive Ability: Analyzing
Client Needs: Physiological Integrity
Clinical Judgment/Cognitive Skills: Generate Solutions
Integrated Process: Clinical Judgment; Nursing Process: Planning
Content Area: Maternity: Antepartum
Health Problems: Newborn: Disorders of Prenatal Development
Priority Concepts: Reproduction; Safety

Answer: 4
Rationale: The first trimester, "organogenesis," is characterized by the differentiation and development of fetal organs, systems, and structures. The effects of alcohol on the developing fetus during this critical period depend not only on the amount of alcohol consumed but also on the interaction of quantity, frequency, type of alcohol, and other drugs that may be abused during this period by the pregnant client. Eliminating consumption of alcohol during this time may promote normal fetal organ development. Although options 1, 2, and 3 may be concerns, they are not specifically associated with the first trimester of pregnancy.
Test-Taking Strategy: Focus on the subject, effects of alcohol on the fetus, and note the strategic word, *immediately*. Recall that during the first trimester, development of fetal organs, tissues, and structures take place.
Priority Nursing Tip: Fetal alcohol syndrome is caused by maternal alcohol use during pregnancy and causes physical and mental retardation.
Reference: McKinney, E. S., et al. (2022). *Maternal child nursing* (6th ed., pp. 241, 273). Elsevier.

301. The nurse is admitting a client with a diagnosis of hypothyroidism. What assessment would the nurse perform to obtain data related to this diagnosis?

1. Inspect facial features.
2. Auscultate lung sounds.
3. Percuss the thyroid gland.
4. Inspect ability to ambulate safely.

Level of Cognitive Ability: Applying
Client Needs: Physiological Integrity
Clinical Judgment/Cognitive Skills: Recognize Cues
Integrated Process: Nursing Process/Assessment
Content Area: Adult Health: Endocrine
Health Problems: Adult Health: Endocrine: Thyroid Disorders
Priority Concepts: Clinical Judgment; Thermoregulation

Answer: 1
Rationale: Inspection of facial features will reveal the characteristic coarse features, presence of edema around the eyes and face, and the blank expression that are characteristics of hypothyroidism. The assessment techniques in options 2, 3, and 4 will not reveal information related to the diagnosis of hypothyroidism.
Test-Taking Strategy: Focus on the subject, hypothyroidism. Eliminate options 2 and 4 because they do not relate to the thyroid gland. From the remaining options, recall that palpation, rather than percussion, of the thyroid is the assessment technique used to evaluate the thyroid gland.
Priority Nursing Tip: Hypothyroidism is characterized by a decreased rate of metabolism. Assessment findings relate to this characteristic.
Reference: Ignatavicius, D., et al. (2021). *Medical-surgical nursing: Concepts for interprofessional collaborative care* (10th ed., pp. 1251–1252). Elsevier.

❖ **302.** The nurse is teaching a client diagnosed with chronic obstructive pulmonary disease (COPD) how to do pursed-lip breathing. Evaluation of understanding is evident if the client performs which action?
1. Loosens the abdominal muscles while breathing out
2. Breathes in and then holds the breath for 30 seconds
3. Inhales with puckered lips and exhales with the mouth open wide
4. Breathes so that expiration is two to three times as long as inspiration

Level of Cognitive Ability: Evaluating
Client Needs: Physiological Integrity
Clinical Judgment/Cognitive Skills: Evaluate Outcomes
Integrated Process: Clinical Judgment; Nursing Process/Evaluation
Content Area: Adult Health: Respiratory
Health Problems: Adult Health: Respiratory: Chronic Obstructive Pulmonary Disease
Priority Concepts: Patient Education; Gas Exchange

Answer: 4
Rationale: COPD is a disease state characterized by airflow obstruction. Prolonging expiration time reduces air trapping caused by airway narrowing that occurs in COPD. The client is not instructed to breathe in and hold the breath for 30 seconds; this action has no useful purpose for the client with COPD. Tightening (not loosening) the abdominal muscles aids in expelling air. Exhaling through pursed lips (not with the mouth wide open) increases the intraluminal pressure and prevents the airways from collapsing.
Test-Taking Strategy: Focus on the subject, pursed-lip breathing in a client with chronic obstructive pulmonary disease (COPD). Visualize each of the actions in the options. Recalling that a major purpose of pursed-lip breathing is to prevent air trapping during exhalation will direct you to the correct option.
Priority Nursing Tip: For the client with chronic obstructive pulmonary disease, the stimulus to breathe is a low arterial Po_2 instead of an increased Pco_2.
Reference: Ignatavicius, D., et al. (2021). *Medical-surgical nursing: Concepts for interprofessional collaborative care* (10th ed., pp. 547–548). Elsevier.

303. While providing care to a client with a head injury, the nurse notes that a client exhibits this posture **(refer to figure)**. What would the nurse document that the client is exhibiting?

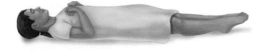

1. Flaccidity
2. Decorticate posturing
3. Decerebrate posturing
4. Rigidity in the upper extremities

Level of Cognitive Ability: Analyzing
Client Needs: Physiological Integrity
Clinical Judgment/Cognitive Skills: Recognize Cues
Integrated Process: Clinical Judgment; Nursing Process/Assessment
Content Area: Adult Health: Neurologic
Health Problems: Adult Health: Neurologic: Head Injury/Trauma
Priority Concepts: Clinical Judgment; Intracranial Regulation

Answer: 2
Rationale: Decortication is abnormal posturing seen in the client with lesions that interrupt the corticospinal pathways. In this posturing, the client's arms, wrists, and fingers are flexed with internal rotation and plantar flexion of the feet and legs extended. Flaccidity indicates weak, soft, and flabby muscles that lack normal muscle tone. Decerebration is abnormal posturing and rigidity characterized by extension of the arms and legs, pronation of the arms, plantar flexion, and opisthotonos. Decerebration is usually associated with dysfunction in the brainstem area. Rigidity indicates hardness, stiffness, or inflexibility. Decerebrate posturing is associated with rigidity.
Test-Taking Strategy: Focus on the subject, posturing. Review the figure and use knowledge regarding the characteristics of posturing to answer the question. First eliminate options 3 and 4 because they are comparable or alike in that decerebrate posturing is associated with rigidity. Next, recalling that flaccidity indicates weak, soft, and flabby muscles that lack normal muscle tone will assist in eliminating option 1.
Priority Nursing Tip: Decorticate posturing is also known as flexor posturing, and decerebrate posturing is also known as extensor posturing.
Reference: Ignatavicius, D., et al. (2021). *Medical-surgical nursing: Concepts for interprofessional collaborative care* (10th ed., p. 833). Elsevier.

❖ **304.** A client prescribed lithium carbonate for the treatment of bipolar disorder has a lithium blood level drawn. Based on the test result, which assessment question would the nurse ask to determine whether the client is experiencing signs of lithium toxicity?

Laboratory Results

Test and Result	Reference Range
Lithium 1.6 mEq/L (1.6 mmol/L)	0.6 to 1.2 mEq/L (0.6 to 1.2 mmol/L)

1. "Do you hear ringing in your ears?"
2. "Have you noted that your vision is blurred?"
3. "Have you fallen recently because you are dizzy?"
4. "Have you been experiencing any nausea, vomiting, or diarrhea?"

Level of Cognitive Ability: Analyzing
Client Needs: Physiological Integrity
Clinical Judgment/Cognitive Skills: Take Action
Integrated Process: Clinical Judgment; Nursing Process/Assessment
Content Area: Pharmacology: Psychotherapeutics: Mood Stabilizers
Health Problems: Mental Health: Mood Disorders
Priority Concepts: Clinical Judgment; Safety

Answer: 4
Rationale: One of the most common early signs of lower level lithium toxicity is gastrointestinal (GI) disturbances such as nausea, vomiting, or diarrhea. The assessment questions in options 1, 2, and 3 are related to the findings in lithium toxicity at higher levels.
Test-Taking Strategy: Focus on the subject, signs of lithium toxicity and toxic lithium levels. Focus on the test result and the reference range. Recalling that GI disturbances are early manifestations will direct you to the correct option.
Priority Nursing Tip: Instruct the client taking lithium carbonate to drink six to eight glasses of water daily and to maintain an adequate intake of salt to prevent lithium toxicity.
Reference: Varcarolis, E., & Fosbre, C. (2021). *Essentials of psychiatric mental health nursing: A communication approach to evidence-based care* (4th ed., pp. 237, 240). Elsevier.

305. A postpartum nurse caring for a client who delivered vaginally 2 hours ago palpates the fundus and notes the character of the lochia. Which characteristic of the lochia would indicate to the nurse that the client's recovery is normal?
1. Pink-colored lochia
2. White-colored lochia
3. Serosanguineous lochia
4. Dark red-colored lochia

Level of Cognitive Ability: Applying
Client Needs: Physiological Integrity
Clinical Judgment/Cognitive Skills: Recognize Cues
Integrated Process: Nursing Process/Assessment
Content Area: Maternity: Postpartum
Health Problems: N/A
Priority Concepts: Health Promotion; Reproduction

Answer: 4
Rationale: When checking the perineum, the nurse monitors the lochia for amount, color, and the presence of clots. The color of the lochia during the fourth stage of labor (the first 1 to 4 hours after birth) is dark red. Options 1, 2, and 3 are not the expected characteristics of lochia at this time period.
Test-Taking Strategy: Focus on the subject, lochia assessment postpartum. Noting that the question refers to a client who delivered 2 hours ago will direct you to the correct option.
Priority Nursing Tip: Lochia discharge should smell like normal menstrual flow. If it has a foul-smelling odor, infection should be suspected.
Reference: McKinney, E. S., et al. (2022). *Maternal child nursing* (6th ed., pp. 329, 400). Elsevier.

❖ **306.** The nurse is performing a prenatal examination on a client in the third trimester. The nurse begins an abdominal examination that includes Leopold maneuvers. What information would the nurse be able to determine after performing the assessment's first maneuver?
1. Fetal descent
2. Placenta previa
3. Fetal lie and presentation
4. Strength of uterine contractions

Level of Cognitive Ability: Analyzing
Client Needs: Physiological Integrity
Clinical Judgment/Cognitive Skills: Recognize Cues
Integrated Process: Nursing Process/Assessment
Content Area: Maternity: Antepartum
Health Problems: N/A
Priority Concepts: Health Promotion; Reproduction

Answer: 3
Rationale: The first maneuver, the fundal grip, determines the contents (size, consistency, shape, and mobility) of the fundus (either the fetal head or breech) and thereby the fetal lie. Fetal descent is determined with the fourth maneuver. Placenta previa is diagnosed by ultrasound and not by palpation. Leopold maneuvers are not performed during a contraction.
Test-Taking Strategy: Focus on the subject, Leopold maneuvers, and this will assist in eliminating options 2 and 4. From the remaining options, it is necessary to know that the first maneuver determines fetal lie.
Priority Nursing Tip: Before performing Leopold maneuvers, the nurse should assist the client in emptying the bladder.
Reference: McKinney, E. S., et al. (2022). *Maternal child nursing* (6th ed., pp. 312–314). Elsevier.

307. The nurse is caring for a client who sustained a spinal cord injury that has resulted in spinal shock. Which assessment will provide relevant information about recovery from spinal shock?
1. Reflexes
2. Pulse rate
3. Temperature
4. Blood pressure

Level of Cognitive Ability: Analyzing
Client Needs: Physiological Integrity
Clinical Judgment/Cognitive Skills: Recognize Cues
Integrated Process: Clinical Judgment; Nursing Process/Assessment
Content Area: Complex Care: Shock
Health Problems: Adult Health: Neurologic: Spinal Cord Injury
Priority Concepts: Mobility; Intracranial Regulation

Answer: 1
Rationale: Areflexia characterizes spinal shock; therefore, reflexes would provide the best information about recovery. Vital sign changes (options 2, 3, and 4) are not consistently affected by spinal shock. Because vital signs are affected by many factors, they do not give reliable information about spinal shock recovery. Blood pressure would provide good information about recovery from other types of shock, but not spinal shock.
Test-Taking Strategy: Focus on the subject, recovery from spinal shock. Note that options 2, 3, and 4 are comparable or alike and are all vital signs. Therefore, eliminate these options.
Priority Nursing Tip: Spinal shock can occur after a spinal cord injury and ends when the reflexes are regained.
Reference: Ignatavicius, D., et al. (2021). *Medical-surgical nursing: Concepts for interprofessional collaborative care* (10th ed., p. 879). Elsevier.

❖ **308.** A hospitalized client awaiting repair of an unruptured cerebral aneurysm is frequently assessed by the nurse. Which assessment finding would the nurse identify as an **early** indication that the aneurysm has ruptured?
1. Widened pulse pressure
2. Unilateral motor weakness
3. Unilateral slowing of pupil response
4. A decline in the level of consciousness

Level of Cognitive Ability: Analyzing
Client Needs: Physiological Integrity
Clinical Judgment/Cognitive Skills: Recognize Cues
Integrated Process: Clinical Judgment; Nursing Process/Assessment
Content Area: Complex Care: Emergency Situations/Management
Health Problems: Adult Health: Neurologic: Aneurysm
Priority Concepts: Clinical Judgment; Intracranial Regulation

Answer: **4**
Rationale: Rupture of a cerebral aneurysm usually results in increased intracranial pressure (ICP). The first sign of pressure in the brain is a change in the level of consciousness. This change in consciousness can be as subtle as drowsiness or restlessness. Because centers that control blood pressure are located lower in the brain than those that control consciousness, blood pressure alteration is a later sign. Slowing of pupil response and motor weakness are also late signs.
Test-Taking Strategy: Focus on the subject, signs of a ruptured cerebral aneurysm. Note the strategic word, *early.* Remember that changes in level of consciousness are the first indication of increased ICP.
Priority Nursing Tip: The level of consciousness is the most sensitive and earliest indicator of a change in the neurologic status.
Reference: Ignatavicius, D., et al. (2021). *Medical-surgical nursing: Concepts for interprofessional collaborative care.* (10th ed., pp. 916–917). Elsevier.

309. The nurse in the mental health unit is preparing to admit a severely depressed client. Which findings on assessment support the diagnosis of this client? **Select all that apply.**
❏ 1. Insomnia
❏ 2. Flat affect
❏ 3. Hypersomnia
❏ 4. Substantial weight loss
❏ 5. Weight gain since onset of depression
❏ 6. Reports, "I don't have any more tears to cry."

Level of Cognitive Ability: Analyzing
Client Needs: Physiological Integrity
Clinical Judgment/Cognitive Skills: Recognize Cues
Integrated Process: Clinical Judgment/Nursing Process/Assessment
Content Area: Mental Health
Health Problems: Mental Health: Mood Disorders
Priority Concepts: Clinical Judgment; Mood and Affect

Answer: **1, 2, 4, 6**
Rationale: In the severely depressed client, loss of weight is typical, whereas the mildly depressed client may experience a gain in weight. Sleep is generally affected in a similar way, with hypersomnia in the mildly depressed client and insomnia in the severely depressed client. The severely depressed client may report that no tears are left for crying. A flat affect may be associated with depression.
Test-Taking Strategy: Focus on the subject, a severely depressed client. Recall that there are varying degrees of depression that can present different physical signs and symptoms. Focusing on severe depression will direct you to the correct option.
Priority Nursing Tip: If the client has depression, always assess the client's risk of harm to self or others.
Reference: Varcarolis, E., & Fosbre, C. (2021). *Essentials of psychiatric mental health nursing: A communication approach to evidence-based care* (4th ed., pp. 203, 208–209). Elsevier.

❖ **310.** A client admitted to the hospital is suspected of having Guillain-Barré syndrome. Which assessment findings would the nurse identify as manifestations of this disorder? **Select all that apply.**
- ❏ 1. Dysphagia
- ❏ 2. Paresthesia
- ❏ 3. Facial weakness
- ❏ 4. Difficulty speaking
- ❏ 5. Hyperactive deep tendon reflexes
- ❏ 6. Descending symmetrical muscle weakness

Level of Cognitive Ability: Analyzing
Client Needs: Physiological Integrity
Clinical Judgment/Cognitive Skills: Recognize Cues
Integrated Process: Clinical Judgment; Nursing Process/Assessment
Content Area: Adult Health: Neurologic
Health Problems: Adult Health: Neurologic: Guillain-Barré Syndrome
Priority Concepts: Clinical Judgment; Mobility

Answer: 1, 2, 3, 4
Rationale: Guillain-Barré syndrome is an acute autoimmune disorder characterized by varying degrees of motor weakness and paralysis. Motor manifestations include ascending symmetric muscle weakness that leads to flaccid paralysis without muscle atrophy, decreased or absent deep tendon reflexes, respiratory compromise and respiratory failure, and loss of bladder and bowel control. Sensory manifestations include pain (cramping) and paresthesia. Cranial nerve manifestations include facial weakness, dysphagia, diplopia, and difficulty speaking. Autonomic manifestations include labile blood pressure, dysrhythmias, and tachycardia.
Test-Taking Strategy: Focus on the subject, Guillain-Barré syndrome, and note that it is an acute autoimmune disorder characterized by varying degrees of motor weakness and paralysis. This will assist in determining that options 1, 2, 3, and 4 are correct.
Priority Nursing Tip: To remember that an ascending progression of paralysis occurs in Guillain-Barré syndrome, think about G to B (Guillain-Barré), from the Ground to the Brain.
Reference: Lewis, S., et al. (2020). *Medical-surgical nursing: Assessment and management of clinical problems* (11th ed., pp. 1424–1425). Elsevier.

311. A visiting home care nurse finds a client unconscious in the bedroom. The client has a history of depression and abusing the selective serotonin reuptake inhibitor, sertraline. The nurse would **immediately** conduct which assessment?
1. Pulse
2. Respirations
3. Blood pressure
4. Urinary output

Level of Cognitive Ability: Analyzing
Client Needs: Physiological Integrity
Clinical Judgment/Cognitive Skills: Prioritize Hypotheses
Integrated Process: Clinical Judgment; Nursing Process/Assessment
Content Area: Complex Care: Emergency Situations/Management
Health Problems: Mental Health: Mood Disorders
Priority Concepts: Clinical Judgment; Safety

Answer: 2
Rationale: In an emergency situation, the nurse would determine breathlessness first and then assess for a pulse. Blood pressure would be assessed after these assessments are performed. Urinary output is also important but is not the priority at this time.
Test-Taking Strategy: Note the strategic word, *immediately*. Use the ABCs—airway, breathing, and circulation—as the guide for answering this question. Respirations specifically relate to airway and breathing.
Priority Nursing Tip: Selective serotonin reuptake inhibitors (SSRIs) can interact with numerous medications. Therefore, it is important to check the client's prescribed medications to determine the potential for an adverse interaction.
Reference: Lewis, S., et al. (2020). *Medical-surgical nursing: Assessment and management of clinical problems* (11th ed., pp. 1392, 1624–1625). Elsevier.

❖ **312.** The nurse checks a unit of blood received from the blood bank and notes the presence of gas bubbles in the bag. What action would the nurse take?

1. Return the bag to the blood bank.
2. Infuse the blood using filter tubing.
3. Add 10 mL normal saline to the bag.
4. Agitate the bag to mix contents gently.

Level of Cognitive Ability: Applying
Client Needs: Physiological Integrity
Clinical Judgment/Cognitive Skills: Take Action
Integrated Process: Nursing Process/Implementation
Content Area: Complex Care: Blood Administration
Health Problems: N/A
Priority Concepts: Clinical Judgment; Safety

Answer: 1
Rationale: The nurse would return the unit of blood to the blood bank because the gas bubbles in the bag indicate possible contamination. Whenever administering blood, the nurse would use filter tubing to trap particulate matter. Although normal saline can be infused concurrently with the blood, normal saline or any other substance should never be added to the blood in a blood bag. The bag should not be agitated because this can harm red blood cells.
Test-Taking Strategy: Focus on the subject, blood administration. Recalling that the presence of gas bubbles indicates potential bacterial growth directs you to the correct option. Remember that, when in doubt, consult with the blood bank.
Priority Nursing Tip: The blood for infusion is always checked for leaks, abnormal color, clots, and bubbles before administration. If any of these are noted, it is not administered and is returned to the blood bank.
Reference: Ignatavicius, D., et al. (2021). *Medical-surgical nursing: Concepts for interprofessional collaborative care* (10th ed., p. 816). Elsevier.

313. What is the smallest gauge catheter that the nurse can use to administer blood to an adult client experiencing hypovolemic shock?

1. 12 gauge
2. 20 gauge
3. 22 gauge
4. 24 gauge

Level of Cognitive Ability: Applying
Client Needs: Physiological Integrity
Clinical Judgment/Cognitive Skills: Generate Solutions
Integrated Process: Nursing Process/Planning
Content Area: Complex Care: Blood Administration
Health Problems: Adult Health: Cardiovascular: Hypovolemic Shock
Priority Concepts: Clinical Judgment; Safety

Answer: 2
Rationale: An intravenous catheter used to infuse blood needs to be at least 20 gauge or larger to help prevent additional hemolysis of red blood cells and to allow infusion of the blood without occluding the IV catheter.
Test-Taking Strategy: Focus on the subject, the smallest gauge catheter that the nurse can use for infusion of blood. This focus will assist in eliminating options 3 and 4. From the remaining options, think about the gauge of IV catheters to direct you to the correct option.
Priority Nursing Tip: Ensure that the client has an adequate and functioning intravenous catheter inserted before obtaining the blood for administration from the blood bank.
Reference: Lewis, S., et al. (2020). *Medical-surgical nursing: Assessment and management of clinical problems* (11th ed., p. 647). Elsevier.

❖ **314.** A client began receiving an intravenous (IV) infusion of packed red blood cells 30 minutes ago. What is the **initial** nursing action when the client reports itching and a tight sensation in the chest?
1. Stop the transfusion.
2. Check client's temperature.
3. Call the physician.
4. Recheck the unit of blood for compatibility.

Level of Cognitive Ability: Applying
Client Needs: Physiological Integrity
Clinical Judgment/Cognitive Skills: Take Action
Integrated Process: Clinical Judgment; Nursing Process/Implementation
Content Area: Complex Care: Blood Administration
Health Problems: Adult Health: Immune: Hypersensitivity Reactions and Allergy
Priority Concepts: Clinical Judgment; Safety

Answer: 1
Rationale: The symptoms reported by the client indicate that the client is experiencing a transfusion reaction. The first action of the nurse when a transfusion reaction is observed is to discontinue the transfusion. The IV of normal saline with new IV tubing is started and the physician is notified. The nurse then checks the client's vital signs: temperature, pulse, and respirations and then rechecks the unit of blood as appropriate for infusion into the client. Depending on agency protocol, the nurse may also obtain a urinalysis, draw a sample of blood, and return the unit of blood and tubing to the blood bank. The nurse also institutes supportive care for the client, which may include administration of antihistamines, crystalloids, epinephrine steroids, or vasopressors as prescribed.
Test-Taking Strategy: Focus on the subject, the action to take if a transfusion reaction occurs. Noting the strategic word, *initial*, will direct you to the correct option. Remember that the first action of the nurse when a transfusion reaction is observed is to discontinue the transfusion.
Priority Nursing Tip: If a blood transfusion reaction occurs, do not leave the client alone and continuously monitor the client for any life-threatening symptoms.
Reference: Lewis, S., et al. (2020). *Medical-surgical nursing: Assessment and management of clinical problems* (11th ed., p. 649). Elsevier.

315. A client has not ingested any food or liquids for 4 hours after two episodes of nausea and vomiting and is dehydrated. What would the nurse offer the client **initially** now that the client is no longer nauseated?
1. Toast
2. Gelatin
3. Dry cereal
4. Ginger ale

Level of Cognitive Ability: Applying
Client Needs: Physiological Integrity
Clinical Judgment/Cognitive Skills: Take Action
Integrated Process: Nursing Process/Implementation
Content Area: Foundations of Care: Therapeutic Diets
Health Problems: Adult Health: Gastrointestinal: Dehydration
Priority Concepts: Clinical Judgment; Nutrition

Answer: 4
Rationale: Clear liquids are best tolerated first after episodes of nausea and vomiting. If the client tolerates sips (20 to 30 mL at a time) of clear liquids, such as water or ginger ale (with the carbonation removed if better tolerated), then the amounts may be increased and gelatin, tea, and broth may be added. Once these are tolerated, solid foods such as toast, cereal, chicken, and other easily digested foods may be tried.
Test-Taking Strategy: Focus on the subject, nausea and vomiting, and the strategic word, *initially*. Begin to answer this question by eliminating options 1 and 3, which identify solid foods and are less well tolerated than liquids. Choose ginger ale over gelatin because it is a liquid at all temperatures.
Priority Nursing Tip: Vomiting places the client at risk for dehydration and metabolic alkalosis.
References: Nix, S. (2022). *Williams' Basic nutrition and diet therapy* (16th ed.). Elsevier; Potter, P., et al. (2021). *Fundamentals of nursing* (10th ed., pp. 1122, 1201). Elsevier.

❖ **316.** A client has just undergone an upper gastro-intestinal (GI) series to rule out peptic ulcer disease. Upon the client's return to the unit, what physician's prescriptions does the nurse expect to note as a part of routine postprocedure care?
  1. Bland diet
  2. NPO status
  3. Mild laxative
  4. Decreased fluids

Level of Cognitive Ability: Applying
Client Needs: Physiological Integrity
Clinical Judgment/Cognitive Skills: Generate Solutions
Integrated Process: Nursing Process/Planning
Content Area: Foundations of Care: Diagnostic Tests
Health Problems: Adult Health: Gastrointestinal: Peptic Ulcer Disease
Priority Concepts: Clinical Judgment; Elimination

Answer: 3
Rationale: Barium sulfate, which is used as a contrast material during an upper GI series, is constipating. If it is not eliminated from the GI tract, it can cause obstruction. Therefore, laxatives or cathartics are administered as part of routine postprocedure care. Increased (not decreased) fluids are also helpful but do not act in the same way as a laxative to eliminate the barium. Options 1 and 2 are not routine postprocedure measures.
Test-Taking Strategy: Focus on the subject, upper GI series, and the words "routine postprocedure." Recalling that barium is used in this diagnostic test will direct you to the correct option.
Priority Nursing Tip: After an upper gastrointestinal (GI) series, instruct the client to increase oral fluid intake to help pass the barium.
Reference: Lewis, S., et al. (2020). *Medical-surgical nursing: Assessment and management of clinical problems* (11th ed., pp. 841, 844). Elsevier.

317. The nurse prepares the client for the removal of a nasogastric tube that was inserted to treat bowel obstruction. During the tube removal, the nurse instructs the client to take which action?
  1. Inhale deeply.
  2. Exhale slowly.
  3. Hold in a deep breath.
  4. Pause between breaths.

Level of Cognitive Ability: Applying
Client Needs: Physiological Integrity
Clinical Judgment/Cognitive Skills: Take Action
Integrated Process: Nursing Process/Implementation
Content Area: Skills: Tube Care
Health Problems: Adult Health: Gastrointestinal: Bowel Obstruction
Priority Concepts: Clinical Judgment; Safety

Answer: 3
Rationale: Just before the tube is removed, the client is asked to take a deep breath and hold it because breath-holding minimizes the risk of aspirating gastric contents spilled from the tube during removal. The maneuver partially occludes the airway during tube removal; afterward, the client exhales as soon as the tube is out and thus avoids drawing the gastric contents into the trachea. The nurse pulls the tube out steadily and smoothly while the client holds the breath. The remaining options are incorrect because options 1 and 2 increase the risk of aspiration, and option 4 is ineffective.
Test-Taking Strategy: Focus on the subject, nasogastric tube removal. Visualize this procedure. Recalling that the airway is partially occluded during tube removal and that the risk of aspiration is present will direct you to the correct option.
Priority Nursing Tip: After removal of a nasogastric tube, monitor the client for abdominal distention and signs of aspiration.
Reference: Potter, P., et al. (2021). *Fundamentals of nursing* (10th ed., p. 1138). Elsevier.

❖ **318.** The nurse is caring for a client being treated for essential fatty-acid deficiency (EFAD) who has a prescription for an intravenous intralipid infusion. What intervention would the nurse implement before hanging the intralipid infusion?
  1. Refrigerate the bottle of solution.
  2. Add 100 mL normal saline to the infusion bottle.
  3. Place an inline filter on the administration tubing.
  4. Check the solution for separation or an oily residue.

Level of Cognitive Ability: Applying
Client Needs: Physiological Integrity
Clinical Judgment/Cognitive Skills: Take Action
Integrated Process: Nursing Process/Implementation
Content Area: Skills: Nutrition
Health Problems: Adult Health: Gastrointestinal: Nutrition/Malabsorption Problems
Priority Concepts: Nutrition; Safety

Answer: 4
Rationale: Intralipids provide nonprotein calories and prevent or correct fatty acid deficiency. The nurse checks the solution for separation or an oily appearance because this can indicate a spoiled or contaminated solution. Refrigeration renders the intralipid solution too thick to administer. Because they can affect the stability of the solution, the nurse avoids injecting additives into the intralipid infusion. Furthermore, an inline filter is not used because it can disrupt the flow of solution by becoming clogged.
Test-Taking Strategy: Focus on the subject, actions to take before administering intralipids. Think about the consistency of this solution to direct you to the correct option.
Priority Nursing Tip: Fat emulsions (lipids) would not be given to a client with an egg allergy because lipids contain egg yolk phospholipids.
Reference: Gahart, B., Nazareno, A., & Ortega, M. (2021). *Gahart's 2021 Intravenous medications: A handbook for nurses and health professionals* (37th ed., pp. 606–607). Elsevier.

319. The nurse creates a discharge plan for a diabetic client diagnosed with peripheral neuropathy of the lower extremities. Which instructions would the nurse include in the plan? **Select all that apply.**
  ❑ 1. Wear support or elastic stockings.
  ❑ 2. Wear well-fitted shoes and walk barefoot when at home.
  ❑ 3. Wear dark-colored stockings or socks and change them daily.
  ❑ 4. Use a heating pad set at low setting on the feet if they feel cold.
  ❑ 5. Apply lanolin or lubricating lotion to the legs and feet once or twice daily.
  ❑ 6. Wash the feet and legs with mild soap and water and rinse and dry them well.

Level of Cognitive Ability: Creating
Client Needs: Physiological Integrity
Clinical Judgment/Cognitive Skills: Generate Solutions
Integrated Process: Clinical Judgment; Nursing Process: Planning
Content Area: Adult Health: Neurologic
Health Problems: Adult Health: Neurologic: Pain
Priority Concepts: Patient Education; Tissue Integrity

Answer: 1, 5, 6
Rationale: Peripheral neuropathy is any functional or organic disorder of the peripheral nervous system. Clinical manifestations can include muscle weakness, stabbing pain, paresthesia or loss of sensation, impaired reflexes, and autonomic manifestations. Home care instructions include wearing support or elastic stockings for dependent edema, applying lanolin or lubricating lotion to the legs and feet once or twice daily, washing the feet and legs with mild soap and water and rinsing and drying them well, inspecting the legs and feet daily and reporting any skin changes or open areas to the physician, wearing white or colorfast stockings or socks and changing them daily, checking the temperature of the bath water with a thermometer before putting the feet into the water, avoiding the use of heat (hot foot soaks, heating pad, hot water bottle) on the feet because of the risk of burning, avoiding the use of sharp devices to cut nails, and wearing well-fitted shoes and avoiding going barefoot.
Test-Taking Strategy: Focus on the subject, peripheral neuropathy. This client will experience paresthesia or loss of sensation. This will assist in eliminating option 4. Finally eliminate option 3 because the client must wear white or colorfast stockings or socks.
Priority Nursing Tip: A complication of diabetes mellitus is peripheral neuropathy. The client experiences decreased sensation and must be cautious about exposure to extreme temperatures and potential injuries.
Reference: Ignatavicius, D., et al. (2021). *Medical-surgical nursing: Concepts for interprofessional collaborative care* (10th ed., pp. 715–716). Elsevier.

❖ **320.** A physician is inserting a chest tube to treat pneumothorax. Which materials would the nurse have available to be used as the first layer of the dressing at the chest tube insertion site?
1. Petrolatum jelly gauze
2. Sterile 4 × 4 gauze pad
3. Absorbent gauze dressing
4. Gauze impregnated with povidone-iodine

Level of Cognitive Ability: Applying
Client Needs: Physiological Integrity
Clinical Judgment/Cognitive Skills: Generate Solutions
Integrated Process: Nursing Process/Planning
Content Area: Skills: Wound Care
Health Problems: Adult Health: Respiratory: Pneumothorax
Priority Concepts: Gas Exchange; Safety

Answer: 1
Rationale: The first layer of the chest tube dressing is petrolatum gauze, which allows for an occlusive seal at the chest tube insertion site. Additional layers of gauze cover this layer, and the dressing is secured with a strong adhesive tape or Elastoplast tape. The items in the remaining options would not be selected as the first protective layer.
Test-Taking Strategy: Focus on the subject, the first layer of the dressing at the chest tube insertion site. Recall that an occlusive seal at the site is needed and think about which dressing material will help achieve this seal.
Priority Nursing Tip: An occlusive sterile dressing is maintained at the chest tube insertion site to prevent an air leak.
Reference: Potter, P., et al. (2021). *Fundamentals of nursing* (10th ed., p. 965). Elsevier.

321. During a follow-up visit 2 weeks after pneumonectomy to treat lung cancer, the client reports numbness and tenderness at the surgical site. Which statement would the nurse make to accurately address the client's concerns?
1. "This is likely to be temporary, but may last for some months."
2. "You are having a severe problem and will probably be re-hospitalized"
3. "This is probably caused by permanent nerve damage as a result of surgery."
4. "This is often the first sign of a wound infection; I will check your temperature."

Level of Cognitive Ability: Applying
Client Needs: Physiological Integrity
Clinical Judgment/Cognitive Skills: Take Action
Integrated Process: Clinical Judgment; Nursing Process/Implementation
Content Area: Adult Health: Respiratory
Health Problems: Adult Health: Cancer: Laryngeal and Lung
Priority Concepts: Gas Exchange; Tissue Integrity

Answer: 1
Rationale: Clients who undergo pneumonectomy or other surgical procedures may experience numbness, altered sensation, or tenderness in the area that surrounds the incision. These sensations may last for months. They are not considered to be a severe problem and are not indicative of a wound infection.
Test-Taking Strategy: Focus on the subject, numbness and tenderness at the surgical site after pneumonectomy. Eliminate option 2 because of the word "severe." Eliminate option 3 because of the word "permanent." Eliminate option 4 because numbness and tenderness are not signs of infection.
Priority Nursing Tip: After pneumonectomy, check the surgeon's prescription regarding client positioning. Avoid complete lateral turning of the client.
Reference: Ignatavicius, D., et al. (2021). *Medical-surgical nursing: Concepts for interprofessional collaborative care* (10th ed., pp. 184–185, 559). Elsevier.

❖ **322.** A client, who was diagnosed with a malignant tumor in the left lung, is scheduled for pneumonectomy and tells the nurse that a friend had lung surgery that required chest tubes. The client asks how long to expect chest tubes to be in place. Which statement by the nurse appropriately educates the client about the presence of a chest tube postpneumonectomy?
1. "They are generally removed after 36 to 48 hours."
2. "Not every lung surgery requires chest tubes to be used."
3. "They usually remain in place for a full week after surgery."
4. "Your type of surgery rarely requires chest tubes to be inserted after surgery."

Level of Cognitive Ability: Applying
Client Needs: Physiological Integrity
Clinical Judgment/Cognitive Skills: Take Action
Integrated Process: Teaching and Learning
Content Area: Adult Health: Respiratory
Health Problems: Adult Health: Cancer: Laryngeal and Lung
Priority Concepts: Patient Education; Gas Exchange

Answer: 4
Rationale: Pneumonectomy involves removal of the entire lung, usually caused by extensive disease such as bronchogenic carcinoma, unilateral tuberculosis, or lung abscess. Chest tubes are not inserted because the cavity is left to fill with serosanguineous fluid, which later solidifies. Therefore, options 1, 2, and 3 are incorrect.
Test-Taking Strategy: Focus on the **subject,** postoperative expectations after pneumonectomy. Recall that the entire lung is removed with this procedure. This would guide you to reason that chest tubes are unnecessary because there is no lung remaining to reinflate to fill the pleural space.
Priority Nursing Tip: After pneumonectomy, serous fluid accumulates in the empty thoracic cavity and eventually consolidates, preventing shifts of the mediastinum, heart, and remaining lung.
Reference: Ignatavicius, D., et al. (2021). *Medical-surgical nursing: Concepts for interprofessional collaborative care* (10th ed., p. 559). Elsevier.

323. The nurse is creating a plan of care for a client diagnosed with a dissecting abdominal aortic aneurysm. Which interventions would be included in the plan of care? **Select all that apply.**
☐ 1. Assess peripheral circulation.
☐ 2. Monitor for abdominal distention.
☐ 3. Educate client that abdominal pain is to be expected.
☐ 4. Assess client for observable ecchymoses on the lower back.
☐ 5. Perform deep palpation of the abdomen to assess the size of the aneurysm.

Level of Cognitive Ability: Creating
Client Needs: Physiological Integrity
Clinical Judgment/Cognitive Skills: Generate Solutions
Integrated Process: Clinical Judgment; Nursing Process/Planning
Content Area: Complex Care: Emergency Situations/Management
Health Problems: Adult Health: Cardiovascular: Vascular Disorders
Priority Concepts: Clinical Judgment; Perfusion

Answer: 1, 2, 4
Rationale: If the client has an abdominal aortic aneurysm, the nurse is concerned about rupture and monitors the client closely. The nurse would assess peripheral circulation and monitor for abdominal distention. The nurse also looks for ecchymoses on the lower back to determine if the aneurysm is leaking. The nurse tells the client to report abdominal pain, or back pain, which may radiate to the groin, buttocks, or legs because this is a sign of rupture. The nurse also avoids deep palpation in the client in whom a dissecting abdominal aortic aneurysm is known or suspected. Doing so could place the client at risk for rupture.
Test-Taking Strategy: Focus on the **subject,** care for a client with a dissecting abdominal aortic aneurysm. Eliminate options 3 and 5 because the presence of abdominal pain is a sign of rupture and deep palpation places the aneurysm at risk for rupture.
Priority Nursing Tip: Systolic bruit heard over the abdominal aorta is a manifestation of an abdominal aortic aneurysm.
Reference: Ignatavicius, D., et al. (2021). *Medical-surgical nursing: Concepts for interprofessional collaborative care* (10th ed., pp. 718–719). Elsevier.

❖ **324.** A client with peripheral vascular disease has undergone angioplasty of the iliac artery. Which technique would the nurse perform to **best** detect bleeding from the angioplasty in the region of the iliac artery?
1. Palpate the pedal pulses.
2. Measure the abdominal girth.
3. Assess client about the level of pain in the area.
4. Auscultate over the iliac area with a Doppler device.

Level of Cognitive Ability: Analyzing
Client Needs: Physiological Integrity
Clinical Judgment/Cognitive Skills: Take Action
Integrated Process: Clinical Judgment; Nursing Process/Assessment
Content Area: Adult Health: Cardiovascular
Health Problems: Adult Health: Cardiovascular: Vascular Disorders
Priority Concepts: Clinical Judgment; Perfusion

Answer: 2
Rationale: Bleeding after iliac artery angioplasty causes blood to accumulate in the retroperitoneal area. This can most directly be detected by measuring abdominal girth. Palpation and auscultation of pulses determine patency. Assessment of pain is routinely done, and mild regional discomfort is expected.
Test-Taking Strategy: Note the strategic word, *best.* Focus on the subject of bleeding from the angioplasty in the region of the iliac artery. Select the option that addresses an abdominal assessment because the iliac arteries are located in the peritoneal cavity. This will direct you to the correct option.
Priority Nursing Tip: After angioplasty, assess the insertion site frequently for the presence of bloody drainage or hematoma formation.
Reference: Ignatavicius, D., et al. (2021). *Medical-surgical nursing: Concepts for interprofessional collaborative care* (10th ed., pp. 630, 1160). Elsevier.

325. A client states, "I'm sure I have restless leg syndrome." The nurse determines that the client is in **need of further teaching** on the condition when the client identifies the presence of which characteristics? **Select all that apply.**
❑ 1. A heavy feeling in the legs
❑ 2. Burning sensations in the limbs
❑ 3. Symptom relief when lying down
❑ 4. Decreased ability to move the legs
❑ 5. Symptoms that are worse in the morning
❑ 6. Feeling the need to move the limbs repeatedly

Level of Cognitive Ability: Evaluating
Client Needs: Physiological Integrity
Clinical Judgment/Cognitive Skills: Evaluate Outcomes
Integrated Process: Clinical Judgment; Nursing Process/Evaluation
Content Area: Adult Health: Neurologic
Health Problems: Adult Health: Neurologic: Restless Legs Syndrome
Priority Concepts: Clinical Judgment; Mobility

Answer: 1, 3, 4, 5
Rationale: Restless leg syndrome is characterized by leg paresthesia associated with an irresistible urge to move. The client complains of intense burning or "crawling-type" sensations in the limbs and subsequently feels the need to move the limbs repeatedly to relieve the symptoms. The symptoms are worse in the evening and night when the client is still.
Test-Taking Strategy: Focus on the subject, manifestations of restless leg syndrome. Note the strategic words, *need for further teaching.* These words indicate a negative event query and the need to select incorrect characteristics. This will assist in eliminating options 2 and 6, which are characteristics of restless leg syndrome.
Priority Nursing Tip: Some nonpharmacologic measures to relieve the symptoms of restless leg syndrome include walking, stretching, moderate exercise, or a warm bath.
Reference: Lewis, S., et al. (2020). *Medical-surgical nursing: Assessment and management of clinical problems* (11th ed., pp. 1365–1366). Elsevier.

❖ **326.** A client with peripheral vascular disease who underwent peripheral arterial bypass surgery 16 hours ago reports that there is increasing pain in the leg that worsens with movement and is accompanied by paresthesia. Based on these data, which action would the nurse take?
1. Call the surgeon.
2. Administer an opioid analgesic.
3. Apply warm moist heat for comfort.
4. Apply ice to minimize any developing swelling.

Level of Cognitive Ability: Applying
Client Needs: Physiological Integrity
Clinical Judgment/Cognitive Skills: Take Action
Integrated Process: Clinical Judgment; Nursing Process/Implementation
Content Area: Adult Health: Cardiovascular
Health Problems: Adult Health: Cardiovascular: Vascular Disorders
Priority Concepts: Clinical Judgment; Perfusion

Answer: 1
Rationale: Compartment syndrome is characterized by increased pressure within a muscle compartment caused by bleeding or excessive edema. It compresses the nerves in the area and can cause vascular compromise. The classic signs of compartment syndrome are pain at rest that intensifies with movement and the development of paresthesia. Compartment syndrome is an emergency, and the physician is notified immediately because the client could require an emergency fasciotomy to relieve the pressure and restore perfusion. Options 2, 3, and 4 are incorrect actions.
Test-Taking Strategy: Focus on the subject, a postoperative client who had peripheral arterial bypass surgery. Note the words "increasing pain." Also note that the surgery was 16 hours ago. The signs and symptoms described indicate a new problem. These factors indicate that the surgeon needs to be notified.
Priority Nursing Tip: After arterial bypass surgery, warmth, redness, and edema of the affected extremity are expected occurrences because of the increased blood flow to the area.
Reference: Ignatavicius, D., et al. (2021). *Medical-surgical nursing: Concepts for interprofessional collaborative care* (10th ed., pp. 715, 1031). Elsevier.

327. The nurse in an ambulatory care clinic takes a client's blood pressure (BP) in the left arm; it is 200/118 mm Hg. Which action would the nurse take **next?**
1. Notify the physician.
2. Inquire about the presence of kidney disorders.
3. Check client's blood pressure in the right arm.
4. Recheck the pressure in the same arm within 30 seconds.

Level of Cognitive Ability: Applying
Client Needs: Physiological Integrity
Clinical Judgment/Cognitive Skills: Take Action
Integrated Process: Clinical Judgment; Nursing Process/Implementation
Content Area: Skills: Vital Signs
Health Problems: Adult Health: Cardiovascular: Hypertension
Priority Concepts: Clinical Judgment; Perfusion

Answer: 3
Rationale: When a high BP reading is noted, the nurse takes the pressure in the opposite arm to see if the blood pressure is elevated in one extremity only. The nurse would also recheck the blood pressure in the same arm but would wait at least 2 minutes between readings. The nurse would inquire about the presence of kidney disorders that could contribute to the elevated blood pressure. The nurse would notify the physician because immediate treatment may be required, but this would not be done without obtaining verification of the elevation.
Test-Taking Strategy: Focus on the subject, hypertension. Note the strategic word, *next*. Eliminate option 4 first because of the time frame, 30 seconds. From the remaining options, select the correct option because it provides verification of the initial reading.
Priority Nursing Tip: Hypertension is a major risk factor for coronary, cerebral, renal, and peripheral vascular disease.
Reference: Lewis, S., et al. (2020). *Medical-surgical nursing: Assessment and management of clinical problems* (11th ed., p. 692). Elsevier.

❖ **328.** A prenatal client is being evaluated for possible gestational diabetes. Which data identified and documented after the nursing assessment would support that diagnosis?
1. 22 years old
2. A gravida 4, para 0, aborta 3
3. 5′ 6″ tall, weighs 130 pounds
4. Stated, "I get really tired after working all day"

Level of Cognitive Ability: Analyzing
Client Needs: Physiological Integrity
Clinical Judgment/Cognitive Skills: Analyze Cues
Integrated Process: Clinical Judgment; Nursing Process/Analysis
Content Area: Maternity: Antepartum
Health Problems: Maternity: Gestational Diabetes Mellitus
Priority Concepts: Glucose Regulation; Reproduction

Answer: 2
Rationale: A history of unexplained stillbirths or miscarriages puts the client at high risk for gestational diabetes. Fatigue is a normal occurrence during pregnancy. The client's height (5′ 6″ tall) and weight (130 pounds) do not meet the criteria of 20% over ideal weight. Therefore, the client is not obese, a possible factor related to gestational diabetes. To be at high risk for gestational diabetes, the maternal age should be greater than 25 years.
Test-Taking Strategy: Focus on the subject, gestational diabetes. Option 4 can be eliminated because fatigue is a normal occurrence during pregnancy. Recalling the risk factors associated with gestational diabetes will indicate that options 1 and 3 do not apply to this client.
Priority Nursing Tip: Pregnant clients should be screened for gestational diabetes between 24 and 28 weeks of pregnancy.
Reference: McKinney, E. S., et al. (2022). *Maternal child nursing* (6th ed., pp. 231, 560–561). Elsevier.

329. The nurse is caring for a client diagnosed with preeclampsia. When the client's condition progresses from preeclampsia to eclampsia, what would the nurse's **first** action be?
1. Prepare to maintain an open airway.
2. Prepare to administer oxygen by face mask.
3. Assess client's blood pressure and fetal heart tones.
4. Administer an intravenous infusion of magnesium sulfate.

Level of Cognitive Ability: Applying
Client Needs: Physiological Integrity
Clinical Judgment/Cognitive Skills: Take Action
Integrated Process: Clinical Judgment; Nursing Process/Implementation
Content Area: Maternity: Antepartum
Health Problems: Maternity: Gestational Hypertension/Preeclampsia and Eclampsia
Priority Concepts: Perfusion; Reproduction

Answer: 1
Rationale: Eclampsia is characterized by the occurrence of seizures. If the client experiences seizures, it is important as a first action to establish and maintain an open airway and prevent injuries to the client. Options 2, 3, and 4 are all interventions that should be done but not initially.
Test-Taking Strategy: Note the strategic word, *first*. Use the ABCs—airway, breathing, and circulation—to direct you to the correct option.
Priority Nursing Tip: The nurse would never leave the client who is having a seizure. The nurse stays with the client, maintaining an open airway and calling for help.
Reference: McKinney, E. S., et al. (2022). *Maternal child nursing* (6th ed., pp. 542, 548–549). Elsevier.

❖ **330.** The nurse admits a client who is bleeding freely from a scalp laceration that resulted from a fall. The nurse would take which action **first** in the care of this wound?
1. Prepare for suturing the area.
2. Determine when client last had a tetanus vaccine.
3. Cleanse the wound by flushing with sterile normal saline.
4. Apply direct pressure to the laceration to stop the bleeding.

Level of Cognitive Ability: Applying
Client Needs: Physiological Integrity
Clinical Judgment/Cognitive Skills: Take Action
Integrated Process: Clinical Judgment; Nursing Process/Implementation
Content Area: Complex Care: Emergency Situations/Management
Health Problems: Adult Health: Neurologic: Head Injury/Trauma
Priority Concepts: Clotting; Tissue Integrity

Answer: 4
Rationale: The initial nursing action is to stop the bleeding, and direct pressure is applied. The nurse will then cleanse the wound thoroughly with sterile normal saline. This action removes dirt or foreign matter in the wound and allows visualization of the size of the wound. If suturing is necessary, the surrounding hair may be shaved per prescription. The date of the client's last tetanus shot is determined, and prophylaxis is given if needed.
Test-Taking Strategy: Note the **strategic word**, *first*, which implies that more than one or all of the options may be partially or totally correct. Focus on **ABCs—airway, breathing, circulation.** This will direct you to the correct option.
Priority Nursing Tip: The nurse must ask the client who sustains a laceration about the date of the last tetanus immunization because the client may need a tetanus injection.
Reference: Ball, J., et al. (2019). *Seidel's Guide to physical examination: An interprofessional approach* (9th ed., p. 636). Elsevier; Lewis, S., et al. (2020). *Medical-surgical nursing: Assessment and management of clinical problems* (11th ed., p. 1311). Elsevier.

331. A client admitted to the nursing unit with a closed head injury 6 hours ago has begun to vomit and reports being dizzy and having a headache. Based on these data, which is the **most important** nursing action?
1. Administering a prescribed antiemetic
2. Having client rate the headache pain on a scale of 1 to 10
3. Notifying the physician of client's condition
4. Reminding client to use the call bell when needing help to the bathroom

Level of Cognitive Ability: Applying
Client Needs: Physiological Integrity
Clinical Judgment/Cognitive Skills: Take Action
Integrated Process: Clinical Judgment; Nursing Process/Implementation
Content Area: Complex Care: Emergency Situations/Management
Health Problems: Adult Health: Neurologic: Head Injury/Trauma
Priority Concepts: Clinical Judgment; Intracranial Regulation

Answer: 3
Rationale: The client with a closed head injury is at risk of developing increased intracranial pressure (ICP). Increased ICP is evidenced by signs and symptoms such as headache, dizziness, confusion, weakness, and vomiting. Because of the implications of the client's manifestations, the most important nursing action is to notify the physician. Although the other nursing actions are not inappropriate, none of them address the critical issue of the potential of the client developing ICP.
Test-Taking Strategy: Note the **strategic words**, *most important*. This directs you to prioritize the possible nursing actions. Considering the client's diagnosis, a closed head injury, and the signs and symptoms, the nurse would suspect increased ICP. The physician needs to be notified.
Priority Nursing Tip: The head of the bed of the client with increased intracranial pressure needs to be elevated 30 to 40 degrees.
Reference: Lewis, S., et al. (2020). *Medical-surgical nursing: Assessment and management of clinical problems* (11th ed., p. 1315). Elsevier.

❖ **332.** A client is brought into the emergency department after sustaining a possible closed head injury. Which assessment would the nurse perform **first**?
  1. Level of consciousness
  2. Pulse and blood pressure
  3. Respiratory rate and depth
  4. Ability to move extremities

Level of Cognitive Ability: Applying
Client Needs: Physiological Integrity
Clinical Judgment/Cognitive Skills: Take Action
Integrated Process: Clinical Judgment; Nursing Process/Implementation
Content Area: Complex Care: Emergency Situations/Management
Health Problems: Adult Health: Neurologic: Head Injury/Trauma
Priority Concepts: Clinical Judgment; Intracranial Regulation

Answer: 3
Rationale: The first action of the nurse is to ensure that the client has an adequate airway and respiratory status. In rapid sequence, the client's circulatory status is evaluated by assessing pulse and blood pressure, followed by evaluation of the status of the cardiovascular and neurologic systems.
Test-Taking Strategy: Note the strategic word, *first.* Use the ABCs—airway, breathing, and circulation. The correct option will most often be the one that deals with the client's airway. Respiratory rate and depth support this action.
Priority Nursing Tip: Complications of a head injury include cerebral bleeding, hematomas, uncontrolled increased intracranial pressure, infections, and seizures.
Reference: Sweet, V., & Foley, P., eds. (2020). *Sheehy's emergency nursing: Principles and practice* (7th ed., p. 407). Elsevier.

333. A client with a spinal cord injury is at risk of developing footdrop. What intervention would the nurse use as a preventive measure?
  1. Moleskin-lined heel protectors
  2. Regular use of posterior splints
  3. Application of pneumatic boots
  4. Avoiding dorsal flexion of the foot

Level of Cognitive Ability: Applying
Client Needs: Physiological Integrity
Clinical Judgment/Cognitive Skills: Take Action
Integrated Process: Clinical Judgment; Nursing Process/Implementation
Content Area: Adult Health: Neurologic
Health Problems: Adult Health: Neurologic: Spinal Cord Injury
Priority Concepts: Clinical Judgment; Mobility

Answer: 2
Rationale: The effective means of preventing footdrop (plantar flexion) is the use of posterior splints or high-top sneakers. Dorsal flexing of the foot would help to counteract the effects of footdrop. Heel protectors protect the skin but do not prevent footdrop. Pneumatic boots prevent deep vein thrombosis but not footdrop.
Test-Taking Strategy: Focus on the subject, preventing footdrop. This guides you to select the option that immobilizes the foot in a functional position while protecting the skin of the extremities.
Priority Nursing Tip: Footdrop is preventable and the nurse needs to be alert to clients at risk for developing footdrop, such as immobile and bedridden clients, and initiate measures to prevent it.
Reference: Lewis, S., et al. (2020). *Medical-surgical nursing: Assessment and management of clinical problems* (11th ed., p. 1459). Elsevier.

❖ **334.** After a cervical spine fracture, this device (**refer to figure**) is placed on the client. The nurse creates a discharge plan for the client to ensure safety and includes which measures? **Select all that apply.**

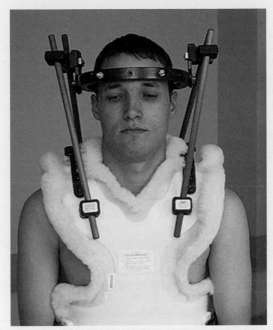

(From Ignatavicius, D., Workman, M. L., & Rebar, C. R. [2018]. *Medical-surgical nursing: Concepts for interprofessional collaborative care* [9th ed.]. Saunders.)

- ❏ 1. Teach the client how to ambulate with a walker.
- ❏ 2. Instruct the client to bend at the waist to pick up needed items.
- ❏ 3. Demonstrate the procedure for scanning the environment for vision.
- ❏ 4. Inform the client about the importance of wearing rubber-soled shoes.
- ❏ 5. Teach the spouse to use the metal frame to assist client to turn in bed.

Level of Cognitive Ability: Creating
Client Needs: Physiological Integrity
Clinical Judgment/Cognitive Skills: Generate Solutions
Integrated Process: Clinical Judgment; Nursing Process/Planning
Content Area: Adult Health: Neurologic
Health Problems: Adult Health: Neurologic: Spinal Cord Injury
Priority Concepts: Clinical Judgment; Safety

Answer: 1, 3, 4
Rationale: The client with a halo fixation device needs to be taught that the use of a walker and rubber-soled shoes may help prevent falls and injury and these are therefore also helpful. It is helpful for the client to scan the environment visually because the client's peripheral vision is diminished from keeping the neck in a stationary position. The client with a halo fixation device needs to avoid bending at the waist because the halo vest is heavy, and the client's trunk is limited in flexibility. The nurse instructs the client and family that the metal frame on the device is never used to move or lift the client because this will disrupt the attachment to the client's skull, which is stabilizing the fracture.
Test-Taking Strategy: Focus on the subject, client instructions for a halo fixation device. Visualize the actions in the options to assist in identifying how injury could be prevented. This will assist in eliminating options 2 and 5.
Priority Nursing Tip: The weight of the halo fixation device can alter the client's balance, and the nurse must teach the client measures that will ensure safety.
Reference: Ignatavicius, D., et al. (2021). *Medical-surgical nursing: Concepts for interprofessional collaborative care* (10th ed., p. 883). Elsevier.

335. To monitor for a temporary but common postsurgical complication of a transsphenoidal resection of the pituitary gland, the nurse would regularly perform which assessment?
1. Pulse rate
2. Temperature
3. Urine output
4. Oxygen saturation

Level of Cognitive Ability: Applying
Client Needs: Physiological Integrity
Clinical Judgment/Cognitive Skills: Take Action
Integrated Process: Clinical Judgment; Nursing Process/Assessment
Content Area: Adult Health: Endocrine
Health Problems: Adult Health: Endocrine: Pituitary Disorders
Priority Concepts: Clinical Judgment; Fluids and Electrolytes

Answer: **3**
Rationale: A common complication of surgery on the pituitary gland is temporary diabetes insipidus. This results from a deficiency in antidiuretic hormone (ADH) secretion as a result of surgical trauma. The nurse measures the client's urine output to determine whether this complication is occurring. Polyuria of 4 to 24 L/day is characteristic of this complication. Options 1, 2, and 4 are not specifically related to a common complication after this surgery.
Test-Taking Strategy: Focus on the subject, transsphenoidal resection of a pituitary adenoma. Recalling that the pituitary gland is responsible for the production of ADH and a deficiency results in diabetes insipidus will direct you to the correct option.
Priority Nursing Tip: After transsphenoidal resection of a pituitary adenoma, monitor the client for postnasal or nasal drainage, which might indicate leakage of cerebrospinal fluid.
Reference: Ignatavicius, D., et al. (2021). *Medical-surgical nursing: Concepts for interprofessional collaborative care* (10th ed., p. 1235). Elsevier.

❖ **336.** Which piece of equipment would the nurse routinely use to assess the fetal heart rate of a client at 16 weeks of gestation?
1. Fetal heart monitor
2. An adult stethoscope
3. Bell of a stethoscope
4. Ultrasound fetoscope

Level of Cognitive Ability: Applying
Client Needs: Physiological Integrity
Clinical Judgment/Cognitive Skills: Take Action
Integrated Process: Nursing Process/Assessment
Content Area: Maternity: Antepartum
Health Problems: N/A
Priority Concepts: Development; Perfusion

Answer: **4**
Rationale: Toward the end of the first trimester, the fetal heart tones can be heard with an ultrasound fetoscope. Options 2 and 3 are not designed to adequately assess the fetal heart rate. A fetal heart monitor is used during labor or in other situations when the fetal heart rate needs continuous monitoring.
Test-Taking Strategy: Focus on the subject, fetal heart assessment. Eliminate options 2 and 3 first because they are comparable or alike. Recalling that a fetal heart monitor is used for continuous monitoring will direct you to the correct option.
Priority Nursing Tip: The normal fetal heart rate is 110 to 160 beats/min.
Reference: McKinney, E. S., et al. (2022). *Maternal child nursing* (6th ed., pp. 336–337). Elsevier.

337. The nurse is creating a discharge plan for a postoperative client who had a unilateral adrenalectomy. What area of instruction would the nurse include in the plan to minimize the client's risk for injury?
1. Teaching client to maintain a diabetic diet
2. Encouraging the adoption of a realistic exercise routine
3. Providing a detailed list of the early signs of a wound infection
4. Explaining the need for lifelong replacement of all adrenal hormones

Level of Cognitive Ability: Creating
Client Needs: Physiological Integrity
Clinical Judgment/Cognitive Skills: Generate Solutions
Integrated Process: Clinical Judgment; Nursing Process/Planning
Content Area: Adult Health: Endocrine
Health Problems: Adult Health: Endocrine: Adrenal Disorders
Priority Concepts: Patient Education; Infection

Answer: **3**
Rationale: A client who had a unilateral adrenalectomy (one adrenal gland was removed) will be placed on corticosteroids temporarily to avoid a cortisol deficiency; lifelong replacement is not necessary. Corticosteroids will be gradually weaned in the postoperative period until they are discontinued. Also, because of the anti-inflammatory properties of corticosteroids produced by the adrenals, clients who undergo an adrenalectomy are at increased risk of developing wound infections. Because of this increased risk of infection, it is important for the client to know measures to prevent infection, early signs of infection, and what to do if an infection seems to be present. The client does not need to maintain a diabetic diet. The importance of regular exercise is not specific to this client.
Test-Taking Strategy: Focus on the subject, unilateral adrenalectomy. Recalling that the hormones from the adrenal glands are needed for proper immune system function will eliminate options 1 and 2. From the remaining options, recalling that one gland can take over the function of two adrenal glands will direct you to the correct option.
Priority Nursing Tip: After adrenalectomy, monitor the client closely for bleeding because the adrenal glands are highly vascular.
Reference: Ignatavicius, D., et al. (2021). *Medical-surgical nursing: Concepts for interprofessional collaborative care* (10th ed., p. 1245). Elsevier.

❖ **338.** The nurse is caring for a client who has undergone transsphenoidal surgery for a pituitary adenoma. In the postoperative period, which information would the nurse provide to the client to minimize the risk for surgery-related injury?
1. Cough and deep breathe hourly.
2. Nasal packing will be removed after 48 hours.
3. Report frequent swallowing or postnasal drip.
4. Acetaminophen is prescribed for severe postsurgical headache.

Level of Cognitive Ability: Applying
Client Needs: Physiological Integrity
Clinical Judgment/Cognitive Skills: Take Action
Integrated Process: Teaching and Learning
Content Area: Adult Health: Neurologic
Health Problems: Adult Health: Endocrine: Pituitary Disorders
Priority Concepts: Patient Education; Intracranial Regulation

Answer: 3
Rationale: The client needs to report frequent swallowing or postnasal drip or nasal drainage after transsphenoidal surgery because it could indicate cerebrospinal fluid (CSF) leakage. The client would deep breathe, but coughing is contraindicated because it could cause increased intracranial pressure. The surgeon removes the nasal packing placed during surgery, usually after 24 hours. The client needs to also report severe headache because it could indicate increased intracranial pressure.
Test-Taking Strategy: Focus on the subject, transsphenoidal surgery. Think about the anatomic location of this surgical procedure. Recalling that the concern is increased intracranial pressure and CSF leakage will direct you to the correct option.
Priority Nursing Tip: After transsphenoidal surgery for a pituitary adenoma, assess nasal drainage for quantity, quality, and the presence of glucose, which indicates that the drainage is cerebrospinal fluid.
Reference: Ignatavicius, D., et al. (2021). *Medical-surgical nursing: Concepts for interprofessional collaborative care* (10th ed., p. 1234). Elsevier.

339. A client is receiving desmopressin intranasally. Which assessment parameters would the nurse monitor to determine the **effectiveness** of this medication?
1. Daily weight
2. Temperature
3. Apical heart rate
4. Pupillary response

Level of Cognitive Ability: Evaluating
Client Needs: Physiological Integrity
Clinical Judgment/Cognitive Skills: Evaluate Outcomes
Integrated Process: Clinical Judgment; Nursing Process/Evaluation
Content Area: Pharmacology: Endocrine: Antidiuretics
Health Problems: Adult Health: Endocrine: Pituitary Disorders
Priority Concepts: Hormonal Regulation; Safety

Answer: 1
Rationale: Desmopressin is an analog of vasopressin (antidiuretic hormone). It is used in the management of diabetes insipidus. The nurse monitors the client's fluid balance to determine the effectiveness of the medication. Fluid status can be evaluated by noting intake and urine output, daily weight, and the presence of edema. The measurements in options 2, 3, and 4 are not related to this medication.
Test-Taking Strategy: Focus on the subject, desmopressin. Note the strategic word, *effectiveness*. Noting the client's diagnosis and recalling the pathophysiology associated with this diagnosis will direct you to the correct option.
Priority Nursing Tip: Monitor the client taking desmopressin for signs of water intoxication (drowsiness, listlessness, shortness of breath, headache), indicating the need to decrease the dosage.
Reference: Ignatavicius, D., et al. (2021). *Medical-surgical nursing: Concepts for interprofessional collaborative care* (10th ed., p. 1236). Elsevier.

❖ **340.** As the nurse begins to administer scheduled doses of furosemide and nifedipine, the client asks for an as needed (PRN) dose of aluminum hydroxide. Which action by the nurse would **best** ensure the **effectiveness** of all the medications?
1. Assess client's immediate need for the antacid.
2. Administer all three medications at the same time.
3. Administer the nifedipine and aluminum hydroxide, then the furosemide 1 hour later.
4. Administer the furosemide and aluminum hydroxide, then the nifedipine 1 hour later.

Level of Cognitive Ability: Analyzing
Client Needs: Physiological Integrity
Clinical Judgment/Cognitive Skills: Take Action
Integrated Process: Clinical Judgment; Nursing Process/Implementation
Content Area: Skills: Medication Administration
Health Problems: N/A
Priority Concepts: Clinical Judgment; Safety

Answer: 1
Rationale: Antacids such as aluminum hydroxide often interfere with the absorption of other medications. For this reason, antacids need to be separated from other medications by at least 1 hour. Because of the diuretic action of the furosemide and the antihypertensive action of the nifedipine, it is important to administer them on time if the client can tolerate waiting for the aluminum hydroxide. The nurse would assess the client to determine the need for the antacid. Therefore, options 2, 3, and 4 are incorrect.
Test-Taking Strategy: Note the strategic words, *best* and *effectiveness*. Recalling that antacids interfere with absorption of other medications will assist in eliminating options 2, 3, and 4. Also recalling that the diuretic and antihypertensive medication need to be administered on time will assist in directing you to the correct option. Additionally, option 1 addresses the first step of the nursing process, assessment.
Priority Nursing Tip: Always check medication interactions before administering medications. Generally, the client should not take an antacid with medication because it will affect the absorption of the medication.
Reference: Ignatavicius, D., et al. (2021). *Medical-surgical nursing: Concepts for interprofessional collaborative care* (10th ed., p. 1097). Elsevier.

341. The nurse monitors the client taking amitriptyline for which common side effect of this antidepressant?
1. Diarrhea
2. Drowsiness
3. Hypertension
4. Increased salivation

Level of Cognitive Ability: Analyzing
Client Needs: Physiological Integrity
Clinical Judgment/Cognitive Skills: Recognize Cues
Integrated Process: Clinical Judgment; Nursing Process/Assessment
Content Area: Pharmacology: Psychotherapeutics: Tricyclic Antidepressants
Health Problems: Mental Health: Mood Disorders
Priority Concepts: Clinical Judgment; Safety

Answer: 2
Rationale: Common side effects of amitriptyline (a tricyclic antidepressant) include the central nervous system effects of drowsiness, fatigue, lethargy, and sedation. Other common side effects include dry mouth or eyes, blurred vision, hypotension, and constipation. The nurse monitors the client for these side effects.
Test-Taking Strategy: Focus on the subject, side effect of amitriptyline. Noting that amitriptyline is an antidepressant will lead you to the correct option.
Priority Nursing Tip: If a tricyclic antidepressant is prescribed, instruct the client to avoid driving or other activities requiring alertness until the response to the medication is known.
Reference: Ignatavicius, D., et al. (2021). *Medical-surgical nursing: Concepts for interprofessional collaborative care* (10th ed., p. 91). Elsevier.

❖ **342.** Which nursing question would elicit the **most** thorough assessment data regarding the client's recent sleeping patterns?
1. "Are you sleeping well at home?"
2. "Did you get much sleep last night?"
3. "May we talk about how you've been sleeping?"
4. "Do you think you get enough sleep on a nightly basis?"

Level of Cognitive Ability: Analyzing
Client Needs: Physiological Integrity
Clinical Judgment/Cognitive Skills: Analyze Cues
Integrated Process: Clinical Judgment; Nursing Process/Analysis
Content Area: Foundations of Care: Sleep and Rest
Health Problems: N/A
Priority Concepts: Clinical Judgment; Communication

Answer: 3
Rationale: Option 3 is a question and provides the client the opportunity to express thoughts and feelings. The remaining options could lead to a one-word answer that would not provide thorough assessment data. Additionally, 1 night of sleep may not tell the nurse how the pattern has been over time. Anyone may or may not sleep well for one night, and that sleep or loss of sleep does not indicate a problem.
Test-Taking Strategy: Focus on the subject, therapeutic communication during a sleeping pattern assessment. Note the strategic word, *most.* Use therapeutic communication techniques. Select the option that is open-ended and allows the client to take the lead in the conversation. This will direct you to the correct option.
Priority Nursing Tip: Sleep patterns tend to change as a person ages. Older people find they have a harder time falling asleep and wake up more often during the night and earlier in the morning.
Reference: Potter, P., et al. (2021). *Fundamentals of nursing* (10th ed., pp. 333–335, 1047). Elsevier.

343. A client is admitted after attempting suicide by ingesting a prescribed antipsychotic medication. What is the **most important** piece of information the nurse would obtain **initially?**
1. Where and when the medication was ingested
2. The name and amount of ingested medication
3. If client continues to have suicidal ideations
4. If there is a history of previous suicidal attempts

Level of Cognitive Ability: Analyzing
Client Needs: Physiological Integrity
Clinical Judgment/Cognitive Skills: Recognize Cues
Integrated Process: Clinical Judgment; Nursing Process/Assessment
Content Area: Complex Care: Emergency Situations/Management
Health Problems: Mental Health: Suicide
Priority Concepts: Clinical Judgment; Safety

Answer: 2
Rationale: In an emergency, lifesaving facts are obtained first. The name of and the amount of medication ingested is of utmost importance in treating this potentially life-threatening situation. The remaining data can be assessed once the client's physical condition is stabilized.
Test-Taking Strategy: Note the strategic words, *most important* and *initially.* Lifesaving treatment cannot begin until the medication and dosage amount are identified.
Priority Nursing Tip: Extrapyramidal side effects can occur in the client taking an antipsychotic medication.
References: Sweet, V., & Foley, P., eds. (2020). *Sheehy's emergency nursing: Principles and practice* (7th ed., p. 399). Elsevier; Varcarolis, E., & Fosbre, C. (2021). *Essentials of psychiatric mental health nursing: A communication approach to evidence-based care* (4th ed., p. 370). Elsevier.

❖ **344.** The nurse determines that a client understands the purpose of a phytonadione injection for the newborn when the client is heard making which statement to the partner?
1. "The baby's liver cannot produce that vitamin."
2. "Most newborns need a supplement of this vitamin."
3. "All newborns lack intestinal bacteria to produce this vitamin."
4. "It's unusual but our baby lack's the vitamin that helps the blood to clot."

Level of Cognitive Ability: Evaluating
Client Needs: Physiological Integrity
Clinical Judgment/Cognitive Skills: Evaluate Outcomes
Integrated Process: Teaching and Learning
Content Area: Pharmacology: Maternity/Newborn: Vitamin K
Health Problems: N/A
Priority Concepts: Clotting; Development

Answer: 3
Rationale: The absence of normal flora needed to synthesize vitamin K (phytonadione) in the normal newborn gut results in low levels of vitamin K and creates a transient blood coagulation deficiency between the second and fifth day of life. From a low point at about 2 to 3 days after birth, these coagulation factors rise slowly but do not approach normal adult levels until 9 months of age or later. Increasing levels of these vitamin K–dependent factors indicate a response to dietary intake and bacterial colonization of the intestines. An injection is administered prophylactically on the day of birth to combat the deficiency. Options 1, 2, and 4 are incorrect.
Test-Taking Strategy: Focus on the subject, the purpose of administering phytonadione injection to a newborn. Recalling the physiology associated with the synthesis of phytonadione in the newborn will direct you to the correct option.
Priority Nursing Tip: In the newborn, phytonadione (vitamin K) is administered in the lateral aspect of the middle third of the vastus lateralis muscle of the thigh.
Reference: McKinney, E. S., et al. (2022). *Maternal child nursing* (6th ed., p. 469). Elsevier.

345. The nurse is assigned to give a child a tepid tub bath to treat hyperthermia. After the bath, which action would the nurse take?
 1. Leave the child uncovered for 15 minutes.
 2. Assist the child to put on a cotton sleep shirt.
 3. Take the child's axillary temperature in 2 hours.
 4. Place the child in bed and cover the child with a blanket.

Level of Cognitive Ability: Applying
Client Needs: Physiological Integrity
Clinical Judgment/Cognitive Skills: Take Action
Integrated Process: Clinical Judgment; Nursing Process/Implementation
Content Area: Pediatrics: Metabolic/Endocrine
Health Problems: Pediatric-Specific: Fever
Priority Concepts: Clinical Judgment; Thermoregulation

Answer: 2
Rationale: Cotton is a lightweight material that will protect the child from becoming chilled after the bath. Option 1 is incorrect because the child should not be left uncovered. Option 3 is incorrect because the child's temperature needs to be reassessed a half hour after the bath. Option 4 is incorrect because a blanket is heavy and may increase the child's body temperature and further increase metabolism.
Test-Taking Strategy: Focus on the subject, to treat hyperthermia. Eliminate option 1 because of the word "uncovered." Eliminate option 3 because of the time frame. Eliminate option 4 because of the word "blanket."
Priority Nursing Tip: Aspirin (acetylsalicylic acid) should not be administered to a child unless specifically prescribed because of the risk of Reye's syndrome.
Reference: Hockenberry, M., Wilson, D., & Rodgers, C. (2019). *Wong's Nursing care of infants and children* (11th ed., p. 694). Elsevier.

❖ **346.** The nurse caring for an infant demonstrating diarrhea would monitor the infant for which **early** sign of dehydration?
 1. Cool extremities
 2. Gray, mottled skin
 3. Capillary refill of 3 seconds
 4. Apical pulse rate of 200 beats/min

Level of Cognitive Ability: Analyzing
Client Needs: Physiological Integrity
Clinical Judgment/Cognitive Skills: Recognize Cues
Integrated Process: Clinical Judgment; Nursing Process/Assessment
Content Area: Pediatrics: Metabolic/Endocrine
Health Problems: Pediatric-Specific: Dehydration
Priority Concepts: Development; Fluids and Electrolytes

Answer: 4
Rationale: Dehydration causes interstitial fluid to shift to the vascular compartment in an attempt to maintain fluid volume. When the body is unable to compensate for fluid lost, circulatory failure occurs. The blood pressure will decrease and the pulse rate will increase. This will be followed by peripheral symptoms. Options 1, 2, and 3 are not early signs, and these assessment findings relate to peripheral circulatory status.
Test-Taking Strategy: Note the strategic word, *early,* and think about the physiology that occurs in dehydration. Also note that options 1, 2, and 3 are comparable or alike and relate directly to peripheral circulatory status.
Priority Nursing Tip: Acute diarrhea is a cause of dehydration, particularly in children younger than 5 years.
Reference: Hockenberry, M., Wilson, D., & Rodgers, C. (2019). *Wong's Nursing care of infants and children* (11th ed., pp. 831, 835). Elsevier.

347. Acetylsalicylic acid (aspirin) is prescribed for a client diagnosed with coronary artery disease before a percutaneous transluminal coronary angioplasty (PTCA). The nurse administers the medication understanding that it is prescribed for what purpose?
1. Relieve postprocedure pain.
2. Prevent thrombus formation.
3. Prevent postprocedure hyperthermia.
4. Prevent inflammation of the puncture site.

Level of Cognitive Ability: Applying
Client Needs: Physiological Integrity
Clinical Judgment/Cognitive Skills: Take Action
Integrated Process: Clinical Judgment; Nursing Process/Implementation
Content Area: Pharmacology: Cardiovascular: Antiplatelets
Health Problems: Adult Health: Cardiovascular: Coronary Artery Disease
Priority Concepts: Clotting; Perfusion

Answer: 2
Rationale: Before PTCA, the client is usually given an anticoagulant, commonly aspirin, to help reduce the risk of occlusion of the artery during the procedure because the aspirin inhibits platelet aggregation. Options 1, 3, and 4 are unrelated to the purpose of administering aspirin to this client.
Test-Taking Strategy: Focus on the subject, aspirin prescribed to a client before percutaneous transluminal coronary angioplasty (PTCA). Think about the potential complications of a PTCA and the action and properties of aspirin to direct you to the correct option.
Priority Nursing Tip: A daily dose of acetylsalicylic acid (aspirin) may be prescribed after percutaneous transluminal coronary angioplasty because of its antiplatelet aggregation properties.
Reference: Ignatavicius, D., et al. (2021). *Medical-surgical nursing: Concepts for interprofessional collaborative care* (10th ed., pp. 759, 761–762). Elsevier.

❖ **348.** The nurse reviews a physician's prescriptions and notes that a topical nitrate is prescribed. The nurse notes that acetaminophen is prescribed to be administered before the nitrate. The nurse implements the prescription with which understanding about why acetaminophen is prescribed?
1. Headache is a common side effect of nitrates.
2. Fever usually accompanies myocardial infarction.
3. Acetaminophen potentiates the therapeutic effect of nitrates.
4. Acetaminophen does not interfere with platelet action as acetylsalicylic acid (aspirin) does.

Level of Cognitive Ability: Applying
Client Needs: Physiological Integrity
Clinical Judgment/Cognitive Skills: Take Action
Integrated Process: Clinical Judgment; Nursing Process/Implementation
Content Area: Pharmacology: Cardiovascular: Vasodilators
Health Problems: Adult Health: Cardiovascular: Coronary Artery Disease
Priority Concepts: Clinical Judgment; Safety

Answer: 1
Rationale: Headache occurs as a side effect of nitrates in many clients. Acetaminophen may be administered before nitrates to prevent headaches or minimize the discomfort from the headaches. Options 2, 3, and 4 are incorrect.
Test-Taking Strategy: Focus on the subject, nitrate administration. Eliminate option 3 first because this is an incorrect statement. Whereas options 2 and 4 are true statements, they do not address the subject of the question. Also recalling that headache is a common side effect of nitrates will direct you to the correct option.
Priority Nursing Tip: Nitrates produce vasodilation, which can cause a headache. Although headaches are a common side effect of nitrates, they may become less frequent with continued use.
Reference: Ignatavicius, D., et al. (2021). *Medical-surgical nursing: Concepts for interprofessional collaborative care* (10th ed., pp. 758–759). Elsevier.

349. The nurse performs an assessment on a client newly diagnosed with rheumatoid arthritis. The nurse expects to note which **early** manifestations of the disease? **Select all that apply.**
- ❏ 1. Fatigue
- ❏ 2. Anorexia
- ❏ 3. Weakness
- ❏ 4. Low-grade fever
- ❏ 5. Joint deformities
- ❏ 6. Joint inflammation

Level of Cognitive Ability: Analyzing
Client Needs: Physiological Integrity
Clinical Judgment/Cognitive Skills: Recognize Cues
Integrated Process: Clinical Judgment; Nursing Process/Assessment
Content Area: Adult Health: Musculoskeletal
Health Problems: Adult Health: Musculoskeletal: Rheumatoid Arthritis and Osteoarthritis
Priority Concepts: Functional Ability; Mobility

Answer: 1, 2, 3, 4, 6
Rationale: Rheumatoid arthritis is a chronic, progressive, systemic inflammatory autoimmune disease process that primarily affects the synovial joints. It also affects other joints and body tissues. Early manifestations include fatigue, anorexia, weakness, joint inflammation, low-grade fever, and paresthesia. Joint deformities are late manifestations.
Test-Taking Strategy: Focus on the subject, manifestations of rheumatoid arthritis and note the strategic word, *early*. Keeping this word in mind will assist in eliminating option 5, because joint deformities are late manifestations.
Priority Nursing Tip: For rheumatoid arthritis, the earlier the treatment is begun, the slower the progression of the disease. Treatment includes exercise, physical therapy, medications, and possibly surgery.
Reference: Ignatavicius, D., et al. (2021). *Medical-surgical nursing: Concepts for interprofessional collaborative care* (10th ed., p. 1018). Elsevier.

❖ **350.** A client with a history of myocardial infarction is prescribed warfarin sodium has been instructed to limit the intake of foods high in vitamin K. The nurse determines that the client understands the instructions if the client indicates that which food items need to be avoided? **Select all that apply.**
- ❏ 1. Tea
- ❏ 2. Turnips
- ❏ 3. Oranges
- ❏ 4. Cabbage
- ❏ 5. Broccoli
- ❏ 6. Strawberries

Level of Cognitive Ability: Evaluating
Client Needs: Physiological Integrity
Clinical Judgment/Cognitive Skills: Evaluate Outcomes
Integrated Process: Clinical Judgment; Nursing Process/Evaluation
Content Area: Pharmacology: Cardiovascular: Anticoagulants
Health Problems: Adult Health: Cardiovascular: Myocardial Infarction
Priority Concepts: Clotting; Nutrition

Answer: 1, 2, 4, 5
Rationale: Warfarin sodium is an anticoagulant that interferes with the hepatic synthesis of vitamin K–dependent clotting factors. The client is instructed to limit the intake of foods high in vitamin K while taking this medication. These foods include coffee or tea (caffeine), turnips, cabbage, broccoli, greens, fish, and liver. Oranges and strawberries are high in vitamin C.
Test-Taking Strategy: Focus on the subject, foods high in vitamin K. Knowledge regarding the foods high in vitamin K is needed to answer correctly. However, note that options 3 and 6 are comparable or alike in that they are both fruits.
Priority Nursing Tip: Warfarin sodium is an anticoagulant and bleeding is a concern when this medication is administered.
References: Ignatavicius, D., et al. (2021). *Medical-surgical nursing: Concepts for interprofessional collaborative care* (10th ed., p. 726). Elsevier; Nix, S. (2022). *Williams' basic nutrition and diet therapy* (16th ed., p. 93). Elsevier.

351. The nurse is caring for a newly delivered infant who is breast-/chest-feeding. Which nursing intervention would **best** prevent jaundice in this infant?
1. Placing the infant under phototherapy
2. Keeping the infant NPO until the second period of reactivity
3. Encouraging the parent to breast-/chest-feed the infant every 2 to 3 hours
4. Encouraging the parent to supplement breast-/chest-feeding with formula

Level of Cognitive Ability: Applying
Client Needs: Physiological Integrity
Clinical Judgment/Cognitive Skills: Take Action
Integrated Process: Teaching and Learning
Content Area: Maternity: Newborn
Health Problems: Newborn: Hyperbilirubinemia
Priority Concepts: Development; Safety

Answer: 3
Rationale: To help prevent jaundice, the parent should feed the infant frequently in the immediate birth period because colostrum is a natural laxative and helps promote the passage of meconium. Breast-/chest-feeding should begin as soon as possible after birth while the infant is in the first period of reactivity. Delaying feeding decreases the production of prolactin, which decreases the parent's milk production. Phototherapy requires a primary health care provider's prescription and is not implemented until bilirubin levels are 12 mg/dL (204 mcmol/L) or higher in the healthy term infant. Offering the infant a formula supplement will cause nipple confusion and decrease the amount of milk produced by the parent.
Test-Taking Strategy: Focus on the subject, newborn jaundice. Recalling the physiology associated with jaundice and noting the strategic word, *best*, will assist in eliminating options 1 and 2. From the remaining options, select the correct option based on the fact that offering a formula supplement will cause nipple confusion.
Priority Nursing Tip: The appearance of jaundice in the first 24 hours of life is abnormal and must be reported to the primary health care provider.
Reference: McKinney, E. S., et al. (2022). *Maternal child nursing* (6th ed., pp. 438, 651). Elsevier.

352. The nurse creates a postoperative plan of care for a client undergoing an arthroscopy. The nurse would include which **priority** action in the plan?
1. Monitor intake and output.
2. Assess the tissue at the surgical site.
3. Monitor the area for numbness or tingling.
4. Assess the complete blood cell count results.

Level of Cognitive Ability: Creating
Client Needs: Physiological Integrity
Clinical Judgment/Cognitive Skills: Prioritize Hypotheses
Integrated Process: Clinical Judgment; Nursing Process/Planning
Content Area: Foundations of Care: Diagnostic Tests
Health Problems: Adult Health: Musculoskeletal: Rheumatoid Arthritis and Osteoarthritis
Priority Concepts: Perfusion; Safety

Answer: 3
Rationale: Arthroscopy provides an endoscopic examination of the joint and is used to diagnose and treat acute and chronic disorders of the joint. The priority nursing action is to monitor the affected area for numbness or tingling. Options 1, 2, and 4 are also components of postoperative care, but from the options presented, they are not the initial priorities.
Test-Taking Strategy: Note the strategic word, *priority*. Use the ABCs—airway, breathing, and circulation—to answer the question. The correct option relates to circulation.
Priority Nursing Tip: Assessment of neurovascular status of an extremity includes checking distal pulses, capillary refill, warmth, presence of pain, color, movement, and sensation.
Reference: Ignatavicius, D., et al. (2021). *Medical-surgical nursing: Concepts for interprofessional collaborative care* (10th ed., pp. 981–982). Elsevier.

353. The nurse is caring for a client diagnosed with active tuberculosis who is prescribed rifampin therapy. The nurse instructs the client to expect which side effect of this medication?
1. Green urine
2. Yellow sclera
3. Orange secretions
4. Clay-colored stools

Level of Cognitive Ability: Applying
Client Needs: Physiological Integrity
Clinical Judgment/Cognitive Skills: Take Action
Integrated Process: Teaching and Learning
Content Area: Pharmacology: Respiratory: Tuberculosis Medications
Health Problems: Adult Health: Respiratory: Tuberculosis
Priority Concepts: Patient Education; Safety

Answer: 3
Rationale: Rifampin is an antituberculosis medication. Secretions will become orange as a result of the rifampin. The client needs to be instructed that this side effect will likely occur and needs to be told that soft contact lenses, if used by the client, will become permanently discolored. Options 1, 2, and 4 are not expected effects.
Test-Taking Strategy: Focus on the **subject**, an expected side effect of rifampin. Eliminate options 1, 2, and 4 because they are **comparable or alike** in that they are all symptoms of intrahepatic obstruction as seen in viral hepatitis.
Priority Nursing Tip: Rifampin is hepatotoxic and the client needs to notify the physician if jaundice (yellow eyes or skin) occurs.
Reference: Ignatavicius, D., et al. (2021). *Medical-surgical nursing: Concepts for interprofessional collaborative care* (10th ed., p. 579). Elsevier.

❖ **354.** The nurse sends a sputum specimen to the laboratory for culture from a client with suspected active tuberculosis (TB). The results report that *Mycobacterium tuberculosis* is cultured. How would the nurse correctly analyze these results?
1. The results are positive for active tuberculosis.
2. The results indicate a less virulent strain of tuberculosis.
3. The results are inconclusive until a repeat sputum specimen is sent.
4. The results are unreliable unless the client has also had a positive tuberculin skin test (TST).

Level of Cognitive Ability: Analyzing
Client Needs: Physiological Integrity
Clinical Judgment/Cognitive Skills: Analyze Cues
Integrated Process: Clinical Judgment; Nursing Process/Analysis
Content Area: Adult Health: Respiratory
Health Problems: Adult Health: Respiratory: Tuberculosis
Priority Concepts: Clinical Judgment; Infection

Answer: 1
Rationale: Culture of *Mycobacterium tuberculosis* from sputum or other body secretions or tissue confirms the diagnosis of active tuberculosis. Options 2 and 3 are incorrect statements. The TST test is performed to assist in diagnosing TB but does not confirm active disease.
Test-Taking Strategy: Focus on the **subject**, tuberculosis. Recall that culture of the bacteria from sputum confirms the diagnosis. Because tuberculosis affects the respiratory system, it would make sense that the bacteria would be found in the sputum if the client had active disease, thereby confirming the diagnosis.
Priority Nursing Tip: The client with active tuberculosis is placed in respiratory isolation precautions in a negative-pressure room.
Reference: Ignatavicius, D., et al. (2021). *Medical-surgical nursing: Concepts for interprofessional collaborative care* (10th ed., pp. 332, 575). Elsevier.

355. A coronary care unit (CCU) nurse is caring for a client admitted with acute myocardial infarction (MI). The nurse would monitor the client for which **most** common complication of MI?
1. Heart failure
2. Cardiogenic shock
3. Cardiac dysrhythmias
4. Recurrent myocardial infarction

Level of Cognitive Ability: Analyzing
Client Needs: Physiological Integrity
Clinical Judgment/Cognitive Skills: Recognize Cues
Integrated Process: Clinical Judgment; Nursing Process/Assessment
Content Area: Complex Care: Emergency Situations/Management
Health Problems: Adult Health: Cardiovascular: Myocardial Infarction
Priority Concepts: Clinical Judgment; Perfusion

Answer: 3
Rationale: Dysrhythmias are the most common complication and cause of death after an MI. Heart failure, cardiogenic shock, and recurrent MI are also complications but occur less frequently.
Test-Taking Strategy: Note the strategic word, *most*. Think about the pathophysiology associated with MI and the complications of MI to direct you to the correct option.
Priority Nursing Tip: Administering morphine sulfate as prescribed is a priority in managing pain in the client having a myocardial infarction. Pain relief increases oxygen supply to the myocardium.
Reference: Lewis, S., et al. (2020). *Medical-surgical nursing: Assessment and management of clinical problems* (11th ed., p. 720). Elsevier.

356. The nurse in the newborn nursery is planning for the admission of a large for gestational age (LGA) infant whose birthing parent is diabetic. In planning care for this infant, the nurse would obtain equipment to perform which diagnostic test?
1. Serum insulin level
2. Heel-stick blood glucose
3. Rh and ABO blood typing
4. Indirect and direct bilirubin levels

Level of Cognitive Ability: Applying
Client Needs: Physiological Integrity
Clinical Judgment/Cognitive Skills: Generate Solutions
Integrated Process: Clinical Judgment; Nursing Process/Planning
Content Area: Maternity: Newborn
Health Problems: Newborn: Newborn of a Diabetic Mother
Priority Concepts: Development; Glucose Regulation

Answer: 2
Rationale: After birth, the most common problem in the LGA infant is hypoglycemia, especially if the birthing parent is diabetic. At delivery when the umbilical cord is clamped and cut, the birthing parent's blood glucose supply is lost. The newborn continues to produce large amounts of insulin, which deplete the infant's blood glucose within the first hours after birth. If immediate identification and treatment of hypoglycemia are not performed, the newborn may suffer central nervous system damage caused by inadequate circulation of glucose to the brain. Serum insulin levels are not helpful because there is no intervention to decrease these levels to prevent hypoglycemia. There is no rationale for prescribing an Rh and ABO blood type unless the birthing parent's blood type is O or Rh negative. Indirect and direct bilirubin levels are usually prescribed after the first 24 hours because jaundice is usually seen at 48 to 72 hours after birth.
Test-Taking Strategy: Focus on the subject, an LGA infant. Recalling that hypoglycemia is the concern will direct you to the correct option.
Priority Nursing Tip: Feedings need to be provided to the LGA newborn soon after birth because of the risk for hypoglycemia in the infant.
Reference: McKinney, E. S., et al. (2022). *Maternal child nursing* (6th ed., pp. 456, 643). Elsevier.

357. The nurse caring for a client receiving intravenous (IV) therapy monitors for which signs of infiltration of an IV infusion? **Select all that apply.**
- ❑ 1. Slowing of the IV rate
- ❑ 2. Tenderness at the insertion site
- ❑ 3. Edema around the insertion site
- ❑ 4. Skin tightness at the insertion site
- ❑ 5. Warmth of skin at the insertion site
- ❑ 6. Fluid leaking from the insertion site

Level of Cognitive Ability: Analyzing
Client Needs: Physiological Integrity
Clinical Judgment/Cognitive Skills: Recognize Cues
Integrated Process: Clinical Judgment; Nursing Process/Assessment
Content Area: Skills: Medication Administration
Health Problems: N/A
Priority Concepts: Tissue Integrity; Safety

Answer: 1, 2, 3, 4, 6
Rationale: Infiltration is the leakage of an IV solution into the extravascular tissue. Manifestations include slowing of the IV rate; burning, tenderness, or general discomfort at the insertion site; increasing edema in or around the catheter insertion site; complaints of skin tightness; blanching or coolness of the skin; and fluid leaking from the insertion site.
Test-Taking Strategy: Focus on the subject, IV infiltration. Read each option, thinking about the characteristics of infiltration. Recalling that infiltration is the leakage of an IV solution into the extravascular tissue will assist in eliminating option 5. Remember that fluid infusing into tissue will result in coolness, not warmth.
Priority Nursing Tip: Infiltration at an IV site produces coolness of the skin, whereas phlebitis at an intravenous site produces warmth of the skin.
Reference: Ignatavicius, D., et al. (2021). *Medical-surgical nursing: Concepts for interprofessional collaborative care* (10th ed., pp. 277, 294). Elsevier.

❖ **358.** A client receiving total parenteral nutrition (TPN) through a subclavian catheter suddenly develops dyspnea, tachycardia, cyanosis, and decreased level of consciousness. Based on these findings, which is the **best** intervention for the nurse to take for the client?
1. Obtain a stat oxygen saturation level.
2. Examine the insertion site for redness.
3. Perform a stat finger-stick glucose level.
4. Turn client to the left side in Trendelenburg's position.

Level of Cognitive Ability: Analyzing
Client Needs: Physiological Integrity
Clinical Judgment/Cognitive Skills: Take Action
Integrated Process: Clinical Judgment; Nursing Process/Implementation
Content Area: Complex Care: Emergency Situations/Management
Health Problems: Adult Health: Respiratory: Pulmonary Embolism
Priority Concepts: Gas Exchange; Perfusion

Answer: 4
Rationale: Clinical indicators of air embolism include chest pain, tachycardia, dyspnea, anxiety, feelings of impending doom, cyanosis, and hypotension. Positioning the client in Trendelenburg's and on the left side helps isolate the air embolism in the right atrium and prevents a thromboembolic event in a vital organ. Monitoring the oxygen saturation is a reasonable nursing response to the client's condition; however, acting to prevent deterioration in the client's condition is more important than obtaining additional client data. Options 2 and 3 are unrelated to the symptoms identified in the question.
Test-Taking Strategy: Focus on the subject, air embolism, and note the strategic word, *best*. Note the assessment findings in the question and recall that the signs of air embolism are similar to those experienced with pulmonary embolism. Then analyze the options to determine the action that is the best in this situation, which will direct you to the correct option.
Priority Nursing Tip: Measures that prevent air embolism from an intravenous (IV) infusion include priming the tubing with fluid before use, securing all connections, and replacing the IV fluid before the container is empty.
Reference: Ignatavicius, D., et al. (2021). *Medical-surgical nursing: Concepts for interprofessional collaborative care* (10th ed., p. 291). Elsevier.

359. The physician orders a serum calcium level on a client and the nurse reviews the test result. Based on the test result, which clinical manifestations would the nurse expect to note on assessment of the client? **Select all that apply.**

Laboratory Results

Test and Result	Reference Range
Calcium 7.5 mg/dL (1.88 mmol/L)	9–10.5 mg/dL (2.25–2.75 mmol/L)

❑ 1. Constipation
❑ 2. Muscle twitches
❑ 3. Negative Chvostek's sign
❑ 4. Positive Trousseau's sign
❑ 5. Hyperactive deep tendon reflexes
❑ 6. Prolonged ST interval on electrocardiogram (ECG)

Level of Cognitive Ability: Analyzing
Client Needs: Physiological Integrity
Clinical Judgment/Cognitive Skills: Recognize Cues
Integrated Process: Clinical Judgment; Nursing Process/Assessment
Content Area: Foundations of Care: Fluids and Electrolytes
Health Problems: N/A
Priority Concepts: Clinical Judgment; Fluids and Electrolytes

Answer: **2, 4, 5, 6**
Rationale: Hypocalcemia is a total serum calcium level less than 9 mg/dL (2.25 mmol/L). Clinical manifestations of hypocalcemia include decreased heart rate, diminished peripheral pulses, hypotension, and prolonged ST interval and QT interval on ECG. Neuromuscular manifestations include anxiety and irritability; paresthesia followed by numbness; muscle twitches, cramps, tetany, and seizures; hyperactive deep tendon reflexes; and positive Trousseau's and Chvostek's signs. Gastrointestinal manifestations include increased gastric motility, hyperactive bowel sounds, abdominal cramping, and diarrhea.
Test-Taking Strategy: Focus on the subject, hypocalcemia. Note the data in the question and the calcium level. First determine that the level is low and the client is experiencing hypocalcemia. Next think about the manifestations associated with hypocalcemia. Remember that hyperactive bowel sounds and diarrhea occur in hypocalcemia.
Priority Nursing Tip: Calcium gluconate 10% may be prescribed to treat acute calcium deficit.
Reference: Ignatavicius, D., et al. (2021). *Medical-surgical nursing: Concepts for interprofessional collaborative care* (10th ed., pp. 256–257). Elsevier.

360. A client is experiencing acute cardiac and cerebral symptoms as a result of excess fluid volume. Which measure would the nurse implement to increase the client's comfort until specific therapy is prescribed by the physician?
1. Cover the client with warm blankets.
2. Minimize visual and auditory stimuli present.
3. Elevate the client's head to at least 45 degrees.
4. Initiate oxygen at 4 L/min by nasal cannula.

Level of Cognitive Ability: Applying
Client Needs: Physiological Integrity
Clinical Judgment/Cognitive Skills: Take Action
Integrated Process: Clinical Judgment; Nursing Process/Implementation
Content Area: Complex Care: Emergency Situations/Management
Health Problems: Adult Health: Cardiovascular: Heart Failure
Priority Concepts: Caregiving; Perfusion

Answer: **3**
Rationale: Elevating the head of the bed to 45 degrees decreases venous return to the heart from the lower body, thus reducing the volume of blood that has to be pumped by the heart. It also promotes venous drainage from the brain, reducing cerebral symptoms. Oxygen is a medication and is not initiated at 4 L without a prescription to do so. Options 1 and 2 are not related to this scenario.
Test-Taking Strategy: Focus on the subject, measures to increase the client's comfort. This tells you that the correct option is one that directly involves care delivery to the client. With this in mind, eliminate options 1 and 2 because they are not associated with the condition of the client. From the remaining options, note that the correct option identifies a nursing measure.
Priority Nursing Tip: A client with kidney failure is at high risk for fluid volume excess.
Reference: Lewis, S., et al. (2020). *Medical-surgical nursing: Assessment and management of clinical problems* (11th ed., pp. 742, 744). Elsevier.

361. The nurse creates a discharge plan for a client who had an abdominal hysterectomy. Which activity instructions would the nurse include in the plan? **Select all that apply.**
❑ **1.** Avoid heavy lifting.
❑ **2.** Sit as much as possible.
❑ **3.** Take baths rather than showers.
❑ **4.** Limit stair climbing to five times a day.
❑ **5.** Gradually increase walking as exercise, but stop before becoming fatigued.
❑ **6.** Avoid jogging, aerobic exercises, sports, or any strenuous exercise for 6 weeks.

Level of Cognitive Ability: Creating
Client Needs: Physiological Integrity
Clinical Judgment/Cognitive Skills: Generate Solutions
Integrated Process: Clinical Judgment; Nursing Process/Planning
Content Area: Adult Health: Reproductive
Health Problems: N/A
Priority Concepts: Patient Education; Safety

Answer: 1, 4, 5, 6
Rationale: After abdominal hysterectomy, the client needs to avoid lifting anything that is heavy and limit stair climbing to five times a day. The client should walk indoors for the first week and then gradually increase walking as exercise, but stop before becoming fatigued. The client needs to avoid jogging, aerobic exercises, sports, or any strenuous exercise for 6 weeks. The client is also told to avoid the sitting position for extended periods, to take showers rather than tub baths, avoid crossing the legs at the knees, and avoid driving for at least 4 weeks or until the surgeon has given permission to do so.
Test-Taking Strategy: Focus on the subject, activity instructions after abdominal hysterectomy. Read each option carefully, focusing on the type and location of the surgery and the importance of protecting the surgical area. This will assist in eliminating options 2 and 3.
Priority Nursing Tip: Monitor vaginal bleeding after hysterectomy. More than one saturated pad per hour may indicate excessive bleeding.
Reference: Ignatavicius, D., et al. (2021). *Medical-surgical nursing: Concepts for interprofessional collaborative care* (10th ed., p. 1457). Elsevier.

❖ **362.** The nurse has a prescription to ambulate a client with a nephrostomy tube four times a day. The nurse determines that the safest way to ambulate the client while maintaining the integrity of the nephrostomy tube is to implement which intervention?
1. Change the drainage bag to a leg collection bag.
2. Tie the drainage bag to the client's waist while ambulating.
3. Use a walker to hang the drainage bag from while ambulating.
4. Tell client to hold the drainage bag higher than the level of the bladder.

Level of Cognitive Ability: Applying
Client Needs: Physiological Integrity
Clinical Judgment/Cognitive Skills: Generate Solutions
Integrated Process: Clinical Judgment; Nursing Process/Planning
Content Area: Skills: Tube Care
Health Problems: Adult Health: Renal and Urinary: Urinary Tract Inflammation/Infection/Trauma
Priority Concepts: Elimination; Safety

Answer: 1
Rationale: The safest approach to protect the integrity and safety of the nephrostomy tube with a mobile client is to attach the tube to a leg collection bag. This allows for greater freedom of movement, while preventing accidental disconnection or dislodgment. The drainage bag is kept below the level of the bladder. Option 3 presents the risk of tension or pulling on the nephrostomy tube by the client during ambulation.
Test-Taking Strategy: Focus on the subject, safety in regard to a nephrostomy tube. Note that options 2, 3, and 4 are comparable or alike because they all indicate placing the drainage bag above the level of the bladder.
Priority Nursing Tip: The total bladder capacity for an adult is 600 to 800 mL, and the normal urine output is 1500 to 2000 mL/day.
Reference: Potter, P., et al. (2021). *Fundamentals of nursing* (10th ed., p. 1188). Elsevier.

363. A client newly diagnosed with polycystic kidney disease asks the nurse to explain again what the **most** serious complication of the disorder might be. The nurse would provide the client with information concerning which condition?
  1. Diabetes insipidus
  2. End-stage renal disease (ESRD)
  3. Chronic urinary tract infection (UTI)
  4. Syndrome of inappropriate antidiuretic hormone (SIADH) secretion

Level of Cognitive Ability: Applying
Client Needs: Physiological Integrity
Clinical Judgment/Cognitive Skills: Take Action
Integrated Process: Teaching and Learning
Content Area: Adult Health: Renal and Urinary
Health Problems: Adult Health: Renal and Urinary: Polycystic Kidney Disease
Priority Concepts: Patient Education; Elimination

Answer: 2
Rationale: In polycystic kidney disease, cystic formation and hypertrophy of the kidneys occur. The most serious complication of polycystic kidney disease is ESRD, which is managed with dialysis or transplant. There is no reliable way to predict who will ultimately progress to ESRD. Chronic UTIs are the most common complication because of the altered anatomy of the kidney and from development of resistant strains of bacteria. Diabetes insipidus and SIADH secretion are unrelated disorders.
Test-Taking Strategy: Note the strategic word, *most*. Also noting the words "end-stage" and recalling that ESRD is life threatening and requires dialysis for treatment will direct you to the correct option.
Priority Nursing Tip: The nurse should discuss the importance of seeking genetic counseling with the client diagnosed with polycystic kidney disease because the disease is hereditary.
Reference: Lewis, S., et al. (2020). *Medical-surgical nursing: Assessment and management of clinical problems* (11th ed., pp. 1041–1042). Elsevier.

❖ **364.** The nurse is creating a plan of care for a client who has returned to the nursing unit after left nephrectomy. Which assessments would the nurse include in the plan of care? **Select all that apply.**
  ❑ 1. Pain level
  ❑ 2. Vital signs
  ❑ 3. Hourly urine output
  ❑ 4. Tolerance for food and fluid intake
  ❑ 5. Ability to cough and deep breathe

Level of Cognitive Ability: Creating
Client Needs: Physiological Integrity
Clinical Judgment/Cognitive Skills: Generate Solutions
Integrated Process: Clinical Judgment; Nursing Process/Planning
Content Area: Adult Health: Renal and Urinary
Health Problems: Adult Health: Renal and Urinary: Urinary Tract Inflammation/Infection/Trauma
Priority Concepts: Clinical Judgment; Elimination

Answer: 1, 2, 3, 5
Rationale: After nephrectomy, it is imperative to measure the urine output on an hourly basis. This is done to monitor the effectiveness of the remaining kidney and detect renal failure early, if it should occur. The client may also experience significant pain after this surgery, which could affect the client's ability to reposition, cough, and deep breathe. Therefore, the next most important measurements are vital signs, pain level, and ability to cough and deep breathe. Food is not given until the client has bowel sounds.
Test-Taking Strategy: Focus on the subject, assessment after nephrectomy. Note the relationship between "nephrectomy" in the question and "urine output" in option 3. Remember that the client may also experience significant pain after surgery, which could affect the client's ability to cough and deep breathe. Therefore, options 1, 2, and 5 (vital signs, pain level, and ability to cough and deep breathe) are necessary assessments after left nephrectomy.
Priority Nursing Tip: After nephrectomy, monitor for a urinary output of 30 to 50 mL/hr.
Reference: Ignatavicius, D., et al. (2021). *Medical-surgical nursing: Concepts for interprofessional collaborative care* (10th ed., p. 1370). Elsevier.

365. The nurse instructs a parent of a child who had a plaster cast applied to the arm about measures that will help the cast dry. Which instructions would the nurse provide to the parent? **Select all that apply.**
- ❏ 1. Lift the cast using the fingertips.
- ❏ 2. Place the child on a firm mattress.
- ❏ 3. Direct a fan toward the cast to facilitate drying.
- ❏ 4. Support the cast and adjacent joints with pillows.
- ❏ 5. Place the extremity with the cast in a dependent position.
- ❏ 6. Reposition the extremity with the cast every 2 to 4 hours.

Level of Cognitive Ability: Applying
Client Needs: Physiological Integrity
Clinical Judgment/Cognitive Skills: Take Action
Integrated Process: Teaching and Learning
Content Area: Pediatrics: Musculoskeletal
Health Problems: Pediatric-Specific: Fractures
Priority Concepts: Patient Education; Mobility

Answer: 2, 3, 4, 6
Rationale: To help the cast dry, the child needs to be placed on a firm mattress. A fan may be directed toward the cast to facilitate drying. Once the cast is dry, the cast will be cool to touch. The cast and adjacent joints need to be elevated and supported with pillows. To ensure thorough drying, the extremity with the cast needs to be repositioned every 2 to 4 hours. The cast is lifted by using the palms of the hands (not the fingertips) to prevent indentation in the wet cast surface. Indentations could possibly cause pressure on the skin under the cast.
Test-Taking Strategy: Focus on the subject, measures that will help the cast dry. Eliminate option 1 because of the word "fingertips" and option 5 because of the word "dependent."
Priority Nursing Tip: Monitor the extremity with a cast for signs of circulatory impairment. If these occur, notify the physician immediately and prepare for bivalving and cutting the cast.
Reference: McKinney, E. S., et al. (2022). *Maternal child nursing* (6th ed., pp. 1219, 1225). Elsevier.

❖ **366.** A client is receiving cisplatin as part of a treatment plan for esophageal cancer. On assessment of the client, which findings indicate that the client is experiencing an adverse effect of the medication?
1. Tinnitus
2. Increased appetite
3. Excessive urination
4. Yellow halos in front of the eyes

Level of Cognitive Ability: Analyzing
Client Needs: Physiological Integrity
Clinical Judgment/Cognitive Skills: Analyze Cues
Integrated Process: Clinical Judgment; Nursing Process/Analysis
Content Area: Pharmacology: Oncology: Alkylating
Health Problems: Adult Health: Cancer: Esophageal/Gastric/Intestinal
Priority Concepts: Cellular Regulation; Safety

Answer: 1
Rationale: Cisplatin is an antineoplastic medication. An adverse effect related to the administration of cisplatin is ototoxicity with hearing loss. The nurse needs to assess for this adverse reaction when administering this medication. Options 2, 3, and 4 are not adverse effects of this medication.
Test-Taking Strategy: Focus on the subject, an adverse effect of cisplatin. Recalling that ototoxicity is an adverse effect will direct you to the correct option, the only option that relates to the ear.
Priority Nursing Tip: Cisplatin, an antineoplastic medication, is a platinum compound and can cause ototoxicity, tinnitus, hypokalemia, hypocalcemia, hypomagnesemia, and nephrotoxicity.
Reference: Kizior, R., & Hodgson, B. (2023). *Saunders Nursing drug handbook 2023* (pp. 238, 240). Elsevier.

367. A child is admitted to the hospital with a diagnosis of nephrotic syndrome. The nurse expects to note documentation of which manifestation in the medical record? **Select all that apply.**
- ❑ 1. Edema
- ❑ 2. Proteinuria
- ❑ 3. Hypertension
- ❑ 4. Abdominal pain
- ❑ 5. Increased weight
- ❑ 6. Hypoalbuminemia

Level of Cognitive Ability: Analyzing
Client Needs: Physiological Integrity
Clinical Judgment/Cognitive Skills: Recognize Cues
Integrated Process: Clinical Judgment; Nursing Process/Assessment
Content Area: Pediatrics: Renal and Urinary
Health Problems: Pediatric-Specific: Nephrotic Syndrome
Priority Concepts: Clinical Judgment; Elimination

Answer: 1, 2, 4, 5, 6
Rationale: Nephrotic syndrome refers to a kidney disorder characterized by edema, proteinuria, and hypoalbuminemia. The child also experiences anorexia, fatigue, abdominal pain, respiratory infection, and increased weight. The child's blood pressure is usually normal or slightly below normal.
Test-Taking Strategy: Focus on the subject, nephrotic syndrome. Recalling that nephrotic syndrome is characterized by proteinuria, hypoalbuminemia, and edema will assist in determining the correct options. Also remember that the blood pressure is usually normal in this condition.
Priority Nursing Tip: For the client with nephrotic syndrome, a regular diet without added salt may be prescribed if the child is in remission; sodium and fluids may be restricted during periods of massive edema.
Reference: McKinney, E. S., et al. (2022). *Maternal child nursing* (6th ed., p. 1023). Elsevier.

❖ **368.** Twelve hours after delivery, the nurse assesses the client for uterine involution. The nurse determines that the uterus is progressing normally toward its prepregnancy state when palpation of the client's fundus is at which level?
1. At the umbilicus
2. One fingerbreadth below the umbilicus
3. Two fingerbreadths below the umbilicus
4. Midway between the umbilicus and the symphysis pubis

Level of Cognitive Ability: Analyzing
Client Needs: Physiological Integrity
Clinical Judgment/Cognitive Skills: Analyze Cues
Integrated Process: Clinical Judgment; Nursing Process/Analysis
Content Area: Maternity: Postpartum
Health Problems: Maternity: Postpartum Uterine Problems
Priority Concepts: Clinical Judgment; Reproduction

Answer: 1
Rationale: The term "involution" is used to describe the rapid reduction in size and the return of the uterus to a normal condition similar to its nonpregnant state. Immediately after the delivery of the placenta, the uterus contracts to the size of a large grapefruit. The fundus is situated in the midline between the symphysis pubis and the umbilicus. Within 6 to 12 hours after birth, the fundus of the uterus rises to the level of the umbilicus. The top of the fundus remains at the level of the umbilicus for about a day and then descends into the pelvis approximately one fingerbreadth on each succeeding day.
Test-Taking Strategy: Focus on the subject, the location of the uterus 12 hours after birth. Visualize the process of assessment of involution and the expected finding at this time to answer the question.
Priority Nursing Tip: By approximately 10 days postpartum, the uterus cannot be palpated abdominally.
Reference: McKinney, E. S., et al. (2022). *Maternal child nursing* (6th ed., pp. 399, 407). Elsevier.

369. A client is scheduled for a subtotal gastrectomy (Billroth II procedure) to treat stomach cancer. The nurse explains that the procedure will have which surgical results?
   1. Proximal end of the distal stomach is anastomosed to the duodenum.
   2. Entire stomach is removed and the esophagus is anastomosed to the duodenum.
   3. Lower portion of the stomach is removed and the remainder is anastomosed to the jejunum.
   4. Antrum of the stomach is removed and the remaining portion is anastomosed to the duodenum.

Level of Cognitive Ability: Applying
Client Needs: Physiological Integrity
Clinical Judgment/Cognitive Skills: Take Action
Integrated Process: Teaching and Learning
Content Area: Adult Health: Gastrointestinal
Health Problems: Adult Health: Cancer: Esophageal/Gastric/Intestinal
Priority Concepts: Patient Education; Safety

Answer: 3
Rationale: In the Billroth II procedure, the lower portion of the stomach is removed and the remainder is anastomosed to the jejunum. The duodenal stump is preserved to permit bile flow to the jejunum. Options 1, 2, and 4 are incorrect descriptions.
Test-Taking Strategy: Focus on the subject, gastrectomy (Billroth II procedure), which indicates removal of the stomach. This will assist in eliminating option 1. From the remaining options, note the word "subtotal" in the question, which indicates "lower and a part of." This should direct you to the correct option.
Priority Nursing Tip: Postoperative complications after gastrectomy procedures include hemorrhage, dumping syndrome, diarrhea, hypoglycemia, and vitamin B_{12} deficiency.
Reference: Ignatavicius, D., et al. (2021). *Medical-surgical nursing: Concepts for interprofessional collaborative care* (10th ed., pp. 1105–1106). Elsevier.

❖ **370.** A client diagnosed with diabetes mellitus receives 8 units of regular insulin subcutaneously at 0730. The nurse would be **most** alert to signs of hypoglycemia at what time during the day?
   1. 1330 to 1530
   2. 1530 to 1730
   3. 0930 to 1130
   4. 1130 to 1330

Level of Cognitive Ability: Analyzing
Client Needs: Physiological Integrity
Clinical Judgment/Cognitive Skills: Recognize Cues
Integrated Process: Nursing Process/Assessment
Content Area: Pharmacology: Endocrine: Insulin
Health Problems: Adult Health: Endocrine: Diabetes Mellitus
Priority Concepts: Clinical Judgment; Glucose Regulation

Answer: 3
Rationale: Regular insulin is a short-acting insulin. Its onset of action occurs in a half hour and peaks in 2 to 4 hours. Its duration of action is 4 to 6 hours. A hypoglycemic reaction will most likely occur at peak time, which in this situation is between 0930 and 1130.
Test-Taking Strategy: Note the strategic word, *most*. Recall knowledge regarding the onset, peak, and duration of action of regular insulin to answer this question. Recalling that regular insulin is a short-acting insulin will direct you to the correct option.
Priority Nursing Tip: Not all types of insulin can be administered by the intravenous route. Regular insulin is one type of insulin that can be administered intravenously.
Reference: Ignatavicius, D., et al. (2021). *Medical-surgical nursing: Concepts for interprofessional collaborative care* (10th ed., p. 1279). Elsevier.

371. The nurse creates a postoperative plan of care for a client scheduled for a hypophysectomy. Which interventions would be included in the plan of care? **Select all that apply.**
- ❑ **1.** Obtain daily weights.
- ❑ **2.** Monitor intake and output.
- ❑ **3.** Elevate the head of the bed.
- ❑ **4.** Use a soft toothbrush for mouth care.
- ❑ **5.** Encourage coughing and deep breathing.

Level of Cognitive Ability: Creating
Client Needs: Physiological Integrity
Clinical Judgment/Cognitive Skills: Generate Solutions
Integrated Process: Clinical Judgment; Nursing Process/Planning
Content Area: Adult Health: Endocrine
Health Problems: Adult Health: Endocrine: Pituitary Disorders
Priority Concepts: Intracranial Regulation; Safety

Answer: 1, 2, 3
Rationale: A hypophysectomy is done to remove a pituitary tumor. Because temporary diabetes insipidus or syndrome of inappropriate antidiuretic hormone can develop after this surgery, obtaining daily weights and monitoring intake and output are important interventions. The head of the bed is elevated to assist in preventing increased intracranial pressure. Tooth brushing, sneezing, coughing, nose blowing, and bending are activities that need to be avoided postoperatively in the client who underwent a hypophysectomy because of the risk of increasing intracranial pressure. These activities interfere with the healing of the incision and can disrupt the graft.
Test-Taking Strategy: Focus on the subject, postoperative care after hypophysectomy. Consider the anatomic location of the surgical procedure and associated complications. Although coughing and deep breathing are usually a normal component of postoperative care, in this situation, coughing is contraindicated. Additionally tooth brushing can interfere with healing.
Priority Nursing Tip: Increased intracranial pressure is a complication of hypophysectomy.
Reference: Ignatavicius, D., et al. (2021). *Medical-surgical nursing: Concepts for interprofessional collaborative care* (10th ed., pp. 1234–1235). Elsevier.

❖ **372.** After undergoing a thyroidectomy, a client is monitored for signs of damage to the parathyroid glands postoperatively. The nurse would determine which finding suggests damage to the parathyroid glands?
1. Fever
2. Neck pain
3. Hoarseness
4. Tingling around the mouth

Level of Cognitive Ability: Analyzing
Client Needs: Physiological Integrity
Clinical Judgment/Cognitive Skills: Recognize Cues
Integrated Process: Clinical Judgment; Nursing Process/Assessment
Content Area: Adult Health: Endocrine
Health Problems: Adult Health: Endocrine: Thyroid Disorders
Priority Concepts: Clinical Judgment; Fluids and Electrolytes

Answer: 4
Rationale: The parathyroid glands can be damaged or their blood supply impaired during thyroid surgery. Hypocalcemia and tetany result when parathyroid hormone (PTH) levels decrease. The nurse monitors for complaints of tingling around the mouth or of the toes or fingers and muscular twitching because these are signs of calcium deficiency. Additional later signs of hypocalcemia are positive Chvostek's and Trousseau's signs. Fever may be expected in the immediate postoperative period but is not an indication of damage to the parathyroid glands. However, if a fever persists the surgeon is notified. Neck pain and hoarseness are expected findings postoperatively.
Test-Taking Strategy: Focus on the subject, damage to the parathyroid glands, and consider the anatomic location of the surgical procedure. Recalling that neck pain and hoarseness are expected findings postoperatively will assist in eliminating options 1 and 2. From the remaining options, focusing on the subject will assist in eliminating option 3. Also, recalling that hypocalcemia results when PTH levels decrease will assist in directing you to the correct option.
Priority Nursing Tip: After thyroidectomy, maintain the client in a semi-Fowler's position to reduce swelling at the operative site.
Reference: Ignatavicius, D., et al. (2021). *Medical-surgical nursing: Concepts for interprofessional collaborative care* (10th ed., p. 1259). Elsevier.

373. The nurse is performing an admission assessment on a client admitted with a diagnosis of Raynaud's disease. The nurse assesses for the associated symptoms by performing which actions?
1. Checking for a rash on the digits
2. Observing for softening of the nails or nail beds
3. Palpating for a rapid or irregular peripheral pulse
4. Palpating for diminished or absent peripheral pulses

Level of Cognitive Ability: Applying
Client Needs: Physiological Integrity
Clinical Judgment/Cognitive Skills: Take Action
Integrated Process: Clinical Judgment; Nursing Process/Assessment
Content Area: Adult Health: Cardiovascular
Health Problems: Adult Health: Cardiovascular: Vascular Disorders
Priority Concepts: Clinical Judgment; Perfusion

Answer: 4
Rationale: Raynaud's disease is vasospasm of the arterioles and arteries of the upper and lower extremities. It produces closure of the small arteries in the distal extremities in response to cold, vibration, or external stimuli. Palpation for diminished or absent peripheral pulses checks for interruption of circulation. Skin changes include hair loss, thinning or tightening of the skin, and delayed healing of cuts or injuries. A rash on the digits is not a characteristic of this disorder. The nails grow slowly, become brittle or deformed, and heal poorly around the nail beds when infected. Although palpation of peripheral pulses is correct, a rapid or irregular pulse would not be noted.
Test-Taking Strategy: Focus on the subject, assessment for Raynaud's disease. Recall the physiologic occurrences in Raynaud's disease. Palpation for diminished or absent peripheral pulses checks for interruption of circulation.
Priority Nursing Tip: Teach the client with Raynaud's disease to avoid smoking; wear warm clothing, socks, and gloves in cold weather; and avoid injuries to the fingers and hands.
Reference: Ignatavicius, D., et al. (2021). *Medical-surgical nursing: Concepts for interprofessional collaborative care* (10th ed., p. 720). Elsevier.

❖ **374.** The nurse teaches a postpartum client about postdelivery lochia. The nurse determines that the education has been **effective** when the client says that on the second day postpartum, the lochia should be which color?
1. Red
2. Pink
3. White
4. Yellow

Level of Cognitive Ability: Evaluating
Client Needs: Physiological Integrity
Clinical Judgment/Cognitive Skills: Evaluate Outcomes
Integrated Process: Teaching and Learning
Content Area: Maternity: Postpartum
Health Problems: N/A
Priority Concepts: Patient Education; Reproduction

Answer: 1
Rationale: The uterus rids itself of the debris that remains after birth through a discharge called lochia, which is classified according to its appearance and contents. Lochia rubra is dark red. It occurs from delivery to 3 days postpartum and contains epithelial cells, erythrocytes, leukocytes, shreds of decidua, and occasionally fetal meconium, lanugo, and vernix caseosa. Lochia serosa is a brownish pink discharge that occurs from days 4 to 10. Lochia alba is a white discharge that occurs from days 10 to 14. Lochia should not be yellow or contain large clots; if it does, the cause needs to be investigated without delay.
Test-Taking Strategy: Focus on the subject, lochia. Note the strategic word, *effective.* Noting the words "second day postpartum" will direct you to the correct option.
Priority Nursing Tip: The amount of lochial discharge may increase with ambulation.
Reference: McKinney, E. S., et al. (2022). *Maternal child nursing* (6th ed., pp. 400, 406). Elsevier.

375. The nurse creates a care plan for a client receiving hemodialysis through an arteriovenous (AV) fistula in the right arm. The nurse includes which interventions in the plan to protect the AV fistula from injury? **Select all that apply.**
- ❑ **1.** Assess pulses and circulation proximal to the fistula.
- ❑ **2.** Palpate for thrills and auscultate for a bruit every 4 hours.
- ❑ **3.** Check for bleeding and infection at hemodialysis needle insertion sites.
- ❑ **4.** Avoid taking blood pressure or performing venipunctures in the extremity.
- ❑ **5.** Instruct client not to carry heavy objects or anything that compresses the extremity.
- ❑ **6.** Instruct client not to sleep in a position that places their body weight on top of the extremity.

Level of Cognitive Ability: Creating
Client Needs: Physiological Integrity
Clinical Judgment/Cognitive Skills: Generate Solutions
Integrated Process: Clinical Judgment; Nursing Process/Planning
Content Area: Adult Health: Renal and Urinary
Health Problems: Adult Health: Renal and Urinary: Acute Kidney Injury and Chronic Kidney Disease
Priority Concepts: Perfusion; Safety

Answer: 2, 3, 4, 5, 6
Rationale: An AV fistula is an internal anastomosis of an artery to a vein and is used as an access for hemodialysis. The nurse would implement the following to protect the fistula: palpate for thrills and auscultate for a bruit every 4 hours, check for bleeding and infection at hemodialysis needle insertion sites, avoid taking blood pressures or performing venipunctures in the extremity, instruct the client not to carry heavy objects or anything that compresses the extremity, instruct the client not to sleep in a position that places the body weight on top of the extremity, and the nurse needs to assess pulses and circulation distal to the fistula.
Test-Taking Strategy: Focus on the subject, protecting the AV fistula. Visualize this vascular access device and read each option carefully. Noting the word *proximal* in option 1 will assist in eliminating this option.
Priority Nursing Tip: Arterial steal syndrome can develop in a client with an arteriovenous fistula. In this condition, too much blood is diverted to the vein, and arterial perfusion to the hand is compromised.
Reference: Ignatavicius, D., et al. (2021). *Medical-surgical nursing: Concepts for interprofessional collaborative care* (10th ed., pp. 1398–1399). Elsevier.

❖ **376.** The newborn nursery nurse is performing an admission assessment on a newborn with the diagnosis of cephalohematoma. Which intervention would the nurse implement to assess for the **primary** symptom associated with subdural hematoma?
- **1.** Monitor the urine for blood.
- **2.** Monitor the urinary output pattern.
- **3.** Test for contractures of the extremities.
- **4.** Test for equality of extremity reflexes.

Level of Cognitive Ability: Analyzing
Client Needs: Physiological Integrity
Clinical Judgment/Cognitive Skills: Take Action
Integrated Process: Clinical Judgment; Nursing Process/Implementation
Content Area: Maternity: Newborn
Health Problems: Newborn: Cephalohematoma
Priority Concepts: Development; Intracranial Regulation

Answer: 4
Rationale: A cephalohematoma can cause pressure on a specific area of the cerebral tissue. This can cause changes in the stimuli responses in the extremities on the opposite side of the body, especially if the newborn is actively bleeding. Options 1 and 2 are incorrect. After delivery, a newborn would normally be incontinent of urine. Blood in the urine would indicate abdominal trauma and would not be a result of the hematoma. Option 3 is incorrect because contractures would not occur this soon after delivery.
Test-Taking Strategy: Note the strategic word, *primary*. Eliminate options 1 and 2 because they are comparable or alike and are similar assessments. Remember that the method of assessing for complications and active bleeding into the cranial cavity is a neurologic assessment. Checking newborn reflexes is a neurologic assessment. Although contractures of extremities could occur as residual effects, this would not occur immediately.
Priority Nursing Tip: With a cephalohematoma, blood collects between the newborn's scalp and the skull. The pooling of blood is the result of blood vessels that are damaged during labor and delivery.
Reference: McKinney, E. S., et al. (2022). *Maternal child nursing* (6th ed., pp. 449–450). Elsevier.

377. A client has received atropine sulfate preoperatively. The nurse monitors the client for which effect of the medication in the immediate postoperative period?
1. Diarrhea
2. Bradycardia
3. Urinary retention
4. Excessive salivation

Level of Cognitive Ability: Applying
Client Needs: Physiological Integrity
Clinical Judgment/Cognitive Skills: Recognize Cues
Integrated Process: Clinical Judgment; Nursing Process/Assessment
Content Area: Pharmacology: Neurologic: Anticholinergics
Health Problems: N/A
Priority Concepts: Clinical Judgment; Safety

Answer: 3
Rationale: Atropine sulfate is an anticholinergic medication that causes tachycardia, drowsiness, blurred vision, dry mouth, constipation, and urinary retention. The nurse needs to monitor the client for any of these effects in the immediate postoperative period. None of the other options relate to this medication.
Test-Taking Strategy: Focus on the subject, effects of atropine sulfate. Recalling that atropine sulfate is an anticholinergic and recalling the effects of an anticholinergic will direct you to the correct option.
Priority Nursing Tip: Anticholinergic medications are contraindicated in the client with glaucoma.
Reference: Skidmore-Roth, L., (2021). *2021 Mosby's nursing drug reference* (34th ed., pp. 116–117). Elsevier.

❖ **378.** A client experiencing calcium oxalate renal calculi is told to limit dietary intake of oxalate. The nurse is confident that the teaching has been **effective** when the client includes which items on a list of foods high in oxalate? **Select all that apply.**
☐ 1. Beets
☐ 2. Spinach
☐ 3. Rhubarb
☐ 4. Black tea
☐ 5. Cantaloupe
☐ 6. Watermelon

Level of Cognitive Ability: Evaluating
Client Needs: Physiological Integrity
Clinical Judgment/Cognitive Skills: Evaluate Outcomes
Integrated Process: Teaching and Learning
Content Area: Adult Health: Renal and Urinary
Health Problems: Adult Health: Renal and Urinary: Calculi
Priority Concepts: Patient Education; Nutrition

Answer: 1, 2, 3, 4
Rationale: Food items that are high in oxalate include beets, spinach, rhubarb, black tea, Swiss chard, cocoa, wheat germ, cashews, almonds, pecans, peanuts, okra, chocolate, and lime peel.
Test-Taking Strategy: Focus on the subject, food high in oxalate. Note the strategic word, *effective.* Knowledge regarding food items high in oxalate is needed to answer this question. Remembering that fruits are generally not sources of dietary oxalate will assist in answering questions similar to this one.
Priority Nursing Tip: Encourage the client with renal calculi to increase fluid intake up to 3000 mL/day, unless contraindicated, to facilitate the passage of the stone and prevent infection.
Reference: Ignatavicius, D., et al. (2021). *Medical-surgical nursing: Concepts for interprofessional collaborative care* (10th ed., p. 1345). Elsevier.

379. The nurse is conducting a health history on a client diagnosed with hyperparathyroidism. Which question asked of the client would elicit information about this condition?
1. "Do you have tremors in your hands?"
2. "Are you experiencing pain in your joints?"
3. "Have you had problems with diarrhea lately?"
4. "Do you notice any swelling in your legs at night?"

Level of Cognitive Ability: Applying
Client Needs: Physiological Integrity
Clinical Judgment/Cognitive Skills: Recognize Cues
Integrated Process: Clinical Judgment; Nursing Process/Assessment
Content Area: Adult Health: Endocrine
Health Problems: Adult Health: Endocrine: Parathyroid Disorders
Priority Concepts: Clinical Judgment; Safety

Answer: 2
Rationale: Hyperparathyroidism causes an oversecretion of parathyroid hormone (PTH), which causes excessive osteoblast growth and activity within the bones. When bone reabsorption is increased, calcium is released from the bones into the blood, causing hypercalcemia. The bones suffer demineralization as a result of calcium loss, leading to bone and joint pain and pathological fractures. Options 1 and 3 relate to assessment of hypoparathyroidism. Option 4 is unrelated to hyperparathyroidism.
Test-Taking Strategy: Focus on the subject, hyperparathyroidism. Knowledge regarding the pathophysiology associated with hyperparathyroidism is required to answer the question. Eliminate options 1 and 3 first because these options provide information about hypoparathyroidism. From the remaining options, it is necessary to know the relationship among hyperparathyroidism, PTH, and joint pain to direct you to the correct option.
Priority Nursing Tip: Safety is a priority in the care of the client with hyperparathyroidism. Move the client slowly and carefully because the client is at risk for pathologic fractures.
Reference: Ignatavicius, D., et al. (2021). *Medical-surgical nursing: Concepts for interprofessional collaborative care* (10th ed., pp. 1262–1263). Elsevier.

❖ 380. A client seeks medical attention for intermittent signs and symptoms that suggest a diagnosis of Raynaud's disease. The nurse would assess the trigger of these signs/symptoms by asking which question?
1. "Does being exposed to heat seem to cause the episodes?"
2. "Do the signs and symptoms occur while you are asleep?"
3. "Does drinking coffee or ingesting chocolate seem related to the episodes?"
4. "Have you experienced any injuries that have limited your activity levels lately?"

Level of Cognitive Ability: Analyzing
Client Needs: Physiological Integrity
Clinical Judgment/Cognitive Skills: Recognize Cues
Integrated Process: Clinical Judgment; Nursing Process/Assessment
Content Area: Adult Health: Cardiovascular
Health Problems: Adult Health: Cardiovascular: Vascular Disorders
Priority Concepts: Clinical Judgment; Perfusion

Answer: 3
Rationale: Raynaud's disease is vasospasm of the arterioles and arteries of the upper and lower extremities. It produces closure of the small arteries in the distal extremities in response to cold, vibration, or external stimuli. Episodes are characterized by pallor, cold, numbness, and possible cyanosis of the fingers, followed by erythema, tingling, and aching pain. Attacks are triggered by exposure to cold, nicotine, caffeine, trauma to the fingertips, and stress. Prolonged episodes of inactivity are unrelated to these episodes.
Test-Taking Strategy: Focus on the subject, precipitating factors for Raynaud's disease. Recalling that symptoms occur with vasoconstriction will assist in eliminating options 1, 2, and 4 because these events are unlikely to cause vasoconstriction.
Priority Nursing Tip: Because stress can trigger vasospasm, the nurse needs to teach the client with Raynaud's disease stress management techniques.
Reference: Ignatavicius, D., et al. (2021). *Medical-surgical nursing: Concepts for interprofessional collaborative care* (10th ed., p. 720). Elsevier.

381. The nurse provides information to a client diagnosed with insulin-dependent diabetes mellitus. Which manifestations resulting from a hypoglycemia event would the nurse include in the information? **Select all that apply.**
- ❑ 1. Hunger
- ❑ 2. Sweating
- ❑ 3. Weakness
- ❑ 4. Nervousness
- ❑ 5. Cool, clammy skin
- ❑ 6. Increased urinary output

Level of Cognitive Ability: Applying
Client Needs: Physiological Integrity
Clinical Judgment/Cognitive Skills: Take Action
Integrated Process: Teaching and Learning
Content Area: Pharmacology: Endocrine: Insulin
Health Problems: Adult Health: Endocrine: Diabetes Mellitus
Priority Concepts: Patient Education; Glucose Regulation

Answer: 1, 2, 3, 4, 5
Rationale: Hypoglycemia is characterized by a blood glucose level less than 70 mg/dL (3.9 mmol/L). Clinical manifestations of hypoglycemia include hunger, sweating, weakness, nervousness, cool clammy skin, blurred vision or double vision, tachycardia, and palpitations. Increased urinary output is a manifestation of hyperglycemia.
Test-Taking Strategy: Focus on the subject, the manifestations of hypoglycemia. Recall that hypoglycemia is characterized by a blood glucose level lower than 70 mg/dL (3.9 mmol/L). Next think about the manifestations that occur when the blood glucose level is low. Also recalling the "3 Ps" associated with hyperglycemia—polyuria, polydipsia, and polyphagia—will assist in eliminating option 6.
Priority Nursing Tip: If the client exhibits signs of a hypoglycemic reaction, perform a finger stick and check the client's glucose level. If hypoglycemia is confirmed, give the client a 10- to 15-g carbohydrate item such as a ½ cup of fruit juice to drink.
Reference: Ignatavicius, D., et al. (2021). *Medical-surgical nursing: Concepts for interprofessional collaborative care* (10th ed., pp. 1289, 1291–1292). Elsevier.

❖ **382.** The ambulatory care nurse is assessing a client with chronic sinusitis. The nurse determines that which manifestations reported by the client are related to this problem? **Select all that apply.**
- ❑ 1. Anosmia
- ❑ 2. Chronic cough
- ❑ 3. Blurry vision
- ❑ 4. Nasal stuffiness
- ❑ 5. Purulent nasal discharge
- ❑ 6. Headache that worsens in the evening

Level of Cognitive Ability: Analyzing
Client Needs: Physiological Integrity
Clinical Judgment/Cognitive Skills: Recognize Cues
Integrated Process: Clinical Judgment; Nursing Process/Assessment
Content Area: Adult Health: Respiratory
Health Problems: Adult Health: Respiratory: Infections of the Upper Airway
Priority Concepts: Clinical Judgment; Inflammation

Answer: 1, 2, 4, 5
Rationale: Chronic sinusitis is characterized by anosmia (loss of smell), a chronic cough resulting from nasal discharge, nasal stuffiness, persistent purulent nasal discharge, and headache that is worse upon arising after sleep. Blurred vision is not associated directly with this condition.
Test-Taking Strategy: Focus on the subject, chronic sinusitis. Think about the pathophysiology associated with this disorder. This will assist in determining the signs and symptoms and will direct you to the correct option. Remember that headache is worse upon arising after sleep.
Priority Nursing Tip: Inhaling steam may be a helpful measure to treat sinusitis, but the nurse must teach the client the safe method to do so because of the risk associated with burns from the steam.
Reference: Lewis, S., et al. (2020). *Medical-surgical nursing: Assessment and management of clinical problems* (11th ed., pp. 485–486). Elsevier.

383. A client is diagnosed with hypothyroidism. The nurse performs an assessment on the client, expecting to note which findings? **Select all that apply.**
- ❑ 1. Weight loss
- ❑ 2. Bradycardia
- ❑ 3. Hypotension
- ❑ 4. Dry, scaly skin
- ❑ 5. Heat intolerance
- ❑ 6. Decreased body temperature

Level of Cognitive Ability: Analyzing
Client Needs: Physiological Integrity
Clinical Judgment/Cognitive Skills: Recognize Cues
Integrated Process: Clinical Judgment; Nursing Process/Assessment
Content Area: Adult Health: Endocrine
Health Problems: Adult Health: Endocrine: Thyroid Disorders
Priority Concepts: Clinical Judgment; Thermoregulation

Answer: 2, 3, 4, 6
Rationale: The manifestations of hypothyroidism are the result of decreased metabolism from low levels of thyroid hormones. Some of these manifestations are bradycardia; hypotension; cool, dry, scaly skin; decreased body temperature; dry, coarse, brittle hair; decreased hair growth; cold intolerance; slowing of intellectual functioning; lethargy; weight gain; and constipation.
Test-Taking Strategy: Focus on the subject, hypothyroidism. Recall that it occurs as the result of decreased metabolism from low levels of thyroid hormones. Correlate *hypo*thyroidism with *decreased* body functioning to assist in answering the question. Weight loss and heat intolerance occur in hyperthyroidism.
Priority Nursing Tip: A severe complication of hypothyroidism is myxedema coma, a rare but serious disorder that results from persistently low thyroid production. It can be caused by acute illness, anesthesia and surgery, hypothermia, and the use of sedatives and opioids.
Reference: Ignatavicius, D., et al. (2021). *Medical-surgical nursing: Concepts for interprofessional collaborative care* (10th ed., p. 1252). Elsevier.

❖ **384.** A client is diagnosed with diabetes insipidus. The nurse would plan interventions to address which manifestations of this disorder? **Select all that apply.**
- ❑ 1. Bradycardia
- ❑ 2. Hypertension
- ❑ 3. Poor skin turgor
- ❑ 4. Increased urinary output
- ❑ 5. Dry mucous membranes
- ❑ 6. Decreased pulse pressure

Level of Cognitive Ability: Applying
Client Needs: Physiological Integrity
Clinical Judgment/Cognitive Skills: Generate Solutions
Integrated Process: Clinical Judgment; Nursing Process/Planning
Content Area: Adult Health: Endocrine
Health Problems: Adult Health: Endocrine: Pituitary Disorders
Priority Concepts: Clinical Judgment; Safety

Answer: 3, 4, 5, 6
Rationale: Diabetes insipidus is a water metabolism problem caused by an antidiuretic hormone (ADH) deficiency (either a decrease in ADH synthesis or an inability of the kidneys to respond to ADH). Clinical manifestations include poor skin turgor, increased urinary output, dry mucous membranes, decreased pulse pressure, tachycardia, hypotension, weak peripheral pulses, and increased thirst.
Test-Taking Strategy: Focus on the subject, diabetes insipidus. Think about the pathophysiology of this disorder and recall that diabetes insipidus is caused by an ADH deficiency. This will assist in eliminating options 1 and 2.
Priority Nursing Tip: Monitor for an electrolyte imbalance and signs of dehydration in the client with diabetes insipidus. If the condition is untreated, the client experiences a urine output of 4 to 24 L/day.
Reference: Ignatavicius, D., et al. (2021). *Medical-surgical nursing: Concepts for interprofessional collaborative care* (10th ed., p. 1236). Elsevier.

385. A client diagnosed with pneumonia reports a decreased sense of taste that has greatly affected the motivation to eat and drink. Which action would the nurse take to help increase the client's appetite?
1. Offer snacks in between meals.
2. Provide three large meals daily.
3. Provide mouth care before meals.
4. Offer to sit with client during meals.

Level of Cognitive Ability: Applying
Client Needs: Physiological Integrity
Clinical Judgment/Cognitive Skills: Take Action
Integrated Process: Nursing Process/Implementation
Content Area: Adult Health: Respiratory
Health Problems: Adult Health: Respiratory: Pneumonia
Priority Concepts: Gas Exchange; Nutrition

Answer: 3
Rationale: The client with pneumonia may experience decreased taste sensation as a result of sputum expectoration. To minimize this adverse effect, the nurse would provide oral hygiene before meals. The client should also have small, frequent meals because of dyspnea. The remaining options will not address the issue of impaired sense of taste.
Test-Taking Strategy: Focus on the subject, anorexia and increasing the client's appetite. Eliminate options 1, 2, and 4 because they are comparable or alike and will not increase the client's appetite. Additionally, as a general measure, small frequent meals are better tolerated than large meals.
Priority Nursing Tip: Unless contraindicated, encourage the client with pneumonia to consume fluids, up to 3 L/day, to thin secretions.
Reference: Lewis, S., et al. (2020). *Medical-surgical nursing: Assessment and management of clinical problems* (11th ed., pp. 507, 509). Elsevier.

❖ 386. The nurse notes that a large number of clients reporting the presence of flulike symptoms are being seen in the clinic. Which recommendations would the nurse provide to these clients? **Select all that apply.**
❑ 1. Get plenty of rest.
❑ 2. Increase intake of liquids.
❑ 3. Get a flu shot immediately.
❑ 4. Take antipyretics for fever.
❑ 5. Consume a well-balanced diet.

Level of Cognitive Ability: Applying
Client Needs: Physiological Integrity
Clinical Judgment/Cognitive Skills: Take Action
Integrated Process: Teaching and Learning
Content Area: Adult Health: Respiratory
Health Problems: Adult Health: Respiratory: Infections of the Lower Airway
Priority Concepts: Patient Education; Infection

Answer: 1, 2, 4, 5
Rationale: Treatment for the flu includes getting rest, drinking fluids, and taking in nutritious foods and beverages. Medications such as antipyretics and analgesics may also be used for symptom management. Immunizations against influenza are a prophylactic measure and are not used to treat flu symptoms.
Test-Taking Strategy: Focus on the subject, interventions for influenza. Recalling that a flu shot is a prophylactic measure will assist in directing you to the correct option.
Priority Nursing Tip: Because the strain of influenza virus is different every year, annual vaccination is recommended.
Reference: Lewis, S., et al. (2020). *Medical-surgical nursing: Assessment and management of clinical problems* (11th ed., pp. 483, 485). Elsevier.

387. The nurse instructing a client with chronic pancreatitis about measures to prevent its exacerbation would provide which information? **Select all that apply.**
- ❏ **1.** Eat bland foods.
- ❏ **2.** Avoid alcohol ingestion.
- ❏ **3.** Avoid cigarette smoking.
- ❏ **4.** Avoid caffeinated beverages.
- ❏ **5.** Eat small meals and snacks high in calories.
- ❏ **6.** Eat high-fat, low-protein, high-carbohydrate meals.

Level of Cognitive Ability: Applying
Client Needs: Physiological Integrity
Clinical Judgment/Cognitive Skills: Generate Solutions
Integrated Process: Teaching and Learning
Content Area: Adult Health: Gastrointestinal
Health Problems: Adult Health: Gastrointestinal: Pancreatitis
Priority Concepts: Nutrition; Inflammation

Answer: 1, 2, 3, 4, 5
Rationale: Chronic pancreatitis is a progressive, destructive disease of the pancreas, characterized by remissions and exacerbations (recurrence). Measures to prevent an exacerbation include eating bland, low-fat, high-protein, moderate-carbohydrate meals; avoiding alcohol ingestion, nicotine, and caffeinated beverages; eating small meals and snacks high in calories; and avoiding gastric stimulants such as spices.
Test-Taking Strategy: Focus on the subject, measures to prevent an exacerbation of chronic pancreatitis. Thinking about the pathophysiology associated with pancreatitis and noting the term *high-fat* in option 6 will direct you to eliminate this option.
Priority Nursing Tip: The pain that is associated with acute pancreatitis is aggravated if the client lies in a recumbent position.
Reference: Lewis, S., et al. (2020). *Medical-surgical nursing: Assessment and management of clinical problems* (11th ed., pp. 996–997). Elsevier.

❖ **388.** The nurse notes this cardiac rhythm on the cardiac monitor **(refer to figure).** What would the nurse interpret that the client is experiencing?

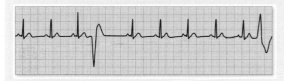

1. Atrial fibrillation
2. Sinus bradycardia
3. Ventricular fibrillation (VF)
4. Premature ventricular contractions (PVCs)

Level of Cognitive Ability: Analyzing
Client Needs: Physiological Integrity
Clinical Judgment/Cognitive Skills: Analyze Cues
Integrated Process: Clinical Judgment; Nursing Process/Analysis
Content Area: Adult Health: Cardiovascular
Health Problems: Adult Health: Cardiovascular: Dysrhythmias
Priority Concepts: Clinical Judgment; Perfusion

Answer: 4
Rationale: PVCs are abnormal ectopic beats (occurring in otherwise normal sinus rhythm) originating in the ventricles. They are characterized by an absence of P waves, wide and bizarre QRS complexes, and a compensatory pause that follows the ectopy. In atrial fibrillation, no definitive P wave usually can be observed; only fibrillatory waves before each QRS complex are observed. In sinus bradycardia, atrial and ventricular rhythms are regular, and the rates are less than 60 beats/min. In ventricular fibrillation, impulses from many irritable foci in the ventricles fire in a totally disorganized manner, which appears as a chaotic rapid rhythm in which the ventricles quiver.
Test-Taking Strategy: Focus on the subject, the cardiac rhythm on the cardiac monitor. Remember that PVCs are characterized by wide and bizarre QRS complexes.
Priority Nursing Tip: The physician is notified if the client experiences premature ventricular contractions so that their cause can be identified and they can be treated.
Reference: Lewis, S., et al. (2020). *Medical-surgical nursing: Assessment and management of clinical problems* (11th ed., pp. 766–767). Elsevier.

389. A client is diagnosed with cholecystitis. The nurse reviews the client's medical record, expecting to note documentation of which manifestations of this disorder? **Select all that apply.**
- ❑ **1.** Dyspepsia
- ❑ **2.** Dark stools
- ❑ **3.** Light-colored and clear urine
- ❑ **4.** Feelings of abdominal fullness
- ❑ **5.** Rebound tenderness in the abdomen
- ❑ **6.** Upper abdominal pain that radiates to the right shoulder

Level of Cognitive Ability: Analyzing
Client Needs: Physiological Integrity
Clinical Judgment/Cognitive Skills: Recognize Cues
Integrated Process: Clinical Judgment; Nursing Process/Assessment
Content Area: Adult Health: Gastrointestinal
Health Problems: Adult Health: Gastrointestinal: Gallbladder Disease
Priority Concepts: Clinical Judgment; Inflammation

Answer: 1, 4, 5, 6
Rationale: Cholecystitis is an inflammation of the gallbladder. Manifestations include dyspepsia; feelings of abdominal fullness; rebound tenderness (Blumberg's sign); upper abdominal pain or discomfort that can radiate to the right shoulder; pain triggered by a high-fat meal; clay-colored stools, dark urine, and possible steatorrhea; anorexia, nausea, and vomiting; eructation; flatulence; fever; and jaundice.
Test-Taking Strategy: Focus on the subject, cholecystitis. Think about the function of the gallbladder and the pathophysiology associated with this disorder. This will assist in eliminating options 2 and 3. Remember that clay-colored stools and dark urine occur in this disorder.
Priority Nursing Tip: Instruct the client with cholecystitis to consume a diet that is low in fat.
Reference: Ignatavicius, D., et al. (2021). *Medical-surgical nursing: Concepts for interprofessional collaborative care* (10th ed., pp. 1178–1179). Elsevier.

❖ **390.** A client is experiencing pulmonary edema as an exacerbation of chronic left-sided heart failure. The nurse would assess the client for what manifestation?
1. Weight loss
2. Bilateral crackles
3. Distended neck veins
4. Peripheral pitting edema

Level of Cognitive Ability: Analyzing
Client Needs: Physiological Integrity
Clinical Judgment/Cognitive Skills: Recognize Cues
Integrated Process: Clinical Judgment; Nursing Process/Assessment
Content Area: Adult Health: Cardiovascular
Health Problems: Adult Health: Cardiovascular: Pulmonary Edema
Priority Concepts: Clinical Judgment; Perfusion

Answer: 2
Rationale: The client with pulmonary edema presents primarily with symptoms that are respiratory in nature because the blood flow is stagnant in the lungs, which lie behind the left side of the heart from a circulatory standpoint. The client would experience weight gain from fluid retention, not weight loss. Distended neck veins and peripheral pitting edema are classic signs of right-sided heart failure.
Test-Taking Strategy: Focus on the subject, pulmonary edema, and note the words "left-sided" heart failure. Knowing that blood flow is stagnant behind the area of failure allows you to eliminate each of the incorrect options. To remember the signs and symptoms of heart failure, remember "left, lungs" and "right, systemic." Option 2 relates to the lungs.
Priority Nursing Tip: If the client develops pulmonary edema, immediately place the client in a high-Fowler's position. The nurse would stay with the client, call for assistance, and ask that the physician be contacted immediately.
Reference: Ignatavicius, D., et al. (2021). *Medical-surgical nursing: Concepts for interprofessional collaborative care* (10th ed., p. 671). Elsevier.

391. A client begins to experience a tonic-clonic seizure. Which actions would the nurse take to ensure client safety? **Select all that apply.**
- ❑ 1. Restrict the client's movements.
- ❑ 2. Turn the supine client to the side.
- ❑ 3. Open the unconscious client's airway.
- ❑ 4. Gently guide the standing client to the floor.
- ❑ 5. Place a padded tongue blade into the client's mouth.
- ❑ 6. Loosen any restrictive clothing that the client is wearing.

Level of Cognitive Ability: Applying
Client Needs: Physiological Integrity
Clinical Judgment/Cognitive Skills: Take Action
Integrated Process: Clinical Judgment; Nursing Process/Implementation
Content Area: Adult Health: Neurologic
Health Problems: Adult Health: Neurologic: Seizure Disorder/Epilepsy
Priority Concepts: Intracranial Regulation; Safety

Answer: 2, 3, 4, 6
Rationale: Precautions are taken to prevent a client from sustaining injury during a seizure. The nurse would maintain the client's airway and turn the client to the side. The nurse would also protect the client from injury, guide the client's movements, and loosen any restrictive clothing. Restraints are never used because they could injure the client during the seizure. A padded tongue blade or any other object is never placed into the client's mouth after a seizure begins because the jaw may clench down.
Test-Taking Strategy: Focus on the subject, a client experiencing seizure activity. Focus on ABCs—airway, breathing, and circulation. Visualize each of the actions to assist in answering correctly. Remember that restraints are never used because they could injure the client, and a padded tongue blade or any other object is never placed into the client's mouth.
Priority Nursing Tip: If a client experiences a seizure while standing or sitting, gently ease the client to the floor and protect the client's head and body.
Reference: Ignatavicius, D., et al. (2021). *Medical-surgical nursing: Concepts for interprofessional collaborative care* (10th ed.). Elsevier.

❖ **392.** The nurse is monitoring a client diagnosed with a ruptured appendix for signs of peritonitis. The nurse would assess for which manifestations of this complication? **Select all that apply.**
- ❑ 1. Bradycardia
- ❑ 2. Distended abdomen
- ❑ 3. Subnormal temperature
- ❑ 4. Rigid, board-like abdomen
- ❑ 5. Diminished bowel sounds
- ❑ 6. Inability to pass flatus or feces

Level of Cognitive Ability: Analyzing
Client Needs: Physiological Integrity
Clinical Judgment/Cognitive Skills: Recognize Cues
Integrated Process: Clinical Judgment; Nursing Process/Assessment
Content Area: Adult Health: Gastrointestinal
Health Problems: Adult Health: Gastrointestinal: Peritonitis
Priority Concepts: Clinical Judgment; Inflammation

Answer: 2, 4, 5, 6
Rationale: Peritonitis is an acute inflammation of the visceral and parietal peritoneum, the endothelial lining of the abdominal cavity. Clinical manifestations include distended abdomen; a rigid, board-like abdomen; diminished bowel sounds; inability to pass flatus or feces; abdominal pain (localized, poorly localized, or referred to the shoulder or thorax); anorexia, nausea, and vomiting; rebound tenderness in the abdomen; high fever; tachycardia; dehydration from the high fever; decreased urinary output; hiccups; and possible compromise in respiratory status.
Test-Taking Strategy: Focus on the subject, signs of peritonitis. Remember that the suffix *-itis* indicates inflammation or infection. This will assist in determining that options 1 and 3 are incorrect. In inflammation, the client would experience an elevated temperature, and tachycardia is a physiologic bodily response to fever.
Priority Nursing Tip: Avoid the application of heat to the abdomen of a client with appendicitis because heat can cause rupture of the appendix leading to peritonitis.
Reference: Ignatavicius, D., et al. (2021). *Medical-surgical nursing: Concepts for interprofessional collaborative care* (10th ed., pp. 1134–1135). Elsevier.

393. While preparing to administer an intravenous (IV) medication, the nurse notes that the medication is incompatible with the IV solution. Which intervention would the nurse take to ensure the client's safety?
1. Ask the provider to prescribe a compatible IV solution.
2. Start a new IV catheter for the incompatible medication.
3. Collaborate with the provider for a new administration route.
4. Flush tubing before and after administering the medication with normal saline.

Level of Cognitive Ability: Applying
Client Needs: Physiological Integrity
Clinical Judgment/Cognitive Skills: Take Action
Integrated Process: Clinical Judgment; Nursing Process/Implementation
Content Area: Skills: Medication Administration
Health Problems: N/A
Priority Concepts: Clinical Judgment; Safety

Answer: 4
Rationale: When giving a medication intravenously, if the medication is incompatible with the IV solution, the tubing is flushed before and after the medication with infusions of normal saline to prevent inline precipitation of the incompatible agents. Starting a new IV, changing the solution, or changing the administration route is unnecessary because a simpler, less risky, viable option exists.
Test-Taking Strategy: Focus on the subject, intravenous medication administration. You can eliminate options 1, 2, and 3 because they are unnecessary; in addition, option 2 increases the risk of infection and is likely to cause the client discomfort.
Priority Nursing Tip: Normal saline is physiologically similar to body fluid and is generally the solution of choice to flush an intravenous line.
Reference: Potter, P., et al. (2021). *Fundamentals of nursing* (10th ed., p. 665). Elsevier.

❖ **394.** The nurse is preparing to administer eardrops to an infant. The nurse would plan to proceed by taking which step to ensure the appropriate instillation of the medication?
1. Pull down and back on the auricle, and direct the solution onto the eardrum.
2. Pull up and back on the earlobe, and direct the solution toward the wall of the ear canal.
3. Pull up and back on the auricle, and direct the solution toward the wall of the ear canal.
4. Pull down and back on the auricle, and direct the solution toward the wall of the ear canal.

Level of Cognitive Ability: Applying
Client Needs: Physiological Integrity
Clinical Judgment/Cognitive Skills: Generate Solutions
Integrated Process: Nursing Process/Planning
Content Area: Skills: Medication Administration
Health Problems: N/A
Priority Concepts: Development; Safety

Answer: 4
Rationale: The infant needs to be turned on the side with the affected ear uppermost. With the nondominant hand, the nurse pulls down and back on the auricle. The wrist of the dominant hand is rested on the infant's head. The medication is administered by aiming it at the wall of the ear canal rather than directly onto the eardrum. The infant needs to be held or positioned with the affected ear uppermost for 10 to 15 minutes to retain the solution. In the adult, the auricle is pulled up and back to straighten the auditory canal.
Test-Taking Strategy: Focus on the subject, administering ear medications. Basic safety principles related to the administration of ear medications will assist in eliminating option 1. Option 3 is eliminated because it is the adult procedure. It would be difficult to pull up and back on an earlobe; therefore, eliminate option 2.
Priority Nursing Tip: For an infant or child younger than 3 years, pull the auricle down and back to administer ear medications. For a child older than 3 years, pull the auricle up and back.
Reference: McKinney, E. S., et al. (2022). *Maternal child nursing* (6th ed., p. 863). Elsevier.

395. A client seeks treatment in an ambulatory clinic for hoarseness that has persisted for 8 weeks. Based on the symptom, the nurse interprets that the client is at risk for which disorder?
1. Thyroid cancer
2. Acute laryngitis
3. Laryngeal cancer
4. Bronchogenic cancer

Level of Cognitive Ability: Analyzing
Client Needs: Physiological Integrity
Clinical Judgment/Cognitive Skills: Analyze Cues
Integrated Process: Clinical Judgment; Nursing Process/Analysis
Content Area: Adult Health: Respiratory
Health Problems: Adult Health: Cancer: Laryngeal and Lung
Priority Concepts: Clinical Judgment; Cellular Regulation

Answer: 3
Rationale: Hoarseness is a common early sign of laryngeal cancer, but not of thyroid or bronchogenic cancer. Hoarseness that persists for 8 weeks is not associated with an acute problem, such as laryngitis.
Test-Taking Strategy: Focus on the **subject**, persistent hoarseness. Begin to answer this question by eliminating option 2, because an acute problem would not generally last for 8 weeks. From the remaining options, recall that the vocal cords are in the larynx when selecting the correct option.
Priority Nursing Tip: Risk factors for laryngeal cancer include smoking, heavy alcohol use, exposure to environmental pollutants such as asbestos or wood dust, and exposure to radiation.
Reference: Ignatavicius, D., et al. (2021). *Medical-surgical nursing: Concepts for interprofessional collaborative care* (10th ed., p. 526). Elsevier.

❖ **396.** A client is admitted to the cardiac intensive care unit after coronary artery bypass graft (CABG) surgery. The nurse notes that in the first hour after admission, the mediastinal chest tube drainage was 75 mL. During the second hour, the drainage has dropped to 5 mL. The nurse interprets this data and implements which intervention?
1. Identifies that the tube is draining normally
2. Assesses the tube to locate a possible occlusion
3. Auscultates the lungs for appropriate bilateral expansion
4. Assists client with frequent coughing and deep breathing

Level of Cognitive Ability: Analyzing
Client Needs: Physiological Integrity
Clinical Judgment/Cognitive Skills: Analyze Cues
Integrated Process: Clinical Judgment; Nursing Process/Analysis
Content Area: Complex Care: Emergency Situations/Management
Health Problems: Adult Health: Cardiovascular: Coronary Artery Disease
Priority Concepts: Clinical Judgment; Safety

Answer: 2
Rationale: After CABG surgery, chest tube drainage should not exceed 100 to 150 mL/hr during the first 2 hours postoperatively, and approximately 500 mL of drainage is expected in the first 24 hours after CABG surgery. The sudden drop in drainage between the first and second hour indicates that the tube is possibly occluded and requires further assessment by the nurse. Options 1, 3, and 4 are incorrect interventions.
Test-Taking Strategy: Focus on the **subject**, chest tube drainage. Eliminate option 3 first because the mediastinal chest tubes remove fluid from the mediastinum and are unrelated to restoration of negative pleural pressure or bilateral expansion. Needing to cough and deep breathe is a response that is unrelated to the client's problem, so option 4 is eliminated next. From the remaining options, knowing that the drainage would not drop so radically in 1 hour in the immediate postoperative period directs you to the correct option.
Priority Nursing Tip: After CABG surgery, monitor the client for hypotension and hypertension. Hypotension can cause collapse of a vein graft. Hypertension causes increased pressure and can promote leakage from the suture line and bleeding.
Reference: Lewis, S., et al. (2020). *Medical-surgical nursing: Assessment and management of clinical problems* (11th ed., pp. 527, 716–717). Elsevier.

397. The nurse is assessing a client diagnosed with pleurisy 48 hours ago. When auscultating the chest, the nurse is unable to detect the pleural friction rub, which was auscultated on admission. This change in the client's condition confirms which event has occurred?

1. The prescribed medication therapy has been effective.
2. The client has been taking deep breaths as instructed.
3. The effects of the inflammatory reaction at the site decreased.
4. There is now an accumulation of pleural fluid in the inflamed area.

Level of Cognitive Ability: Analyzing
Client Needs: Physiological Integrity
Clinical Judgment/Cognitive Skills: Analyze Cues
Integrated Process: Clinical Judgment; Nursing Process/Analysis
Content Area: Adult Health: Respiratory
Health Problems: Adult Health: Respiratory: Pleurisy
Priority Concepts: Clinical Judgment; Gas Exchange

Answer: 4
Rationale: Pleurisy is the inflammation of the visceral and parietal membranes. These membranes rub together during respiration and cause pain. Pleural friction rub is auscultated early in the course of pleurisy, before pleural fluid accumulates. Once fluid accumulates in the inflamed area, there is less friction between the visceral and parietal lung surfaces, and the pleural friction rub disappears. Options 1, 2, and 3 are incorrect interpretations.
Test-Taking Strategy: Focus on the subject, pleurisy and pleural friction rub. Options 1 and 3 are comparable or alike, and because the question states that the problem was diagnosed 48 hours ago, these options should be eliminated. Eliminate option 2 because deep breaths would intensify the pain. Remember that fluid accumulation in the area provides a buffer between the lung and chest wall surfaces, which resolves the friction rub.
Priority Nursing Tip: Instruct the client with pleurisy to lie on the affected side to splint the chest. This will ease the pain when coughing and deep breathing.
Reference: Lewis, S., et al. (2020). *Medical-surgical nursing: Assessment and management of clinical problems* (11th ed., pp. 506, 509). Elsevier.

❖ **398.** The nurse provides information to a client with a colostomy resulting from treatment for cancer. When discussing measures to help manage colostomy odors, the nurse will encourage the client to regularly consume which foods? **Select all that apply.**

❏ 1. Parsley
❏ 2. Yogurt
❏ 3. Buttermilk
❏ 4. Cucumbers
❏ 5. Cauliflower
❏ 6. Cranberry juice

Level of Cognitive Ability: Applying
Client Needs: Physiological Integrity
Clinical Judgment/Cognitive Skills: Generate Solutions
Integrated Process: Teaching and Learning
Content Area: Foundations of Care: Therapeutic Diets
Health Problems: Adult Health: Cancer: Esophageal/Gastric/Intestinal
Priority Concepts: Nutrition; Elimination

Answer: 1, 2, 3, 6
Rationale: The nurse would provide information about foods and measures that will prevent odor from a colostomy. Parsley, yogurt, buttermilk, and cranberry juice will prevent odor. Charcoal filters, pouch deodorizers, ostomy bags with a vent and a deodorizing filter, or placement of a breath mint in the pouch will also eliminate odors. Foods should be avoided that cause flatus and thus odor, including broccoli, Brussels sprouts, cabbage, cauliflower, cucumbers, mushrooms, and peas.
Test-Taking Strategy: Focus on the subject, foods to control odor. Eliminate options 4 and 5 using basic knowledge regarding nutrition because these foods cause flatus.
Priority Nursing Tip: Body image is a concern for a client with a colostomy, and the nurse needs to be sensitive to the client when discussing this concern with the client.
Reference: Ignatavicius, D., et al. (2021). *Medical-surgical nursing: Concepts for interprofessional collaborative care* (10th ed., pp. 1122–1123). Elsevier; United Ostomy Associations of America. https://www.uoaa.org

399. When a client experiences frequent runs of ventricular tachycardia, the physician prescribes flecainide. Because of the effects of the medication, which nursing intervention is specific to this client's safety?
1. Monitor client's urinary output.
2. Assess client for neurologic problems.
3. Ensure that the bed rails remain in the up position.
4. Monitor client's vital signs and electrocardiogram (ECG) frequently.

Level of Cognitive Ability: Analyzing
Client Needs: Physiological Integrity
Clinical Judgment/Cognitive Skills: Take Action
Integrated Process: Clinical Judgment; Nursing Process/Implementation
Content Area: Pharmacology: Cardiovascular: Antidysrhythmics
Health Problems: Adult Health: Cardiovascular: Dysrhythmias
Priority Concepts: Perfusion; Safety

Answer: 4
Rationale: Flecainide is an antidysrhythmic medication that slows conduction and decreases excitability, conduction velocity, and automaticity. However, the nurse must monitor for the development of a new or worsening dysrhythmia. Options 1, 2, and 3 are components of standard care but are not specific to this medication.
Test-Taking Strategy: Focus on the subject, flecainide. Note the relation of the information in the question (the client has a dysrhythmia) and the nursing action in the correct option. Select the option that relates to cardiac status monitoring.
Priority Nursing Tip: Monitor the client receiving flecainide for an increase and severity of dysrhythmias. This adverse effect may warrant a decrease in dosage or discontinuation of the medication.
Reference: Ignatavicius, D., et al. (2021). *Medical-surgical nursing: Concepts for interprofessional collaborative care* (10th ed., pp. 650–651). Elsevier.

❖ **400.** The nurse provides information to a client diagnosed with gastroesophageal reflux disease (GERD). Which foods would the nurse mention that contribute to decreased lower esophageal sphincter (LES) pressure and thus worsen the condition? **Select all that apply.**
1. Alcohol
2. Fatty foods
3. Citrus fruits
4. Baked potatoes
5. Caffeinated beverages
6. Tomatoes and tomato products

Level of Cognitive Ability: Applying
Client Needs: Physiological Integrity
Clinical Judgment/Cognitive Skills: Take Action
Integrated Process: Teaching and Learning
Content Area: Adult Health: Gastrointestinal
Health Problems: Adult Health: Gastrointestinal: Gastroesophageal Reflux Disease
Priority Concepts: Patient Education; Nutrition

Answer: 1, 2, 3, 5, 6
Rationale: GERD occurs as a result of the backward flow (reflux) of gastrointestinal contents into the esophagus. The most common cause of GERD is inappropriate relaxation of the LES, which allows the reflux of gastric contents into the esophagus and exposes the esophageal mucosa to gastric contents. Factors that influence the tone and contractility of the LES and lower LES pressure include alcohol; fatty foods; citrus fruits; caffeinated beverages such as coffee, tea, and cola; tomatoes and tomato products; chocolate; nicotine in cigarette smoke; calcium channel blockers; nitrates; anticholinergics; high levels of estrogen and progesterone; peppermint and spearmint; and nasogastric tube placement. Baked potatoes would not contribute to worsening the problem.
Test-Taking Strategy: Note the client's diagnosis of GERD and focus on the subject, factors that contribute to decreased lower esophageal sphincter (LES) pressure. Read each option and consider whether the item will aggravate the client's condition. The only item that will not is option 4, baked potatoes.
Priority Nursing Tip: Teach the client with GERD to avoid lying down with a full stomach and avoid eating within 2 to 3 hours of bedtime; to avoid wearing tight-fitting clothing, particularly around the waist; and to sleep with the head of the bed raised at least 6 to 8 inches.
Reference: Ignatavicius, D., et al. (2021). *Medical-surgical nursing: Concepts for interprofessional collaborative care* (10th ed., p. 1081). Elsevier.

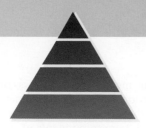

CHAPTER 7

Safe and Effective Care Environment Practice Questions

1. The nurse is developing an educational session on client advocacy for the nursing staff. The nurse would include which interventions as examples of the nurse acting as a client advocate? **Select all that apply.**
   - ❑ 1. Obtaining an informed consent for a surgical procedure
   - ❑ 2. Providing information necessary for a client to make informed decisions
   - ❑ 3. Providing assistance in asserting the client's human and legal rights if the need arises
   - ❑ 4. Including the client's religious or cultural beliefs when assisting the client in making an informed decision
   - ❑ 5. Defending the client's rights by speaking out against policies or actions that might endanger the client's well-being

Level of Cognitive Ability: Applying
Client Needs: Safe and Effective Care Environment
Clinical Judgment/Cognitive Skills: Generate Solutions
Integrated Process: Teaching and Learning
Content Area: Leadership/Management: Ethical/Legal
Health Problems: N/A
Priority Concepts: Caregiving; Professional Identity

Answer: 2, 3, 4, 5
Rationale: In the role of client advocate, the nurse protects the client's human and legal rights and provides assistance in asserting those rights if the need arises. The nurse advocates for the client by providing information needed so that the client can make an informed decision. The nurse needs to consider the client's religion and culture when functioning as an advocate and when providing care. The nurse would include the client's religious or cultural beliefs in discussions about treatment plans so that an informed decision can be made. The nurse also defends clients' rights in a general way by speaking out against policies or actions that might endanger the client's well-being or conflict with the client's rights. Informed consent is part of the primary health care provider–client relationship; in most situations, obtaining the client's informed consent does not fall within the nursing duty. Even though the nurse assumes the responsibility for witnessing the client's signature on the consent form, the nurse does not legally assume the duty of obtaining informed consent.
Test-Taking Strategy: Focus on the subject, examples of the nurse acting as a client advocate. Read each option carefully and recall the definition of a client advocate. Remembering that in this role the nurse protects the client's human and legal rights and provides assistance in asserting those rights if the need arises will assist in selecting the correct examples.
Priority Nursing Tip: The nurse is a care provider who spends a significant amount of time with the client and, therefore, is in a critical position to act as a client advocate.
Reference: Potter, P., et al. (2021). *Fundamentals of nursing.* (10th ed.,p. 296). Elsevier.

❖ **2.** The registered nurse (RN) planning the assignments for the day is leading a team comprised of a licensed practical nurse (LPN) and an unlicensed assistive personnel (UAP). Based on licensure, which client is **most appropriate** to assign to the LPN?
1. A client diagnosed with dementia
2. A 1-day postoperative mastectomy client
3. A client who requires some assistance with bathing
4. A client who requires some assistance with ambulation

Level of Cognitive Ability: Applying
Client Needs: Safe and Effective Care Environment
Clinical Judgment/Cognitive Skills: Generate Solutions
Integrated Process: Clinical Judgment; Nursing Process/Planning
Content Area: Leadership/Management: Delegating/Supervising
Health Problems: N/A
Priority Concepts: Care Coordination; Leadership

Answer: 2
Rationale: Assignment of tasks must be implemented based on the job description of the LPN and UAP, the level of education and clinical competence, and state law. The 1-day postoperative mastectomy client will need care that requires the skill of a licensed nurse. The UAP has the skills to care for a client requiring noninvasive care, such as a client with dementia, a client who requires some assistance with bathing, and a client who requires some assistance with ambulation.
Test-Taking Strategy: Note the strategic words, *most appropriate*. Also, focus on the subject, client assignments for the LPN and UAP. Think about the needs of each client to assist in determining the assignment. Remember that the LPN will be performing at a higher skill level than the UAP.
Priority Nursing Tip: Do not delegate an activity to anyone who has never performed the task. Perform the activity with the individual and teach about the procedure for performing it; this ensures client safety. Clients who are potentially unstable or complicated need to be assigned to licensed staff.
Reference: Potter, P., et al. (2021). *Fundamentals of nursing* (10th ed., pp. 289–290). Elsevier.

3. The nurse is delegating unit nursing tasks for the day. Which tasks would the nurse delegate to the unlicensed assistive personnel (UAP)? **Select all that apply.**
❑ 1. Deliver fresh water to clients.
❑ 2. Empty urine out of urinary catheter bags.
❑ 3. Take temperatures, pulses, respirations, and blood pressures.
❑ 4. Count the substance control medications in the opioid medication supply.
❑ 5. Check the crash cart (cardiopulmonary resuscitation cart) for necessary supplies using a checklist.
❑ 6. Check all intravenous (IV) solution bags on clients receiving IV therapy for the remaining amounts of solution in the bags.

Level of Cognitive Ability: Applying
Client Needs: Safe and Effective Care Environment
Clinical Judgment/Cognitive Skills: Generate Solutions
Integrated Process: Clinical Judgment; Nursing Process/Planning
Content Area: Leadership/Management: Delegating/Supervising
Health Problems: N/A
Priority Concepts: Care Coordination; Leadership

Answer: 1, 2, 3
Rationale: Delegation is the transfer of responsibility for the performance of an activity or task while retaining accountability for the outcome. When delegating an activity, the nurse must consider the educational preparation and experience of the individual. The UAP is trained to perform noninvasive tasks and those that meet basic client needs. The UAP is also trained to take vital signs. Therefore, the appropriate activities to assign to the UAP would be to deliver fresh water to clients; empty urine out of urinary catheter bags; and take temperatures, pulses, respirations, and blood pressures. Although the UAP is trained in performing cardiopulmonary resuscitation, the UAP is not trained to check a crash cart, and this activity must be assigned to a licensed nurse. Any activities related to medications and IV therapy must be delegated to a licensed nurse.
Test-Taking Strategy: Focus on the subject, activities to be delegated to a UAP. Recalling that a UAP is trained to perform noninvasive tasks and that medication and IV therapy and any activity that requires critical thinking skills must be delegated to a licensed nurse will assist in answering this question.
Priority Nursing Tip: To ensure client safety, it is very important for the nurse to delegate appropriately to the UAP. Most tasks that are noninvasive can be assigned to the UAP.
Reference: Lewis, S., et al. (2020). *Medical-surgical nursing: Assessment and management of clinical problems* (11th ed., pp. 9–10). Elsevier.

Client Needs

4. In the middle of bathing a client, the unit secretary notifies the nurse that there is an emergency telephone call. Which action would the nurse implement to **best** ensure client safety?

1. Quickly finish the bath before answering the call.
2. Immediately leave the client's room and answer the call.
3. Cover the client, place the call light within reach, and then leave to answer the call.
4. Leave the door open and ask staff to monitor the client, and then leave to answer the call.

Level of Cognitive Ability: Applying
Client Needs: Safe and Effective Care Environment
Clinical Judgment/Cognitive Skills: Take Action
Integrated Process: Nursing Process/Implementation
Content Area: Foundations of Care: Safety
Health Problems: N/A
Priority Concepts: Clinical Judgment: Safety

Answer: 3
Rationale: Because the telephone call is an emergency, the nurse may need to answer it. To maintain privacy and safety, the nurse covers the client and places the call light within the client's reach. Additionally, the client's door needs to be closed or the room curtains pulled around the bathing area. The other appropriate action is to ask another nurse to accept the call. This, however, is not one of the options. None of the other options effectively meet the client's safety needs.
Test-Taking Strategy: Note the strategic word, *best*. Focus on the subject, the need for the nurse to respond to an emergency call. Eliminate option 1 because this delays the nurse responding. Eliminate option 2 because this action does not provide client safety. From the remaining options, recalling the rights of the client and the principles related to safety will assist in eliminating option 4.
Priority Nursing Tip: If it is necessary to leave the client's bedside, return the bed to low position, elevate side rails as appropriate per state and agency policies, place the call light in the client's reach, and ensure that the client knows how to use it.
Reference: Potter, P., et al. (2021). *Fundamentals of nursing* (10th ed., pp. 404, 873). Elsevier.

5. The nurse manager reviewing the purposes for applying restraints to a client determines that **further education is necessary** when a nursing staff member makes which statement supporting the use of a restraint?

1. "It limits movement of a limb during a painful procedure."
2. "It prevents the violent client from injuring self and others."
3. "At night it keeps the client in bed instead of wandering about."
4. "It is useful in preventing the client from pulling out intravenous lines."

Level of Cognitive Ability: Evaluating
Client Needs: Safe and Effective Care Environment
Clinical Judgment/Cognitive Skills: Evaluate Outcomes
Integrated Process: Nursing Process/Evaluation
Content Area: Foundations of Care: Safety
Health Problems: N/A
Priority Concepts: Health Care Law; Safety

Answer: 3
Rationale: Wrist and ankle restraints are devices used to limit the client's movement in situations when it is necessary to immobilize a limb. Restraints are not applied to keep a client in bed at night and are never used as a form of punishment. Restraints are applied to prevent the client from injuring self or others; pulling out intravenous lines, catheters, or tubes; or removing dressings. Restraints also may be used to keep children still and from injuring themselves during treatments and diagnostic procedures. A physician's prescription is required for the use of restraints, and state and agency procedures are always followed when restraints are used.
Test-Taking Strategy: Note the strategic words, *further education is necessary.* These words indicate a negative event query and the need to select the option that identifies an inaccurate use for restraints. Eliminate options 1 and 4 first because they are comparable or alike. From the remaining options, read each option carefully. Recalling the guidelines for the use of restraints will direct you to the correct option.
Priority Nursing Tip: Assess the client with restraints applied continuously to determine if the restraints remain necessary.
Reference: Potter, P., et al. (2019). *Essentials for nursing practice* (9th ed., p. 417). Elsevier.

6. A client diagnosed with epilepsy has a prescription for valproic acid 250 mg once daily. To maximize the client's safety, which time is **best** for the nurse to schedule administration of the medication?
1. With lunch
2. With breakfast
3. Before breakfast
4. At bedtime with a snack

Level of Cognitive Ability: Applying
Client Needs: Safe and Effective Care Environment
Clinical Judgment/Cognitive Skills: Take Action
Integrated Process: Nursing Process/Implementation
Content Area: Pharmacology: Neurologic: Antiseizure
Health Problems: Adult Health: Neurologic: Seizure Disorder/Epilepsy
Priority Concepts: Clinical Judgment; Safety

Answer: **4**
Rationale: Valproic acid is an anticonvulsant that causes central nervous system (CNS) depression. For this reason, the side and adverse effects include sedation, dizziness, ataxia, and confusion. When the client is taking this medication as a single daily dose, administering it at bedtime negates the risk of injury from sedation and enhances client safety. Otherwise, it may be given after meals to avoid gastrointestinal upset. Carbonated beverages need to be avoided with its administration, and the client needs to follow the physician's prescription regarding its administration.
Test-Taking Strategy: Note the strategic word, *best*. Recalling that this medication is an anticonvulsant with CNS depressant properties and that sedation can occur will direct you to option 4. Administration at bedtime allows the sedative effects of the medication to occur at a time when the client is sleeping. Also note that options 1 and 3 are comparable or alike in that they indicate administering the medication with meals.
Priority Nursing Tip: If the client is taking a CNS depressant, inform the client that sedation can occur and of the measures that ensure safety.
Reference: Lilley, L., Rainforth Collins, S., & Snyder, J. (2020). *Pharmacology and the nursing process* (9th ed., pp. 226–227). Elsevier.

7. Which findings documented in the history of an older adult client would require the nurse to implement an accident prevention protocol? **Select all that apply.**
☐ 1. Range of motion is limited.
☐ 2. Peripheral vision is decreased.
☐ 3. Transmission of hot impulses is delayed.
☐ 4. The client reports incidences of nocturia.
☐ 5. High-frequency hearing tones are perceptible.
☐ 6. Voluntary and autonomic reflexes are slowed.

Level of Cognitive Ability: Analyzing
Client Needs: Safe and Effective Care Environment
Clinical Judgment/Cognitive Skills: Recognize Cues
Integrated Process: Clinical Judgment; Nursing Process/Assessment
Content Area: Foundations of Care: Safety
Health Problems: N/A
Priority Concepts: Development; Safety

Answer: **1, 2, 3, 4, 6**
Rationale: The physiologic changes that occur during the aging process increase the client's risk for accidents. Musculoskeletal changes include a decrease in muscle strength and function, lessened joint mobility, and limited range of motion. Sensory changes include a decrease in peripheral vision and lens accommodation, delayed transmission of hot and cold impulses, and impaired hearing as high-frequency tones become less perceptible. Nervous system changes include slowed voluntary and autonomic reflexes. Genitourinary changes may include nocturia.
Test-Taking Strategy: Focus on the subject, accident prevention in an older client. Reading each option carefully and keeping in mind the factors that affect client safety will assist in answering the question.
Priority Nursing Tip: Age-related changes occur on an individual basis, and one client may experience an age-related change to a lesser extent than another client. The nurse must gather baseline data and then assess for changes and determine the appropriate course of action to compensate to promote client safety.
Reference: Potter, P., et al. (2021). *Fundamentals of nursing* (10th ed., pp. 179, 181). Elsevier.

8. Which actions would the nurse take when obtaining a sputum culture from a client with a diagnosis of pneumonia? **Select all that apply.**

☐ **1.** Explain the procedure to the client.
☐ **2.** Obtain the specimen early in the morning.
☐ **3.** Have the client brush their teeth before expectoration.
☐ **4.** Instruct the client to take deep breaths before coughing.
☐ **5.** Place the lid of the culture container face down on the bedside table.

Level of Cognitive Ability: Applying
Client Needs: Safe and Effective Care Environment
Clinical Judgment/Cognitive Skills: Take Action
Integrated Process: Nursing Process/Implementation
Content Area: Skills: Specimen Collection
Health Problems: Adult Health: Respiratory: Pneumonia
Priority Concepts: Clinical Judgment; Infection

Answer: 1, 2, 3, 4
Rationale: The nurse always explains a procedure to the client. The specimen is obtained early in the morning whenever possible because increased amounts of sputum collect in the airways during sleep. The client needs to rinse the mouth or brush the teeth before specimen collection to avoid contaminating the specimen. The client would take deep breaths before expectoration for best sputum production. Placing the lid face down on the bedside table contaminates the lid and could result in inaccurate findings.
Test-Taking Strategy: Focus on the subject, the procedure for obtaining a sputum culture. Read each option carefully. Visualizing the procedures for using the basic principles of aseptic technique will direct you to eliminate option 5.
Priority Nursing Tip: Any specimen for culture needs to be collected via sterile technique because contamination of the specimen invalidates the results.
Reference: Pagana, K., Pagana, T., & Pagana, T. N. (2021). *Mosby's Diagnostic and laboratory test reference* (15th ed., pp. 830–831). Elsevier.

---

9. The nurse would wear this protective device when caring for hospitalized clients with which diagnosed disorders? **(Refer to the figure.) Select all that apply.**

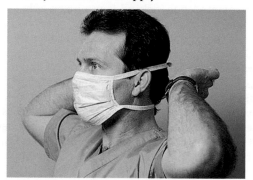

(From Potter, P., Perry, A., Stockert, P., & Hall, A. [2017]. *Fundamentals of nursing* [9th ed.]. Mosby.)

☐ **1.** Scabies
☐ **2.** Tuberculosis
☐ **3.** Hepatitis A virus
☐ **4.** Pharyngeal diphtheria
☐ **5.** Streptococcal pharyngitis
☐ **6.** Meningococcal pneumonia

Level of Cognitive Ability: Applying
Client Needs: Safe and Effective Care Environment
Clinical Judgment/Cognitive Skills: Take Action
Integrated Process: Nursing Process/Implementation
Content Area: Foundations of Care: Infection Prevention and Control
Health Problems: N/A
Priority Concepts: Infection; Safety

Answer: 4, 5, 6
Rationale: A standard surgical mask is used as part of droplet precautions to protect the nurse from acquiring the client's infection. Droplet precautions refer to precautions used for organisms that can spread through the air but are unable to remain in the air farther than 3 feet. Many respiratory viral infections such as respiratory viral influenza require the use of a standard surgical mask when caring for the client. Some other disorders requiring the use of a standard surgical mask include pharyngeal diphtheria; rubella; streptococcal pharyngitis; pertussis; mumps; pneumonia, including meningococcal pneumonia; and the pneumonic plague. Scabies and hepatitis A are transmitted by direct contact with an infected person and require the use of contact precautions for protection. Tuberculosis requires the use of airborne precautions and the use of an individually fitted particulate filter mask. A standard surgical mask would not protect the nurse from *Mycobacterium tuberculosis*.
Test-Taking Strategy: Focus on the subject, the need to wear a standard mask. This indicates the need for nurses to protect themselves from inhaling an organism. You can eliminate option 2 by recalling that tuberculosis requires the use of an individually fitted particulate filter mask. Next eliminate options 1 and 3 by recalling that these infections are not transmitted by the respiratory route. Noting that options 4, 5, and 6 are respiratory disorders will assist in answering correctly.
Priority Nursing Tip: Infection control is very important to implement when caring for clients. Nosocomial, or hospital-acquired, infections, can be prevented if these practices are properly implemented. In-service educational sessions are effective ways to remind health care workers of proper precautionary procedures.
References: Ignatavicius, D., et al. (2021). *Medical-surgical nursing: Concepts for interprofessional collaborative care* (10th ed., p. 410). Elsevier; Potter, P., et al. (2021). *Fundamentals of nursing* (10th ed., p. 438). Elsevier.

❖ **10.** The nurse is developing a hospital policy on guidelines for telephone and verbal prescriptions. Which guidelines would the nurse include in the policy? **Select all that apply.**
- ❑ 1. Avoid using all abbreviations.
- ❑ 2. Verbal prescriptions are rarely acceptable.
- ❑ 3. Clarify any questions with the physician.
- ❑ 4. Repeat the prescribed prescriptions back to the physician.
- ❑ 5. If the prescriber is the client's physician, documentation is unnecessary.

Level of Cognitive Ability: Applying
Client Needs: Safe and Effective Care Environment
Clinical Judgment/Cognitive Skills: Take Action
Integrated Process: Nursing Process/Implementation
Content Area: Leadership/Management: Ethical/Legal
Health Problems: N/A
Priority Concepts: Communication; Safety

Answer: 3, 4
Rationale: To avoid misunderstandings, the nurse would always clarify a telephone or verbal prescription with the physician if the nurse had any questions about the prescription, and the nurse would repeat any prescriptions back to the physician. A telephone order (TO) or prescription involves a physician stating a prescribed therapy over the phone to the nurse. TOs are frequently given at night or during an emergency and need to be given only when absolutely necessary. Likewise, a verbal order (VO) or prescription is acceptable when there is no opportunity for the physician to write the prescription such as in an emergency situation. Additional guidelines for telephone and verbal prescriptions include the following: clearly determine the client's name, room number, and diagnosis; indicate TO or VO, including the date and time, name of the client, complete prescription, name of the physician giving the prescription, and nurse taking the prescription; and have the physician cosign the prescription within the time frame designated by the health care agency (usually 24 hours). There are some abbreviations that are acceptable, and documentation is necessary regardless of the prescriber.
Test-Taking Strategy: Focus on the subject, guidelines for taking TOs and VOs. Eliminate option 1 because of the closed-ended word, *all* and option 5 because of the words *is unnecessary.* Next, reading the remaining options carefully and thinking about the legal issues related to physicians' prescriptions will assist you in answering correctly.
Priority Nursing Tip: The nurse plays a vital role in maintaining the safety of the client. The nurse is considered the "last line of defense" for clients in terms of noting a prescription that may be harmful to them.
Reference: Potter, P., et al. (2021). *Fundamentals of nursing* (10th ed., pp. 376, 602). Elsevier.

11. The nurse employed in a preschool agency is planning a staff education program to prevent the spread of an intestinal parasitical disease. Which prevention measure would the nurse include in the educational session?
1. All food will be cooked before eating.
2. Only bottled water will be used for drinking.
3. All toileting areas will be cleansed daily with soap and water.
4. Standard precautions will be used when assisting children with toileting.

Level of Cognitive Ability: Applying
Client Needs: Safe and Effective Care Environment
Clinical Judgment/Cognitive Skills: Generate Solutions
Integrated Process: Teaching and Learning
Content Area: Foundations of Care: Infection Control
Health Problems: Pediatric-Specific: Intestinal Parasites
Priority Concepts: Infection; Safety

Answer: 4
Rationale: The fecal-oral route is the mode of transmission of an intestinal parasitical disease. Standard precautions prevent the transmission of infection. Some fresh foods do not need to be cooked as long as they are washed well and were not grown in soil contaminated with human feces. Water and fresh foods can be vehicles for transmission, but municipal water sources are usually safe. Cleaning with soap and water is not as effective as the use of bleach.
Test-Taking Strategy: Focus on the subject, preventing the spread of an intestinal parasitical infection. Option 4 addresses the subject of the question and is the umbrella option, addressing standard precautions. Also, note that options 1, 2, and 3 contain the closed-ended words "all" and "only."
Priority Nursing Tip: Regardless of the infectious agent, infection control measures are essential to protect health care providers and clients.
Reference: Hockenberry, M., Wilson, D., & Rodgers, C. (2019). *Wong's Nursing care of infants and children* (11th ed., pp. 169–170, 192). Elsevier.

❖ **12.** A client has arrived at the labor and delivery unit in active labor. The nursing assessment reveals a recurrent history of diagnosed genital herpes and the presence of lesions in the genital tract. Which intervention would the nurse initiate?
  1. Limiting visitors
  2. Maintaining reverse isolation
  3. Preparing for a cesarean delivery
  4. Preparing for the artificial membrane rupturing

Level of Cognitive Ability: Applying
Client Needs: Safe and Effective Care Environment
Clinical Judgment/Cognitive Skills: Take Action
Integrated Process: Clinical Judgment; Nursing Process/Implementation
Content Area: Maternity: Intrapartum
Health Problems: Maternity: Infections/Inflammations
Priority Concepts: Infection; Reproduction

Answer: 3
Rationale: A cesarean delivery can reduce the risk of neonatal infection with a client in labor who has herpetic genital tract lesions. There is no need to limit visitors or maintain isolation, although standard precautions need to be maintained. A vaginal delivery presents a risk of transmitting the disease to the neonate. Intact membranes provide another barrier to transmitting the disease to the neonate.
Test-Taking Strategy: Focus on the subject, the presence of genital herpes lesions. Eliminate option 4 first because this action would place the neonate in contact with the lesions. From the remaining options, consider the risks to the neonate to direct you to the correct option.
Priority Nursing Tip: No vaginal examinations are performed on a pregnant client who has active vaginal herpetic lesions.
Reference: McKinney, E. S., et al. (2022). *Maternal child nursing* (6th ed., p. 392). Elsevier.

13. Which interventions would the nurse perform when inserting an indwelling urinary catheter in order to maintain both the integrity of the catheter and the client's safety? **Select all that apply.**
  ❑ 1. Use strict aseptic technique.
  ❑ 2. Place the drainage bag lower than the bladder level.
  ❑ 3. Inflate the balloon 4 to 5 mL beyond its capacity.
  ❑ 4. Swab the urinary catheter with sterile water before inserting.
  ❑ 5. Advance the catheter 1 to 2 inches after urine appears in the tubing.

Level of Cognitive Ability: Applying
Client Needs: Safe and Effective Care Environment
Clinical Judgment/Cognitive Skills: Take Action
Integrated Process: Nursing Process/Implementation
Content Area: Skills: Elimination
Health Problems: N/A
Priority Concepts: Clinical Judgment; Safety

Answer: 1, 2, 5
Rationale: The nurse would use strict aseptic technique to insert the catheter. The drainage bag is placed lower than bladder level to ensure drainage, prevent retrograde flow of urine, and reduce the risk of infection. Advancing the catheter 1 to 2 inches beyond the point where the flow of urine is first noted is also good practice because this ensures that the catheter balloon is completely in the bladder before it is inflated. The nurse risks rupturing the catheter's balloon by overinflating it; therefore, the nurse inflates the balloon with the specified volume for the catheter because inflating the balloon 4 to 5 mL beyond its capacity is unsafe. The urinary catheter is sterile, so it is inappropriate and unnecessary to swab it with sterile water before inserting.
Test-Taking Strategy: Focus on the subject, the procedure for inserting a urinary catheter, visualizing the procedure to answer correctly. Noting the words *beyond its capacity* in option 3 will assist in eliminating this option. Recalling that the urinary catheter is sterile will assist in eliminating option 4.
Priority Nursing Tip: When preparing to insert a urinary catheter, it is advisable to bring an extra urinary catheter, an extra pair of gloves, and a flashlight along with the regular urinary catheter insertion equipment to the client's room.
Reference: Potter, P., et al. (2021). *Fundamentals of nursing* (10th ed., pp. 1181, 1186, 1188). Elsevier.

14. A client admitted 2 days ago with a diagnosis of moderate depression begins smiling and reporting that the crisis is over. Which **priority** modification to the treatment plan would occur based on the behavioral cues of the client?
1. Allowing off-unit privileges PRN
2. Suggesting a reduction of medication
3. Allowing increased "in-room" activities
4. Increasing the level of suicide precautions

Level of Cognitive Ability: Analyzing
Client Needs: Safe and Effective Care Environment
Clinical Judgment/Cognitive Skills: Analyze Cues
Integrated Process: Clinical Judgment; Nursing Process/Analysis
Content Area: Mental Health
Health Problems: Mental Health: Mood Disorders
Priority Concepts: Mood and Affect; Safety

Answer: 4
Rationale: A client who is diagnosed as moderately depressed and has only been hospitalized 2 days is unlikely to have such a dramatic cure. When a mood suddenly lifts, it is likely that the client may have made the decision to cause self-harm. Suicide precautions are necessary to keep the client safe. Options 1 and 2 are incorrect because they support a "quick" cure. In-room activities do not encourage social interaction; social interaction would be a desired outcome for a moderately depressed client.
Test-Taking Strategy: Note the strategic word, *priority*. Focus on the subject, client diagnosed with moderate depression, and recall that depression does not resolve in 2 days. Options 1 and 2 support the client's notion that a cure has occurred. Option 3 allows the client to increase isolation. Recalling that safety is of the utmost importance will direct you to option 4.
Priority Nursing Tip: When a client diagnosed with moderate depression at risk for suicide displays increased alertness and energy, suicide precautions need to be continued. These observations are an indication that the client has the energy to perform the act of suicide.
Reference: Varcarolis, E., & Fosbre, C. (2021). *Essentials of psychiatric mental health nursing: A communication approach to evidence-based care* (4th ed., pp. 209–210). Elsevier.

15. The nurse is planning care for a client admitted with suicidal ideations. To **best** ensure client safety the nurse would implement additional precautions during which time period?
1. During the day shift
2. On weekday evenings
3. Between 0800 and 1000
4. During the unit shift change

Level of Cognitive Ability: Applying
Client Needs: Safe and Effective Care Environment
Clinical Judgment/Cognitive Skills: Generate Solutions
Integrated Process: Nursing Process/Planning
Content Area: Mental Health
Health Problems: Mental Health: Suicide
Priority Concepts: Mood and Affect; Safety

Answer: 4
Rationale: At shift change, there is often less availability of staff. The psychiatric nurse and staff need to increase precautions for suicidal clients at that time. The night shift also presents a high-risk time, as do weekends, not weekdays.
Test-Taking Strategy: Note the strategic word, *best*. Options 1, 2, and 3 are comparable or alike since they represent predictable times and can be eliminated. Remember that the nurse needs to anticipate that times with less supervision of the client could be times of increased risks.
Priority Nursing Tip: Provide one-on-one supervision at all times for a client at risk for suicide.
Reference: Varcarolis, E., & Fosbre, C. (2021). *Essentials of psychiatric mental health nursing: A communication approach to evidence-based care* (4th ed., p. 372). Elsevier.

❖ **16.** The nurse is assisting with the transfer of a client from the operating room table to a stretcher. Which interventions would the nurse implement to ensure client safety? **Select all that apply.**
   ❑ 1. Check the client's level of consciousness.
   ❑ 2. Check wheel locks of the operating room table.
   ❑ 3. Complete the client transfer as quickly as possible.
   ❑ 4. Tell the client to move self from the table to the stretcher.
   ❑ 5. Raise side rails after the client is positioned on the stretcher per agency policy.

Level of Cognitive Ability: Applying
Client Needs: Safe and Effective Care Environment
Clinical Judgment/Cognitive Skills: Take Action
Integrated Process: Nursing Process/Implementation
Content Area: Foundations of Care: Safety
Health Problems: N/A
Priority Concepts: Clinical Judgment; Safety

Answer: 1, 2, 5
Rationale: As part of the safe transfer of a client after a surgical procedure, the nurse would assess the client's level of consciousness and, if appropriate, let the client know that they will be transferred from the operating room table to the stretcher. The nurse checks the wheel locks of the table and the stretcher to prevent any movement during the transfer. In addition, the nurse raises the side rails per agency policy to prevent the client from falling off the stretcher. This is important because the client is likely to be sedated or disoriented and unable to protect themselves from falling. Personnel avoid hurried movements and rapid changes in position because hurried movements predispose the client to hypotension; moreover, secure, deliberate movement increases the security of the client. Because the client remains affected by anesthesia, the client should not move themself.
Test-Taking Strategy: Focus on the subject, safety during client transfer. Note the word *quickly* in option 3; this is likely to increase the risk of client injury. Option 4 is unsuitable because of the residual effects of anesthesia and also increases the risk of client injury.
Priority Nursing Tip: The nurse would always obtain additional nursing staff assistance when moving a client or transferring a client from a bed to a stretcher or other location.
Reference: Potter, P., et al. (2021). *Fundamentals of nursing* (10th ed., pp. 813–814). Elsevier.

17. The nurse is planning care for a suicidal client who is hallucinating and delusional. Which intervention would the nurse incorporate into the nursing care plan to **best** ensure client safety?
   1. Check the client's location every 15 minutes.
   2. Begin suicide precautions with 30-minute checks.
   3. Initiate one-to-one suicide precautions immediately.
   4. Ask the client to report suicidal thoughts immediately.

Level of Cognitive Ability: Applying
Client Needs: Safe and Effective Care Environment
Clinical Judgment/Cognitive Skills: Generate Solutions
Integrated Process: Clinical Judgment; Nursing Process/Planning
Content Area: Mental Health
Health Problems: Mental Health: Suicide
Priority Concepts: Mood and Affect; Safety

Answer: 3
Rationale: One-to-one suicide precautions are required for the client rescued from a suicide attempt. In this situation, additional significant information is that the client is delusional and hallucinating. Both of these factors increase the risk of unpredictable behavior, compromised judgment, and the risk of suicide. Options 1, 2, and 4 do not provide the constant supervision necessary for this client.
Test-Taking Strategy: Note the strategic word, *best*. Focusing on the subject, suicide attempt with hallucinations and delusions, will direct you to option 3, the intervention that will provide the most supervision.
Priority Nursing Tip: Never leave a client at risk for suicide alone.
Reference: Varcarolis, E., & Fosbre, C. (2021). *Essentials of psychiatric mental health nursing: A communication approach to evidence-based care* (4th ed., p. 372). Elsevier.

18. The nurse is planning care for a client with a prescription for an anticoagulant agent as part of treatment for a deep vein thrombosis. Which would the nurse identify as a potential concern for this client?
1. Fatigue
2. Bruising
3. Infection
4. Dehydration

Level of Cognitive Ability: Analyzing
Client Needs: Safe and Effective Care Environment
Clinical Judgment/Cognitive Skills: Prioritize Hypotheses
Integrated Process: Clinical Judgment; Nursing Process/Analysis
Content Area: Pharmacology: Cardiovascular: Anticoagulants
Health Problems: Adult Health: Cardiovascular: Deep Vein Thrombosis
Priority Concepts: Clotting; Safety

Answer: 2
Rationale: Anticoagulant therapy predisposes the client to injury because of the agent's inhibitory effects on the body's normal blood clotting mechanism. Bruising, bleeding, and hemorrhage may occur in the course of activities of daily living and with other activities. Options 1, 3, and 4 are unrelated to this form of therapy.
Test-Taking Strategy: Focus on the subject, risks associated with anticoagulant therapy. Recalling that anticoagulants present a risk for bleeding will assist in directing you to option 2.
Priority Nursing Tip: Teach the client taking warfarin sodium to avoid consuming green, leafy vegetables and foods high in vitamin K because they interact with the action of the medication.
Reference: Lewis, S., et al. (2020). *Medical-surgical nursing: Assessment and management of clinical problems* (11th ed., pp. 820–821). Elsevier.

19. A client reporting abdominal pain has a diagnosis of acute abdominal syndrome, but the cause has not been determined. Which prescription would the nurse question at this time?
1. Clear liquid diet only
2. Insertion of a nasogastric tube
3. Administration of an analgesic
4. Insertion of an intravenous (IV) line

Level of Cognitive Ability: Analyzing
Client Needs: Safe and Effective Care Environment
Clinical Judgment/Cognitive Skills: Take Action
Integrated Process: Clinical Judgment; Nursing Process/Implementation
Content Area: Adult Health: Gastrointestinal
Health Problems: Adult Health: Neurologic: Pain
Priority Concepts: Clinical Judgment; Safety

Answer: 1
Rationale: Until the cause of the acute abdominal syndrome is determined and a decision about the need for surgery is made, the nurse would question a prescription to give a clear liquid diet. The nurse can expect the client to be placed on nothing by mouth (NPO) status and to have an IV line inserted. Insertion of a nasogastric tube may be helpful to provide decompression of the stomach. Pain management with medications that do not alter level of consciousness can decrease diffuse abdominal pain and rigidity, help with localizing the pain, and lead to more prompt diagnosis and treatment.
Test-Taking Strategy: Focus on the subject, undetermined abdominal pain and the prescription that the nurse would question. Think about the client's diagnosis. Recalling that surgery may be a necessary intervention will help direct you to the correct option.
Priority Nursing Tip: Signs of perforation and peritonitis include restlessness, guarding of the abdomen, distention and a rigid abdomen, increased fever, chills, tachycardia, and tachypnea.
Reference: Lewis, S., et al. (2020). *Medical-surgical nursing: Assessment and management of clinical problems* (11th ed., pp. 934–935, 938). Elsevier.

❖ **20.** A friend of the parents of a newborn with a diagnosis of congenital tracheoesophageal fistula contacts the home health nurse with an offer to help. Which is the **best** nursing action at this time to address the needs and rights of the family?
  1. Advise the friend to contact the family directly and offer assistance to them.
  2. Request that the friend come to the client's home during the next home health visit.
  3. Report the friend's call to the nurse manager for referral to the client's social worker.
  4. Assure the friend that there is no need for assistance since the nurse is visiting daily.

Level of Cognitive Ability: Applying
Client Needs: Safe and Effective Care Environment
Clinical Judgment/Cognitive Skills: Take Action
Integrated Process: Nursing Process/Implementation
Content Area: Leadership/Management: Ethical/Legal
Health Problems: Pediatric-Specific: Disorders of Prenatal Development
Priority Concepts: Ethics; Health Care Law

Answer: 1
Rationale: The nurse must uphold the client's rights and does not give any information regarding a client's care needs to anyone who is not directly involved in the client's care. To request that the friend come for teaching is a direct violation of the client's right to privacy. There is no information in the question to indicate that the family desires assistance from the friend. To refer the call to the nurse manager and social worker again assumes that the friend's assistance and involvement are desired by the family. Informing the friend that the nurse is visiting daily is providing information that is considered confidential. Option 1 directly refers the friend to the family.
Test-Taking Strategy: Note the strategic word, *best*. Focus on the subject, confidentiality and the client's right to privacy. Option 1 is the only option that upholds the client's rights.
Priority Nursing Tip: The nurse must protect client confidentiality at all times.
Reference: Potter, P., et al. (2021). *Fundamentals of nursing* (10th ed., p. 296). Elsevier.

21. The home health nurse is not willing to care for a client who identifies as a homosexual and is diagnosed with human immunodeficiency virus (HIV) because of religious beliefs and objections. The nurse then leaves the client's home. Which statement accurately identifies the nurse's rights and actions? **Select all that apply.**
  ❑ 1. The nurse has the moral right to leave the client's home at any time.
  ❑ 2. The nurse has a legal right to inform the client of any barriers to providing care.
  ❑ 3. The nurse has a duty to protect self from client care situations that are morally repellent.
  ❑ 4. The nurse has a duty to provide competent care to assigned clients in a nondiscriminatory manner.
  ❑ 5. The nurse has the right to refuse to care for any client on religious grounds if competent care coverage is arranged.

Level of Cognitive Ability: Understanding
Client Needs: Safe and Effective Care Environment
Clinical Judgment/Cognitive Skills: Take Action
Integrated Process: Nursing Process/Implementation
Content Area: Leadership/Management: Ethical/Legal
Health Problems: Adult Health: Immune: Immunodeficiency Syndrome
Priority Concepts: Ethics; Health Care Law

Answer: 4, 5
Rationale: The nurse has a duty to provide care to all clients in a nondiscriminatory manner. Personal autonomy does not apply if it interferes with the rights of the client. Refusal to provide care may be acceptable if that refusal does not put the client's safety at risk and the refusal is primarily associated with religious objections, not personal objection, to lifestyle or medical diagnosis. There is no legal obligation to inform the client of the nurse's personal objections to the client. The nurse also has an obligation to observe the principle of nonmaleficence (neither causing nor allowing harm to befall the client).
Test-Taking Strategy: Focus on the subject, client's rights and the nurse's ethical and legal responsibilities. Recognize that refusal to care for a client on religious grounds is permitted if client coverage is arranged. Note the words *competent care* and *nondiscriminatory* in the correct choices. The remaining options are incorrect related to the client's rights and the nurse's moral, religious, and legal obligations.
Priority Nursing Tip: The client always has the right to considerate and respectful care.
Reference: Potter, P., et al. (2021). *Fundamentals of nursing* (10th ed., pp. 294–295). Elsevier.

❖ **22.** The nurse is preparing to administer prescribed heparin sodium 5000 units subcutaneously for deep vein thrombosis prophylaxis. Which action would the nurse take to safely administer the medication?
1. Inject via an infusion device.
2. Inject within 1 inch of the umbilicus.
3. Massage the injection site after administration for a full minute.
4. Change the needle on the syringe after withdrawing the medication from the vial.

Level of Cognitive Ability: Applying
Client Needs: Safe and Effective Care Environment
Clinical Judgment/Cognitive Skills: Take Action
Integrated Process: Nursing Process/Implementation
Content Area: Skills: Medication Administration
Health Problems: Adult Health: Cardiovascular: Deep Vein Thrombosis
Priority Concepts: Clinical Judgment; Safety

Answer: 4
Rationale: After withdrawal of heparin from the vial, the needle is changed before injection to prevent leakage of medication along the needle tract. Heparin administered subcutaneously does not require an infusion device. The injection site is located in the abdominal fat layer. It is not injected within 2 inches of the umbilicus or into any scar tissue. The needle is withdrawn rapidly, pressure is applied, and the area is not massaged. Injection sites are rotated.
Test-Taking Strategy: Focus on the subject, heparin administration. Noting that the heparin is to be administered subcutaneously will assist in eliminating option 1. From the remaining options, recall that heparin is an anticoagulant. This will assist in eliminating options 2 and 3.
Priority Nursing Tip: Monitor the client receiving an anticoagulant for bleeding, such as bleeding gums, bruises, nosebleeds, hematuria, hematemesis, petechiae, and occult blood in the stool.
Reference: Lilley, L., Rainforth Collins, S., & Snyder, J. (2020). *Pharmacology and the nursing process* (9th ed., pp. 113, 421). Elsevier.

23. A client asks the nurse to act as a witness for an advance directive. Which is the **best** intervention for the nurse to implement?
1. Suggest the nurse manager as a witness.
2. Agree to sign the document as a witness.
3. Notify the physician of the client's request.
4. Help the client find an unrelated third party.

Level of Cognitive Ability: Applying
Client Needs: Safe and Effective Care Environment
Clinical Judgment/Cognitive Skills: Take Action
Integrated Process: Nursing Process/Implementation
Content Area: Leadership/Management: Ethical/Legal
Health Problems: N/A
Priority Concepts: Ethics; Health Care Law

Answer: 4
Rationale: An advance directive addresses the withdrawal or withholding of life-sustaining interventions that can prolong life and identifies the person who will make care decisions if the client becomes incompetent. Two people unrelated to the client witness the client's signature and then sign the document signifying that the client signed the advance directive authentically. Nurses or employees of a facility in which the client is receiving care and beneficiaries of the client should not serve as a witness because of conflict of interest concerns. There is no reason to call the physician unless the absence of the advance directive interferes with client care.
Test-Taking Strategy: Note the strategic word, *best*. Focus on the subject, witness for a legal document. Eliminate option 1 because it demonstrates the nurse's reluctance to serve as the client's advocacy. Examine the remaining options and recall the nurse's role as a witness of a legal document.
Priority Nursing Tip: If the client signs an advance directive at the time of hospital admission, it must be documented in the client's medical record.
Reference: Zerwekh, J., & Zerwekh Garneau, A. (2021). *Nursing today: Transition and trends* (10th ed., pp. 436, 490–491). Elsevier.

❖ **24.** The nurse provides home care instructions to the parent of a child with a diagnosis of chickenpox about preventing the transmission of the virus. Which is the **best** statement for the nurse to include in the instructions?
1. Isolate the child until the skin vesicles have dried and crusted.
2. Ensure that the child uses a separate bathroom for elimination.
3. Bring all household members to the clinic for a varicella vaccine.
4. Request a prescription for antibiotics for all household members.

Level of Cognitive Ability: Applying
Client Needs: Safe and Effective Care Environment
Clinical Judgment/Cognitive Skills: Take Action
Integrated Process: Teaching and Learning
Content Area: Foundations of Care: Infection Prevention and Control
Health Problems: Pediatric-Specific: Communicable Diseases
Priority Concepts: Patient Education; Infection

Answer: 1
Rationale: Chickenpox is caused by the varicella-zoster virus. The communicable period is from 1 to 2 days before the onset of the rash to 6 days after the first crop of vesicles, when crusts have formed. Transmission occurs by direct contact with secretions from the vesicles or contaminated objects and via respiratory tract secretions. It is not transmitted via urine or feces. The recommended preventative schedule for receiving the varicella vaccine is at 12 to 15 months of age (first dose) and 4 to 6 years of age (second dose). It is not administered at the time of exposure to the virus. Antibiotics are not used to treat a viral infection. Rather, they are used for treating bacterial infections.
Test-Taking Strategy: Note the strategic word, *best*. Focus on the subject, preventing the transmission of chickenpox. Eliminate option 4 first, recalling that antibiotics are not used to treat a viral infection. Eliminate option 3, recalling that recommended schedule for the administration of the varicella vaccine. Next, eliminate option 2, recalling the mode of transmission of the virus.
Priority Nursing Tip: The skin is the first line of defense against infection. Altered skin integrity can lead to a skin or systemic infection.
Reference: McKinney, E. S., et al. (2022, pp. 916–918). *Maternal child nursing* (6th ed.). Elsevier.

25. An older adult client has been identified as a victim of psychological abuse. Which action by the nurse is the **priority** nursing intervention?
1. Obtaining mental health treatment for the client
2. Adhering to federal mandatory abuse reporting laws
3. Notifying the case worker to intervene in the family situation
4. Removing the client from any situation that presents immediate danger

Level of Cognitive Ability: Applying
Client Needs: Safe and Effective Care Environment
Clinical Judgment/Cognitive Skills: Take Action
Integrated Process: Nursing Process/Implementation
Content Area: Mental Health
Health Problems: Mental Health: Abuse/Neglect
Priority Concepts: Interpersonal Violence; Safety

Answer: 4
Rationale: The priority nursing intervention is to remove the abused victim from the abusive environment. Options 1, 2, and 3 may be appropriate interventions but are not the priority.
Test-Taking Strategy: Note the strategic word, *priority*. Use Maslow's Hierarchy of Needs theory, remembering that if a physiologic need is not present, then safety is the priority. Option 4 is the only option that directly addresses immediate client safety.
Priority Nursing Tip: Older clients most at risk for abuse include individuals who are dependent because of illness, immobility, or altered mental status.
Reference: Lewis, S., et al. (2020). *Medical-surgical nursing: Assessment and management of clinical problems* (11th ed., pp. 66–67). Elsevier.

❖ **26.** A client with a diagnosis of leukemia asks the nurse questions about preparing a living will. Which recommendation from the nurse would be the **best** method of preparing this document?
1. Talk to the hospital chaplain.
2. Obtain advice from an attorney.
3. Consult the American Cancer Society.
4. Discuss the request with the physician.

Level of Cognitive Ability: Applying
Client Needs: Safe and Effective Care Environment
Clinical Judgment/Cognitive Skills: Generate Solutions
Integrated Process: Nursing Process/Planning
Content Area: Leadership/Management: Ethical/Legal
Health Problems: Adult Health: Cancer: Leukemia
Priority Concepts: Ethics; Health Care Law

Answer: 4
Rationale: Living wills are legal documents known as advance directives wherein the client delineates the withdrawal or withholding of treatment when the client is incompetent. Living wills should not be confused with a will that bequeaths personal property and specifies other actions at the time of the client's death. The client starts the process of writing a living will by discussing treatment options and other related issues with the physician. In addition, the client should discuss this issue with the family. Although options 1 and 2 may be helpful, contacting them is not the initial step because both professionals lack the medical information the client needs to make an informed decision; however, the lawyer may be involved after discussion with the physician and family. The American Cancer Society may have pertinent information on living wills; however, the information is not individualized to the client's needs.
Test-Taking Strategy: Note the strategic word, *best.* This indicates an initial step. Remembering that the physician is the primary care person will assist in directing you to the correct option. Contacts addressed in options 1, 2, and 3 may follow the discussion with the provider.
Priority Nursing Tip: A living will lists the medical treatment that a client chooses to omit or refuse if the client becomes unable to make decisions and is terminally ill.
Reference: Lewis, S., et al. (2020). *Medical-surgical nursing: Assessment and management of clinical problems* (11th ed., pp. 133–134). Elsevier.

27. Which clinical situation would the nurse identify as an example of slander?
1. The physician tells a client that the nurse "does not know anything."
2. The nurse tells a client that a nasogastric tube will be inserted if client continues to refuse to eat.
3. The nurse restrains a client at bedtime because the client gets up during the night and wanders around.
4. The laboratory technician restrains the arm of a client refusing to have blood drawn so that the specimen can be obtained.

Level of Cognitive Ability: Understanding
Client Needs: Safe and Effective Care Environment
Clinical Judgment/Cognitive Skills: Recognize Cues
Integrated Process: Nursing Process/Assessment
Content Area: Leadership/Management: Ethical/Legal
Health Problems: N/A
Priority Concepts: Ethics; Health Care Law

Answer: 1
Rationale: Defamation takes place when a falsehood is said (slander) or written (libel) about a person that results in injury to that person's good name and reputation. Battery involves offensive touching or the use of force by a perpetrator without the permission of the victim. An assault occurs when a person puts another person in fear of a harmful or offensive act.
Test-Taking Strategy: Focus on the subject, the situation that constitutes slander. Read the situation presented in each option carefully. Recalling that slander constitutes verbal defamation will direct you to the correct option.
Priority Nursing Tip: A tort is a civil wrong, other than a breach of contract, in which the law allows an injured person to seek damages from a person who caused the injury.
Reference: Potter, P., et al. (2021). *Fundamentals of nursing* (10th ed., pp. 314–315). Elsevier.

❖ **28.** A client with a diagnosis of subarachnoid hemorrhage secondary to ruptured cerebral aneurysm has been placed on aneurysm precautions. To promote safety, the nurse would ensure that which intervention is provided to the client?
   1. Liquid diet
   2. Enemas as needed
   3. Help with ambulation
   4. Daily stool softeners

Level of Cognitive Ability: Applying
Client Needs: Safe and Effective Care Environment
Clinical Judgment/Cognitive Skills: Generate Solutions
Integrated Process: Nursing Process/Planning
Content Area: Adult Health: Neurologic
Health Problems: Adult Health: Neurologic: Aneurysm
Priority Concepts: Intracranial Regulation; Safety

Answer: 4
Rationale: Aneurysm precautions include a variety of measures designed to decrease stimuli that could increase the client's intracranial pressure. Stool softeners should be provided, but enemas need to be avoided. Straining at stool is contraindicated because it increases intracranial pressure. Other measures to decrease stimuli include instituting dim lighting and reducing environmental noise and stimuli. The remaining options are not related to minimizing stimulation.
Test-Taking Strategy: Focus on the subject, ruptured cerebral aneurysm with subarachnoid hemorrhage. With this condition, there is a need to reduce environmental stimuli and prevent increased intracranial pressure. Options 1 and 3 can be eliminated first because these items will not effectively minimize stimulating the client. From the remaining options, eliminate option 2 because administration of an enema will increase intracranial pressure.
Priority Nursing Tip: An early sign of increased intracranial pressure is a change in the level of consciousness.
Reference: Lewis, S., et al. (2020). *Medical-surgical nursing: Assessment and management of clinical problems* (11th ed., pp. 725, 1311). Elsevier.

29. The nurse is about to administer a prescribed intravenous dose of tobramycin when the client reports vertigo and ringing in the ears. Which action would the nurse take **next**?
   1. Check the client's pupillary responses.
   2. Hang the dose of medication immediately.
   3. Give a dose of droperidol with the tobramycin.
   4. Hold the dose and call the physician.

Level of Cognitive Ability: Analyzing
Client Needs: Safe and Effective Care Environment
Clinical Judgment/Cognitive Skills: Take Action
Integrated Process: Nursing Process/Implementation
Content Area: Pharmacology: Immune: Aminoglycosides
Health Problems: N/A
Priority Concepts: Clinical Judgment; Safety

Answer: 4
Rationale: Tobramycin is an antibiotic (aminoglycoside). Ringing in the ears and vertigo are two symptoms that may indicate dysfunction of the eighth cranial nerve. The nurse would hold the dose and notify the physician. Ototoxicity is an adverse effect of therapy with aminoglycosides and could result in permanent hearing loss. There is no need to check the pupillary response. Administering the dose would be an unsafe response.
Test-Taking Strategy: Note the strategic word, *next*. Focus on the client's complaints, and recall that ototoxicity can occur with this medication. Recalling that the physician is notified if toxicity is suspected will direct you to option 4.
Priority Nursing Tip: The client with vertigo is at risk for injury; therefore, safety is a priority.
Reference: Gahart, B., Nazareno, A., & Ortega, M. (2021). *Gahart's 2021 Intravenous medications: a handbook for nurses and health professionals* (37th ed., p. 1289). Elsevier.

❖ **30.** The nurse is preparing to administer prescribed amiodarone intravenously. To provide a safe environment, the nurse would ensure that which specific safety consideration is in place for the client before administering the medication?
1. Oxygen therapy
2. Oxygen saturation monitor
3. Continuous cardiac monitoring
4. Noninvasive blood pressure cuff

Level of Cognitive Ability: Applying
Client Needs: Safe and Effective Care Environment
Clinical Judgment/Cognitive Skills: Take Action
Integrated Process: Nursing Process/Implementation
Content Area: Pharmacology: Cardiovascular: Antidysrhythmics
Health Problems: Adult Health: Cardiovascular: Dysrhythmias
Priority Concepts: Caregiving; Safety

Answer: 3
Rationale: Amiodarone is an antidysrhythmic used to treat life-threatening ventricular dysrhythmias. The client needs to have continuous cardiac monitoring in place for safety, and the medication needs to be infused by intravenous pump. Although options 1, 2, and 4 may be in place for the client, they are not specific items needed for the administration of this medication.
Test-Taking Strategy: Focus on the subject, care to the client receiving amiodarone. Recalling that this medication is an antidysrhythmic will direct you to continuous cardiac monitoring.
Priority Nursing Tip: Electrolyte and mineral imbalances can cause cardiac electrical instability that can result in life-threatening dysrhythmias.
Reference: Gahart, B., Nazareno, A., & Ortega, M. (2021). *Gahart's 2021 Intravenous medications: a handbook for nurses and health professionals* (37th ed., p. 76). Elsevier.

31. During the admission process of a client being admitted for surgery, the client asks the nurse if a living will, prepared 3 years ago, remains in effect. Which response is **most appropriate** for the nurse to provide the client?
1. "Yes, a living will never expires."
2. "You need to speak with an attorney."
3. "I will call someone to answer your question."
4. "Yes, if it accurately reflects your situation and wishes."

Level of Cognitive Ability: Applying
Client Needs: Safe and Effective Care Environment
Clinical Judgment/Cognitive Skills: Take Action
Integrated Process: Nursing Process/Implementation
Content Area: Leadership/Management: Ethical/Legal
Health Problems: N/A
Priority Concepts: Ethics; Health Care Law

Answer: 4
Rationale: The client needs to discuss the living will with the physician on a regular basis to ensure that it contains the client's current wishes and desires based on the client's current health status. Option 1 is incorrect. Although the client can consult an attorney if the living will must be changed, the accurate nursing response is to tell the client that a living will needs to be reviewed. Option 3 is not at all helpful to the client and is, in fact, a communication block and places the client's question on hold.
Test-Taking Strategy: Note the strategic words, *most appropriate*. Eliminate options 1 and 3 first because they are nontherapeutic and place the client's question on hold. Also note the closed-ended word "never" in option 1. From the remaining options, it is necessary to know that the document is reviewed on a regular basis with the physician.
Priority Nursing Tip: On admission to a health care facility, the nurse needs to determine whether an advance directive exists and ensure that it is part of the client's medical record.
Reference: Zerwekh, J., & Zerwekh Garneau, A. (2021). *Nursing today: Transition and trends* (10th ed., pp. 436, 490–491). Elsevier.

❖ **32.** The nurse reviews wound culture results and learns that an assigned client has methicillin-resistant *Staphylococcus aureus* (MRSA) in a wound bed. Which type of transmission-based precautions would the nurse implement for this client?
1. Enteric precautions
2. Droplet precautions
3. Contact precautions
4. Airborne precautions

Level of Cognitive Ability: Applying
Client Needs: Safe and Effective Care Environment
Clinical Judgment/Cognitive Skills: Take Action
Integrated Process: Nursing Process/Implementation
Content Area: Foundations of Care: Infection Prevention and Control
Health Problems: Adult Health: Integumentary: Wounds
Priority Concepts: Infection; Safety

Answer: 3
Rationale: Contact precautions include standard precautions and require the use of barrier precautions such as gloves and goggles. Contact precautions are used for clients who have diarrhea, draining wounds, or methicillin-resistant infections. The goal of these precautions is to eliminate disease transmission resulting either from direct contact with the client or from indirect contact through inanimate objects or surfaces that the pathogen has contaminated, such as instruments, linens, dressing materials, or hands. Enteric precautions are initiated if the organism is transmitted via the gastrointestinal tract. Droplet and airborne precautions are used if the organism is transmitted via the respiratory tract.
Test-Taking Strategy: Focus on the subject, the client's diagnosis (MRSA), which can be transmitted by contact with the infecting organism. Note the location of the pathogen to decide how its transmission can be prevented to assist in answering the question. Recall that *enteric* refers to the gastrointestinal tract and eliminate option 1. Eliminate options 2 and 4 because they are comparable or alike and unrelated to a wound bed.
Priority Nursing Tip: Handle all blood and body fluids from all clients as if they were contaminated.
Reference: Ignatavicius, D., et al. (2021). *Medical-surgical nursing: Concepts for interprofessional collaborative care* (10th ed., pp. 408, 410). Elsevier.

33. The nurse is caring for a client immediately after a bronchoscopy. The client received intravenous sedation and a topical anesthetic for the procedure. Which **priority** nursing intervention would the nurse perform to provide a safe environment for the client at this time?
1. Place pads on the side rails.
2. Connect the client to a bedside ECG.
3. Remove all food or fluids within the client's reach.
4. Place a water-seal chest drainage set at the bedside.

Level of Cognitive Ability: Applying
Client Needs: Safe and Effective Care Environment
Clinical Judgment/Cognitive Skills: Take Action
Integrated Process: Nursing Process/Implementation
Content Area: Foundations of Care: Diagnostic Tests
Health Problems: N/A
Priority Concepts: Gas Exchange; Safety

Answer: 3
Rationale: After this procedure, the client remains on nothing by mouth (NPO) status until the cough, gag, and swallow reflexes have returned, which is usually in 1 to 2 hours. Once the client can swallow and the gag reflex has returned, oral intake may begin with ice chips and small sips of water. No information in the question suggests that the client is at risk for a seizure. Even though the client is monitored for signs of any distress, seizures would not be anticipated. No data are given to support that the client is at increased risk for cardiac dysrhythmias. A pneumothorax is a possible complication of this procedure, and the nurse needs to monitor the client for signs of distress. However, a water-seal chest drainage set would not be placed routinely at the bedside.
Test-Taking Strategy: Note the strategic word, *priority.* Consider that this client is sedated and has received a topical anesthetic. Use the ABCs—airway, breathing, and circulation—to direct you to the correct option.
Priority Nursing Tip: Complications after bronchoscopy include bronchospasm or bronchial perforation indicated by facial or neck crepitus, dysrhythmias, hemorrhage, hypoxemia, and pneumothorax.
Reference: Pagana, K., Pagana, T., & Pagana, T. N. (2021). *Mosby's Diagnostic and laboratory test reference* (15th ed., p. 188). Elsevier.

❖ **34.** A client with a history of silicosis is admitted, diagnosed with respiratory distress and impending respiratory failure. The nurse would plan to have which supplies/equipment readily available at the client's bedside to ensure a safe environment?
1. Code cart
2. Intubation tray
3. Thoracentesis tray
4. Chest tube and drainage system

Level of Cognitive Ability: Applying
Client Needs: Safe and Effective Care Environment
Clinical Judgment/Cognitive Skills: Generate Solutions
Integrated Process: Nursing Process/Planning
Content Area: Complex Care: Acute Respiratory Failure
Health Problems: Adult Health: Respiratory: Environmental
Priority Concepts: Gas Exchange; Safety

Answer: 2
Rationale: Respiratory failure occurs when insufficient oxygen is transported to the blood or inadequate carbon dioxide is removed from the lungs and the client's compensatory mechanisms fail. The client with impending respiratory failure may need intubation and mechanical ventilation. The nurse ensures that an intubation tray is readily available. The other items are not needed at the client's bedside. A code cart is used for resuscitation. A thoracentesis tray contains the necessary items for performing a thoracentesis. A chest tube drainage system is used to treat a pneumothorax.
Test-Taking Strategy: Focus on the subject, impending respiratory failure. Use the ABCs—airway, breathing, and circulation—to direct you to the correct option.
Priority Nursing Tip: For the client with respiratory failure, mechanical ventilation is needed if supplemental oxygen cannot maintain acceptable Pao_2 and $Paco_2$ levels.
Reference: Lewis, S., et al. (2020). *Medical-surgical nursing: Assessment and management of clinical problems* (11th ed., p. 1594). Elsevier.

35. The nurse is preparing to administer a first dose of prescribed pentamidine isethionate intravenously to a client diagnosed with pneumonia. Before administering the dose, which safety measure would the nurse plan for this client?
1. Assign to a private room.
2. Establish a supine position.
3. Place on respiratory precautions.
4. Assist to a semi-Fowler's position.

Level of Cognitive Ability: Applying
Client Needs: Safe and Effective Care Environment
Clinical Judgment/Cognitive Skills: Generate Solutions
Integrated Process: Nursing Process/Planning
Content Area: Pharmacology: Immune: Antifungals
Health Problems: Adult Health: Respiratory: Pneumonia
Priority Concepts: Clinical Judgment; Safety

Answer: 2
Rationale: Pentamidine isethionate is an anti-infective medication and can cause severe and sudden hypotension, even with administration of a single dose. The client needs to be lying down during administration of this medication. The blood pressure is monitored frequently during administration. Assigning to a private room, instituting respiratory precautions, or assisting to a semi-Fowler's position are all unnecessary interventions.
Test-Taking Strategy: Focus on the subject, an adverse effect of pentamidine isethionate. It is necessary to know these adverse effects to answer correctly. Recalling that the medication causes hypotension will direct you to the correct option.
Priority Nursing Tip: Pentamidine isethionate may be prescribed to treat opportunistic infections such as *Pneumocystis jiroveci* pneumonia.
Reference: Gahart, B., Nazareno, A., & Ortega, M. (2021). *Gahart's 2021 Intravenous medications: a handbook for nurses and health professionals* (37th ed., p. 1081). Elsevier.

❖ **36.** The nurse is administering a dose of prescribed intravenous hydralazine to a client. To provide a safe environment, the nurse would ensure that which safety measure is in place before injecting the medication?
   1. Central line
   2. Thermometer
   3. Indwelling urinary catheter
   4. Blood pressure cuff

Level of Cognitive Ability: Applying
Client Needs: Safe and Effective Care Environment
Clinical Judgment/Cognitive Skills: Generate Solutions
Integrated Process: Nursing Process/Planning
Content Area: Pharmacology: Cardiovascular: Vasodilators
Health Problems: Adult Health: Cardiovascular: Hypertension
Priority Concepts: Clinical Judgment; Safety

Answer: 4
Rationale: Hydralazine is an antihypertensive medication used in the management of moderate to severe hypertension. The blood pressure and pulse need to be monitored frequently after administration, so a blood pressure cuff is the item to have in place. Although intravenous access is needed, a central line is unnecessary. The other options are also unnecessary and are unrelated to the administration of this medication.
Test-Taking Strategy: Focus on the subject, hydralazine. Read about common antihypertensive medications. Also, use of the ABCs—airway, breathing, and circulation—will direct you to the correct option.
Priority Nursing Tip: Safety is a priority when an antihypertensive medication is administered because of the risk for hypotension after administration.
Reference: Gahart, B., Nazareno, A., & Ortega, M. (2021). *Gahart's 2021 Intravenous medications: a handbook for nurses and health professionals* (37th ed., p. 712). Elsevier.

37. A hospitalized client is found lying on the floor next to the bed. Once the client is cared for, the nurse completes an incident report. Which written statements exemplify correct documentation on the report? **(Refer to exhibit.)** **Select all that apply.**

INCIDENT REPORT
☐ 1. The client fell out of bed.
☐ 2. No bruises or injuries are noted on the client.
☐ 3. The client apparently climbed over the side rails when the nurse was out of the room.
☐ 4. The health care provider was notified that the client was found lying on the floor next to the bed.
☐ 5. The client is alert and oriented and stated the need to "go to the bathroom and didn't want to bother the nurse."
☐ 6. Vital signs are temperature: 98.6° F (37° C); pulse 78 beats per minute and regular; respirations 16 breaths per minute and regular; blood pressure 188/78 mm Hg.

Level of Cognitive Ability: Applying
Client Needs: Safe and Effective Care Environment
Clinical Judgment/Cognitive Skills: Take Action
Integrated Process: Communication and Documentation
Content Area: Leadership/Management: Informatics and Health Care Technologies
Health Problems: N/A
Priority Concepts: Communication; Safety

Answer: 2, 4, 5, 6
Rationale: An incident report is a tool used by health care facilities to document situations that have caused harm or have the potential to cause harm to clients, employees, or visitors. The nurse who identifies the situation initiates the report. The report identifies the people involved in the incident, including witnesses; describes the event; and records the date, time, location, factual findings, actions taken, and any other relevant information. The primary health care provider is notified of the incident and completes the report after examining the client. Documentation on the report needs to always be as factual as possible and needs to avoid accusations. Because the client was found lying on the floor, it is unknown whether the client actually fell out of bed. Additionally, the nurse does not know that the client climbed over the side rails when the nurse was out of the room.
Test-Taking Strategy: Focus on the subject, correct documentation on the incident report. Recalling that documentation on the report needs to always be as factual as possible and must avoid accusations will assist in answering this question.
Priority Nursing Tip: An incident (unusual occurrence) report is considered a legal document and should not be placed in the client's chart after completion. It needs to be maintained and filed in a designated area as determined by agency procedure.
Reference: Potter, P., et al. (2021). *Fundamentals of nursing* (10th ed., p. 376). Elsevier.

❖ **38.** A home care nurse is visiting an older client recovering from stroke affecting the left side. The client lives alone but receives regular assistance from their two adult children, who both live within 10 miles. To assess for risk factors related to safety, which actions would the nurse take? **Select all that apply.**
- ❏ 1. Assess the client's visual acuity.
- ❏ 2. Observe the client's gait and posture.
- ❏ 3. Evaluate the client's muscle strength.
- ❏ 4. Look for any hazards in the home care environment.
- ❏ 5. Ask a family member to move in with the client until recovery is complete.
- ❏ 6. Request that the client transfer to an assisted living environment for at least 1 month.

Level of Cognitive Ability: Analyzing
Client Needs: Safe and Effective Care Environment
Clinical Judgment/Cognitive Skills: Take Action
Integrated Process: Clinical Judgment; Nursing Process/Implementation
Content Area: Foundations of Care: Safety
Health Problems: Adult Health: Neurologic: Stroke
Priority Concepts: Clinical Judgment; Safety

Answer: 1, 2, 3, 4
Rationale: To conduct a thorough client assessment, the nurse assesses for possible risk factors related to safety. The assessment needs to include visual acuity, gait and posture, and muscle strength because alterations in these areas place the client at risk for falls and injury. The nurse needs to also assess the home environment, looking for any hazards or obstacles that would affect safety. Asking a family member to move in with the client until recovery is complete and requesting that the client transfer to an assisted living environment for at least 1 month are not assessment activities. Additionally, nothing in the question indicates that these actions are necessary; therefore, these options are unrealistic and unreasonable.
Test-Taking Strategy: Focus on the subject, assessing for risk factors related to safety after a stroke. Note that options 5 and 6 are unrelated to the subject of the question.
Priority Nursing Tip: Age-related changes occur on an individual basis, and one client may experience an age-related change to a lesser extent than another client. The older client who has suffered a stroke will be at a higher risk for injury related to age-related changes.
Reference: Potter, P., et al. (2021). *Fundamentals of nursing* (10th ed., pp. 399, 401). Elsevier.

39. Which medical asepsis actions would the nurse implement to reduce and prevent the spread of microorganisms? **Select all that apply.**
- ❏ 1. Practicing hand hygiene
- ❏ 2. Reapplying a sterile dressing
- ❏ 3. Sterilizing contaminated items
- ❏ 4. Applying a sterile gown and gloves
- ❏ 5. Routinely cleaning the hospital environment
- ❏ 6. Wearing clean gloves to prevent direct contact with blood or body fluids

Level of Cognitive Ability: Applying
Client Needs: Safe and Effective Care Environment
Clinical Judgment/Cognitive Skills: Take Action
Integrated Process: Nursing Process/Implementation
Content Area: Foundations of Care: Infection Control
Health Problems: N/A
Priority Concepts: Infection; Safety

Answer: 1, 5, 6
Rationale: Medical asepsis, or clean technique, includes procedures to reduce and prevent the spread of microorganisms. Practicing hand hygiene, routinely cleaning the hospital environment, and wearing clean gloves to prevent direct contact with blood or body fluids are examples of medical asepsis. Surgical asepsis involves the use of sterile technique. Examples of surgical asepsis include reapplying a sterile dressing, sterilization of contaminated items, and applying a sterile gown and gloves.
Test-Taking Strategy: Focus on the subject, medical asepsis. Recalling the definition of medical asepsis and that it involves clean techniques will assist in answering this question. Also note the word *sterile* in options 2 and 4, and the word *sterilizing* in option 3. These words indicate surgical asepsis.
Priority Nursing Tip: Medical asepsis is intended to reduce and prevent the spread of microorganisms, whereas surgical asepsis aims to eliminate all microorganisms in a particular environment.
Reference: Potter, P., et al. (2021). *Fundamentals of nursing* (10th ed., pp. 435, 440). Elsevier.

❖ **40.** The nurse is caring for a hospitalized client who is having a prescribed dosage of clonazepam adjusted. Because of the adjustment in the medication administration, which **priority** safety activity would the nurse plan to implement?

1. Weigh the client daily.
2. Assess for ecchymoses.
3. Institute seizure precautions.
4. Monitor blood glucose levels.

Level of Cognitive Ability: Analyzing
Client Needs: Safe and Effective Care Environment
Clinical Judgment/Cognitive Skills: Generate Solutions
Integrated Process: Nursing Process/Planning
Content Area: Pharmacology: Psychiatric: Barbiturate and Sedative-Hypnotics
Health Problems: Adult Health: Neurologic: Seizure Disorder/Epilepsy
Priority Concepts: Clinical Judgment; Safety

Answer: **3**
Rationale: Clonazepam is a benzodiazepine that is used as an anticonvulsant. During initial therapy and periods of dosage adjustment, the nurse needs to initiate seizure precautions for the client. This medication does not cause weight gain or loss, bleeding or bruising, or fluctuations in blood glucose levels.
Test-Taking Strategy: Note the strategic word, *priority.* Focus on the subject, clonazepam, and think about its classification. Recalling that this medication is an anticonvulsant will direct you to the correct option.
Priority Nursing Tip: Flumazenil reverses the effects of benzodiazepines.
Reference: Kizior, R., & Hodgson, B. (2023). *Saunders Nursing drug handbook 2023* (p. 253). Elsevier.

41. The nurse is planning to obtain an arterial blood gas (ABG) from the radial artery of a client with a diagnosis of chronic obstructive pulmonary disease (COPD). To prevent bleeding after the procedure, which **priority** activity would the nurse plan time for after the arterial blood is drawn?

1. Holding a warm compress over the puncture site for 5 minutes
2. Encouraging the client to open and close the hand rapidly for 2 minutes
3. Applying pressure to the puncture site by applying a 2 × 2 gauze for 5 minutes
4. Having the client keep the radial pulse puncture site in a dependent position for 5 minutes

Level of Cognitive Ability: Applying
Client Needs: Safe and Effective Care Environment
Clinical Judgment/Cognitive Skills: Generate Solutions
Integrated Process: Nursing Process/Planning
Content Area: Skills: Specimen Collection
Health Problems: Adult Health: Respiratory: Chronic Obstructive Pulmonary Disease
Priority Concepts: Clotting; Safety

Answer: **3**
Rationale: Applying pressure over the puncture site for 5 to 10 minutes reduces the risk of hematoma formation and damage to the artery. A cold compress would aid in limiting blood flow; a warm compress would increase blood flow. Keeping the extremity still and out of a dependent position will aid in the formation of a clot at the puncture site.
Test-Taking Strategy: Note the strategic word, *priority.* Focus on the subject, preventing bleeding following an ABG draw. Eliminate options 1, 2, and 4 because these activities promote bleeding. Option 3, applying pressure, aids in the prevention of bleeding into the surrounding tissues.
Priority Nursing Tip: Before drawing blood for an ABG analysis, perform the Allen's test to determine the presence of collateral circulation.
Reference: Pagana, K., Pagana, T., & Pagana, T. N. (2021). *Mosby's Diagnostic and laboratory test reference* (15th ed., p. 109). Elsevier.

❖ **42.** The nurse is admitting a client with an arteriovenous (AV) fistula in the right arm for hemodialysis. Which strategy would the nurse plan to implement to **best** prevent injury to the AV fistula site?

1. Applying an allergy bracelet to the right arm
2. Placing an alert bracelet per agency procedure on the client's right arm
3. Putting a large note about the access site on the front of the medical record
4. Telling the client to inform all caregivers who enter the room about the presence of the access site

Level of Cognitive Ability: Applying
Client Needs: Safe and Effective Care Environment
Clinical Judgment/Cognitive Skills: Generate Solutions
Integrated Process: Nursing Process/Planning
Content Area: Foundations of Care: Safety
Health Problems: Adult Health: Renal and Urinary: Acute Kidney Injury and Chronic Kidney Disease
Priority Concepts: Clinical Judgment; Safety

Answer: 2
Rationale: No venipunctures or blood pressure measurements are done in the extremity with a hemodialysis access device. This is commonly communicated to all caregivers by placing an alert bracelet on the arm that needs to be protected. This alert bracelet prompts health care providers to investigate the need for the bracelet. The use of an alert wrist bracelet (rather than a visibly posted note or sign) also maintains client confidentiality. Agency procedure is always followed. An allergy bracelet is placed on the client with an allergy. Placing a note on the front of the medical record does not ensure that everyone caring for the client is aware of the access device. The client should not be responsible for informing the caregivers.
Test-Taking Strategy: Note the strategic word, *best*. Eliminate option 1 because an allergy bracelet is used for a client with an allergy. Eliminate option 3 because placing a note on the client chart does not ensure that all caregivers will have access to this information in a timely manner. Eliminate option 4 next because this responsibility should not be placed on the client. Option 2 best informs those caring for the client of the presence of the fistula.
Priority Nursing Tip: To assess for patency of the AV fistula, feel for a thrill and listen for a bruit. The physician is notified immediately if disruption of patency is suspected.
Reference: Ignatavicius, D., et al. (2021). *Medical-surgical nursing: Concepts for interprofessional collaborative care* (10th ed., p. 1399). Elsevier.

43. Regular insulin by continuous intravenous (IV) infusion is prescribed for a client diagnosed with diabetes mellitus, and the nurse checks the client's most recent blood glucose result. How would the nurse administer this medication safely?

Laboratory Results

Test and Results	Reference Range
Blood glucose 700 mg/dL (40 mmol/L)	70–99 mg/dL (3.9–5.5 mmol/L)

1. Mix the solution in 5% dextrose.
2. Change the solution every 6 hours.
3. Infuse the medication via an electronic infusion pump.
4. Titrate the infusion according to the client's urine glucose levels.

Level of Cognitive Ability: Applying
Client Needs: Safe and Effective Care Environment
Clinical Judgment/Cognitive Skills: Take Action
Integrated Process: Clinical Judgment; Nursing Process/Implementation
Content Area: Pharmacology: Endocrine: Insulin
Health Problems: Adult Health: Endocrine: Diabetes Mellitus
Priority Concepts: Glucose Regulation; Safety

Answer: 3
Rationale: Insulin is administered via an infusion pump to prevent inadvertent overdose and subsequent hypoglycemia. Dextrose is added to the IV infusion once the serum glucose level reaches 250 mg/dL (14.2 mmol/L) to prevent the occurrence of hypoglycemia. Administering dextrose to a client with a serum glucose level of 700 mg/dL (40 mmol/L) would counteract the beneficial effects of insulin in reducing the glucose level. There is no reason to change the solution every 6 hours. Glycosuria is not a reliable indicator of the actual serum glucose levels because many factors affect the renal threshold for glucose loss in the urine.
Test-Taking Strategy: Focus on the subject, administration of IV insulin to the client with severe blood glucose elevation. Eliminate option 1, knowing that dextrose would not be administered to a client with a blood glucose of 700 mg/dL (40 mmol/L). Eliminate option 2 because there is no need to change the solution every 6 hours. Eliminate option 4, knowing that urine glucose levels do not provide an accurate indication of the client's status. Insulin needs to be administered with an electronic infusion pump.
Priority Nursing Tip: Regular insulin is a type of insulin that can be given by the intravenous route. When administering intravenous insulin, monitor the blood glucose level and the potassium levels closely.
Reference: Lewis, S., et al. (2020). *Medical-surgical nursing: Assessment and management of clinical problems* (11th ed., pp. 1116–1117). Elsevier.

❖ **44.** Which action demonstrates a situational leadership style by the nurse manager?
1. The nurse manager delegates tasks to each team member.
2. The nurse manager allows team members to work without supervision.
3. The nurse manager invites team members to provide input about a unit problem.
4. The nurse manager quickly delegates activities to team members during an emergency situation.

Level of Cognitive Ability: Applying
Client Needs: Safe and Effective Care Environment
Clinical Judgment/Cognitive Skills: Take Action
Integrated Process: Nursing Process/Implementation
Content Area: Leadership/Management: Management of Care
Health Problems: N/A
Priority Concepts: Leadership; Professional Identity

Answer: 4
Rationale: The situational leadership style uses a style depending on the situation and events. This type of leadership style is used in emergency situations when the nurse manager needs to quickly delegate activities to achieve a successful outcome for the situation. A laissez-faire leader abdicates leadership and responsibilities, allowing staff to work without assistance, direction, or supervision. Participative leadership demonstrates an "in-between" style, neither authoritarian nor democratic. In participative leadership, the manager presents an analysis of problems and proposals for actions to team members, inviting critique and comments. The participative leader then analyzes the comments and makes the final decision. The autocratic style of leadership is task oriented and directive.
Test-Taking Strategy: Focus on the subject, style of leadership, noting the words *situational leadership*. Recalling that a situational leadership style uses a style depending on the situation and events will direct you to the correct option.
Priority Nursing Tip: The nurse is always responsible for their actions when providing care to a client.
Reference: Zerwekh, J., & Zerwekh Garneau, A. (2021). *Nursing today: Transition and trends* (10th ed., p. 224). Elsevier.

45. The clinic nurse wants to develop a teaching program for clients with a diagnosis of diabetes mellitus. Which strategy would the nurse initiate **first** in order to **best** meet the clients' needs?
1. Assess the clients' functional abilities.
2. Ensure that insurance will pay for participation in the program.
3. Discuss the focus of the program with the multidisciplinary team.
4. Include everyone who comes into the clinic in the teaching sessions.

Level of Cognitive Ability: Applying
Client Needs: Safe and Effective Care Environment
Clinical Judgment/Cognitive Skills: Take Action
Integrated Process: Teaching and Learning
Content Area: Foundations of Care: Client Teaching
Health Problems: Adult Health: Endocrine: Diabetes Mellitus
Priority Concepts: Patient Education; Health Promotion

Answer: 1
Rationale: Nurse-managed clinics focus on individualized disease prevention and health promotion and maintenance. Therefore, the nurse must first assess the clients and their needs to effectively plan the program. Options 2, 3, and 4 do not address the clients' needs related to the diagnosis.
Test-Taking Strategy: Note the strategic words, *first* and *best*. Use the steps of the nursing process. Remember that the first step is assessment. Option 1 reflects assessment.
Priority Nursing Tip: When determining priorities for client teaching, identify the client's immediate learning needs, as well as what the client perceives as important.
Reference: Potter, P., et al. (2021). *Fundamentals of nursing* (10th ed., p. 351). Elsevier.

❖ **46.** The nurse notes that a postoperative client has not been obtaining relief from pain with the prescribed opioid analgesics when a particular licensed coworker is assigned to the client. Which action is **most appropriate** for the nurse to implement **initially?**
1. Reassign the coworker to the care of clients not receiving opioids.
2. Notify the physician that the client needs an increase in opioid dosage.
3. Review the client's medication administration record immediately, and discuss the observations with the nursing supervisor.
4. Confront the coworker with the information about the client having pain control problems, and ask if the coworker is using the opioids personally.

Level of Cognitive Ability: Applying
Client Needs: Safe and Effective Care Environment
Clinical Judgment/Cognitive Skills: Take Action
Integrated Process: Nursing Process/Implementation
Content Area: Leadership/Management: Ethical/Legal
Health Problems: Adult Health: Neurologic: Pain
Priority Concepts: Ethics; Professional Identity

Answer: 3
Rationale: In this situation, the nurse has noted an unusual occurrence, but before deciding what action to take next, the nurse needs more data than just suspicion. This can be obtained by reviewing the client's record. State and federal labor and opioid regulations, as well as institutional policies and procedures, must be followed. It is, therefore, most appropriate that the nurse discuss the situation with the nursing supervisor before taking further action. To reassign the coworker to clients not receiving opioids ignores the issue. The client does not need an increase in opioids. A confrontation is not the most advisable action because it could result in an argumentative situation.
Test-Taking Strategy: Focus on the subject, suspicion of substance abuse in another nurse. Note the strategic words, *most appropriate* and *initially*. Recall knowledge regarding the roles and responsibilities of the nurse in a situation in which another nurse may be abusing the client's medication and the organizational channels of communication that need to be used. Option 3 is the only option that includes consultation with an authority figure, the nursing supervisor.
Priority Nursing Tip: If the nurse suspects that a coworker is abusing chemicals and potentially jeopardizing a client's safety, the nurse must report the individual to nursing administration in a confidential manner.
Reference: Zerwekh, J., & Zerwekh Garneau, A. (2021). *Nursing today: Transition and trends* (10th ed., pp. 473–474). Elsevier.

47. The medication nurse is supervising a newly hired licensed practical nurse (LPN) during the administration of prescribed oral pyridostigmine bromide to a client with a diagnosis of myasthenia gravis. Which observation by the medication nurse indicates safe practice by the LPN?
1. Asking the client to take sips of water
2. Asking the client to lie down on the right side
3. Asking the client to look up at the ceiling for 30 seconds
4. Instructing the client to void before taking the medication

Level of Cognitive Ability: Evaluating
Client Needs: Safe and Effective Care Environment
Clinical Judgment/Cognitive Skills: Evaluate Outcomes
Integrated Process: Nursing Process/Evaluation
Content Area: Pharmacology: Neurologic: Antimyasthenic
Health Problems: Adult Health: Neurologic: Myasthenia Gravis
Priority Concepts: Clinical Judgment; Safety

Answer: 1
Rationale: Myasthenia gravis can affect the client's ability to swallow. The primary assessment is to determine the client's ability to handle oral medications or any oral substance. Options 2 and 3 are not appropriate. Option 2 could result in aspiration, and option 3 has no useful purpose. There is no specific reason for the client to void before taking this medication.
Test-Taking Strategy: Focus on the subject, myasthenia gravis. Recalling that myasthenia gravis affects the client's ability to swallow will direct you to the correct option, assessing for the ability to swallow oral medication. Also, note the relation between the words *oral* in the question and *sips of water* in the correct option.
Priority Nursing Tip: To assess the client's ability to swallow, elevate the head of the bed to high-Fowler's position, and ask the client to sit up straight in bed before swallowing.
Reference: Lewis, S., et al. (2020). *Medical-surgical nursing: Assessment and management of clinical problems* (11th ed., p. 1378). Elsevier; Skidmore-Roth, L. (2021). *2021 Mosby's Nursing drug reference* (34th ed., p. 1061). Elsevier.

❖ **48.** The nurse does not intervene when a client becomes hypotensive after surgery. As a result, the client requires emergency surgery to stop postoperative bleeding later that night. The nurse could potentially face which types of prosecution for failing to act? **Select all that apply.**
   - ❑ 1. Felony
   - ❑ 2. Tort law
   - ❑ 3. Malpractice
   - ❑ 4. Statutory law
   - ❑ 5. Misdemeanor

Level of Cognitive Ability: Understanding
Client Needs: Safe and Effective Care Environment
Clinical Judgment/Cognitive Skills: Recognize Cues
Integrated Process: Nursing Process/Assessment
Content Area: Leadership/Management: Ethical/Legal
Health Problems: Adult Health: Cardiovascular: Hypovolemic Shock
Priority Concepts: Ethics; Health Care Law

Answer: 2, 3
Rationale: Tort law deals with wrongful acts intentionally or unintentionally committed against a person or the person's property. The nurse commits a tort offense by failing to act when the client became hypotensive. Malpractice occurs when a duty to the client is established and the nurse neglects to act responsibly. Options 1 and 5 are offenses under criminal law. Option 4 describes laws enacted by state, federal, or local governments.
Test-Taking Strategy: Focus on the subject, laws applying to failure to meet standards of care. Recalling that both a tort and malpractice refer to wrongful acts will direct you to options 2 and 3.
Priority Nursing Tip: Malpractice is negligence on the part of the nurse. The nurse who does not meet appropriate standards of care may be held liable.
Reference: Potter, P., et al. (2021). *Fundamentals of nursing* (10th ed., pp. 314–315). Elsevier.

49. The nurse gives medical information regarding the client's condition to a person who is assumed to be a family member. Later the nurse discovers that this person is not a family member and realizes that this violated which legal concepts of the nurse–client relationship? **Select all that apply.**
   - ❑ 1. Duty to provide care
   - ❑ 2. Client's right to privacy
   - ❑ 3. Client's right of autonomy
   - ❑ 4. Client's right to confidentiality
   - ❑ 5. Duty to comply with nursing standards

Level of Cognitive Ability: Understanding
Client Needs: Safe and Effective Care Environment
Clinical Judgment/Cognitive Skills: Recognize Cues
Integrated Process: Nursing Process/Assessment
Content Area: Leadership/Management: Ethical/Legal
Health Problems: N/A
Priority Concepts: Ethics; Health Care Law

Answer: 2, 4
Rationale: Discussing a client's condition without client permission violates a client's rights to privacy and confidentiality and places the nurse in legal jeopardy. This action by the nurse is both an invasion of privacy and affects the confidentiality issue with client rights. Options 1, 3, and 5 do not represent violation of the situation presented.
Test-Taking Strategy: Focus on the subject, sharing of client information. Sharing information constitutes an invasion of privacy and violates maintenance of confidentiality.
Priority Nursing Tip: Leaving the curtains or room door open while a treatment or procedure is being performed constitutes an invasion of client privacy.
Reference: Potter, P., et al. (2021). *Fundamentals of nursing* (10th ed., pp. 308, 314). Elsevier.

❖ **50.** In which situation is the nurse manager using an autocratic leadership style?
1. The nurse manager provides the solution for a unit problem.
2. The nurse manager allows the staff to solve their own unit problem.
3. The nurse manager proposes several alternatives and has the unit staff vote on the best proposal.
4. The nurse manager arranges for a staff meeting where all unit employees can share proposals to solve a problem.

Level of Cognitive Ability: Applying
Client Needs: Safe and Effective Care Environment
Clinical Judgment/Cognitive Skills: Take Action
Integrated Process: Nursing Process/Implementation
Content Area: Leadership/Management: Management of Care
Health Problems: N/A
Priority Concepts: Leadership; Professional Identity

Answer: 1
Rationale: The autocratic style of leadership is task oriented and directive. The leader uses their power and position in an authoritarian manner to set and implement organizational goals or solutions. Decisions are made without input from the staff. The situational leadership style uses a style depending on the situation and events. Democratic styles best empower staff toward excellence because this style of leadership allows nurses to provide input regarding the decision-making process and an opportunity to grow professionally. Participatory leadership encourages input from the staff.
Test-Taking Strategy: Focus on the subject, autocratic leadership. Recall the definition of this style of leadership to answer correctly. Also note that all the remaining options are comparable or alike in that they all deal with staff input.
Priority Nursing Tip: Leadership is an interpersonal process that involves influencing others (followers) to achieve goals.
Reference: Zerwekh, J., & Zerwekh Garneau, A. (2021). *Nursing today: Transition and trends* (10th ed., pp. 221–222). Elsevier.

51. The nurse performing an admission assessment notes that a client diagnosed with gastroesophageal reflux disease (GERD) has been prescribed metoclopramide for a prolonged period. The nurse would **immediately** call the primary health care provider if which signs/symptoms were then noted by the nurse?
1. Dry mouth
2. Anxiety or irritability
3. Excessive drowsiness
4. Uncontrolled rhythmic movements of the face or limbs

Level of Cognitive Ability: Analyzing
Client Needs: Safe and Effective Care Environment
Clinical Judgment/Cognitive Skills: Recognize Cues
Integrated Process: Clinical Judgment; Nursing Process/Assessment
Content Area: Pharmacology: Gastrointestinal: Antiemetics
Health Problems: Adult Health: Gastrointestinal: Gastroesophageal Reflux Disease
Priority Concepts: Clinical Judgment; Safety

Answer: 4
Rationale: If the client experiences tardive dyskinesia (rhythmic movements of the face or limbs), the nurse needs to call the primary health care provider because these adverse effects may be irreversible. The medication would be discontinued, and no further doses would be given by the nurse. Anxiety, irritability, and dry mouth are mild side effects that do not harm the client.
Test-Taking Strategy: Note that the question contains the strategic word, *immediately*, which guides you to select the most harmful option. Recalling that this medication causes tardive dyskinesia will direct you to option 4.
Priority Nursing Tip: Metoclopramide stimulates the motility of the upper gastrointestinal tract and is contraindicated in clients with mechanical obstruction, perforation, or gastrointestinal hemorrhage.
Reference: Lewis, S., et al. (2020). *Medical-surgical nursing: Assessment and management of clinical problems* (11th ed., pp. 890, 899). Elsevier.

❖ **52.** Which clinical situation would justifiably be viewed as an assault?
1. The nurse threatens to apply restraints to a client who is exhibiting aggressive behavior.
2. The client requests a medical discharge, but the nurse physically forces the client to stay.
3. The charge nurse sends an email to a staff member that includes a poor performance evaluation about another person.
4. The nurse overhears the physician making derogatory remarks to the client about the nurse's level of competency.

Level of Cognitive Ability: Understanding
Client Needs: Safe and Effective Care Environment
Clinical Judgment/Cognitive Skills: Recognize Cues
Integrated Process: Nursing Process/Assessment
Content Area: Leadership/Management: Ethical/Legal
Health Problems: N/A
Priority Concepts: Ethics; Health Care Law

Answer: 1
Rationale: An assault occurs when a person puts another person in fear of a harmful or offensive act. Battery involves offensive touching or the use of force by a perpetrator without the permission of the victim. Defamation takes place when a falsehood is said (slander) or written (libel) about a person that results in injury to that person's good name and reputation.
Test-Taking Strategy: Focus on the subject, an assault. Eliminate option 2, noting the words *physically forces;* this constitutes battery. Next eliminate options 3 and 4 because they address written and verbal information that can be harmful to another.
Priority Nursing Tip: False imprisonment occurs when a client is not allowed to leave a health care facility when there is no legal justification to detain the client.
Reference: Potter, P., et al. (2021). *Fundamentals of nursing* (10th ed., p. 314). Elsevier.

53. After finding a client sitting on the floor, the nurse ensures the client's safety, completes an incident report, and notifies the physician of the incident. Which action would the nurse implement **next**?
1. Staple the incident report in the client's medical record.
2. Document the client events and follow-up nursing actions.
3. Provide a copy of the incident report to the physician and family.
4. Document that a copy of the report was sent to risk management.

Level of Cognitive Ability: Applying
Client Needs: Safe and Effective Care Environment
Clinical Judgment/Cognitive Skills: Take Action
Integrated Process: Nursing Process/Implementation
Content Area: Leadership/Management: Quality Improvement
Health Problems: N/A
Priority Concepts: Communication; Health Care Law

Answer: 2
Rationale: The nurse documents the incident completely and objectively in the client's record to communicate client data to the health care team. The incident report is a confidential, privileged, and internal document used to improve client safety and quality of care and, therefore, would not be copied, stapled, or placed in the chart. Furthermore, the nurse avoids referring to the incident report in the client's record, such as recording that the incident report has been sent to another department. These actions are necessary because any mention of an incident report in the medical record allows the plaintiff's attorney access to the document through discovery.
Test-Taking Strategy: Note the strategic word, *next.* Focus on the subject, an incident report. Eliminate options 1 and 4 first because incident reports are neither stapled nor referred to in the medical record. From the remaining options, recall that an incident report is an internal, confidential document that is not intended for the family and is never copied, eliminating option 3.
Priority Nursing Tip: An incident report is used as a means of identifying risk situations and improving client care.
Reference: Potter, P., et al. (2021). *Fundamentals of nursing* (10th ed., p. 376). Elsevier.

❖ **54.** A client had a colon resection made necessary by a cancer diagnosis. A nasogastric tube was in place when a regular diet was brought to the client's room. The client did not want to eat solid food and asked that the physician be called. The nurse insisted that the solid food was the correct diet. The client ate and subsequently required additional surgery as a result of complications. The determination of negligence is based on which premise in this situation?

1. The nurse's persistence
2. A duty existed that was breached
3. Not notifying the physician
4. The dietary department sending the wrong food

Level of Cognitive Ability: Analysis
Client Needs: Safe and Effective Care Environment
Clinical Judgment/Cognitive Skills: Analyze Cues
Integrated Process: Nursing Process/Analysis
Content Area: Leadership/Management: Ethical/Legal
Health Problems: Adult Health: Cancer: Esophageal/Gastric/Intestinal
Priority Concepts: Clinical Judgment; Health Care Law

Answer: 2
Rationale: For negligence to be proved, there must be a duty and then a breach of duty; the breach of duty must cause the injury, and damages or injury must be experienced. Options 1, 3, and 4 do not fall under the criteria for negligence. Option 2 is the only option that fits the criteria of negligence.
Test-Taking Strategy: Focus on the subject, negligence. Options 1, 3, and 4 do not directly support the subject of negligence because it would be difficult to determine that these elements caused injury. The focus relates to the responsibility of the nurse.
Priority Nursing Tip: Negligence is conduct that falls below the standard of care.
Reference: Potter, P., et al. (2021). *Fundamentals of nursing* (10th ed., pp. 315, 318). Elsevier.

55. The nurse is caring for a child with a diagnosis of intussusception. During care, the child passes a formed brown stool. Which action is **most appropriate** for the nurse to take at this time?

1. Note the child's physical symptoms.
2. Prepare the child for hydrostatic reduction.
3. Prepare the child and parents for the possibility of surgery.
4. Report the passage of a normal brown stool to the pediatrician.

Level of Cognitive Ability: Applying
Client Needs: Safe and Effective Care Environment
Clinical Judgment/Cognitive Skills: Take Action
Integrated Process: Nursing Process/Implementation
Content Area: Pediatrics: Gastrointestinal
Health Problems: Pediatric-Specific: Intussusception
Priority Concepts: Clinical Judgment; Elimination

Answer: 4
Rationale: Intussusception is the telescoping of one portion of the bowel into another portion. Passage of a normally formed brown stool usually indicates that the intussusception has reduced itself. This is immediately reported to the pediatrician, who may choose to alter the diagnostic or therapeutic plan of care. Although the nurse would note the child's physical symptoms, based on the data in the question, option 4 is the appropriate action. Hydrostatic reduction and surgery may not be necessary.
Test-Taking Strategy: Note the strategic words, *most appropriate*. Focus on the subject, intussusception. Note the similarity between the information in the question and the correct option. Also, recalling the physiology associated with intussusception will direct you to the correct option.
Priority Nursing Tip: Currant jelly–like stools that contain blood and mucus are characteristic of intussusception.
Reference: McKinney, E. S., et al. (2022). *Maternal child nursing* (6th ed., pp. 990–992). Elsevier.

❖ **56.** The nurse caring for a client with a diagnosis of end-stage kidney failure is asked by a family member about advance directives. Which statements would the nurse plan to include when discussing advance directives with the client's family member? **Select all that apply.**

❑ **1.** A health care proxy can write a living will for a client if the client becomes incompetent and unable to do so.

❑ **2.** Two witnesses, either a relative or physician, are needed when the client signs a living will.

❑ **3.** The determination of decisional capacity of a client is usually made by the physician and family.

❑ **4.** Living wills are written documents that direct treatment in accordance with a client's wishes in the event of a terminal illness or condition.

❑ **5.** Under the Patient Self-Determination Act (PSDA), it must be documented in the client's record whether the client has signed an advance directive.

❑ **6.** For advance directives to be enforceable, the client must be legally incompetent or lack decisional capacity to make decisions regarding health care treatment.

Level of Cognitive Ability: Applying
Client Needs: Safe and Effective Care Environment
Clinical Judgment/Cognitive Skills: Generate Solutions
Integrated Process: Nursing Process/Planning
Content Area: Leadership/Management: Ethical/Legal
Health Problems: Adult Health: Renal and Urinary: Acute Kidney Injury and Chronic Kidney Disease
Priority Concepts: Ethics; Health Care Law

Answer: 3, 4, 5, 6
Rationale: The two basic advance directives are living wills and durable powers of attorney for health care. Under the PSDA, it must be documented in the client's record whether the client has signed an advance directive. For living wills or durable powers of attorney for health care to be enforceable, the client must be legally incompetent or lack decisional capacity to make decisions regarding health care treatment. The determination of decisional capacity is usually made by the physician and family, whereas the determination of legal competency is made by a judge. Living wills are written documents that direct treatment in accordance with a client's wishes in the event of a terminal illness or condition. Generally, two witnesses, neither of whom can be a relative or physician, are needed when the client signs the document. A durable power of attorney for health care designates an agent, surrogate, or proxy to make health care decisions if and when the client is no longer able to make decisions on their own behalf; however, a health care proxy cannot legally write a living will for a client.
Test-Taking Strategy: Focus on the subject, the characteristics of advance directives. Read each option carefully. Recalling that these are legal documents based on the client's wishes will assist in determining the correct options.
Priority Nursing Tip: Advance directives are used so that health care professionals can make decisions that are based on the client's wishes if the client is unable to make them. They clearly delineate end-of-life care decisions ahead of time so that appropriate action can be taken.
Reference: Zerwekh, J., & Zerwekh Garneau, A. (2021). *Nursing today: Transition and trends* (10th ed., pp. 436, 490–491). Elsevier.

57. A client asks the nurse how to become an organ donor. Which information would the nurse include in the discussion?

1. The client can donate by written consent.
2. A family member must witness the consent.
3. The donor must be older than 21 years of age.
4. A family member must be present when a client consents to organ donation.

Level of Cognitive Ability: Applying
Client Needs: Safe and Effective Care Environment
Clinical Judgment/Cognitive Skills: Take Action
Integrated Process: Teaching and Learning
Content Area: Leadership/Management: Ethical/Legal
Health Problems: N/A
Priority Concepts: Health Policy; Health Care Law

Answer: 1
Rationale: The client has the right to donate their own organs for transplantation, and any person who is 18 years of age or older may become an organ donor by written consent without the permission or presence of the family. In the absence of suitable documentation, a family member or legal guardian can authorize donation of the decedent's organs.
Test-Taking Strategy: Focus on the subject, organ donation and issues related to client rights. This will direct you to the correct option. Also note the closed-ended word "must" in all of the incorrect options.
Priority Nursing Tip: Requests to the deceased's family for organ donation usually are made by the physician or nurse or designated person specially trained for making such requests.
Reference: Lewis, S., et al. (2020). *Medical-surgical nursing: Assessment and management of clinical problems* (11th ed., p. 133). Elsevier.

❖ **58.** A registered nurse (RN) is providing postmortem care for a deceased client whose eyes will be donated. Which measure would the nurse anticipate will **most likely** be prescribed that will provide appropriate care of the client's body?
1. Closing the eyes with paper tape
2. Maintaining the client in a supine position
3. Placing gauze pads wet with saline covered by a small ice pack on the eyes
4. Placing the client in a lateral recumbent position, rotating right and left sides

Level of Cognitive Ability: Applying
Client Needs: Safe and Effective Care Environment
Clinical Judgment/Cognitive Skills: Generate Solutions
Integrated Process: Nursing Process/Planning
Content Area: Developmental Stages: End-of-Life
Health Problems: Adult Health: Immune: Transplantation
Priority Concepts: Safety; Tissue Integrity

Answer: 3
Rationale: When a corneal donor dies, the eyes are closed and usually the primary health care provider prescribes placing gauze pads wet with saline over them with a small ice pack. Within 2 to 4 hours the eyes are enucleated, and the corneas are usually transplanted within 24 to 48 hours. The head of the bed needs to be elevated. With the head of the bed elevated, the eyes will likely remain closed.
Test-Taking Strategy: Focus on the subject, donation of the eyes. Also note the strategic words, *most likely,* in the question. These words indicate that a procedure specific to eye harvesting is necessary to preserve the cornea. Visualize each option and think about the subject of preserving the eyes. This will direct you to option 3. Also note that the positions identified in the incorrect options are comparable or alike.
Priority Nursing Tip: Donor eyes are obtained from cadavers and must be enucleated soon after death because of rapid endothelial cell death.
Reference: Ignatavicius, D., et al. (2021). *Medical-surgical nursing: Concepts for interprofessional collaborative care* (10th ed., p. 948). Elsevier.

59. A clinical nurse manager conducts an educational session for the staff nurses about case management. Which premise regarding case management, if stated by one of the staff nurses, would necessitate a **need for further teaching**?
1. Manages client care by managing the client care environment
2. Maximizes hospital revenues while providing for optimal client care
3. Represents a primary health prevention focus managed by a single case manager
4. Is designed to promote appropriate use of hospital personnel and material resources

Level of Cognitive Ability: Evaluating
Client Needs: Safe and Effective Care Environment
Clinical Judgment/Cognitive Skills: Evaluate Outcomes
Integrated Process: Teaching and Learning
Content Area: Leadership/Management: Management of Care
Health Problems: N/A
Priority Concepts: Care Coordination; Professional Identity

Answer: 3
Rationale: Case management represents an interdisciplinary health care delivery system to promote appropriate use of hospital personnel and material resources to maximize hospital revenues while providing for optimal client care. It manages client care by managing the client care environment and includes assessment and development of a plan of care, coordination of all services, referral, and follow-up.
Test-Taking Strategy: Note the strategic words, *need for further teaching.* These words indicate a negative event query and the need to select the option that is an incorrect characteristic of case management. Noting the word *single* in option 3 will direct you to this option.
Priority Nursing Tip: Case management involves consultation and collaboration with an interprofessional health care team.
Reference: Zerwekh, J., & Zerwekh Garneau, A. (2021). *Nursing today: Transition and trends* (10th ed., pp. 350–351). Elsevier.

❖ **60.** A registered nurse is delegating activities to the nursing staff. Which activities can be safely assigned to the unlicensed assistive personnel (UAP)? **Select all that apply.**
☐ 1. Collecting a urine specimen from a client
☐ 2. Obtaining frequent oral temperatures on a client
☐ 3. Assessing a client who returned from the recovery room 6 hours ago
☐ 4. Assisting a post–cardiac catheterization client who needs to lie flat to eat lunch
☐ 5. Accompanying a client being discharged to meet spouse at the hospital exit door

Level of Cognitive Ability: Applying
Client Needs: Safe and Effective Care Environment
Clinical Judgment/Cognitive Skills: Generate Solutions
Integrated Process: Nursing Process/Planning
Content Area: Leadership/Management: Delegating/Supervising
Health Problems: N/A
Priority Concepts: Leadership; Safety

Answer: 1, 2, 5
Rationale: Work that is delegated to others must be consistent with the individual's level of expertise and licensure, if any. Options 1, 2, and 5 do not include situations that indicate that these activities carry foreseeable risk. The least appropriate activities for the UAP would be assessing a client and assisting the post–cardiac catheterization client. The UAP is not trained or educated to safely and accurately perform an assessment on a client. Because the post–cardiac catheterization client needs to eat while lying flat, the client is at risk for aspiration.
Test-Taking Strategy: Focus on the subject, delegation to the UAP. Use the ABCs—airway, breathing, and circulation—to assist in eliminating option 4. Next note the word *assessing* in option 3, and recall that the UAP is not educated to assess a client.
Priority Nursing Tip: Generally, noninvasive interventions, such as skin care, range-of-motion exercises, ambulation, grooming, and hygiene measures, can be assigned to UAP.
Reference: Lewis, S., et al. (2020). *Medical-surgical nursing: Assessment and management of clinical problems* (11th ed., pp. 9–11). Elsevier.

61. The nurse manager is reviewing the critical paths of the clients on the nursing unit. The nurse manager collaborates with each nurse assigned to the clients and performs a variance analysis. Which finding would indicate the **need for further assessment and analysis?**
1. A client is performing their own colostomy care.
2. A 1-day postoperative client has a temperature of 98.8° F (37.1° C).
3. A 2-day post abdominal hysterectomy client has drainage noted from the incision.
4. A client newly diagnosed with diabetes mellitus is preparing their own insulin for injection.

Level of Cognitive Ability: Evaluating
Client Needs: Safe and Effective Care Environment
Clinical Judgment/Cognitive Skills: Evaluate Outcomes
Integrated Process: Clinical Judgment; Nursing Process/Evaluation
Content Area: Leadership/Management: Quality Improvement
Health Problems: N/A
Priority Concepts: Health Care Quality; Leadership

Answer: 3
Rationale: Variances are actual deviations or detours from the critical paths. Option 3 is the only option that identifies the need for further action. Variances can be either positive or negative or avoidable or unavoidable and can be caused by a variety of things. Positive variance occurs when the client achieves maximum benefit and is discharged earlier than anticipated. Negative variance occurs when untoward events prevent a timely discharge. Variance analysis occurs continually to anticipate and recognize negative variance early so that appropriate action can be taken.
Test-Taking Strategy: Note the strategic words, *need for further assessment and analysis.* These words indicate a negative event query and the need to identify the negative variance. Options 1, 2, and 4 identify positive outcomes. Option 3 identifies a negative outcome.
Priority Nursing Tip: Variation analysis is a continuous process that the case manager and other caregivers conduct by comparing the specific client outcomes with expected outcomes.
Reference: Potter, P., et al. (2021). *Fundamentals of nursing* (10th ed., pp. 377–378). Elsevier.

❖ **62.** Which client would the nurse safely assign to the unlicensed assistive personnel (UAP)?
1. A client requiring dressing changes
2. A client requiring frequent ambulation
3. A client on a bowel management program requiring rectal suppositories
4. A client newly admitted with nausea, vomiting, and moderate neck pain

Level of Cognitive Ability: Applying
Client Needs: Safe and Effective Care Environment
Clinical Judgment/Cognitive Skills: Generate Solutions
Integrated Process: Nursing Process/Planning
Content Area: Leadership/Management: Delegating/Supervising
Health Problems: N/A
Priority Concepts: Leadership; Safety

Answer: 2
Rationale: Assignment of tasks to the UAP needs to be made based on job description, level of clinical competence, and state law. The client described in option 2 has needs, frequent ambulation, that can be met by the UAP. Options 1, 3, and 4 involve care that requires the skill of a licensed nurse.
Test-Taking Strategy: Focus on the subject, the assignment to the UAP. Think about the tasks that a UAP can safely perform, and match the client's needs with these tasks. Eliminate options 1, 3, and 4 because these clients require care that needs to be provided by a licensed nurse. Remember that a UAP can perform noninvasive tasks.
Priority Nursing Tip: Client safety is the priority when determining which tasks can be delegated and to whom.
Reference: Zerwekh, J., & Zerwekh Garneau, A. (2021). *Nursing today: Transition and trends* (10th ed., pp. 264–265). Elsevier.

63. A client with a diagnosis of schizophrenia and psychosis is pacing, agitated, and presenting with aggressive gestures. The client's speech pattern is rapid, and the client's affect is belligerent. Which **priority** nursing intervention based on these objective data would the nurse implement?
1. Provide safety for the client and other clients on the unit.
2. Bring the client to a less stimulated area to regain control.
3. Provide the clients on the unit with a sense of comfort and safety.
4. Assist the staff in caring for the client in a controlled environment.

Level of Cognitive Ability: Analyzing
Client Needs: Safe and Effective Care Environment
Clinical Judgment/Cognitive Skills: Take Action
Integrated Process: Clinical Judgment; Nursing Process/Implementation
Content Area: Mental Health
Health Problems: Mental Health: Schizophrenia
Priority Concepts: Clinical Judgment; Safety

Answer: 1
Rationale: If a client is exhibiting signs that indicate loss of control, the nurse's immediate priority is to ensure safety for all clients. Option 1 is the only option that addresses the client's and other clients' safety needs. Option 2 addresses the client's needs. Option 3 addresses other clients' needs. Option 4 is not client centered.
Test-Taking Strategy: Focus on the data in the question. Note the subject of the question, safety. Note the strategic word, priority. Option 1 is an umbrella option and addresses the safety of all.
Priority Nursing Tip: Encourage the client who is agitated to talk out instead of acting out feelings of frustration and aggression.
Reference: Varcarolis, E., & Fosbre, C. (2021). *Essentials of psychiatric mental health nursing: A communication approach to evidence-based care* (4th ed., pp. 253, 259). Elsevier.

❖ **64.** The nurse manager is developing an educational session for nursing staff on the components of informed consent and the information to be shared with a client to obtain informed consent. Which information would the nurse manager include in the session? **Select all that apply.**
- ❑ 1. The client needs to be informed of the prognosis if the test, procedure, or treatment is refused.
- ❑ 2. The client cannot refuse a test, procedure, or treatment once the test, procedure, or treatment is started.
- ❑ 3. The name(s) of the persons performing the test or procedure or providing treatment needs to be documented on the informed consent form.
- ❑ 4. A description of the complications and risks of the test, procedure, or treatment, as well as anticipated pain or discomfort, needs to be explained to the client.
- ❑ 5. The nurse is responsible for obtaining the client's signature on an informed consent form even if the client has questions about the test, procedure, or treatment to be performed.

Level of Cognitive Ability: Applying
Client Needs: Safe and Effective Care Environment
Clinical Judgment/Cognitive Skills: Generate Solutions
Integrated Process: Teaching and Learning
Content Area: Leadership/Management: Ethical/Legal
Health Problems: N/A
Priority Concepts: Health Care Law; Health Policy

Answer: 1, 3, 4
Rationale: Informed consent is a person's agreement to allow something to happen based on full disclosure of risks, benefits, alternatives, and consequences of refusal. The physician is responsible for conveying information and obtaining the informed consent. The nurse may be the person who actually ensures that the client signs the informed consent form; however, the nurse does this only after the physician has instructed the client and it has been determined that the client has understood the information. The following factors are required for informed consent: a brief, complete explanation of the test, procedure, or treatment; names and qualifications of persons performing and assisting in the test, procedure, or treatment; a description of the complications and risks, as well as anticipated pain or discomfort; an explanation of alternative therapies to the proposed test, procedure, or treatment, as well as the risks of doing nothing; and the client's right to refuse the test, procedure, or treatment even after it has been started.
Test-Taking Strategy: Focus on the subject, informed consent. To answer this question correctly, there are two primary factors to bear in mind. The first factor is that the physician is responsible for conveying information and obtaining the informed consent. The second factor is that the client has the right to be fully informed. Bearing these factors in mind will assist in answering this question and other questions related to informed consent.
Priority Nursing Tip: An informed consent is a legal document. The client needs to be a participant in decisions regarding health care and can withdraw consent at any time.
Reference: Zerwekh, J., & Zerwekh Garneau, A. (2021). *Nursing today: Transition and trends* (10th ed., pp. 489–490). Elsevier.

65. Wrist restraints have been prescribed for a client who is continuously pulling at the gastrostomy tube placed as part of the treatment for esophageal cancer. The nurse develops a care plan and would determine that which findings would be negative outcomes related to the use of restraints? **Select all that apply.**
- ❑ 1. The client is increasingly agitated.
- ❑ 2. The client's left hand is pale and cold.
- ❑ 3. The client's skin under the restraint is red.
- ❑ 4. The client verbalizes the reason for the restraints.
- ❑ 5. The client is unable to reach the gastrostomy tube with their hands.
- ❑ 6. The client demonstrates behavior that includes biting the attending staff.

Level of Cognitive Ability: Evaluating
Client Needs: Safe and Effective Care Environment
Clinical Judgment/Cognitive Skills: Evaluate Outcomes
Integrated Process: Clinical Judgment; Nursing Process/Evaluation
Content Area: Foundations of Care: Safety
Health Problems: Adult Health: Cancer: Esophageal/Gastric/Intestinal
Priority Concepts: Health Care Law; Safety

Answer: 1, 2, 3, 6
Rationale: A physical restraint is a mechanical or physical device used to immobilize a client or extremity. The restraint restricts freedom of movement. Negative outcomes in the use of restraints include signs of impaired skin integrity such as redness or skin breakdown; altered neurovascular status such as cyanosis, pallor, or coldness of the skin or complaints of tingling, numbness, or pain; increased confusion, disorientation, or agitation; or injuring staff. Client verbalization of the reason for the restraints and the client's inability to reach the gastrostomy tube with their hands are expected outcomes.
Test-Taking Strategy: Focus on the subject, use of restraints. Recognize that the words *negative outcomes* asks you to select the options that indicate undesirable effects of the use of the restraints. Focusing on the data in the question and recalling the nursing responsibilities related to care of a client in restraints will assist in answering the question.
Priority Nursing Tip: If the restraints are placed on a client during a period in which the behavior cannot be controlled or in an emergency situation, a physician's prescription for the restraints must be obtained in a timely manner. Additionally, the continued need for restraints needs to be assessed regularly according to agency policy.
Reference: Potter, P., et al. (2021). *Fundamentals of nursing* (10th ed., pp. 414–415, 417). Elsevier.

❖ **66.** The nurse is discussing accident prevention with the family of a client who is being discharged from the hospital after having hip surgery. Which physical factors place the client at risk for injury in the home? **Select all that apply.**
- ❑ 1. A night-light in the bathroom
- ❑ 2. Elevated toilet seat with armrests
- ❑ 3. Cooking equipment such as a stove
- ❑ 4. Smoke and carbon monoxide detectors
- ❑ 5. Objects such as a doormat and scatter rugs
- ❑ 6. A low thermostat setting on the water heater

Level of Cognitive Ability: Analyzing
Client Needs: Safe and Effective Care Environment
Clinical Judgment/Cognitive Skills: Recognize Cues
Integrated Process: Clinical Judgment; Nursing Process/Assessment
Content Area: Leadership/Management: Management of Care
Health Problems: Adult Health: Musculoskeletal: Skeletal Injury
Priority Concepts: Patient Education; Safety

Answer: 3, 5
Rationale: Physical hazards in the environment place the client at risk for accidental injury and death. Injuries in the home frequently result from tripping over or coming into contact with common household objects such as a doormat, small rugs on the floor or stairs, or clutter around the house. Adequate lighting such as night-lights in dark hallways and bathrooms reduces the physical hazard by illuminating areas in which a person moves about. An elevated toilet seat with armrests and nonslip strips on the floor in front of the toilet are useful in reducing falls in the bathroom. Cooking equipment and appliances, particularly stoves, can be a main source for in-home fires and fire injuries. Smoke and carbon monoxide detectors need to be placed throughout the home to alert members of the household of a potential danger. A low thermostat setting on the water heater reduces the risk of burns during water use such as bathing or showering.
Test-Taking Strategy: Focus on the subject, the physical factors that place the client at risk for injury at home. Next think about whether the factor is safe or presents a potential for injury; this will assist in answering the question.
Priority Nursing Tip: A client with peripheral neuropathy (decreased sensation in the extremities), such as the client with diabetes mellitus, is at a high risk for injury such as falls, cuts, or burns because of the inability to sense objects or high temperatures.
Reference: Potter, P., et al. (2021). *Fundamentals of nursing* (10th ed., pp. 397, 403). Elsevier.

67. The nurse is caring for a client receiving total parenteral nutrition (TPN). Which action is **most appropriate** for the nurse to implement in order to decrease the risk of infection?
1. Assess vital signs at 4-hour intervals.
2. Administer prophylactic antimicrobial agents.
3. Check the solution's label against the prescription.
4. Use aseptic technique in handling the TPN solution.

Level of Cognitive Ability: Applying
Client Needs: Safe and Effective Care Environment
Clinical Judgment/Cognitive Skills: Take Action
Integrated Process: Nursing Process/Implementation
Content Area: Skills: Nutrition
Health Problems: N/A
Priority Concepts: Infection; Safety

Answer: 4
Rationale: Clients receiving TPN are at high risk for developing infection because the concentrated glucose solutions are an excellent medium for bacterial growth. The nurse reduces the client's risk of infection by using aseptic technique when handling all equipment and solutions related to the TPN infusion (option 4). Option 1 is a reasonable intervention for early detection of infection but does not prevent infection. Prophylactic antibiotics are not indicated for TPN infusions and can contribute to the development of secondary infections. The nurse implements option 3 to ensure that the client receives the correct infusion, but it is not relevant to decreasing the risk of infection.
Test-Taking Strategy: Note the strategic words, *most appropriate.* Focus on the subject, TPN and decreasing the risk for infection. Option 1 relates to early detection of infection, option 2 is not indicated, and option 3 does not relate to the subject. Remember that aseptic technique is critical to prevent infection.
Priority Nursing Tip: TPN is the least desirable form of providing nutrition and is used when there is no other nutritional alternative.
Reference: Potter, P., et al. (2021). *Fundamentals of nursing* (10th ed., pp. 435, 447, 999). Elsevier.

❖ **68.** To ensure that the client diagnosed with cancer has adequate and safe pain control, which plan would the nurse implement?
1. Rely primarily on prescription and over-the-counter medications to relieve pain.
2. Keep a baseline level of pain so that the client does not become sedated or addicted.
3. Try multiple medication modalities for pain relief to get the maximum pain relief effect.
4. Start with low doses of medication and gradually increase to a safe dose that relieves pain.

Level of Cognitive Ability: Applying
Client Needs: Safe and Effective Care Environment
Clinical Judgment/Cognitive Skills: Generate Solutions
Integrated Process: Nursing Process/Planning
Content Area: Adult Health: Oncology
Health Problems: Adult Health: Neurologic: Pain
Priority Concepts: Pain; Safety

Answer: 4
Rationale: Safe pain control includes starting with low doses and working up to a dose of medication that relieves the pain. Option 1 does not take into account other nursing interventions that may relieve pain, such as massage, therapeutic touch, or music. Maintaining a baseline level of pain to avoid sedation or addiction is not appropriate practice unless the client requests this, and this information has not been provided in the case situation. Interventions using multiple medication modalities can be unsafe and ineffective.
Test-Taking Strategy: Focus on the subject, safe and effective pain management for the cancer client. Option 1 uses the word *primarily* and does not allow for any alternative interventions. Option 3 uses the word *multiple*, which is not appropriate in this instance; mixing of multiple medications may be unsafe. Option 2 can be eliminated because it is inaccurate information. Option 4 is the only safe, effective approach.
Priority Nursing Tip: Pain is what the client describes or says that it is. Do not undermedicate the cancer client who is in pain.
Reference: Lewis, S., et al. (2020). *Medical-surgical nursing: Assessment and management of clinical problems* (11th ed., pp. 261–263). Elsevier.

69. To ensure that the client self-administers medications safely in the home, which action would the nurse implement?
1. Perform a pill count of each prescription bottle at every home visit.
2. Provide information on the purpose of all the prescribed medications.
3. Instruct the client to double up on a medication when a dose is missed.
4. Ask the client to explain and demonstrate self-administration procedures.

Level of Cognitive Ability: Applying
Client Needs: Safe and Effective Care Environment
Clinical Judgment/Cognitive Skills: Take Action
Integrated Process: Teaching and Learning
Content Area: Foundations of Care: Communication
Health Problems: N/A
Priority Concepts: Patient Education; Safety

Answer: 4
Rationale: To ensure safe administration of medication, the nurse asks the client to explain and demonstrate correct self-administration of medication procedures because demonstrating the proper procedure for the client does not ensure that the client can safely perform any procedure. Usually it is not acceptable to double up on missed medication, and conducting a pill count on each visit is unrealistic and disrespectful.
Test-Taking Strategy: Focus on the subject, safe administration of medication. Eliminate options 1, 2, and 3 because these are unlikely to ensure correct client practices. Option 4 is the only client-centered choice.
Priority Nursing Tip: Determine the client's readiness to learn before implementing a teaching plan. If the client is not ready to learn, learning will not take place.
Reference: Potter, P., et al. (2021). *Fundamentals of nursing* (10th ed., pp. 607, 612–613). Elsevier.

❖ **70.** A client remains in diagnosed atrial fibrillation with rapid ventricular response despite prescribed pharmacologic intervention. Synchronous cardioversion is scheduled to convert the rapid rhythm. Which action would the nurse plan to take to ensure safety and prevent complications of this procedure?
1. Cardiovert the client at 360 joules.
2. Sedate the client before cardioversion.
3. Ensure that emergency equipment is available.
4. Check that the defibrillator is set on the synchronous mode.

Level of Cognitive Ability: Applying
Client Needs: Safe and Effective Care Environment
Clinical Judgment/Cognitive Skills: Generate Solutions
Integrated Process: Clinical Judgment; Nursing Process/Planning
Content Area: Complex Care: Emergency Situations/Management
Health Problems: Adult Health: Cardiovascular: Dysrhythmias
Priority Concepts: Clinical Judgment; Safety

Answer: 4
Rationale: Cardioversion is similar to defibrillation with two major exceptions: the countershock is synchronized to occur during ventricular depolarization (QRS complex), and less energy is used for the countershock. The rationale for delivering the shock during the QRS complex is to prevent the shock from being delivered during repolarization (T wave), often termed the *vulnerable period*. If the shock is delivered during this period, the resulting complication is ventricular fibrillation. It is crucial that the defibrillator is set on the "synchronous" mode for a successful cardioversion. Cardioversion usually begins with 50 to 100 joules. Options 2 and 3 will not prevent complications.
Test-Taking Strategy: Focus on the *subject*, ensuring safety and preventing complications with synchronous cardioversion. Note that the question denotes *synchronous* cardioversion and its relationship to the information in option 4.
Priority Nursing Tip: Indicators of a successful response to cardioversion include conversion of the dysrhythmia to sinus rhythm, strong peripheral pulses, an adequate blood pressure, and an adequate urine output.
Reference: Ignatavicius, D., et al. (2021). *Medical-surgical nursing: Concepts for interprofessional collaborative care* (10th ed., p. 654). Elsevier.

71. A client with a diagnosis of thrombophlebitis is being treated with prescribed heparin sodium therapy. In planning a safe environment, the nurse would ensure that which medication is available if the client develops a significant bleeding problem?
1. Reteplase
2. Phytonadione
3. Protamine sulfate
4. Fresh frozen plasma

Level of Cognitive Ability: Applying
Client Needs: Safe and Effective Care Environment
Clinical Judgment/Cognitive Skills: Generate Solutions
Integrated Process: Nursing Process/Planning
Content Area: Pharmacology: Cardiovascular: Anticoagulants
Health Problems: Adult Health: Cardiovascular: Deep Vein Thrombosis
Priority Concepts: Perfusion; Safety

Answer: 3
Rationale: Protamine sulfate is the antidote for heparin sodium. Fresh frozen plasma may be used for bleeding related to warfarin therapy. Reteplase is a thrombolytic agent used to dissolve blood clots. Phytonadione is the antidote for warfarin.
Test-Taking Strategy: Focus on the *subject*, planning a safe environment for the client receiving heparin. It is necessary to recall that the antidote for heparin sodium is protamine sulfate to answer correctly.
Priority Nursing Tip: To maintain a therapeutic level of anticoagulation when a client is receiving a continuous infusion of heparin sodium, the activated partial thromboplastin time (aPTT) needs to be 1.5 to 2.5 times the normal value.
Reference: Gahart, B., Nazareno, A., & Ortega, M. (2021). *Gahart's 2021 Intravenous medications: A handbook for nurses and health professionals* (37th ed., p. 708). Elsevier.

❖ **72.** The nurse is teaching a client with a diagnosis of cardiomyopathy about home care safety measures. Which instruction is **most important** for the nurse to include?
1. Reporting pain
2. Appropriate vasodilator administration
3. Avoiding over-the-counter medications
4. Moving slowly from a sitting to a standing position

Level of Cognitive Ability: Applying
Client Needs: Safe and Effective Care Environment
Clinical Judgment/Cognitive Skills: Generate Solutions
Integrated Process: Teaching and Learning
Content Area: Adult Health: Cardiovascular
Health Problems: Adult Health: Cardiovascular: Inflammatory and Structural Heart Disorders
Priority Concepts: Perfusion; Safety

Answer: 4
Rationale: Orthostatic changes can occur in the client with cardiomyopathy as a result of venous return obstruction. Sudden changes in blood pressure may lead to falls. Reporting pain, while important, is not directly related to the issue of safety. Vasodilators are not normally prescribed for the client with cardiomyopathy. Option 3, although important, is not directly related to the issue of safety.
Test-Taking Strategy: Focus on the subject, to ensure client safety at home, and note the strategic words, *most important.* Recalling that blood pressure changes occur in cardiomyopathy will direct you to option 4.
Priority Nursing Tip: Treatment for cardiomyopathy is palliative, not curative, and the client needs to deal with numerous lifestyle changes and a shortened life span.
Reference: Ignatavicius, D., et al. (2021). *Medical-surgical nursing: Concepts for interprofessional collaborative care* (10th ed., p. 693). Elsevier.

73. The nurse instructs a client with a diagnosis of atrial fibrillation who has been prescribed warfarin to use an electric razor for shaving. Which premise **best** supports the rationale for this instruction?
1. Cuts need to be avoided.
2. Any cut may cause infection.
3. Electric razors can be disinfected.
4. All straight razors contain bacteria.

Level of Cognitive Ability: Applying
Client Needs: Safe and Effective Care Environment
Clinical Judgment/Cognitive Skills: Take Action
Integrated Process: Teaching and Learning
Content Area: Pharmacology: Cardiovascular: Anticoagulants
Health Problems: Adult Health: Cardiovascular: Dysrhythmias
Priority Concepts: Perfusion; Safety

Answer: 1
Rationale: Clients with atrial fibrillation are placed on anticoagulants to prevent thrombus formation and possible stroke. Therefore, measures to prevent bleeding need to be taught to the client. The importance of use of an electric razor is to prevent cuts and possible bleeding. Not all cuts cause infection. Electric razors can be cleaned but usually cannot be disinfected. Not all straight razors contain bacteria. Additionally, options 2, 3, and 4 are all unrelated to the subject of bleeding; rather, they relate to infection.
Test-Taking Strategy: Note the strategic word, *best.* Recalling that the client with atrial fibrillation will be prescribed anticoagulants will assist in answering the question. Note that options 2, 3, and 4 are comparable or alike and relate to infection. Additionally, options 2 and 4 can be eliminated because of the words "any" and "all," which are closed-ended words. Option 1 relates to bleeding.
Priority Nursing Tip: In atrial fibrillation, usually no definitive P wave can be observed, only fibrillatory waves before each QRS.
Reference: Ignatavicius, D., et al. (2021). *Medical-surgical nursing: Concepts for interprofessional collaborative care* (10th ed., p. 724). Elsevier.

❖ **74.** A cardiac catheterization, using the femoral artery approach, is performed to assess the degree of coronary artery thrombosis in a client. Which **priority** safety actions would the nurse implement in the postprocedure period? **Select all that apply.**
☐ 1. Restricting visitors
☐ 2. Checking the client's groin for bleeding
☐ 3. Encouraging the client to increase fluid intake
☐ 4. Placing the client's bed in the high-Fowler's position
☐ 5. Instructing the client to move the toes when checking circulation, motion, and sensation

Level of Cognitive Ability: Applying
Client Needs: Safe and Effective Care Environment
Clinical Judgment/Cognitive Skills: Take Action
Integrated Process: Nursing Process/Implementation
Content Area: Adult Health: Cardiovascular
Health Problems: Adult Health: Cardiovascular: Coronary Artery Disease
Priority Concepts: Perfusion; Safety

Answer: 2, 3, 5
Rationale: Immediately after a cardiac catheterization with the femoral artery approach, the client should not flex or hyperextend the affected leg to avoid blood vessel occlusion or hemorrhage. The groin is checked for bleeding, and, if any occurs, the nurse immediately places pressure on the site and asks another staff member to contact the cardiologist. Fluids are encouraged to assist in removing the contrast medium from the body. Asking the client to move the toes is done to assess motion, which could be impaired if a hematoma or thrombus was developing. There is no need to restrict visitors. Placing the client in the high-Fowler's position (flexion) increases the risk of occlusion or hemorrhage.
Test-Taking Strategy: Note the strategic word, *priority*. Focus on the subject, cardiac catheterization. Also note the words *femoral artery approach*. Recalling that flexion or hyperextension is avoided after this procedure will assist in determining that option 4 is incorrect. There is no useful or helpful reason for restricting visitors, so eliminate option 1.
Priority Nursing Tip: Inform the client undergoing a cardiac catheterization that they may experience a fluttery feeling as the catheter is passed through the heart, a flushed warm feeling when the dye is injected, a desire to cough, and palpitations caused by heart irritability.
Reference: Ignatavicius, D., et al. (2021). *Medical-surgical nursing: Concepts for interprofessional collaborative care* (10th ed., pp. 628–630). Elsevier.

75. The nurse is reviewing general injury prevention guidelines with the pediatric department staff in the hospital. Which interventions aimed at promoting safety specifically for infants and toddlers would the nurse include in this review? **Select all that apply.**
☐ 1. Ensure that crib sides are up.
☐ 2. Place large, soft pillows in the crib.
☐ 3. Use large, soft toys without small parts.
☐ 4. Attach a pacifier to a stretchable piece of ribbon and pin to the infant's clothing.
☐ 5. Allow a toddler who is toilet training privacy in the bathroom to promote autonomy.
☐ 6. Ensure that an infant or toddler is never left unattended while lying on a changing table.

Level of Cognitive Ability: Applying
Client Needs: Safe and Effective Care Environment
Clinical Judgment/Cognitive Skills: Generate Solutions
Integrated Process: Teaching and Learning
Content Area: Foundations of Care: Safety
Health Problems: N/A
Priority Concepts: Health Promotion; Safety

Answer: 1, 3, 6
Rationale: To promote safety for infants and toddlers, crib sides are never left down because the child could roll and fall. Large, soft toys without small parts need to be used because small parts can become dislodged and choking and aspiration may occur. For this same reason, an infant or toddler is never left unattended while lying on a changing table. Pillows, stuffed toys, comforters, or other objects are not placed in the crib because the child can become entwined in these items and suffocate. Pacifiers would not be attached to string or ribbon because of the risk associated with choking. The child is never left alone in the bathroom, in the tub, or near any other water source because of the risk of drowning.
Test-Taking Strategy: Focus on the subject, safety measures specific for infants and toddlers. Read each option carefully, thinking about the subject of the question and how the intervention may present a risk to the child. This will assist in answering correctly.
Priority Nursing Tip: The nurse needs to educate the parents about baby-proofing the home.
Reference: Hockenberry, M., Wilson, D., & Rodgers, C. (2019). *Wong's Nursing care of infants and children* (11th ed., pp. 694–695). Elsevier.

❖ **76.** Which scenarios demonstrate a participative style of leadership? **Select all that apply.**

❑ 1. The nurse manager presents a problem to the staff and tells the staff to solve the problem.

❑ 2. The nurse manager arranges unit meetings for all shifts to deal with an identified problem.

❑ 3. The nurse manager assesses a problem and informs the staff of the solution to be implemented.

❑ 4. The nurse manager proposes several methods of dealing with a problem and invites team input.

❑ 5. The nurse manager proposes several solutions to a problem and has the unit staff vote on the best option.

❑ 6. The nurse manager considers staff input related to a problem but makes the final decision on implementation of the solution.

Level of Cognitive Ability: Understanding
Client Needs: Safe and Effective Care Environment
Clinical Judgment/Cognitive Skills: Recognize Cues
Integrated Process: Nursing Process/Assessment
Content Area: Leadership/Management: Management of Care
Health Problems: N/A
Priority Concepts: Leadership; Professional Identity

Answer: 2, 4, 6
Rationale: Participative leadership demonstrates an "in-between" style, neither authoritarian nor democratic. In participative leadership, the manager presents an analysis of problems and proposals for actions to team members, inviting critique and comments. The participative leader then analyzes the comments and makes the final decision. The autocratic style of leadership is task oriented and directive. A laissez-faire leader abdicates leadership and responsibilities, allowing staff to work without assistance, direction, or supervision. The democratic style of leadership involves a majority rule.
Test-Taking Strategy: Focus on the subject, participative leadership. Options 2, 4, and 6 involve staff input to the nurse manager. The remaining options reflect other forms of leadership that do not seek staff input.
Priority Nursing Tip: The nurse is always responsible for their actions when providing care to a client.
Reference: Zerwekh, J., & Zerwekh Garneau, A. (2021). *Nursing today: Transition and trends* (10th ed., p. 419). Elsevier.

77. A physician prescribes 1000 mL of 0.45% normal saline solution to run over 8 hours. The drop factor is 15 drops/mL. The nurse adjusts the flow rate to how many drops per minute to safely administer this intravenous (IV) solution? **Fill in the blank and round answer to the nearest whole number.**

Answer: _____ gtt/min

Level of Cognitive Ability: Applying
Client Needs: Safe and Effective Care Environment
Clinical Judgment/Cognitive Skills: Generate Solutions
Integrated Process: Nursing Process/Planning
Content Area: Skills: Dosage Calculations
Health Problems: N/A
Priority Concepts: Clinical Judgment; Safety

Answer: 31
Rationale: The prescribed 1000 mL is to be infused over 8 hours. Follow the formula for calculating IV flow rates and multiply 1000 mL by 15 (drop factor). Then divide the result by 480 minutes (8 hours × 60 minutes). The infusion is to run at 31.2 or 31 drops/min.
Formula:

$$\frac{\text{Total volume in mL} \times \text{drop factor}}{\text{Time in minutes}} = \text{Flow rate in drops/min}$$

$$\frac{1000 \text{ mL} \times 15 \text{ drop per mL}}{480 \text{ minutes}} = \frac{15,000}{480} = 31.2, \text{or } 31 \text{ drops/min}$$

Test-Taking Strategy: Focus on the subject, IV flow rate calculation. Recall the formula for calculating the infusion rate for an IV and be certain to change 8 hours to 480 minutes. After you have performed the calculation, verify your answer using a calculator.
Priority Nursing Tip: Most intravenous flow rate calculations involve changing the time for infusion from hours to minutes.
Reference: Potter, P., et al. (2021). *Fundamentals of nursing* (10th ed., pp. 1022–1023). Elsevier.

❖ **78.** A client diagnosed with terminal liver cancer asks the home care nurse to witness the client's signature on a living will with the client's attorney in attendance. Which action is **most appropriate** for the nurse to implement?
1. Decline to witness the signature on the living will.
2. Sign the living will as a witness to the signature only.
3. Notify the supervisor that a living will is being witnessed.
4. Sign the living will with identifying credentials and employment agency.

Level of Cognitive Ability: Applying
Client Needs: Safe and Effective Care Environment
Clinical Judgment/Cognitive Skills: Take Action
Integrated Process: Nursing Process/Implementation
Content Area: Leadership/Management: Ethical/Legal
Health Problems: Adult Health: Cancer: Liver
Priority Concepts: Ethics; Health Care Law

Answer: 1
Rationale: Living wills are written documents and need to be signed by the client. The client's signature must be either witnessed by nonagency individuals or notarized; thus, the nurse would decline to sign the will to avoid a conflict of interest. There is no need to contact the supervisor or sign the living will with or without credentials because the nurse cannot sign this document as a witness. Therefore, options 2, 3, and 4 are incorrect.
Test-Taking Strategy: Note the strategic words, *most appropriate.* Eliminate options 2, 3, and 4 because they are comparable or alike and indicate that the nurse will sign the will as a witness.
Priority Nursing Tip: A living will is a type of advance directive, and all health care workers must follow the directions of an advance directive to ensure that the client's wishes are implemented and to be safe from liability.
Reference: Lewis, S., et al. (2020). *Medical-surgical nursing: Assessment and management of clinical problems* (11th ed., pp. 133–134). Elsevier; Potter, P., et al. (2021). *Fundamentals of nursing* (10th ed., p. 310). Elsevier.

79. The nurse notices old and new ecchymotic areas on an older adult client's arms and buttocks upon admission. The client states to the nurse in confidence that "the family members frequently hit me." Which therapeutic statement would the nurse communicate in response?
1. "I have a legal obligation to report this type of abuse."
2. "Let's get these treated, and I will maintain confidence."
3. "Let's talk about ways to prevent someone from hitting you."
4. "If this happens again, you must call the emergency department."

Level of Cognitive Ability: Applying
Client Needs: Safe and Effective Care Environment
Clinical Judgment/Cognitive Skills: Take Action
Integrated Process: Nursing Process/Implementation
Content Area: Leadership/Management: Ethical/Legal
Health Problems: Mental Health: Abuse/Neglect
Priority Concepts: Interpersonal Violence; Safety

Answer: 1
Rationale: The nurse would inform the client that nurses cannot maintain confidence about alleged abusive behavior and that the nurse must report situations related to abuse. The nurse avoids bargaining with the client about treatment to maintain a confidence that the nurse is legally bound to report. Options 3 and 4 delay protective action and place the client at risk for future abuse.
Test-Taking Strategy: Focus on the subject, elder abuse. The nurse is legally obligated to report the occurrence of elder abuse. Option 2 can be eliminated first because this action does not protect the client from injury. Options 3 and 4 would be eliminated next because they place the client at risk for future abuse.
Priority Nursing Tip: Victims of abuse may attempt to dismiss injuries as accidental, and abusers may prevent victims from receiving proper medical care to avoid discovery.
Reference: Ignatavicius, D., et al. (2021). *Medical-surgical nursing: Concepts for interprofessional collaborative care* (10th ed., pp. 64–65). Elsevier.

❖ **80.** At the scene of a train crash, the nurse triages the victims. Which clients would be coded for triage as **most** urgent or the **first** priority? Refer to chart. Select all that apply.

VICTIMS
- ☐ **1.** Is dead
- ☐ **2.** Has chest pain
- ☐ **3.** Has a leg sprain
- ☐ **4.** Has a chest wound
- ☐ **5.** Has multiple fractures
- ☐ **6.** Has full-thickness burns over 30% of the body

Level of Cognitive Ability: Analyzing
Client Needs: Safe and Effective Care Environment
Clinical Judgment/Cognitive Skills: Analyze Cues
Integrated Process: Clinical Judgment; Nursing Process/Analysis
Content Area: Leadership/Management: Mass Casualty Preparedness and Response
Health Problems: N/A
Priority Concepts: Clinical Judgment; Safety

Answer: 2, 4, 6
Rationale: In a disaster situation, saving the greatest number of lives is the most important goal. During a disaster the nurse would triage the victims to maximize the number of survivors and sort the treatable from the untreatable victims. Prioritizing victims can be done in many ways, and many communities use a color-coding system. First priority victims (most urgent and coded red) have life-threatening injuries and are experiencing hypoxia or near hypoxia. Examples of injuries in this category are shock, chest wounds, internal hemorrhage, head injuries producing loss of consciousness, partial- or full-thickness burns over 20% of the body surface, and chest pain. Second priority victims (urgent and coded yellow) have injuries with systemic effects but are not yet hypoxic or in shock and can withstand a 2-hour wait without immediate risk (e.g., a victim with multiple fractures). Third priority victims (coded green) have minimal injuries unaccompanied by systemic complications and can wait for more than 2 hours for treatment without risk (leg sprain). Dying or dead victims have catastrophic injuries, and the dying victims would not survive under the best of circumstances (coded black).
Test-Taking Strategy: Note the strategic words, *most* and *first priority.* Read each option carefully and recall that, in a disaster situation, saving the greatest number of lives is the most important goal and that the nurse would triage the victims to maximize the number of survivors. Also, use of the ABCs—airway, breathing, and circulation—will direct you to the correct options.
Priority Nursing Tip: As a first responder to the scene of a disaster, think survivability. The priority victim is the one whose life can be saved.
Reference: Ignatavicius, D., et al. (2021). *Medical-surgical nursing: Concepts for interprofessional collaborative care* (10th ed., pp. 228–229). Elsevier.

81. A client tells the home care nurse of a personal decision to refuse external cardiac resuscitation measures. Which is the **most appropriate initial** nursing action?
1. Discuss the client's request with the client's family.
2. Document the client's request in the home care nursing care plan.
3. Notify the client's physician of the client's request.
4. Conduct a client conference with the home care staff to share the client's request.

Level of Cognitive Ability: Applying
Client Needs: Safe and Effective Care Environment
Clinical Judgment/Cognitive Skills: Take Action
Integrated Process: Nursing Process/Implementation
Content Area: Leadership/Management: Ethical/Legal
Health Problems: N/A
Priority Concepts: Health Care Law; Palliative Care

Answer: 3
Rationale: External cardiac resuscitation is a lifesaving treatment that a client may refuse. The most appropriate initial nursing action is to notify the physician because a written "do not resuscitate" (DNR) prescription from the physician is needed to ensure that the client's wishes are followed. The DNR prescription must be reviewed or renewed on a regular basis per agency policy. Although options 1, 2, and 4 may be appropriate, remember that obtaining a written physician's DNR prescription must be completed first.
Test-Taking Strategy: Note the strategic words, *most appropriate initial.* The strategic words indicate that more than one option may be correct, but there is only one initial action. Although options 1, 2, and 4 may be appropriate, remember that first a written physician's prescription is necessary.
Priority Nursing Tip: All health care personnel must know whether a client has a DNR prescription.
Reference: Potter, P., et al. (2021). *Fundamentals of nursing* (10th ed., p. 310). Elsevier.

❖ **82.** The nurse prepares a client for discharge who is prescribed intermittent antibiotic infusions through a peripherally inserted central catheter (PICC) line for a foot infection. Which instruction would the nurse include in client teaching about necessary daily infusion care in the home?
1. Keep the affected arm immobilized.
2. Aspirate 3 mL of blood from the line daily.
3. Maintain a continuous intravenous infusion.
4. Check the insertion site for redness and swelling.

Level of Cognitive Ability: Applying
Client Needs: Safe and Effective Care Environment
Clinical Judgment/Cognitive Skills: Generate Solutions
Integrated Process: Nursing Process/Planning
Content Area: Skills: Medication Administration
Health Problems: Adult Health: Integumentary: Inflammations/Infections
Priority Concepts: Patient Education; Safety

Answer: 4
Rationale: A PICC line is designed for long-term intravenous infusions and usually is inserted into the median cubital vein with the terminal end of the catheter in the superior vena cava. Although the risk of infection is less with a PICC line than with a central venous catheter, it is possible for phlebitis or infection to develop. Clients must inspect the insertion site and affected arm daily and report any discharge, redness, swelling, or pain to the nurse or physician immediately. A PICC line does not require the affected arm to be immobilized. Although a PICC line can be used to obtain a blood specimen, the risk of occlusion from aspirating blood as part of the related daily care is greater than any potential benefit. The PICC line can be used for intermittent or continuous fluid infusion.
Test-Taking Strategy: Focus on the subject, daily infusion care for a PICC line. Basic principles of infection control lead you to choose option 4. Additionally, option 4 represents the first step of the nursing process, assessment. Eliminate option 1 because this action can be appropriate for a short-length peripheral intravenous catheter if placed in a movable or vulnerable spot (such as the wrist). Eliminate option 2 because it is contraindicated; the risks of aspirating blood from the catheter are greater than the potential benefit, and this practice is not recommended as routine care. Because the nature of a PICC line allows for either continuous or intermittent infusions, option 3 is also incorrect.
Priority Nursing Tip: A small amount of bleeding may occur at the time of insertion of a PICC line and may continue for 24 hours, but bleeding thereafter is not expected.
References: Ignatavicius, D., et al. (2021). *Medical-surgical nursing: Concepts for interprofessional collaborative care* (10th ed., pp. 281–283, 294). Elsevier; Potter, P., et al. (2021). *Fundamentals of nursing* (10th ed., p. 1005). Elsevier.

83. The nurse is preparing the client assignments for the day to a licensed practical nurse (LPN) and an unlicensed assistive personnel (UAP). Which clients would the nurse assign to the LPN because of client needs that cannot be met by a UAP? **Select all that apply.**
❑ 1. Client requiring frequent suctioning
❑ 2. Client requiring a dressing change to the foot
❑ 3. Client requiring range-of-motion exercises twice daily
❑ 4. Client requiring reinforcement of teaching about a diabetic diet
❑ 5. Client on bed rest requiring vital sign measurement every 4 hours
❑ 6. Client requiring collection of a urine specimen for urinalysis testing

Level of Cognitive Ability: Analyzing
Client Needs: Safe and Effective Care Environment
Clinical Judgment/Cognitive Skills: Generate Solutions
Integrated Process: Nursing Process/Planning
Content Area: Leadership/Management: Delegating/Supervising
Health Problems: N/A
Priority Concepts: Care Coordination; Leadership

Answer: 1, 2, 4
Rationale: Delegation is the transferring to a competent individual the authority to perform a nursing task. When the nurse plans client assignments, the nurse needs to consider the educational level and experience of the individual and the needs of the client. The LPN is trained to perform all the tasks indicated in the options; the clients who have needs that cannot be met by the UAP are those requiring suctioning, a dressing change, and reinforcement of teaching about a diabetic diet. UAPs are trained to perform range-of-motion exercises, measure vital signs, and collect a urine specimen.
Test-Taking Strategy: Focus on the subject, client needs that cannot be met by the UAP. Read each option carefully and consider the needs of the client. Recalling that the UAP can be assigned activities that are noninvasive will assist in answering the question.
Priority Nursing Tip: The safety of the client is always the nurse's primary concern when delegating nursing tasks.
Reference: Zerwekh, J., & Zerwekh Garneau, A. (2021). *Nursing today: Transition and trends* (10th ed., pp. 264, 324–325). Elsevier.

84. A charge nurse observes that a staff nurse is not able to meet client needs in a reasonable time frame, does not problem-solve situations, and does not prioritize nursing care. Which strategy is **most appropriate** for the charge nurse to employ?

1. Ask other staff members to help the staff nurse get the work done.
2. Supervise the staff nurse more closely so that tasks are completed.
3. Provide support and identify the underlying cause of the staff nurse's problem.
4. Report the staff nurse to the supervisor so that remediation to resolve the problem occurs.

Level of Cognitive Ability: Analyzing
Client Needs: Safe and Effective Care Environment
Clinical Judgment/Cognitive Skills: Generate Solutions
Integrated Process: Nursing Process/Planning
Content Area: Leadership/Management: Delegating/Supervising
Health Problems: N/A
Priority Concepts: Leadership; Professional Identity

Answer: 3
Rationale: Option 3 empowers the charge nurse to assist the staff nurse while trying to identify and reduce the behaviors that make it difficult for the staff nurse to function. Options 1, 2, and 4 are punitive actions, shift the burden to other workers, and do not solve the problem.
Test-Taking Strategy: Note the strategic words, *most appropriate.* Remember that assessment is the first step of the nursing process. The charge nurse needs to gather information before making any decisions or deciding on a course of action. Identifying the underlying cause of the problem is a process of assessment.
Priority Nursing Tip: Problem-solving involves obtaining information and using it to reach an acceptable solution to a problem.
Reference: Zerwekh, J., & Zerwekh Garneau, A. (2021). *Nursing today: Transition and trends* (10th ed., p. 235). Elsevier.

85. A registered nurse is a preceptor for a new nurse and is observing the new nurse organize the client assignments and prioritize daily tasks. The registered nurse would intervene if the new nurse implements which action?

1. Provides times for staff meals
2. Gathers the supplies needed for a task
3. Combines all tasks for clients in one list
4. Documents task completions at the end of the day

Level of Cognitive Ability: Applying
Client Needs: Safe and Effective Care Environment
Clinical Judgment/Cognitive Skills: Take Action
Integrated Process: Teaching and Learning
Content Area: Leadership/Management: Delegating/Supervising
Health Problems: N/A
Priority Concepts: Leadership; Professional Identity

Answer: 4
Rationale: The nurse needs to document task completion continuously throughout the day. Options 1, 2, and 3 identify accurate components of time management.
Test-Taking Strategy: Note the word *intervene,* and focus on the subject, the incorrect component of time management. Recalling that the nurse needs to document client data and task completion continuously throughout the day will direct you to option 4.
Priority Nursing Tip: Time management involves efficiency in completing tasks safely as quickly as possible and effectiveness in deciding on the most important task to do (prioritizing) and doing it correctly.
Reference: Zerwekh, J., & Zerwekh Garneau, A. (2021). *Nursing today: Transition and trends* (10th ed., pp. 261–263). Elsevier.

86. The registered nurse instructs the new nurse that a variance analysis is performed on all clients with respect to which time frame?
1. Continuously
2. Daily during hospitalization
3. Every third day of hospitalization
4. Every other day of hospitalization

Level of Cognitive Ability: Understanding
Client Needs: Safe and Effective Care Environment
Clinical Judgment/Cognitive Skills: Take Action
Integrated Process: Teaching and Learning
Content Area: Leadership/Management: Quality Improvement
Health Problems: N/A
Priority Concepts: Health Care Quality; Leadership

Answer: 1
Rationale: Variance analysis occurs continuously as the case manager and other caregivers monitor client outcomes against critical paths. The goal of critical paths is to anticipate and recognize negative variance early so that appropriate action can be taken. A negative variance occurs when untoward events preclude a timely discharge and the length of stay is longer than planned for a client on a specific critical path. Options 2, 3, and 4 are incorrect.
Test-Taking Strategy: Focus on the subject, critical paths and variance analysis. Recall that the goal of critical paths is to recognize negative variance early. This will direct you to option 1. Remember that it is best to monitor a client continuously.
Priority Nursing Tip: Variance analysis is a continuous process that the case manager and other caregivers conduct by comparing the specific client outcomes with the expected outcomes described on the critical pathway.
Reference: Potter, P., et al. (2021). *Fundamentals of nursing* (10th ed., pp. 377–378). Elsevier.

87. When the nurse manager encourages staff to provide input in the decision-making process, which leadership style is being demonstrated?
1. Autocratic
2. Situational
3. Democratic
4. Laissez-faire

Level of Cognitive Ability: Understanding
Client Needs: Safe and Effective Care Environment
Clinical Judgment/Cognitive Skills: Recognize Cues
Integrated Process: Teaching and Learning
Content Area: Leadership/Management: Management of Care
Health Problems: N/A
Priority Concepts: Leadership; Professional Identity

Answer: 3
Rationale: The democratic style of leadership best empowers staff toward excellence because this style of leadership allows nurses to provide input regarding the decision-making process and an opportunity to grow professionally. The autocratic style of leadership is task oriented and directive. The leader uses their power and position in an authoritarian manner to set and implement organizational goals. Decisions are made without input from the staff. The situational leadership style uses a style depending on the situation and events. The laissez-faire style allows staff to work without assistance, direction, or supervision.
Test-Taking Strategy: Focus on the subject, the type of leadership employed. Note the words, *encourages staff to provide input.* This will assist in directing you to the correct option.
Priority Nursing Tip: A democratic leader acts primarily as a facilitator and resource person and is concerned about the ideas and input that each member of the group offers. This style is based on the belief that every group member would have input into the development of goals and problem-solving.
Reference: Zerwekh, J., & Zerwekh Garneau, A. (2021). *Nursing today: Transition and trends* (10th ed., p. 222). Elsevier.

❖ **88.** A hospital administrator has implemented a change in the method of assigning nurses to client care units. A group of registered nurses is resistant to the change, and the nursing administrator anticipates that the nurses will not facilitate the process of change. Which approach is **best** for the administrator to take **initially** in dealing with the resistance?
1. Cancel the implementation of the change.
2. Implement the change first on a trial basis.
3. Delay implementing the change for a few weeks.
4. Encourage the nurses to verbalize feelings regarding the change.

Level of Cognitive Ability: Applying
Client Needs: Safe and Effective Care Environment
Clinical Judgment/Cognitive Skills: Take Action
Integrated Process: Teaching and Learning
Content Area: Leadership/Management: Quality Improvement
Health Problems: N/A
Priority Concepts: Collaboration; Leadership

Answer: 4
Rationale: Face-to-face meetings to address the issue at hand will allow verbalization of feelings, identification of problems and issues, and the development of strategies to solve the problem. Option 1 will not address the problem. Option 2 is not the initial intervention. Option 3 may provide a temporary solution to the resistance but will not specifically address the concern.
Test-Taking Strategy: Note the strategic words, *best* and *initially*. Focus on the subject, resistance to change. Options 1 and 2 can be easily eliminated first because these actions do not address the problem and may produce additional resistance. From the remaining options, select option 4 because this option specifically addresses the subject and would provide problem-solving measures.
Priority Nursing Tip: Resistance to change by staff occurs when an individual(s) rejects proposed new ideas without critically thinking about the proposal. The nurse leader would describe the proposed new idea and focus on the benefits of the idea in relation to improvement in client care.
Reference: Zerwekh, J., & Zerwekh Garneau, A. (2021). *Nursing today: Transition and trends* (10th ed., pp. 241–242). Elsevier.

89. Which situation represents the primary nursing care delivery model?
1. The registered nurse (RN) performs all tasks needed by the individual client to optimize health.
2. The RN provides care to four clients, while the unlicensed assistive personnel (UAP) is assigned to care for two clients.
3. The RN develops a plan of care for each client and collaborates with other staff members assigned to the same group of clients.
4. The UAP is assigned to make beds and fill water pitchers. The RN is assigned to administer medications.

Level of Cognitive Ability: Understanding
Client Needs: Safe and Effective Care Environment
Clinical Judgment/Cognitive Skills: Generate Solutions
Integrated Process: Nursing Process/Planning
Content Area: Leadership/Management: Management of Care
Health Problems: N/A
Priority Concepts: Clinical Judgment; Leadership

Answer: 1
Rationale: In primary nursing, option 1, concern is with keeping the nurse at the bedside actively involved in care, providing goal-directed and individualized client care. Option 2 does not follow the guidelines for any specific type of nursing care delivery approach. Team nursing, option 3, is characterized by a high degree of communication and collaboration among members. The team is generally led by an RN who is responsible for assessing, developing nursing diagnoses, planning, and evaluating each client's plan of care. The functional model of care involves an assembly line approach to client care, with major tasks being delegated by the charge nurse to individual staff members.
Test-Taking Strategy: Focus on the subject, primary nursing care delivery model. Read each option carefully and note the words *individual client* in the correct option.
Priority Nursing Tip: The functional model of nursing care delivery focuses on the delegated task rather than the total client. This can result in fragmentation of care and lack of accountability by the health care member.
Reference: Zerwekh, J., & Zerwekh Garneau, A. (2021). *Nursing today: Transition and trends* (10th ed., p. 361). Elsevier.

❖ **90.** The nurse assesses a client 24 hours following an above-the-knee amputation. Which action would the nurse take to ensure that the client's residual limb is placed in the **most appropriate** position?
   1. Elevate the foot of the bed.
   2. Put the bed in reverse Trendelenburg's.
   3. Position the residual limb flat on the bed.
   4. Keep the residual limb slightly elevated with the client lying on the operative side.

Level of Cognitive Ability: Applying
Client Needs: Safe and Effective Care Environment
Clinical Judgment/Cognitive Skills: Take Action
Integrated Process: Clinical Judgment; Nursing Process/Implementation
Content Area: Skills: Activity/Mobility
Health Problems: Adult Health: Musculoskeletal: Amputation
Priority Concepts: Mobility; Tissue Integrity

Answer: 3
Rationale: Some (not all) surgeons may prescribe elevation of the residual limb for the first 24 hours following amputation to control edema. If elevation is allowed, after the first 24 hours the residual limb is usually placed flat on the bed (as prescribed) to reduce hip contracture. Edema is also controlled by residual limb wrapping techniques. Reverse Trendelenburg's is an inappropriate position and may cause pressure on the diaphragm, affecting breathing.
Test-Taking Strategy: Note the strategic words, *most appropriate*. Eliminate options 1 and 4 first because they are comparable or alike positions. To select from the remaining options, note that the client is 24 hours postoperative. Recalling that hip contracture is a concern will assist in directing you to option 3.
Priority Nursing Tip: After amputation, assess the client for phantom limb sensation and pain. Explain these feelings of sensation and pain to the client, and medicate the client as prescribed.
Reference: Ignatavicius, D., et al. (2021). *Medical-surgical nursing: Concepts for interprofessional collaborative care* (10th ed., pp. 1049–1050). Elsevier.

91. An emergency department nurse is a member of an all-hazards disaster preparedness planning group. The group is developing a specific emergency response plan in the event that a client with smallpox arrives in the emergency department. Which interventions would **initially** be included in the plan? **Select all that apply.**
   ☐ 1. Isolate the client.
   ☐ 2. Don protective equipment immediately.
   ☐ 3. Notify infectious disease specialists, public health officials, and the police.
   ☐ 4. Lock down the emergency department and the entire hospital immediately.
   ☐ 5. Identify all client contacts, including transport services to the emergency department and clients in the waiting room.
   ☐ 6. Administer smallpox vaccines to all hospital staff, client contacts, and clients sitting in the emergency department waiting room immediately.

Level of Cognitive Ability: Analyzing
Client Needs: Safe and Effective Care Environment
Clinical Judgment/Cognitive Skills: Generate Solutions
Integrated Process: Nursing Process/Planning
Content Area: Leadership/Management: Mass Casualty Preparedness and Response
Health Problems: Adult Health: Respiratory: Infections of the Upper Airway
Priority Concepts: Infection; Safety

Answer: 1, 2, 3, 5
Rationale: An all-hazards disaster preparedness group is a multifaceted internal and external disaster preparedness group that establishes action plans for every type of disaster or combination of disaster events. In the event of emergency department exposure to a communicable disease such as smallpox, the client would be isolated immediately and the staff would immediately don protective equipment. The emergency department would be locked down immediately. Locking down the entire hospital may not be necessary, and infectious disease specialists and public health officials will determine whether it is necessary to take this action. Infectious disease specialists, public health officials, and the police are notified. All client contacts (name, addresses, telephone numbers), including transport services to the emergency department and clients in the waiting room, would be identified so that the public health department can follow through on notifying and treating these individuals appropriately. Although getting the vaccine within 3 days after exposure will help prevent the disease or make it less severe, it is unreasonable and unnecessary to administer smallpox vaccines to all hospital staff, client contacts, and clients sitting in the emergency department waiting room.
Test-Taking Strategy: Note the strategic word, *initially*. Focus on the subject, a client with smallpox in the emergency department. Next read each option carefully, noting that the client is in the emergency department. Eliminate option 4 because of the words *entire hospital* and option 6 because of the words *all hospital staff*.
Priority Nursing Tip: Smallpox is transmitted in air droplets and by handling contaminated materials and is highly contagious.
Reference: Sweet, V., & Foley, P., eds. (2020). *Sheehy's Emergency nursing: Principles and practice* (7th ed., pp. 175–176). Elsevier; The Federal Emergency Management Agency (http://www.fema.gov).

❖ **92.** A pregnant client tests positive for the hepatitis B virus. The client asks the nurse about being able to breast-feed/chest-feed the baby as planned after delivery. Which therapeutic response would the nurse communicate to the client?
1. "You will not be able to breast-feed/chest-feed the baby until 6 months after delivery."
2. "Breast-feeding/chest-feeding is not advised, and you need to seriously consider bottle-feeding the baby."
3. "Breast-feeding/chest-feeding is not a problem, and you will be able to breast-feed/chest-feed immediately after delivery."
4. "Breast-feeding/chest-feeding is allowed if the baby receives prophylaxis treatment at birth and scheduled immunizations."

Level of Cognitive Ability: Applying
Client Needs: Safe and Effective Care Environment
Clinical Judgment/Cognitive Skills: Take Action
Integrated Process: Teaching and Learning
Content Area: Maternity: Antepartum
Health Problems: Maternity: Infections/Inflammations
Priority Concepts: Patient Education; Infection

Answer: 4
Rationale: The pregnant client who tests positive for hepatitis B virus needs to be reassured that breast-feeding/chest-feeding is not contraindicated if the infant receives prophylaxis at birth and remains on the schedule for immunizations. Therefore, options 1, 2, and 3 are incorrect.
Test-Taking Strategy: Eliminate options 1, 2, and 3 because of the closed-ended word "not" in these options. Also, use therapeutic communication techniques to direct you to option 4.
Priority Nursing Tip: Hepatitis is transmitted through blood, saliva, vaginal secretions, semen, human milk, and across the placental barrier.
Reference: McKinney, E. S., et al. (2022). *Maternal child nursing* (6th ed., pp. 573, 1001). Elsevier.

93. The nurse manager is planning to implement needed changes in the method of the documentation system for the nursing unit. Which would be the **initial** step in the process of change for the nurse manager?
1. Plan strategies to implement the change.
2. Set goals and priorities regarding the change process.
3. Identify the inefficiency that needs improvement or correction.
4. Identify potential solutions and strategies for the change process.

Level of Cognitive Ability: Applying
Client Needs: Safe and Effective Care Environment
Clinical Judgment/Cognitive Skills: Generate Solutions
Integrated Process: Nursing Process/Planning
Content Area: Leadership/Management: Informatics and Health Care Technologies
Health Problems: N/A
Priority Concepts: Leadership; Professional Identity

Answer: 3
Rationale: When beginning the change process, the nurse needs to identify and define the problem that needs improvement or correction. This important first step can prevent many future problems because, if the problem is not correctly identified, a plan for change may be aimed at the wrong problem. This is followed by goal setting, prioritizing, and identifying potential solutions and strategies to implement the change.
Test-Taking Strategy: Note the strategic word, *initial*. Eliminate options 1 and 4 because they are comparable or alike. Next use the steps of the nursing process and knowledge regarding the change process to answer this question. This will direct you to the correct option.
Priority Nursing Tip: When implementing change, evaluate the change process on an ongoing basis, and keep everyone involved in the process informed of the progress.
Reference: Zerwekh, J., & Zerwekh Garneau, A. (2021). *Nursing today: Transition and trends* (10th ed., pp. 241–242, 244). Elsevier.

❖ **94.** A delivery room nurse is preparing a client for a cesarean delivery to facilitate the birth of triplets. Which position will promote maximum uteroplacental perfusion during this surgery?
1. Prone position
2. Semi-Fowler's position
3. Trendelenburg's position
4. Supine position with a wedged right hip

Level of Cognitive Ability: Understanding
Client Needs: Safe and Effective Care Environment
Clinical Judgment/Cognitive Skills: Generate Solutions
Integrated Process: Nursing Process/Planning
Content Area: Maternity: Intrapartum
Health Problems: N/A
Priority Concepts: Reproduction; Safety

Answer: 4
Rationale: Vena cava and descending aorta compression by the pregnant uterus impede blood return from the lower trunk and extremities, thereby decreasing cardiac return, cardiac output, and blood flow to the uterus and subsequently the fetus. The best position to prevent this would be side-lying with the uterus displaced off the abdominal vessels. Positioning for abdominal surgery necessitates a supine position, so a wedge placed under the right hip provides displacement of the uterus off of the vena cava. A semi-Fowler's or prone position is not practical for this type of abdominal surgery. Trendelenburg's positioning places pressure from the pregnant uterus on the diaphragm and lungs, decreasing respiratory capacity and oxygenation.
Test-Taking Strategy: Focus on the subject, positioning for a cesarean delivery. Visualize each of the positions in the options. Recalling the concern in the pregnant client related to vena cava and descending aorta compression will direct you to the correct option.
Priority Nursing Tip: Vena cava syndrome, also known as *supine hypotension*, occurs when the venous return to the heart is impaired by the weight of the pregnant uterus on the vena cava.
Reference: McKinney, E. S., et al. (2022). *Maternal child nursing* (6th ed., p. 395). Elsevier.

95. The nurse in the day care center is told that a child with a diagnosis of autism will be attending the center. The nurse collaborates with the staff of the day care center and plans activities that will meet the child's needs. Which **priority** consideration would the nurse incorporate in planning activities for this child?
1. Safety
2. Verbal stimulation
3. Social interactions
4. Familiarity and orientation

Level of Cognitive Ability: Applying
Client Needs: Safe and Effective Care Environment
Clinical Judgment/Cognitive Skills: Generate Solutions
Integrated Process: Clinical Judgment; Nursing Process/Planning
Content Area: Pediatrics: Neurologic
Health Problems: Pediatric-Specific: Autism Spectrum Disorders
Priority Concepts: Functional Ability; Safety

Answer: 1
Rationale: The child with autism is unable to anticipate danger, has a tendency for self-mutilation, and has sensory perceptual deficits. Safety with activities is a priority in planning activities with the child. Although verbal communications, social interactions, and providing familiarity and orientation are also appropriate interventions, the priority is safety.
Test-Taking Strategy: Note the strategic word, *priority*. Use Maslow's Hierarchy of Needs theory to answer this question. Physiologic needs take priority. When a physiologic need does not exist, safety needs are the priority. None of the options addresses a physiologic need. Option 1 addresses the safety need. Options 2, 3, and 4 address psychosocial needs.
Priority Nursing Tip: For a child with an autism spectrum disorder, the nurse needs to plan care so that disruption in the child's normal routines does not occur. A child with autism spectrum disorder is usually unable to tolerate even the slightest change in routine and may withdraw or become self-abusive or violent if their routine is altered.
Reference: McKinney, E. S., et al. (2022). *Maternal child nursing* (6th ed., pp. 1360–1362). Elsevier.

❖ **96.** The registered nurse (RN) is reviewing a plan of care developed by a new nurse for a child who is being admitted to the pediatric unit with a diagnosis of seizures. The RN determines that the new nurse **needs further teaching** and needs to revise the plan of care if which incorrect intervention is documented?

1. Maintain the bed in a low position.
2. Immobilize the child if a seizure occurs.
3. Place padding on the side rails of the bed.
4. Place the child in a side-lying lateral position postseizure.

Level of Cognitive Ability: Evaluating
Client Needs: Safe and Effective Care Environment
Clinical Judgment/Cognitive Skills: Evaluate Outcomes
Integrated Process: Teaching and Learning
Content Area: Pediatrics: Neurologic
Health Problems: Pediatric-Specific: Seizures
Priority Concepts: Intracranial Regulation; Safety

Answer: 2
Rationale: Restraints (immobilization) are not to be applied to a child with a seizure because they could cause injury to the child. The bed is maintained in low position to provide safety in the event that the child has a seizure. The side rails of the bed are padded to prevent injury. Positioning the child on their side will prevent aspiration as the saliva drains out of the child's mouth during the seizure.
Test-Taking Strategy: Note the strategic words, *needs further teaching,* and the words *revise* and *incorrect* in the question. These indicate a negative event query and the need to select the incorrect intervention. Focus on safety to eliminate the appropriate interventions, and recall that restraints are not to be used.
Priority Nursing Tip: If a child is experiencing a seizure, do not restrain the child, place anything in the child's mouth, or give any foods or liquids to the child.
Reference: McKinney, E. S., et al. (2022). *Maternal child nursing* (6th ed., pp. 1309–1310). Elsevier.

97. The nurse is caring for the body and personal belongings of a client who died as a result of multiple gunshot wounds. Which actions would the nurse take to properly secure and handle legal evidence? **Select all that apply.**

❑ 1. Place paper bags on the hands and feet.
❑ 2. Give the clothing and wallet to the family.
❑ 3. Cut clothing along the seams, avoiding bullet holes.
❑ 4. Collect all personal items, including items from clothing pockets.
❑ 5. Place wet clothing and personal belongings in a labeled, sealed plastic bag.
❑ 6. Do not allow family members, significant others, or friends to be alone with the client.

Level of Cognitive Ability: Applying
Client Needs: Safe and Effective Care Environment
Clinical Judgment/Cognitive Skills: Take Action
Integrated Process: Clinical Judgment; Nursing Process/Implementation
Content Area: Leadership/Management: Ethical/Legal
Health Problems: N/A
Priority Concepts: Evidence; Health Care Law

Answer: 1, 3, 4, 6
Rationale: Basic rules for securing and handling evidence include minimally handling the body of a deceased person; placing paper bags on the hands and feet and possibly over the head of a deceased person (protects trace evidence and residue); placing clothing and personal items in paper bags (plastic bags can destroy items because items can sweat in plastic); cutting clothes along seams, avoiding areas where there are obvious holes or tears; and collecting all personal items, including items from clothing pockets. Evidence is never released to the family to take home, and family members, significant others, or friends are not allowed to be alone with the client because of the possibility of jeopardizing any existing legal evidence.
Test-Taking Strategy: Focus on the subject, proper securing and handling of legal evidence. Read each option carefully and visualize and think about how the action may or may not preserve evidence. This strategy will direct you to the correct actions.
Priority Nursing Tip: Nurses are required to report certain communicable diseases or criminal activities such as child or elder abuse or domestic violence; a dog bite or other animal bite; gunshot or stab wounds, assaults, or homicides; and suicides to the appropriate authorities.
Reference: Sweet, V., & Foley, P., eds. (2020). *Sheehy's Emergency nursing: Principles and practice* (7th ed., pp. 481, 596). Elsevier.

❖ **98.** The nurse prepares for the admission of the child with a diagnosis of tonic-clonic seizures and plans to place which items at the bedside?
1. A tracheotomy set and oxygen
2. Suction apparatus and oxygen
3. An endotracheal tube and an airway
4. An emergency cart and laryngoscope

Level of Cognitive Ability: Applying
Client Needs: Safe and Effective Care Environment
Clinical Judgment/Cognitive Skills: Generate Solutions
Integrated Process: Nursing Process/Planning
Content Area: Pediatrics: Neurologic
Health Problems: Pediatric-Specific: Seizures
Priority Concepts: Intracranial Regulation; Safety

Answer: 2
Rationale: Tonic-clonic seizures cause tightening of all body muscles followed by tremors. Obstructed airway and increased oral secretions are the major complications during and after a seizure. Suction is helpful to prevent choking, and oxygen is helpful to prevent cyanosis. Options 1 and 3 are incorrect because inserting an endotracheal tube or a tracheotomy is not performed. It is not necessary to have an emergency cart (which contains a laryngoscope) at the bedside, but a cart needs to be available in the treatment room or on the nursing unit.
Test-Taking Strategy: Focus on the subject, tonic-clonic seizures. Recalling that tonic-clonic seizures produce excessive oral secretions and airway obstruction will assist in selecting the correct option.
Priority Nursing Tip: If a child is experiencing a seizure, the priority is to ensure a patent airway.
Reference: McKinney, E. S., et al. (2022). *Maternal child nursing* (6th ed., p. 1309). Elsevier.

99. The nurse is admitting a 56-year-old client with a diagnosis of exacerbation of chronic obstructive pulmonary disease (COPD) and learns that the client received immunization for pneumococcal pneumonia 6 years ago. Which consideration is **essential** to include in the plan of care during the client's hospital admission?
1. Offer revaccination to the client.
2. Document the previous immunization on the client record.
3. Instruct the client that this vaccine provides lifelong immunity.
4. Explain to the client that revaccinations can only be given during the fall months.

Level of Cognitive Ability: Applying
Client Needs: Safe and Effective Care Environment
Clinical Judgment/Cognitive Skills: Generate Solutions
Integrated Process: Nursing Process/Planning
Content Area: Adult Health: Respiratory
Health Problems: Adult Health: Respiratory: Chronic Obstructive Pulmonary Disease
Priority Concepts: Clinical Judgment; Health Promotion

Answer: 1
Rationale: During the history-taking of a client diagnosed with a respiratory disorder, the nurse would ask if the client had been previously vaccinated for influenza (flu) and had received pneumococcal pneumonia vaccine. Revaccination with pneumococcal pneumonia vaccine is currently advised in a client with COPD if the client received the vaccine more than 5 years previously and if the client was younger than 65 years of age at the time of vaccination. Although documentation would be completed, this is not the essential action at this time. This vaccine does not provide lifelong immunity in a 56-year-old client who received the vaccine 6 years ago. The pneumococcal pneumonia vaccine is administered any time during the year.
Test-Taking Strategy: Note the strategic word, *essential*, and focus on the subject, pneumococcal pneumonia vaccination. Recognize that this client does not have lifelong immunity and some type of intervention besides documentation is needed. Eliminate options 3 and 4, knowing that pneumococcal pneumonia vaccine can be administered any time of the year and does not provide lifelong immunity to this client.
Priority Nursing Tip: Because the strain of the influenza virus is different every year, annual vaccination is recommended (usually in October or November).
References: Lewis, S., et al. (2020). *Medical-surgical nursing: Assessment and management of clinical problems* (11th ed., p. 507). Elsevier; Lilley, L., Rainforth Collins, S., & Snyder, J. (2020). *Pharmacology and the nursing process* (9th ed., pp. 774, 778). Elsevier.

❖ **100.** The nurse in a well-baby clinic is providing safety instructions to the parent of a 1-month-old infant. Which safety instructions are **most appropriate** to include at this age? **Select all that apply.**
  ❏ **1.** Lock up all poisons.
  ❏ **2.** Cover electrical outlets.
  ❏ **3.** Never shake the infant's head.
  ❏ **4.** Place the infant on the back to sleep.
  ❏ **5.** Remove hazardous objects from low places.

Level of Cognitive Ability: Applying
Client Needs: Safe and Effective Care Environment
Clinical Judgment/Cognitive Skills: Take Action
Integrated Process: Teaching and Learning
Content Area: Developmental Stages: Infant
Health Problems: N/A
Priority Concepts: Health Promotion; Safety

Answer: 3, 4
Rationale: The age-appropriate instructions that are most important are to instruct the parent not to shake or vigorously jiggle the baby's head and to place the infant on their back to sleep. Options 1, 2, and 5 are important instructions to provide to the parents as the child reaches the age of 6 months and begins to explore the environment.
Test-Taking Strategy: Note the strategic words, *most appropriate*. Focus on the subject, safety and the 1-month-old infant. A 1-month-old is not at a developmental level to explore the environment, which will assist in eliminating options 1, 2, and 5.
Priority Nursing Tip: Shaken baby syndrome is caused by the violent shaking of an infant younger than 1 year and results in intracranial (usually subdural hemorrhage) trauma; this can lead to cerebral edema and death.
Reference: McKinney, E. S., et al. (2022). *Maternal child nursing* (6th ed., p. 93). Elsevier.

101. A registered nurse (RN) in charge of the client care unit is preparing the assignments for the day. The RN assigns an unlicensed assistive personnel (UAP) to make beds and bathe one of the clients on the unit and assigns an additional UAP to fill the water pitchers and serve juice to all of the clients. Another RN is assigned to administer all medications. Based on the assignments designed by the RN in charge, which nursing care delivery model is being implemented?
  1. Team
  2. Primary
  3. Functional
  4. Exemplary

Level of Cognitive Ability: Applying
Client Needs: Safe and Effective Care Environment
Clinical Judgment/Cognitive Skills: Take Action
Integrated Process: Nursing Process/Implementation
Content Area: Leadership/Management: Management of Care
Health Problems: N/A
Priority Concepts: Clinical Judgment; Leadership

Answer: 3
Rationale: The functional model of care involves an assembly line approach to client care, with major tasks being delegated by the charge nurse to individual staff members. Team nursing is characterized by a high degree of communication and collaboration among members. The team is generally led by an RN, who is responsible for assessing, developing nursing diagnoses, planning, and evaluating each client's plan of care. In primary nursing, concern is with keeping the nurse at the bedside actively involved in care, providing goal-directed and individualized client care. In an exemplary model of team nursing, each staff member works fully within the realm of educational and clinical experience in an effort to provide comprehensive individualized client care. Each staff member is accountable for client care and outcomes of care.
Test-Taking Strategy: Focus on the subject, nursing care delivery systems. Noting that each staff member is assigned a specific task will direct you to option 3.
Priority Nursing Tip: The functional model of nursing care delivery focuses on the delegated task rather than the total client. This can result in fragmentation of care and lack of accountability by the health care member.
Reference: Zerwekh, J., & Zerwekh Garneau, A. (2021). *Nursing today: Transition and trends* (10th ed., pp. 359–360.). Elsevier.

❖ **102.** A client who is immunosuppressed is being admitted to the hospital on neutropenic precautions. Which nursing interventions would be implemented to protect the client from infection? **Select all that apply.**

❑ 1. Restrict all visitors.
❑ 2. Admit the client to a private room.
❑ 3. Place a mask on the client if the client leaves the room.
❑ 4. Use strict aseptic technique for all invasive procedures.
❑ 5. Place a "See the Nurse Before Entering" sign on the door to the room.
❑ 6. Remove a vase with fresh flowers in the room that was left by a previous client.

Level of Cognitive Ability: Applying
Client Needs: Safe and Effective Care Environment
Clinical Judgment/Cognitive Skills: Take Action
Integrated Process: Nursing Process/Implementation
Content Area: Foundations of Care: Infection Control
Health Problems: Adult Health: Immune: Immunodeficiency Syndrome
Priority Concepts: Infection; Safety

Answer: 2, 3, 4, 5, 6
Rationale: The client needs to wear a mask for protection from exposure to microorganisms whenever leaving the room. The client who is on neutropenic precautions is immunosuppressed and, therefore, is admitted to a private room on the nursing unit. The use of strict aseptic technique is necessary with all invasive procedures to prevent infection. A sign indicating "See the Nurse Before Entering" needs to be placed on the door to the client's room so that the nurse can ensure that neutropenic precautions are implemented by anyone entering the room. Sources of standing water and fresh flowers need to be removed to decrease the microorganism count. Not all visitors must be restricted; however, visitors need to be restricted to healthy adults and must perform strict hand washing procedures and don a mask before entering the client's room.
Test-Taking Strategy: Focus on the subject, an immunosuppressed client and neutropenic precautions. Read each option carefully and recall that the client is at risk for contracting infection. Select the options that protect the client from infection.
Priority Nursing Tip: Neutropenia can be caused by chemotherapy and places the cancer client at risk for a life-threatening infection. White blood cell counts and differentials are monitored closely, and the client is placed on neutropenic precautions if the counts decrease.
Reference: Ignatavicius, D., et al. (2021). *Medical-surgical nursing: Concepts for interprofessional collaborative care* (10th ed., p. 388). Elsevier.

103. A home care nurse is providing instructions to the parent of a toddler regarding safety measures in the home to prevent an accidental burn injury. Which statement by the parent indicates a **need for further instruction?**

1. "I need to use the back burners for cooking."
2. "I need to remain in the kitchen when I prepare meals."
3. "I need to be sure to place my cup of coffee on the counter."
4. "I need to turn pot handles inward and to the middle of the stove."

Level of Cognitive Ability: Evaluating
Client Needs: Safe and Effective Care Environment
Clinical Judgment/Cognitive Skills: Evaluate Outcomes
Integrated Process: Teaching and Learning
Content Area: Foundations of Care: Safety
Health Problems: Pediatric-Specific: Burns
Priority Concepts: Patient Education; Safety

Answer: 3
Rationale: Toddlers, with their increased mobility and developing motor skills, can reach hot water or hot objects placed on counters and open fires or burners on stoves above their eye level. The parent's statement in option 3 does not indicate an adequate understanding of the principles of safety. Hot liquids would never be left unattended, and the toddler would always be supervised. Parents need to be encouraged to use the back burners on the stove, remain in the kitchen when preparing a meal, and turn pot handles inward and toward the middle of the stove.
Test-Taking Strategy: Note the strategic words, *need for further instruction.* These words indicate a negative event query and the need to select the option that identifies an incorrect statement by the parent. Options 1, 2, and 4 can be eliminated because they identify basic safety principles. Also recalling that the toddler is in the stage of developing motor skills will assist in directing you to option 3.
Priority Nursing Tip: Toddlers are eager to explore the environment around them, and they need to be supervised at all times to ensure safety.
Reference: McKinney, E. S., et al. (2022). *Maternal child nursing* (6th ed., p. 123). Elsevier.

104. The nurse prepares a client with the diagnosis of right pleural effusion for a thoracentesis; however, the client experiences severe dizziness when sitting upright. Into which alternate position would the nurse assist the client to maintain safety during the procedure?
1. Right side-lying with the head of the bed flat
2. Prone with the head turned toward the affected side
3. Left side-lying with the head of the bed elevated 45 degrees
4. Modified left lateral position with the head of the bed elevated 45 degrees

Level of Cognitive Ability: Applying
Client Needs: Safe and Effective Care Environment
Clinical Judgment/Cognitive Skills: Take Action
Integrated Process: Nursing Process/Implementation
Content Area: Foundations of Care: Diagnostic Tests
Health Problems: Adult Health: Respiratory: Pleural Effusion
Priority Concepts: Gas Exchange; Safety

Answer: 3
Rationale: A thoracentesis is a procedure in which fluid or air is removed from the pleural space via a transthoracic aspiration. Positioning can help isolate the fluid in a pleural effusion; generally, the client sits at the edge of the bed, leaning over the bedside table, allowing the fluid to collect in a dependent body area. If the client is unable to sit up, the nurse turns the client to the unaffected side and elevates the head of the bed 30 to 45 degrees. Turning to the affected side, the prone, and the modified left lateral positions are unsuitable positions for this procedure because these do not facilitate fluid removal.
Test-Taking Strategy: Focus on the subject, alternate position for thoracentesis procedure. Eliminate option 1 because lying on the affected side makes it difficult to perform the procedure. Eliminate option 2 because prone positioning does not facilitate fluid removal, and eliminate option 4 because the modified left lateral position is used for rectal enemas or irrigations primarily.
Priority Nursing Tip: After a thoracentesis, monitor the client for signs of pneumothorax, air embolism, and pulmonary edema.
Reference: Ignatavicius, D., et al. (2021). *Medical-surgical nursing: Concepts for interprofessional collaborative care* (10th ed., pp. 492–493). Elsevier; Pagana, K., Pagana, T., & Pagana, T. N. (2021). *Mosby's Diagnostic and laboratory test reference* (15th ed., p. 858). Elsevier.

105. A physician has written a prescription to administer methylergonovine maleate to a postpartum client. The nurse would contact the physician to verify the prescription if which condition is present in the client?
1. Hypertension
2. Excessive lochia
3. Difficulty locating the uterine fundus
4. Excessive bleeding and saturation of more than one peri-pad per hour

Level of Cognitive Ability: Analyzing
Client Needs: Safe and Effective Care Environment
Clinical Judgment/Cognitive Skills: Analyze Cues
Integrated Process: Clinical Judgment; Nursing Process/Analysis
Content Area: Pharmacology: Maternity/Newborn: Ergot Alkaloids
Health Problems: Maternity: Postpartum Uterine Problems
Priority Concepts: Clinical Judgment; Safety

Answer: 1
Rationale: Methylergonovine maleate is an ergot alkaloid used to treat uterine atony. It is contraindicated for the hypertensive individual, individuals with severe hepatic or renal disease, and during the third stage of labor. Excessive lochia, a uterine fundus that is difficult to locate, and excessive bleeding are clinical manifestations of uterine atony indicating the need for methylergonovine.
Test-Taking Strategy: Eliminate options 2, 3, and 4 because they are comparable or alike in that they are clinical manifestations of uterine atony.
Priority Nursing Tip: Methylergonovine maleate is an ergot alkaloid that produces vasoconstriction. The client's blood pressure needs to be monitored closely, and if an increase is noted, the medication is withheld and the primary health care provider is notified.
Reference: McKinney, E. S., et al. (2022). *Maternal child nursing* (6th ed., p. 605). Elsevier.

❖ **106.** After receiving detailed information about a colonoscopy from the physician, the nurse asks the client to sign the informed consent form and discovers that the client cannot write. Which is the **best** intervention for the nurse to implement?
1. Contact the physician to obtain informed consent.
2. Obtain a verbal informed consent from the client.
3. Have two nurses witness the client sign with an X.
4. Clarify information to the client with another nurse.

Level of Cognitive Ability: Applying
Client Needs: Safe and Effective Care Environment
Clinical Judgment/Cognitive Skills: Take Action
Integrated Process: Nursing Process/Implementation
Content Area: Leadership/Management: Ethical/Legal
Health Problems: N/A
Priority Concepts: Ethics; Health Care Law

Answer: 3
Rationale: Nurses are responsible to ensure that the signed informed consent form is in the client's medical record before a procedure and for clarifying facts that have already been presented by the physician. Nonetheless, the person performing the procedure obtains informed consent and provides the explanations to the client. Informed consent can be obtained verbally, but that is also the responsibility of the physician. Clients who cannot write may sign an informed consent with an X in the presence of two witnesses. Nurses can serve as a witness to the client's signature but not to the fact that the client is informed.
Test-Taking Strategy: Note the strategic word, *best.* Focus on the subject, inability to sign an informed consent form. Eliminate options 1, 2, and 4 because they are unnecessary, and the physician has already provided detailed information to the client.
Priority Nursing Tip: A client who has been medicated with sedating medications or any other medications that can affect the client's cognitive abilities would not be asked to sign an informed consent.
Reference: Ignatavicius, D., et al. (2021). *Medical-surgical nursing: Concepts for interprofessional collaborative care* (10th ed., pp. 161–162). Elsevier.

107. A child diagnosed with a malignant brain tumor is admitted for removal of the tumor. The nurse would include which action in the plan of care to ensure a safe environment for the child?
1. Initiating seizure precautions
2. Using a wheelchair for out-of-bed activities
3. Assisting the child with ambulation at all times
4. Minimizing contact with other children on the nursing unit

Level of Cognitive Ability: Applying
Client Needs: Safe and Effective Care Environment
Clinical Judgment/Cognitive Skills: Generate Solutions
Integrated Process: Nursing Process/Planning
Content Area: Pediatrics: Neurologic
Health Problems: Pediatric-Specific: Cancers
Priority Concepts: Intracranial Regulation; Safety

Answer: 1
Rationale: Seizure precautions need to be implemented for any child with a brain tumor, both preoperatively and postoperatively. Options 2 and 3 are not required unless functional deficits exist. Based on the child's diagnosis, option 4 is not necessary.
Test-Taking Strategy: Focus on the subject, safe environment for a child with a brain tumor. Eliminate options 2 and 3 first because they are comparable or alike. Additionally, note the closed-ended word "all" in option 3. From the remaining options, eliminate option 4 because there is no reason for the child to avoid contact with other children.
Priority Nursing Tip: Monitor the child with a brain tumor or a child who has had a craniotomy for signs of increased intracranial pressure (ICP). If signs of increased ICP occur, notify the physician immediately.
Reference: McKinney, E. S., et al. (2022). *Maternal child nursing* (6th ed., p. 1166). Elsevier.

❖ **108.** The nurse caring for a chronically ill client with a poor prognosis shows an understanding of the basic values that guide the implementation of a living will by asking which questions? **Select all that apply.**

❑ 1. "Are you planning to become an organ donor?"

❑ 2. "Do you feel the need to discuss your end-of-life decisions with your family?"

❑ 3. "Did you have the discussion with your children about being your health care surrogate?"

❑ 4. "Can we discuss what will happen if you decide to refuse antibiotics if you get an infection?"

❑ 5. "Have you given thought to whether you want cardiopulmonary resuscitation (CPR) measures if your condition worsens?"

Level of Cognitive Ability: Understanding
Client Needs: Safe and Effective Care Environment
Clinical Judgment/Cognitive Skills: Recognize Cues
Integrated Process: Nursing Process/Assessment
Content Area: Leadership/Management: Ethical/Legal
Health Problems: N/A
Priority Concepts: Health Care Law; Palliative Care

Answer: 2, 4, 5
Rationale: A living will lists the treatment that a client chooses to omit or refuse if the client becomes unable to make decisions and is terminally ill. The client may want to discuss their decisions with the family. Although both the living will and durable powers of attorney for health care are based on values of informed consent, autonomy over end-of-life decisions, and control over the dying process, living wills do not involve health care surrogates or the decision to donate organs.
Test-Taking Strategy: Focus on the subject, living will. Understanding the purpose and components of a living will direct you to the correct options 2, 4, and 5. Remember that living wills do not involve health care surrogates or the decision to donate organs.
Priority Nursing Tip: A living will is based on the client's decisions regarding end-of-life wishes related to health care.
Reference: Potter, P., et al. (2021). *Fundamentals of nursing* (10th ed., pp. 310–311). Elsevier.

109. The nurse is reviewing the results of the rubella screening (titer) with a pregnant client. The test results are positive, and the client asks if it is safe for the toddler to receive the vaccine. Which response by the nurse is **most appropriate?**

1. "Most children do not receive the vaccine until they are 5 years of age."

2. "You are still susceptible to rubella, so your toddler should receive the vaccine."

3. "It is not advised for children of pregnant persons to be vaccinated during their parent's pregnancy."

4. "Your titer supports your immunity to rubella, and it is safe for your toddler to receive the vaccine."

Level of Cognitive Ability: Applying
Client Needs: Safe and Effective Care Environment
Clinical Judgment/Cognitive Skills: Take Action
Integrated Process: Nursing Process/Implementation
Content Area: Maternity: Antepartum
Health Problems: Maternity: Infections/Inflammations
Priority Concepts: Immunity; Safety

Answer: 4
Rationale: All pregnant individuals need to be screened for prior rubella exposure. A positive titer indicates that a significant antibody titer has developed in response to a prior exposure to the *Rubivirus*. All children of pregnant persons need to receive their immunizations according to schedule. Additionally, no definitive evidence suggests that the rubella vaccine virus is transmitted from person to person.
Test-Taking Strategy: Note the strategic words, *most appropriate*. Focus on the subject, administration of rubella vaccine to a toddler whose parent is pregnant. Recalling that a positive titer indicates immunity will direct you to option 4.
Priority Nursing Tip: Rubella vaccine is not administered to a pregnant individual because the live attenuated virus may cross the placenta and present a risk to the developing fetus.
Reference: McKinney, E. S., et al. (2022). *Maternal child nursing* (6th ed., pp. 405, 571–572). Elsevier.

110. After delivery, the postpartum nurse instructs the client with known cardiac disease to call for the nurse when needing to get out of bed or when planning to care for the newborn infant. Which rationale is the basis for these instructions?

1. Help the birthing parent assume the parenting role.
2. Minimize the potential of postpartum hemorrhage.
3. Provide an opportunity for the nurse to teach newborn infant care techniques.
4. Avoid birthing parent or infant injury caused by the potential for syncope or overexertion.

Level of Cognitive Ability: Applying
Client Needs: Safe and Effective Care Environment
Clinical Judgment/Cognitive Skills: Generate Solutions
Integrated Process: Teaching and Learning
Content Area: Maternity: Postpartum
Health Problems: Maternity: Cardiac Disease
Priority Concepts: Patient Education; Safety

Answer: 4
Rationale: The immediate postpartum period is associated with increased risks for the cardiac client. Hormonal changes and fluid shifts from extravascular tissues to the circulatory system cause additional stress on cardiac functioning. Although options 1, 2, and 3 are appropriate nursing concerns during the postpartum period, the primary concern for the cardiac client is to maintain a safe environment because of the potential for cardiac compromise.
Test-Taking Strategy: Focus on the subject, safety for the postpartum client with cardiac disease. Option 4 is the only option that relates directly to the subject of safety.
Priority Nursing Tip: Monitor the postpartum client with cardiac disease closely for signs and symptoms of cardiac stress and decompensation. These include cough, fatigue, dyspnea, chest pain, and tachycardia.
Reference: McKinney, E. S., et al. (2022). *Maternal child nursing* (6th ed., pp. 566–567). Elsevier.

111. The nurse is assessing a client with a lower leg cast who has just been measured and fitted for crutches. Which observation would help the nurse determine if the client's crutches are fitted correctly?

1. The top of the crutch is even with the axilla.
2. The elbow is straight when the hand is on the handgrip.
3. The client's axilla is resting on the crutch pad during ambulation.
4. The elbow is at a 30-degree angle when the hand is on the handgrip.

Level of Cognitive Ability: Evaluating
Client Needs: Safe and Effective Care Environment
Clinical Judgment/Cognitive Skills: Evaluate Outcomes
Integrated Process: Nursing Process/Evaluation
Content Area: Skills: Activity/Mobility
Health Problems: Adult Health: Musculoskeletal: Skeletal Injury
Priority Concepts: Mobility; Safety

Answer: 4
Rationale: When using crutches, for optimal upper extremity leverage, the elbow needs to be at approximately 30 degrees of flexion when the hand is resting on the handgrip. The top of the crutch needs to be two to three fingerbreadths lower than the axilla. When crutch walking, all weight needs to be on the hands to prevent nerve palsy from pressure on the axilla. Therefore, options 1, 2, and 3 are incorrect.
Test-Taking Strategy: Options 1 and 3 are comparable or alike and can be eliminated first. Visualize the mechanics of crutch walking to assist in selecting from the remaining options. If the weight needs to be resting on the hands, then there needs to be some flexion to push off from during ambulation.
Priority Nursing Tip: An accurate measurement of the client for crutches is important because an incorrect measurement could damage the brachial plexus.
Reference: Potter, P., et al. (2021). *Fundamentals of nursing* (10th ed., pp. 797–798). Elsevier.

112. When assessing the client with a wrist restraint at the beginning of the day shift, which observation by the charge nurse would indicate that the nurse who placed the restraint on the client failed to follow safety guidelines?
1. The client was toileted frequently.
2. The wrist restraint was applied snugly.
3. The call bell was placed within easy reach.
4. A slip knot was used to secure the restraint.

Level of Cognitive Ability: Evaluating
Client Needs: Safe and Effective Care Environment
Clinical Judgment/Cognitive Skills: Evaluate Outcomes
Integrated Process: Nursing Process/Evaluation
Content Area: Foundations of Care: Safety
Health Problems: N/A
Priority Concepts: Clinical Judgment; Safety

Answer: 2
Rationale: A restraint is never applied snugly because it could impair circulation. A slip knot may be used on the client because it can easily be released in an emergency. The call bell must always be within the client's reach. The client must be toileted frequently to provide comfort.
Test-Taking Strategy: Focus on the subject, safety with the use of restraints. The words *failed to follow safety guidelines* indicate the need to select the unsafe action performed by the nurse. Noting the word *snugly* in option 2 will direct you to this option.
Priority Nursing Tip: A physician's prescription for the use of a restraint (security device) is needed.
Reference: Potter, P., et al. (2021). *Fundamentals of nursing* (10th ed., p. 417). Elsevier.

113. The nurse documents a written entry regarding client care in the client's medical record. When checking the entry, the nurse notices that some of the documented information was incorrect. Which action would the nurse implement at this time?
1. Obliterate the incorrect information with a black marker.
2. Use correction fluid to cover up the incorrect information.
3. Erase the error completely and write in the correct information.
4. Draw a line through the incorrect information and initial the change.

Level of Cognitive Ability: Applying
Client Needs: Safe and Effective Care Environment
Clinical Judgment/Cognitive Skills: Take Action
Integrated Process: Communication and Documentation
Content Area: Leadership/Management: Informatics and Health Care Technologies
Health Problems: N/A
Priority Concepts: Communication; Health Care Law

Answer: 4
Rationale: To correct a written error documented in a medical record, the nurse draws one line through the incorrect information and then initials the error. The information remains visible and properly labeled as incorrect. Errors are never erased, and correction fluid or markers that cover the information are never used on a legal document such as the medical record.
Test-Taking Strategy: Focus on the subject, correcting a written error documented in a medical record. Note that options 1, 2, and 3 are comparable or alike in that they indicate completely covering up or eliminating the incorrect information.
Priority Nursing Tip: Documentation in a client's medical record is legally required by accrediting agencies, state licensing laws, and state nurse and medical practice acts.
Reference: Potter, P., et al. (2021). *Fundamentals of nursing* (10th ed., p. 367). Elsevier.

114. A client receiving chemotherapy to treat lung cancer has an extremely low white blood cell count and is immediately placed on neutropenic precautions that include a low-bacteria diet. Which food items is the client now allowed to consume? **Select all that apply.**

- ❏ 1. Raw celery
- ❏ 2. Fresh apple
- ❏ 3. Italian bread
- ❏ 4. Tossed salad
- ❏ 5. Baked chicken
- ❏ 6. Well-cooked cheeseburger

Level of Cognitive Ability: Applying
Client Needs: Safe and Effective Care Environment
Clinical Judgment/Cognitive Skills: Generate Solutions
Integrated Process: Nursing Process/Planning
Content Area: Foundations of Care: Infection Control
Health Problems: Adult Health: Cancer: Laryngeal and Lung
Priority Concepts: Infection; Safety

Answer: 3, 5, 6
Rationale: An extremely low white blood cell count places the client at risk for infection. In the immunocompromised client, a low-bacteria diet is implemented. Italian bread, baked chicken, and a well-done cheeseburger are acceptable to consume because all products are thoroughly cooked. The client avoids eating fresh fruits and vegetables. Fresh fruits and vegetables harbor organisms and place the client at risk for infection.
Test-Taking Strategy: Focus on the subject, a low-bacteria diet. Read each option carefully and think about the food items that harbor bacteria. Recalling that fresh fruits and vegetables are restricted from a low-bacteria diet will assist in selecting the correct items.
Priority Nursing Tip: Most antineoplastic medications cause neutropenia and thrombocytopenia. Monitor the white blood cell count and the platelet count closely for indications of these adverse effects.
References: Ignatavicius, D., et al. (2021). *Medical-surgical nursing: Concepts for interprofessional collaborative care* (10th ed., p. 388). Elsevier; Nix, S. (2022). *Williams' Basic nutrition and diet therapy* (16th ed., p. 440). Elsevier.

115. When teaching a competent postoperative client about a patient-controlled analgesia (PCA) pump, the nurse would include which instructions to the client? **Select all that apply.**

- ❏ 1. Report the inability to void.
- ❏ 2. Report any nausea and vomiting.
- ❏ 3. Push the button before the pain becomes too great.
- ❏ 4. Inform the nurse about the pain levels being experienced.
- ❏ 5. Ask the family to assume management when the client is sleeping.

Level of Cognitive Ability: Applying
Client Needs: Safe and Effective Care Environment
Clinical Judgment/Cognitive Skills: Take Action
Integrated Process: Teaching and Learning
Content Area: Pharmacology: Pain Medications: Opioid Analgesics
Health Problems: Adult Health: Neurologic: Pain
Priority Concepts: Patient Education; Pain

Answer: 1, 2, 3, 4
Rationale: PCA pumps have opioid medications infusing. Opioids can have an effect on the parasympathetic nervous system causing nausea, vomiting, and an inability to void and defecate; these occurrences need to be reported. The nurse must be kept informed about the pain relief achieved by the client and if there is any breakthrough pain. The client needs to be instructed to push the button before the pain becomes too great. Because the client is competent and there is a basal dose being administered, there is no need for the family to push the buttons for pain relief. In addition, no one other than the client should touch the pump unless instructed to do so.
Test-Taking Strategy: Focus on the subject, teaching regarding a PCA pump. A PCA pump is designed for clients to administer their own dose of pain medication within the parameters set by the physician. Use these guidelines to assist in answering. Also, note that the incorrect option addresses the family, not the client.
Priority Nursing Tip: Patient-controlled analgesia pumps are very effective in controlling client pain. A basal dose is given continuously so that if a client falls asleep or naps, they do not wake in excruciating pain. When a PCA pump administers a basal rate, it is imperative that the nurse monitors the client's vital signs, especially respiratory rate. The demand rate is just that; it is the dose the client receives when pressing the button on the PCA pump. Both the basal and demand rates are set by the physician to prevent overdose.
Reference: Potter, P., et al. (2021). *Fundamentals of nursing* (10th ed., pp. 1086–1087). Elsevier.

116. The nurse observes that a postoperative client has episodes of extreme agitation. Which is the **best** nursing measure to implement to prevent escalating the agitation?
1. Gently hold the client's hand while speaking.
2. Wait to approach until the client's agitation has subsided.
3. Speak in a calm tone while moving slowly toward the client.
4. Communicate with the client from the entrance to the room.

Level of Cognitive Ability: Applying
Client Needs: Safe and Effective Care Environment
Clinical Judgment/Cognitive Skills: Generate Solutions
Integrated Process: Nursing Process/Planning
Content Area: Foundations of Care: Communication
Health Problems: Mental Health: Violence
Priority Concepts: Mood and Affect; Safety

Answer: 3
Rationale: Speaking and moving slowly toward the client will prevent the client from becoming further agitated because any sudden moves or speaking too quickly may cause the client to have a violent episode. Holding the client's hand can be misinterpreted by a client to mean restraint. If the client's agitation is not addressed, it is likely to increase; therefore, waiting for the agitation to subside is not a suitable option. Remaining at the entrance of the room can make the client feel alienated.
Test-Taking Strategy: Note the strategic word, *best*. Focus on the subject, agitated client. Remember that one of the most basic principles in preventing episodes of agitation or violent episodes is to avoid further agitation. Remember to be empathetic to the client while avoiding actions that potentially startle the client. These principles will direct you to the correct option.
Priority Nursing Tip: Client safety is always the priority. Protect the client and remove any objects in the environment that could be potentially harmful to the client.
Reference: Varcarolis, E., & Fosbre, C. (2021). *Essentials of psychiatric mental health nursing: A communication approach to evidence-based care* (4th ed., pp. 381–382). Elsevier.

117. A 17-year-old client is discharged to home with the client's newborn baby after the nurse provides information about home safety for children. Which statement by the client would alert the nurse that **further teaching is required** regarding home safety?
1. "I can keep my aluminum pots and pans in my lower cabinets."
2. "I will not use the microwave oven to heat my baby's formula."
3. "I have locks on all my cabinets that contain my cleaning supplies."
4. "I have a car seat that I will put in the front seat to keep my baby safe."

Level of Cognitive Ability: Evaluating
Client Needs: Safe and Effective Care Environment
Clinical Judgment/Cognitive Skills: Evaluate Outcomes
Integrated Process: Teaching and Learning
Content Area: Maternity: Postpartum
Health Problems: N/A
Priority Concepts: Patient Education; Safety

Answer: 4
Rationale: A baby car seat is never placed in the front seat because of the potential for life-threatening injury on impact. It is perfectly safe to leave pots and pans in the lower cabinets for a child to investigate, as long as they are not made of glass, which would harm the baby if broken. Microwave ovens are not used to heat formula because the formula heats unevenly, and it could burn and even scald the baby's mouth. Even though the bottle may feel warm, it could contain hot spots that could severely damage the baby's mouth. Any cabinets that contain dangerous items that a baby or child could swallow need to be locked.
Test-Taking Strategy: Note the strategic words, *further teaching is required*. These words indicate a negative event query and the need to select the incorrect client statement. Remember that a baby car seat is never placed in the front seat because of the potential for injury on impact.
Priority Nursing Tip: Teach parents that when traveling with a child, always lock the car doors. Four-door cars need to be equipped with child safety locks on the back doors.
References: McKinney, E. S., et al. (2022). *Maternal child nursing* (6th ed., pp. 122, 483). Elsevier; American Academy of Pediatrics (2023). Car seats: Information for families. https://www.healthychildren.org/English/safety-prevention/on-thego/Pages/Car-Safety-Seats-Information-for-Families.aspx.

118. The nurse, after administering an injection to a client, accidentally drops the syringe on the floor. Which nursing action is **most appropriate** in this situation?
1. Obtain a dustpan and mop to sweep up the syringe.
2. Call the housekeeping department to pick up the syringe.
3. Carefully pick up the syringe from the floor and gently recap the needle.
4. Carefully pick up the syringe from the floor and dispose of it in a sharps container.

Level of Cognitive Ability: Applying
Client Needs: Safe and Effective Care Environment
Clinical Judgment/Cognitive Skills: Take Action
Integrated Process: Nursing Process/Implementation
Content Area: Foundations of Care: Safety
Health Problems: N/A
Priority Concepts: Clinical Judgment; Safety

Answer: 4
Rationale: Used syringes need to always be placed in a sharps container immediately after use to prevent injury. A syringe is not swept up because this action poses an additional risk for getting pricked. It is not the responsibility of the housekeeping department to pick up the syringe. Syringes are never to be recapped under any circumstances because of the risk of getting pricked with a contaminated needle.
Test-Taking Strategy: Note the strategic words, *most appropriate*. Focus on the subject, procedure for disposal of a used needle. Recall basic principles related to the safe disposal of syringes to answer the question. Remember that recapping a needle places the nurse at risk for injury and that the needle is always disposed of in a sharps container.
Priority Nursing Tip: Sharps, such as needles, are disposed of immediately after use in closed, puncture-resistant disposal containers that are leak proof and labeled or color coded.
Reference: Potter, P., et al. (2021). *Fundamentals of nursing* (10th ed., pp. 636–637). Elsevier.

119. The nurse is assigned to care for a client who is in traction. Which intervention by the nurse would ensure a safe environment for the client?
1. Making sure that the knots are at the pulley sites
2. Checking the weights to be sure that they are off the floor
3. Making sure that the head of the bed is kept at a 90-degree angle
4. Monitoring the weights to be sure that they are resting on a firm surface

Level of Cognitive Ability: Applying
Client Needs: Safe and Effective Care Environment
Clinical Judgment/Cognitive Skills: Take Action
Integrated Process: Nursing Process/Implementation
Content Area: Adult Health: Musculoskeletal
Health Problems: Adult Health: Musculoskeletal: Skeletal Injury
Priority Concepts: Mobility; Safety

Answer: 2
Rationale: To achieve proper traction, weights need to be free-hanging, with knots kept away from the pulleys. The head of the bed is usually kept low to provide countertraction. Weights are not to be kept resting on a firm surface.
Test-Taking Strategy: Focus on the subject, traction. Visualize the traction, recalling that there must be weight to exert the pull from the traction setup. This concept will assist in eliminating options 1 and 4. Recalling that countertraction is needed will assist in eliminating option 3.
Priority Nursing Tip: For a client in traction, the nurse needs to frequently monitor color, motion, and sensation of the affected extremity.
Reference: Ignatavicius, D., et al. (2021). *Medical-surgical nursing: Concepts for interprofessional collaborative care* (10th ed., p. 1037). Elsevier.

120. The nurse is observing a client using a walker after experiencing a stroke. Which observation by the nurse would determine that the client is using the walker correctly?
  1. Puts weight on the hand pieces, slides the walker forward, and then walks into it
  2. Puts weight on the hand pieces, moves the walker forward, and then walks into it
  3. Puts all four points of the walker flat on the floor, puts weight on the hand pieces, and then walks into it
  4. Walks into the walker, puts weight on the hand pieces, and then puts all four points of the walker flat on the floor

Level of Cognitive Ability: Evaluating
Client Needs: Safe and Effective Care Environment
Clinical Judgment/Cognitive Skills: Evaluate Outcomes
Integrated Process: Nursing Process/Evaluation
Content Area: Skills: Activity/Mobility
Health Problems: Adult Health: Neurologic: Stroke
Priority Concepts: Mobility; Safety

Answer: **3**
Rationale: When the client uses a walker, the nurse stands adjacent to the affected side. The client is instructed to put all four points of the walker 2 feet forward flat on the floor before putting weight on the hand pieces. This will ensure client safety and prevent stress cracks in the walker. The client is then instructed to move the walker forward and walk into it. Therefore, options 1, 2, and 4 are incorrect procedures for using a walker.
Test-Taking Strategy: Focus on the subject, correct use of a walker. Visualize each of the options. Options 1 and 2 can be eliminated because putting weight on the hand pieces initially would cause an unsafe situation. From the remaining options, recalling that the walker is placed on all four points first will direct you to option 3.
Priority Nursing Tip: Safety is a priority concern when the client uses an assistive device for ambulating. Be certain that the client can demonstrate correct use of the device.
Reference: Potter, P., et al. (2021). *Fundamentals of nursing* (10th ed., p. 797). Elsevier.

121. A client is admitted to the labor and delivery unit for a labor induction to help manage gestational hypertension. The physician has prescribed oxytocin to be initiated by piggyback at an initial rate of 2 milliunits/min and increased by a rate of 2 milliunits/min every 30 minutes until contractions are 2 to 3 minutes apart, lasting 80 to 90 seconds. How many mL/hr will the nurse initially set the infusion pump if the dilution of the oxytocin is 10 units of oxytocin in 1000 mL of 0.225% normal saline? **Fill in the blank.**
Answer: _____ mL/hr
Level of Cognitive Ability: Applying
Client Needs: Safe and Effective Care Environment
Clinical Judgment/Cognitive Skills: Generate Solutions
Integrated Process: Nursing Process/Planning
Content Area: Pharmacology: Maternity/Newborn: Uterine Stimulants
Health Problems: Maternity: Gestational Hypertension/Preeclampsia and Eclampsia
Priority Concepts: Clinical Judgment; Safety

Answer: **12**
Rationale: Use the medication calculation formula to calculate the correct dose.

Formula:
10 units of oxytocin in 1000 mL of 0.225% normal saline
= 10,000 milliunits per 1000 mL or 10 milliunits per 1 mL.
Solve by the ratio proportion method.

$$10 \text{ milliunits} : 1 \text{ mL} :: 2 \text{ milliunits} : x \text{ mL/min} =$$
$$10x = 2$$
$$x = 2 \text{ divided by } 10$$
$$x = 0.2 \text{ mL/min}$$

Multiply by 60 minutes to get the amount infused per hour:

$$0.2 \times 60 = 12 \text{ mL/hr}$$

Test-Taking Strategy: Focus on the subject, a medication calculation. Use ratio and proportion method to perform the calculation. Follow the formula for the calculation of the correct dose. Once you have performed the calculation, verify your answer using a calculator and make sure that the answer is reasonable.
Priority Nursing Tip: Oxytocin stimulates the smooth muscle of the uterus and increases the force, frequency, and duration of uterine contractions.
Reference: Potter, P., et al. (2021). *Fundamentals of nursing* (10th ed., pp. 638–639). Elsevier.

122. The nurse is caring for an adolescent client with a diagnosis of conjunctivitis. Which instruction is **most appropriate** for the nurse to relate to the adolescent?
  1. Avoid using all eye makeup to prevent possible reinfection.
  2. Apply hot compresses to decrease pain and lessen irritation.
  3. Obtain a new set of contact lenses for use after the infection clears.
  4. Isolate for 3 days after beginning antibiotic eye drops to avoid the spread of infection.

Level of Cognitive Ability: Applying
Client Needs: Safe and Effective Care Environment
Clinical Judgment/Cognitive Skills: Take Action
Integrated Process: Teaching and Learning
Content Area: Pediatrics: Eye/Ear
Health Problems: Pediatric-Specific: Conjunctivitis
Priority Concepts: Patient Education; Infection

Answer: 3
Rationale: Conjunctivitis is inflammation of the conjunctiva. A new set of contact lenses needs to be obtained. If the client has conjunctivitis, eye makeup needs to be replaced but can still be worn. Cool compresses decrease pain and irritation. Isolation for 24 hours after antibiotics are initiated is necessary.
Test-Taking Strategy: Focus on the strategic words, *most appropriate.* Eliminate option 1 because of the closed-ended word "all." Recalling the principles related to the effectiveness of antibiotics will assist in eliminating option 4. From the remaining options, noting the word *hot* in option 2 will assist in eliminating this option.
Priority Nursing Tip: Chlamydial conjunctivitis is rare in older children. If diagnosed in a child who is not sexually active, the child needs to be assessed for possible sexual abuse.
Reference: McKinney, E. S., et al. (2022). *Maternal child nursing* (6th ed., pp. 1372–1373). Elsevier.

123. A client who has experienced a stroke has partial hemiplegia of the left leg. The straight-leg cane formerly used by the client is not sufficient to provide support. The nurse determines that the client could benefit from the greater support, stability, and safety provided by which devices? **Select all that apply.**
  ❑ 1. Walker
  ❑ 2. Wheelchair
  ❑ 3. Tripod cane
  ❑ 4. Wooden crutch
  ❑ 5. Quadripod cane
  ❑ 6. Lofstrand crutch

Level of Cognitive Ability: Analyzing
Client Needs: Safe and Effective Care Environment
Clinical Judgment/Cognitive Skills: Analyze Cues
Integrated Process: Nursing Process/Assessment
Content Area: Skills: Activity/Mobility
Health Problems: Adult Health: Neurologic: Stroke
Priority Concepts: Mobility; Safety

Answer: 1, 3, 5
Rationale: A tripod or quadripod cane may be prescribed for the client who requires greater support and stability than is provided by a straight-leg cane. The tripod or quadripod cane provides multiple points of support and is indicated for use by clients with partial or complete hemiplegia. A walker may potentially be needed by this client, if only for a short duration, and still encourages some client mobility. Neither wheelchair nor crutches are indicated for use with a client such as described in this question. A Lofstrand crutch is useful for clients with bilateral weakness.
Test-Taking Strategy: Focus on the subject, support device for the client with hemiplegia. Providing a wheelchair to a client with partial hemiplegia is excessive and is eliminated first. Wooden crutches are not indicated because there is no restriction in weight bearing. Lofstrand crutches (forearm crutches) are useful for bilateral weakness.
Priority Nursing Tip: A quadripod cane provides more security to the client than a single-tipped cane.
Reference: Potter, P., et al. (2021). *Fundamentals of nursing* (10th ed., p. 797). Elsevier.

124. A postoperative client begins to drain small amounts of bright red blood from the tracheostomy tube 24 hours after a laryngectomy. Which **priority** action would the nurse implement?
1. Notify the surgeon.
2. Increase the frequency of suctioning.
3. Add moisture to the oxygen delivery system.
4. Document the character and amount of drainage.

Level of Cognitive Ability: Applying
Client Needs: Safe and Effective Care Environment
Clinical Judgment/Cognitive Skills: Take Action
Integrated Process: Clinical Judgment; Nursing Process/Implementation
Content Area: Complex Care: Emergency Situations/Management
Health Problems: Adult Health: Respiratory: Artificial Airways
Priority Concepts: Clinical Judgment; Safety

Answer: 1
Rationale: Immediately after laryngectomy, a small amount of bleeding occurs from the tracheostomy that resolves within the first few hours. Otherwise, bleeding that is bright red may be a sign of impending rupture of a vessel. The bleeding in this instance represents a potential life-threatening situation, and the surgeon is notified to further evaluate the client and suture or repair the bleed. The other options do not address the urgency of the problem. Failure to notify the surgeon places the client at risk.
Test-Taking Strategy: Note the strategic word, *priority.* The additional information provided—*bright red blood* and *24 hours after the surgery*—would indicate that a potential complication exists and directs you to the correct option.
Priority Nursing Tip: The presence of bright red bleeding indicates active bleeding and is always a cause for concern, indicating the need to notify the surgeon.
Reference: Ignatavicius, D., et al. (2021). *Medical-surgical nursing: Concepts for interprofessional collaborative care* (10th ed., p. 527). Elsevier.

125. The nurse needs to withdraw a prescribed 7000 units from the medication vial for administration. For a safe dose of medication, how many milliliters would the nurse withdraw? **(Refer to the figure.) Fill in the blank and record your answer using one decimal place.**
Answer: _____ mL

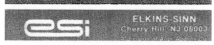

Each mL contains heparin sodium 5000 USP units, sodium chloride 7 mg and benzyl alcohol 0.01 mL in Water for Injection. pH 5.0-7.5; sodium hydroxide and/or hydrochloric acid added, if needed, for pH adjustment.

esi
10 mL
MULTIPLE DOSE Vial
NDC 0641-2460-41

HEPARIN
SODIUM INJECTION, USP
5000 USP units / 1 mL
FOR INTRAVENOUS OR SUBCUTANEOUS USE

DERIVED FROM PORCINE INTESTINES

Caution: Federal law prohibits dispensing without prescription. SAMPLE COPY

esi
ELKINS-SINN
Cherry Hill NJ 08003

(From Kee, J., & Marshall, S. [2013]. *Clinical calculations: With applications to general and specialty areas.* [7th ed.]. Saunders.)
Level of Cognitive Ability: Applying
Client Needs: Safe and Effective Care Environment
Clinical Judgment/Cognitive Skills: Generate Solutions
Integrated Process: Nursing Process/Planning
Content Area: Skills: Dosage Calculations
Health Problems: N/A
Priority Concepts: Clinical Judgment; Safety

Answer: 1.4
Rationale: Use the medication calculation formula.
Formula:
$$\frac{Desired \times Volume}{Available} = mL/dose$$
$$\frac{7000\ units \times 1\ mL}{5000\ units} = 1.4\ mL/dose$$

Test-Taking Strategy: Focus on the subject, medication administration, and focus on the data on the medication label. Follow the formula for calculating the correct dose. Once you have performed the calculation, recheck your work with a calculator, and make certain that the answer makes sense.
Priority Nursing Tip: It is important for the nurse to check the expiration date on a medication label. Medications that have expired lose their potency and may not be effective any longer.
Reference: Potter, P., et al. (2021). *Fundamentals of nursing.* (10th ed., pp. 599–601). Elsevier.

❖ **126.** The nurse assists a postoperative appendectomy client from a lying to a sitting position to prepare for ambulation. Which nursing action is **most appropriate initially** to maintain the safety of the client?
1. Assess the client for signs of dizziness and hypotension.
2. Be sure that the client is wearing slippers with nonslip soles.
3. Secure the assistance of at least one additional staff member to help with the ambulation.
4. Encourage the client to support the abdomen with a small pillow while walking.

Level of Cognitive Ability: Applying
Client Needs: Safe and Effective Care Environment
Clinical Judgment/Cognitive Skills: Take Action
Integrated Process: Nursing Process/Implementation
Content Area: Skills: Activity/Mobility
Health Problems: Adult Health: Gastrointestinal: Appendicitis
Priority Concepts: Clinical Judgment; Safety

Answer: 1
Rationale: Early ambulation should not exceed the client's tolerance. The client needs to be assessed for dizziness and hypotension before ambulation begins. Nonslip soles are appropriate but not the initial intervention. The situation does not indicate the need for either of the remaining interventions.
Test-Taking Strategy: Focus on the strategic words, *most appropriate* and *initially.* Eliminate options 2, 3, and 4 because they do not support safety of the client being assisted to a sitting position on the side of the bed. Additionally, option 1 is the only option that reflects assessment, the first step of the nursing process.
Priority Nursing Tip: When moving a client from a lying to a sitting position, monitor for signs of orthostatic hypotension. If the client complains of dizziness, lightheadedness, or nausea, place the client back into the lying position and check the blood pressure and pulse.
Reference: Ignatavicius, D., et al. (2021). *Medical-surgical nursing: Concepts for interprofessional collaborative care* (10th ed., pp. 125, 247). Elsevier.

127. The nurse would implement which safety measures to prevent an electrical shock when using electrical equipment? **Select all that apply.**
☐ 1. Use a two-prong outlet.
☐ 2. Check the electrical cord for fraying.
☐ 3. Keep the electrical cord away from the sink.
☐ 4. Place the excess electrical cord under a small carpet.
☐ 5. Grasp the electrical cord when unplugging the equipment.
☐ 6. Disconnect the electrical cord from the wall socket when cleaning the equipment.

Level of Cognitive Ability: Applying
Client Needs: Safe and Effective Care Environment
Clinical Judgment/Cognitive Skills: Take Action
Integrated Process: Nursing Process/Implementation
Content Area: Foundations of Care: Safety
Health Problems: N/A
Priority Concepts: Clinical Judgment; Safety

Answer: 2, 3, 6
Rationale: The nurse needs to implement measures to prevent an electrical shock when using electrical equipment. These measures include using a three-prong plug that is grounded, checking the electrical cord for fraying or other damage, keeping the electrical cord away from the sink or other sources of water, using electrical tape to secure the excess electrical cord to the floor where it will not be stepped on (the cord would not be placed under carpet), grasping the plug (not the electrical cord) when unplugging the equipment, and disconnecting the electrical cord from the wall socket when cleaning the equipment.
Test-Taking Strategy: Focus on the subject, electrical safety. Read each option carefully and visualize how the measure may or may not prevent an electrical shock.
Priority Nursing Tip: Any electrical equipment that a client brings into a health care facility, such as an electric shaver, needs to be inspected for safety before use.
Reference: Potter, P., et al. (2021). *Fundamentals of nursing* (10th ed., pp. 403, 407). Elsevier.

❖ **128.** Upon transfer from the post-anesthesia care unit (PACU) after spinal fusion, which technique would the nurse use to transfer the client from the stretcher to the bed?

1. A bath blanket and the assistance of at least two people
2. A bath blanket and the assistance of at least three people
3. A transfer board and the assistance of at least two people
4. A transfer board and the assistance of at least three people

Level of Cognitive Ability: Applying
Client Needs: Safe and Effective Care Environment
Clinical Judgment/Cognitive Skills: Take Action
Integrated Process: Nursing Process/Implementation
Content Area: Skills: Activity/Mobility
Health Problems: Adult Health: Musculoskeletal: Skeletal Injury
Priority Concepts: Mobility; Safety

Answer: 4
Rationale: After spinal fusion, with or without instrumentation, the client is transferred from the stretcher to the bed using a transfer board and the assistance of at least three people. This permits optimal stabilization and support of the spine while allowing the client to be moved smoothly and gently. Therefore, the remaining options are incorrect and unsafe.
Test-Taking Strategy: Focus on the subject, transfer of the client with spinal fusion. Think about the level of comfort and stability provided to the client's spine with the amounts of assistance given in each option. Using this approach will assist in eliminating the incorrect options.
Priority Nursing Tip: Physical stress for the health care provider can be decreased significantly by the use of a transfer board. In addition, the use of a transfer board prevents friction on the client's skin during the move.
Reference: Potter, P., et al. (2021). *Fundamentals of nursing* (10th ed., pp. 783, 814–815). Elsevier.

129. Which actions are **most appropriate** for the nurse to take in the event of an accidental poisoning of a child? **Select all that apply.**

☐ 1. Save vomitus for laboratory analysis.
☐ 2. Place the child in a flat supine position.
☐ 3. Induce vomiting if a household cleaner was ingested.
☐ 4. Assess for airway patency, breathing, and circulation.
☐ 5. Determine the type and amount of substance ingested.
☐ 6. Remove any visible materials from the nose and mouth.

Level of Cognitive Ability: Applying
Client Needs: Safe and Effective Care Environment
Clinical Judgment/Cognitive Skills: Take Action
Integrated Process: Clinical Judgment; Nursing Process/Implementation
Content Area: Complex Care: Emergency Situations/Management
Health Problems: Pediatric-Specific: Poisoning
Priority Concepts: Clinical Judgment; Safety

Answer: 1, 4, 5, 6
Rationale: In the event of accidental poisoning, the poison control center is called before attempting any interventions. Additional interventions in an accidental poisoning include saving vomitus for laboratory analysis, which may assist with further treatment; assessing for airway patency, breathing, and circulation; determining the type and amount of substance ingested if possible to identify an antidote; removing any visible materials from the nose and mouth to terminate exposure; and positioning the victim with the head to the side to prevent aspiration of vomitus and assist in keeping the airway open. Vomiting is never induced in an unconscious person or one who is experiencing seizures because of the risk of aspiration. Additionally, vomiting is not induced if lye, household cleaners, hair care products, grease or petroleum products, or furniture polish was ingested because of the risk of internal burns.
Test-Taking Strategy: Note the strategic words, *most appropriate.* Focus on the subject, accidental poisoning. Visualize each of the interventions and how they may be helpful in treating the poisoning. Use of the ABCs—airway, breathing, and circulation—will assist in determining the correct interventions. Also remember that any substances that are caustic can result in further injury to the client.
Priority Nursing Tip: In the event of a poisoning, the poison control center is contacted immediately.
Reference: McKinney, E. S., et al. (2022). *Maternal child nursing* (6th ed., pp. 123–124, 774). Elsevier.

130. The nurse inserts an indwelling urinary catheter into a client being prepared for surgery to remove a kidney stone. As the catheter moves into the bladder, urine begins to flow into the tubing. Which action would the nurse implement **next?**
1. Inflate the balloon with water.
2. Secure the catheter to the client.
3. Measure the initial urine output.
4. Advance the catheter 2.5 to 5 cm.

Level of Cognitive Ability: Applying
Client Needs: Safe and Effective Care Environment
Clinical Judgment/Cognitive Skills: Take Action
Integrated Process: Nursing Process/Implementation
Content Area: Skills: Elimination
Health Problems: Adult Health: Renal and Urinary: Calculi
Priority Concepts: Elimination; Safety

Answer: 4
Rationale: The balloon of a urinary catheter is behind the opening at the insertion tip, so the nurse inserts the catheter 2.5 to 5 cm further after urine begins to flow so as to provide sufficient space to inflate the balloon. The balloon is not inflated as soon as urine appears because the balloon could be located in the urethra. After the insertion procedure and inflation of the balloon, the nurse secures the catheter to the client's leg and then measures the initial urine output.
Test-Taking Strategy: Note the strategic word, *next.* Visualize the procedure described in the question and the effects of each description in the options to direct you to the correct option.
Priority Nursing Tip: Strict aseptic technique is required when inserting a urinary catheter into a client.
Reference: Potter, P., et al. (2021). *Fundamentals of nursing* (10th ed., p. 1186). Elsevier.

131. The nurse is preparing to administer oxygen to a client with a diagnosis of chronic obstructive pulmonary disease (COPD) and is at risk for carbon dioxide narcosis. The nurse would check to see that the oxygen flow rate is prescribed at which rate?
1. 2 to 4 L/min
2. 4 to 5 L/min
3. 6 to 8 L/min
4. 8 to 10 L/min

Level of Cognitive Ability: Applying
Client Needs: Safe and Effective Care Environment
Clinical Judgment/Cognitive Skills: Take Action
Integrated Process: Nursing Process/Implementation
Content Area: Adult Health: Respiratory
Health Problems: Adult Health: Respiratory: Chronic Obstructive Pulmonary Disease
Priority Concepts: Clinical Judgment; Safety

Answer: 1
Rationale: In carbon dioxide narcosis, the central chemoreceptors lose their sensitivity to increased levels of carbon dioxide and no longer respond by increasing the rate and depth of respiration. For these clients, the stimulus to breathe is a decreased arterial oxygen concentration. In the client with COPD, a low arterial oxygen level is the client's primary drive for breathing. If high levels of oxygen are administered, the client may lose the respiratory drive, and respiratory failure results. Thus, the nurse checks the flow of oxygen to see that it does not exceed 2 to 4 L/min unless a specific physician prescription indicates a different flow of the oxygen.
Test-Taking Strategy: Focus on the subject, COPD. Recalling the pathophysiology that occurs in COPD and that a low arterial oxygen level is the client's primary drive for breathing will direct you to the option with the lowest oxygen liter flow.
Priority Nursing Tip: The chest x-ray for a client with COPD typically reveals hyperinflation.
Reference: Ignatavicius, D., et al. (2021). *Medical-surgical nursing: Concepts for interprofessional collaborative care* (10th ed., pp. 546, 548). Elsevier.

❖ **132.** A client undergoes a subtotal thyroidectomy. The nurse ensures that which **priority** item is at the client's bedside upon arrival from the postanesthesia care unit (PACU)?
1. An apnea monitor
2. A suction unit and oxygen
3. A blood transfusion warmer
4. An ampule of phytonadione

Level of Cognitive Ability: Applying
Client Needs: Safe and Effective Care Environment
Clinical Judgment/Cognitive Skills: Generate Solutions
Integrated Process: Nursing Process/Planning
Content Area: Adult Health: Endocrine
Health Problems: Adult Health: Endocrine: Thyroid Disorders
Priority Concepts: Gas Exchange; Safety

Answer: 2
Rationale: After thyroidectomy, respiratory distress can occur from tetany, tissue swelling, or hemorrhage. It is important to have oxygen and suction equipment readily available and in working order if such an emergency were to arise. Apnea is not a problem associated with thyroidectomy unless the client experienced respiratory arrest. Blood transfusions can be administered without a warmer, if necessary. Phytonadione would not be administered for a client who is hemorrhaging unless deficiencies in clotting factors warrant its administration.
Test-Taking Strategy: Note the strategic word, *priority.* Recall the anatomic location of the thyroid gland and its proximity to the trachea. Use the ABCs—airway, breathing, and circulation—to direct you to the correct option.
Priority Nursing Tip: After thyroidectomy, the client needs to be maintained in a semi-Fowler's position to prevent edema at the surgical site.
Reference: Ignatavicius, D., et al. (2021). *Medical-surgical nursing: Concepts for interprofessional collaborative care* (10th ed., p. 1259). Elsevier.

133. The nurse places a hospitalized client with a diagnosis of active tuberculosis in a private, well-ventilated isolation room. In addition, which action would the nurse take before entering the client's room?
1. Wash the hands.
2. Wash the hands and wear a gown and gloves.
3. Wash the hands and place a high-efficiency particulate air (HEPA) respirator over the nose and mouth.
4. The nurse needs no special precautions, but the client is instructed to cover their mouth and nose when coughing or sneezing.

Level of Cognitive Ability: Applying
Client Needs: Safe and Effective Care Environment
Clinical Judgment/Cognitive Skills: Take Action
Integrated Process: Nursing Process/Implementation
Content Area: Foundations of Care: Infection Control
Health Problems: Adult Health: Respiratory: Tuberculosis
Priority Concepts: Infection; Safety

Answer: 3
Rationale: Tuberculosis is a highly communicable disease caused by *Mycobacterium tuberculosis.* The nurse wears a HEPA respirator when caring for a client with active tuberculosis. Hands are always thoroughly washed before and after caring for the client. Option 1 is an incomplete action. Option 2 is also inaccurate and incomplete. Gowning is only indicated when there is a possibility of contaminating clothing. Option 4 is an incorrect statement because special precautions are needed.
Test-Taking Strategy: Focus on the subject, caring for the client with tuberculosis. Recalling the route of transmission and the need for airborne precautions will direct you to the correct option.
Priority Nursing Tip: A positive tuberculin skin test reaction does not mean that active tuberculosis is present, but it does indicate previous exposure to tuberculosis or the presence of inactive (dormant) disease.
Reference: Ignatavicius, D., et al. (2021). *Medical-surgical nursing: Concepts for interprofessional collaborative care* (10th ed., pp. 409, 580). Elsevier.

❖ **134.** The nurse is assigned to care for a hospitalized toddler. Which measure would the nurse plan to implement as the **highest priority** of care?
1. Providing a consistent caregiver
2. Protecting the toddler from injury
3. Adapting the toddler to the hospital routine
4. Allowing the toddler to participate in play and diversional activities

Level of Cognitive Ability: Applying
Client Needs: Safe and Effective Care Environment
Clinical Judgment/Cognitive Skills: Prioritize Hypotheses
Integrated Process: Nursing Process/Planning
Content Area: Foundations of Care: Safety
Health Problems: N/A
Priority Concepts: Development; Safety

Answer: 2
Rationale: The toddler is at high risk for injury as a result of developmental abilities and an unfamiliar environment. Although consistency, adaptation, and diversion are important, protection from injury is the highest priority.
Test-Taking Strategy: Note the strategic words, *highest priority*. Use Maslow's Hierarchy of Needs theory. Physiologic needs come first, followed by safety. Because no physiologic needs are addressed, the safety option of preventing injury takes priority.
Priority Nursing Tip: Although safety is the highest priority, the nurse must remember that hospitalization, with its own set of rituals and routines, can severely disrupt the life of a toddler.
Reference: McKinney, E. S., et al. (2022). *Maternal child nursing* (6th ed., pp. 789–790). Elsevier.

135. A client suspected of having developed tuberculosis is to undergo pleural biopsy at the bedside. Knowing the potential complications of the procedure, what equipment would the nurse plan to have available at the bedside?
1. Intubation tray
2. Morphine sulfate injection
3. Portable chest x-ray machine
4. Chest tube and drainage system

Level of Cognitive Ability: Applying
Client Needs: Safe and Effective Care Environment
Clinical Judgment/Cognitive Skills: Generate Solutions
Integrated Process: Nursing Process/Planning
Content Area: Foundations of Care: Diagnostic Tests
Health Problems: Adult Health: Respiratory: Tuberculosis
Priority Concepts: Gas Exchange; Safety

Answer: 4
Rationale: Complications after pleural biopsy include hemothorax, pneumothorax, and temporary pain from intercostal nerve injury. The nurse has a chest tube and drainage system available at the bedside for use if hemothorax or pneumothorax develops. An intubation tray is not indicated. The client needs to be premedicated before the procedure, or a local anesthetic is used. A portable chest x-ray machine would be called for to verify placement of a chest tube if one was inserted, but it is unnecessary to have at the bedside before the procedure.
Test-Taking Strategy: Focus on the subject, pleural biopsy. Think about how this procedure is done. Recalling the complications of this procedure and noting the relation of this procedure to the correct option will direct you to this option.
Priority Nursing Tip: Absence of breath sounds on the affected side of the lungs is a manifestation of pneumothorax.
References: Lewis, S., et al. (2020). *Medical-surgical nursing: Assessment and management of clinical problems* (11th ed., pp. 474, 530). Elsevier; Pagana, K., Pagana, T., & Pagana, T. N. (2021). *Mosby's Diagnostic and laboratory test reference* (15th ed., pp. 857–858). Elsevier.

Client Needs

❖ **136.** The nurse manager of a hemodialysis unit observes a new nurse preparing hemodialysis on a client with a diagnosis of chronic kidney disease. The nurse manager would note that the new nurse **needs further teaching** and would intervene if which action is carried out by the new nurse?
1. Uses sterile technique for needle insertion
2. Wears full protective clothing such as goggles, mask, gown, and gloves
3. Covers the connection site with a bath blanket to enhance extremity warmth
4. Puts on a mask and gives one to the client to wear during connection to the machine

Level of Cognitive Ability: Evaluating
Client Needs: Safe and Effective Care Environment
Clinical Judgment/Cognitive Skills: Evaluate Outcomes
Integrated Process: Teaching and Learning
Content Area: Foundations of Care: Infection Control
Health Problems: Adult Health: Renal and Urinary: Acute Kidney Injury and Chronic Kidney Disease
Priority Concepts: Infection; Safety

Answer: 3
Rationale: While the client is receiving hemodialysis, the connection site should not be covered, and it needs to be visible so that the nurse can assess for bleeding, ischemia, and infection at the site during the procedure. Infection is a major concern with hemodialysis. For that reason, the use of sterile technique and the application of a face mask for both the nurse and client are extremely important. It is also imperative that standard precautions be followed, which includes the use of goggles, a mask, gloves, and a gown.
Test-Taking Strategy: Note the strategic words, *needs further teaching* and *intervene*. These words indicate a negative event query and require you to select the option that indicates an incorrect nursing action. Eliminate the remaining options because they are comparable or alike in that they relate to infection control and standard precautions.
Priority Nursing Tip: The nurse needs to assess the client for fluid overload before hemodialysis and fluid volume deficit after hemodialysis.
Reference: Ignatavicius, D., et al. (2021). *Medical-surgical nursing: Concepts for interprofessional collaborative care* (10th ed., p. 1399). Elsevier.

137. The nurse is going to suction an adult client with a tracheostomy who has respiratory secretions. Which intervention would the nurse implement to perform this procedure safely?
1. Occluding the Y-port of the suction catheter while advancing it
2. Applying continuous suction in the airway for up to 20 seconds
3. Setting the suction pressure range between 160 and 180 mm Hg
4. Hyperoxygenating the client by asking the client to take four to five deep breaths

Level of Cognitive Ability: Applying
Client Needs: Safe and Effective Care Environment
Clinical Judgment/Cognitive Skills: Take Action
Integrated Process: Nursing Process/Implementation
Content Area: Skills: Oxygenation
Health Problems: Adult Health: Respiratory: Artificial Airways
Priority Concepts: Gas Exchange; Safety

Answer: 4
Rationale: To perform suctioning, the nurse hyperoxygenates the client by asking client to take four to five deep breaths, using a manual resuscitation bag or using the sigh mechanism if the client is on a mechanical ventilator. The safe suction range for an adult is 100 to 120 mm Hg. The nurse uses intermittent suction in the airway for up to 10 to 15 seconds. The nurse advances the suction catheter into the tracheostomy without occluding the Y-port; suction is never applied while introducing the catheter because it would traumatize mucosa and remove oxygen from the respiratory tract.
Test-Taking Strategy: Visualize this procedure. Recalling that suction is applied intermittently and on catheter withdrawal only will eliminate options 2 and 3. From the remaining options, use the ABCs—airway, breathing, and circulation—to direct you to the correct option.
Priority Nursing Tip: To perform suctioning, the client is assisted to a sitting upright position such as semi-Fowler's with the head hyperextended (unless contraindicated).
Reference: Ignatavicius, D., et al. (2021). *Medical-surgical nursing: Concepts for interprofessional collaborative care* (10th ed., p. 509). Elsevier.

❖ **138.** The nurse is collecting a sputum specimen for culture and sensitivity testing from a client who has a productive cough suspected of having pneumonia. Which intervention would the nurse implement to obtain the specimen?
1. Ask the client to obtain the specimen after breakfast.
2. Use a sterile plastic container for obtaining the specimen.
3. Provide tissues for expectoration and obtaining the specimen.
4. Ask the client to expectorate a small amount of sputum into the emesis basin.

Level of Cognitive Ability: Applying
Client Needs: Safe and Effective Care Environment
Clinical Judgment/Cognitive Skills: Take Action
Integrated Process: Nursing Process/Implementation
Content Area: Skills: Specimen Collection
Health Problems: Adult Health: Respiratory: Pneumonia
Priority Concepts: Infection; Safety

Answer: 2
Rationale: Sputum specimens for culture and sensitivity testing need to be obtained using sterile techniques because the test is done to determine the presence of organisms. If the procedure for obtaining the specimen is not sterile, then the specimen would be contaminated and the results of the test would be invalid. A first-morning specimen is preferred because it represents overnight secretions of the tracheobronchial tree.
Test-Taking Strategy: Focus on the subject, sputum specimen for culture and sensitivity. The words *culture and sensitivity* tell you that the test is being done to identify the presence of microorganisms. Recalling that microorganisms will multiply in the specimen and that accurate identification of organisms is needed to determine treatment will direct you to the correct option. Also, noting the word *sterile* in the correct option will direct you to this option.
Priority Nursing Tip: Always collect a specimen for culture and sensitivity before prescribed antibiotics are initiated because the antibiotic may alter the testing by affecting the organism count.
Reference: Pagana, K., Pagana, T., & Pagana, T. N. (2021). *Mosby's Diagnostic and laboratory test reference* (15th ed., pp. 830–831). Elsevier.

139. The post-myocardial infarction client is scheduled for a technetium-99m ventriculography (multigated acquisition [MUGA] scan). The nurse would ensure that which item is in place before the procedure?
1. An indwelling urinary catheter
2. Signed informed consent
3. A central venous pressure (CVP) line
4. Notation of allergies to iodine or shellfish

Level of Cognitive Ability: Applying
Client Needs: Safe and Effective Care Environment
Clinical Judgment/Cognitive Skills: Take Action
Integrated Process: Nursing Process/Implementation
Content Area: Foundations of Care: Diagnostic Tests
Health Problems: Adult Health: Cardiovascular: Myocardial Infarction
Priority Concepts: Perfusion; Safety

Answer: 2
Rationale: MUGA is a radionuclide study used to detect myocardial infarction and decreased myocardial blood flow and to determine left ventricular function. A radioisotope is injected intravenously. Therefore, a signed informed consent is necessary. An indwelling urinary catheter and CVP line are not required. The procedure does not use radiopaque dye; therefore, allergy to iodine and shellfish is not a concern.
Test-Taking Strategy: Focus on the subject, MUGA scan. Think about how the procedure is performed. Recalling that the procedure involves injection of a radioisotope will direct you to the correct option.
Priority Nursing Tip: The left ventricular ejection fraction (LVEF) should be above 55%.
Reference: Pagana, K., Pagana, T., & Pagana, T. N. (2021). *Mosby's Diagnostic and laboratory test reference* (15th ed., p. 210). Elsevier.

❖ **140.** Which interventions would the emergency department nurse implement during the management of a client suspected of exposure to anthrax? **Select all that apply.**
- ❑ 1. Handle clothing minimally.
- ❑ 2. Store contaminated clothing in a labeled paper bag.
- ❑ 3. Instruct the client to remove contaminated clothing.
- ❑ 4. Wear sterile gloves when handling contaminated items.
- ❑ 5. Instruct the client to shower thoroughly using soap and water.
- ❑ 6. Consult with the physician regarding postexposure prophylaxis with oral fluoroquinolones for the client.

Level of Cognitive Ability: Applying
Client Needs: Safe and Effective Care Environment
Clinical Judgment/Cognitive Skills: Take Action
Integrated Process: Nursing Process/Implementation
Content Area: Leadership/Management: Mass Casualty Preparedness and Response
Health Problems: Adult Health: Integumentary: Inflammations/Infections
Priority Concepts: Clinical Judgment; Safety

Answer: 1, 3, 5, 6
Rationale: An important aspect of care for a client who has a bioterrorism-related illness is postexposure management. Decontamination and exposure management of the client suspected of anthrax exposure includes instructing the client to remove contaminated clothing and store contaminated clothing in a labeled plastic (not paper) bag; handling clothing minimally to avoid agitation; instructing the client to shower thoroughly using soap and water; and using standard precautions and wearing appropriate protective barriers when handling contaminated clothing or other items. Postexposure prophylaxis with oral fluoroquinolones for the client is also recommended. The use of sterile gloves is unnecessary.
Test-Taking Strategy: Focus on the subject, a client suspected of exposure to anthrax. Read each option carefully. Recalling that postexposure management involves decontamination will assist in selecting the correct interventions. Remember that preventing exposure is a critical intervention.
Priority Nursing Tip: Anthrax is transmitted by direct contact with bacteria and spores and can be contracted through the digestive system, abrasions in the skin, or inhalation through the lungs.
Reference: Sweet, V., & Foley, P., eds. (2020). *Sheehy's Emergency nursing: Principles and practice* (7th ed., p. 174). Elsevier; Federal Emergency Management Agency (online). Official website of the United States Government. http://fema.gov/.

141. Which statements describe characteristics of case management? **Select all that apply.**
- ❑ 1. A case manager usually does not provide direct care.
- ❑ 2. Critical pathways and CareMaps are types of case management.
- ❑ 3. A case manager does not need to be concerned with standards of cost management.
- ❑ 4. A case manager collaborates with other staff members and actively coordinates client discharge planning.
- ❑ 5. The evaluation process involves continuous monitoring and analysis of the needs of the client and services provided.
- ❑ 6. A case manager coordinates a hospitalized client's acute care and follows up with the client after discharge to home.

Level of Cognitive Ability: Understanding
Client Needs: Safe and Effective Care Environment
Clinical Judgment/Cognitive Skills: Generate Solutions
Integrated Process: Nursing Process/Planning
Content Area: Leadership/Management: Management of Care
Health Problems: N/A
Priority Concepts: Care Coordination; Health Care Quality

Answer: 1, 4, 5, 6
Rationale: Case management is a care management approach that coordinates health care services to clients and their families while maintaining quality of care and minimizing health care costs. Case managers usually do not provide direct care; instead, they collaborate with other staff members and actively coordinate client discharge planning. A case manager is usually held accountable for some standard of cost management. A case manager coordinates a hospitalized client's acute care, follows up with the client after discharge to home, and is responsible and accountable for appraising the overall usefulness and effectiveness of the case-managed services. This evaluation process involves continuous monitoring and analysis of the client's needs and services provided. Critical pathways or CareMaps are not types of case management; rather, they are multidisciplinary treatment plans used in a case management delivery system to implement timely interventions in a coordinated care plan.
Test-Taking Strategy: Focus on the subject, the characteristics of case management, and read each option carefully. Recall that case management is a care management approach that coordinates health care services to clients and their families while maintaining quality of care and keeping health care costs at a minimum. This will assist in selecting the correct options.
Priority Nursing Tip: Case management requires the nurse to analyze a client's situation from a holistic perspective and determine the client's needs. The nurse then consults the appropriate disciplines to meet these needs.
Reference: Potter, P., et al. (2021). *Fundamentals of nursing* (10th ed., pp. 283, 377–378). Elsevier.

❖ **142.** A client is being admitted to the hospital following insertion of a radiation implant after being diagnosed with cervical cancer. Which **priority** action would the nurse implement in the care of this client?

1. Encourage the family to visit.
2. Admit the client to a private room.
3. Place the client on protective isolation.
4. Encourage the client to take frequent rest periods.

Level of Cognitive Ability: Applying
Client Needs: Safe and Effective Care Environment
Clinical Judgment/Cognitive Skills: Take Action
Integrated Process: Nursing Process/Implementation
Content Area: Adult Health: Oncology
Health Problems: Adult Health: Cancer: Cervical/Uterine/Ovarian
Priority Concepts: Clinical Judgment; Safety

Answer: 2
Rationale: The client who has a radiation implant is placed in a private room and has limited visitors. This reduces the exposure of others to the radiation. Protective isolation is unnecessary; rather, individuals other than the client need to be protected. Frequent rest periods are a helpful general intervention but are not a priority for the client in this situation.
Test-Taking Strategy: Note the strategic word, *priority*, and focus on the subject, radiation implant. Recalling the concepts related to environmental safety and that other individuals need to have limited exposure to clients with radiation implants will direct you to the correct option.
Priority Nursing Tip: Pregnant individuals and any individual younger than 16 years old are not allowed in the room of a client with a radiation implant.
Reference: Ignatavicius, D., et al. (2021). *Medical-surgical nursing: Concepts for interprofessional collaborative care* (10th ed., p. 381). Elsevier.

143. The client with a diagnosis of bladder cancer is to undergo weekly intravesical chemotherapy for the next 8 weeks. Which statement by the client would indicate to the nurse that the client understands how to manage urine as a biohazard?

1. Void into a bedpan and then empty the urine into the toilet.
2. Purchase extra bottles of scented disinfectant for daily bathroom cleansing.
3. Have one bathroom strictly set aside for the client's use for the next 8 weeks.
4. Disinfect the toilet with household bleach after voiding for 6 hours after a treatment.

Level of Cognitive Ability: Evaluating
Client Needs: Safe and Effective Care Environment
Clinical Judgment/Cognitive Skills: Evaluate Outcomes
Integrated Process: Clinical Judgment; Teaching and Learning
Content Area: Foundations of Care: Safety
Health Problems: Adult Health: Cancer: Bladder and Kidney
Priority Concepts: Patient Education; Safety

Answer: 4
Rationale: Intravesical instillation involves instilling a chemotherapeutic agent into the bladder via a urethral catheter. This method of treatment provides a concentrated topical treatment with minimal systemic absorption. The client retains the medication for approximately 2 hours. After intravesical chemotherapy, the client treats the urine as a biohazard. This involves disinfecting the toilet after voiding with household bleach for 6 hours after a treatment. There is no value in using a bedpan for voiding. Scented disinfectants are of no particular use. The client does not need to have a separate bathroom for personal use.
Test-Taking Strategy: Focus on the subject, intravesical instillation with a chemotherapeutic agent. Option 1 has no value and is eliminated first. Because scented disinfectants also have no value, option 2 is eliminated next. Also, option 3 is unnecessary and may be unrealistic for many clients. Knowing that the urine and toilet need special treatment for 6 hours after intravesical chemotherapy directs you to the correct option.
Priority Nursing Tip: After intravesical instillation with a chemotherapeutic agent to treat bladder cancer, the client is instructed to increase fluid intake to flush the bladder.
Reference: Ignatavicius, D., et al. (2021). *Medical-surgical nursing: Concepts for interprofessional collaborative care* (10th ed., pp. 1350–1351). Elsevier.

❖ **144.** A client who is admitted to the hospital for an unrelated medical problem is diagnosed with urethritis caused by chlamydial infection. The unlicensed assistive personnel (UAP) assigned to the client asks the nurse what measures are necessary to prevent contraction of the infection during care. The nurse tells the UAP that which intervention is needed for infection control?

1. Enteric precautions need to be instituted for the client.
2. Gloves and mask need to be used when in the client's room.
3. Contact isolation needs to be initiated because the disease is highly contagious.
4. Standard precautions are sufficient because the disease is transmitted sexually.

Level of Cognitive Ability: Applying
Client Needs: Safe and Effective Care Environment
Clinical Judgment/Cognitive Skills: Take Action
Integrated Process: Teaching and Learning
Content Area: Foundations of Care: Infection Control
Health Problems: Adult Health: Renal and Urinary: Inflammation/Infections
Priority Concepts: Infection; Safety

Answer: 4
Rationale: *Chlamydia* is a sexually transmitted infection. Caregivers cannot acquire the disease during administration of care, and standard precautions are the only measure that needs to be used. Recognizing the necessary precautions will help you in identifying the remaining options as incorrect.
Test-Taking Strategy: Focus on the subject, infection control for a *Chlamydia* infection. Recall that this infection is sexually transmitted. Also, note that the correct option is the umbrella option.
Priority Nursing Tip: A pregnant client with a chlamydial infection can transmit the infection to the neonate during a vaginal birth. This occurrence can result in neonatal conjunctivitis or pneumonitis.
Reference: Ignatavicius, D., et al. (2021). *Medical-surgical nursing: Concepts for interprofessional collaborative care* (10th ed., pp. 410, 1515). Elsevier.

145. The nurse manager is reviewing the principles of surgical asepsis with the nursing staff. In which situations would the nurse manager communicate to the staff that it is necessary to use the principles of surgical asepsis? **Select all that apply.**

❑ 1. Removing a dressing
❑ 2. Reapplying sterile dressings
❑ 3. Inserting an intravenous (IV) line
❑ 4. Inserting an indwelling urinary catheter
❑ 5. Suctioning the tracheobronchial airway
❑ 6. Caring for an immunosuppressed client

Level of Cognitive Ability: Applying
Client Needs: Safe and Effective Care Environment
Clinical Judgment/Cognitive Skills: Take Action
Integrated Process: Teaching and Learning
Content Area: Leadership/Management: Interprofessional Collaboration
Health Problems: Adult Health: Immune: Sepsis
Priority Concepts: Infection; Safety

Answer: 2, 3, 4, 5
Rationale: Surgical asepsis involves the use of sterile technique. Some examples of procedures in which surgical asepsis is necessary include reapplying sterile dressings, inserting an IV or urinary catheter, and suctioning the tracheobronchial airway. Medical asepsis, or clean technique, includes procedures to reduce and prevent the spread of microorganisms. Removing a dressing can be done by clean technique using clean gloves (although reapplying the dressing requires surgical asepsis). Caring for an immunosuppressed client requires medical asepsis techniques.
Test-Taking Strategy: Focus on the subject, surgical asepsis. Recalling the definitions of medical and surgical asepsis and thinking about the invasiveness of each activity in the options will assist in answering this question.
Priority Nursing Tip: Medical and surgical asepsis are measures instituted to protect both the client and health care workers. Medical asepsis is intended to reduce and prevent the spread of microorganisms, whereas surgical asepsis aims to eliminate all microorganisms in a particular environment.
Reference: Potter, P., et al. (2019). *Essentials for nursing practice* (9th ed., pp. 446–447). Elsevier.

❖ **146.** The nurse is preparing the client's morning prescribed NPH insulin dose and notices a clumpy precipitate inside the insulin vial. Which action would the nurse take?
1. Draw the dose from a new vial.
2. Draw up and administer the dose.
3. Shake the vial in an attempt to disperse the clumps.
4. Warm the bottle under running water to dissolve the clump.

Level of Cognitive Ability: Applying
Client Needs: Safe and Effective Care Environment
Clinical Judgment/Cognitive Skills: Take Action
Integrated Process: Nursing Process/Implementation
Content Area: Skills: Medication Administration
Health Problems: Adult Health: Endocrine: Diabetes Mellitus
Priority Concepts: Clinical Judgment; Safety

Answer: 1
Rationale: The nurse needs to always inspect the vial of insulin before use for solution changes that may signify loss of potency. NPH insulin is normally uniformly cloudy. Clumping, frosting, and precipitates are signs of insulin damage. In this situation, because potency is questionable, it is safer to discard the vial and draw up the dose from a new vial.
Test-Taking Strategy: Focus on the subject, NPH insulin. Remember that NPH insulin is cloudy but not clumpy. This will direct you to the correct option, the safest action. Remember that when in doubt, throw it out.
Priority Nursing Tip: NPH insulin is an intermediate-acting insulin whose onset of action is 1.5 hours, peak time is 4 to 12 hours, and duration of action is approximately 16 to 24 hours.
Reference: Ignatavicius, D., et al. (2021). *Medical-surgical nursing: Concepts for interprofessional collaborative care* (10th ed., p. 1280). Elsevier.

147. The nurse is preparing the bedside for a postoperative parathyroidectomy client. The nurse would ensure that which specific **priority** item is at the client's bedside?
1. Cardiac monitor
2. Tracheotomy set
3. Intermittent gastric suction
4. Underwater seal chest drainage system

Level of Cognitive Ability: Applying
Client Needs: Safe and Effective Care Environment
Clinical Judgment/Cognitive Skills: Take Action
Integrated Process: Nursing Process/Implementation
Content Area: Adult Health: Endocrine
Health Problems: Adult Health: Endocrine: Parathyroid Disorders
Priority Concepts: Clinical Judgment; Safety

Answer: 2
Rationale: Respiratory distress caused by hemorrhage, swelling, and compression of the trachea is a primary concern for the nurse managing the care of a postoperative parathyroidectomy client. An emergency tracheotomy set is always routinely placed at the bedside of the client with this type of surgery in anticipation of this potential complication. Although a cardiac monitor may be attached to the client in the postoperative period, it is not specific to this type of surgery. Options 3 and 4 also are not specifically needed with the surgical procedure.
Test-Taking Strategy: Note the strategic word, *priority*. Focus on the subject, specific equipment needed after parathyroidectomy. Think about the location of the surgical incision and what potential problems might occur from that location. This will direct you to the correct option.
Priority Nursing Tip: After parathyroidectomy, monitor the client for hypocalcemic crisis, as evidenced by tingling and twitching in the extremities and face.
Reference: Ignatavicius, D., et al. (2021). *Medical-surgical nursing: Concepts for interprofessional collaborative care* (10th ed., pp. 1259, 1263). Elsevier.

❖ **148.** The nurse has a prescription to administer foscarnet sodium intravenously to a client with a diagnosis of acquired immunodeficiency syndrome (AIDS). Before administering this medication, which measure would the nurse implement?
1. Obtain a sputum culture.
2. Obtain folic acid as an antidote.
3. Place the solution on a controlled infusion pump.
4. Ensure that liver enzyme levels have been drawn as a baseline.

Level of Cognitive Ability: Applying
Client Needs: Safe and Effective Care Environment
Clinical Judgment/Cognitive Skills: Take Action
Integrated Process: Nursing Process/Implementation
Content Area: Pharmacology: Immune: Antivirals
Health Problems: Adult Health: Immune: Immunodeficiency Syndrome
Priority Concepts: Immunity; Safety

Answer: 3
Rationale: Foscarnet sodium is an antiviral agent used to treat cytomegalovirus (CMV) retinitis in clients with AIDS. Because of the potential toxicity of the medication, it is administered with the use of a controlled infusion device. A sputum culture is not necessary. Folic acid is not an antidote. Foscarnet sodium is highly toxic to the kidneys, and serum creatinine levels are measured frequently during therapy, not liver enzymes.
Test-Taking Strategy: Focus on the subject, administration of foscarnet sodium. Eliminate option 1 because the medication is usually indicated in the treatment of CMV retinitis, not respiratory infection. Additionally, no data in the question indicate the need for a sputum culture. Option 2 is eliminated next because folic acid is not an antidote. From the remaining options, it is necessary to know that the medication can be toxic and cannot be infused too quickly. This will direct you to option 3. Also, recalling that the medication is toxic to the kidneys, not the liver, will direct you to the correct option.
Priority Nursing Tip: The client with human immunodeficiency virus (HIV) or AIDS is at high risk for the development of opportunistic infections.
Reference: Gahart, B., Nazareno, A., & Ortega, M. (2021). *Gahart's 2021 Intravenous medications: A handbook for nurses and health professionals* (37th ed., p. 652). Elsevier.

149. An adult client who has a severe neurocognitive impairment is scheduled for gallbladder surgery. With regard to the informed consent, which would the nurse implement **first** to facilitate the scheduled surgery?
1. Check for the identity of the client's legal guardian.
2. Inform the legal guardian about advance directives.
3. Arrange for the surgeon to provide informed consent.
4. Ensure that the legal guardian signed the informed consent.

Level of Cognitive Ability: Applying
Client Needs: Safe and Effective Care Environment
Clinical Judgment/Cognitive Skills: Take Action
Integrated Process: Nursing Process/Implementation
Content Area: Leadership/Management: Ethical/Legal
Health Problems: Mental Health: Neurocognitive Impairment
Priority Concepts: Ethics; Health Care Law

Answer: 1
Rationale: A client with a neurocognitive impairment is not competent to sign an informed consent, so the nurse would first check the identity of the client's legal guardian. This action fulfills part of the nurse's duty in informed consent, helps avoid improperly signed documents, and directs the surgeon to the legal representatives of the client's interests. The client and/or legal guardian is asked about the existence of an advance directive at the time of admission, so this would have already been done, making option 2 incorrect. The surgeon is responsible for obtaining the informed consent, but based on the options provided, option 3 is not the first nursing action. Likewise, option 4 is not the first action; the nurse checks identity of the legal guardian first.
Test-Taking Strategy: Note the strategic word, *first*, and focus on the subject, obtaining permission for the surgical procedure for a client who is mentally impaired. To ensure safe, effective care, the nurse ensures the identity of the client's legal guardian before checking any other aspect of obtaining informed consent.
Priority Nursing Tip: A mentally or emotionally incompetent client is an individual who has been declared incompetent, is unconscious, is under the influence of chemical agents such as alcohol or drugs, or has chronic dementia or another mental deficiency that impairs thought processes and the ability to make decisions.
Reference: Potter, P., et al. (2021). *Fundamentals of nursing* (10th ed., pp. 312–313). Elsevier.

❖ **150.** A client with a diagnosis of an acute respiratory infection and sinus tachycardia is admitted to the hospital. The nurse would develop a plan of care for the client and include which intervention?
1. Limiting oral and intravenous fluids
2. Measuring the client's pulse once each shift
3. Providing the client with short, frequent walks
4. Eliminating sources of caffeine from meal trays

Level of Cognitive Ability: Applying
Client Needs: Safe and Effective Care Environment
Clinical Judgment/Cognitive Skills: Generate Solutions
Integrated Process: Nursing Process/Planning
Content Area: Adult Health: Respiratory
Health Problems: Adult Health: Respiratory: Infections of the Upper Airway
Priority Concepts: Perfusion; Safety

Answer: 4
Rationale: In sinus tachycardia, the heart rate is greater than 100 beats per minute. Sinus tachycardia is often caused by fever, physical and emotional stress, heart failure, hypovolemia, certain medications, nicotine, caffeine, and exercise. Fluid restriction and exercise will not alleviate tachycardia and could exacerbate the condition. Measuring the client's pulse during each shift will not decrease the heart rate. Additionally, the pulse needs to be taken more frequently than once each shift.
Test-Taking Strategy: Focus on the subject, sinus tachycardia. Recalling the causes of tachycardia will direct you to the correct option. Remember that caffeine is a stimulant and will increase the heart rate.
Priority Nursing Tip: If the client experiences sinus tachycardia, the physician is notified. The cause is identified, and the heart rate is decreased to normal by treating the underlying cause.
Reference: Ignatavicius, D., et al. (2021). *Medical-surgical nursing: Concepts for interprofessional collaborative care* (10th ed., p. 646). Elsevier.

151. Which action would the nurse implement to obtain a urine specimen for a urinalysis from a client with an indwelling urinary catheter recovering from prostate surgery?
1. Cleanse the perineum.
2. Detach the tubing of the drainage bag.
3. Use a sterile container for the specimen.
4. Aspirate the urine from the drainage bag port.

Level of Cognitive Ability: Applying
Client Needs: Safe and Effective Care Environment
Clinical Judgment/Cognitive Skills: Take Action
Integrated Process: Nursing Process/Implementation
Content Area: Skills: Specimen Collection
Health Problems: Adult Health: Renal and Urinary: Obstructive Problems
Priority Concepts: Elimination; Infection

Answer: 4
Rationale: A specimen for urinalysis does not need to be sterile; however, the indwelling urinary catheter system must remain sterile to reduce the risk of infection. Therefore, the nurse obtains the specimen using sterile technique and obtains a fresh specimen by aspirating urine from the drainage bag port after sanitizing the port and inserting a sterile needle. The nurse avoids breaking the integrity of the urinary collection system to prevent contamination. The nurse also avoids taking urine from the urinary drainage bag because the urine is less likely to reflect the current client status and because urine undergoes chemical changes and particulate matter settles over time. A sterile container is unnecessary for a urinalysis, and because the client has an indwelling catheter, perineal cleansing before obtaining a urine specimen is unnecessary.
Test-Taking Strategy: Focus on the subject of obtaining a urine specimen for urinalysis. Basic principles of asepsis direct you to eliminate options 2 and 3. Eliminate option 1 because the client has an indwelling catheter.
Priority Nursing Tip: Specimens need to be labeled properly and placed in a biohazard bag for transport to the laboratory. Specific agency procedure is always followed.
Reference: Potter, P., et al. (2021). *Fundamentals of nursing* (10th ed., pp. 1170, 1179). Elsevier.

Client Needs

152. An unlicensed assistive personnel (UAP) is caring for a client who has an indwelling urinary catheter as part of treatment for renal calculi. Which direction would the registered nurse provide to the UAP regarding urinary catheter care?
1. Loop the tubing under the client's leg.
2. Place the tubing below the client's knee.
3. Use soap and water to cleanse the perineal area.
4. Keep the drainage bag above the level of the bladder.

Level of Cognitive Ability: Applying
Client Needs: Safe and Effective Care Environment
Clinical Judgment/Cognitive Skills: Take Action
Integrated Process: Teaching and Learning
Content Area: Skills: Elimination
Health Problems: Adult Health: Renal and Urinary: Calculi
Priority Concepts: Elimination; Care Coordination

Answer: 3
Rationale: Proper care of an indwelling urinary catheter is especially important to prevent infection. The perineal area is cleansed thoroughly using mild soap and water at least three times a day and after a bowel movement. The drainage tubing is not placed or looped under the client's leg because this would inhibit the flow of urine. The drainage bag is kept below the level of the bladder to prevent urine from being trapped in the bladder. The tubing must drain freely at all times.
Test-Taking Strategy: Eliminate options 1 and 2 first because they are comparable or alike in that they both address the tubing. From the remaining options, noting the word *above* in option 4 will assist in eliminating this option. Also, note that option 3 relates to preventing infection.
Priority Nursing Tip: If permitted, the client with a urinary catheter needs to consume a daily fluid intake of 2000 to 2500 mL.
Reference: Potter, P., et al. (2021). *Fundamentals of nursing* (10th ed., pp. pp. 1189–1191). Elsevier.

153. The nurse is assigned to care for a client with a diagnosis of preeclampsia. The nurse would plan to implement which action to provide a safe environment?
1. Maintain fluid and sodium restrictions.
2. Take the client's vital signs every 4 hours.
3. Turn off the room lights and draw the window shades.
4. Encourage visits from family and friends for psychosocial support.

Level of Cognitive Ability: Applying
Client Needs: Safe and Effective Care Environment
Clinical Judgment/Cognitive Skills: Generate Solutions
Integrated Process: Nursing Process/Planning
Content Area: Maternity: Antepartum
Health Problems: Maternity: Gestational Hypertension/Preeclampsia and Eclampsia
Priority Concepts: Reproduction; Safety

Answer: 3
Rationale: Clients with preeclampsia are at risk of developing eclampsia (seizures). Bright lights and sudden loud noises may initiate seizures in this client. A client with preeclampsia needs to be placed in a dimly lighted, quiet, private room. Clients with preeclampsia have decreased plasma volume, and adequate fluid and sodium intake is necessary to maintain fluid volume and tissue perfusion. Vital signs need to be monitored more frequently than every 4 hours when preeclampsia is present. Visitors need to be limited to allow for rest and to prevent overstimulation.
Test-Taking Strategy: Focus on the subject, preeclampsia. Eliminate option 4 because it is not a physiologic need and provides too much stimulation for this client. Eliminate option 2 next because vital signs need to be monitored more frequently than every 4 hours. From the remaining options, knowing that seizures may be precipitated by sudden loud noises and bright lights will assist in directing you to the correct option.
Priority Nursing Tip: The signs of preeclampsia are hypertension and proteinuria. Swelling (edema), particularly in the face and hands, often accompanies preeclampsia but is not considered a reliable sign of preeclampsia, however, because it also occurs in many normal pregnancies.
Reference: McKinney, E. S., et al. (2022). *Maternal child nursing* (6th ed., p. 545). Elsevier.

❖ **154.** The client being treated for possible lung cancer is scheduled for a bronchoscopy. Which **priority** action would the nurse plan to implement?
1. Confirm informed consent.
2. Ask the client about allergies to shellfish.
3. Restrict the diet to clear liquids on the day of the test.
4. Administer preprocedure antibiotics prophylactically.

Level of Cognitive Ability: Applying
Client Needs: Safe and Effective Care Environment
Clinical Judgment/Cognitive Skills: Generate Solutions
Integrated Process: Nursing Process/Planning
Content Area: Foundations of Care: Diagnostic Tests
Health Problems: Adult Health: Cancer: Laryngeal and Lung
Priority Concepts: Ethics; Health Care Law

Answer: 1
Rationale: Bronchoscopy is a procedure in which the physician uses a fiber-optic bronchoscope for direct visualization of the larynx, trachea, and bronchi. Because the procedure is invasive, it requires obtaining informed consent from the client. It is unnecessary to inquire about allergies to shellfish before this procedure because contrast dye is not injected. The client is kept on nothing by mouth (NPO) status for at least 6 hours before the procedure. There is also no need for prophylactic antibiotics.
Test-Taking Strategy: Note the strategic word, *priority*. Focus on the subject, bronchoscopy. Recalling that bronchoscopy is an invasive procedure and requires an informed consent will direct you to the correct option.
Priority Nursing Tip: Any procedure that is invasive requires an informed consent from the client.
Reference: Pagana, K., Pagana, T., & Pagana, T. N. (2021). *Mosby's Diagnostic and laboratory test reference* (15th ed., p. 186). Elsevier.

155. The nurse hangs a 1000-mL intravenous (IV) solution of D_5W (5% dextrose in water) at 0900 and sets the infusion rate to administer 100 mL/hr. On assessment of the IV infusion, the nurse expects that the remaining amount of solution in the IV bag at 1400 will be represented at which level? **Fill in the blank.**
Answer: _____ mL
Level of Cognitive Ability: Evaluating
Client Needs: Safe and Effective Care Environment
Clinical Judgment/Cognitive Skills: Evaluate Outcomes
Integrated Process: Nursing Process/Evaluation
Content Area: Skills: Dosage Calculations
Health Problems: N/A
Priority Concepts: Clinical Judgment; Safety

Answer: 500
Rationale: The nurse hangs an IV solution at 0900 and sets the IV solution to infuse at 100 mL/hr. A total of 500 mL will be infused in the 5 elapsed hours. At 1400 the nurse would expect 500 mL of solution to be safely infused and 500 mL to be remaining.
Test-Taking Strategy: Focus on the subject, infusion of an IV at 100 mL/hr. In a 5-hour period, 500 mL of fluid will infuse for a solution infusing at 100 mL/hr.
Priority Nursing Tip: Monitor IV flow rates frequently (per agency policy) even if the IV solution is being administered via an electronic infusion device.
Reference: Potter, P., et al. (2021). *Fundamentals of nursing* (10th ed., pp. 1022–1023). Elsevier.

❖ **156.** The nurse is planning care for a client with a diagnosis of acute glomerulonephritis. Which action would the nurse instruct the unlicensed assistive personnel (UAP) to implement in the care of the client?
1. Ambulate the client frequently.
2. Encourage a diet that is high in protein.
3. Monitor the temperature every 2 hours.
4. Remove the water pitcher from the bedside.

Level of Cognitive Ability: Applying
Client Needs: Safe and Effective Care Environment
Clinical Judgment/Cognitive Skills: Take Action
Integrated Process: Nursing Process/Implementation
Content Area: Leadership/Management: Delegating/Supervising
Health Problems: Adult Health: Renal and Urinary: Urinary Tract Inflammation/Infection/Trauma
Priority Concepts: Fluids and Electrolytes; Care Coordination

Answer: 4
Rationale: A client with acute glomerulonephritis commonly experiences fluid volume excess and fatigue. Interventions include fluid restriction, as well as monitoring weight and intake and output. The client may be placed on bed rest or at least encouraged to rest because a direct correlation exists among proteinuria, hematuria, edema, and increased activity levels. The diet is high in calories but low in protein. It is unnecessary to monitor the temperature as frequently as every 2 hours.
Test-Taking Strategy: Focus on the subject, acute glomerulonephritis. Knowing that the client needs rest eliminates option 1. The question provides no information about the client's actual temperature, so option 3 is eliminated next. From the remaining options, it is necessary to know either that fluid is restricted or protein is limited.
Priority Nursing Tip: A cause of glomerulonephritis is infection of the pharynx with group A beta-hemolytic streptococcus.
Reference: Ignatavicius, D., et al. (2021). *Medical-surgical nursing: Concepts for interprofessional collaborative care* (10th ed., pp. 1360–1361). Elsevier.

157. The nurse is caring for a client with a diagnosis of a C6 spinal cord injury during the spinal shock phase. Which action would the nurse implement when preparing the client to sit in a chair?
1. Apply knee splints to stabilize the joints during transfer.
2. Teach the client to lock the knees during the pivoting stage of the transfer.
3. Administer a vasodilator in order to improve circulation of the lower limbs.
4. Raise the head of the bed slowly to decrease orthostatic hypotensive episodes.

Level of Cognitive Ability: Applying
Client Needs: Safe and Effective Care Environment
Clinical Judgment/Cognitive Skills: Take Action
Integrated Process: Nursing Process/Implementation
Content Area: Complex Care: Trauma
Health Problems: Adult Health: Neurologic: Spinal Cord Injury
Priority Concepts: Mobility; Safety

Answer: 4
Rationale: Spinal shock is a sudden depression of reflex activity in the spinal cord that occurs below the level of injury (areflexia). It is often accompanied by vasodilation in the lower limbs, which results in a fall in blood pressure upon rising. The client can have dizziness and feel faint. The nurse would provide for a gradual progression in head elevation while monitoring the blood pressure. The use of splints would impair the transfer. Clients with cervical cord injuries cannot lock their knees. A vasodilator would exacerbate the problem.
Test-Taking Strategy: Focusing on the subject, spinal cord injury during spinal shock phase, will assist in eliminating options 1 and 2. From the remaining options, recalling that spinal shock is accompanied by vasodilation will direct you to the correct option.
Priority Nursing Tip: Spinal shock is also called *spinal shock syndrome.* It occurs immediately as the cord's response to the injury. The client develops complete but temporary loss of motor, sensory, reflex, and autonomic function. This often lasts less than 48 hours but may continue for several weeks.
Reference: Lewis, S., et al. (2020). *Medical-surgical nursing: Assessment and management of clinical problems* (11th ed., pp. 1404, 1410). Elsevier.

❖ **158.** The nurse checks the lithium level result on a client taking lithium. Based on the test result, which **priority** intervention would the nurse implement?

Laboratory Results

Test and Results	Reference Range
Lithium 3.9 mEq/L (3.9 mmol/L)	0.6 to 1.2 mEq/L (0.6 to 1.2 mmol/L)

1. Determining visual acuity
2. Assisting with ambulation
3. Monitoring intake and output
4. Instituting seizure precautions

Level of Cognitive Ability: Analyzing
Client Needs: Safe and Effective Care Environment
Clinical Judgment/Cognitive Skills: Take Action
Integrated Process: Nursing Process/Implementation
Content Area: Pharmacology: Psychotherapeutics: Mood Stabilizers
Health Problems: Mental Health: Mood Disorders
Priority Concepts: Clinical Judgment; Safety

Answer: 4
Rationale: The lithium level must be monitored closely in a client taking lithium. A therapeutic regimen is designed to attain a serum lithium level of 0.6 to 1.2 mEq/L (0.6 to 1.2 mmol/L) for maintenance treatment. This client's lithium level is in the toxic range, and seizures may occur at levels of 3.5 mEq/L (3.5 mmol/L) and higher. While the remaining options are appropriate interventions, they are not the priority because they are not related to the possibility of toxicity.
Test-Taking Strategy: Note the strategic word, *priority*. Focus on the medication name and recall that it can cause toxicity. Next, recall the manifestations that occur in a toxic lithium level. This will direct you to option 4.
Priority Nursing Tip: The nurse would instruct the client prescribed lithium to maintain a fluid intake of six to eight glasses of water a day and an adequate salt intake to prevent lithium toxicity.
Reference: Varcarolis, E. & Fosbre, C. (2021). *Essentials of psychiatric mental health nursing: A communication approach to evidence-based care* (4th ed., pp. 240–241). Elsevier.

159. When a hospitalized child develops a rash that covers the trunk and extremities, the nurse notes in the history that the child was exposed to varicella 2 weeks ago. Which nursing intervention has **priority**?
1. Immediately reassign the child's roommate.
2. Place the child in a private room on strict isolation.
3. Confirm the exposure occurred with the child's parent.
4. Assess the progression of the rash and report it to the pediatrician.

Level of Cognitive Ability: Applying
Client Needs: Safe and Effective Care Environment
Clinical Judgment/Cognitive Skills: Take Action
Integrated Process: Nursing Process/Implementation
Content Area: Foundations of Care: Infection Control
Health Problems: Pediatric-Specific: Communicable Diseases
Priority Concepts: Infection; Safety

Answer: 2
Rationale: The child with undiagnosed rash needs to be placed on strict isolation. Varicella causes a profuse rash on the trunk with a sparse rash on the extremities. The incubation period is 14 to 21 days. It is important to prevent the spread of this communicable disease by placing the child in isolation until further diagnosis and treatment are made. None of the other options address the need to prevent the spread of the disease.
Test-Taking Strategy: Noting the strategic word, *priority*, and the subject, exposure to varicella, will direct you to option 2. This action will prevent exposure of this communicable disease to others.
Priority Nursing Tip: Varicella-zoster virus can be transmitted via direct contact, droplet (airborne) spread, or contaminated objects.
Reference: McKinney, E. S., et al. (2022). *Maternal child nursing* (6th ed., p. 918). Elsevier.

❖ **160.** The nurse manager is observing the interaction between a new staff nurse and a client currently receiving hemodialysis. Which intervention would the nurse manager implement when the nurse and client are both drinking coffee and discussing the client's feeling about the procedure?
1. Getting a cup of coffee and joining in on the conversation
2. Determining whether or not the client should be drinking coffee
3. Complementing the staff nurse on the development of a good therapeutic relation
4. Asking the staff nurse to refrain from eating and drinking in the hemodialysis area

Level of Cognitive Ability: Applying
Client Needs: Safe and Effective Care Environment
Clinical Judgment/Cognitive Skills: Take Action
Integrated Process: Nursing Process/Implementation
Content Area: Foundations of Care: Infection Control
Health Problems: Adult Health: Renal and Urinary: Acute Kidney Injury and Chronic Kidney Disease
Priority Concepts: Infection; Safety

Answer: 4
Rationale: The nurse manager would ask the second nurse to stop eating and drinking in the client area. A potential complication of hemodialysis is the acquisition of dialysis-associated hepatitis B. This is a concern for clients (who may carry the virus), client families (at risk from contact with the client and with environmental surfaces), and staff (who may acquire the virus from contact with the client's blood). This risk is minimized by the use of standard precautions; appropriate hand washing and sterilization procedures; and the prohibition of eating, drinking, or other hand-to-mouth activity in the hemodialysis unit. None of the remaining options relate to management of this potential complication.
Test-Taking Strategy: Focus on the subject, hemodialysis. Recall the complications associated with hemodialysis and principles related to standard precautions to direct you to the correct option.
Priority Nursing Tip: The nurse needs to measure the client's weight before and after the hemodialysis procedure to determine the amount of fluid removed during the procedure.
Reference: Ignatavicius, D., et al. (2021). *Medical-surgical nursing: Concepts for interprofessional collaborative care* (10th ed., pp. 1399–1400). Elsevier.

161. A new nurse is learning the functions of the unit's nurse manager. Which functions are included? **Select all that apply.**
☐ 1. Recruiting new employees
☐ 2. Conducting regular staff meetings
☐ 3. Assisting staff in meeting annual goals
☐ 4. Monitoring professional standards of practice on the nursing unit
☐ 5. Delegating problem-solving of client or family complaints to all nursing staff
☐ 6. Writing prescriptions for the physician when conducting rounds

Level of Cognitive Ability: Applying
Client Needs: Safe and Effective Care Environment
Clinical Judgment/Cognitive Skills: Take Action
Integrated Process: Nursing Process/Implementation
Content Area: Leadership/Management: Management of Care
Health Problems: N/A
Priority Concepts: Leadership; Professional Identity

Answer: 1, 2, 3, 4
Rationale: Responsibilities of the nurse manager (middle manager) include recruiting new employees (interviewing and hiring), conducting regular staff meetings, assisting staff in meeting annual goals for the unit and systems needed to accomplish goals, monitoring professional standards of practice on the nursing unit, developing an ongoing staff development plan, conducting routine staff evaluations, acting as a role model, submitting staff schedules for the unit, conducting regular client rounds and problem-solving client and family complaints, establishing and implementing a unit quality improvement plan, and conducting rounds with physicians. The nurse is not responsible for writing prescriptions for physicians when conducting rounds; the physician is responsible for writing prescriptions.
Test-Taking Strategy: Focus on the subject, the responsibilities of the nurse manager. Recalling that the nurse manager functions in the role of a leader and facilitator and recalling the legal issues relating to physicians' prescriptions will assist in answering the question. Also, option 5 can be eliminated because of the closed-ended word "all."
Priority Nursing Tip: An effective leader and manager is visible to employees, is flexible, and provides guidance, assistance, and feedback to employees.
Reference: Zerwekh, J., & Zerwekh Garneau, A. (2021). *Nursing today: Transition and trends* (10th ed., pp. 150, 218–220). Elsevier.

❖ **162.** Which statements describe the characteristics of team nursing? **Select all that apply.**

☐ 1. A registered nurse (RN) leads a team of staff members.

☐ 2. Each nurse assumes responsibility for a specific task.

☐ 3. Team members provide direct care to groups of clients.

☐ 4. Unlicensed assistive personnel (UAP) are given a client assignment.

☐ 5. The RN assumes responsibility for a caseload of clients over time.

☐ 6. Team nursing maintains continuity of care across nursing shifts, days, and home care visits.

Level of Cognitive Ability: Understanding
Client Needs: Safe and Effective Care Environment
Clinical Judgment/Cognitive Skills: Generate Solutions
Integrated Process: Nursing Process/Planning
Content Area: Leadership/Management: Management of Care
Health Problems: N/A
Priority Concepts: Caregiving; Leadership

Answer: 1, 3, 4
Rationale: In team nursing, an RN leads a team that is comprised of other RNs, licensed practical or licensed vocational nurses, and UAPs and technicians. The team members provide direct client care to groups of clients under the direct supervision of the RN team leader. In this model, UAPs are given client assignments rather than being assigned particular nursing tasks. In functional nursing, tasks are divided, with one nurse assuming responsibility for specific tasks. Primary nursing is a model in which the RN assumes responsibility for a caseload of clients over time. In primary nursing, continuity of care across nursing shifts, days, and home care visits is maintained.
Test-Taking Strategy: Focus on the subject, the characteristics of team nursing. Thinking about the definition of and the concepts related to the word *team* will assist in answering the question.
Priority Nursing Tip: In team nursing, the team leader determines the work assignment. Each staff member works fully within the realm of their educational and clinical expertise and job description.
Reference: Zerwekh, J., & Zerwekh Garneau, A. (2021). *Nursing today: Transition and trends* (10th ed., pp. 359–360). Elsevier.

---

163. The nurse is creating a discharge teaching plan for a client who sustained a spinal cord injury. To provide for a safe environment regarding home care, which option would be the **priority** in the discharge teaching plan?

1. Assisting the client to deal with long-term care placement

2. Including the client's significant others in the teaching session

3. Following up on laboratory and diagnostic tests that were prescribed

4. Including information the primary health care provider has indicated

Level of Cognitive Ability: Analyzing
Client Needs: Safe and Effective Care Environment
Clinical Judgment/Cognitive Skills: Generate Solutions
Integrated Process: Clinical Judgment; Nursing Process/Planning
Content Area: Adult Health: Neurologic
Health Problems: Adult Health: Neurologic: Spinal Cord Injury
Priority Concepts: Patient Education; Safety

Answer: 2
Rationale: Involving the client's significant others in discharge teaching is a priority in planning for the client with a spinal cord injury. The client will need the support of the significant others. Knowledge and understanding of what to expect will help both the client and significant others deal with the client's limitations. Long-term placement is not the only option for a client with a spinal cord injury. Laboratory and diagnostic testing are not priority discharge instructions for this client. A primary health care provider's prescription is not necessary for discharge planning and teaching; this is an independent nursing action.
Test-Taking Strategy: Note the strategic word, *priority*. Focus on the subject, a safe home care environment for a client with a spinal cord injury. Eliminate option 4 because, although the primary health care provider's prescriptions need to be addressed, teaching is an independent nursing action. Eliminate option 1 because long-term placement is not the only choice for a client with a spinal cord injury. There is no indication that laboratory or diagnostic tests have been imminently prescribed. Remember that home care and support will be needed.
Priority Nursing Tip: Involving the client's significant others in discharge teaching will assist in ensuring support for the client. However, the client needs to be consulted about the inclusion of others in the teaching process before initiating the plan.
Reference: Ignatavicius, D., et al. (2021). *Medical-surgical nursing: Concepts for interprofessional collaborative care* (10th ed., pp. 885–886). Elsevier.

❖ **164.** The nurse observes a client looking frightened and reporting "feeling out of control." Which therapeutic approach by the nurse is **most appropriate** to maintain a safe environment?
1. Administer a PRN antianxiety medication immediately.
2. Provide isolation for the client in the unit's "time-out" room.
3. Observe the client in an ongoing manner, but do not intervene.
4. Encourage the client to talk about their feelings in a quiet setting.

Level of Cognitive Ability: Analyzing
Client Needs: Safe and Effective Care Environment
Clinical Judgment/Cognitive Skills: Generate Solutions
Integrated Process: Clinical Judgment; Nursing Process/Planning
Content Area: Mental Health
Health Problems: Mental Health: Coping
Priority Concepts: Anxiety; Communication

Answer: 4
Rationale: The anxiety symptoms demonstrated by this client require some form of intervention. Moving the client to a quiet setting decreases environmental stimuli. Talking provides the nurse an opportunity to assess the cause of the client's feelings and identify appropriate interventions. Medication is used only when other noninvasive approaches have been unsuccessful. Isolation is appropriate if a client is a danger to self or others.
Test-Taking Strategy: Use therapeutic communication techniques. Focus on the strategic words, *most appropriate.* Option 4 is the only choice that addresses the client's feelings. Remember that a client's feelings are most important.
Priority Nursing Tip: The nurse would not leave a client who feels "out of control." The nurse needs to be sure that the client is in a quiet area, encourage the client to talk about their feelings, and determine what the client considers to be their own needs.
Reference: Varcarolis, E. & Fosbre, C. (2021). *Essentials of psychiatric mental health nursing: A communication approach to evidence-based care* (4th ed., pp. 142, 145, 147). Elsevier.

165. A client with a diagnosis of urolithiasis is scheduled for extracorporeal shock wave lithotripsy. Which information would the nurse provide to ensure that the client understands the procedure?
1. There is usually no discomfort involved with this procedure.
2. Hematuria is not a side effect associated with this procedure.
3. The stone granules are passed in the urine within a few days after the procedure.
4. The stone is broken up by a vibrating needle that is inserted into the urinary tract.

Level of Cognitive Ability: Applying
Client Needs: Safe and Effective Care Environment
Clinical Judgment/Cognitive Skills: Take Action
Integrated Process: Teaching and Learning
Content Area: Foundations of Care: Diagnostic Tests
Health Problems: Adult Health: Renal and Urinary: Calculi
Priority Concepts: Patient Education; Elimination

Answer: 3
Rationale: In extracorporeal shock wave lithotripsy, a noninvasive procedure, shock waves are administered that shatter the stone without damaging the surrounding tissues. The stone is broken into fine sand, which is passed in the client's urine within a few days after the procedure. The client may feel some discomfort from the shock waves. Hematuria is common after the procedure. The presence of clots in the urine needs to be reported to the primary health care provider. Clots could indicate a complication such as a hematoma.
Test-Taking Strategy: Eliminate options 1 and 2 first because of the closed-ended words "no" and "not" in these options. From the remaining options, recalling that the procedure is noninvasive and is done via shock waves (not a vibrating needle) will direct you to the correct option.
Priority Nursing Tip: After extracorporeal shock wave lithotripsy, the client is instructed to increase fluid intake to flush out stone fragments.
Reference: Ignatavicius, D., et al. (2021). *Medical-surgical nursing: Concepts for interprofessional collaborative care* (10th ed., pp. 1348–1349). Elsevier.

❖ **166.** To maintain a safe environment, the nurse would determine which clients require contact precautions based on the modes of disease transmission? **(Refer to chart.) Select all that apply.**

CLIENTS
- ☐ **1.** A child with mumps
- ☐ **2.** A client with scabies
- ☐ **3.** A child with streptococcal pharyngitis
- ☐ **4.** A client with pulmonary tuberculosis
- ☐ **5.** A child with respiratory syncytial virus (RSV)
- ☐ **6.** A client infected with a multi–drug–resistant organism

Level of Cognitive Ability: Applying
Client Needs: Safe and Effective Care Environment
Clinical Judgment/Cognitive Skills: Generate Solutions
Integrated Process: Clinical Judgment; Nursing Process/Planning
Content Area: Foundations of Care: Infection Control
Health Problems: N/A
Priority Concepts: Infection; Safety

Answer: 2, 5, 6
Rationale: Contact precautions are initiated when disease transmission occurs from direct contact with the client or the client's environment. Diseases that require the use of contact precautions include colonization or infection with multi-drug–resistant organisms, respiratory syncytial virus, shigella and other enteric pathogens, wound infections, herpes simplex, scabies, and disseminated varicella zoster. Clients with mumps or streptococcal pharyngitis require droplet precautions. A client with pulmonary tuberculosis requires airborne precautions.
Test-Taking Strategy: Focus on the **subject,** clients who require contact precautions. Read each client diagnosis. Determining the mode of transmission for each illness will assist in answering this question correctly.
Priority Nursing Tip: Contact precautions require placing the client in a private room or with a cohort client in certain situations.
Reference: Potter, P., et al. (2021). *Fundamentals of nursing* (10th ed., p. 438). Elsevier.

167. The emergency room nurse is planning the discharge instructions for an adult client who is a victim of family violence. The nurse would understand that it is **most important** that which information is included in the discharge plans?
1. Instructions to call the police the next time the abuse occurs
2. Exploration of the pros and cons of remaining with the abusive family member
3. Specific information regarding "safe havens" or shelters in the client's neighborhood
4. Specific information about current opportunities to enroll in local self-defense classes

Level of Cognitive Ability: Applying
Client Needs: Safe and Effective Care Environment
Clinical Judgment/Cognitive Skills: Generate Solutions
Integrated Process: Nursing Process/Planning
Content Area: Mental Health
Health Problems: Mental Health: Violence
Priority Concepts: Interpersonal Violence; Safety

Answer: 3
Rationale: For the victim of family violence, any of the options might be included in the discharge plan at some point if long-term therapy or a long-term relationship with the nurse is established. The question refers to an emergency department setting. It is most important to assist victims of abuse with identifying a plan for how to remove self from harmful situations should they arise again. An abused person is usually reluctant to call the police. It is not the best time for the nurse to explore the pros and cons of remaining with the abusive family member; additionally, this action does not ensure safety for the victim. Teaching the victim to fight back (as in the use of self-defense) is not the best action when dealing with a violent person.
Test-Taking Strategy: Note the strategic words, *most important.* Use Maslow's Hierarchy of Needs theory. Remember that if a physiologic need is not present, then safety is the priority. This will direct you to the correct option.
Priority Nursing Tip: In a victim of violence, self-esteem becomes diminished with chronic abuse. Victims may blame themselves for the violence and be unable to see a way out of the situation.
Reference: Varcarolis, E., & Fosbre, C. (2021). *Essentials of psychiatric mental health nursing: A communication approach to evidence-based care* (4th ed., pp. 349–350). Elsevier.

❖ **168.** During an emergency code situation, a physician about to defibrillate a client diagnosed in ventricular fibrillation says in a loud voice, "CLEAR!" Which action would the nurse **immediately** implement?
   1. Shut off the mechanical ventilator.
   2. Shut off the intravenous infusion going into the client's arm.
   3. Place the conductive gel pads for defibrillation on the client's chest.
   4. Step away from the bed and make sure that all others have done the same.

Level of Cognitive Ability: Applying
Client Needs: Safe and Effective Care Environment
Clinical Judgment/Cognitive Skills: Take Action
Integrated Process: Clinical Judgment; Nursing Process/Implementation
Content Area: Complex Care: Emergency Situations/Management
Health Problems: Adult Health: Cardiovascular: Dysrhythmias
Priority Concepts: Perfusion; Safety

Answer: 4
Rationale: For the safety of all personnel, when the defibrillator paddles are being discharged, all personnel must stand back and be clear of all contact with the client or the client's bed. It is the primary responsibility of the person defibrillating to communicate the "clear" message loudly enough for all to hear and ensure their compliance. All personnel must immediately comply with this command. Stepping back from the bed prevents the nurse or others from being defibrillated along with the client. A ventilator is not in use during a code; rather, an Ambu (resuscitation) bag is used. Shutting off the intravenous infusion has no useful purpose. The gel pads should have been placed on the client's chest before the defibrillator paddles were applied.
Test-Taking Strategy: Focus on the subject, the procedure for defibrillation. Note the strategic word, *immediately*. Recalling the risks associated with this procedure and noting the word *clear* in the question will direct you to the correct option.
Priority Nursing Tip: To perform defibrillation, one paddle is placed at the third intercostal space to the right of the sternum; the other is placed at the fifth intercostal space on the left midaxillary line.
Reference: Lewis, S., et al. (2020). *Medical-surgical nursing: Assessment and management of clinical problems* (11th ed., p. 769). Elsevier.

169. A client with a diagnosis of chronic kidney disease has an indwelling peritoneal catheter in the abdomen for peritoneal dialysis. While bathing, the client spills water on the abdominal dressing. Which action would the nurse perform to **best** ensure client safety?
   1. Change the dressing.
   2. Reinforce the dressing.
   3. Flush the peritoneal dialysis catheter.
   4. Scrub the catheter with povidone-iodine.

Level of Cognitive Ability: Applying
Client Needs: Safe and Effective Care Environment
Clinical Judgment/Cognitive Skills: Take Action
Integrated Process: Nursing Process/Implementation
Content Area: Skills: Wound Care
Health Problems: Adult Health: Renal and Urinary: Acute Kidney Injury and Chronic Kidney Disease
Priority Concepts: Clinical Judgment; Safety

Answer: 1
Rationale: Clients with peritoneal dialysis catheters are at high risk for infection. A dressing that is wet is a conduit for bacteria to reach the catheter insertion site. The nurse ensures that the dressing is kept dry at all times. Reinforcing the dressing is not a safe practice to prevent infection in this circumstance. Flushing the catheter is not indicated. Scrubbing the catheter with povidone-iodine is done at the time of connection or disconnection of peritoneal dialysis.
Test-Taking Strategy: Note the strategic word, *best*. Focus on the subject, a wet dressing to a peritoneal catheter. The correct option would focus on the dressing, not the catheter. Therefore, eliminate options 3 and 4. Knowing that it is better to change a wet dressing than reinforce it will direct you to the correct option.
Priority Nursing Tip: If the outflow of the peritoneal dialysis solution is cloudy or opaque, the nurse would suspect peritonitis.
Reference: Ignatavicius, D., et al. (2021). *Medical-surgical nursing: Concepts for interprofessional collaborative care* (10th ed., pp. 290, 1404). Elsevier.

❖ **170.** The nurse manager is providing an educational session to the nursing staff on the safe use of physical restraints. Which are examples of safety guidelines when using physical restraints? **Select all that apply.**
- ☐ 1. Restraints need to be secured with a quick-release tie.
- ☐ 2. A physician's prescription is required.
- ☐ 3. Restraints are secured to side rails so that they can be easily removed as necessary.
- ☐ 4. Restraints are used when other measures have failed to prevent self-injury or injury to others.
- ☐ 5. Restraints can be used as a usual part of treatment plans, as indicated by client's condition or symptoms.
- ☐ 6. The use of restraints can be prescribed PRN (as needed) as long as the nurse performs a thorough assessment before applying them.

Level of Cognitive Ability: Applying
Client Needs: Safe and Effective Care Environment
Clinical Judgment/Cognitive Skills: Generate Solutions
Integrated Process: Teaching and Learning
Content Area: Foundations of Care: Safety
Health Problems: N/A
Priority Concepts: Leadership; Safety

Answer: 1, 2, 4
Rationale: A physical restraint is a mechanical or physical device that is used to immobilize a client or extremity. It restricts the freedom of movement or normal access to a client's body. A physician's prescription is required for the use of restraints. Restraints need to be secured with a quick-release tie so that they can be easily removed in an emergency. Restraints are considered for use only when other measures have failed to prevent self-injury or injury to others. Restraints are secured to the bed frame, not the side rails, because the client may be injured if the side rail is lowered. Restraints, not a usual part of treatment plans, may be indicated by the person's condition or symptoms and are not prescribed on a PRN basis.
Test-Taking Strategy: Focus on the subject, guidelines for the safe use of physical restraints. Read each option and carefully think about two issues: client safety and the legalities related to the use of restraints. This will assist in answering the question.
Priority Nursing Tip: The reason for using a restraint needs to be given to the client and the family, and their permission needs to be sought.
Reference: Potter, P., et al. (2021). *Fundamentals of nursing* (10th ed., pp. 414–415). Elsevier.

171. The nurse is planning activities for a client diagnosed with depression who was just admitted to the hospital. Which therapeutic action would the nurse implement as part of the plan?
1. Provide an activity that is quiet and solitary in nature.
2. Plan nothing until the client asks to participate in the milieu.
3. Offer the client a menu of activities and insist that the client participate in all of them.
4. Provide a structured daily program of activities and encourage the client to participate.

Level of Cognitive Ability: Applying
Client Needs: Safe and Effective Care Environment
Clinical Judgment/Cognitive Skills: Take Action
Integrated Process: Nursing Process/Implementation
Content Area: Mental Health
Health Problems: Mental Health: Mood Disorders
Priority Concepts: Functional Ability; Mood and Affect

Answer: 4
Rationale: A depressed person is often withdrawn. In addition, the person experiences difficulty concentrating, loss of interest or pleasure, low energy and fatigue, and feelings of worthlessness and poor self-esteem. The plan of care needs to provide stimulation in a structured environment. Options 1 and 2 are restrictive and offer little or no structure and stimulation. The nurse would not insist that a client participate in all activities.
Test-Taking Strategy: Focus on the subject, a depressed client. Eliminate option 3 first because of the word *insist* and the closed-ended word "all." From the remaining options, noting the word *structured* in option 4 will direct you to this option.
Priority Nursing Tip: For the client with depression, the nurse would provide gentle encouragement to participate in activities of daily living and unit therapies.
Reference: Varcarolis, E., & Fosbre, C. (2021). *Essentials of psychiatric mental health nursing: A communication approach to evidence-based care* (4th ed., p. 210). Elsevier.

Client Needs

❖ **172.** An older client had an open reduction with internal fixation (ORIF) for a hip fracture 4 days ago. Which measure would the nurse implement to provide safe care?
1. Provide ice chips instead of drinking water.
2. Instruct the client to call for help before getting up.
3. Minimize opioid administration to prevent dizziness.
4. Tell the client to roll to the affected side first before getting up.

Level of Cognitive Ability: Applying
Client Needs: Safe and Effective Care Environment
Clinical Judgment/Cognitive Skills: Take Action
Integrated Process: Nursing Process/Implementation
Content Area: Foundations of Care: Safety
Health Problems: Adult Health: Musculoskeletal: Skeletal Injury
Priority Concepts: Mobility; Safety

Answer: 2
Rationale: The nurse instructs the client to call for help before getting up because the client has multiple risk factors for falls, is of older age, has postoperative status, and may also be receiving opioid analgesia. Restricting fluid intake with ice chips is not indicated; besides, adequate hydration is important for maintaining cardiac output and renal function, for keeping respiratory secretions thin, and in preventing constipation. The nurse administers opioid analgesics as indicated and fulfills the nurse's duty owed to the client by acting to resolve pain. The nurse instructs the client to roll to the unaffected side to get up to prevent excessive stress on the fragile surgical wound.
Test-Taking Strategy: Focusing on the **subject,** preventing injury, will direct you to the correct option. Restricting fluid, inadequate pain control, and inaccurate mobility instructions prevent the nurse from fulfilling the duty owed to the client to prevent safe and effective care.
Priority Nursing Tip: The nurse would assign a client at risk for falling to a room near the nurses' station.
Reference: Ignatavicius, D., et al. (2021). *Medical-surgical nursing: Concepts for interprofessional collaborative care* (10th ed., pp. 1043–1044). Elsevier.

173. The nurse assisting in the care of a client who is to be cardioverted would set the monophasic defibrillator to which starting energy levels range, depending on the specific primary health care provider prescription?
1. 50 to 100 joules
2. 200 to 250 joules
3. 250 to 300 joules
4. 350 to 400 joules

Level of Cognitive Ability: Applying
Client Needs: Safe and Effective Care Environment
Clinical Judgment/Cognitive Skills: Take Action
Integrated Process: Nursing Process/Implementation
Content Area: Complex Care: Emergency Situations/Management
Health Problems: Adult Health: Cardiovascular: Dysrhythmias
Priority Concepts: Perfusion; Safety

Answer: 1
Rationale: Cardioversion is synchronized countershock to convert an undesirable rhythm to a stable rhythm. Cardioversion is usually started at 50 to 100 joules. When a client is cardioverted, the defibrillator is charged to the energy level prescribed by the primary health care provider, and the remaining options identify energy levels that are too high for cardioversion.
Test-Taking Strategy: Focus on the **subject,** cardioversion. Remember that, in instances in which cardioversion is used, an underlying cardiac rhythm needs to be converted to a better rhythm; therefore, lower voltages are used.
Priority Nursing Tip: When cardioversion is performed, the defibrillator is synchronized to the client's R wave to avoid discharging the shock during the vulnerable period (T wave).
Reference: Lewis, S., et al. (2020). *Medical-surgical nursing: Assessment and management of clinical problems* (11th ed., p. 770). Elsevier.

174. The nurse has a prescription to get the client out of bed to a chair on the first postoperative day after total knee replacement surgery. Which action is **most appropriate** for the nurse to plan to implement to protect the knee joint?

1. Applying both ice and a compression dressing to the knee while sitting
2. Obtaining a walker to minimize weight bearing by the client on the affected leg
3. Applying a knee immobilizer and then elevating the affected leg while sitting
4. Lifting the client to the bedside chair, leaving the continuous passive motion (CPM) machine in place

Level of Cognitive Ability: Applying
Client Needs: Safe and Effective Care Environment
Clinical Judgment/Cognitive Skills: Generate Solutions
Integrated Process: Nursing Process/Planning
Content Area: Adult Health: Musculoskeletal
Health Problems: Adult Health: Musculoskeletal: Skeletal Injury
Priority Concepts: Mobility; Safety

Answer: 3
Rationale: After a total knee replacement, as prescribed, the nurse assists the client to get out of bed on the first postoperative day after putting a knee immobilizer on the affected joint to provide stability. The leg is elevated while the client is sitting in the chair to minimize edema. A compression dressing should already be in place on the wound. Ice is not used unless prescribed. The surgeon prescribes the weight-bearing limits on the affected leg. A CPM machine is used only while the client is in bed and is initiated when prescribed.
Test-Taking Strategy: Note the strategic words, *most appropriate.* Focus on the subject, transfer of a client with a new total knee replacement. Note the relation between the subject, the words *protect the knee joint* in the question and *knee immobilizer* in option 3.
Priority Nursing Tip: The nurse instructs the client who has had a total knee replacement to avoid leg dangling.
Reference: Lewis, S., et al. (2020). *Medical-surgical nursing: Assessment and management of clinical problems* (11th ed., p. 1473). Elsevier.

175. A client is admitted to the psychiatric unit after a suicide attempt. The nurse would plan which intervention as the **most important** to maintain client safety?

1. Assigning a staff member to remain with the client at all times
2. Requesting that the client promise to alert staff of suicidal thoughts
3. Removing the client's personal clothing and replacing them with a hospital gown
4. Placing the client in a seclusion room where all dangerous articles are removed

Level of Cognitive Ability: Applying
Client Needs: Safe and Effective Care Environment
Clinical Judgment/Cognitive Skills: Generate Solutions
Integrated Process: Nursing Process/Planning
Content Area: Mental Health
Health Problems: Mental Health: Suicide
Priority Concepts: Mood and Affect; Safety

Answer: 1
Rationale: The plan of care must reflect the action that will promote the client's safety. Constant observation by a staff member is necessary. It is not advisable to rely on the client to report suicidal thoughts at this point in the treatment. Removing one's clothing does not maximize all possible safety strategies. Placing the client in seclusion further isolates the client.
Test-Taking Strategy: Focus on the subject, attempted suicide. Note the strategic words, *most important.* Recalling that one-to-one supervision is necessary will direct you to the correct option.
Priority Nursing Tip: The nurse who is caring for a client with a diagnosis of depression needs to always consider the client's risk for attempting suicide.
Reference: Varcarolis, E., & Fosbre, C. (2021). *Essentials of psychiatric mental health nursing: A communication approach to evidence-based care* (4th ed., p. 372). Elsevier.

❖ **176.** The nurse receives a telephone call from a client who states, "I want to kill myself and I have a loaded gun on the table." Which intervention **best** ensures the client's safety?
1. Encouraging the client to unload the gun and go to the hospital
2. Telling the client that suicide is not the way to deal with a problem
3. Using therapeutic communication techniques, especially the reflection of feelings
4. Engaging the client while another staff member contacts the police for their assistance

Level of Cognitive Ability: Applying
Client Needs: Safe and Effective Care Environment
Clinical Judgment/Cognitive Skills: Take Action
Integrated Process: Nursing Process/Implementation
Content Area: Mental Health
Health Problems: Mental Health: Suicide
Priority Concepts: Clinical Judgment; Safety

Answer: 4
Rationale: In a crisis, the nurse must take an authoritative, active role to promote the client's safety. A loaded gun in the home of a client who states, "I want to kill myself" is a crisis. The client's safety is of prime concern. Keeping the client on the phone and getting help to the client is the best intervention. Option 1 lacks the authoritative action stance of securing the client's safety. Option 2 is not a helpful strategy and may block communication. Using therapeutic communication techniques is important, but overuse of reflection may sound uncaring or superficial and is lacking direction and a solution to the immediate problem of the client's safety.
Test-Taking Strategy: Focus on the subject, the potential for suicide. Note the strategic word, *best*. Using Maslow's Hierarchy of Needs theory, recognize that safety is the priority. The only choice that will provide direct help is option 4.
Priority Nursing Tip: Assessment of the client at risk for suicide includes determining if the client has a plan, determining the lethality of the plan, and if the client has a means of carrying out the plan.
Reference: Varcarolis, E., & Fosbre, C. (2021). *Essentials of psychiatric mental health nursing: A communication approach to evidence-based care* (4th ed., p. 370). Elsevier.

177. A client has become physically aggressive toward staff and other clients. What action by the nurse will **best** ensure the safety of the milieu while preserving the client's rights?
1. Sedating the client
2. Applying wrist restraints
3. Contacting the client's physician
4. Considering all possible alternative measures

Level of Cognitive Ability: Applying
Client Needs: Safe and Effective Care Environment
Clinical Judgment/Cognitive Skills: Take Action
Integrated Process: Nursing Process/Implementation
Content Area: Mental Health
Health Problems: Mental Health: Violence
Priority Concepts: Health Care Law; Safety

Answer: 4
Rationale: Before applying restraints, the nurse must exhaust alternative measures to restraints such as a bed alarm, distraction, and a sitter. If the nurse determines that a restraint is necessary, its use is discussed with the client and family, and a prescription is obtained from the physician. The nurse would explain carefully to the client and family the indications for the restraint, the type of restraint selected, and the anticipated duration for its use. Sedation can be considered as a chemical restraint.
Test-Taking Strategy: Focus on the subject, use of restraints. Note the strategic word, *best*. Recall principles and concepts related to ethical and legal issues. Eliminate options 1 and 2 because they both involve the use of restraints. Eliminate option 3, which is not the best action because alternative measures need to be implemented before contacting the physician.
Priority Nursing Tip: If a restraint is used on a client, it must not interfere with any treatments or affect the client's health problem.
Reference: Varcarolis, E., & Fosbre, C. (2021). *Essentials of psychiatric mental health nursing: A communication approach to evidence-based care* (4th ed., pp. 64–65, 385). Elsevier.

❖ **178.** The nurse prepares a client diagnosed with chronic bronchitis who is being discharged from the hospital to receive oxygen therapy at home. Which action would the nurse include in client teaching about oxygen safety?
1. Holding the oxygen tank on your lap when traveling
2. Checking the oxygen level of the tank on a regular basis
3. Lighting candles at least a few feet away from the oxygen tank
4. Reporting low oxygen levels in the tank to the physician

Level of Cognitive Ability: Applying
Client Needs: Safe and Effective Care Environment
Clinical Judgment/Cognitive Skills: Generate Solutions
Integrated Process: Teaching and Learning
Content Area: Skills: Oxygenation
Health Problems: Adult Health: Respiratory: Infections of the Lower Airway
Priority Concepts: Patient Education; Safety

Answer: 2
Rationale: The nurse instructs the client and family to check the oxygen level in the tank on a regular basis to prevent the oxygen from running out. When traveling, the oxygen tank needs to be secured in place to prevent tank damage and a potentially devastating injury from a moving tank. Oxygen is a highly combustible gas, and, although it will not spontaneously burn or cause an explosion, it contributes to a fire if it contacts a spark from a cigarette, burning candle, or electrical equipment. The nurse instructs the client to contact the oxygen supplier about low oxygen levels in the tank; contacting the physician is likely to delay prompt replacement of the oxygen tank.
Test-Taking Strategy: Focus on the subject, safe administration of oxygen. Eliminate option 1 by visualizing travel with an oxygen tank. A heavy metal tank can cause injury if it is not secured in place. Recall that oxygen is a highly combustible gas to eliminate option 3, and recall that oxygen is not supplied by the physician to eliminate option 4.
Priority Nursing Tip: An "Oxygen in Use" sign needs to be placed at the bedside of the client using the oxygen. For the client at home who uses oxygen, the sign needs to be placed in an area that is visible to all, such as the front window.
Reference: Potter, P., et al. (2021). *Fundamentals of nursing* (10th ed., p. 942). Elsevier.

179. Which measure would the nurse implement to ensure electrical safety for a home care client who needs to receive intravenous (IV) pain medication therapy via an IV pump?
1. Keep the pump on at all times.
2. Use an extension cord during ambulation.
3. Obtain a three-pronged grounded plug adapter.
4. Keep the pump plugged in the wall at all times.

Level of Cognitive Ability: Applying
Client Needs: Safe and Effective Care Environment
Clinical Judgment/Cognitive Skills: Take Action
Integrated Process: Nursing Process/Implementation
Content Area: Foundations of Care: Safety
Health Problems: Adult Health: Neurologic: Pain
Priority Concepts: Clinical Judgment; Safety

Answer: 3
Rationale: Electrical equipment requires grounding to prevent static, sparks, and uninterrupted operation. Extension cords are never recommended; instead, the nurse suggests that the client sit close to a three-pronged outlet during therapy. The pump should not be left "on" at all times, and plugging into wall power at all times may be unnecessary because many pump batteries recharge during operation of the pump. Keeping the pump plugged into the wall also can create a trip hazard.
Test-Taking Strategy: Read each option carefully. Focus on the subject, basic electrical safety, to direct you to the correct option. Remember that a three-pronged grounded plug adapter needs to be used.
Priority Nursing Tip: Teach the client and family that electrical equipment would never be used near sinks, bathtubs, or other water sources.
Reference: Potter, P., et al. (2021). *Fundamentals of nursing* (10th ed., p. 403). Elsevier.

❖ **180.** The home care nurse assesses the client's environment for potential safety hazards related to mobility issues causes by osteoarthritis. Which observation requires the nurse to counsel the client and family about the potential for injury?
1. Fluorescent light bulbs in every table lamp
2. Trash can next to the client's favorite chair
3. Stairway with a landing that leads to bedrooms
4. Extension cord tucked away between the seating area and wall

Level of Cognitive Ability: Analyzing
Client Needs: Safe and Effective Care Environment
Clinical Judgment/Cognitive Skills: Recognize Cues
Integrated Process: Nursing Process/Assessment
Content Area: Foundations of Care: Safety
Health Problems: Adult Health: Musculoskeletal: Rheumatoid Arthritis and Osteoarthritis
Priority Concepts: Patient Education; Safety

Answer: 3
Rationale: The stairway creates a potential hazard for the client because stairs are associated with an increased risk of falls. Options 1 and 2 do not represent potential hazards for the client. An extension cord tucked away from a traffic area is not a potential hazard as long as a suitable electrical demand is drawn on the cord, the cord is grounded properly, and the cord does not traverse a pathway.
Test-Taking Strategy: Focus on the subject, potential environmental hazards. Recalling that stairs are associated with an increased risk of falls will direct you to the correct option.
Priority Nursing Tip: The nurse needs to inform the client and family of potential environmental hazards for falling, such as clutter and physical obstacles.
Reference: Potter, P., et al. (2021). *Fundamentals of nursing* (10th ed., pp. 387, 397). Elsevier.

181. A hospitalized client diagnosed with chronic depression wants to leave the hospital before being discharged by the physician. Which action would be the **next** intervention for the nurse to implement?
1. Notify the nursing supervisor of the client's plans to leave.
2. Ask the client about transportation plans from the hospital.
3. Arrange medication prescriptions at the client's preferred pharmacy.
4. Discuss the potential consequences of the plans for leaving with the client.

Level of Cognitive Ability: Applying
Client Needs: Safe and Effective Care Environment
Clinical Judgment/Cognitive Skills: Take Action
Integrated Process: Clinical Judgment; Nursing Process/Implementation
Content Area: Leadership/Management: Management of Care
Health Problems: Mental Health: Mood Disorders
Priority Concepts: Ethics; Health Care Law

Answer: 1
Rationale: The nurse notifies the nursing supervisor of the client's plan to leave without the physician's approval to ensure client safety and to help the nurse manage the situation. This will help the nurse manage the situation in a thoughtful, comprehensive manner and complete nursing interventions that include asking about transportation, arranging medication prescriptions, and discussing the risks and benefits of leaving or remaining in the hospital. The physician needs to be contacted and the client encouraged to remain until the physician arrives. The nurse avoids coercion, restraint, or security measures meant to prohibit the client's exit to prevent claims of false imprisonment.
Test-Taking Strategy: Note the strategic word, *next*. This indicates that one intervention is most important. Review the options for the choice that offers the most potential for a positive outcome. Note that option 1 offers the nurse assistance in a difficult situation involving client safety.
Priority Nursing Tip: False imprisonment occurs when a client is not allowed to leave a health care facility when there is no legal justification to detain the client.
Reference: Varcarolis, E., & Fosbre, C. (2021). *Essentials of psychiatric mental health nursing: A communication approach to evidence-based care* (4th ed., pp. 67, 69). Elsevier.

❖ **182.** The nurse is in the cafeteria and communicates to a physical therapist about a client who is physically abused. During the next visit to physical therapy, the client discovers that the nurse told the therapist about the abuse and is emotionally harmed. As a result of the events in the cafeteria, which ramification do the nurse and physical therapist potentially face? **Select all that apply.**
- ❑ 1. They can be charged with libel.
- ❑ 2. They can be charged with slander.
- ❑ 3. They can be charged with battery.
- ❑ 4. They can be terminated by the facility.
- ❑ 5. They can be charged with a HIPAA (Health Insurance Portability and Accountability Act) violation.

Level of Cognitive Ability: Understanding
Client Needs: Safe and Effective Care Environment
Clinical Judgment/Cognitive Skills: Analyze Cues
Integrated Process: Nursing Process/Analysis
Content Area: Leadership/Management: Interprofessional Collaboration
Health Problems: Mental Health: Abuse/Neglect
Priority Concepts: Ethics; Health Care Law

Answer: 2, 4, 5
Rationale: Defamation of a client occurs when information is communicated to a third party that causes damage to the client's reputation either verbally (slander) or in writing (libel). In addition, this situation violates the client's right to confidentiality as defined by HIPAA. Common examples of slander are discussing information about a client in public areas or speaking negatively about coworkers. Such actions can result in being terminated as an employee of the facility. Both the nurse and the therapist can receive privileged information about the client but not in this manner because communicating aspects of the medical record should not occur in a public setting. The nurse and therapist do not know with certainty that the conversation was not overheard by another person.
Test-Taking Strategy: Focus on the subject, client rights and confidentiality, and the health care team's responsibilities with privileged information. Recall that slander constitutes verbal discussion regarding a client and that client information is protected under HIPAA. Recall that such behavior would likely result in the termination of employment. Eliminate libel and battery because they do not apply to the given situation.
Priority Nursing Tip: The nurse is bound to protect client confidentiality. Disclosure of confidential information exposes the nurse to liability.
Reference: Potter, P., et al. (2021). *Fundamentals of nursing* (10th ed., pp. 314–315). Elsevier.

183. A registered nurse (RN) delegates the changing of a client's colostomy bag to a licensed practical nurse (LPN) who has never performed the procedure on a client. Which is the **most appropriate** action for the RN to implement?
1. Perform the procedure with the LPN.
2. Request that the LPN observe another LPN perform the procedure.
3. Ask the LPN to review the materials from the in-service before performing the procedure.
4. Instruct the LPN to review the procedure in the hospital manual and use the written procedure as a reference.

Level of Cognitive Ability: Applying
Client Needs: Safe and Effective Care Environment
Clinical Judgment/Cognitive Skills: Take Action
Integrated Process: Teaching and Learning
Content Area: Leadership/Management: Delegating/Supervising
Health Problems: N/A
Priority Concepts: Leadership; Safety

Answer: 1
Rationale: The RN must remember that, even though a task may be delegated to someone, the nurse who delegates maintains accountability for the overall nursing care of the client. Only the task, not the ultimate accountability, may be delegated to another. The RN is responsible for ensuring that competent and accurate care is delivered to the client. Because colostomy bag change is a new procedure for this LPN, the RN would accompany the LPN, provide guidance, and answer questions after the procedure. Requesting that the LPN observe another LPN perform the procedure does not ensure that the procedure will be done correctly. Although it is appropriate to review the in-service materials and the hospital procedure manual, it is best for the RN to accompany the LPN to perform the procedure.
Test-Taking Strategy: Focus on the subject, delegation. Note the strategic words, *most appropriate*. Eliminate options 3 and 4 first because they are comparable or alike in that they both involve a review of in-service materials and the hospital procedure manual. From the remaining options, select option 1 because option 2 does not ensure that another LPN will perform this procedure appropriately. Additionally, it is the RN's responsibility to educate.
Priority Nursing Tip: The five rights to delegation include the right task, right circumstances, right person, right direction/communication, and right supervision/evaluation.
Reference: Zerwekh, J., & Zerwekh Garneau, A. (2021). *Nursing today: Transition and trends* (10th ed., pp. 322–323). Elsevier.

❖ **184.** The nurse has applied the patch electrodes of an automatic external defibrillator (AED) to the chest of a client who is pulseless. The defibrillator has interpreted the rhythm to be ventricular fibrillation. Which **priority** action would the nurse implement **next?**
   1. Administer rescue breathing during the defibrillation.
   2. Perform cardiopulmonary resuscitation (CPR) for 1 minute before defibrillating.
   3. Charge the machine and immediately push the "discharge" buttons on the console.
   4. Order any personnel away from the client, charge the machine, and defibrillate through the console.

Level of Cognitive Ability: Applying
Client Needs: Safe and Effective Care Environment
Clinical Judgment/Cognitive Skills: Take Action
Integrated Process: Clinical Judgment; Nursing Process/Implementation
Content Area: Complex Care: Cardiopulmonary Resuscitation/Cardiac Arrest
Health Problems: Adult Health: Cardiovascular: Dysrhythmias
Priority Concepts: Clinical Judgment; Safety

Answer: 4
Rationale: If the AED advises to defibrillate, the nurse or rescuer orders all persons away from the client, charges the machine, and pushes both of the "discharge" buttons on the console at the same time. The charge is delivered through the patch electrodes, and this method is known as "hands-off" defibrillation, which is safest for the rescuer. The sequence of charges is similar to that of conventional defibrillation. Option 1 is contraindicated for the safety of any rescuer. Performing CPR delays the defibrillation attempt.
Test-Taking Strategy: Note the strategic words, *priority* and *next*. Focus on the subject, defibrillation and recall the guidelines related to defibrillation using an AED. Recalling the need to avoid contact with the client during this procedure will direct you to the correct option.
Priority Nursing Tip: An AED is used by laypersons and emergency medical technicians for prehospital cardiac arrest situations.
Reference: Ignatavicius, D., et al. (2021). *Medical-surgical nursing: Concepts for interprofessional collaborative care* (10th ed., p. 661). Elsevier.

185. The nurse is planning care for a client with the diagnosis of deep vein thrombosis (DVT) of the left leg. The client is experiencing severe edema and pain in the affected extremity. Which interventions would the nurse plan to implement in the care of this client? **Select all that apply.**
   ❑ 1. Elevate the left leg.
   ❑ 2. Apply moist heat to the left leg.
   ❑ 3. Administer acetaminophen as prescribed.
   ❑ 4. Ambulate in the hall three times per shift.
   ❑ 5. Administer anticoagulation as prescribed.

Level of Cognitive Ability: Applying
Client Needs: Safe and Effective Care Environment
Clinical Judgment/Cognitive Skills: Generate Solutions
Integrated Process: Clinical Judgment; Nursing Process/Planning
Content Area: Adult Health: Cardiovascular
Health Problems: Adult Health: Cardiovascular: Deep Vein Thrombosis
Priority Concepts: Clinical Judgment; Safety

Answer: 1, 2, 3, 5
Rationale: Management of the client with DVT who is experiencing severe edema and pain includes bed rest; limb elevation; relief of discomfort with warm, moist heat and analgesics as needed; anticoagulant therapy; and monitoring for signs of pulmonary embolism. In current practice, activity restriction may not be prescribed if the client is receiving low-molecular-weight anticoagulation; however, some physicians may still prefer bed rest for the client.
Test-Taking Strategy: Focus on the subject, deep vein thrombosis (DVT). Noting that the client is experiencing severe edema and pain and recalling the complications associated with DVT will direct you to the correct options.
Priority Nursing Tip: The client with DVT is at risk for pulmonary embolism.
Reference: Ignatavicius, D., et al. (2021). *Medical-surgical nursing: Concepts for interprofessional collaborative care* (10th ed., p. 722). Elsevier.

❖ **186.** The nurse is caring for a pregnant client with preeclampsia who is receiving a prescribed intravenous (IV) infusion of magnesium sulfate. To provide a safe environment, the nurse would ensure that which **priority** item is available?
1. Tongue blade
2. Percussion hammer
3. Calcium gluconate injection
4. Potassium chloride injection

Level of Cognitive Ability: Applying
Client Needs: Safe and Effective Care Environment
Clinical Judgment/Cognitive Skills: Generate Solutions
Integrated Process: Nursing Process/Planning
Content Area: Pharmacology: Maternity/Newborn: Magnesium Sulfate
Health Problems: Maternity: Gestational Hypertension/Preeclampsia and Eclampsia
Priority Concepts: Clinical Judgment; Safety

Answer: 3
Rationale: Magnesium sulfate is a central nervous system depressant and relaxes smooth muscle. Toxic effects of magnesium sulfate may cause loss of deep tendon reflexes, heart block, respiratory paralysis, and cardiac arrest. The antidote for magnesium sulfate is calcium gluconate and needs to be available. An airway rather than a tongue blade is also an appropriate item. A percussion hammer may be important to assess reflexes but is not the priority item. Potassium chloride is not related to the administration of magnesium sulfate.
Test-Taking Strategy: Note the strategic word, *priority*. This indicates that more than one or all of the options may be correct but that you need to identify the most important one. Remember that the percussion hammer would identify the decrease in deep tendon reflexes, but the calcium gluconate is required to treat the life-threatening condition that can occur.
Priority Nursing Tip: An IV controller device is always used when administering magnesium sulfate. Respiratory depression is a concern with the administration of magnesium sulfate, and the physician is notified if respirations are less than 12 breaths per minute.
Reference: McKinney, E. S., et al. (2022). *Maternal child nursing* (6th ed., p. 545). Elsevier.

187. The nurse administers digoxin 0.25 mg by mouth rather than the prescribed dose of 0.125 mg to the client. After assessing the client and notifying the physician, which action would the nurse implement **first**?
1. Write an incident report.
2. Administer digoxin immune Fab.
3. Tell the client about the medication error.
4. Tell the client about the adverse effects of digoxin.

Level of Cognitive Ability: Applying
Client Needs: Safe and Effective Care Environment
Clinical Judgment/Cognitive Skills: Take Action
Integrated Process: Nursing Process/Implementation
Content Area: Pharmacology: Cardiovascular: Antidysrhythmics
Health Problems: Adult Health: Cardiovascular: Dysrhythmias
Priority Concepts: Ethics; Safety

Answer: 1
Rationale: According to agency policy, the nurse would file an incident report when a medication error occurs to accurately document the facts. The nurse would assess the client first and then contact the physician because in this situation the client received too much medication. The client needs to be informed of the error and the adverse effects in a professional manner to avoid alarm and concern. However, in many situations, the physician prefers to discuss this with the client. Digoxin immune Fab is reserved for extreme toxicity and requires a prescription and may be prescribed depending on the client's response and the serum digoxin level.
Test-Taking Strategy: Note the strategic word, *first*. Eliminate options 3 and 4 because the physician usually prefers to inform the client of the error. Eliminate option 2 because a physician's prescription is needed for its administration. Remember, after assessing the client and notifying the physician, to complete an incident report when an error occurs.
Priority Nursing Tip: The nurse always counts the client's apical heart rate for 1 full minute before administering digoxin to an adult client. If the rate is less than 60 beats per minute for an adult, the digoxin is withheld and the physician is notified.
Reference: Potter, P., et al. (2021). *Fundamentals of nursing* (10th ed., p. 376). Elsevier

❖ **188.** When planning the discharge of a client with a diagnosis of chronic anxiety, the nurse develops client goals to promote a safe environment at home. Which topic is an appropriate maintenance goal for the client to focus on?
1. Identifying anxiety-producing situations
2. Maintaining contact with a crisis counselor
3. Techniques for ignoring feelings of anxiety
4. Eliminating all anxiety from daily situations

Level of Cognitive Ability: Applying
Client Needs: Safe and Effective Care Environment
Clinical Judgment/Cognitive Skills: Generate Solutions
Integrated Process: Nursing Process/Planning
Content Area: Mental Health
Health Problems: Mental Health: Anxiety Disorder
Priority Concepts: Anxiety; Safety

Answer: 1
Rationale: Recognizing situations that produce anxiety allows the client to prepare to cope with anxiety or avoid a specific stimulus. Counselors will not be available for all anxiety-producing situations. Additionally, this option does not encourage the development of internal strengths. Ignoring feelings will not resolve anxiety. It is impossible to eliminate all anxiety from life.
Test-Taking Strategy: Focus on the subject, the client experiencing anxiety. Eliminate option 4 first because of the closed-ended word "all." Eliminate option 3 next because feelings should not be ignored. From the remaining choices, select option 1 because it is more client-centered and provides preparation for the client to deal with anxiety if it occurs.
Priority Nursing Tip: The immediate nursing action for a client with anxiety is to decrease stimuli in the environment and provide a calm and quiet environment.
Reference: Varcarolis, E., & Fosbre, C. (2021). *Essentials of psychiatric mental health nursing: A communication approach to evidence-based care* (4th ed., pp. 145–147). Elsevier.

189. The nurse is planning to instruct a client with a diagnosis of chronic vertigo about safety measures to prevent exacerbation of symptoms or injury. Which instruction is **most important** for the nurse to incorporate in a teaching plan?
1. Turn the head slowly when spoken to.
2. Remove throw rugs and clutter in the home.
3. Drive at times when the client does not feel dizzy.
4. Walk to the bedroom and lie down when vertigo is experienced.

Level of Cognitive Ability: Applying
Client Needs: Safe and Effective Care Environment
Clinical Judgment/Cognitive Skills: Generate Solutions
Integrated Process: Teaching and Learning
Content Area: Adult Health: Ear
Health Problems: Adult Health: Ear: Vertigo/Tinnitus
Priority Concepts: Safety; Sensory Perception

Answer: 2
Rationale: The client needs to maintain the home in a clutter-free state and have throw rugs removed because the effort of trying to regain balance after slipping could trigger the onset of vertigo. To further prevent vertigo attacks, the client needs to change position slowly and needs to turn the entire body, not just the head, when spoken to. The client with chronic vertigo needs to use public transportation and avoid driving. The sudden movements involved in each could precipitate an attack. If vertigo does occur, the client needs to immediately sit down or lie down (rather than walking to the bedroom) or grasp the nearest piece of furniture.
Test-Taking Strategy: Focus on the subject, chronic vertigo and preventing injury. Note the strategic words, *most important*. Eliminate options 3 and 4 first because they put the client at greatest risk of injury secondary to vertigo. From the remaining options, recalling that the client is taught to turn the entire body, not just the head, will direct you to option 2.
Priority Nursing Tip: The inner ear contains the sensory receptors for sound and equilibrium. Provide safety measures for the client with an inner ear disorder because the client may experience vertigo.
Reference: Ignatavicius, D., et al. (2021). *Medical-surgical nursing: Concepts for interprofessional collaborative care* (10th ed., pp. 967–968). Elsevier.

❖ **190.** The nurse checks the activated partial thromboplastin time (aPTT) result for a client receiving heparin therapy for a diagnosis of an acute myocardial infarction. Before reporting the laboratory result to the physician, the nurse verifies that which medication is available for use if prescribed?

Laboratory Results

Test and Results	Reference Range
aPTT 100 seconds	30–40 sec (30–40 sec)

1. Vitamin K
2. Vitamin B$_{12}$
3. Methylene blue
4. Protamine sulfate

Level of Cognitive Ability: Applying
Client Needs: Safe and Effective Care Environment
Clinical Judgment/Cognitive Skills: Take Action
Integrated Process: Nursing Process/Implementation
Content Area: Pharmacology: Cardiovascular: Anticoagulants
Health Problems: Adult Health: Cardiovascular: Myocardial Infarction
Priority Concepts: Clinical Judgment; Safety

Answer: 4
Rationale: Heparin is an anticoagulant. Therapeutic values of the aPTT for clients on heparin range between 60 and 70 seconds, depending on the control value. A value of 100 seconds indicates that the client has received too much heparin and is at risk for bleeding. The antidote for heparin overdosage is protamine sulfate and may be prescribed. Vitamin K is the antidote for warfarin sodium overdosage. Methylene blue is an antidote for cyanide poisoning. Vitamin B$_{12}$ is used to treat clients with pernicious anemia.
Test-Taking Strategy: Focus on the **subject**, heparin therapy and aPTT results. Recalling that protamine sulfate is the antidote for heparin will direct you to the correct option.
Priority Nursing Tip: For a client receiving heparin therapy, as prescribed, if the aPTT value is too long, longer than 80 seconds, the heparin dosage would need to be lowered. If the aPTT is too short, less than 60 seconds, the dosage would need to be increased.
Reference: Kizior, R., & Hodgson, B. (2023). *Saunders Nursing drug handbook 2023* (p. 561). Elsevier.

191. A client who had expressed suicidal ideations upon admission is being discharged home with family. Which statement by a family member might constitute criteria for delaying discharge?

1. The client's partner asks, "Does my spouse know that I've already moved out and filed for a divorce?"
2. The client's adult child states, "I've decided to postpone my wedding until my parent is feeling better."
3. The client's adult child states, "One of my parent's coworkers visited last week to tell us their union is out on strike."
4. The client's family member asks, "Will my sibling be able to continue as executor of our parent's trust?"

Level of Cognitive Ability: Analyzing
Client Needs: Safe and Effective Care Environment
Clinical Judgment/Cognitive Skills: Recognize Cues
Integrated Process: Nursing Process/Assessment
Content Area: Mental Health
Health Problems: Mental Health: Suicide
Priority Concepts: Mood and Affect; Safety

Answer: 1
Rationale: Single, divorced, and widowed clients have suicide rates that are greater than those who are married. Although the client might feel responsible for the postponement of the wedding, if presented as an action to include the client, the client will feel loved and cared for. Although the situation of the strike is stressful, the client will probably receive a portion of wages and can derive hope and a sense of belonging from being a member of the union. Although being suicidal may reduce the ability to concentrate, if the client perceives the executorship positively, taking the role away reinforces the client's low self-esteem and self-worth. This statement by the client's family member also indicates a need for the client's family member to be educated about depressive illness.
Test-Taking Strategy: Focus on the **subject**, delaying discharge in a suicidal client. Read each option carefully. Recalling the risks associated with suicidal intention will direct you to the correct option.
Priority Nursing Tip: One clue that the client is suicidal is when the client at risk gives away personal, special, and prized possessions.
Reference: Varcarolis, E., & Fosbre, C. (2021). *Essentials of psychiatric mental health nursing: A communication approach to evidence-based care* (4th ed., p. 367). Elsevier.

❖ **192.** The nurse is preparing to ambulate a client with a diagnosis of Parkinson's disease who has recently been prescribed levodopa. Which information is **most important** for the nurse to assess before ambulating the client?
1. The client's history of falls
2. Assistive devices used by the client
3. The client's postural (orthostatic) vital signs
4. The degree of intention tremors exhibited by the client

Level of Cognitive Ability: Analyzing
Client Needs: Safe and Effective Care Environment
Clinical Judgment/Cognitive Skills: Recognize Cues
Integrated Process: Clinical Judgment; Nursing Process/Assessment
Content Area: Pharmacology: Neurologic: Antiparkinsonians
Health Problems: Adult Health: Neurologic: Parkinson's Disease
Priority Concepts: Clinical Judgment; Safety

Answer: 3
Rationale: Clients diagnosed with Parkinson's disease are at risk for postural (orthostatic) hypotension from the disease. This problem is exacerbated with the introduction of levodopa, which can also cause postural hypotension. Although knowledge of the client's risk for falls and the client's use of assistive devices are helpful, it is not the most important piece of assessment data, based on the wording of this question. Clients with Parkinson's disease generally have resting, not intention, tremors.
Test-Taking Strategy: Focus on the strategic words, *most important*. Postural hypotension presents the greatest safety risk to the client. Also, use of the ABCs—airway, breathing, and circulation—will direct you to the correct option. Checking postural vital signs is one way to assess circulation.
Priority Nursing Tip: Foods high in pyridoxine must be avoided with the use of some antiparkinsonian medications, such as levodopa, because the vitamin blocks the effects of the medications.
Reference: Lewis, S., et al. (2020). *Medical-surgical nursing: Assessment and management of clinical problems* (11th ed., pp. 1374–1375). Elsevier.

193. The nurse prepares to transfer a client who has residual right-sided weakness as a result of a stroke from the bed to the wheelchair. With the client dangling on the side of the bed, which location would the nurse **best** position the wheelchair in for safety?
1. Directly in front of the client
2. At a right angle to the client's left leg
3. Ninety degrees to the client's right leg
4. At a right angle to the client's right leg

Level of Cognitive Ability: Applying
Client Needs: Safe and Effective Care Environment
Clinical Judgment/Cognitive Skills: Take Action
Integrated Process: Nursing Process/Implementation
Content Area: Skills: Activity/Mobility
Health Problems: Adult Health: Neurologic: Stroke
Priority Concepts: Mobility; Safety

Answer: 2
Rationale: When a client has a weakened lower extremity, movement needs to occur toward the client's unaffected (strong) side, the left side. This wheelchair position allows the client to use the unaffected leg effectively and safely to stand, pivot, and sit in the wheelchair. Placing the wheelchair in front of the client directly increases the risk to the client because the client must pivot 180 degrees to the wheelchair in this position.
Test-Taking Strategy: Note the strategic word, *best*. Focus on the subject, a safe transfer technique with right-sided weakness. Visualize each option to direct you to option 2. Positioning the wheelchair next to the client's unaffected leg allows the client to use the stronger leg more effectively for a safe transfer. Also, eliminate options 3 and 4 because they are comparable or alike as they both involve the same leg.
Priority Nursing Tip: Safety is the priority concern when transferring a client from the bed to a chair. Always obtain ample assistance to transfer the client, especially if the client's ability to participate in the transfer is unknown.
Reference: Potter, P., et al. (2021). *Fundamentals of nursing* (10th ed., pp. 809–811). Elsevier.

194. The nurse is caring for a client determined to be brain dead who is a potential organ donor. Before approaching the family to discuss organ donation, the nurse reviews the client's medical record for potential contraindications to organ donation. Which finding would the nurse recognize as a contraindication to organ donation?
1. Allergy to penicillin
2. Hepatitis B infection
3. Older than 20 years old
4. History of foreign travel

Level of Cognitive Ability: Analyzing
Client Needs: Safe and Effective Care Environment
Clinical Judgment/Cognitive Skills: Recognize Cues
Integrated Process: Nursing Process/Assessment
Content Area: Developmental Stages: End-of-Life Care
Health Problems: N/A
Priority Concepts: Ethics; Health Care Law

Answer: 2
Rationale: A decedent who had a hepatitis B infection cannot donate organs because the organ recipient may contract the infection. Contraindications to organ donation do not include penicillin allergies or foreign travel. Although foreign travel increases the risk of contracting certain communicable diseases, foreign travel alone does not constitute a contraindication. Age may or may not be a contraindication, depending on the organ involved.
Test-Taking Strategy: Focus on the subject, contraindications to organ donations. Noting the word *infection* will direct you to the correct option.
Priority Nursing Tip: Individuals who are at least 18 years old may indicate a wish to become a donor on their driver's license (state-specific) or in an advance directive.
Reference: Lewis, S., et al. (2020). *Medical-surgical nursing: Assessment and management of clinical problems* (11th ed., p. 1081). Elsevier.

195. The nurse monitors a client who has been diagnosed with brain death as a result of a severe head injury and is a potential organ donor. Which client assessment data would indicate to the nurse that the standard of care as an organ donor has been maintained?
1. Urine output: 100 mL/hr
2. Capillary refill: 5 seconds
3. Blood pressure: 90/48 mm Hg
4. Heart rate: 60 beats per minute

Level of Cognitive Ability: Evaluating
Client Needs: Safe and Effective Care Environment
Clinical Judgment/Cognitive Skills: Evaluate Outcomes
Integrated Process: Nursing Process/Evaluation
Content Area: Developmental Stages: End-of-Life Care
Health Problems: Adult Health: Neurologic: Head Injury/Trauma
Priority Concepts: Clinical Judgment; Palliative Care

Answer: 1
Rationale: Urine output at 100 mL/hr indicates adequate renal perfusion and that care standards as an organ donor are maintained. Clinical indicators of care below the standard include a heart rate of 60 beats per minute, which is too slow; capillary refill at 5 seconds, which is also too slow; and hypotension, indicating an inadequate cardiac output. Guidelines that may be used and are helpful in determining organ viability are the "rule of 100s" in which the systolic blood pressure is maintained at 100 mm Hg, urine output at 100 mL/hr, heart rate at 100 beats per minute, and PO_2 at 100 mm Hg.
Test-Taking Strategy: Focus on the subject, organ donation. Eliminate options 2, 3, and 4 because they are comparable or alike because the listed criteria are below optimal values.
Priority Nursing Tip: A client has a right to decide to become an organ donor and a right to refuse organ transplantation as a treatment option.
References: Lewis, S., et al. (2020). *Medical-surgical nursing: Assessment and management of clinical problems* (11th ed., pp. 1082, 1084). Elsevier; Urden, L., Stacy, K., & Lough, M. (2022). *Critical care nursing: Diagnosis and management* (9th ed., pp. 895–896). Elsevier.

❖ **196.** A client diagnosed with brain death as a result of a severe head injury had received vigorous treatment to control cerebral edema. Which intervention would the nurse plan to implement as a **priority** to maintain viability of the kidneys before organ donation?
1. Screen the donor for infection.
2. Administer intravenous (IV) fluids.
3. Maintain ventilation and oxygenation.
4. Administer vasopressors intravenously.

Level of Cognitive Ability: Analyzing
Client Needs: Safe and Effective Care Environment
Clinical Judgment/Cognitive Skills: Prioritize Hypotheses
Integrated Process: Clinical Judgment; Nursing Process/Analysis
Content Area: Developmental Stages: End-of-Life Care
Health Problems: Adult Health: Neurologic: Head Injury/Trauma
Priority Concepts: Palliative Care; Perfusion

Answer: 2
Rationale: The kidneys require a minimum perfusion pressure of 80 mm Hg to produce urine and maintain renal function, and because of the aggressive treatment for cerebral edema, the client is likely to have a fluid volume deficiency. Therefore, the nurse restores the intravascular blood volume to maintain the blood pressure and renal perfusion pressure. The nurse screens the donor for infections because diseases such as hepatitis B and human immunodeficiency virus contraindicate organ donation; however, this option is unrelated to viability of the kidneys. Ventilation and oxygenation are important factors in tissue viability; however, the organ must be perfused adequately, first, to deliver any blood. The nurse administers vasopressors with caution to help maintain the donor's blood pressure; however, vasopressors potentially contribute to tissue destruction.
Test-Taking Strategy: Note the strategic word, *priority*. Focus on the subject, maintenance of kidney viability before organ donation. Note that this client has had *treatment to control cerebral edema*, which may impact the level of hydration. Next, note the relation between the subject and the correct option.
Priority Nursing Tip: The most desirable source of kidneys for transplantation is living related donors whose tissues closely match the client.
Reference: Urden, L., Stacy, K., & Lough, M. (2022). *Critical care nursing: Diagnosis and management* (9th ed., p. 895). Elsevier.

197. The nurse is working in the emergency department of a small local hospital when a client with multiple stab wounds arrives by ambulance. Which action by the nurse is contraindicated when handling potential legal evidence?
1. Initiating a chain of custody log
2. Giving clothing and wallet to the family
3. Cutting clothing along seams, avoiding stab holes
4. Placing personal belongings in a labeled, sealed paper bag

Level of Cognitive Ability: Applying
Client Needs: Safe and Effective Care Environment
Clinical Judgment/Cognitive Skills: Take Action
Integrated Process: Nursing Process/Implementation
Content Area: Leadership/Management: Ethical/Legal
Health Problems: Adult Health: Integumentary: Wounds
Priority Concepts: Ethics; Health Care Law

Answer: 2
Rationale: Potential evidence is never released to the family to take home. Basic rules for handling evidence include initiating a chain of custody log to track handling and movement of evidence, limiting the number of people with access to the evidence, and carefully removing clothing and placing personal belongings in a labeled, sealed paper bag to avoid destroying evidence. This also usually includes cutting clothes along seams, while avoiding areas where there are obvious holes or tears.
Test-Taking Strategy: Focus on the subject, client with multiple stab wounds. Note the word *contraindicated*; this requires you to select the option that identifies an incorrect nursing action. Use knowledge of basic emergency care principles related to a potential crime to eliminate each of the incorrect options. Remember that giving the client's belongings to the family may be giving up evidence.
Priority Nursing Tip: Family members, significant others, or friends of a client who is the victim of a crime, such as a stabbing or gunshot incident, are not allowed to be alone with the client because of the possibility of jeopardizing any existing legal evidence.
Reference: Sweet, V., & Foley, P., eds. (2020). *Sheehy's Emergency nursing: Principles and practice* (7th ed., pp. 394, 596–597). Elsevier.

❖ **198.** The nurse working on a medical nursing unit during an external disaster is called to assist with care for clients coming into the emergency department. Using principles of triage, the nurse would implement **immediate** care for a client with which injury?
1. Fractured tibia
2. Penetrating abdominal injury
3. Bright red bleeding from a neck wound
4. Open massive head injury, resulting in deep coma

Level of Cognitive Ability: Applying
Client Needs: Safe and Effective Care Environment
Clinical Judgment/Cognitive Skills: Take Action
Integrated Process: Clinical Judgment; Nursing Process/Implementation
Content Area: Leadership/Management: Mass Casualty Preparedness and Response
Health Problems: Adult Health: Cardiovascular: Hypovolemic Shock
Priority Concepts: Clinical Judgment; Safety

Answer: 3
Rationale: The client with bright red (arterial) bleeding from a neck wound is in "immediate" need of treatment to save the client's life. This client is classified as an emergent (life-threatening) client and would wear a red tag from the triage process. A green or "minimal" (nonurgent) designation would be given to the client with a fractured tibia, who requires intervention but who can provide self-care if needed. The client with a penetrating abdominal injury would be tagged yellow and classified as "urgent," requiring intervention within 60 to 120 minutes. A designation of "expectant" would be applied to the client with massive injuries and minimal chance of survival. This client would be color-coded black in the triage process. The client who is color-coded black is given supportive care and pain management but is given definitive treatment last.
Test-Taking Strategy: Focus on the strategic word, *immediate*. Use the principles of triage and prioritize. Noting the words *bright red* will direct you to the correct option.
Priority Nursing Tip: The purpose of primary assessment for triage in an emergency department is to identify any client problems that pose an immediate or potential threat to life.
Reference: Ignatavicius, D., et al. (2021). *Medical-surgical nursing: Concepts for interprofessional collaborative care* (10th ed., p. 228). Elsevier.

199. The nurse working on an adult nursing unit is told to review the client census to determine which clients could be discharged if there are a large number of admissions from a newly declared disaster. The nurse determines that the clients with which medical situations would need to remain hospitalized? **Select all that apply.**
❑ 1. Laparoscopic cholecystectomy
❑ 2. Fractured hip, pinned 5 days ago
❑ 3. Diabetes mellitus with blood glucose at 180 mg/dL (10.2 mmol/L)
❑ 4. Ongoing ventricular dysrhythmias while receiving procainamide
❑ 5. Newly delivered postpartal client with a blood pressure of 146/94 mm Hg and 2 + proteinuria.

Level of Cognitive Ability: Analyzing
Client Needs: Safe and Effective Care Environment
Clinical Judgment/Cognitive Skills: Analyze Cues
Integrated Process: Clinical Judgment; Nursing Process/Analysis
Content Area: Leadership/Management: Mass Casualty Preparedness and Response
Health Problems: N/A
Priority Concepts: Clinical Judgment; Safety

Answer: 4, 5
Rationale: The client with ongoing ventricular dysrhythmias requires ongoing medical evaluation and treatment because of potentially lethal complications of the problem. The newly delivered postpartal client is showing classic signs for mild preeclampsia. This condition would need to be reversed before discharge. Each of the other problems listed may be managed at home with appropriate agency referrals for home care services and support from the family at home.
Test-Taking Strategy: Use the principles of triage. Severity of illness usually guides the determination of who requires ongoing monitoring and care. The use of the ABCs—airway, breathing, and circulation—will direct you to option 4. Use of the steps of the nursing process indicates that the newly delivered postpartal client has not been stabilized and requires further assessment.
Priority Nursing Tip: The nurse can use the ABCs—airway, breathing, and circulation—as a guide in assessing a client's needs and their severity.
Reference: Ignatavicius, D., et al. (2021). *Medical-surgical nursing: Concepts for interprofessional collaborative care* (10th ed., p. 231). Elsevier.

Client Needs

❖ **200.** A registered nurse (RN) is orienting an unlicensed assistive personnel (UAP) to the clinical nursing unit. The RN determines that the UAP **needs further teaching** if which action is performed by the UAP during a routine handwashing procedure?

1. Keeps hands lower than elbows
2. Dries from forearm down to fingers
3. Washes continuously for 10 to 15 seconds
4. Uses 3 to 5 mL of soap from the dispenser

Level of Cognitive Ability: Evaluating
Client Needs: Safe and Effective Care Environment
Clinical Judgment/Cognitive Skills: Evaluate Outcomes
Integrated Process: Nursing Process/Evaluation
Content Area: Foundations of Care: Infection Control
Health Problems: N/A
Priority Concepts: Leadership; Safety

Answer: 2
Rationale: Proper handwashing procedure involves wetting the hands and wrists and keeping the hands lower than the forearms so that water flows toward the fingertips. The nurse uses 3 to 5 mL of soap and scrubs for 10 to 15 seconds, using rubbing and circular motions. The hands are rinsed and then dried, moving from the fingers to the forearms. The paper towel is then discarded, and a second one is used to turn off the faucet to avoid hand contamination.
Test-Taking Strategy: Note the strategic words, *needs further teaching*. These words indicate a negative event query and require you to select the option that identifies an incorrect action by the UAP. Use basic principles of medical asepsis and visualize each of the actions in the options to assist in directing you to the correct option.
Priority Nursing Tip: The nurse is a supervisor and educator, and a primary responsibility is to ensure client safety. If the nurse observes a health care worker performing a procedure incorrectly, the nurse must intervene and teach the health care worker how to perform the procedure correctly and safely.
Reference: Potter, P., et al. (2021). *Fundamentals of nursing* (10th ed., pp. 451–452.). Elsevier.

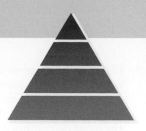

Health Promotion and Maintenance Practice Questions

1. The nurse caring for a client in labor who has been diagnosed with gestational diabetes would assess the fetal heart rate (FHR) at which specific times? **Select all that apply.**
- ❑ **1.** Before ambulation
- ❑ **2.** After vaginal examination
- ❑ **3.** After rupture of the membranes
- ❑ **4.** Before turning the client on the side
- ❑ **5.** Before the administration of oxytocin

Level of Cognitive Ability: Analyzing
Client Needs: Health Promotion and Maintenance
Clinical Judgment/Cognitive Skills: Take Action
Integrated Process: Clinical Judgment; Nursing Process/Analysis
Content Area: Maternity: Intrapartum
Health Problems: Maternity: Gestational Diabetes Mellitus
Priority Concepts: Perfusion; Reproduction

Answer: 1, 2, 3, 5
Rationale: Assessment of the birthing parent and fetus is continuous during the process of labor. However, for all clients, the FHR needs to be assessed before ambulation; immediately after vaginal examinations, rupture of the membranes, or any other invasive procedure; and before the administration of oxytocin because these activities or situations can cause alterations in the FHR. The FHR is also assessed in between contractions, during the contraction, and for at least 30 seconds after the contraction. It is not necessary to assess the FHR before turning the client on the side.
Test-Taking Strategy: Note the subject of the question relates to the times at which FHR monitoring is necessary. Read each option and think about the effect that the activity or situation has on the FHR. Eliminate option 4 (before turning the client on the side) because this activity will not affect the FHR.
Priority Nursing Tip: Electronic fetal heart monitoring is performed during labor to monitor the well-being of the fetus. The normal fetal heart rate at term is 120 to 160 beats/min.
Reference: McKinney, E. S., et al. (2022). *Maternal child nursing* (6th ed., pp. 311, 559). Elsevier.

2. A parent of a 3-year-old child asks the nurse what personal and social developmental milestones can be expected in the child. The nurse would plan to tell the parent to expect which findings? **Select all that apply.**
- ❑ **1.** Begins problem-solving
- ❑ **2.** Exhibits sexual curiosity
- ❑ **3.** May begin to masturbate
- ❑ **4.** Notices gender differences
- ❑ **5.** Develops a sense of initiative
- ❑ **6.** Develops positive self-esteem through skill acquisition

Level of Cognitive Ability: Applying
Client Needs: Health Promotion and Maintenance
Clinical Judgment/Cognitive Skills: Generate Solutions
Integrated Process: Clinical Judgment; Nursing Process/Planning
Content Area: Developmental Stages: Early Childhood
Health Problems: N/A
Priority Concepts: Development; Health Promotion

Answer: 2, 3, 4
Rationale: Personal and social developmental milestones of the 3-year-old child include exhibiting sexual curiosity; possibly beginning to masturbate; noticing gender differences and identifying with children of like gender; putting on articles of clothing; brushing teeth with help; washing and drying hands using soap and water; knowing own name; and understanding the need to take turns and share with others but perhaps not being ready to do so. Developmental milestones for the 4- and 5-year-old child include developing a sense of initiative and beginning to problem-solve. Developing positive self-esteem through skill acquisition and task completion is characteristic of a 6- to 8-year-old child.
Test-Taking Strategy: Focus on the subject, the developmental milestones of a 3-year-old. Read each option carefully, thinking about what can be expected of a child at this age. This will assist in eliminating these answer options: begins problem-solving, develops a sense of initiative, and develops self-esteem through skill acquisition. (These are higher-level abilities.)
Priority Nursing Tip: A major socializing mechanism of a toddler is parallel play; therapeutic play can also begin at this age.
Reference: McKinney, E. S., et al. (2022). *Maternal child nursing* (6th ed., p. 126). Elsevier.

3. The nurse has taught a client with a below-the-knee amputation about home care and about monitoring for and preventing complications related to prosthesis and residual limb care. The nurse determines that the client has understood the instructions if the client stated that which action needs to be taken?
1. Wear a clean nylon sock over the residual limb every day.
2. Use a mirror to inspect all areas of the residual limb each day.
3. Toughen the skin of the residual limb by rubbing it with alcohol.
4. Prevent cracking of the skin of the residual limb by applying lotion daily.

Level of Cognitive Ability: Evaluating
Client Needs: Health Promotion and Maintenance
Clinical Judgment/Cognitive Skills: Evaluate Outcomes
Integrated Process: Clinical Judgment; Nursing Process/Evaluation
Content Area: Adult Health: Musculoskeletal
Health Problems: Adult Health: Musculoskeletal: Amputation
Priority Concepts: Patient Education; Tissue Integrity

Answer: 2
Rationale: The client needs to inspect all surfaces of the residual limb daily for irritation, blisters, and breakdown. The client needs to wear a clean woolen (not nylon) sock each day. The residual limb is cleansed daily with a gentle soap and water and dried carefully. Alcohol is avoided because it could cause drying or cracking of the skin. Oils and creams are also avoided because they are too softening to the skin for safe prosthesis use.
Test-Taking Strategy: Focus on the subject, prosthesis and residual limb care. Recall that nylon is a synthetic material that does not allow for the best air circulation and holds in moisture; therefore, nylon is incorrect. Alcohol and lotion can interfere with the natural condition of the skin, thus increasing the likelihood of breakdown either from drying or excess moisture; therefore, eliminate alcohol and lotion.
Priority Nursing Tip: Encourage the client who underwent an amputation to verbalize feelings regarding the loss of the body part and assist the client to identify coping mechanisms to deal with the loss.
Reference: Ignatavicius, D., et al. (2021). *Medical-surgical nursing: Concepts for interprofessional collaborative care* (10th ed., p. 1049). Elsevier.

 4. The nurse is teaching a client with a right leg fracture who has a prescription for partial weight-bearing status how to ambulate with crutches. The nurse determines that the client demonstrates compliance with this restriction to prevent complications of the fracture if the client follows which direction?
1. Allows the right foot to only touch the floor
2. Does not bear any weight on the right leg/foot
3. Puts 30% to 50% of the weight on the right leg/foot
4. Puts 60% to 80% of the weight on the right leg/foot

Level of Cognitive Ability: Evaluating
Client Needs: Health Promotion and Maintenance
Clinical Judgment/Cognitive Skills: Evaluate Outcomes
Integrated Process: Clinical Judgment; Nursing Process/Evaluation
Content Area: Skills: Activity/Mobility
Health Problems: Adult Health: Musculoskeletal: Skeletal Injury
Priority Concepts: Mobility; Safety

Answer: 3
Rationale: The client who has partial weight-bearing status is allowed to place 30% to 50% of the body weight on the affected limb. Touchdown weight bearing allows the client to let the limb touch the floor but not to bear weight. Non–weight-bearing status does not allow the client to let the limb touch the floor. There is no classification for 60% to 80% weight-bearing status. Full weight-bearing status involves placing full weight on the limb.
Test-Taking Strategy: Focus on the subject, partial weight-bearing status. Eliminate option 1 because of the closed-ended word "only." Think about the description of what partial weight bearing means. Weight bearing of 30% to 50% is the only choice that fits the definition of partial weight bearing.
Priority Nursing Tip: Instruct the client with crutches never to rest the axillae on the axillary bars because of the risk of damaging the brachial plexus.
Reference: Ignatavicius, D., et al. (2021). *Medical-surgical nursing: Concepts for interprofessional collaborative care* (10th ed., pp. 1040, 1045). Elsevier.

5. To promote client self-care, the nurse is planning to teach a client in skeletal leg traction about measures to increase bed mobility. Which item is **most** helpful for this client for achievement of this goal?
   1. Fracture bedpan
   2. Overhead trapeze
   3. Isometric exercises
   4. Range-of-motion exercises

Level of Cognitive Ability: Applying
Client Needs: Health Promotion and Maintenance
Clinical Judgment/Cognitive Skills: Generate Solutions
Integrated Process: Teaching and Learning
Content Area: Skills: Activity/Mobility
Health Problems: Adult Health: Musculoskeletal: Skeletal Injury
Priority Concepts: Mobility; Safety

Answer: 2
Rationale: The use of an overhead trapeze is extremely helpful for assisting a client with moving about in bed and getting on and off the bedpan. This device has the greatest value for increasing overall bed mobility. A fracture bedpan is useful for reducing discomfort with elimination. Isometric exercises will not increase bed mobility and could be harmful for a client in skeletal traction. Range-of-motion exercises can also be harmful to a client in skeletal traction and would not be initiated unless there are specific prescriptions to do so.
Test-Taking Strategy: Note the strategic word, *most*, and focus on the subject, promoting self-care and increased bed mobility. Eliminate isometric and range-of-motion exercises first because they can be harmful to a client in skeletal traction. To select from the remaining options, note that the only one that helps with bed mobility is the trapeze.
Priority Nursing Tip: Monitor the color, motion, and sensation of the affected extremity for a client in traction. If the client is in skeletal traction, also monitor insertion sites for redness, swelling, drainage, or increased pain.
Reference: Potter, P., et al. (2021). *Fundamentals of nursing* (10th ed., p. 844). Elsevier.

6. The nurse at a community health care clinic is teaching parents about measures to take to prevent and manage obesity in children. The nurse determines that the parents **need additional teaching** if they indicate that they will implement which measures? **Select all that apply.**
   1. Use food as a reward.
   2. Offer options of healthy foods.
   3. Avoid eating at fast-food restaurants.
   4. Maintain healthy, personal eating habits.
   5. Allow eating in-between meals and snack times.
   6. Establish consistent times for meals and snacks.

Level of Cognitive Ability: Evaluating
Client Needs: Health Promotion and Maintenance
Clinical Judgment/Cognitive Skills: Evaluate Outcomes
Integrated Process: Clinical Judgment; Nursing Process/Evaluation
Content Area: Foundations of Care: Community / Public/Population Health
Health Problems: Pediatric-Specific: Childhood Obesity
Priority Concepts: Patient Education; Health Promotion

Answer: 1, 5
Rationale: Parents can implement several measures to prevent and manage obesity in their children. These measures include not using food as a reward; establishing consistent times for meals and snacks, and not allowing eating in-between; offering only healthy food options; minimizing trips to fast-food restaurants; keeping unhealthy food out of the house; acting as a role model for children; encouraging the child to do fun, physical activities with the family; and praising the child for making appropriate food choices and increasing physical activity levels.
Test-Taking Strategy: Note the strategic words, *need additional teaching*. These words indicate a negative event query and ask you to select the options that are incorrect statements. Read each option and think about its effect on preventing and managing obesity; this will direct you to the correct options.
Priority Nursing Tip: Obesity places a person at risk for hypertension, hyperlipidemia, myocardial infarction, stroke (brain attack), diabetes mellitus, cancer, and other health conditions.
Reference: McKinney, E. S., et al. (2022). *Maternal child nursing* (6th ed., pp. 147, 149). Elsevier.

7. The nurse is percussing the anterior thorax and the abdomen for tones and expects to note dullness in which anatomic location? **(Refer to figure.)**

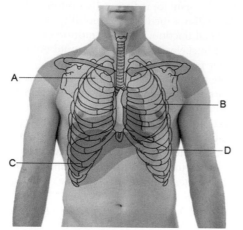

(From Wilson, S., & Giddens, J. [2013]. *Health assessment for nursing practice* [5th ed.]. Mosby.)

1. A
2. B
3. C
4. D

Level of Cognitive Ability: Applying
Client Needs: Health Promotion and Maintenance
Clinical Judgment/Cognitive Skills: Recognize Cues
Integrated Process: Nursing Process/Assessment
Content Area: Health Assessment/Physical Exam: Thorax and Lungs
Health Problems: N/A
Priority Concepts: Clinical Judgment; Health Promotion

Answer: 3
Rationale: Percussion involves tapping the body with the fingertips to set the underlying structures in motion and thus produce a sound. Dullness will be noted over the liver, located in the upper right quadrant of the abdomen and beneath the lower ribs on the right side. Tympany is the most common percussion tone heard in the abdomen and is caused by the presence of gas. Resonance is the percussion tone heard between the ribs.
Test-Taking Strategy: Focus on the subject, the anatomic location in which dullness would be percussed. Look at the figure. Recalling that dullness on percussion indicates the presence of an organ will assist in answering the question.
Priority Nursing Tip: The presence of an abnormal mass would produce dullness on percussion.
Reference: Jarvis, C. (2020). *Physical examination and health assessment* (8th ed., p. 542). Elsevier.

8. The home care nurse visits an older client diagnosed with Parkinson's disease who requires instillation of multiple eye drops. Which instruction for the administration of eye drops would the nurse provide to this client?
1. Administer the eye drops rapidly.
2. Have a family member instill the eye drops.
3. Lie down on a bed or sofa to instill the eye drops.
4. Keep the eye drops in the refrigerator so that they will thicken.

Level of Cognitive Ability: Applying
Client Needs: Health Promotion and Maintenance
Clinical Judgment/Cognitive Skills: Take Action
Integrated Process: Teaching and Learning
Content Area: Skills: Medication Administration
Health Problems: Adult Health: Neurologic: Parkinson's Disease
Priority Concepts: Patient Education; Safety

Answer: 3
Rationale: Older adults diagnosed with Parkinson's disease will experience tremors, making it more difficult to instill eye drops. The older client is instructed to lie down on a bed or sofa to instill the eye drops to provide control and allow the drops to be administered more easily. If multiple eye drops are needed, there should be a wait time of 3 to 4 minutes between drops. It is unreasonable to expect a family member to be available consistently to instill the eye drops. Additionally, this discourages client independence. Placing the eye drops in the refrigerator should not be done unless specifically prescribed.
Test-Taking Strategy: Focus on the subject, Parkinson's disease and safety when administering eye medications. Eliminate refrigeration of the medication first because eye medication should not be refrigerated unless specifically prescribed. Eliminate administering the eye drops rapidly as eye medications typically have a 3- to 4-minute wait between eye drops. Considering the need to promote client independence and the fact that the question does not provide data regarding the client's family, eliminate family participation. From the remaining choices, select lying down on a bed or sofa because this action provides environmental control and greater safety for the older client.
Priority Nursing Tip: If both an eye drop and eye ointment are scheduled to be administered at the same time, administer the eye drop first.
Reference: Lilley, L., Rainforth Collins, S., & Snyder J. (2020). *Pharmacology and the nursing process* (9th ed., pp. 127–128). Elsevier.

9. A client at the family planning clinic requests a prescription for oral contraceptives from the nurse who is performing an assessment. After reviewing the client's chart, the nurse determines that oral contraceptives are contraindicated because of which documented item? **(Refer to medical record.)**

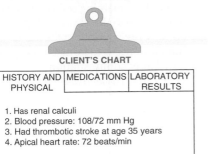

CLIENT'S CHART

HISTORY AND PHYSICAL	MEDICATIONS	LABORATORY RESULTS
1. Has renal calculi 2. Blood pressure: 108/72 mm Hg 3. Had thrombotic stroke at age 35 years 4. Apical heart rate: 72 beats/min		

Level of Cognitive Ability: Analyzing
Client Needs: Health Promotion and Maintenance
Clinical Judgment/Cognitive Skills: Analyze Cues
Integrated Process: Clinical Judgment; Nursing Process/Analysis
Content Area: Pharmacology: Reproductive: Contraceptives
Health Problems: Adult Health: Reproductive: Menstruation Problems/Fertility/Infertility
Priority Concepts: Reproduction; Safety

Answer: 3
Rationale: Oral contraceptives are contraindicated in those with a history of thrombophlebitis and thromboembolic disorders; cardiovascular or cerebrovascular diseases (including stroke); any estrogen-dependent cancer or breast cancer, or benign or malignant liver tumors; impaired liver function; hypertension; or diabetes mellitus with vascular involvement. Adverse effects of oral contraceptives include increased risk of superficial and deep vein thrombosis, pulmonary embolism, thrombotic stroke (or other types of strokes), myocardial infarction, and acceleration of preexisting breast tumors.
Test-Taking Strategy: Focus on the **subject,** the item that is a contraindication to the use of oral contraceptives. Eliminate options that present normal findings. To select from the remaining choices, remember that oral contraceptives are contraindicated in cardiovascular or cerebrovascular disorders.
Priority Nursing Tip: Antibiotics may decrease the absorption and effectiveness of contraceptives.
References: Burchum, J., & Rosenthal, L. (2022). *Lehne's Pharmacology for nursing care* (11th ed., p. 746). Elsevier; Lewis, S., et al. (2020). *Medical-surgical nursing: Assessment and management of clinical problems* (11th ed., p. 663). Elsevier.

10. The nurse provides dietary instruction to the parents of a child with a diagnosis of cystic fibrosis. The nurse would tell the parents that which diet plan needs to be followed?
1. Fat free
2. Low in protein
3. Low in sodium
4. High in calories

Level of Cognitive Ability: Applying
Client Needs: Health Promotion and Maintenance
Clinical Judgment/Cognitive Skills: Take Action
Integrated Process: Clinical Judgment; Teaching and Learning
Content Area: Skills: Nutrition
Health Problems: Pediatric-Specific: Cystic Fibrosis
Priority Concepts: Patient Education; Nutrition

Answer: 4
Rationale: Children with cystic fibrosis are managed with a high-calorie, high-protein diet; pancreatic enzyme replacement therapy; fat-soluble vitamin supplements; and, if nutritional problems are severe, nighttime gastrostomy feedings or parental nutrition. Fats are not restricted unless steatorrhea cannot be controlled by increased pancreatic enzymes. Sodium intake is unrelated to this disorder.
Test-Taking Strategy: Focus on the **subject,** diet for the child with cystic fibrosis. Think about the pathophysiology associated with cystic fibrosis. Select the high-calorie diet because children require calories for growth and development and because this choice is the **umbrella option.**
Priority Nursing Tip: The child with cystic fibrosis needs to be monitored closely for signs/symptoms of failure to thrive.
Reference: McKinney, E. S., et al. (2022). *Maternal child nursing* (6th ed., p. 1077). Elsevier.

11. A clinic nurse providing home care instructions to an adolescent diagnosed with iron-deficiency anemia concentrates on the administration of oral iron preparations. The nurse would tell the adolescent that it is **best** to take the iron with which liquid?

1. Cola
2. Soda
3. Water
4. Tomato juice

Level of Cognitive Ability: Applying
Client Needs: Health Promotion and Maintenance
Clinical Judgment/Cognitive Skills: Generate Solutions
Integrated Process: Clinical Judgment; Teaching and Learning
Content Area: Developmental Stages: Adolescent
Health Problems: Pediatric-Specific: Anemias
Priority Concepts: Patient Education; Health Promotion

Answer: 4
Rationale: Iron needs to be administered with vitamin C–rich fluids because vitamin C enhances the absorption of the iron preparation. Tomato juice has a high ascorbic acid (vitamin C) content, whereas cola, soda, and water do not contain vitamin C.
Test-Taking Strategy: Note the strategic word, *best*. Eliminate cola and soda first because they are comparable or alike because both are sweetened carbonated beverages. From the remaining choices, recall that vitamin C increases the absorption of iron to direct you to tomato juice.
Priority Nursing Tip: Liquid iron preparations stain the teeth. Teach the child and parents that liquid iron needs to be taken through a straw, and the teeth need to be brushed after administration.
Reference: McKinney, E. S., et al. (2022). *Maternal child nursing* (6th ed., p. 1128). Elsevier.

❖ **12.** The nurse is performing an assessment on an older client. Which signs/symptoms are age-related changes in the eye? **Select all that apply.**

❑ 1. Clear sclera
❑ 2. Blurred vision
❑ 3. Protruding cornea
❑ 4. Increased tear production
❑ 5. Diminished pupillary adaptation to darkness
❑ 6. Increased ability to discriminate among colors

Level of Cognitive Ability: Understanding
Client Needs: Health Promotion and Maintenance
Clinical Judgment/Cognitive Skills: Recognize Cues
Integrated Process: Nursing Process/Assessment
Content Area: Developmental Stages: Later Adulthood
Health Problems: Adult Health: Eye: Visual Problems/Refractive Errors
Priority Concepts: Development; Sensory Perception

Answer: 2, 5
Rationale: Age-related changes in the eye include flattening of the cornea, which causes blurred vision; poor pupillary adaptation to darkness; yellowing sclera; a sunken appearance; diminished tear production; diminished ability to discriminate among colors; and reduced ocular muscle strength.
Test-Taking Strategy: Focus on the subject, age-related changes in the eye. Eliminate tear production and ability to discriminate colors because of the word *increased*. Noting the words *blurred* and *diminished* will direct you to these choices.
Priority Nursing Tip: The client experiencing age-related changes in the eye is at risk for injury; therefore, it is important for the nurse to teach the client about ways to compensate for these changes.
Reference: Ignatavicius, D., et al. (2021). *Medical-surgical nursing: Concepts for interprofessional collaborative care* (10th ed., p. 933). Elsevier.

13. The nurse has given the client with a nephrostomy tube instructions to follow after hospital discharge to prevent complications. The nurse determines that the client understands the instructions if the client verbalizes the need to drink how many glasses of water per day?
1. 1 to 3
2. 6 to 8
3. 10 to 12
4. 14 to 16

Level of Cognitive Ability: Evaluating
Client Needs: Health Promotion and Maintenance
Clinical Judgment/Cognitive Skills: Evaluate Outcomes
Integrated Process: Clinical Judgment; Nursing Process/Evaluation
Content Area: Adult Health: Renal and Urinary
Health Problems: Adult Health: Renal and Urinary: Urinary Tract Inflammation/Infection/Trauma
Priority Concepts: Patient Education; Elimination

Answer: 2
Rationale: The client with a nephrostomy tube needs to have adequate fluid intake to dilute urinary particles that could cause calculus and provide good mechanical flushing of the kidney and the tube. The nurse encourages the client to take in 2000 mL of fluid per day, which is roughly equivalent to 6 to 8 glasses of water. One to three glasses of water is an inadequate amount. Amounts over 10 glasses of water could distend the renal pelvis.
Test-Taking Strategy: Focus on the subject, fluid intake for a client with a nephrostomy tube. Recall that the client needs 2 L of fluid per day. This will direct you to select 6 to 8 glasses of water/day. Also, avoid options in the much higher range because these are unnecessary and could possibly place undue distention on the renal pelvis.
Priority Nursing Tip: If the client has a ureteral or nephrostomy tube, monitor the output closely; urine output of less than 30 mL/hr or lack of output for more than 15 minutes needs to be reported to the surgeon immediately.
Reference: Lewis, S., et al. (2020). *Medical-surgical nursing: Assessment and management of clinical problems* (11th ed., pp. 341, 1053). Elsevier.

14. The nurse provides home care instructions to a client who has been diagnosed with recurrent trichomoniasis. The nurse determines the **need for follow-up** teaching if the client indicates taking which action?
1. Avoid sexual intercourse.
2. Perform good perineal hygiene.
3. Use the metronidazole as prescribed.
4. Discontinue treatment during menstruation.

Level of Cognitive Ability: Evaluating
Client Needs: Health Promotion and Maintenance
Clinical Judgment/Cognitive Skills: Evaluate Outcomes
Integrated Process: Clinical Judgment; Nursing Process/Evaluation
Content Area: Foundations of Care: Infection Control
Health Problems: Adult Health: Reproductive: Inflammatory/Infectious Problems
Priority Concepts: Patient Education; Infection

Answer: 4
Rationale: Treatment for a recurrent vaginal trichomoniasis infection continues through the menstrual period because the vagina is more alkaline during menses and a flare-up is more likely to occur. While the infection remains active, the client needs to refrain from sexual intercourse or instruct the partner to wear a condom. To help break the chain of infection, the nurse directs the client to perform perineal hygiene after each voiding and each bowel movement. Metronidazole must be taken as prescribed.
Test-Taking Strategy: Note the strategic words, *need for follow-up*. These words indicate a negative event query and that the answer will be a client misunderstanding about self-care while treating this infection. Recall the basic principles related to infection control for vaginal fungal infections and medication administration to direct you to the correct option.
Priority Nursing Tip: Trichomoniasis is a sexually transmitted infection and is associated during the maternity cycle with premature rupture of the membranes and postpartum endometritis.
Reference: Lewis, S., et al. (2020). *Medical-surgical nursing: Assessment and management of clinical problems* (11th ed., p. 1216). Elsevier.

15. Which problems would the nurse counsel adoptive parents about encountering? **Select all that apply.**

❑ 1. Setting unrealistically high standard for themselves
❑ 2. Lacking basic knowledge about the child's biological health history
❑ 3. Having difficulty assimilating if the child is adopted from another country
❑ 4. Having difficulty deciding when and how to tell the child about being adopted
❑ 5. Feeling the need for more assistance and support in child-rearing than biological parents do
❑ 6. Dealing with feelings of loss and grief in the child regarding family social history and traditions

Level of Cognitive Ability: Analyzing
Client Needs: Health Promotion and Maintenance
Clinical Judgment/Cognitive Skills: Prioritize Hypotheses
Integrated Process: Clinical Judgment; Nursing Process/Analysis
Content Area: Adult Health: Reproductive
Health Problems: Mental Health: Coping
Priority Concepts: Family Dynamics; Reproduction

Answer: 1, 2, 3, 4, 6
Rationale: Adoptive parents may add pressure to themselves by setting unrealistically high standards for themselves as parents. Additional problems adoptive families may face include possible lack of knowledge about the child's biological health history, difficulty assimilating if the child is adopted from another country, difficulty deciding when and how to tell the child about being adopted, and dealing with social and traditional issues of the biological family. Otherwise, most problems faced by adoptive parents are no different from those encountered by natural parents. All parents want to be good parents. Both adoptive parents and biological parents need information, support, and guidance to prepare them to care for their child.
Test-Taking Strategy: Focus on the subject, problems that adoptive parents may encounter. Read each option and determine if the information distinctively relates to adoption. Remember that both biological parents and adoptive parents need assistance with child rearing and frequently face similar problems. This will assist in answering the question.
Priority Nursing Tip: In adoption, all rights and responsibilities that belonged to the original parent or parents are legally transferred to the person(s) who becomes the new parent(s).
Reference: McKinney, E. S., et al. (2022). *Maternal child nursing* (6th ed., pp. 35, 522–523). Elsevier.

❖ **16.** A client with a history of depression will be participating in cognitive therapy for health maintenance. The client asks the nurse, "How does this treatment work?" Which statement is **most appropriate** for the nurse to make to the client?

1. "This treatment helps you relax and develop new coping skills."
2. "This treatment helps you confront your fears by gradually exposing you to them."
3. "This treatment helps you examine how your past life has contributed to your problems."
4. "This treatment helps examine how your thoughts and feelings contribute to your difficulties."

Level of Cognitive Ability: Applying
Client Needs: Health Promotion and Maintenance
Clinical Judgment/Cognitive Skills: Take Action
Integrated Process: Nursing Process/Implementation
Content Area: Mental Health
Health Problems: Mental Health: Mood Disorders
Priority Concepts: Health Promotion; Mood and Affect

Answer: 4
Rationale: Cognitive therapy is frequently used with clients who have depression. This type of therapy is based on exploring the client's personal experience. It includes examining the client's thoughts and feelings about situations and how these thoughts and feelings contribute to and perpetuate the client's difficulties and mood. The development of new coping skills, gradually confronting fears, and reviewing one's past life in relation to your current problems are not characteristics of cognitive therapy.
Test-Taking Strategy: Note the strategic words, *most appropriate*, and focus on the subject, a description of cognitive therapy. Note the relationship between the word *cognitive* in the question and the word *thoughts* in option 4. This will lead you to select the correct option.
Priority Nursing Tip: Cognitive therapy is based on the principle that how individuals feel and behave is determined by how they think about the world and their place in it.
Reference: Varcarolis, E., & Fosbre, C. (2021). *Essentials of psychiatric mental health nursing: A communication approach to evidence-based care* (4th ed., pp. 24, 214). Elsevier.

17. A client diagnosed with acquired immunodeficiency syndrome (AIDS) has a problem with nutrition, resulting in a weight loss. The nurse has instructed the client regarding methods of increasing weight for health maintenance. The nurse determines that there is a **need for further instruction** if the client states the need to implement which measure?

1. Eat low-calorie snacks between meals.
2. Eat small, frequent meals throughout the day.
3. Consume nutrient-dense foods and beverages.
4. Keep easy-to-prepare foods available in the home.

Level of Cognitive Ability: Evaluating
Client Needs: Health Promotion and Maintenance
Clinical Judgment/Cognitive Skills: Evaluate Outcomes
Integrated Process: Clinical Judgment; Nursing Process/Evaluation
Content Area: Adult Health: Immune
Health Problems: Adult Health: Immune: Immunodeficiency Syndrome
Priority Concepts: Patient Education; Nutrition

Answer: 1
Rationale: The client who has a problem with nutrition and is losing weight should take in nutrient-dense and high-calorie meals and snacks. The client should also eat small, frequent meals throughout the day. The client is encouraged to eat favorite foods to keep intake up and plan meals that are easy to prepare. The client should also avoid taking fluids with meals in order to increase food intake before satiety occurs.
Test-Taking Strategy: Note the strategic words, *need for further instruction.* These words indicate a negative event query and ask you to select an option that is an incorrect statement. Also focus on the data in the question, and note that the client has a problem with nutrition and is losing weight. Recalling that the client should choose snacks that are high in calories (rather than low in calories) will direct you to the correct option.
Priority Nursing Tip: Acquired immunodeficiency syndrome is manifested by opportunistic infections and neoplasms.
Reference: Ignatavicius, D., et al. (2021). *Medical-surgical nursing: Concepts for interprofessional collaborative care* (10th ed., p. 340). Elsevier.

❖ **18.** A school nurse is performing screening examinations for scoliosis. Which signs of scoliosis would the nurse assess for? **Select all that apply.**

❑ 1. Chest asymmetry
❑ 2. Equal waist angles
❑ 3. Unequal rib heights
❑ 4. Equal rib prominences
❑ 5. Equal shoulder heights
❑ 6. Lateral deviation and rotation of each vertebra

Level of Cognitive Ability: Applying
Client Needs: Health Promotion and Maintenance
Clinical Judgment/Cognitive Skills: Recognize Cues
Integrated Process: Clinical Judgment; Nursing Process/Assessment
Content Area: Health Assessment/Physical Exam: Musculoskeletal
Health Problems: Pediatric-Specific: Scoliosis
Priority Concepts: Health Promotion; Mobility

Answer: 1, 3, 6
Rationale: Scoliosis is a lateral curvature of the spine. To ensure early detection and treatment, children aged 9 through 15 years need to be screened for scoliosis; those at greatest risk are girls from 10 years of age through adolescence. The child needs to be unclothed or wearing only underpants so that the chest, back, and hips can be clearly seen. The child would stand with the weight equally on both feet, legs straight, and arms hanging loosely at the sides. The nurse then observes for the signs of scoliosis. These signs include nonpainful lateral curvature of the spine, a curve with one turn (C curve) or two compensating curves (S curve), lateral deviation and rotation of each vertebra, unequal shoulder heights, unequal waist angles, unequal rib prominences and chest asymmetry, and unequal rib heights.
Test-Taking Strategy: Focus on the subject, the signs of scoliosis, and recall the definition of scoliosis, a lateral curvature of the spine. Visualize this disorder and note the word "equal" in the incorrect choices.
Priority Nursing Tip: If scoliosis is suspected, radiographs will be done to confirm the diagnosis.
Reference: McKinney, E. S., et al. (2022). *Maternal child nursing* (6th ed., pp. 714, 1232). Elsevier.

19. The nurse is teaching a client diagnosed with histoplasmosis infection about the prevention of future exposure to infectious sources. The nurse determines that the client **needs further instruction** if the client states that which is a potential source of this infection?
1. Grape arbors
2. Bird droppings
3. Mushroom cellars
4. Floors of chicken houses

Level of Cognitive Ability: Evaluating
Client Needs: Health Promotion and Maintenance
Clinical Judgment/Cognitive Skills: Evaluate Outcomes
Integrated Process: Clinical Judgment; Nursing Process/Evaluation
Content Area: Foundations of Care: Infection Control
Health Problems: Adult Health: Respiratory: Infections of the Lower Airway
Priority Concepts: Patient Education; Infection

Answer: 1
Rationale: Grape arbors do not harbor the causative organism for histoplasmosis. The client diagnosed with histoplasmosis is taught to avoid exposure to potential sources of the fungus, including bird droppings (especially those of starlings and blackbirds), mushroom cellars, and the floors of chicken houses and bat caves.
Test-Taking Strategy: Note the strategic words, *needs further instruction*. These words indicate a negative event query and ask you to select an option that is an incorrect statement. Eliminate bird droppings and floors of chicken houses first because they are comparable or alike in that both are associated with birds. Because histoplasmosis is a fungus, recall that there is increased exposure to areas in which the fungus thrives. Therefore, the least likely option is the grape arbor, which is above ground and is not in a dark and damp area.
Priority Nursing Tip: Transmission of histoplasmosis occurs by the inhalation of spores commonly found in contaminated soil.
Reference: Ignatavicius, D., et al. (2021). *Medical-surgical nursing: Concepts for interprofessional collaborative care* (10th ed., p. 583). Elsevier.

❖ **20.** Which factors increase the risk for hypothermia in an older client? **Select all that apply.**
❑ 1. Burns
❑ 2. Anemia
❑ 3. Alcohol abuse
❑ 4. Hypoglycemia
❑ 5. Hyperthyroidism
❑ 6. Poor thermoregulation

Level of Cognitive Ability: Analyzing
Client Needs: Health Promotion and Maintenance
Clinical Judgment/Cognitive Skills: Recognize Cues
Integrated Process: Clinical Judgment; Nursing Process/Assessment
Content Area: Adult Health: Neurologic
Health Problems: Adult Health: Neurologic: Thermoregulation
Priority Concepts: Development; Thermoregulation

Answer: 1, 2, 3, 4, 6
Rationale: The median oral temperature of an older client is 96.8° F (36° C). Environmental temperatures below 65° F (18° C) may cause a serious drop in core body temperature to 95° F (35° C) or less in the older client. Numerous factors increase the risk of hypothermia in the older client, including conditions that increase heat loss (e.g., burns); conditions that decrease heat production such as hypothyroidism, hypoglycemia, or anemia; medications or substances that interfere with thermoregulation, such as alcohol; or thermoregulatory impairment (failure to sense cold).
Test-Taking Strategy: Focus on the subject, the risks associated with hypothermia. Recall that hypothermia is an abnormally dangerous and low body temperature. Next think about the pathophysiology or effects of each item in the options to answer correctly.
Priority Nursing Tip: Hypothermia can lead to hypoxia and subsequently insufficient circulation, which can be fatal. Early signs include shivering and mental confusion.
Reference: Ignatavicius, D., et al. (2021). *Medical-surgical nursing: Concepts for interprofessional collaborative care* (10th ed., p. 216). Elsevier.

21. The nurse is assigned to care for a client being admitted with a diagnosis of cirrhosis and ascites. Which dietary measure would the nurse expect to be prescribed for the client?
1. Sodium restriction
2. Increased fat intake
3. Decreased carbohydrates
4. Calorie restriction of 1500 daily

Level of Cognitive Ability: Analyzing
Client Needs: Physiological Integrity
Clinical Judgment/Cognitive Skills: Recognize Cues
Integrated Process: Clinical Judgment; Nursing Process/Assessment
Content Area: Adult Health: Gastrointestinal
Health Problems: Adult Health: Gastrointestinal: Cirrhosis
Priority Concepts: Fluids and Electrolytes; Nutrition

Answer: 1
Rationale: If the client has ascites, sodium and possibly fluids would be restricted in the diet. The client should maintain a normal amount of fat intake. The diet needs to supply sufficient carbohydrates to maintain weight and spare protein. The total daily calories range should be between 2000 and 3000. The diet needs to provide ample protein to rebuild tissue but not an amount that will precipitate hepatic encephalopathy.
Test-Taking Strategy: Focus on the **subject**, cirrhosis and ascites. Recalling that ascites refers to the accumulation of body fluid will direct you to the correct option.
Priority Nursing Tip: For the client with cirrhosis, protein may not be restricted in the diet if ascites and edema are absent and the client does not exhibit signs of impending coma.
References: Ignatavicius, D., et al. (2021). *Medical-surgical nursing: Concepts for interprofessional collaborative care* (10th ed., p. 1165). Elsevier; Lewis, S., et al. (2020, pp. 980, 986–987). *Medical-surgical nursing: Assessment and management of clinical problems* (11th ed.). Elsevier.

❖ **22.** The nurse reviews the pattern of a nonstress test performed on a pregnant client and interprets the finding as which result? **(Refer to the figure.)**

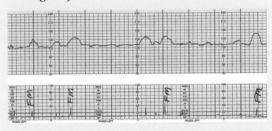

1. Reactive
2. Abnormal
3. Nonreactive
4. Nonreassuring

Level of Cognitive Ability: Analyzing
Client Needs: Health Promotion and Maintenance
Clinical Judgment/Cognitive Skills: Analyze Cues
Integrated Process: Clinical Judgment; Nursing Process/Analysis
Content Area: Maternity: Antepartum
Health Problems: N/A
Priority Concepts: Health Promotion; Reproduction

Answer: 1
Rationale: A nonstress test assesses fetal well-being and evaluates the ability of the fetal heart to accelerate, often in association with fetal movement. Accelerations of the fetal heart rate are associated with adequate oxygenation, a healthy neural pathway, and the fetal heart's ability to respond to stimuli. A reactive test is described as at least two fetal heart rate accelerations, with or without fetal movement, occurring within a 20-minute period and peaking at least 15 beats/min above the baseline and lasting 15 seconds from baseline to baseline. This recording (see figure) identifies a reactive nonstress test. The fetal heart rate acceleration peaks at least 15 beats/min and lasts for at least 15 seconds in response to fetal movement. A nonreactive test is an abnormal or nonreassuring test. In a nonreactive test, the recording does not demonstrate the required characteristics of a reactive test within a 40-minute period.
Test-Taking Strategy: Note the accelerations identified in the figure. Also note that abnormal, nonreactive, and nonreassuring results are **comparable or alike** in that they all indicate an abnormal or nonreactive test results.
Priority Nursing Tip: A nonstress test is a noninvasive measure of fetal well-being. A contraction stress test is performed if the nonstress test is abnormal and involves exposing the fetus to the stress of contractions using a dilute dose of oxytocin.
Reference: McKinney, E. S., et al. (2022). *Maternal child nursing* (6th ed., p. 286). Elsevier.

23. A client is diagnosed with hyperphosphatemia caused by hypoparathyroidism. To prevent worsening of the condition, the nurse would instruct the client to avoid which food selections? **Select all that apply.**

- ❑ 1. Fish
- ❑ 2. Eggs
- ❑ 3. Coffee
- ❑ 4. Grapes
- ❑ 5. Bananas
- ❑ 6. Whole-grain breads

Level of Cognitive Ability: Applying
Client Needs: Health Promotion and Maintenance
Clinical Judgment/Cognitive Skills: Generate Solutions
Integrated Process: Clinical Judgment; Teaching and Learning
Content Area: Skills: Nutrition
Health Problems: Adult Health: Endocrine: Parathyroid Disorders
Priority Concepts: Health Promotion; Nutrition

Answer: 1, 2, 6
Rationale: Food items and liquids that are naturally high in phosphates include fish, eggs, milk products, whole grains, vegetables, and carbonated beverages, and they need to be avoided by the client with hyperphosphatemia. Coffee, grapes, and bananas are acceptable for this client to consume because their phosphate levels are not significant.
Test-Taking Strategy: Focus on the subject, hyperphosphatemia, and the items to avoid because they will worsen the condition. Eliminate grapes and bananas because they are comparable or alike as both are fruits. Coffee does not contain a high phosphate level. Recalling the phosphate content of foods and fluids will assist in answering correctly.
Priority Nursing Tip: The reference range for phosphorus (phosphate) level is 3.0 to 4.5 mg/dL (0.97 to 1.45 mmol/L).
Reference: Lewis, S., et al. (2020). *Medical-surgical nursing: Assessment and management of clinical problems* (11th ed., p. 283). Elsevier.

❖ 24. The community health nurse provides an educational session regarding the risk factors for cervical cancer to people in the local community. The nurse determines that **further teaching is needed** if a person attending the session identifies which as a risk factor for this type of cancer?

1. Smoking tobacco
2. Single sex partner
3. Early age of first intercourse
4. Human papillomavirus (HPV) infection

Level of Cognitive Ability: Evaluating
Client Needs: Health Promotion and Maintenance
Clinical Judgment/Cognitive Skills: Evaluate Outcomes
Integrated Process: Clinical Judgment; Nursing Process/Evaluation
Content Area: Foundations of Care: Community / Public/Population Health
Health Problems: Adult Health: Cancer: Cervical/ Uterine/Ovarian
Priority Concepts: Patient Education; Health Promotion

Answer: 2
Rationale: Having a single sex partner is not a risk factor for cervical cancer. Some risk factors for cervical cancer include having multiple sexual partners or a partner who had multiple sexual partners, smoking tobacco, early age of first intercourse, and HPV infection.
Test-Taking Strategy: Note the strategic words, *further teaching is needed*. These words indicate a negative event query and ask you to select an option that is an incorrect risk factor. Noting the word "single" will direct you to this option.
Priority Nursing Tip: Premalignant changes for cervical cancer are described on a continuum from dysplasia, which is the earliest premalignancy change, to carcinoma in situ, the most advanced premalignant change.
Reference: Ignatavicius, D., et al. (2021). *Medical-surgical nursing: Concepts for interprofessional collaborative care* (10th ed., pp. 373, 1463). Elsevier.

25. The community health nurse teaches a group of clients how to prevent pelvic inflammatory disease (PID). What instruction would the nurse include?
1. To douche monthly
2. To avoid unprotected intercourse
3. To use only ultra-low dose oral contraceptive pills
4. To consult with a gynecologist regarding the placement of an intrauterine device (IUD)

Level of Cognitive Ability: Applying
Client Needs: Health Promotion and Maintenance
Clinical Judgment/Cognitive Skills: Generate Solutions
Integrated Process: Clinical Judgment; Teaching and Learning
Content Area: Foundations of Care: Community / Public/Population Health
Health Problems: Adult Health: Reproductive: Inflammatory/Infectious Problems
Priority Concepts: Patient Education; Health Promotion

Answer: **2**
Rationale: PID is an infection of the pelvis. The primary prevention of PID includes avoiding unprotected intercourse. Douching leads to a higher risk for PID. It is believed that high hormonal doses may decrease risk of PID, but ultra-low doses will not. The use of an IUD may also increase the risk for PID.
Test-Taking Strategy: Focus on the subject, preventing PID. Eliminate option 3 first because of the closed-ended word "only." Next, recall the principle of the exposure of the pelvic area to factors that cause infection. With this concept in mind, eliminate monthly douching and using an IUD. The only safe measure to take to avoid PID is avoiding unprotected intercourse.
Priority Nursing Tip: Pelvic inflammatory disease occurs when organisms from the lower genital tract invade the uterine cavity and the fallopian tubes.
Reference: Ignatavicius, D., et al. (2021). *Medical-surgical nursing: Concepts for interprofessional collaborative care* (10th ed., p. 1519). Elsevier.

❖ **26.** The nurse provides discharge teaching to a client after a vasectomy. Which statement by the client indicates the **need for further teaching?**
1. "I can use a scrotal support if I need to."
2. "I don't need to practice birth control any longer."
3. "I can resume sexual intercourse whenever I want."
4. "I can use an ice bag and take an analgesic for pain or swelling."

Level of Cognitive Ability: Evaluating
Client Needs: Health Promotion and Maintenance
Clinical Judgment/Cognitive Skills: Evaluate Outcomes
Integrated Process: Clinical Judgment; Nursing Process/Evaluation
Content Area: Adult Health: Reproductive
Health Problems: Adult Health: Reproductive: Menstruation Problems/Fertility/Infertility
Priority Concepts: Patient Education; Reproduction

Answer: **2**
Rationale: After vasectomy, the client must continue to practice a method of birth control until the follow-up semen analysis shows azoospermia. Live sperm may be present in the vas deferens after this procedure. Using scrotal support, resuming sexual activity, and promoting pain relief with ice and taking an analgesic such as acetaminophen are appropriate client statements.
Test-Taking Strategy: Note the strategic words, *need for further teaching.* These words indicate a negative event query and ask you to select an option that is an incorrect statement. Thinking about the purpose of a vasectomy will assist in answering correctly. Scrotal support, ice, and acetaminophen analgesic can be eliminated because these measures assist with alleviating discomfort and swelling after the procedure. There would be no reason to avoid sexual intercourse unless the client was experiencing discomfort.
Priority Nursing Tip: A vasectomy is a surgical procedure performed to prevent the release of sperm during ejaculation. It is a method of birth control.
Reference: Lewis, S., et al. (2020). *Medical-surgical nursing: Assessment and management of clinical problems* (11th ed., p. 1273). Elsevier.

27. A nursing instructor asks a student to identify risk factors for and methods of preventing prostate cancer. Which statement by the student indicates the **need for further teaching?**
1. "Smoking increases the risk for this type of cancer."
2. "A high-fat diet will assist in preventing this type of cancer."
3. "A history of a sexually transmitted infection is a risk for this disease."
4. "Those greater than 50 years old need to be monitored with a yearly digital rectal exam."

Level of Cognitive Ability: Evaluating
Client Needs: Health Promotion and Maintenance
Clinical Judgment/Cognitive Skills: Evaluate Outcomes
Integrated Process: Clinical Judgment; Nursing Process/Evaluation
Content Area: Adult Health: Oncology
Health Problems: Adult Health: Cancer: Prostate
Priority Concepts: Clinical Judgment; Health Promotion

Answer: 2
Rationale: Smoking, history of a sexually transmitted infection, and yearly digital examinations are accurate statements regarding the risks and prevention measures related to this type of cancer. Prostate cancer is a slow-growing malignancy of the prostate gland. A high intake of dietary fat is a risk factor for prostate cancer.
Test-Taking Strategy: Note the strategic words, *need for further teaching.* These words indicate a negative event query and ask you to select an option that is an incorrect statement. Recalling the general principles related to cancer prevention will direct you to the correct option.
Priority Nursing Tip: The risk of prostate cancer increases with each decade after the age of 50 years.
References: Ignatavicius, D., et al. (2021). *Medical-surgical nursing: Concepts for interprofessional collaborative care* (10th ed., p. 1470). Elsevier; Lewis, S., et al. (2020). *Medical-surgical nursing: Assessment and management of clinical problems* (11th ed., p. 1262). Elsevier.

 28. A clinic nurse provides information to a married couple regarding measures to prevent infertility. Which statement made by the couple indicates the **need for further education?**
1. "Eating a nutritious diet is most important."
2. "It's necessary to avoid the excessive intake of alcohol."
3. "We need to decrease exposure to environmental hazards."
4. "We need to maintain warmth to the scrotum by taking hot baths frequently."

Level of Cognitive Ability: Evaluating
Client Needs: Health Promotion and Maintenance
Clinical Judgment/Cognitive Skills: Evaluate Outcomes
Integrated Process: Clinical Judgment; Nursing Process/Evaluation
Content Area: Adult Health: Reproductive
Health Problems: Adult Health: Reproductive: Menstruation Problems/Fertility/Infertility
Priority Concepts: Patient Education; Reproduction

Answer: 4
Rationale: Keeping the testes cool by avoiding hot baths and tight clothing appears to improve the sperm count. Avoiding factors that depress spermatogenesis (such as the use of drugs, alcohol, and marijuana), maintaining good nutrition, and limiting exposure to occupational and environmental hazards are vital components of preventing infertility.
Test-Taking Strategy: Note the strategic words, *need for further education.* These words indicate a negative event query and ask you to select an option that is an incorrect statement. Eliminate option 1 first because the maintenance of a nutritious diet is important in all situations. From the remaining options, recalling that heat decreases the motility of sperm will assist with directing you to the correct option.
Priority Nursing Tip: Infertility is the involuntary inability to conceive when desired. Several diagnostic tests are available to determine the probable cause of infertility, and the therapy recommended may depend on the cause.
Reference: Lewis, S., et al. (2020). *Medical-surgical nursing: Assessment and management of clinical problems* (11th ed., pp. 1275–1276). Elsevier.

29. The nurse is teaching a client who is preparing for discharge from the hospital after a total hip arthroplasty. Which statement by the client indicates the **need for further teaching?**

1. "I need to avoid twisting my body when I am standing."
2. "I need to check my incision every day for signs of infection."
3. "I should not sit in one position for a prolonged period of time."
4. "I can cross my legs if it is more comfortable for me when I sit."

Level of Cognitive Ability: Evaluating
Client Needs: Health Promotion and Maintenance
Clinical Judgment/Cognitive Skills: Evaluate Outcomes
Integrated Process: Clinical Judgment; Nursing Process/Evaluation
Content Area: Adult Health: Musculoskeletal
Health Problems: Adult Health: Musculoskeletal: Skeletal Injury
Priority Concepts: Patient Education; Health Promotion

Answer: **4**
Rationale: After total hip arthroplasty, there are several measures that the client needs to take to ensure healing and protection and safety to the surgical site. Some hip precautions include not standing or sitting for prolonged periods of time, avoiding crossing the legs beyond the midline of the body, avoiding bending the hips more than 90 degrees, and avoiding twisting the body when standing. The client is also instructed to check the incision site daily for signs of infection (redness, heat, or drainage) and to contact the surgeon if signs of infection are noted.
Test-Taking Strategy: Note the strategic words, *need for further teaching.* These words indicate a negative event query and ask you to select an option that is an incorrect statement. Recalling standard measures related to the postoperative period will assist you in eliminating monitoring for signs of infection. To select from the remaining options, think about this surgical procedure and the measures that will protect the surgical site; this will direct you to the correct option.
Priority Nursing Tip: In the postoperative period after total hip arthroplasty, an important nursing intervention is to perform frequent neurovascular assessments of the affected extremity by checking color, pulses, capillary refill, movement, and sensation.
Reference: Ignatavicius, D., et al. (2021). *Medical-surgical nursing: Concepts for interprofessional collaborative care* (10th ed., p. 1012). Elsevier.

❖ **30.** The nurse is working at an osteoporosis screening clinic and is interviewing and performing health assessments on clients. Which clients are at greatest risk for developing osteoporosis? **Select all that apply.**

☐ 1. An older adult client
☐ 2. A large-boned, dark-skinned client
☐ 3. A client who started menopause early
☐ 4. A client with a family history of the disease
☐ 5. A client who has a physically active lifestyle
☐ 6. A client with an inadequate intake of calcium and vitamin D

Level of Cognitive Ability: Analyzing
Client Needs: Health Promotion and Maintenance
Clinical Judgment/Cognitive Skills: Recognize Cues
Integrated Process: Clinical Judgment; Nursing Process/Assessment
Content Area: Health Assessment/Physical Exam: Health History
Health Problems: Adult Health: Musculoskeletal: Osteoporosis
Priority Concepts: Health Promotion; Mobility

Answer: **1, 3, 4, 6**
Rationale: Osteoporosis is a disorder characterized by abnormal loss of bone density and deterioration of bone tissue, with an increased fracture risk. Asian, white, small-boned, and fair-skinned persons are at greatest risk for osteoporosis. Other risk factors include early menopause, a family history of the disease, and a sedentary lifestyle. Inadequate intake of calcium and vitamin D is a major risk factor because it results in abnormal loss of bone density and deterioration of bone tissue. Those who smoke, drink alcohol, or take corticosteroids or anticonvulsants, as well as those who consume excessive amounts of caffeine, also have increased risk for osteoporosis.
Test-Taking Strategy: Focus on the subject, the risk factors for osteoporosis. Recalling that osteoporosis is characterized by an abnormal loss of bone density and deterioration of bone tissue will assist in identifying the risk factors. Also remember that small-boned, fair-skinned, white and Asian persons are at greatest risk for osteoporosis.
Priority Nursing Tip: A client with osteoporosis is at risk for pathologic fractures.
Reference: Ignatavicius, D., et al. (2021). *Medical-surgical nursing: Concepts for interprofessional collaborative care* (10th ed., p. 985). Elsevier.

31. The clinic nurse instructs a client diagnosed with type 1 diabetes mellitus about preventing diabetic ketoacidosis on days when the client is feeling ill. Which statement by the client indicates the **need for further teaching?**
  1. "I need to stop my insulin if I am vomiting."
  2. "I need to call my doctor if I am ill for more than 24 hours."
  3. "I need to eat 10 to 15 g of carbohydrates every 1 to 2 hours."
  4. "I need to drink small quantities of fluid every 15 to 30 minutes."

Level of Cognitive Ability: Evaluating
Client Needs: Health Promotion and Maintenance
Clinical Judgment/Cognitive Skills: Evaluate Outcomes
Integrated Process: Clinical Judgment; Nursing Process/Evaluation
Content Area: Adult Health: Endocrine
Health Problems: Adult Health: Endocrine: Diabetes Mellitus
Priority Concepts: Patient Education; Glucose Regulation

Answer: 1
Rationale: Diabetic ketoacidosis is a life-threatening complication of type 1 diabetes mellitus that develops when a severe insulin deficiency occurs. The client needs to be instructed to take insulin, even if the client is vomiting and unable to eat. It is important to self-monitor blood glucose more frequently during illness (every 2 to 4 hours). If the pre-meal blood glucose is more than 250 mg/dL (13.9 mmol/L), the client needs to test for urine ketones and contact the primary health care provider. All the remaining options are accurate interventions.
Test-Taking Strategy: Note the strategic words, *need for further teaching*. These words indicate a negative event query and ask you to select an option that is an incorrect statement. Recalling that insulin must be taken every day will assist with directing you to the correct option.
Priority Nursing Tip: The primary clinical manifestations of diabetic ketoacidosis include hyperglycemia, dehydration, ketosis, and acidosis. The client will have a "fruity" breath odor.
Reference: Ignatavicius, D., et al. (2021). *Medical-surgical nursing: Concepts for interprofessional collaborative care* (10th ed., p. 1294). Elsevier.

❖ **32.** The nurse is instructing a client with diabetes mellitus regarding hypoglycemia. Which statement by the client indicates the **need for further teaching?**
  1. "Hypoglycemia can occur at any time of the day or night."
  2. "I need to drink 6 to 8 ounces of milk if hypoglycemia occurs."
  3. "If I feel sweaty or shaky, I might be experiencing hypoglycemia."
  4. "If hypoglycemia occurs, I need to take my regular insulin as prescribed."

Level of Cognitive Ability: Evaluating
Client Needs: Health Promotion and Maintenance
Clinical Judgment/Cognitive Skills: Evaluate Outcomes
Integrated Process: Clinical Judgment; Nursing Process/Evaluation
Content Area: Adult Health: Endocrine
Health Problems: Adult Health: Endocrine: Diabetes Mellitus
Priority Concepts: Patient Education; Glucose Regulation

Answer: 4
Rationale: Hypoglycemia can occur when the blood glucose level falls below 70 mg/dL (3.9 mmol/L). Insulin is not taken as a treatment for hypoglycemia because the insulin will lower the blood glucose level. Hypoglycemic reactions can occur at any time of the day or night. If a hypoglycemic reaction occurs, the client will need to consume 10 to 15 g of carbohydrate; 6 to 8 ounces of milk, for example, contain this amount of carbohydrate. Tremors and diaphoresis are signs of mild hypoglycemia.
Test-Taking Strategy: Note the strategic words, *need for further teaching*. These words indicate a negative event query and ask you to select an option that is an incorrect statement. Remember that the blood glucose level is lowered in clients with hypoglycemia. Insulin also lowers blood glucose; therefore, it would seem reasonable that insulin is not a treatment for this condition.
Priority Nursing Tip: Never attempt to administer food or fluids to a client experiencing a severe hypoglycemic reaction who is semiconscious or unconscious and is unable to swallow because the client is at risk for aspiration.
References: Ignatavicius, D., et al. (2021). *Medical-surgical nursing: Concepts for interprofessional collaborative care* (10th ed., p. 984). Elsevier; Lewis, S., et al. (2020). *Medical-surgical nursing: Assessment and management of clinical problems* (11th ed., pp. 1134–1135). Elsevier.

33. A client diagnosed with nephrolithiasis arrives at the clinic for a follow-up visit. The laboratory analysis of the stone that the client passed 1 week ago indicates that the stone is composed of calcium oxalate. On the basis of this analysis, the nurse would tell the client that it is **best** to avoid which food to minimize the risk of recurrence?

1. Pasta
2. Lentils
3. Lettuce
4. Spinach

Level of Cognitive Ability: Applying
Client Needs: Health Promotion and Maintenance
Clinical Judgment/Cognitive Skills: Take Action
Integrated Process: Clinical Judgment; Teaching and Learning
Content Area: Adult Health: Renal and Urinary
Health Problems: Adult Health: Renal and Urinary: Calculi
Priority Concepts: Patient Education; Health Promotion

Answer: 4
Rationale: Many kidney stones are composed of calcium oxalate. Foods that raise urinary oxalate excretion and predispose to stone formation include spinach, rhubarb, strawberries, chocolate, wheat bran, nuts, beets, almonds, cashews, and tea.
Test-Taking Strategy: Note the strategic word, *best*, and the subject, the food to avoid, and focus on the type of stone and that it is composed of calcium oxalate. Recalling that foods such as spinach raise urinary oxalate excretion will direct you to the correct option.
Priority Nursing Tip: Renal colic originates in the lumbar region and radiates around the side and down to the testicles and to the bladder. Ureteral colic radiates toward the genitalia and thighs.
Reference: Ignatavicius, D., et al. (2021). *Medical-surgical nursing: Concepts for interprofessional collaborative care* (10th ed., p. 1345). Elsevier.

 34. The nurse provides instructions to a new parent who is about to breast-feed/chest-feed the newborn infant. The nurse observes the new parent while breast-feeding/chest-feeding for the first time and determines the **need for further teaching** if the new parent applies which technique?

1. Turns the newborn infant on the side, facing the parent
2. Tilts up the nipple or squeezes the areola, pushing it into the newborn's mouth
3. Draws the newborn the rest of the way onto the breast/chest when the newborn opens the mouth
4. Places a clean finger in the side of the newborn's mouth to break the suction before removing the newborn from the breast/chest

Level of Cognitive Ability: Evaluating
Client Needs: Health Promotion and Maintenance
Clinical Judgment/Cognitive Skills: Evaluate Outcomes
Integrated Process: Clinical Judgment; Teaching and Learning
Content Area: Maternity: Postpartum
Health Problems: N/A
Priority Concepts: Patient Education; Health Promotion

Answer: 2
Rationale: The parent is instructed to avoid tilting up the nipple or squeezing the areola and pushing it into the newborn's mouth; doing so leads to improper latch or difficulties with the flow of milk. Side-lying position, bringing the newborn to the breast/chest, and correctly breaking suction are appropriate interventions for breast-feeding/chest-feeding.
Test-Taking Strategy: Note the strategic words, *need for further teaching*. This creates a negative event query and asks you to select the incorrect client action. Visualize the descriptions in each of the options. This will eliminate options 1, 3, and 4. Also, carefully reading option 2 and noting the word *pushing*, which suggests force or resistance, will assist with directing you to this option.
Priority Nursing Tip: A breast-fed/chest-fed infant's stools are usually light yellow, seedy, watery, and frequent.
Reference: McKinney, E. S., et al. (2022). *Maternal child nursing* (6th ed., pp. 493–495). Elsevier.

35. The clinic nurse provides home care instructions to a parent regarding the care of the child who is diagnosed with croup. Which statement by the parent indicates the **need for further instructions?**
1. "I will give Tylenol for the fever."
2. "I will give cough syrup every night at bedtime."
3. "Sips of warm fluids during a croup attack will help."
4. "I will place a cool-mist humidifier next to my child's bed."

Level of Cognitive Ability: Evaluating
Client Needs: Health Promotion and Maintenance
Clinical Judgment/Cognitive Skills: Evaluate Outcomes
Integrated Process: Clinical Judgment; Nursing Process/Evaluation
Content Area: Pediatrics: Throat/Respiratory
Health Problems: Pediatric-Specific: Croup
Priority Concepts: Patient Education; Health Promotion

Answer: 2
Rationale: The parent needs to be instructed that cough syrup and cold medicines should not be administered because they may dry and thicken secretions. Acetaminophen (Tylenol) will reduce the fever. Sips of warm fluid will relax the vocal cords and thin the mucus. A cool-mist humidifier rather than a steam vaporizer is recommended because of the danger of the child pulling the machine over and causing a burn.
Test-Taking Strategy: Note the strategic words, *need for further instructions.* These words indicate a negative event query and ask you to select an option that is an incorrect statement. Recalling that cough syrup dries secretions will assist with directing you to select this option for additional instruction. Administration of acetaminophen can be eliminated first, recalling that this medication is normally prescribed to reduce a fever. Recalling that warm fluids will thin secretions will assist you in eliminating this option.
Priority Nursing Tip: Monitor the child with croup for signs/symptoms of respiratory distress, including nasal flaring, sternal retraction, and inspiratory stridor.
Reference: McKinney, E. S., et al. (2022) *Maternal child nursing* (6th ed., p. 1051). Elsevier.

❖ **36.** A client diagnosed with anxiety disorder is prescribed buspirone orally. When the client reports that it is difficult to swallow the tablets, the nurse provides which instruction to promote compliance?
1. Crush the tablets before taking them.
2. Mix the tablets uncrushed in applesauce.
3. Purchase the liquid preparation with the next refill.
4. Call the physician for a change in medication.

Level of Cognitive Ability: Applying
Client Needs: Health Promotion and Maintenance
Clinical Judgment/Cognitive Skills: Take Action
Integrated Process: Clinical Judgment; Nursing Process/Implementation
Content Area: Pharmacology: Psychotherapeutics: Antianxiety/Anxiolytics
Health Problems: Mental Health: Anxiety Disorder
Priority Concepts: Adherence; Patient Education

Answer: 1
Rationale: Buspirone tablets may be crushed and administered without regard to meals. Mixing the tablet uncrushed in applesauce will not ensure ease of swallowing. This medication is not available in liquid form. It is premature to advise the client to call the physician for a change in medication without first trying alternative interventions.
Test-Taking Strategy: Focus on the subject, difficulty swallowing buspirone. Eliminate notifying the physician because, in most situations, a nursing intervention can be instituted first before calling the physician. Next, eliminate mixing the uncrushed tablet in applesauce because this instruction will not ensure ease of swallowing. This medication is not available in liquid form.
Priority Nursing Tip: Most tablets can be crushed if needed to facilitate administration. Enteric-coated and sustained-release tablets are not to be crushed. Additionally, capsules are not to be crushed.
References: Kizior, R., & Hodgson, B. (2023). *Saunders Nursing drug handbook 2023* (p. 165). Elsevier; Skidmore-Roth, L. (2021). *2021 Mosby's Nursing drug reference* (34th ed., p. 201). Elsevier.

37. The nurse caring for a child with congestive heart failure who will be discharged to home provides instructions to the parents regarding the administration of digoxin. Which statement by the parent indicates a **need for further teaching?**
1. "I will mix the medication with food."
2. "I will check my child's pulse before giving the medication."
3. "If my child vomits after I give the medication, I will not repeat the dose."
4. "I will check the dose of medication with my spouse before I give the medication."

Level of Cognitive Ability: Evaluating
Client Needs: Health Promotion and Maintenance
Clinical Judgment/Cognitive Skills: Evaluate Outcomes
Integrated Process: Clinical Judgment; Nursing Process/Evaluation
Content Area: Pharmacology: Cardiovascular: Cardiac Glycosides
Health Problems: Pediatric-Specific: Congenital Cardiac Defects
Priority Concepts: Patient Education; Safety

Answer: 1
Rationale: Digoxin is a cardiac glycoside. The medication should not be mixed with food or formula because this method would not ensure that the child receives the entire dose of medication. Checking the child's pulse, not repeating the dose following vomiting, and having a second medication check are correct interventions. Additionally, if a dosage is missed and this is not identified until 4 or more hours later, the dose is not administered. If more than one consecutive dose is missed, the physician needs to be notified.
Test-Taking Strategy: Note the strategic words, *need for further teaching.* These words indicate a negative event query and ask you to select an option that is an incorrect statement. General principles regarding medication administration to children will assist with directing you to the correct option. Mixing medications with formula or food may alter the effectiveness of the medication. More important, if the child does not consume all of the formula or food, the total dosage may not be administered.
Priority Nursing Tip: Signs of digoxin toxicity in an infant include poor feeding and vomiting.
Reference: McKinney, E. S., et al. (2022). *Maternal child nursing* (6th ed., p. 1094). Elsevier.

❖ **38.** The nurse provides discharge instructions to the parent of a child who was hospitalized for heart surgery. Which instruction would the nurse provide to the parent?
1. The child can play outside for short periods of time.
2. After bathing the child, rub lotion and sprinkle powder on the incision.
3. The child may return to school 1 week after hospital discharge.
4. Notify the surgeon if the child develops a fever greater than 100.5° F (38° C).

Level of Cognitive Ability: Applying
Client Needs: Health Promotion and Maintenance
Clinical Judgment/Cognitive Skills: Take Action
Integrated Process: Clinical Judgment; Teaching and Learning
Content Area: Pediatrics: Cardiovascular
Health Problems: Pediatric-Specific: Congenital Cardiac Defects
Priority Concepts: Patient Education; Safety

Answer: 4
Rationale: After the child has heart surgery, the surgeon must be notified if the child develops a fever of more than 100.5° F (38° C). The parent is instructed to not allow the child to play outside for several weeks. No creams, lotions, or powders should be placed on the incision until it is completely healed and without scabs. The child should not return to school until 3 weeks after hospital discharge, at which time the child would go to school for half days for the first few days.
Test-Taking Strategy: Note the subject, a child who was hospitalized for heart surgery. Keep in mind the potential for infection in this child. Eliminate outside play because this can expose the child to infection and the risk of injury. Basic principles related to incision care will assist you in eliminating application of lotion and powder. Eliminate early return to school because of the time frame of only 1 week.
Priority Nursing Tip: Immunizations, dental visits, and invasive procedures must be avoided for 2 months in the child who had cardiac surgery.
Reference: McKinney, E. S., et al. (2022). *Maternal child nursing* (6th ed., p. 1111). Elsevier.

39. The clinic nurse provides instructions to a client who will begin taking oral contraceptives. Which statement by the client indicates the **need for further teaching?**
1. "I will take one pill daily at the same time every day."
2. "If I miss a pill, I must take it as soon as I remember."
3. "I will not need to use an additional birth control method after I start these pills."
4. "If I miss two pills, I will take them both as soon as I remember, and then two pills the next day."

Level of Cognitive Ability: Evaluating
Client Needs: Health Promotion and Maintenance
Clinical Judgment/Cognitive Skills: Evaluate Outcomes
Integrated Process: Clinical Judgment; Nursing Process/Evaluation
Content Area: Pharmacology: Reproductive: Contraceptives
Health Problems: Adult Health: Reproductive: Menstruation Problems/Fertility/Infertility
Priority Concepts: Patient Education; Reproduction

Answer: 3
Rationale: The client must be instructed to use a second birth control method during the first pill cycle of contraceptives. Taking the pill at the same time each day, taking a missed pill as soon as it is remembered, and taking 2 missed pills as soon as remembered and doubling up the next day are correct responses. Additionally, the client must be instructed that, if three pills are missed, the client will need to discontinue pill use for that cycle and use another birth control method.
Test-Taking Strategy: Note the strategic words, *need for further teaching.* These words indicate a negative event query and ask you to select an option that is an incorrect statement. It would seem reasonable that, during the first pill cycle, a second birth control method would need to be used to prevent conception.
Priority Nursing Tip: Contraceptives provide reversible prevention of pregnancy.
Reference: Lilley, L., Rainforth Collins, S., & Snyder J. (2020). *Pharmacology and the nursing process* (9th ed., p. 535). Elsevier.

❖ **40.** The nurse is providing home care dietary instructions to a client who has been hospitalized for pancreatitis. Which food would the nurse instruct the client to avoid to prevent recurrence?
1. Chili
2. Bagels
3. Lentil soup
4. Watermelon

Level of Cognitive Ability: Applying
Client Needs: Health Promotion and Maintenance
Clinical Judgment/Cognitive Skills: Take Action
Integrated Process: Clinical Judgment; Teaching and Learning
Content Area: Adult Health: Gastrointestinal
Health Problems: Adult Health: Gastrointestinal: Pancreatitis
Priority Concepts: Patient Education; Inflammation

Answer: 1
Rationale: Pancreatitis is the acute or chronic inflammation of the pancreas with the associated escape of pancreatic enzymes into surrounding tissue. The client must avoid spicy foods such as chili, alcohol, coffee, tea, and heavy meals because they stimulate pancreatic secretions and produce attacks of pancreatitis. The client is instructed regarding the benefit of eating small, frequent meals that are high in protein, low in fat, and moderate to high in carbohydrates.
Test-Taking Strategy: Focus on the subject, the food item to avoid to prevent recurrence of pancreatitis. Note that bagels, lentil soup, and watermelon are foods that are moderately bland. Option 1 is different in that chili is a spicy food.
Priority Nursing Tip: Cullen's sign is the discoloration of the abdomen and periumbilical area. Turner's sign is the bluish coloration of the flanks. Both are signs indicative of pancreatitis.
Reference: Ignatavicius, D., et al. (2021). *Medical-surgical nursing: Concepts for interprofessional collaborative care* (10th ed., p. 1187). Elsevier.

41. The home care nurse visits a client who was recently diagnosed with cirrhosis and provides home care management instructions to the client. Which statement by the client indicates the **need for further teaching?**

1. "I will obtain adequate rest."
2. "I need to monitor my weight regularly."
3. "I will take acetaminophen if I get a headache."
4. "I need to include sufficient carbohydrates in my diet."

Level of Cognitive Ability: Evaluating
Client Needs: Health Promotion and Maintenance
Clinical Judgment/Cognitive Skills: Evaluate Outcomes
Integrated Process: Clinical Judgment; Nursing Process/Evaluation
Content Area: Adult Health: Gastrointestinal
Health Problems: Adult Health: Gastrointestinal: Cirrhosis
Priority Concepts: Patient Education; Safety

Answer: 3
Rationale: Cirrhosis is a chronic progressive disease of the liver characterized by diffuse degeneration and destruction of hepatocytes. Acetaminophen is avoided because it can cause fatal liver damage in the client with cirrhosis. Adequate rest and nutrition are important. The client's weight needs to be monitored regularly. The diet needs to supply sufficient carbohydrates with a total daily intake of 2000 to 3000 calories.
Test-Taking Strategy: Note the strategic words, *need for further teaching.* These words indicate a negative event query and ask you to select an option that is an incorrect statement. Recalling that acetaminophen is a hepatotoxic agent will assist with directing you to option 3 as the one needing further teaching.
Priority Nursing Tip: In cirrhosis, the repeated destruction of hepatic cells causes the formation of scar tissue.
Reference: Ignatavicius, D., et al. (2021). *Medical-surgical nursing: Concepts for interprofessional collaborative care* (10th ed., p. 1165). Elsevier.

 42. A client has a history of urolithiasis related to hyperuricemia. To prevent the formation of future stones, the nurse instructs the client to avoid which food?

1. Liver
2. Carrots
3. White rice
4. Skim milk

Level of Cognitive Ability: Applying
Client Needs: Health Promotion and Maintenance
Clinical Judgment/Cognitive Skills: Take Action
Integrated Process: Teaching and Learning
Content Area: Adult Health: Renal and Urinary
Health Problems: Adult Health: Renal and Urinary: Calculi
Priority Concepts: Patient Education; Health Promotion

Answer: 1
Rationale: Because the client has a high level of uric acid in the blood and a history of kidney stones from crystallized uric acid in the renal pelvis, the nurse instructs the client to avoid foods that contain high amounts of purines because these foods contain a high concentration of uric acid. This includes limiting or avoiding organ meats, such as liver, brain, heart, and kidney. Other foods to avoid include sweetbreads, herring, sardines, anchovies, meat extracts, consommés, and gravies. Foods that are low in purines include all fruits, many vegetables, milk, cheese, eggs, refined cereals, coffee, tea, chocolate, and carbonated beverages.
Test-Taking Strategy: Focus on the subject, the client's diagnosis of urolithiasis related to hyperuricemia. Also note the word *avoid.* Because purines are end products of protein metabolism, eliminate carrots and white rice first. From the remaining options, recall that organ meats such as liver provide a greater quantity of protein than milk does.
Priority Nursing Tip: Allopurinol is a medication that may be prescribed to lower uric acid levels.
Reference: Ignatavicius, D., et al. (2021). *Medical-surgical nursing: Concepts for interprofessional collaborative care* (10th ed., p. 1345). Elsevier.

43. A client recovering from an appendectomy tells the nurse about getting dizzy and lightheaded with each use of the incentive spirometer. The nurse asks the client to demonstrate the use of the device. Which action would the nurse determine to be a contributing factor in this client's symptoms?
1. Inhaling too slowly
2. Exhaling too slowly
3. Not resting adequately between breaths
4. Not forming a tight seal around the mouthpiece

Level of Cognitive Ability: Evaluating
Client Needs: Health Promotion and Maintenance
Clinical Judgment/Cognitive Skills: Evaluate Outcomes
Integrated Process: Clinical Judgment; Nursing Process/Evaluation
Content Area: Skills: Oxygenation
Health Problems: Adult Health: Gastrointestinal: Appendicitis
Priority Concepts: Patient Education; Gas Exchange

Answer: 3
Rationale: Hyperventilation is the most common cause of respiratory alkalosis, which is characterized by lightheadedness and dizziness. If the client does not breathe normally between incentive spirometer breaths, hyperventilation and fatigue can result.
Test-Taking Strategy: Focus on the subject, the cause of the lightheadedness and dizziness when using an incentive spirometer. Think about each of the actions described in the options to direct you to inadequately resting between breaths. Inhaling or exhaling too slowly or not forming a tight seal around the mouthpiece would result in ineffective use but would not cause dizziness and lightheadedness.
Priority Nursing Tip: Instruct the client to assume a sitting or upright position when using an incentive spirometer.
Reference: Ignatavicius, D., et al. (2021). *Medical-surgical nursing: Concepts for interprofessional collaborative care* (10th ed., pp. 166, 168). Elsevier.

44. The community health nurse is conducting a health screening clinic. The nurse interprets that which client participating in the screening is the **highest priority** client to provide instruction to lower the risk of developing respiratory disease?
1. A smoker who works in an acute care hospital
2. A person who works with lawn care pesticides
3. A person who has done woodworking as a hobby for 8 years
4. A smoker who has cracked asbestos lining on the basement pipes

Level of Cognitive Ability: Analyzing
Client Needs: Health Promotion and Maintenance
Clinical Judgment/Cognitive Skills: Recognize Cues
Integrated Process: Clinical Judgment; Nursing Process/Assessment
Content Area: Foundations of Care: Community/Public/Population Health
Health Problems: Adult Health: Respiratory: Environmental
Priority Concepts: Clinical Judgment; Gas Exchange

Answer: 4
Rationale: Smoking greatly enhances the client's risk of developing some form of respiratory disease. Other risk factors include exposure to harmful chemicals, airborne toxins, and dust or fumes. For the options provided, the client who is at the greatest risk has two identified risk factors, one of which is smoking.
Test-Taking Strategy: Note the strategic words, *highest priority.* Eliminate working with pesticides or having a woodworking hobby first because the most harmful risk factor for the respiratory system is smoking. From the remaining options, select option 4 because it contains two high risk factors—smoking and asbestos exposure—whereas other choices contain only one high risk factor. Asbestos is toxic to the lungs if its particles are inhaled.
Priority Nursing Tip: Risk factors for respiratory disorders include smoking and the use of chewing tobacco, allergies, crowded living conditions, exposure to chemicals and environmental pollutants, family history of infectious diseases, frequent respiratory illnesses and viral syndromes, surgery, and travel to foreign countries.
Reference: Lewis, S., et al. (2020). *Medical-surgical nursing: Assessment and management of clinical problems* (11th ed., p. 503). Elsevier.

45. The nurse has conducted teaching, with a client who experienced pulmonary embolism, about methods to prevent recurrence after discharge. Which client statement demonstrates understanding of the teaching?
1. "I will limit the intake of fluids."
2. "I will sit down whenever possible."
3. "I am planning to continue to wear supportive stockings."
4. "I will cross my legs only at the ankle and not at the knees."

Level of Cognitive Ability: Evaluating
Client Needs: Health Promotion and Maintenance
Clinical Judgment/Cognitive Skills: Evaluate Outcomes
Integrated Process: Clinical Judgment; Nursing Process/Evaluation
Content Area: Adult Health: Respiratory
Health Problems: Adult Health: Respiratory: Pulmonary Embolism
Priority Concepts: Patient Education; Gas Exchange

Answer: 3
Rationale: The recurrence of pulmonary embolism can be minimized with wearing elastic or supportive stockings, if prescribed, because these enhance venous return. The client needs to take in sufficient fluids to prevent hemoconcentration and hypercoagulability. The client also enhances venous return by interspersing periods of sitting with walking, avoiding crossing the legs at the knees or ankles, and doing active foot and ankle exercises.
Test-Taking Strategy: Note the **subject**, preventing reoccurrence of pulmonary embolism. Recalling that promoting venous return will prevent pulmonary embolism will direct you to the correct option.
Priority Nursing Tip: Pulmonary embolism occurs when a thrombus forms (most commonly in a deep vein), detaches, travels to the right side of the heart, and then lodges in a branch of the pulmonary artery.
Reference: Lewis, S., et al. (2020). *Medical-surgical nursing: Assessment and management of clinical problems* (11th ed., pp. 534, 816). Elsevier.

❖ **46.** A client is being discharged from the hospital to home with an indwelling urinary catheter after the surgical repair of the bladder after trauma. The nurse determines that the client understands the principles of catheter management to prevent complications if the client states to follow which instruction?
1. Cleanse the perineal area with soap and water once a day.
2. Keep the drainage bag lower than the level of the bladder.
3. Limit fluid intake so that the bag will not become full so quickly.
4. Coil the tubing and place it under the thigh when sitting to avoid tugging on the bladder.

Level of Cognitive Ability: Evaluating
Client Needs: Health Promotion and Maintenance
Clinical Judgment/Cognitive Skills: Evaluate Outcomes
Integrated Process: Clinical Judgment; Nursing Process/Evaluation
Content Area: Skills: Tube Care
Health Problems: Adult Health: Renal and Urinary: Urinary Tract Inflammation/Infection/Trauma
Priority Concepts: Patient Education; Elimination

Answer: 2
Rationale: The drainage bag of an indwelling urinary catheter needs to be lower than the level of the bladder, and the tubing needs to be free of kinks and compression. The perineal area needs to be cleansed twice daily and after each bowel movement with soap and water. Adequate fluid intake is necessary to prevent infection and provide natural irrigation of the catheter from increased urine flow. Coiling the tubing and placing it under the thigh can compress the tube.
Test-Taking Strategy: Note the **subject**, a client with an indwelling urinary catheter. Coiling and tucking catheter tubing is eliminated first because sitting on coiled tubing could cause compression and obstruct drainage. Decreasing fluid intake is eliminated next because increased fluids are important. From the remaining options, noting the words *once a day* will assist you in eliminating this option.
Priority Nursing Tip: The total bladder capacity is 1 L. The normal adult urine output is 1500 mL/day.
References: Ignatavicius, D., et al. (2021). *Medical-surgical nursing: Concepts for interprofessional collaborative care* (10th ed., p. 1335). Elsevier; Potter, P., et al. (2021). *Fundamentals of nursing* (10th ed., pp. 1245–1246). Elsevier.

47. A client with a family history of heart disease presents to the primary health care provider's office asking to begin oral contraceptive therapy for birth control. What important topic would the nurse ask the client about **next**?
1. Smoking
2. Regular exercise
3. A low-cholesterol diet
4. Alternative birth control methods

Level of Cognitive Ability: Applying
Client Needs: Health Promotion and Maintenance
Clinical Judgment/Cognitive Skills: Take Action
Integrated Process: Clinical Judgment; Nursing Process/Assessment
Content Area: Pharmacology: Reproductive: Contraceptives
Health Problems: Adult Health: Reproductive: Menstruation Problems/Fertility/Infertility
Priority Concepts: Health Promotion; Reproduction

Answer: 1
Rationale: Oral contraceptive use is a risk factor for heart disease, particularly when it is combined with cigarette smoking. Regular exercise and keeping total cholesterol levels less than 200 mg/dL (<5 mmol/L) are general measures to decrease cardiovascular risk.
Test-Taking Strategy: Note the strategic word, *next.* Remember that smoking is the item that is linked to oral contraceptive use to make it a risk factor for cardiovascular disease. This will direct you to the correct option.
Priority Nursing Tip: Oral contraceptives are usually taken for 21 consecutive days and stopped for 7 days; the administration cycle is then repeated.
Reference: Lilley, L., Rainforth Collins, S., & Snyder J. (2020). *Pharmacology and the nursing process* (9th ed., p. 535). Elsevier.

48. The nurse is teaching a client diagnosed with atrial fibrillation about the need to begin long-term anticoagulant therapy. Which explanation would the nurse use to **best** describe the reasoning for this therapy?
1. "Because of this dysrhythmia, blood backs up in the legs and puts you at risk for blood clots."
2. "This dysrhythmia decreases the volume of blood flowing from the heart, which can lead to blood clots forming in the brain."
3. "The antidysrhythmic medications you are taking cause blood clots as a side effect, so you need this medication to prevent them."
4. "Because the atria are quivering, blood flows sluggishly through them, and clots can form along the heart wall, which could then loosen and travel to the lungs or brain."

Level of Cognitive Ability: Applying
Client Needs: Health Promotion and Maintenance
Clinical Judgment/Cognitive Skills: Take Action
Integrated Process: Clinical Judgment; Teaching and Learning
Content Area: Pharmacology: Cardiovascular: Anticoagulants
Health Problems: Adult Health: Cardiovascular: Dysrhythmias
Priority Concepts: Patient Education; Perfusion

Answer: 4
Rationale: A severe complication of atrial fibrillation is the development of mural thrombi. The blood stagnates in the "quivering" atria because of the loss of organized atrial muscle contraction and "atrial kick." The blood that pools in the atria can then clot, which increases the risk of pulmonary and cerebral emboli. Options 1, 2, and 3 do not provide accurate descriptions of the purpose for anticoagulant therapy.
Test-Taking Strategy: Note the strategic word, *best.* Also, note the subject, a client with atrial fibrillation beginning long-term anticoagulant therapy. Note the relationship between the client's diagnosis of atrial fibrillation and the words *atria are quivering* in the correct option.
Priority Nursing Tip: On a cardiac monitor, atrial fibrillation can be easily recognized because usually there is no definitive P wave; fibrillatory waves before each QRS are noted.
Reference: Ignatavicius, D., et al. (2021). *Medical-surgical nursing: Concepts for interprofessional collaborative care* (10th ed., pp. 653–654). Elsevier.

49. The clinic nurse is providing instructions to a client in the third trimester of pregnancy regarding relief measures for heartburn. Which instruction would the nurse provide to the client?
1. Sip on milk or hot tea.
2. Use antacids that contain sodium.
3. Eat fatty foods once a day in the morning only.
4. Eat three large meals a day rather than small, frequent meals.

Level of Cognitive Ability: Applying
Client Needs: Health Promotion and Maintenance
Clinical Judgment/Cognitive Skills: Take Action
Integrated Process: Clinical Judgment; Teaching and Learning
Content Area: Maternity: Antepartum
Health Problems: Maternity: Discomforts of Pregnancy
Priority Concepts: Patient Education; Health Promotion

Answer: 1
Rationale: Measures to provide relief of heartburn include frequent sips of milk or hot tea; avoiding fatty and fried foods, coffee, and cigarettes; and eating small, frequent meals. Mild antacids can be used if they do not contain aspirin or sodium.
Test-Taking Strategy: Note the subject, teaching a pregnant client how to avoid heartburn. Eliminate antacids that contain sodium first because increased sodium intake will lead to edema, and edema needs to be avoided, especially during pregnancy. Eliminate consuming fatty foods in the morning next on the basis of basic nutritional principles that fatty and fried foods need to be avoided. Eating large, heavy meals will not reduce the amount of heartburn that the client is experiencing. Recalling that milk and hot tea can be soothing to the gastrointestinal tract will assist you in selecting the correct option.
Priority Nursing Tip: In pregnancy, heartburn most often occurs in the second and third trimesters and results from increased progesterone levels, decreased gastrointestinal motility, esophageal reflux, and displacement of the stomach by the enlarging uterus.
Reference: McKinney, E. S., et al. (2022). *Maternal child nursing* (6th ed., p. 237). Elsevier.

50. The nurse provides instructions regarding home care to a parent of a 3-year-old child who has been hospitalized with hemophilia. Which statement by the parent indicates the **need for further teaching**?
1. "I should not leave my child unattended."
2. "I need to pad table corners in my home."
3. "My child cannot have any immunizations."
4. "I need to remove household items that can tip over."

Level of Cognitive Ability: Evaluating
Client Needs: Health Promotion and Maintenance
Clinical Judgment/Cognitive Skills: Evaluate Outcomes
Integrated Process: Clinical Judgment; Teaching and Learning
Content Area: Pediatrics: Hematologic
Health Problems: Pediatric-Specific: Bleeding Disorders
Priority Concepts: Patient Education; Clotting

Answer: 3
Rationale: Hemophilia refers to a group of bleeding disorders resulting from a deficiency of specific coagulation proteins. The nurse must stress the importance of immunizations, dental hygiene, and routine well-child care. Not leaving a young child unattended and modifying the environment for safety are appropriate. The parent also needs to be instructed regarding measures to implement if blunt trauma occurs (especially trauma involving the joints) and how to apply prolonged pressure to superficial wounds until the bleeding has stopped.
Test-Taking Strategy: Note the strategic words, *need for further teaching*. These words indicate a negative event query and ask you to select an option that is an incorrect statement. Recalling that bleeding is a concern in clients with this disorder will assist you in eliminating options that include measures of protection and safety for the child. Recalling the importance of immunizations will direct you to the correct option.
Priority Nursing Tip: Bleeding is a primary concern for the child with hemophilia. Teach the parents about safety measures to implement to prevent injury such as wearing protective devices (helmets and knee and elbow pads) when participating in sports such as bicycling.
Reference: McKinney, E. S., et al. (2022). *Maternal child nursing* (6th ed., p. 1140). Elsevier.

Client Needs

51. The nurse provides instructions to the client taking clorazepate for the management of an anxiety disorder. What information related to this medication would the nurse provide to the client?
1. Dizziness is a side effect.
2. Smoking increases the effectiveness of the medication.
3. If drowsiness occurs, call the primary health care provider.
4. If gastrointestinal disturbances occur, discontinue the medication.

Level of Cognitive Ability: Applying
Client Needs: Health Promotion and Maintenance
Clinical Judgment/Cognitive Skills: Take Action
Integrated Process: Teaching and Learning
Content Area: Pharmacology: Psychotherapeutics: Benzodiazepines
Health Problems: Mental Health: Anxiety Disorder
Priority Concepts: Patient Education; Safety

Answer: 1
Rationale: Dizziness is a side effect of this medication. The client needs to be instructed, if dizziness occurs, to change positions slowly from lying to sitting to standing. Drowsiness is also a side effect that diminishes with continued therapy and does not warrant the need to contact the primary health care provider. Smoking reduces medication effectiveness. Gastrointestinal disturbance is an occasional side effect, and the medication can be given with food if this occurs.
Test-Taking Strategy: Note the subject, clorazepate. Eliminate discontinuing the medication first because the client would not be instructed to discontinue the medication without the primary health care provider's approval. Eliminate drowsiness because this side effect commonly occurs with antianxiety medications. Eliminate smoking next because smoking reduces medication effectiveness.
Priority Nursing Tip: Clorazepate is a benzodiazepine. Abrupt withdrawal of benzodiazepines can be potentially life-threatening, and withdrawal needs to occur only under medical supervision.
Reference: Lilley, L., Rainforth Collins, S., & Snyder J. (2020). *Pharmacology and the nursing process* (9th ed., p. 279). Elsevier.

52. The client diagnosed with prostatitis asks the nurse, "Why do I need to take a stool softener? The problem is with my urine, not my bowels!" Which response would the nurse make to the client?
1. "This is a standard medication prescription for anyone with a urine problem."
2. "This will keep the bowel free of feces, which helps decrease the swelling inside."
3. "Being constipated puts you at more risk for developing complications of prostatitis."
4. "This will help you prevent constipation because straining is painful with prostatitis."

Level of Cognitive Ability: Applying
Client Needs: Health Promotion and Maintenance
Clinical Judgment/Cognitive Skills: Take Action
Integrated Process: Teaching and Learning
Content Area: Adult Health: Renal and Urinary
Health Problems: Adult Health: Renal and Urinary: Urinary Tract Inflammation/Infection/Trauma
Priority Concepts: Patient Education; Inflammation

Answer: 4
Rationale: Prostatitis is an inflammation of the prostate gland. Stool softeners are prescribed for the client with prostatitis to prevent constipation, which can be painful. Stool softeners are not a standard prescription for "anyone with a urine problem." Stool softeners have no direct effect on decreasing swelling. Constipation does not cause complications of prostatitis.
Test-Taking Strategy: Note the subject, a client with prostatitis taking a stool softener. Recalling the purpose and use of stool softeners to prevent constipation and pain from straining will direct you to the correct option.
Priority Nursing Tip: Bacterial prostatitis occurs as a result of an organism reaching the prostate via the urethra, bladder, bloodstream, or lymphatic channels. The bacterial type usually occurs after a viral illness or a decrease in sexual activity.
Reference: Lewis, S., et al. (2020). *Medical-surgical nursing: Assessment and management of clinical problems* (11th ed., pp. 931, 1269–1270). Elsevier.

53. A client diagnosed with Parkinson's disease has begun therapy with levodopa. The nurse determines that the client understands the action of the medication if the client verbalizes that results may not be apparent for what period of time?
1. 1 week
2. 24 hours
3. 5 to 7 days
4. 2 to 3 weeks

Level of Cognitive Ability: Evaluating
Client Needs: Health Promotion and Maintenance
Clinical Judgment/Cognitive Skills: Evaluate Outcomes
Integrated Process: Clinical Judgment; Nursing Process/Evaluation
Content Area: Pharmacology: Neurologic: Antiparkinsonians
Health Problems: Adult Health: Neurologic: Parkinson's Disease
Priority Concepts: Patient Education; Safety

Answer: 4
Rationale: Parkinson's disease is a degenerative illness caused by the depletion of dopamine. Signs and symptoms of Parkinson's disease usually begin to resolve within 2 to 3 weeks after starting therapy, although in some clients, marked improvement may not be seen for up to 6 months. Clients must understand this concept to aid in their compliance with medication therapy.
Test-Taking Strategy: Note the subject, levodopa, and recall knowledge regarding this medication. Eliminate 1 week and 5 to 7 days because they involve comparable or alike time frames. From the remaining options, eliminate 24 hours as it is unlikely that results would be noted that quickly.
Priority Nursing Tip: Levodopa taken with a monoamine oxidase inhibitor antidepressant can cause a hypertensive crisis.
Reference: Lilley, L., Rainforth Collins, S., & Snyder J. (2020). *Pharmacology and the nursing process* (9th ed., pp. 233–234). Elsevier.

❖ **54.** The nurse provides information to a client about performing a breast self-examination (BSE). The nurse determines that the client **needs further teaching** if the client makes which statements? **Select all that apply.**
❑ 1. "The BSE must be done monthly."
❑ 2. "Lumps in my armpit area are normal."
❑ 3. "I can palpate my breasts with soapy water while showering."
❑ 4. "I need to perform the examination on the day that I start my period."
❑ 5. "When I squeeze my nipples, I should expect to note some discharge."
❑ 6. "I need to stand before a mirror and inspect each breast for anything unusual."

Level of Cognitive Ability: Evaluating
Client Needs: Health Promotion and Maintenance
Clinical Judgment/Cognitive Skills: Evaluate Outcomes
Integrated Process: Clinical Judgment; Nursing Process/Evaluation
Content Area: Health Assessment/Physical Exam: Breasts
Health Problems: Adult Health: Cancer: Breast
Priority Concepts: Patient Education; Health Promotion

Answer: 2, 4, 5
Rationale: Any lumps (including lumps in the armpit) and nipple discharge are abnormal and must be reported to the primary health care provider immediately. The examination is performed 2 or 3 days after menstruation ends, when the breasts are least likely to be tender and swollen. The client is taught that BSE needs to be done once a month so that the client becomes familiar with the usual feel and appearance of the breasts. The client is taught to palpate each breast and axillary area; this part of the examination can be performed in the shower using soap, which allows the fingers to glide easily over the skin. The client is taught to also stand before a mirror and inspect each breast for anything unusual.
Test-Taking Strategy: Note the strategic words, *needs further teaching.* These words indicate a negative event query and ask you to select the options that are incorrect statements. Read each option carefully, and remember that the examination is performed 2 or 3 days after menstruation ends, when the breasts are least likely to be tender and swollen. Also, recalling that any lumps (including lumps in the armpit) and nipple discharge are abnormal will assist in answering correctly.
Priority Nursing Tip: Postmenopausal clients or clients who have had a hysterectomy need to select a specific day of the month and perform BSE monthly on that day.
Reference: Ignatavicius, D., et al. (2021). *Medical-surgical nursing: Concepts for interprofessional collaborative care* (10th ed., pp. 1436–1437). Elsevier.

55. A client is being discharged to home after prostatectomy for treatment of benign prostatic hyperplasia. Which instruction would the nurse plan to provide to the client as part of the discharge teaching?
1. Mowing the lawn is allowed after 1 week.
2. Avoid lifting more than 50 pounds for 4 to 6 weeks after surgery.
3. Drink at least 15 glasses of water a day to minimize clot formation.
4. Notify the surgeon if fever, increased pain, or an inability to void occurs.

Level of Cognitive Ability: Applying
Client Needs: Health Promotion and Maintenance
Clinical Judgment/Cognitive Skills: Generate Solutions
Integrated Process: Clinical Judgment; Teaching and Learning
Content Area: Adult Health: Renal and Urinary
Health Problems: Adult Health: Renal and Urinary: Urinary Tract Inflammation/Infection/Trauma
Priority Concepts: Patient Education; Health Promotion

Answer: 4
Rationale: The client needs to notify the surgeon if there are any signs/symptoms of infection, bleeding, increased pain, or urinary obstruction. Strenuous activities that could increase intra-abdominal tension are restricted, such as mowing the lawn. Lifting more than 20 (not 50) pounds is prohibited for 4 to 6 weeks after surgery. The client needs to take in 6 to 8 glasses of water or nonalcoholic beverages per day to minimize the risk of clot formation (15 glasses a day is excessive).
Test-Taking Strategy: Focus on the **subject**, discharge teaching for a client after prostatectomy. Eliminate 15 glasses of water first as an excessive fluid intake. Noting that the activities of mowing the lawn and lifting close to 50 pounds are also excessive activities postoperatively should assist you in eliminating these choices.
Priority Nursing Tip: Sterility is a possible occurrence after prostatectomy.
Reference: Ignatavicius, D., et al. (2021). *Medical-surgical nursing: Concepts for interprofessional collaborative care* (10th ed., pp. 1477–1478). Elsevier.

❖ **56.** The nurse is teaching a client with acute kidney injury to include proteins in the diet that are considered high-quality or complete proteins. The nurse determines that the client **needs further teaching** if the client indicates that which food item is considered high quality?
1. Fish
2. Eggs
3. Chicken
4. Broccoli

Level of Cognitive Ability: Evaluating
Client Needs: Health Promotion and Maintenance
Clinical Judgment/Cognitive Skills: Evaluate Outcomes
Integrated Process: Clinical Judgment; Nursing Process/Evaluation
Content Area: Adult Health: Renal and Urinary
Health Problems: Adult Health: Renal and Urinary: Acute Kidney Injury and Chronic Kidney Disease
Priority Concepts: Patient Education; Nutrition

Answer: 4
Rationale: High-quality or complete proteins come from animal sources and include such foods as eggs, chicken, meat, and fish. Low-quality or incomplete proteins are derived from plant sources and include vegetables and foods made from grains. Because the renal diet is limited in protein, it is important that the proteins ingested are of high quality.
Test-Taking Strategy: Note the **strategic words**, *needs further teaching*. These words indicate a **negative event query** and the need to select the food that is low-quality protein. When comparing the choices, note that option 4 is the only item that is not derived from an animal source. Fish, eggs, and chicken are from animal sources, whereas broccoli is a plant.
Priority Nursing Tip: High-quality proteins or complete proteins contain adequate amounts of essential amino acids.
Reference: Nix, S. (2022). *Williams' basic nutrition and diet therapy* (16th ed., p. 398). Elsevier.

57. The home care nurse visits a client who had a stroke with resultant unilateral neglect who was recently discharged from the hospital. Which instruction would the nurse provide to the family regarding care?
1. Assist the client from the affected side.
2. Place personal items directly in front of the client.
3. Discourage the client from scanning the environment.
4. Assist the client with grooming the unaffected side first.

Level of Cognitive Ability: Applying
Client Needs: Health Promotion and Maintenance
Clinical Judgment/Cognitive Skills: Take Action
Integrated Process: Clinical Judgment; Teaching and Learning
Content Area: Adult Health: Neurologic
Health Problems: Adult Health: Neurologic: Stroke
Priority Concepts: Patient Education; Safety

Answer: 1
Rationale: Unilateral neglect is a pattern of a lack of awareness of body parts such as paralyzed arms or legs. Initially the environment is adapted to the deficit by focusing on the client's unaffected side, and the client's personal items are placed on the unaffected side; gradually the client's attention is focused on the affected side to promote awareness of that side. Therefore, the family is taught to assist the client from the affected side, and the client grooms the affected side first. The client needs to scan the entire environment.
Test-Taking Strategy: Note the client's diagnosis of unilateral neglect and the subject, home care instructions. Recalling the physiologic alteration that occurs with unilateral neglect and that it involves a pattern of a lack of awareness of body parts will direct you to the correct option.
Priority Nursing Tip: Cerebral anoxia lasting longer than 10 minutes causes cerebral infarction with irreversible change.
Reference: Ignatavicius, D., et al. (2021). *Medical-surgical nursing: Concepts for interprofessional collaborative care* (10th ed., p. 549). Elsevier.

58. The nurse has completed discharge teaching with a client who has had surgery for lung cancer. The nurse determines that the client **needs additional teaching** about the elements of home management if the client verbalizes the need to follow which instruction?
1. Avoid exposure to crowds.
2. Deal with any increases in pain independently.
3. Sit up and lean forward to breathe more easily.
4. Call the surgeon if shortness of breath occurs.

Level of Cognitive Ability: Evaluating
Client Needs: Health Promotion and Maintenance
Clinical Judgment/Cognitive Skills: Evaluate Outcomes
Integrated Process: Clinical Judgment; Nursing Process/Evaluation
Content Area: Adult Health: Oncology
Health Problems: Adult Health: Cancer: Laryngeal and Lung
Priority Concepts: Patient Education; Health Promotion

Answer: 2
Rationale: The client who just had surgery for lung cancer would not be expected to deal with increases in pain independently. Health teaching includes avoiding exposure to crowds or persons with respiratory infections and reporting signs and symptoms of respiratory infection or increases in pain. The client would also use positions that facilitate respiration, such as sitting up and leaning forward.
Test-Taking Strategy: Note the strategic words, *needs additional teaching.* These words indicate a negative event query and ask you to select an option that is an incorrect statement. Focusing on the client's diagnosis of lung cancer will direct you to the correct option.
Priority Nursing Tip: Pain is a very individualized experience. It is what the client describes or says it is.
Reference: Ignatavicius, D., et al. (2021). *Medical-surgical nursing: Concepts for interprofessional collaborative care* (10th ed., pp. 562–563). Elsevier.

59. A client weighs 165 pounds (75 kg) at admission. During hospitalization, the nurse determines that the client is maintaining adequate nutritional status if the client's weight is how many pounds?
1. 153 pounds (69.5 kg)
2. 155 pounds (70.4 kg)
3. 157 pounds (71.3 kg)
4. 160 pounds (72.7 kg)

Level of Cognitive Ability: Evaluating
Client Needs: Health Promotion and Maintenance
Clinical Judgment/Cognitive Skills: Evaluate Outcomes
Integrated Process: Clinical Judgment; Nursing Process/Evaluation
Content Area: Skills: Nutrition
Health Problems: Adult Health: Gastrointestinal: Nutrition/Malabsorption Problems
Priority Concepts: Health Promotion; Nutrition

Answer: 4
Rationale: The nurse determines that the client has maintained adequate nutritional status if the client maintains the baseline body weight or loses no more than 5 pounds. The client's baseline weight is 165 pounds (75 kg), so the acceptable range for the client's postoperative weight is 160 (72.7 kg) to 165 pounds (75 kg).
Test-Taking Strategy: Focus on the subject, maintaining adequate nutritional status. In this situation, it is best to select the option that identifies the least amount of weight loss; this will direct you to the correct option.
Priority Nursing Tip: To obtain the most accurate weight, the client needs to be weighed in the morning at the same time of day as previous weights have been measured and with the same amount of clothing. The client should also void before the weight measurement.
Reference: Ignatavicius, D., et al. (2021). *Medical-surgical nursing: Concepts for interprofessional collaborative care* (10th ed., p. 1200). Elsevier.

❖ **60.** The nurse has given the client with a nonplaster (fiberglass) leg cast instructions regarding cast care at home. The nurse determines that the client **needs further teaching** if the client makes which statement?
1. "I need to avoid walking on wet, slippery floors."
2. "I'm not supposed to scratch the skin underneath the cast."
3. "It's all right to wipe dirt off of the top of the cast with a damp cloth."
4. "If the cast gets wet, I can dry it with a hair dryer turned to the hot setting."

Level of Cognitive Ability: Evaluating
Client Needs: Health Promotion and Maintenance
Clinical Judgment/Cognitive Skills: Evaluate Outcomes
Integrated Process: Clinical Judgment; Nursing Process/Evaluation
Content Area: Adult Health: Musculoskeletal
Health Problems: Adult Health: Musculoskeletal: Skeletal Injury
Priority Concepts: Patient Education; Mobility

Answer: 4
Rationale: If the cast gets wet, it can be dried with a hair dryer set to a cool setting. The client is instructed to avoid walking on wet, slippery floors to prevent falls. If the skin under the cast itches, cool air from a hair dryer may be used to relieve it. The client should never scratch under the cast because of the risk of skin breakdown and infection. Surface soil on a cast may be removed with a damp cloth.
Test-Taking Strategy: Note the strategic words, *needs further teaching.* These words indicate a negative event query and ask you to select an option that is an incorrect statement. Noting the word *hot* will direct you to this option.
Priority Nursing Tip: Monitor a casted extremity for circulatory impairment such as pain, swelling, discoloration, tingling, numbness, coolness, or diminished pulse.
Reference: Lewis, S., et al. (2020). *Medical-surgical nursing: Assessment and management of clinical problems* (11th ed., p. 1458). Elsevier.

61. A child exposed to the human immunodeficiency virus (HIV) is seen in the health care clinic and tested for the virus. Which home care instruction would the nurse provide to the parents of the child?
   1. Avoid sharing toothbrushes.
   2. Avoid all immunizations until the diagnosis is established.
   3. Wipe up any blood spills with a rag, and allow them to air-dry.
   4. Wash your hands with half-strength bleach if they come in contact with the child's blood.

Level of Cognitive Ability: Applying
Client Needs: Health Promotion and Maintenance
Clinical Judgment/Cognitive Skills: Take Action
Integrated Process: Teaching and Learning
Content Area: Foundations of Care: Infection Control
Health Problems: Pediatric-Specific: Immunodeficiency Disease
Priority Concepts: Patient Education; Infection

Answer: 1
Rationale: Parents are instructed that toothbrushes are not to be shared. Immunizations must be kept up to date. Blood spills are wiped up with a paper towel; the area is then washed with soap and water, rinsed with bleach and water, and allowed to air-dry. Hands are washed with soap and water if they come in contact with blood.
Test-Taking Strategy: Note the subject, a child exposed to HIV infection. Eliminate avoiding all immunizations first because of the closed-ended word "all." Eliminate wiping up the blood spill with a rag and air-drying next on the basis of the knowledge that blood spills must be cleaned with a bleach solution. Eliminate using half-strength bleach to wash hands because bleach would be irritating and caustic to the skin.
Priority Nursing Tip: Human immunodeficiency virus infects CD4+ T cells. A gradual decrease in the count occurs, and this results in a progressive immunodeficiency. The risk for opportunistic infections is present.
Reference: McKinney, ES., et al. (2022). *Maternal Child Nursing* (6th ed., pp. 949–950). St. Louis: Elsevier.

62. The nurse prepares a postoperative client who is ready for discharge for care at home. The client must receive continued intravenous (IV) therapy, so the nurse provides the client with instructions on caring for the IV site to prevent infection. Which is the **best** method of evaluating the client's ability to care for the IV site?
   1. Have the client role-play an IV dressing change.
   2. Have the client change the IV dressing unaided.
   3. Direct the client to explain IV site care completely.
   4. Ask the client to provide self-care before being discharged.

Level of Cognitive Ability: Evaluating
Client Needs: Health Promotion and Maintenance
Clinical Judgment/Cognitive Skills: Evaluate Outcomes
Integrated Process: Clinical Judgment; Nursing Process/Evaluation
Content Area: Skills: Infection Control
Health Problems: N/A
Priority Concepts: Patient Education; Safety

Answer: 2
Rationale: The best method for the nurse to use to evaluate the client's acquisition of psychomotor skills is a teach back method to observe the client performing the skill; in this case, it is an IV dressing change. Role-playing is a suitable method of rehearsing a skill, but actual performance of the skill is best. Explanations are suitable to evaluate client knowledge of a skill, but they will not draw attention to the client's physical inability to perform the psychomotor function. If the nurse was evaluating client self-care, having the client function independently before discharge is suitable; however, the question is asking about IV site care.
Test-Taking Strategy: Use teaching and learning principles to answer the question, and note the strategic word, *best.* This means that all options may be correct, but you must choose the option that is the best choice. The correct option must identify some type of active client participation in skill performance. This concept will direct you to the correct option.
Priority Nursing Tip: Aseptic technique must be used when performing IV therapy procedures.
Reference: Potter, P., et al. (2023). *Fundamentals of nursing* (11th ed., p. 1093). Elsevier.

63. The nurse provides home care instructions to a client diagnosed with advanced breast cancer who has an implanted vascular access port. Which statement by the client indicates the **need for further teaching?**
1. "I need to keep the site clean and dry."
2. "If the site becomes red, I will notify my doctor."
3. "I need to pump the port daily to maintain patency."
4. "The port will need to be flushed with saline to maintain patency."

Level of Cognitive Ability: Evaluating
Client Needs: Health Promotion and Maintenance
Clinical Judgment/Cognitive Skills: Evaluate Outcomes
Integrated Process: Clinical Judgment; Nursing Process/ Evaluation
Content Area: Skills: Tube Care
Health Problems: Adult Health: Cancer: Breast
Priority Concepts: Patient Education; Safety

Answer: 3
Rationale: An implanted vascular access port does not need to be pumped to maintain patency. The site will need to be kept clean and dry, and the primary health care provider needs to be notified about signs/symptoms of infection. Saline is usually used to flush the site to maintain patency; however, agency procedures should always be followed (some agencies use heparin as the flush solution).
Test-Taking Strategy: Note the strategic words, *need for further teaching*. These words indicate a negative event query and ask you to select an option that is an incorrect statement. Using the principles related to vascular access ports and care of an intravenous line will direct you to the correct option.
Priority Nursing Tip: For accessing an implanted vascular access port, the port requires palpation and injection through the skin into the self-sealing port with a noncoring needle such as a Huber-point needle.
Reference: Ignatavicius, D., et al. (2021). *Medical-surgical nursing: Concepts for interprofessional collaborative care* (10th ed., pp. 279–280). Elsevier.

64. The nurse is caring for a client who is a survivor of a disaster event. The client begins to display behaviors not demonstrated before. Which manifestations would indicate to the nurse that the client may be experiencing post-traumatic stress disorder (PTSD)? **Select all that apply.**
1. Irritability and sleep disturbances
2. Flashbacks or recollections of the disaster
3. Regression to an earlier developmental stage
4. A feeling of estrangement or detachment from others
5. Consistent discussion and rationalizing as to why the disaster occurred
6. Repression or the inability to remember an important aspect associated with the disaster

Level of Cognitive Ability: Analyzing
Client Needs: Health Promotion and Maintenance
Clinical Judgment/Cognitive Skills: Analyze Cues
Integrated Process: Clinical Judgment; Nursing Process/Assessment
Content Area: Leadership/Management: Mass Casualty Preparedness and Response
Health Problems: Mental Health: Post-traumatic Stress Disorder
Priority Concepts: Anxiety; Mood and Affect

Answer: 1, 2, 4, 6
Rationale: PTSD is characterized by a sustained maladaptive response to a traumatic event. In this condition, the client experiences recurrent and intrusive recollections of the event (flashbacks), has recurrent dreams of the event, acts or feels as though the event were recurring, and experiences psychological distress when internal or external cues resemble the event. The individual avoids stimuli associated with the trauma or event (thoughts, feelings, conversations about the event, and persons or places that evoke memories of the event) and is likely to experience estrangement and detachment from others. The individual also is unable to remember an important aspect of the event (repression) and experiences somatic symptoms such as irritability and sleep disturbances. Regression to an earlier developmental stage and consistent discussion and rationalizing as to why the disaster occurred are not characteristics of PTSD.
Test-Taking Strategy: Focus on the subject, PTSD, and recall that PTSD is a condition characterized by a sustained maladaptive response to a traumatic event. Read each option and associate the manifestation with the description of the disorder to answer correctly.
Priority Nursing Tip: In PTSD the individual is prone to reexperience the traumatic event and have recurrent and intrusive dreams or flashbacks.
Reference: Varcarolis, E., & Fosbre, C. (2021). *Essentials of psychiatric mental health nursing: A communication approach to evidence-based care* (4th ed., p. 126). Elsevier.

❖ 65. The nurse has completed instructions regarding diet and fluid restriction for the client diagnosed with chronic kidney disease. The nurse determines that the client understands the information presented if the client selected which dessert from the dietary menu?
   1. Jell-O
   2. Sherbet
   3. Ice cream
   4. Angel food cake

Level of Cognitive Ability: Evaluating
Client Needs: Health Promotion and Maintenance
Clinical Judgment/Cognitive Skills: Evaluate Outcomes
Integrated Process: Clinical Judgment; Nursing Process/
Evaluation
Content Area: Foundations of Care: Therapeutic Diets
Health Problems: Adult Health: Renal and Urinary:
Acute Kidney Injury and Chronic Kidney Disease
Priority Concepts: Patient Education; Fluids and
Electrolytes

Answer: 4
Rationale: For clients on a fluid-restricted diet, it is helpful to avoid "hidden" fluids to whatever extent possible. This allows the client to take in more fluid by drinking, which can help alleviate thirst. Dietary fluid includes anything that is liquid at room temperature. This includes items such as Jell-O, sherbet, and ice cream.
Test-Taking Strategy: Note the **subject,** a client diagnosed with chronic kidney disease, and the words *fluid restriction*. Recalling that dietary fluid includes anything that is liquid at room temperature will direct you to the angel food cake.
Priority Nursing Tip: Acute kidney injury is the rapid loss of kidney function from renal cell damage. Chronic kidney disease is a slow, progressive, irreversible loss in kidney function.
References: Ignatavicius, D., et al. (2021). *Medical-surgical nursing: Concepts for interprofessional collaborative care* (10th ed., pp. 1391–1392). Elsevier; Nix, S. (2022). *Williams' Basic nutrition and diet therapy* (16th ed., p. 382). Elsevier.

❖ 66. The nurse has given instructions to the client diagnosed with chronic kidney disease about reducing pruritus from uremia. The nurse determines that the client **needs further teaching** if the client states the intention to use which item for skin care?
   1. Mild soap
   2. Oil in the bathwater
   3. Lanolin-based lotion
   4. Alcohol cleansing pads

Level of Cognitive Ability: Evaluating
Client Needs: Health Promotion and Maintenance
Clinical Judgment/Cognitive Skills: Evaluate Outcomes
Integrated Process: Clinical Judgment; Nursing
Process/Evaluation
Content Area: Adult Health: Renal and Urinary
Health Problems: Adult Health: Renal and Urinary:
Acute Kidney Injury and Chronic Kidney Disease
Priority Concepts: Patient Education; Tissue Integrity

Answer: 4
Rationale: The client diagnosed with chronic kidney disease often has dry skin that is accompanied by itching (pruritus) from uremia. Products that contain perfumes or alcohol increase skin dryness and pruritus, and these need to be avoided. The client should use mild soaps, bath oils, and lotions to reduce dryness without increasing skin irritation.
Test-Taking Strategy: Focus on the **subject,** reducing pruritus, and note the **strategic words,** *needs further teaching*. These words indicate a **negative event query** and ask you to select an incorrect statement. Eliminate oil in the bathwater and lanolin-based lotion first because they are **comparable or alike** as both are forms of lubricants. From the remaining options, eliminate mild soap, knowing that the client needs to avoid putting irritating products such as alcohol on the skin.
Priority Nursing Tip: Uremic syndrome is the accumulation of nitrogenous waste products in the blood caused by the kidneys' inability to filter out these waste products.
Reference: Ignatavicius, D., et al. (2021). *Medical-surgical nursing: Concepts for interprofessional collaborative care* (10th ed., p. 448). Elsevier.

67. A battered victim seen in the emergency department requires tertiary intervention because of repeated abuse. Which nursing interventions are appropriate to include in the plan of care? **Select all that apply.**

❑ 1. Report the abuse to the police.
❑ 2. Provide medications to relieve pain and anxiety.
❑ 3. Explore family and friends as support possibilities.
❑ 4. Focus on the victim's strengths, endurance, and abilities.
❑ 5. Avoid discussing the implications of pressing charges against the batterer.
❑ 6. Discourage the victim from discussing the events leading to past and present abuse situations.

Level of Cognitive Ability: Applying
Client Needs: Health Promotion and Maintenance
Clinical Judgment/Cognitive Skills: Generate Solutions
Integrated Process: Clinical Judgment; Nursing Process/Planning
Content Area: Mental Health
Health Problems: Mental Health: Abuse/Neglect
Priority Concepts: Clinical Judgment; Interpersonal Violence

Answer: 1, 2, 3, 4
Rationale: Tertiary prevention is necessary when a person has been repeatedly abused. The focus is on helping the abused person overcome the physical and psychological effects of the abuse and preventing future abuse. Some of the interventions include reporting the abuse to the police to provide for safety; providing medications to relieve pain and anxiety; exploring family and friends as support possibilities to increase the victim's awareness of potential support; focusing on the victim's strengths, endurance, and abilities to increase self-esteem; discussing the implications of pressing charges against the batterer to increase their awareness of abuse implications; and encouraging the victim to discuss the events leading to past and present abuse situations (this helps reduce guilt and shame).
Test-Taking Strategy: Focus on the subject, tertiary intervention for abuse. Recall that the focus of tertiary prevention is on helping the abused victim overcome the physical and psychological effects of the abuse and preventing future abuse. Next read and visualize each intervention and relate it to the focus of tertiary intervention to select correctly.
Priority Nursing Tip: A victim of abuse may feel trapped in the situation, dependent, helpless, and powerless.
Reference: Potter, P., et al. (2023). *Fundamentals of nursing* (11th ed., pp. 17, 80). Elsevier.

❖ **68.** The nurse provides information to a client who is scheduled for the implantation of an implantable cardioverter defibrillator (ICD) regarding care after implantation. The nurse tells the client that there is a need to keep a diary. What information would the nurse provide concerning the **primary** purpose of the diary?

1. Analyze which activities to avoid.
2. Document events that precipitate a countershock.
3. Provide a count of the number of shocks delivered.
4. Record a variety of data that are useful for the primary health care provider during medical management.

Level of Cognitive Ability: Applying
Client Needs: Health Promotion and Maintenance
Clinical Judgment/Cognitive Skills: Take Action
Integrated Process: Teaching and Learning
Content Area: Adult Health: Cardiovascular
Health Problems: Adult Health: Cardiovascular: Dysrhythmias
Priority Concepts: Patient Education; Perfusion

Answer: 4
Rationale: The client with an ICD maintains a log or diary of a variety of data. This includes recording the date and time of the shock, any activity that took place before the shock, any symptoms experienced, the number of shocks delivered, and how the client felt after the shock. The information is used by the primary health care provider to adjust the medical regimen and especially the medication therapy, which must be maintained after ICD insertion.
Test-Taking Strategy: Note the strategic word, *primary*. Each of the incorrect options lists one of the items that should be logged in the diary, but the correct option is the only one that could be considered a "primary" purpose. Recording a variety of data is also the umbrella option.
Priority Nursing Tip: The client with an ICD needs to be taught to wear loose-fitting clothing over the ICD generator site and avoid contact sports to prevent trauma to the ICD generator and lead wires.
Reference: Ignatavicius, D., et al. (2021). *Medical-surgical nursing: Concepts for interprofessional collaborative care* (10th ed., p. 662). Elsevier.

69. The nurse is evaluating a hypertensive client's understanding of dietary modifications to control the disease process. The nurse determines that the client's understanding is satisfactory if the client made which meal selections?
1. Corned beef, fresh carrots, boiled potato
2. Hot dog on a bun, sauerkraut, baked beans
3. Turkey, baked potato, salad with oil and vinegar
4. Scallops, french fries, salad with bleu cheese dressing

Level of Cognitive Ability: Evaluating
Client Needs: Health Promotion and Maintenance
Clinical Judgment/Cognitive Skills: Evaluate Outcomes
Integrated Process: Clinical Judgment; Nursing Process/Evaluation
Content Area: Foundations of Care: Therapeutic Diets
Health Problems: Adult Health: Cardiovascular: Hypertension
Priority Concepts: Health Promotion; Perfusion

Answer: 3
Rationale: The client with hypertension needs to avoid foods that are high in sodium. Foods from the meat group that are higher in sodium include bacon, hot dogs, luncheon meat, chipped or corned beef, Kosher meat, smoked or salted meat or fish, peanut butter, and a variety of shellfish. Processed foods are also high in sodium.
Test-Taking Strategy: Note the subject, a hypertensive client making dietary modifications. Eliminate corned beef and hot dog menus because they are highly processed meats that would be high in sodium. From the remaining options, recalling that shellfish, french fries, and commercial salad dressing are high in sodium will assist you in eliminating this choice.
Priority Nursing Tip: In addition to limiting sodium intake, the client with hypertension needs to reduce fat intake to prevent the development of atherosclerosis.
Reference: Ignatavicius, D., et al. (2021). *Medical-surgical nursing: Concepts for interprofessional collaborative care* (10th ed., pp. 700–701). Elsevier.

70. The nurse has completed instructions with a client diagnosed with atrial fibrillation who will be taking warfarin sodium indefinitely. Which statement by the client indicates the **need for further teaching?**
1. "I need to use a soft toothbrush."
2. "I need to avoid drinking alcohol while taking this medication."
3. "I can continue to take my NSAIDs as previously prescribed."
4. "I need to carry identification regarding the medication being taken."

Level of Cognitive Ability: Evaluating
Client Needs: Health Promotion and Maintenance
Clinical Judgment/Cognitive Skills: Evaluate Outcomes
Integrated Process: Clinical Judgment; Nursing Process/Evaluation
Content Area: Pharmacology: Cardiovascular: Anticoagulants
Health Problems: Adult Health: Cardiovascular: Dysrhythmias
Priority Concepts: Clotting; Safety

Answer: 3
Rationale: Client instructions for oral anticoagulant therapy include reporting any signs/symptoms of bleeding and implementing measures to prevent bleeding, taking the medication only as prescribed and at the same time each day, avoiding other medications (including over-the-counter medications and nonsteroidal antiinflammatory drugs [NSAIDs]) without physician approval, avoiding alcohol, notifying all caregivers about the medication, carrying a Medic-Alert bracelet or card, and adhering to the schedule for follow-up blood work.
Test-Taking Strategy: Note the strategic words, *need for further teaching*. These words indicate a negative event query and ask you to select an option that is an incorrect statement. Recalling that warfarin sodium is an anticoagulant and that the client is at risk for bleeding will direct you to the fact that NSAIDs may lead to gastrointestinal bleeding when administered with this medication.
Priority Nursing Tip: The antidote for warfarin sodium is vitamin K.
Reference: Ignatavicius, D., et al. (2021). *Medical-surgical nursing: Concepts for interprofessional collaborative care* (10th ed., pp. 726, 864). Elsevier.

71. The home care nurse has given instructions to a client who was recently discharged from the hospital regarding the care of an arterial ischemic leg ulcer. The nurse determines that there is a **need for further teaching** if the client makes which statement?
1. "I need to inspect my feet daily."
2. "I need to wear shoes and socks."
3. "I need to cut my toenails straight across."
4. "I need to raise my legs above the level of my heart periodically."

Level of Cognitive Ability: Evaluating
Client Needs: Health Promotion and Maintenance
Clinical Judgment/Cognitive Skills: Evaluate Outcomes
Integrated Process: Clinical Judgment; Nursing Process/Evaluation
Content Area: Adult Health: Cardiovascular
Health Problems: Adult Health: Cardiovascular: Vascular Disorders
Priority Concepts: Patient Education; Perfusion

Answer: 4
Rationale: Foot care instructions for the client with peripheral arterial ischemia are the same instructions given to the client with diabetes mellitus. The client with arterial disease, however, needs to avoid raising the legs above heart level unless instructed to do so as part of an exercise program (such as Buerger's postural exercises) or if venous stasis is also present. Daily foot inspection, wearing shoes and socks, and cutting toenails straight across are accurate client statements.
Test-Taking Strategy: Note the strategic words, *need for further teaching*. These words indicate a negative event query and ask you to select an option that is an incorrect statement. Note that the client has an arterial disorder. Recalling the anatomy of the blood vessels and the pattern of blood flow in the arteries will direct you to option 4.
Priority Nursing Tip: A manifestation of peripheral arterial disease is intermittent claudication (pain in the muscles resulting from an inadequate blood supply).
Reference: Ignatavicius, D., et al. (2021). *Medical-surgical nursing: Concepts for interprofessional collaborative care* (10th ed., p. 712). Elsevier.

 72. A client diagnosed with chronic kidney disease is about to begin hemodialysis therapy. The client asks the nurse about the frequency and scheduling of hemodialysis treatments. What information would the nurse provide to the client regarding the typical hemodialysis schedule?
1. It is 2 hours of treatment 6 days per week.
2. It is 5 hours of treatment 2 days per week.
3. It is 2 to 3 hours of treatment 5 days per week.
4. It is 3 to 4 hours of treatment 3 days per week.

Level of Cognitive Ability: Applying
Client Needs: Health Promotion and Maintenance
Clinical Judgment/Cognitive Skills: Take Action
Integrated Process: Clinical Judgment; Nursing Process/Implementation
Content Area: Adult Health: Renal and Urinary
Health Problems: Adult Health: Renal and Urinary: Acute Kidney Injury and Chronic Kidney Disease
Priority Concepts: Patient Education; Fluids and Electrolytes

Answer: 4
Rationale: The typical schedule for hemodialysis is 3 to 4 hours of treatment 3 days per week. Individual adjustments may be made according to certain variables, such as the size of the client, the type of dialyzer, the rate of blood flow, and personal client preference.
Test-Taking Strategy: Focus on the subject, the "typical" hemodialysis schedule. Recalling that the client receives dialysis 3 days per week will direct you to the correct option.
Priority Nursing Tip: Monitor the client's vital signs before, during, and after dialysis. The client's temperature may elevate because of slight warming of the blood from the dialysis machine. However, the primary health care provider needs to be notified if temperature elevations are excessive because this could indicate sepsis.
Reference: Ignatavicius, D., et al. (2021). *Medical-surgical nursing: Concepts for interprofessional collaborative care* (10th ed., pp. 1396–1397). Elsevier.

73. The nurse prepares a client receiving treatment for a relapse of their multiple melanoma with a peripheral intravenous (IV) site for home IV therapy for discharge. Which measure would the nurse include in the teaching plan that would help prevent phlebitis and infiltration?
1. Massage the IV site daily.
2. Immobilize the extremity.
3. Stabilize the cannula with tape.
4. Cleanse the site daily with alcohol.

Level of Cognitive Ability: Applying
Client Needs: Health Promotion and Maintenance
Clinical Judgment/Cognitive Skills: Generate Solutions
Integrated Process: Teaching and Learning
Content Area: Skills: Tube Care
Health Problems: Adult Health: Cancer: Multiple Myeloma
Priority Concepts: Patient Education; Safety

Answer: 3
Rationale: Providing IV therapy at home involves the same principles as are used in the hospital. Protecting the IV site and securing it with tape are extremely important to ensure that the IV site remains immobile to reduce the risk of phlebitis and infiltration; however, the extremity does not need to be immobilized. Massaging the site potentially contributes to catheter movement and tissue damage. Immobilization devices such as arm boards are used if a site is near a joint and the IV flow rate is affected by joint movement. Alcohol skin preparation is used during the catheter insertion; because of the potential for excessive drying and client discomfort, alcohol is not used in IV site care.
Test-Taking Strategy: Focus on the subject, preventing phlebitis and infiltration. Eliminate options 1, 2, and 4 because of the words *massage, immobilize,* and *alcohol,* respectively.
Priority Nursing Tip: Signs/symptoms of phlebitis include a sluggish intravenous infusion and heat, redness, and tenderness at the intravenous site. The area is not usually swollen or hard.
Reference: Ignatavicius, D., et al. (2021). *Medical-surgical nursing: Concepts for interprofessional collaborative care* (10th ed., p. 280). Elsevier.

74. The nurse is teaching a client how to stand on crutches. What information would the nurse give the client related to placement of the crutches?
1. Place the crutches 3 inches to the front and side of the toes.
2. Place the crutches 6 inches to the front and side of the toes.
3. Place the crutches 15 inches to the front and side of the toes.
4. Place the crutches 20 inches to the front and side of the toes.

Level of Cognitive Ability: Applying
Client Needs: Health Promotion and Maintenance
Clinical Judgment/Cognitive Skills: Take Action
Integrated Process: Nursing Process/Implementation
Content Area: Skills: Activity/Mobility
Health Problems: Adult Health: Musculoskeletal: Skeletal Injury
Priority Concepts: Patient Education; Safety

Answer: 2
Rationale: The classic tripod position is taught to the client before instructions regarding gait are given. The crutches are placed anywhere from 6 to 10 inches in front of and to the side of the client's toes, depending on the client's body size. This provides a wide enough base of support for the client and improves balance. The other options provide improper distances for crutch placement.
Test-Taking Strategy: Note the subject, teaching a client how to stand on crutches. Three inches (option 1) and 20 inches (option 4) seem excessively short and long, respectively, and these options should be eliminated first. From the remaining options, visualize this procedure. Six inches seems more in keeping with the normal length of a stride than 15 inches.
Priority Nursing Tip: The nurse needs to instruct the client using crutches to look up and outward when ambulating.
Reference: Potter, P., et al. (2023). *Fundamentals of nursing* (11th ed., p. 852). Elsevier.

❖ **75.** The nurse is giving instructions to an adult client diagnosed with heart failure who is beginning therapy with digoxin. To detect **early** complications of therapy, which action would the nurse teach the client to perform?
   1. Take the pulse daily.
   2. Have electrolyte levels drawn weekly.
   3. Monitor the blood pressure once a week.
   4. Measure the weight each morning before breakfast.

Level of Cognitive Ability: Applying
Client Needs: Health Promotion and Maintenance
Clinical Judgment/Cognitive Skills: Take Action
Integrated Process: Teaching and Learning
Content Area: Pharmacology: Cardiovascular: Cardiac Glycosides
Health Problems: Adult Health: Cardiovascular: Heart Failure
Priority Concepts: Patient Education; Safety

Answer: 1
Rationale: Digoxin is a cardiac glycoside. Adult clients taking digoxin need to measure the pulse each day and notify the primary health care provider if the heart rate is less than 60 beats/min or more than 100 beats/min. Having weekly electrolyte levels drawn, monitoring weekly blood pressure, and weighing each morning are not necessary interventions for the client taking digoxin.
Test-Taking Strategy: Note the strategic word, *early*. Focus on the medication identified in the question. Recalling that digoxin is a cardiac medication will direct you to the correct option.
Priority Nursing Tip: Before administering digoxin to a client, the nurse needs to measure the client's apical heart rate for 1 full minute.
Reference: Ignatavicius, D., et al. (2021). *Medical-surgical nursing: Concepts for interprofessional collaborative care* (10th ed., p. 681). Elsevier.

❖ **76.** The nurse has completed teaching with a hemodialysis client regarding the self-monitoring of the fluid status between hemodialysis treatments. The nurse determines that the client understands the information given if the client states the need to record which item(s) on a daily basis?
   1. Activity
   2. Pulse and respiratory rate
   3. Intake, output, and weight
   4. Blood urea nitrogen and creatinine levels

Level of Cognitive Ability: Evaluating
Client Needs: Health Promotion and Maintenance
Clinical Judgment/Cognitive Skills: Evaluate Outcomes
Integrated Process: Clinical Judgment; Nursing Process/Evaluation
Content Area: Adult Health: Renal and Urinary
Health Problems: Adult Health: Renal and Urinary: Acute Kidney Injury and Chronic Kidney Disease
Priority Concepts: Patient Education; Fluids and Electrolytes

Answer: 3
Rationale: The client receiving hemodialysis needs to monitor fluid status between hemodialysis treatments. This can be done by recording intake and output and measuring weight on a daily basis. Ideally the hemodialysis client should not gain more than 0.5 kg of weight per day. It is not necessary to record activity, pulse and respiratory rate, and blood urea nitrogen (BUN) and creatinine levels daily.
Test-Taking Strategy: Immediately eliminate BUN and creatinine because it would not be the client's responsibility to obtain or record this information. Next note the words *daily basis*. Focusing on these words and the subject, a hemodialysis client self-monitoring fluid status, will direct you to monitoring intake, output, and weight.
Priority Nursing Tip: The nurse needs to weigh the client receiving hemodialysis before and after the treatment to determine fluid loss that occurred.
Reference: Ignatavicius, D., et al. (2021). *Medical-surgical nursing: Concepts for interprofessional collaborative care* (10th ed., pp. 1382–1383, 1408). Elsevier.

77. Diltiazem hydrochloride is prescribed for the client with Prinzmetal angina. The nurse provides instructions to the client regarding this medication. Which statement by the client indicates the **need for further teaching**?
1. "I will take the medication after meals."
2. "I will call the physician if shortness of breath occurs."
3. "I will rise slowly when getting out of bed in the morning."
4. "I will avoid activities that require alertness until my body gets used to the medication."

Level of Cognitive Ability: Evaluating
Client Needs: Health Promotion and Maintenance
Clinical Judgment/Cognitive Skills: Evaluate Outcomes
Integrated Process: Clinical Judgment; Nursing Process/Evaluation
Content Area: Pharmacology: Cardiovascular: Calcium Channel Blockers
Health Problems: Adult Health: Cardiovascular: Coronary Artery Disease
Priority Concepts: Patient Education; Safety

Answer: 1
Rationale: Diltiazem hydrochloride is a calcium channel blocker. It is administered before meals and at bedtime, as prescribed. Hypotension can occur, and the client is instructed to rise slowly. The client needs to call the physician if an irregular heartbeat, shortness of breath, pronounced dizziness, nausea, or constipation occurs. The client needs to avoid tasks that require alertness until a response to the medication is established.
Test-Taking Strategy: Note the strategic words, *need for further teaching.* These words indicate a negative event query and ask you to select an option that is an incorrect statement. Focusing on the client's diagnosis of Prinzmetal angina will assist you in eliminating rising slowly when getting out of bed, contacting the physician when shortness of breath occurs, and avoiding activities requiring alertness until adaptation to the medication has occurred as anticipated interventions.
Priority Nursing Tip: Calcium channel blockers promote vasodilation of the coronary and peripheral vessels and are used to treat angina, certain dysrhythmias, or hypertension. They need to be used with caution in clients with heart failure, bradycardia, or atrioventricular block.
Reference: Skidmore-Roth, L. (2021). *2021 Mosby's Nursing drug reference* (34th ed., p. 400). Elsevier.

 78. The nurse has provided instructions to a client being discharged from the hospital to home after an abdominal aortic aneurysm (AAA) resection. The nurse determines that the client understands the instructions if the client states that which is an appropriate activity?
1. Mowing the lawn
2. Playing a game of 18-hole golf
3. Lifting objects up to 30 pounds
4. Walking as tolerated, including outdoors

Level of Cognitive Ability: Evaluating
Client Needs: Health Promotion and Maintenance
Clinical Judgment/Cognitive Skills: Evaluate Outcomes
Integrated Process: Clinical Judgment; Nursing Process/Evaluation
Content Area: Adult Health: Cardiovascular
Health Problems: Adult Health: Cardiovascular: Vascular Disorders
Priority Concepts: Perfusion; Safety

Answer: 4
Rationale: The client can walk as tolerated after the repair or resection of an AAA, including walking outdoors. The client is not to engage in any activities that involve pushing, pulling, or straining, and the client is not to lift objects that weigh more than 15 to 20 pounds for 6 to 12 weeks. Driving is also prohibited for several weeks.
Test-Taking Strategy: Note the subject, a client being discharged after AAA resection, and the words *understands the instructions.* Evaluate each option in terms of the strain that it could put on the sutured graft. This will direct you to the option.
Priority Nursing Tip: An AAA resection is the surgical resection of the aneurysm. The excised section is replaced with a graft that is sewn end-to-end. In the postoperative period, graft occlusion is a concern, so it is important for the nurse to monitor peripheral pulses distal to the graft.
Reference: Ignatavicius, D., et al. (2021). *Medical-surgical nursing: Concepts for interprofessional collaborative care* (10th ed., pp. 718–719). Elsevier.

79. The nurse is planning dietary counseling for the client diagnosed with chronic heart failure taking triamterene. The nurse plans to include which item in a list of foods that are acceptable?
1. Bananas
2. Oranges
3. Baked potato
4. Canned pears

Level of Cognitive Ability: Applying
Client Needs: Health Promotion and Maintenance
Clinical Judgment/Cognitive Skills: Generate Solutions
Integrated Process: Teaching and Learning
Content Area: Pharmacology: Cardiovascular: Diuretics
Health Problems: Adult Health: Cardiovascular: Heart Failure
Priority Concepts: Patient Education; Nutrition

Answer: 4
Rationale: Triamterene is a potassium-sparing diuretic, and clients taking this medication need to be cautioned against eating foods that are high in potassium, including many vegetables, fruits, and fresh meats. Bananas, oranges, and potatoes are high in potassium. Because potassium is very soluble in water, foods that are prepared in cans are often lower in potassium (although some canned foods can be higher in sodium).
Test-Taking Strategy: Focus on the subject, triamterene, and note the words *foods that are acceptable*. Recall that triamterene is a potassium-sparing diuretic. Next, review the options, identifying the food item that is lowest in potassium.
Priority Nursing Tip: Instruct the client taking a potassium-sparing diuretic to avoid using salt substitutes because they contain potassium.
References: Burchum, J., & Rosenthal, L. (2022). *Lehne's Pharmacology for nursing care* (11th ed., pp. 464–465). Elsevier; Nix, S. (2022). *Williams' Basic nutrition and diet therapy* (16th ed., pp. 122, 528). Elsevier.

❖ **80.** Cyclophosphamide is prescribed for the client diagnosed with breast cancer, and the nurse provides instructions to the client regarding the medication. Which statement by the client indicates the **need for further teaching?**
1. "If I lose my hair, it will grow back."
2. "If I develop a sore throat, I need to notify the doctor."
3. "I need to limit my fluid intake while taking this medication."
4. "I need to avoid contact with anyone who recently received a live virus vaccine."

Level of Cognitive Ability: Evaluating
Client Needs: Health Promotion and Maintenance
Clinical Judgment/Cognitive Skills: Evaluate Outcomes
Integrated Process: Clinical Judgment; Nursing Process/ Evaluation
Content Area: Pharmacology: Oncology: Alkylating Agents
Health Problems: Adult Health: Cancer: Breast
Priority Concepts: Patient Education; Safety

Answer: 3
Rationale: Hemorrhagic cystitis is an adverse reaction associated with cyclophosphamide. The client needs to be instructed to consume copious amounts of fluid during therapy. The client's hair will grow back, although it may have a different color and texture. A sore throat may be an indication of an infection, and it must be reported to the primary health care provider. Avoiding contact with anyone who recently received a live virus vaccine is important because cyclophosphamide produces immunosuppression, thus placing the client at risk for infection.
Test-Taking Strategy: Note the strategic words, *need for further teaching*. These words indicate a negative event query and ask you to select an option that is an incorrect statement. Eliminate developing a sore throat and making contact with anyone receiving live virus immunizations because they are comparable or alike in that they both relate to the risk of infection. From the remaining options, recalling that hemorrhagic cystitis is an adverse effect of cyclophosphamide will direct you to the correct option.
Priority Nursing Tip: The client taking cyclophosphamide must be encouraged to consume 2 to 3 L of fluid per day (unless contraindicated) to prevent hemorrhagic cystitis.
Reference: Skidmore-Roth, L., (2021). *2021 Mosby's Nursing drug reference* (34th ed., p. 332). Elsevier.

81. The community health nurse has reviewed information about the population of a local community and has determined that there are groups in the population that are at high risk for infection with tuberculosis (TB). The nurse targets which high-risk group for screening?
1. French Canadians
2. White, Anglo-Saxon Americans
3. Older clients in long-term care facilities
4. Adolescents between the ages of 13 and 17 years

Level of Cognitive Ability: Applying
Client Needs: Health Promotion and Maintenance
Clinical Judgment/Cognitive Skills: Recognize Cues
Integrated Process: Clinical Judgment; Nursing Process/Assessment
Content Area: Foundations of Care: Community/Public/Population Health
Health Problems: Adult Health: Respiratory: Tuberculosis
Priority Concepts: Health Promotion; Infection

Answer: 3
Rationale: Older clients, particularly those in long-term care facilities, are at high risk for infection with TB. Other people at risk include children who are 5 years old and younger, the malnourished, the immunosuppressed, the economically disadvantaged, foreign-born persons, and persons of a minority race who formerly lived in a place where TB is common, such as Asia or the Pacific islands. Therefore, French Canadians, White Anglo-Saxon Americans, and adolescents between the ages of 13 and 17 are not high-risk persons.
Test-Taking Strategy: Focus on the subject, those at risk for TB. Recalling high-risk factors will direct you to option 3, older adults residing in a group setting. Remember that the very young and the very old often fall into high-risk categories.
Priority Nursing Tip: Improper or noncompliant use of treatment programs for TB may cause the development of mutations in the tubercle bacilli, resulting in a multidrug-resistant strain of tuberculosis (MDR-TB).
Reference: Ignatavicius, D., et al. (2021). *Medical-surgical nursing: Concepts for interprofessional collaborative care* (10th ed., p. 576). Elsevier.

82. A toddler with suspected conjunctivitis is crying and refuses to sit still during the eye examination. Which is the **most appropriate** statement for the nurse to make to the child?
1. "Would you like to see my flashlight?"
2. "Don't be scared, the light won't hurt you."
3. "If you will sit still, the exam will be over soon."
4. "I know you are upset. We can do this exam later."

Level of Cognitive Ability: Applying
Client Needs: Health Promotion and Maintenance
Clinical Judgment/Cognitive Skills: Take Action
Integrated Process: Communication and Documentation
Content Area: Pediatrics: Eye/Ear
Health Problems: Pediatric-Specific: Conjunctivitis
Priority Concepts: Development; Health Promotion

Answer: 1
Rationale: Fears in this age-group can be decreased by getting the child actively involved in the examination. Telling a young child to "not be scared" is telling the toddler how to feel. Telling the toddler to sit still ignores the toddler's feelings. Although option 4 acknowledges the toddler's feelings, it falsely puts off the inevitable.
Test-Taking Strategy: Note the strategic words, *most appropriate*. Use knowledge regarding the stages of growth and development, noting that the child is a toddler. The use of therapeutic communication techniques will direct you to the correct option.
Priority Nursing Tip: When approaching the toddler, the nurse should learn the words the toddler uses for common items and use them in conversations. The examiner needs to also use short, concrete terms and use play for demonstrations.
Reference: McKinney, E. S., et al. (2022). *Maternal child nursing* (6th ed., pp. 52–53, 733). Elsevier.

83. The parent of a teenage client diagnosed with an anxiety disorder is concerned about the teenager's progress after discharge. The parent states that the teenager "stashes food, eats all the wrong things that causes hyperactivity," and "hangs out with the wrong crowd." To assist the parent with preparing for the teenager's discharge, the nurse advises the parent to implement which action in order to promote optimal health?

1. Restrict the teenager's socializing time with school friends.
2. Consider taking time off to help the teenager readjust to the home environment.
3. Limit the amount of chocolate and caffeine products that are available in the home.
4. Keep the teenager out of school until the teenager can prove the ability to adjust to the school environment.

Level of Cognitive Ability: Applying
Client Needs: Health Promotion and Maintenance
Clinical Judgment/Cognitive Skills: Take Action
Integrated Process: Teaching and Learning
Content Area: Mental Health
Health Problems: Mental Health: Anxiety Disorder
Priority Concepts: Anxiety; Patient Education

Answer: **3**
Rationale: Clients diagnosed with anxiety disorders are advised to limit their intake of caffeine, chocolate, and alcohol because these products have the potential to increase anxiety. Restricting peer contact and avoiding school for a prolonged period of time are unreasonable and involve unhealthy approaches. In addition, it may not be realistic for a family member to take time off from work.
Test-Taking Strategy: Note the teenager's diagnosis of anxiety, and focus on the **subject**, to promote health. Restricting peer contact, limiting the environment, and avoiding school for a prolonged period of time are **comparable or alike**, as these options are concerned with monitoring or curtailing the teenager's physical activities, whereas making dietary adjustments focuses on the **subject**.
Priority Nursing Tip: The immediate nursing action for a client experiencing anxiety is to decrease stimuli in the environment and provide a calm and quiet environment.
References: Hockenberry, M., Wilson, D., & Rodgers, C. (2019). *Wong's Nursing care of infants and children* (11th ed.). St. Louis: Elsevier. pp. 541, 548. Lilley, L., Rainforth Collins, S., & Snyder J. (2020). *Pharmacology and the nursing process* (9th ed., p. 207). Elsevier.

❖ **84.** The nurse assesses a client with hepatic encephalopathy for the presence of asterixis. What would the nurse do to appropriately test for asterixis?

1. Examine the client's handwriting movements.
2. Check the stool for clay-colored pigmentation.
3. Ask the client to extend the wrist and the fingers.
4. Check the serum bilirubin and liver enzyme levels.

Level of Cognitive Ability: Applying
Client Needs: Health Promotion and Maintenance
Clinical Judgment/Cognitive Skills: Recognize Cues
Integrated Process: Clinical Judgment; Nursing Process/Assessment
Content Area: Health Assessment/Physical Exam: Abdomen
Health Problems: Adult Health: Gastrointestinal: Cirrhosis
Priority Concepts: Clinical Judgment; Health Promotion

Answer: **3**
Rationale: Asterixis is a rapid, nonrhythmic, abnormal muscle tremor of the wrists and fingers that is commonly associated with hepatic encephalopathy and referred to as "liver flap." Handwriting is a nonspecific and insensitive test of motor function, so the nurse avoids using this to assess for asterixis. Clients with hepatic encephalopathy can experience changes in bowel habits and flatulence but should not experience a color change. The nurse expects the liver function studies of a client with hepatic encephalopathy to have above-normal results.
Test-Taking Strategy: Focus on the **subject**, asterixis. Specific knowledge of the definition and manifestations of asterixis is needed to answer this question. Also recalling the signs and symptoms of hepatic encephalopathy will direct you to the correct option.
Priority Nursing Tip: The nurse would monitor the client with cirrhosis for signs associated with hepatic encephalopathy such as asterixis (rapid, nonrhythmic, abnormal muscle tremor of the wrists and fingers) and fetor hepaticus (fruity and musty breath odor).
Reference: Lewis, S., et al. (2020). *Medical-surgical nursing: Assessment and management of clinical problems* (11th ed., p. 984). Elsevier.

85. The nurse assesses cranial nerve XII in the client who sustained a stroke. To assess this cranial nerve, which action would the nurse ask the client to perform?

1. Extend the arms.
2. Extend the tongue.
3. Turn the head toward the nurse's arm.
4. Focus the eyes on an object held by the nurse.

Level of Cognitive Ability: Applying
Client Needs: Health Promotion and Maintenance
Clinical Judgment/Cognitive Skills: Take Action
Integrated Process: Clinical Judgment; Nursing Process/Assessment
Content Area: Health Assessment/Physical Exam: Neurologic
Health Problems: Adult Health: Neurologic: Stroke
Priority Concepts: Health Promotion; Intracranial Regulation

Answer: 2
Rationale: Impairment of cranial nerve XII can occur with a stroke. To assess the function of cranial nerve XII (hypoglossal), the nurse would assess the client's ability to extend the tongue. Extending the arms, turning the head toward the nurse's arm, and focusing the eyes on an object do not test the function of cranial nerve XII.
Test-Taking Strategy: Focus on the subject, the procedure for checking cranial nerve XII. Recalling that cranial nerve XII is the hypoglossal nerve will direct you to extending the tongue, option 2.
Priority Nursing Tip: The hypoglossal nerve (cranial nerve XII) controls the tongue movements involved with swallowing and speech. If the function of this nerve is affected, the client could have difficulty speaking and difficulty swallowing food and fluids, placing the client at risk for aspiration.
Reference: Ignatavicius, D., et al. (2021). *Medical-surgical nursing: Concepts for interprofessional collaborative care* (10th ed., p. 829). Elsevier.

❖ **86.** A client diagnosed with type 2 diabetes mellitus is being discharged from the hospital after an occurrence of hyperglycemic hyperosmolar state (HHS). The nurse creates a discharge teaching plan for the client and identifies which intervention as a **priority**?

1. Exercise routines
2. Controlling dietary intake
3. Keeping follow-up appointments
4. Monitoring for signs/symptoms of dehydration

Level of Cognitive Ability: Creating
Client Needs: Health Promotion and Maintenance
Clinical Judgment/Cognitive Skills: Prioritize Hypotheses
Integrated Process: Clinical Judgment; Teaching and Learning
Content Area: Adult Health: Endocrine
Health Problems: Adult Health: Endocrine: Diabetes Mellitus
Priority Concepts: Patient Education; Glucose Regulation

Answer: 4
Rationale: Clients at risk for HHS need to report signs and symptoms of dehydration to primary health care providers. Dehydration can be severe, and it may progress rapidly. Although exercising, dietary modifications, and follow-up appointments are components of the teaching plan, for the client diagnosed with HHS, dehydration is the priority.
Test-Taking Strategy: Note the strategic word, *priority*. Look at each option in terms of its seriousness, and recall that dehydration can rapidly progress to HHS.
Priority Nursing Tip: Hyperglycemic hyperosmolar state most often occurs in individuals with type 2 diabetes mellitus. The major difference between HHS and diabetic ketoacidosis is that ketosis and acidosis do not occur with HHS.
Reference: Ignatavicius, D., et al. (2021). *Medical-surgical nursing: Concepts for interprofessional collaborative care* (10th ed., pp. 1268, 1283). Elsevier.

87. The nurse creates a plan of care for an older client diagnosed with diabetes mellitus. It is important that the nurse plans to complete which action **first**?
  1. Structure menus for adherence to diet.
  2. Teach with videotapes showing, insulin administration to ensure competence.
  3. Encourage dependence on others to prepare the client for the chronicity of the disease.
  4. Assess the client's ability to read label markings on syringes and blood glucose monitoring equipment.

Level of Cognitive Ability: Creating
Client Needs: Health Promotion and Maintenance
Clinical Judgment/Cognitive Skills: Generate Solutions
Integrated Process: Clinical Judgment; Nursing Process/Planning
Content Area: Adult Health: Endocrine
Health Problems: Adult Health: Endocrine: Diabetes Mellitus
Priority Concepts: Clinical Judgment; Glucose Regulation

Answer: 4
Rationale: The nurse first assesses the client's ability for self-care. Structuring menus for the client promotes dependence. Allowing the client to have hands-on experience rather than teaching with videos is more effective. Independence should be encouraged.
Test-Taking Strategy: Note the strategic word, *first*. Use the steps of the nursing process. Determining the client's visual acuity reflects assessment, which is the first step of the nursing process.
Priority Nursing Tip: There are several components to a teaching plan for a client diagnosed with diabetes mellitus, including diet, exercise, and medication. Before implementing the plan, the nurse must perform an assessment to determine the client's specific learning needs.
Reference: Ignatavicius, D., et al. (2021). *Medical-surgical nursing: Concepts for interprofessional collaborative care* (10th ed., pp. 1282–1283, 1291). Elsevier.

❖ **88.** The nurse is conducting a health screening on a client with a family history of hypertension. Which assessment finding would alert the nurse to the **need for further teaching** related to stroke prevention?
  1. Eats high-fiber grain cereal with skim milk for breakfast
  2. Has a blood pressure of 118/78 mm Hg and has lost 10 pounds recently
  3. Uses condoms for pregnancy and disease prevention and jogs 2 miles daily
  4. Uses oral contraceptives for pregnancy prevention and works as a manager of a busy medical-surgical unit

Level of Cognitive Ability: Evaluating
Client Needs: Health Promotion and Maintenance
Clinical Judgment/Cognitive Skills: Evaluate Outcomes
Integrated Process: Clinical Judgment; Nursing Process/Evaluation
Content Area: Adult Health: Neurologic
Health Problems: Adult Health: Neurologic: Stroke
Priority Concepts: Patient Education; Health Promotion

Answer: 4
Rationale: Oral contraceptive use is discouraged in some clients because of the adverse effect of clot formation. The use of oral contraceptives, obesity, hypertension, hypercholesterolemia, and smoking are all modifiable risk factors for stroke. Low-fat diet and stress-reduction methods are encouraged and identified in options 1 and 3. In option 2, the client has a normal blood pressure and has lost weight.
Test-Taking Strategy: Note the strategic words, *need for further teaching*. These words indicate a negative event query and ask you to select the option that is a risk factor for stroke. Noting the words *oral contraceptives* in option 4 will direct you to this option.
Priority Nursing Tip: A transient ischemic attack may be a warning sign of a stroke.
Reference: Ignatavicius, D., et al. (2021). *Medical-surgical nursing: Concepts for interprofessional collaborative care* (10th ed., p. 700). Elsevier.

89. The nurse is reviewing the assessment data of a client. Which finding is **most important** for the client to modify to lessen the risk for coronary artery disease (CAD)?
1. Elevated triglyceride levels
2. Elevated serum lipase levels
3. Elevated serum testosterone level
4. Elevated low-density lipoprotein (LDL) levels

Level of Cognitive Ability: Analyzing
Client Needs: Health Promotion and Maintenance
Clinical Judgment/Cognitive Skills: Prioritize Hypotheses
Integrated Process: Clinical Judgment; Nursing Process/Analysis
Content Area: Health Assessment/Physical Exam: Heart and Peripheral Vascular
Health Problems: Adult Health: Cardiovascular: Coronary Artery Disease
Priority Concepts: Health Promotion; Perfusion

Answer: 4
Rationale: LDLs are more directly associated with CAD than are other lipoproteins. LDL levels, along with levels of cholesterol, have a higher predictive association with CAD than levels of triglycerides. Lipase is a digestive enzyme that breaks down ingested fats in the gastrointestinal tract. Low rather than high levels of testosterone have a significant negative influence on CAD.
Test-Taking Strategy: Note the strategic words, *most important.* Focus on the subject, the risk factor related to CAD. Recalling that LDL is the "bad" cholesterol will direct you to the correct option.
Priority Nursing Tip: Coronary artery narrowing is significant if the lumen diameter of the left main artery is reduced at least 50% or if any major branch is reduced at least 75%.
Reference: Ignatavicius, D., et al. (2021). *Medical-surgical nursing: Concepts for interprofessional collaborative care* (10th ed., pp. 622–623, 754). Elsevier.

❖ **90.** The nurse is assessing a client who is suspected of having a diagnosis of testicular cancer. Which data will be **most** helpful for determining the client's risk for this type of cancer?
1. Race
2. Marital status
3. Number of children
4. Number of sexual partners

Level of Cognitive Ability: Analyzing
Client Needs: Health Promotion and Maintenance
Clinical Judgment/Cognitive Skills: Analyze Cues
Integrated Process: Clinical Judgment; Nursing Process/Analysis
Content Area: Adult Health: Oncology
Health Problems: Adult Health: Cancer: Testicular
Priority Concepts: Cellular Regulation; Health Promotion

Answer: 1
Rationale: Two basic but important risk factors for testicular cancer are race and age. The incidence of testicular cancer is 4 times higher among white persons than persons of color. It is the most common type of cancer to occur in persons between the ages of 15 and 34 years. Other risk factors include a history of an undescended testis and a family history of testicular cancer. Marital status and the number of children are not risk factors for testicular cancer.
Test-Taking Strategy: Note the strategic word, *most.* Use your knowledge of the risk factors associated with this type of cancer to answer the question. Recalling that testicular cancer most often occurs in persons of white color will direct you to the correct option.
Priority Nursing Tip: Monthly testicular self-examination is the method of early detection of testicular cancer. The nurse needs to teach the client the procedure for performing this self-examination.
Reference: Ignatavicius, D., et al. (2021). *Medical-surgical nursing: Concepts for interprofessional collaborative care* (10th ed., p. 1485). Elsevier.

91. The nurse instructs a perinatal client about measures to prevent urinary tract infections. Which statement by the client indicates an understanding of these measures?
1. "I can wear my tight-fitting jeans."
2. "I should always use scented toilet paper."
3. "I should choose underwear with a cotton panel liner."
4. "I can take a bubble bath as long as the soap doesn't contain any oils."

Level of Cognitive Ability: Evaluating
Client Needs: Health Promotion and Maintenance
Clinical Judgment/Cognitive Skills: Evaluate Outcomes
Integrated Process: Clinical Judgment; Nursing Process/Evaluation
Content Area: Maternity: Antepartum
Health Problems: Maternity: Infections/Inflammations
Priority Concepts: Patient Education; Infection

Answer: 3
Rationale: Wearing items with a cotton panel liner allows for air movement in and around the genital area. Wearing tight clothes irritates the genital area and does not allow for air circulation. Harsh, scented, or printed toilet paper may cause irritation. Bubble bath or other bath oils need to be avoided because these may be irritating to the urethra and lead to a urinary tract infection.
Test-Taking Strategy: Note the words *indicates an understanding.* Eliminate scented toilet paper because of the closed-ended word "always" and wearing jeans because of the words *tight-fitting.* From the remaining options, recall that bubble baths need to be avoided.
Priority Nursing Tip: Measures to treat a urinary tract infections include taking the prescribed medication for the entire time prescribed and drinking at least 2500 to 3000 mL of fluid each day to help dilute the bacteria and flush infection from bladder.
References: Lowdermilk, D., et al. (2020). *Maternity & women's health care* (12th ed., p. 138). Elsevier; Potter, P., et al. (2023). *Fundamentals of nursing* (11th ed., p. 1246). Elsevier.

❖ **92.** The nurse instructs a client with mild preeclampsia about home care measures. Which statement by the client indicates to the nurse that the teaching has been **effective** concerning the assessment of complications for preeclampsia?
1. "I need to check my weight every day at different times during the day."
2. "I need to take my blood pressure each morning and alternate arms each time."
3. "I need to check my urine with a dipstick every day for protein and call the doctor if it is 2+ or more."
4. "As long as the home care nurse is visiting me daily, I do not have to keep my next doctor's appointment."

Level of Cognitive Ability: Evaluating
Client Needs: Health Promotion and Maintenance
Clinical Judgment/Cognitive Skills: Evaluate Outcomes
Integrated Process: Clinical Judgment; Nursing Process/Evaluation
Content Area: Maternity: Antepartum
Health Problems: Maternity: Gestational Hypertension/Preeclampsia and Eclampsia
Priority Concepts: Patient Education; Reproduction

Answer: 3
Rationale: Classic signs of preeclampsia include hypertension and proteinuria. The client diagnosed with preeclampsia needs to be instructed to report any increases in blood pressure; 2+ proteinuria; weight gain of more than 1 pound per week; the presence of edema in the face, hands, and sacral area; and decreased fetal activity to the physician immediately to prevent worsening of the preeclamptic condition. The weight needs to be checked at the same time each day, after voiding, before breakfast, and with the client wearing the same clothes in order to obtain reliable weight readings. Blood pressure measurements need to be taken in the same arm every day in a sitting position to obtain consistent and accurate readings. It is important to keep physician appointments even if the client is receiving visits from a home care nurse.
Test-Taking Strategy: Note the strategic word, *effective.* Basic principles related to health care teaching and focusing on the specific subject, mild preeclampsia, will assist with directing you to evaluating protein in the urine.
Priority Nursing Tip: Predisposing conditions for the development of gestational hypertension include primigravida, those younger than 19 years or older than 40 years, chronic kidney disease, chronic hypertension, diabetes mellitus, Rh incompatibility, and history or family history of gestational hypertension.
Reference: McKinney, E. S., et al. (2022). *Maternal child nursing* (6th ed., p. 549). Elsevier.

❖ **93.** The nurse is providing instructions to a client and family regarding home care after left-eye cataract removal. The nurse tells the client and family about assuming which position during the postoperative period?
   1. Sleep only on the left side.
   2. Sleep on the right side or the back.
   3. Bend below the waist as often as you are able.
   4. Lower the head between the knees 3 times a day.

Level of Cognitive Ability: Applying
Client Needs: Health Promotion and Maintenance
Clinical Judgment/Cognitive Skills: Take Action
Integrated Process: Clinical Judgment; Teaching and Learning
Content Area: Adult Health: Eye
Health Problems: Adult Health: Eye: Cataracts
Priority Concepts: Patient Education; Safety

Answer: 2
Rationale: After cataract surgery, the client is instructed to sleep on the nonoperative side or the back. The client is taught to not sleep on the operative side to prevent the development of edema. The client is also taught to avoid bending below the level of the waist or lowering the head because these actions will increase intraocular pressure.
Test-Taking Strategy: Bending below the waist and lowering the head between the knees several times per day should be eliminated first because these options are comparable or alike and indicate that lowering the head below waist level is acceptable. From the remaining options, remembering that the client needs to be instructed to remain off of the operative side will direct you to option 2.
Priority Nursing Tip: Blurred vision and decreased color perception are early signs/symptoms of a cataract.
Reference: Ignatavicius, D., et al. (2021). *Medical-surgical nursing: Concepts for interprofessional collaborative care* (10th ed., p. 941). Elsevier.

❖ **94.** The nurse has provided instructions to a new birthing parent with a urinary tract infection regarding foods and fluids to consume that will acidify the urine. The nurse determines that **further teaching is needed** if the birthing parent indicates that which fluid will acidify the urine?
   1. Prune juice
   2. Apricot juice
   3. Cranberry juice
   4. Carbonated drinks

Level of Cognitive Ability: Evaluating
Client Needs: Health Promotion and Maintenance
Clinical Judgment/Cognitive Skills: Evaluate Outcomes
Integrated Process: Clinical Judgment; Nursing Process/Evaluation
Content Area: Maternity: Postpartum
Health Problems: Maternity: Infections/Inflammations
Priority Concepts: Patient Education; Infection

Answer: 4
Rationale: Acidification of the urine inhibits the multiplication of bacteria. Carbonated drinks need to be avoided because they increase urine alkalinity. Fluids that acidify the urine include prune, apricot, and cranberry juice.
Test-Taking Strategy: Note the strategic words, *further teaching is needed*. These words indicate a negative event query and ask you to select the fluid item that will not acidify the urine. Note the similarity between prune, apricot, and cranberry juices as all are fruit juices. This will assist with directing you to the correct option.
Priority Nursing Tip: In addition to apricots, prunes, and cranberries, other foods that acidify the urine include tomatoes, meat, fish, oysters, poultry, corn, legumes, cheese, eggs, and whole grains.
Reference: McKinney, E. S., et al. (2022). *Maternal child nursing* (6th ed., p. 617). Elsevier.

95. A postpartum nurse taught a new birthing parent how to bathe their newborn. The nurse demonstrates the procedure to the birthing parent and, on the following day, asks the birthing parent to perform the procedure. Which observation by the nurse indicates that the birthing parent is performing the procedure correctly?
1. Cleans the ears and then moves to the eyes and the face
2. Begins to wash the newborn infant by starting with the eyes and face
3. Washes the arms, chest, and back followed by the neck, arms, and face
4. Washes the entire newborn infant's body and then washes the eyes, face, and scalp

Level of Cognitive Ability: Evaluating
Client Needs: Health Promotion and Maintenance
Clinical Judgment/Cognitive Skills: Evaluate Outcomes
Integrated Process: Clinical Judgment; Nursing Process/Evaluation
Content Area: Skills: Hygiene
Health Problems: N/A
Priority Concepts: Development; Safety

Answer: 2
Rationale: Bathing needs to start at the eyes and face and with the cleanest area first. Next, the external ears and behind the ears are cleaned. The newborn infant's neck needs to be washed because formula, lint, and breast milk will often accumulate in the folds of the neck. The hands and arms are then washed. The newborn infant's legs are washed next, with the diaper area being washed last.
Test-Taking Strategy: Note the subject, bathing a newborn. Use the basic techniques and principles of bathing a newborn to answer this question. Remember to always start with the cleanest area of the body and proceed to the dirtiest area. This principle will direct you to the correct option.
Priority Nursing Tip: Teach the parents to gather all of the necessary equipment needed for the bath before bathing the infant. The infant or child is never left alone during bathing.
Reference: McKinney, E. S., et al. (2022). *Maternal child nursing* (6th ed., pp. 481, 827–828). Elsevier.

96. The nurse is teaching umbilical cord care to a new birthing parent. What information would the nurse provide to the parent related to cord care?
1. Alcohol is the only agent to use to clean the cord.
2. Cord care is done only at birth to control bleeding.
3. It takes at least 21 days for the cord to dry up and fall off.
4. The process of keeping the cord clean and dry will decrease bacterial growth.

Level of Cognitive Ability: Applying
Client Needs: Health Promotion and Maintenance
Clinical Judgment/Cognitive Skills: Take Action
Integrated Process: Teaching and Learning
Content Area: Maternity: Newborn
Health Problems: Newborn: Infections
Priority Concepts: Patient Education; Infection

Answer: 4
Rationale: The cord needs to be kept clean and dry to decrease bacterial growth. It needs to be cleansed 2 to 3 times a day with a prescribed agent. Usually the cord is cleansed with mild soap and water around base of the cord where it joins the skin. The primary health care provider is notified of any odor, discharge, or skin inflammation. The diaper should not cover the cord because a wet or soiled diaper will slow or prevent drying of the cord and foster infection. Cord care is required until the cord dries up and falls off between 7 and 14 days after birth.
Test-Taking Strategy: Eliminate options 1 and 2 first because of the closed-ended word "only." From the remaining options, recalling the purpose of cord care will direct you to the correct option.
Priority Nursing Tip: Note any bleeding or drainage from the umbilical cord in a newborn. If symptoms of infection occur, notify the primary health care provider and use antibiotic prescription as prescribed.
Reference: McKinney, E. S., et al. (2022). *Maternal child nursing* (6th ed., pp. 475, 481). Elsevier.

97. Which event would the nurse identify as a situational crisis? **Select all that apply.**
- ❑ **1.** Divorce
- ❑ **2.** Retirement
- ❑ **3.** Loss of a job
- ❑ **4.** An earthquake
- ❑ **5.** The birth of a child
- ❑ **6.** Death of a loved one

Level of Cognitive Ability: Understanding
Client Needs: Health Promotion and Maintenance
Clinical Judgment/Cognitive Skills: Recognize Cues
Integrated Process: Nursing Process/Assessment
Content Area: Mental Health
Health Problems: Mental Health: Crisis
Priority Concepts: Anxiety; Clinical Judgment

Answer: 1, 3, 6

Rationale: A situational crisis arises from an external rather than an internal source and often is unanticipated. Examples of external situations that can precipitate a situational crisis include divorce, the loss of a job, the death of a loved one, an abortion, a change in job, a change in financial status, and severe physical or mental illness. A maturational crisis occurs at a developmental stage; examples include marriage, the birth of a child, and retirement. An adventitious crisis, or crisis of disaster, is not a part of everyday life and is unplanned or accidental. This type of crisis can result from a natural disaster (flood, fire, earthquake), a national disaster (acts of terrorism, war, riots, airplane crashes), or a crime of violence (rape, assault, murder, bombing, spousal or child abuse).

Test-Taking Strategy: Focus on the **subject**, a situational crisis. Read each option and recall that a situational crisis arises from an external rather than an internal source and often is unanticipated. This will assist in selecting the correct answers.

Priority Nursing Tip: For crisis management, treatment is immediate, supportive, and directly responsive to the immediate crisis.

Reference: Varcarolis, E., & Fosbre, C. (2021). *Essentials of psychiatric mental health nursing: A communication approach to evidence-based care* (4th ed., p. 333). Elsevier.

---

98. The nurse creates a teaching plan regarding the administration of eardrops for the parents of a 6-year-old child. The nurse tells the parents that, when administering the drops, which action is appropriate?
1. Wear gloves.
2. Pull the ear up and back.
3. Hold the child in a sitting position.
4. Position the child so that the affected ear is facing downward.

Level of Cognitive Ability: Creating
Client Needs: Health Promotion and Maintenance
Clinical Judgment/Cognitive Skills: Take Action
Integrated Process: Clinical Judgment; Teaching and Learning
Content Area: Skills: Medication Administration
Health Problems: Pediatric-Specific: Otitis Externa
Priority Concepts: Patient Education; Development

Answer: 2

Rationale: To administer eardrops in a child who is more than 3 years old, the ear is pulled upward and back. The ear is pulled down and back in children less than 3 years old. Gloves do not need to be worn by the parents, but hands must be washed before and after the procedure. The child needs to be in a side-lying position with the affected ear facing upward to facilitate the flow of medication down the ear canal with the help of gravity.

Test-Taking Strategy: Focus on the **subject**, the administration of eardrops to a 6-year-old child. Visualizing this procedure will assist you in eliminating wearing gloves, holding the child in a sitting position, or placing the affected ear downward. Also recalling the anatomy of the child's ear canal and noting the age of the child will direct you to the correct option.

Priority Nursing Tip: When administering the eardrops, the child needs to remain lying down with the affected ear upward for 1 to 2 minutes so that medication can be absorbed.

Reference: McKinney, E. S., et al. (2022). *Maternal child nursing* (6th ed., p. 863). Elsevier.

❖ **99.** The nurse is providing discharge instructions to the parent of an 8-year-old child who had a tonsillectomy. The parent tells the nurse that the child loves tacos and asks when the child can safely eat one. To prevent complications of the surgical procedure, what would be the appropriate response to the parent?
1. "In 1 week"
2. "In 3 weeks"
3. "Six days after surgery"
4. "When the surgeon says it is okay"

Level of Cognitive Ability: Applying
Client Needs: Health Promotion and Maintenance
Clinical Judgment/Cognitive Skills: Take Action
Integrated Process: Clinical Judgment; Nursing Process/Take Action
Content Area: Pediatrics: Throat/Respiratory
Health Problems: Pediatric-Specific: Tonsillitis and Adenoiditis
Priority Concepts: Patient Education; Safety

Answer: 2
Rationale: Rough or scratchy foods, as well as spicy foods, are to be avoided for 3 weeks after a tonsillectomy. Citrus juices that irritate the throat need to be avoided for 10 days. Red liquids are avoided because they will give the appearance of blood if the child vomits. The parent is instructed to add full liquids on the second day and soft foods as the child tolerates them.
Test-Taking Strategy: Eliminate 1 week and 6 days first because they are comparable or alike and identify similar time frames. Eliminate waiting for a response from the surgeon because it places the parent's question on hold.
Priority Nursing Tip: After tonsillectomy, position the child prone or side-lying to facilitate drainage.
Reference: McKinney, E. S., et al. (2022). *Maternal child nursing* (6th ed., p. 1048). Elsevier.

❖ **100.** After a cleft lip repair, the nurse instructs the parents about cleaning of the lip repair site. The nurse would plan to use which solution when demonstrating this procedure to the parents?
1. Tap water
2. Sterile water
3. Full-strength hydrogen peroxide
4. Half-strength hydrogen peroxide

Level of Cognitive Ability: Applying
Client Needs: Health Promotion and Maintenance
Clinical Judgment/Cognitive Skills: Generate Solutions
Integrated Process: Clinical Judgment; Teaching and Learning
Content Area: Pediatrics: Gastrointestinal
Health Problems: Pediatric-Specific: Disorders of Prenatal Development
Priority Concepts: Patient Education; Infection

Answer: 2
Rationale: After cleft lip repair, the site is cleansed with sterile water using a cotton swab after feeding and as prescribed. Agency procedure also needs to be followed. The parents need to be instructed to use a rolling motion starting at the suture line and rolling out. Tap water is not a sterile solution. Hydrogen peroxide may disrupt the integrity of the site.
Test-Taking Strategy: Eliminate full-strength and half-strength hydrogen peroxide first because these solutions are comparable or alike except for strength. From the remaining options, recall the importance of asepsis when treating a surgical site to direct you to the correct option.
Priority Nursing Tip: After cleft lip repair, avoid positioning the infant on the side of the repair or in the prone position because these positions can cause rubbing of the surgical site on the mattress.
Reference: McKinney, E. S., et al. (2022). *Maternal child nursing* (6th ed., p. 968). Elsevier.

101. A child with a diagnosis of umbilical hernia has been scheduled for surgical repair in 2 weeks. The clinic nurse instructs the parents about the signs of possible hernia strangulation. The nurse tells the parents that which sign requires physician notification?
1. Fever
2. Diarrhea
3. Vomiting
4. Constipation

Level of Cognitive Ability: Applying
Client Needs: Health Promotion and Maintenance
Clinical Judgment/Cognitive Skills: Take Action
Integrated Process: Clinical Judgment; Teaching and Learning
Content Area: Pediatrics: Gastrointestinal
Health Problems: Pediatric-Specific: Developmental GI Defects
Priority Concepts: Patient Education; Safety

Answer: 3
Rationale: The parents of a child with an umbilical hernia need to be instructed regarding the signs/symptoms of strangulation, which include vomiting, pain, and an irreducible mass at the umbilicus. Fever, diarrhea, and constipation are not signs of hernia strangulation. The parents need to be instructed to contact the physician immediately if strangulation is suspected.
Test-Taking Strategy: Note the subject, hernia strangulation. Recall the definition of the word *strangulation* to assist you in eliminating fever and diarrhea. From the remaining options, think about the anatomy of the body and the expected occurrence if strangulation developed to direct you to the correct option.
Priority Nursing Tip: An umbilical hernia is a soft swelling or protrusion around the umbilicus that is usually reducible with the finger.
Reference: McKinney, E. S., et al. (2022). *Maternal child nursing* (6th ed., p. 973). Elsevier.

102. A client with a compound (open) fracture of the radius has a plaster cast applied in the emergency department. The nurse provides home care instructions and tells the client to seek medical attention if which finding occurs?
1. Numbness and tingling are felt in the fingers.
2. The cast feels heavy and damp after 24 hours of application.
3. The entire cast feels warm during the first 24 hours after application.
4. Slightly bloody drainage is noted on the cast during the first 6 hours after application.

Level of Cognitive Ability: Applying
Client Needs: Health Promotion and Maintenance
Clinical Judgment/Cognitive Skills: Generate Solutions
Integrated Process: Teaching and Learning
Content Area: Adult Health: Musculoskeletal
Health Problems: Adult Health: Musculoskeletal: Skeletal Injury
Priority Concepts: Perfusion; Safety

Answer: 1
Rationale: A limb encased in a cast is at risk for nerve damage and diminished circulation from increased pressure caused by edema. Signs/symptoms of increased pressure from the cast include numbness, tingling, and increased pain. A cast can take up to 48 hours to dry and generates heat while drying. Some drainage may occur initially with a compound (open) fracture.
Test-Taking Strategy: Note the words *compound (open)* in the question. These words and the use of the ABCs—airway, breathing, and circulation—will direct you to the correct option.
Priority Nursing Tip: Monitor the client with a cast for signs and symptoms of infection under the cast, which include an increased temperature, hot spots on the cast, a foul odor, or changes in pain.
Reference: Ignatavicius, D., et al. (2021). *Medical-surgical nursing: Concepts for interprofessional collaborative care* (10th ed., pp. 1041–1042). Elsevier.

103. The parent of a child with celiac disease asks the nurse how long a special diet is necessary. The nurse provides which instruction to the parent to promote dietary compliance?
1. A gluten-free diet will need to be followed for life.
2. A lactose-free diet will need to be followed temporarily.
3. Added dietary sodium will help prevent episodes of celiac crisis.
4. Supplemental vitamins, iron, and folate will prevent complications.

Level of Cognitive Ability: Applying
Client Needs: Health Promotion and Maintenance
Clinical Judgment/Cognitive Skills: Generate Solutions
Integrated Process: Clinical Judgment; Teaching and Learning
Content Area: Pediatrics: Gastrointestinal
Health Problems: Pediatric-Specific: Nutrition Problems
Priority Concepts: Adherence; Patient Education

Answer: 1
Rationale: Celiac disease is characterized by intolerance to gluten, the protein component of wheat, barley, rye, and oats. The main nursing consideration with celiac disease is helping the child adhere to dietary management. The treatment of celiac disease consists primarily of dietary management with a gluten-free diet. Options 2 and 4 are true statements, but they do not answer the question that the client is asking. Children with untreated celiac disease may have lactose intolerance, which usually improves with gluten withdrawal. Additional sodium does not prevent celiac crisis. Low levels of potassium, calcium, and magnesium are most likely to be present. Nutritional deficiencies resulting from malabsorption are treated with appropriate supplements.
Test-Taking Strategy: Focus on the **subject**, the length of time that a special diet is necessary. Although the remaining options are all true about celiac disease, they do not answer the question that the client is asking. The correct option relates directly to this **subject**.
Priority Nursing Tip: For the client with celiac disease, strict dietary avoidance of gluten minimizes the risk of developing malignant lymphoma of the small intestine and other gastrointestinal malignancies.
Reference: McKinney, E. S., et al. (2022). *Maternal child nursing* (6th ed., p. 997). Elsevier.

❖ **104.** The nurse teaches the parent of a newly circumcised infant about post-circumcision care. Which statement by the parent indicates an understanding of the care required?
1. "I need to clean the penis every hour with baby wipes."
2. "I need to check for bleeding every hour for the first 12 hours."
3. "My baby will not urinate for the next 24 hours because of swelling."
4. "I need to wrap the penis completely in dry sterile gauze, making sure that it is dry when I change the diaper."

Level of Cognitive Ability: Evaluating
Client Needs: Health Promotion and Maintenance
Clinical Judgment/Cognitive Skills: Evaluate Outcomes
Integrated Process: Clinical Judgment; Nursing Process/Evaluation
Content Area: Maternity: Newborn
Health Problems: Newborn: Circumcision
Priority Concepts: Patient Education; Infection

Answer: 2
Rationale: After the circumcision, the parent needs to be taught to observe for bleeding and assess the site hourly for 8 to 12 hours. Water is used for cleaning because soap or baby wipes may irritate the area and cause discomfort. Voiding needs to be assessed. The parent needs to call the surgeon if the baby has not urinated within 24 hours because swelling or damage may obstruct urine output. When the diaper is changed, Vaseline gauze should be reapplied (if prescribed). Frequent diaper changing prevents contamination of the site.
Test-Taking Strategy: Focus on the **subject**, circumcision care. Eliminate option 1 because baby wipes will cause stinging of the newly circumcised penis. Eliminate option 3 because penile swelling that prevents voiding needs to be reported to the primary health care provider. Eliminate option 4 because gauze will stick to the penis if it is completely dry.
Priority Nursing Tip: The nurse should inform the parents that a milky covering over the glans penis is normal and should not be disrupted.
Reference: McKinney, E. S., et al. (2022). *Maternal child nursing* (6th, p. 479). Elsevier.

❖ **105.** The nurse would tell the client to avoid which item while taking phenelzine sulfate?
   1. Blueberries
   2. Vasodilators
   3. Aged cheeses
   4. Digitalis preparations

Level of Cognitive Ability: Applying
Client Needs: Health Promotion and Maintenance
Clinical Judgment/Cognitive Skills: Take Action
Integrated Process: Teaching and Learning
Content Area: Pharmacology: Psychotherapeutics: Monoamine Oxidase Inhibitors (MAOIs)
Health Problems: Mental Health: Mood Disorders
Priority Concepts: Patient Education; Safety

Answer: 3
Rationale: Phenelzine sulfate is in the MAOI class of antidepressant medications. An individual taking an MAOI must avoid aged cheeses, alcoholic beverages, avocados, bananas, and caffeine drinks. There are also other food items to avoid, including chocolate, meat tenderizers, pickled herring, raisins, sour cream, yogurt, and soy sauce. Medications that need to be avoided include amphetamines, antiasthmatics, and certain antidepressants. The client needs to also avoid vasoconstrictors because their concurrent use can cause hypertensive crisis.
Test-Taking Strategy: Focus on the subject, the item to avoid while taking phenelzine sulfate. Recalling that phenelzine sulfate is an MAOI and recalling the foods that need to be avoided will direct you to the correct option.
Priority Nursing Tip: The client taking an MAOI needs to avoid foods containing tyramine. Consuming tyramine-containing foods when taking an MAOI can cause hypertensive crisis.
Reference: Lilley, L., Rainforth Collins, S., & Snyder J. (2020). *Pharmacology and the nursing process* (9th ed., p. 256). Elsevier.

❖ **106.** A pregnant client, suspected of being physically abused by the partner, is brought to the emergency department by a neighbor after being found bleeding from the head. In evaluating the crisis situation, which questions would the nurse specifically ask to assess the client's perception of the precipitating event? **Select all that apply.**
   ❑ 1. Where do you go to worship?
   ❑ 2. Who is available to help you?
   ❑ 3. How does this situation affect your life?
   ❑ 4. Describe how you are feeling right now.
   ❑ 5. To whom do you talk with when you are upset?
   ❑ 6. How do you see this event as affecting your future?

Level of Cognitive Ability: Applying
Client Needs: Health Promotion and Maintenance
Clinical Judgment/Cognitive Skills: Recognize Cues
Integrated Process: Nursing Process/Assessment
Content Area: Mental Health
Health Problems: Mental Health: Crisis
Priority Concepts: Clinical Judgment; Interpersonal Violence

Answer: 3, 4, 6
Rationale: In a crisis situation, the nurse's initial task is to assess the individual or family and the problem. Assessing the client's perception of the precipitating event will assist in clearly defining the problem, which will result in identifying a more effective solution. Examples of some questions that the nurse can ask to assess the client's perception of the precipitating event include the following: How does this situation affect your life? Describe how you are feeling right now. How do you see this event as affecting your future? Has anything particularly upsetting happened to you within the past few days or weeks? What was happening in your life before you started to feel this way? What leads you to seek help now? What would need to be done to resolve this situation? The other questions listed—Where do you go to worship? Who is available to help you? To whom do you talk with when you are upset?—assess situational supports, not the client's perception of the precipitating event.
Test-Taking Strategy: Focus on the subject, a pregnant client suspected of being physically abused by the partner. The question is asking the client's perception of the precipitating event. This will assist in determining the correct questions to ask the client. The incorrect options assess situational supports, not the client's perception of the precipitating event.
Priority Nursing Tip: If the nurse suspects that a client is a victim of abuse, it is the nurse's responsibility to report the suspicion to the appropriate authorities. Additionally, the nurse must ensure confidentiality for the client and family as the appropriate procedures are carried out.
Reference: Varcarolis, E., & Fosbre, C. (2021). *Essentials of psychiatric mental health nursing: A communication approach to evidence-based care* (4th ed., pp. 346, 349). Elsevier.

107. Which action by the client would lead the nurse to determine the **need for further teaching** regarding the use of the incentive spirometer?
  1. Inhales slowly
  2. Breathes through the nose
  3. Removes the mouthpiece to exhale
  4. Forms a tight seal around the mouthpiece with the lips

Level of Cognitive Ability: Evaluating
Client Needs: Health Promotion and Maintenance
Clinical Judgment/Cognitive Skills: Evaluate Outcomes
Integrated Process: Clinical Judgment; Nursing Process/Evaluation
Content Area: Skills: Oxygenation
Health Problems: Adult Health: Respiratory: Infections of the Lower Airway
Priority Concepts: Patient Education; Gas Exchange

Answer: 2
Rationale: Incentive spirometry is ineffective if the client breathes through the nose. The client should exhale, form a tight seal around the mouthpiece, inhale slowly, hold to the count of 5, and remove the mouthpiece to exhale. The client should repeat the exercise approximately 10 times every hour for best results.
Test-Taking Strategy: Note the strategic words, *need for further teaching.* These words indicate a negative event query and ask you to select the option that identifies an incorrect client action. Visualizing the use of this device will direct you to the correct option.
Priority Nursing Tip: Use of an incentive spirometer will assist in preventing respiratory complications such as atelectasis in the postoperative client.
Reference: Ignatavicius, D., et al. (2021). *Medical-surgical nursing: Concepts for interprofessional collaborative care* (10th ed., pp. 166, 168). Elsevier.

❖ **108.** The nurse is giving a client with chronic obstructive pulmonary disease (COPD) information related to the positions used to breathe more easily. The nurse teaches the client to assume which position?
  1. Sit bolt upright in bed with the arms crossed over the chest.
  2. Lie on the side with the head of the bed at a 45-degree angle.
  3. Sit in a reclining chair tilted slightly back with the feet elevated.
  4. Sit on the edge of the bed with the arms leaning on an overbed table.

Level of Cognitive Ability: Applying
Client Needs: Health Promotion and Maintenance
Clinical Judgment/Cognitive Skills: Take Action
Integrated Process: Teaching and Learning
Content Area: Skills: Oxygenation
Health Problems: Adult Health: Respiratory: Chronic Obstructive Pulmonary Disease
Priority Concepts: Patient Education; Gas Exchange

Answer: 4
Rationale: Proper positioning can decrease episodes of dyspnea in a client with COPD. Appropriate positions include sitting upright while leaning on an overbed table, sitting upright in a chair with the arms resting on the knees, and leaning against a wall while standing. Sitting bolt upright with arms folded across the chest restricts the movement of the anterior and posterior walls of the lung, and side-lying with the head of bed raised to a 45-degree position restricts the expansion of the lateral wall of the lung. Option 3 restricts posterior lung expansion.
Test-Taking Strategy: Note the subject, a client with COPD. Visualize each of the positions described in the options, and think about how each position affects lung expansion to direct you to the correct option.
Priority Nursing Tip: The arterial blood gas levels on a client with COPD usually indicate respiratory acidosis and hypoxemia.
Reference: Ignatavicius, D., et al. (2021). *Medical-surgical nursing: Concepts for interprofessional collaborative care* (10th ed., pp. 547–548.). Elsevier.

109. The nurse has taught the client diagnosed with pleurisy about measures to promote comfort during recuperation. The nurse determines that the client has understood the information if the client states the need to follow which instruction?
1. Try to take only small, shallow breaths.
2. Take as much pain medication as possible.
3. Lie on the unaffected side as much as possible.
4. Splint the chest wall during coughing and deep breathing.

Level of Cognitive Ability: Evaluating
Client Needs: Health Promotion and Maintenance
Clinical Judgment/Cognitive Skills: Evaluate Outcomes
Integrated Process: Clinical Judgment; Nursing Process/Evaluation
Content Area: Adult Health: Respiratory
Health Problems: Adult Health: Respiratory: Pleurisy
Priority Concepts: Patient Education; Gas Exchange

Answer: 4
Rationale: The client with pleurisy needs to splint the chest wall during coughing and deep breathing. Taking small, shallow breaths promotes atelectasis. The client needs to take medication cautiously so that adequate coughing and deep breathing are performed and an adequate level of comfort is maintained. The client may also lie on the affected side to minimize the movement of the affected chest wall.
Test-Taking Strategy: Focus on the **subject**, client understanding of measures to promote comfort with pleurisy. Eliminate taking small, shallow breaths because of the **closed-ended word** "only." From the remaining options, noting the word *splint* will direct you to the correct option.
Priority Nursing Tip: The client with pleurisy experiences a knife like pain that is aggravated on deep-breathing and coughing. A pleural friction rub is heard on auscultation of the lungs.
Reference: Lewis, S., et al. (2020). *Medical-surgical nursing: Assessment and management of clinical problems* (11th ed., p. 531). Elsevier.

110. A client with a diagnosis of trigeminal neuralgia is started on a regimen of carbamazepine. The nurse provides instructions to the client about the medication. What statement by the client indicates that the client understands the instructions?
1. "I will report a fever or sore throat to my doctor."
2. "Some joint pain is expected and is nothing to worry about."
3. "I must brush my teeth frequently to avoid damage to my gums."
4. "My urine may turn red but this is nothing to be concerned about."

Level of Cognitive Ability: Evaluating
Client Needs: Health Promotion and Maintenance
Clinical Judgment/Cognitive Skills: Evaluate Outcomes
Integrated Process: Clinical Judgment; Nursing Process/Evaluation
Content Area: Pharmacology: Neurologic: Antiseizure
Health Problems: Adult Health: Neurologic: Trigeminal Neuralgia
Priority Concepts: Patient Education; Safety

Answer: 1
Rationale: Carbamazepine is an anticonvulsant medication and is also used to alleviate the pain associated with trigeminal neuralgia. Agranulocytosis is an adverse effect of carbamazepine, and it places the client at risk for infection. If the client develops a fever or a sore throat, the primary health care provider needs to be notified. Unusual bruising and bleeding are also adverse effects of the medication, and they need to be reported to the primary health care provider if they occur.
Test-Taking Strategy: Eliminate option 3 because of the **closed-ended word** "must." Next, eliminate options 2 and 4 as they are **comparable or alike** and both indicate that the development of an adverse effect is "nothing to be concerned about." Recalling that agranulocytosis is an adverse effect will direct you to the correct option.
Priority Nursing Tip: Trigeminal neuralgia is a sensory disorder of the trigeminal (5th cranial) nerve that results in severe, recurrent, sharp facial pain along the trigeminal nerve.
Reference: Kizior, R., & Hodgson, B. (2023). *Saunders Nursing drug handbook 2023* (pp. 182, 184). Elsevier.

Client Needs

111. The nurse teaches a preoperative client about the nasogastric (NG) tube that will be inserted in preparation for surgery. The nurse determines that the client understands when the tube will be removed during the postoperative period based on which statement by the client?
1. "When my doctor says so."
2. "When I can tolerate food without vomiting."
3. "When my gastrointestinal (GI) system is healed."
4. "When my bowels begin to function again and I begin to pass gas."

Level of Cognitive Ability: Evaluating
Client Needs: Health Promotion and Maintenance
Clinical Judgment/Cognitive Skills: Evaluate Outcomes
Integrated Process: Clinical Judgment; Nursing Process/Evaluation
Content Area: Adult Health: Gastrointestinal
Health Problems: Adult Health: Gastrointestinal: Nutrition/Malabsorption Problems
Priority Concepts: Patient Education; Health Promotion

Answer: 4
Rationale: NG tubes are discontinued when normal function returns to the GI tract. Although the surgeon determines when the NG tube will be removed, "When my doctor says so" does not determine the effectiveness of teaching. Food would not be administered unless bowel function returns. The tube will be removed well before GI healing occurs.
Test-Taking Strategy: Focus on the subject, the client's knowledge about NG tube removal. "When my doctor says so" can be easily eliminated first because it does not determine the effectiveness of teaching. Eliminate GI tract healed next, considering the time factor associated with the healing of the GI tract. From the remaining options, recalling that food would not be administered unless bowel function returns will assist you in eliminating consuming food without vomiting.
Priority Nursing Tip: When removing an NG tube, ask the client to take a deep breath and hold; then remove the tube slowly and evenly over the course of 3 to 6 seconds (coil the tube around the hand while removing it).
Reference: Ignatavicius, D., et al. (2021). *Medical-surgical nursing: Concepts for interprofessional collaborative care* (10th ed., p. 176). Elsevier.

❖ 112. A client is receiving lipids (fat emulsion) intravenously at home, and the client's spouse manages the infusion. The home care nurse makes a visit and discusses potential side and adverse effects of the therapy with the client and the spouse. After the discussion, the nurse expects the spouse to verbalize that, in case of a suspected adverse effect, which action is the **priority?**
1. Stop the infusion.
2. Contact the nurse.
3. Take the client's blood pressure.
4. Contact the local area emergency response team.

Level of Cognitive Ability: Evaluating
Client Needs: Health Promotion and Maintenance
Clinical Judgment/Cognitive Skills: Evaluate Outcomes
Integrated Process: Clinical Judgment; Teaching and Learning
Content Area: Adult Health: Gastrointestinal
Health Problems: Adult Health: Gastrointestinal: Nutrition/Malabsorption Problems
Priority Concepts: Patient Education; Safety

Answer: 1
Rationale: Signs/symptoms of an adverse effect to lipids (fat emulsion) include chest and back pain, chills, vertigo, cyanosis, diaphoresis, dyspnea, fever, flushing, headache, nausea and vomiting, pressure over the eyes, and thrombophlebitis of the vein. The priority action is to stop the infusion to limit the adverse response. Although contacting the nurse, taking the client's blood pressure, and contacting the local emergency response team are correct interventions, the priority is to stop the infusion.
Test-Taking Strategy: Note the strategic word, *priority*. Remembering that the priority action if an adverse effect occurs when fat emulsion is infusing is to stop the infusion will direct you to the correct option.
Priority Nursing Tip: Usually a 1.2-mm filter or larger is used when administering lipids (fat emulsion).
Reference: Gahart, B., Nazareno, A., & Ortega, M. (2021). *Gahart's 2021 Intravenous medications: A handbook for nurses and health professionals* (37th ed., p. 608). Elsevier.

113. The home care nurse suspects that a client's spouse is experiencing caregiver strain. Which action would the nurse take to assess for this condition?
1. Referring the family to a social services agency
2. Gathering data from the caregiver and the client
3. Waiting for the caregiver to talk about the stress
4. Obtaining feedback from the client about the caregiver

Level of Cognitive Ability: Applying
Client Needs: Health Promotion and Maintenance
Clinical Judgment/Cognitive Skills: Take Action
Integrated Process: Caring
Content Area: Mental Health
Health Problems: Mental Health: Coping
Priority Concepts: Caregiving; Coping

Answer: 2
Rationale: Caregiver strain can occur when a client is significantly dependent on the caregiver for personal and health care needs. The nurse gathers data from the client and the caregiver to determine the caregiver's stressors and coping abilities and withholds making any referrals until the assessment is complete and the plan of care is in place. Because the nurse suspects caregiver strain, the nurse fulfills the duty to the client and family by approaching the family with the concern, gathering assessment data, and planning care. The nurse would not expect the client to assess the coping abilities of the caregiver.
Test-Taking Strategy: Use the steps of the nursing process to eliminate options 1 and 4. From the remaining options, eliminate option 3 because it breaches the duty that the nurse owes to the family; however, the nurse begins to fulfill that duty by performing a comprehensive assessment that addresses both the client and the caregiver.
Priority Nursing Tip: The nurse needs to ensure that the client and family are familiar with the appropriate and available support services in the community.
Reference: Potter, P., et al. (2023). *Fundamentals of nursing* (11th ed., p. 134). Elsevier.

114. A client being discharged from the hospital will be taking warfarin sodium at home on a daily basis. The nurse has provided instructions to the client about the medication and determines that **further teaching is needed** if the client makes which statement?
1. "I need to have a prothrombin time checked in 2 weeks."
2. "This medicine thins my blood and allows me to clot more slowly."
3. "I need to increase the intake of foods high in vitamin K in my diet."
4. "If I notice any increased bleeding or bruising, I need to call my doctor."

Level of Cognitive Ability: Evaluating
Client Needs: Health Promotion and Maintenance
Clinical Judgment/Cognitive Skills: Evaluate Outcomes
Integrated Process: Clinical Judgment; Nursing Process/Evaluation
Content Area: Pharmacology: Cardiovascular: Anticoagulants
Health Problems: Adult Health: Hematologic: Bleeding/Clotting Disorders
Priority Concepts: Clotting; Safety

Answer: 3
Rationale: Warfarin sodium is an oral anticoagulant that is used mainly to prevent thrombotic events, such as thrombophlebitis, pulmonary embolism, and embolism formation caused by atrial fibrillation or other disorders. Oral anticoagulants prolong the clotting time and are monitored by the prothrombin time and the international normalized ratio (INR). Client education needs to include signs and symptoms of adverse effects and dietary limitations such as limiting foods high in vitamin K (e.g., leafy green vegetables, liver, cheese, egg yolks) as prescribed because these increase clotting times.
Test-Taking Strategy: Note the strategic words, *further teaching is needed*. These words indicate a negative event query and ask you to select an option that is an incorrect statement. Recalling that warfarin sodium is an anticoagulant will assist you in eliminating evaluating prothrombin time, recognizing clotting changes, and identifying additional bruising or bleeding. Also, remembering the role that vitamin K plays in the clotting mechanism will direct you to the option that will need further teaching.
Priority Nursing Tip: The INR is used to monitor warfarin therapy. The normal INR is 1.3 to 2.0. An INR of 2 to 3 is appropriate for most clients, although for some clients the target INR is 3 to 4.5.
Reference: Ignatavicius, D., et al. (2021). *Medical-surgical nursing: Concepts for interprofessional collaborative care* (10th ed., p. 726). Elsevier.

115. A teenager returns to the gynecologic clinic for a follow-up visit for a sexually transmitted infection (STI). Which statement by the teenager indicates the **need for further teaching?**
1. "I know you won't tell my parents I'm sick."
2. "I finished all of the antibiotics, just like you said."
3. "I always make sure that my partner uses a condom."
4. "My partner doesn't have to come in for treatment, right?"

Level of Cognitive Ability: Evaluating
Client Needs: Health Promotion and Maintenance
Clinical Judgment/Cognitive Skills: Evaluate Outcomes
Integrated Process: Clinical Judgment; Nursing Process/Evaluation
Content Area: Foundations of Care: Infection Control
Health Problems: Adult Health: Reproductive: Inflammatory/Infectious Problems
Priority Concepts: Infection; Sexuality

Answer: 4
Rationale: When STIs are treated, all of the client's sexual contacts must be contacted and treated with medication. The treatment of a teenager for an STI is confidential, and parents will not be contacted, even if the client is less than 18 years old. Clients need to always finish the course of antibiotics prescribed by the primary health care provider. Clients should always use a condom with any sexual contact.
Test-Taking Strategy: Note the strategic words, *need for further teaching.* These words indicate a negative event query and ask you to select an option that is an incorrect statement. Recalling the concepts related to safe sex, the treatment of STIs in the teenager, and the principles related to antibiotic therapy will direct you to the correct option.
Priority Nursing Tip: Normally parental or guardian consent is needed before providing treatment to an adolescent. An exception is treatment of a minor for a STI. In this situation, the minor can legally provide consent.
Reference: Ignatavicius, D., et al. (2021). *Medical-surgical nursing: Concepts for interprofessional collaborative care* (10th ed., pp. 1507–1508). Elsevier.

❖ **116.** The nurse is teaching a client who had been newly diagnosed with diabetes mellitus about blood glucose monitoring. With knowledge that the reference range for the blood glucose is 70 to 99 mg/dL (3.9 to 5.5 mmol/L), the nurse would teach the client to report glucose results that consistently exceed which level?
1. 150 mg/dL (8.35 mmol/L)
2. 200 mg/dL (11.14 mmol/L)
3. 250 mg/dL (13.92 mmol/L)
4. 350 mg/dL (19.5 mmol/L)

Level of Cognitive Ability: Applying
Client Needs: Health Promotion and Maintenance
Clinical Judgment/Cognitive Skills: Take Action
Integrated Process: Clinical Judgment; Teaching and Learning
Content Area: Foundations of Care: Diagnostic Tests
Health Problems: Adult Health: Endocrine: Diabetes Mellitus
Priority Concepts: Patient Education; Glucose Regulation

Answer: 3
Rationale: The reference range for the blood glucose is 70 to 99 mg/dL (3.9 to 5.5 mmol/L), or as designated and preferred by the primary health care provider. The client with diabetes mellitus needs to be taught to report blood glucose levels that exceed 250 mg/dL (13.92 mmol/L), unless otherwise instructed by the primary health care provider. Options 1 and 2 are high levels but do not require primary health care provider notification. Option 4 is a high value; the client needs to report an elevated level before it reaches this point.
Test-Taking Strategy: Note the subject, the glucose level that needs to be reported in a client with diabetes mellitus. Recalling the basic principles related to diabetic home care instructions for a client with diabetes mellitus will direct you to the correct option.
Priority Nursing Tip: Self-monitoring of the blood glucose level for the client diagnosed with diabetes mellitus provides the client with current information about the level and information that will assist in maintaining good glycemic control.
Reference: Ignatavicius, D., et al. (2021). *Medical-surgical nursing: Concepts for interprofessional collaborative care* (10th ed., p. 1267). Elsevier.

117. A client diagnosed with gastritis asks the nurse at a screening clinic about analgesics that will not cause epigastric distress. The nurse would tell the client to take which medication?
1. Aspirin
2. Naproxen
3. Ibuprofen
4. Acetaminophen

Level of Cognitive Ability: Applying
Client Needs: Health Promotion and Maintenance
Clinical Judgment/Cognitive Skills: Take Action
Integrated Process: Teaching and Learning
Content Area: Adult Health: Gastrointestinal
Health Problems: Adult Health: Gastrointestinal: Gastritis/Gastroenteritis
Priority Concepts: Patient Education; Safety

Answer: 4
Rationale: The client needs to be advised to take analgesics that do not contain aspirin, such as acetaminophen. Aspirin is irritating to the gastrointestinal tract of the client with a history of gastritis. Other medications that are irritating to the gastrointestinal tract are the nonsteroidal antiinflammatory drugs naproxen and ibuprofen.
Test-Taking Strategy: Focus on the **subject**, an analgesic that does not cause gastrointestinal bleeding and distress. Eliminate aspirin, naproxen, and ibuprofen because they are very irritating to the stomach lining.
Priority Nursing Tip: The client with gastritis needs to avoid irritating foods, fluids, and other substances, such as spicy and highly seasoned foods, caffeine, alcohol, and nicotine.
Reference: Lewis, S., et al. (2020). *Medical-surgical nursing: Assessment and management of clinical problems* (11th ed., pp. 916–917, 920). Elsevier.

118. A client is diagnosed with thromboangiitis obliterans (Buerger's disease). The nurse places **priority** on teaching the client about modifications of which risk factor related to this disorder?
1. Exposure to heat
2. Cigarette smoking
3. Diet low in vitamin C
4. Excessive water intake

Level of Cognitive Ability: Applying
Client Needs: Health Promotion and Maintenance
Clinical Judgment/Cognitive Skills: Prioritize Hypotheses
Integrated Process: Clinical Judgment; Teaching and Learning
Content Area: Adult Health: Cardiovascular
Health Problems: Adult Health: Cardiovascular: Vascular Disorders
Priority Concepts: Patient Education; Perfusion

Answer: 2
Rationale: Buerger's disease is an occlusive disease of the median small arteries and veins. It occurs predominantly among those who are more than 40 years old who smoke cigarettes. A familial tendency is noted, but cigarette smoking is consistently a risk factor. Symptoms of the disease improve with smoking cessation. Exposure to heat, diet low in vitamin C, and excessive water intake are not risk factors.
Test-Taking Strategy: Note the **strategic word**, *priority*. Recalling the pathophysiology related to this disorder and that it is an occlusive disease of the median small arteries and veins will direct you to the correct option.
Priority Nursing Tip: The client with Buerger's disease is at risk for the development of ulcerations in the extremities.
Reference: Ignatavicius, D., et al. (2021). *Medical-surgical nursing: Concepts for interprofessional collaborative care* (10th ed., p. 720). Elsevier.

119. A client has a new prescription for timolol, and the nurse provides medication instructions to the client. Which statement by the client indicates a **need for further teaching** regarding the instructions?

1. "I need to change positions slowly."
2. "I need to report shortness of breath to the doctor."
3. "I need to taper or discontinue the medication when I feel well."
4. "I have enough medication on hand to last through weekends and vacations."

Level of Cognitive Ability: Evaluating
Client Needs: Health Promotion and Maintenance
Clinical Judgment/Cognitive Skills: Evaluate Outcomes
Integrated Process: Clinical Judgment; Nursing Process/Evaluation
Content Area: Pharmacology: Cardiovascular: Beta Blockers
Health Problems: Adult Health: Eye: Glaucoma
Priority Concepts: Patient Education; Safety

Answer: 3
Rationale: Timolol is a beta-adrenergic blocking agent. The client would not discontinue or change the medication dose. Common client teaching points about beta-adrenergic blocking agents include taking the pulse daily, holding it if the rate is less than 60 beats/min (and notifying the physician); changing positions slowly; and reporting shortness of breath. The client is also instructed to keep enough medication on hand, not take over-the-counter medications (especially decongestants, cough, and cold preparations) without consulting the physician, and carry medical identification that states that a beta blocker is being taken.
Test-Taking Strategy: Note the strategic words, *need for further teaching*. These words indicate a negative event query and ask you to select an option that is an incorrect statement. Noting the word *discontinue* will direct you to this option.
Priority Nursing Tip: Monitor the client taking a beta blocker for signs/symptoms of respiratory distress because these medications can cause bronchospasm.
Reference: Skidmore-Roth, L. (2021). *2021 Mosby's Nursing drug reference* (34th ed., pp. 1224–1225). Elsevier.

❖ **120.** The nurse has completed giving medication instructions to a client receiving benazepril to treat hypertension. Which statement made by the client indicates to the nurse that the client **needs further teaching**?

1. "I need to change positions slowly."
2. "I need to monitor my blood pressure every week."
3. "I need to use salt moderately in cooking and on foods."
4. "I need to report signs and symptoms of infection to my doctor."

Level of Cognitive Ability: Evaluating
Client Needs: Health Promotion and Maintenance
Clinical Judgment/Cognitive Skills: Evaluate Outcomes
Integrated Process: Clinical Judgment; Nursing Process/Evaluation
Content Area: Pharmacology: Cardiovascular: Angiotensin-Converting Enzyme (ACE) Inhibitors
Health Problems: Adult Health: Cardiovascular: Hypertension
Priority Concepts: Patient Education; Safety

Answer: 3
Rationale: Benazepril is an angiotensin-converting enzyme (ACE) inhibitor. The client taking an ACE inhibitor is instructed to avoid the use of salt. The medication needs to be taken exactly as prescribed. The client needs to change positions slowly to avoid orthostatic hypotension, monitor the blood pressure weekly, and continue with other lifestyle changes to control hypertension. The client needs to report fever, mouth sores, and sore throats to the primary health care provider (neutropenia).
Test-Taking Strategy: Note the strategic words, *needs further teaching*. These words indicate a negative event query and ask you to select an option that is an incorrect statement. Noting that the medication is prescribed to treat hypertension will assist you in eliminating changing positions slowly, monitoring blood pressure weekly, and reporting signs/symptoms of infection.
Priority Nursing Tip: Hyperkalemia is a side effect/adverse effect of an ACE inhibitor. Therefore, the client taking an ACE inhibitor would avoid the use of potassium supplements and would not take potassium-sparing diuretics when taking an ACE inhibitor.
Reference: Ignatavicius, D., et al. (2021). *Medical-surgical nursing: Concepts for interprofessional collaborative care* (10th ed., pp. 702–703). Elsevier.

121. The nurse has given medication instructions to a client receiving lovastatin. The nurse determines that the client understands the effects of the medication if the client stated the need to adhere to the periodic evaluation of which laboratory test?
1. Bleeding times
2. Creatinine levels
3. Blood glucose levels
4. Liver function studies

Level of Cognitive Ability: Evaluating
Client Needs: Health Promotion and Maintenance
Clinical Judgment/Cognitive Skills: Evaluate Outcomes
Integrated Process: Nursing Process/Evaluation
Content Area: Pharmacology: Cardiovascular: Antilipemics
Health Problems: Adult Health: Cardiovascular: Coronary Artery Disease
Priority Concepts: Patient Education; Safety

Answer: 4
Rationale: Lovastatin is an HMG-CoA reductase inhibitor used to treat hyperlipidemia. It results in an increase in high-density lipoprotein cholesterol and a decrease in triglycerides and low-density lipoprotein cholesterol. This medication is converted by the liver to active metabolites and therefore is not used in clients with active hepatic disease or elevated transaminase levels. For this reason, it is recommended that clients have periodic liver function studies. Periodic cholesterol levels are also needed to monitor the effectiveness of therapy.
Test-Taking Strategy: Focus on the subject, a client taking lovastatin. Recalling that medication names that end with the letters "-statin" are cholesterol-lowering medications and that cholesterol is synthesized in the liver will direct you to the correct option.
Priority Nursing Tip: Instruct the client taking an antilipemic medication to report any unexplained muscular pain to the primary health care provider.
Reference: Lewis, S., et al. (2020). *Medical-surgical nursing: Assessment and management of clinical problems* (11th ed., p. 707). Elsevier.

122. Clonazepam has been prescribed for the client, and the nurse teaches the client about the medication. Which statement by the client indicates **a need for further teaching**?
1. "If I experience slurred speech, it will disappear in about 8 weeks."
2. "My drowsiness will decrease over time with continued treatment."
3. "I need to take my medicine with food to decrease stomach problems."
4. "I can take my medicine at bedtime if it tends to make me feel drowsy."

Level of Cognitive Ability: Evaluating
Client Needs: Health Promotion and Maintenance
Clinical Judgment/Cognitive Skills: Evaluate Outcomes
Integrated Process: Clinical Judgment; Nursing Process/Evaluation
Content Area: Pharmacology: Psychotherapeutics: Barbiturates and Sedative-Hypnotics
Health Problems: N/A
Priority Concepts: Patient Education; Safety

Answer: 1
Rationale: Clonazepam is a benzodiazepine. Clients who experience signs/symptoms of toxicity with the administration of clonazepam exhibit slurred speech, sedation, confusion, respiratory depression, hypotension, and eventually coma. Some drowsiness may occur, but it will decrease with continued use. The medication may be taken with food to decrease gastrointestinal irritation. The medication may be taken at bedtime if drowsiness does occur. Options 2, 3, and 4 are correct and show an accurate understanding of the medication.
Test-Taking Strategy: Note the strategic words, *a need for further teaching*. These words indicate a negative event query and ask you to select an incorrect statement. Recalling the toxic effects that can occur with the use of this medication will direct you to the correct option. Remember that slurred speech indicates toxicity.
Priority Nursing Tip: Benzodiazepines have anxiety-reducing, sedative-hypnotic, muscle-relaxing, and anticonvulsant actions.
Reference: Kizior, R., & Hodgson, B. (2023). *Saunders Nursing drug handbook 2023* (pp. 252–253). Elsevier.

123. Dipyridamole has been prescribed for the client who underwent a valve replacement, and the nurse has provided teaching to the client about the medication. Which statement indicates that the client understands the medication instructions?
1. "This medication will prevent a stroke."
2. "This medication will prevent a heart attack."
3. "This medicine will protect my artificial heart valve."
4. "This medication will help me keep my blood pressure down."

Level of Cognitive Ability: Evaluating
Client Needs: Health Promotion and Maintenance
Clinical Judgment/Cognitive Skills: Evaluate Outcomes
Integrated Process: Clinical Judgment; Nursing Process/Evaluation
Content Area: Pharmacology: Cardiovascular: Antiplatelets
Health Problems: Adult Health: Cardiovascular: Vascular Disorders
Priority Concepts: Patient Education; Safety

Answer: 3
Rationale: Dipyridamole is an antiplatelet medication. It may be administered in combination with warfarin sodium to protect the client's artificial heart valves. Dipyridamole does not prevent stroke or heart attacks. It is an antiplatelet medication rather than an antihypertensive.
Test-Taking Strategy: Focus on the **subject**, client instructions about dipyridamole. Recalling that this medication is an antiplatelet medication rather than an antihypertensive will assist you in eliminating reducing blood pressure as a correct response. Noting the word *prevent* in the stroke and heart attack choices will assist you in eliminating these options.
Priority Nursing Tip: Antiplatelet medications prolong the bleeding time and are contraindicated in those with bleeding disorders.
Reference: Lilley, L., Rainforth Collins, S., & Snyder J. (2020). *Pharmacology and the nursing process* (9th ed., p. 123). Elsevier.

❖ **124.** The nurse is preparing to care for the birthing parent of a preterm infant. When would the nurse plan to begin discharge planning?
1. When the discharge date is set
2. When the birthing parent is in labor
3. After stabilization of the infant during the early stages of hospitalization
4. When the parents feel comfortable with and can demonstrate adequate care of the infant

Level of Cognitive Ability: Applying
Client Needs: Health Promotion and Maintenance
Clinical Judgment/Cognitive Skills: Generate Solutions
Integrated Process: Clinical Judgment; Nursing Process/Planning
Content Area: Maternity: Newborn
Health Problems: Newborn: Preterm and Postterm Newborn
Priority Concepts: Clinical Judgment; Collaboration

Answer: 3
Rationale: Discharge planning begins at admission of the preterm infant. The determination of the services, needs, supplies, and equipment requirements should not be made on the day of discharge. Beginning planning during labor is incorrect because the outcome of the delivery is not known. At discharge or when the parents feel comfortable caring for their infant are incorrect because these times are much too late to make the plans that need to be made.
Test-Taking Strategy: Note the **subject**, discharge planning for the birthing parent of a preterm infant. Remember that discharge planning always begins at admission to the hospital. Noting the words *early stages of hospitalization* will direct you to the correct option.
Priority Nursing Tip: A case manager is the nurse who assumes responsibility for coordinating the client's care at admission and after discharge.
Reference: McKinney, E. S., et al. (2022). *Maternal child nursing* (6th ed., pp. 425, 625). Elsevier.

125. The nurse is providing home care instructions to a client recovering from an acute inferior myocardial infarction (MI) with recurrent angina. What instruction would the nurse provide to this client?
   1. Avoid sexual intercourse for at least 4 months.
   2. Replace sublingual nitroglycerin tablets yearly.
   3. Participate in an exercise program that includes overhead lifting and reaching.
   4. Recognize the adverse effects of acetylsalicylic acid (aspirin), which include tinnitus and hearing loss.

Level of Cognitive Ability: Applying
Client Needs: Health Promotion and Maintenance
Clinical Judgment/Cognitive Skills: Take Action
Integrated Process: Teaching and Learning
Content Area: Adult Health: Cardiovascular
Health Problems: Adult Health: Cardiovascular: Myocardial Infarction
Priority Concepts: Patient Education; Safety

Answer: 4
Rationale: After an acute MI, many clients are instructed to take an aspirin daily. Adverse effects include tinnitus, hearing loss, epigastric distress, gastrointestinal bleeding, and nausea. Sexual intercourse usually can be resumed in 4 to 8 weeks after an acute MI if the primary health care provider agrees and if the client has been able to achieve traditional parameters such as climbing two flights of steps without chest pain or dyspnea. Clients need to be advised to purchase a new supply of nitroglycerin tablets every 6 months. Expiration dates on the medication bottle also need to be checked. Activities that include lifting and reaching over the head should be avoided because they reduce cardiac output.
Test-Taking Strategy: Focus on the subject, a client recovering from an acute inferior MI with recurrent angina. Noting the time limits in options 1 and 2 ("4 months" and "yearly," respectively) will assist you in eliminating these options. From the remaining options, "overhead lifting and reaching" in option 3 indicates that this is incorrect.
Priority Nursing Tip: Acetylsalicylic acid (aspirin) is an antiplatelet medication that inhibits the aggregation of platelets in the clotting process, thereby prolonging the bleeding time.
Reference: Ignatavicius, D., et al. (2021). *Medical-surgical nursing: Concepts for interprofessional collaborative care* (10th ed., p. 772). Elsevier.

❖ **126.** The nurse is reviewing home care instructions with a client who has been diagnosed with type 1 diabetes mellitus and has a history of diabetic ketoacidosis (DKA). The client's spouse is present when the instructions are given. Which statement by the spouse indicates that there is **a need for further teaching?**
   1. "If my spouse is vomiting, I shouldn't give any insulin."
   2. "I need to bring my spouse to the doctor if a fever develops."
   3. "If our grandchildren are sick, they probably shouldn't come to visit."
   4. "I need to call the doctor if my spouse has nausea or abdominal pain lasting for more than 1 or 2 days."

Level of Cognitive Ability: Evaluating
Client Needs: Health Promotion and Maintenance
Clinical Judgment/Cognitive Skills: Evaluate Outcomes
Integrated Process: Clinical Judgment; Nursing Process/Evaluation
Content Area: Adult Health: Endocrine
Health Problems: Adult Health: Endocrine: Diabetes Mellitus
Priority Concepts: Patient Education; Glucose Regulation

Answer: 1
Rationale: DKA is a life-threatening complication of type 1 diabetes mellitus that develops when a severe insulin deficiency occurs. Infection and the stopping of insulin are precipitating factors for DKA. Nausea and abdominal pain that last more than 1 or 2 days need to be reported to the primary health care provider because these signs/symptoms may be indicative of DKA.
Test-Taking Strategy: Note the strategic words, *a need for further teaching.* These words indicate a negative event query and ask you to select an option that is an incorrect statement. Eliminate options 2 and 3 first because they are comparable or alike in that both relate to infection. From the remaining options, recalling the causes of DKA will direct you to the correct option.
Priority Nursing Tip: Monitor the potassium level closely when the client with DKA receives treatment for dehydration and acidosis because the serum potassium level will decrease and potassium replacement may be required.
Reference: Ignatavicius, D., et al. (2021). *Medical-surgical nursing: Concepts for interprofessional collaborative care* (10th ed., pp. 1290–1292). Elsevier.

127. The nurse is performing an assessment on a primigravida client who has been a marathon runner for several years. The client verbalizes concern because of being no longer able to run in marathons and is concerned about the brown discoloration on the face and increasing size. Which statements by the nurse are therapeutic? **Select all that apply.**

❑ 1. "I can see you're disappointed at not being able to run."

❑ 2. "Tell me how you are feeling about the changes in your body."

❑ 3. "Don't worry. Your body will go back to normal after delivery."

❑ 4. "You need to ask your obstetrician about whether or not you can run."

❑ 5. "Wait and see. You will be back to marathon running after delivery before you know it."

❑ 6. "Some of the changes in pregnancy are permanent and that is the price that you have to pay for that bundle of joy."

Level of Cognitive Ability: Applying
Client Needs: Health Promotion and Maintenance
Clinical Judgment/Cognitive Skills: Take Action
Integrated Process: Communication and Documentation
Content Area: Maternity: Antepartum
Health Problems: Maternity: Discomforts of Pregnancy
Priority Concepts: Communication; Reproduction

Answer: 1, 2
Rationale: The client is concerned about the body changes and life changes being experienced as a result of pregnancy. Therapeutic communication techniques include focusing on the client's feelings and concerns and acknowledging these concerns by the techniques of clarifying and encouraging discussion of feelings. Telling a client "not to worry," placing the client's feelings on hold, and avoiding discussion of the client's feelings are nontherapeutic communication techniques.
Test-Taking Strategy: Read each statement carefully. Knowledge of therapeutic communication techniques will assist in determining the correct nursing statements.
Priority Nursing Tip: Chloasma (mask of pregnancy) is a blotchy brownish hyperpigmentation that occurs over the forehead, cheeks, and nose. It is a normal occurrence during pregnancy.
Reference: McKinney, E. S., et al. (2022). *Maternal child nursing* (6th ed., pp. 27, 225). Elsevier.

❖ **128.** The nurse is performing a socioeconomic assessment on a client. Which questions are appropriate for the nurse to ask? **Select all that apply.**

❑ 1. "What do you do for a living?"

❑ 2. "How much money do you make yearly?"

❑ 3. "Do you have a primary health care provider?"

❑ 4. "How many years of school did you complete?"

❑ 5. "How different is your life here from in your homeland?"

❑ 6. "What type of work did you do back in your homeland?"

Level of Cognitive Ability: Applying
Client Needs: Health Promotion and Maintenance
Clinical Judgment/Cognitive Skills: Recognize Cues
Integrated Process: Clinical Judgment; Nursing Process/Assessment
Content Area: Foundations of Care: Spirituality, Culture, and Ethnicity
Health Problems: N/A
Priority Concepts: Culture; Health Promotion

Answer: 1, 3, 4, 5, 6
Rationale: Aspects to include in a cultural assessment include biocultural history and socioeconomic status (distinct health risks can be attributed to the ecologic and socioeconomic context of the culture) and the client's country of origin. Other aspects to assess include religious and spiritual beliefs (to determine major influences in the client's worldview about health and illness, pain and suffering, and life and death), communication patterns (which reflect core cultural values of a society), time orientation (this information can be useful in planning a day of care, setting up appointments for procedures, and helping a client plan self-care activities in the home), caring beliefs and practices (to identify the central values of a culture), and previous experiences with professional health care (which may have implications for adherence to therapies and continuing access of services). Some specific questions to ask when performing a socioeconomic assessment are noted in the correct options. Asking the client about their early income is inappropriate, unnecessary, and unrelated to health care resources.
Test-Taking Strategy: Focus on the subject, a socioeconomic assessment. Read each assessment question and think about its effect with regard to health risks, health care, and health care resources. This will assist in determining the correct assessment questions.
Priority Nursing Tip: Cultural assessment is a systematic and comprehensive examination of the cultural care values, beliefs, and practices of individuals, families, and communities and is important to the total care of any client.
Reference: Ignatavicius, D., et al. (2021). *Medical-surgical nursing: Concepts for interprofessional collaborative care* (10th ed., p. 123). Elsevier.

129. The nurse is creating a teaching plan for the client diagnosed with Raynaud's disease. Which instruction would the nurse include?
1. Daily cool baths will provide an analgesic effect.
2. A high-protein diet will minimize tissue malnutrition.
3. Vitamin K administration will prevent tendencies toward bleeding.
4. Keeping the hands and feet warm and dry will prevent vasoconstriction.

Level of Cognitive Ability: Creating
Client Needs: Health Promotion and Maintenance
Clinical Judgment/Cognitive Skills: Generate Solutions
Integrated Process: Clinical Judgment; Nursing Process/Planning
Content Area: Adult Health: Cardiovascular
Health Problems: Adult Health: Cardiovascular: Vascular Disorders
Priority Concepts: Patient Education; Perfusion

Answer: 4
Rationale: Raynaud's disease is a vasospasm of the arterioles and arteries of the upper and lower extremities. The use of measures to prevent vasoconstriction is helpful for the management of Raynaud's disease. The hands and feet need to be kept dry. Gloves and warm fabrics need to be worn in cold weather, and the client needs to avoid exposure to nicotine and caffeine. The avoidance of situations that trigger stress is also helpful. Taking daily cool baths, maintaining a high-protein diet, and administering vitamin K are not components of the treatment for this disorder.
Test-Taking Strategy: Focus on the subject, a teaching plan for the client with Raynaud's disease. Recalling the pathophysiology of the disorder and the need to promote vasodilation will direct you to the correct option.
Priority Nursing Tip: The attacks that occur in Raynaud's disease are intermittent, occur with exposure to cold or stress, and primarily affect the fingers, toes, ears, and cheeks.
Reference: Ignatavicius, D., et al. (2021). *Medical-surgical nursing: Concepts for interprofessional collaborative care* (10th ed., p. 720). Elsevier.

❖ **130.** A client with peripheral arterial disease has received instructions from the nurse about how to limit the progression of the disease. The nurse determines that the client **needs further teaching** if which statement was made by the client?
1. "I need to eat a balanced diet."
2. "A heating pad on my leg will help soothe the leg pain."
3. "I need to take special care of my feet to prevent injury."
4. "I should walk daily to increase the circulation to my legs."

Level of Cognitive Ability: Evaluating
Client Needs: Health Promotion and Maintenance
Clinical Judgment/Cognitive Skills: Evaluate Outcomes
Integrated Process: Clinical Judgment; Nursing Process/Evaluation
Content Area: Adult Health: Cardiovascular
Health Problems: Adult Health: Cardiovascular: Vascular Disorders
Priority Concepts: Perfusion; Safety

Answer: 2
Rationale: The application of heat directly to the extremity is contraindicated. The limb may have decreased sensitivity and be more at risk for burns. Additionally, the direct application of heat raises the oxygen and nutritional requirements of the tissue even further. The long-term management of peripheral arterial disease consists of measures that increase peripheral circulation (exercise), promote vasodilation (warmth), relieve pain, and maintain tissue integrity (foot care and nutrition).
Test-Taking Strategy: Focus on the client's diagnosis of peripheral arterial disease, and note the strategic words, *needs further teaching*. These words indicate a negative event query and ask you to select an option that is an incorrect statement. Noting the word *heating* in option 2 will direct you to the correct option.
Priority Nursing Tip: In severe cases of peripheral arterial disease, clients with edema may sleep with the affected limb hanging from the bed or they may sit upright (without leg elevation) in a chair for comfort.
Reference: Ignatavicius, D., et al. (2021). *Medical-surgical nursing: Concepts for interprofessional collaborative care* (10th ed., p. 716). Elsevier.

131. The nurse is teaching a client diagnosed with hypertension about items that contain sodium and reviews a written list of items sent from the cardiac rehabilitation department. The nurse tells the client that which item is lowest in sodium content?
1. Antacids
2. Laxatives
3. Toothpaste
4. Demineralized water

Level of Cognitive Ability: Applying
Client Needs: Health Promotion and Maintenance
Clinical Judgment/Cognitive Skills: Take Action
Integrated Process: Teaching and Learning
Content Area: Adult Health: Cardiovascular
Health Problems: Adult Health: Cardiovascular: Hypertension
Priority Concepts: Patient Education; Health Promotion

Answer: 4
Rationale: Water that is bottled, distilled, deionized, or demineralized may be used for drinking and cooking. Clients are advised to read labels for sodium content. Sodium intake can be increased with the use of several types of products, including toothpaste and mouthwashes; over-the-counter medications such as analgesics, antacids, cough remedies, laxatives, and sedatives; and softened water, as well as some mineral waters.
Test-Taking Strategy: Focus on the subject, the item that is lowest in sodium. Noting the word *demineralized,* which means having the minerals taken out of, will direct you to option 4.
Priority Nursing Tip: The laboratory reference range for sodium is 135 to 145 mEq (135 to 145 mmol/L). A sodium imbalance is usually associated with a fluid volume imbalance.
References: Lewis, S., et al. (2020). *Medical-surgical nursing: Assessment and management of clinical problems* (11th ed., pp. 691–693). Elsevier; Nix, S. (2022). *Williams' Basic nutrition and diet therapy* (16th ed., pp. 358–360). Elsevier.

❖ **132.** The school nurse provides teaching about the hazards of smoking to a group of high school students. Which comment by a student indicates the **need for further teaching?**
1. "Chewing tobacco is much safer than is smoking tobacco."
2. "Smoking during pregnancy increases the risk of stillbirth."
3. "My health is at risk when my family smokes in the house."
4. "Inhaling smoke from other people is a public health issue."

Level of Cognitive Ability: Evaluating
Client Needs: Health Promotion and Maintenance
Clinical Judgment/Cognitive Skills: Evaluate Outcomes
Integrated Process: Clinical Judgment; Nursing Process/Evaluation
Content Area: Foundations of Care: Community/Public/Population Health
Health Problems: N/A
Priority Concepts: Patient Education; Health Promotion

Answer: 1
Rationale: All forms of tobacco use, including chewing tobacco, are health hazards. Smoking during pregnancy, smoking in a household, and second-hand smoke all present health hazards of tobacco use.
Test-Taking Strategy: Note the strategic words, *need for further teaching.* These words indicate a negative event query and ask you to select an option that is an incorrect statement. This will direct you to the correct option that chewing tobacco is not any safer than smoking.
Priority Nursing Tip: Cigarette smoking and exposure to passive smoke are causes of lung cancer.
Reference: Lewis, S., et al. (2020). *Medical-surgical nursing: Assessment and management of clinical problems* (11th ed., pp. 143–144). Elsevier.

133. The nurse is developing goals for the postpartum client who is at risk for uterine infection. Which goal is **most appropriate** for this client?
1. Client will verbalize a reduction of pain.
2. Client will report how to treat an infection.
3. Client will be able to identify measures to prevent infection.
4. Client will identify the presence of Braxton Hicks contractions.

Level of Cognitive Ability: Analyzing
Client Needs: Health Promotion and Maintenance
Clinical Judgment/Cognitive Skills: Generate Solutions
Integrated Process: Clinical Judgment; Nursing Process/Planning
Content Area: Maternity: Postpartum
Health Problems: Maternity: Infections/Inflammations
Priority Concepts: Infection; Reproduction

Answer: 3
Rationale: The uterus is theoretically sterile during pregnancy until the membranes rupture. However, it is capable of being invaded by pathogens after membrane rupture. The reduction of pain and Braxton Hicks contractions that occur during pregnancy are unrelated to the subject of infection. Reporting the treatment of infection indicates that an infection is present. Preventing an infection is a goal for the client who is at risk for infection.
Test-Taking Strategy: Focus on the strategic words, *most appropriate,* and focus on the subject, a client at risk for uterine infection. Reduction of pain and Braxton Hicks contractions are unrelated to the subject of the question. Reporting how to treat an infection implies that an infection has been diagnosed. Noting the word *prevent* in option 3 will direct you to this option.
Priority Nursing Tip: In the postpartum client, a temperature of 100.4° F (38° C) or greater after 24 hours postpartum indicates infection.
Reference: McKinney, E. S., et al. (2022). *Maternal child nursing* (6th ed., pp. 618–619). Elsevier.

❖ **134.** A nurse working in the neonatal intensive care unit (NICU) teaches handwashing techniques to the parents of an infant who is receiving antibiotic treatment for a neonatal infection. The nurse determines that the parents understand the **primary** purpose of handwashing if which statement is made?
1. "It is primarily done to reduce their fears."
2. "It is primarily done to minimize the spread of infection to other siblings."
3. "It is primarily done to allow them an opportunity to communicate with each other and staff."
4. "It is primarily done to reduce the possibility of transmitting an environmental infection to the infant."

Level of Cognitive Ability: Evaluating
Client Needs: Health Promotion and Maintenance
Clinical Judgment/Cognitive Skills: Evaluate Outcomes
Integrated Process: Clinical Judgment; Nursing Process/Evaluation
Content Area: Foundations of Care: Infection Control
Health Problems: Newborn: Infections
Priority Concepts: Patient Education; Infection

Answer: 4
Rationale: Appropriate handwashing by staff and parents has been effective for the prevention of nosocomial infections in nursery units. This action also promotes parents taking an active part in the care of their infant. Reducing fears and encouraging communication are not the primary reasons to perform handwashing. Because the infant already has an infection and is in the NICU, transference to siblings is not the best choice.
Test-Taking Strategy: Note the strategic word, *primary,* to assist you in eliminating reducing fear and promoting communication. Noting that the infant is in the NICU will assist you in eliminating transference of the infection to siblings.
Priority Nursing Tip: Handwashing is the first line of defense against the spread of microorganisms.
Reference: McKinney, E. S., et al. (2022). *Maternal child nursing* (6th ed., p. 827). Elsevier.

135. The nurse monitors a client for brachial plexus compromise after shoulder arthroplasty and is checking the status of the ulnar nerve. Which technique would the nurse use to assess the status of this nerve?
1. Ask the client to raise the forearm above the head.
2. Have the client spread all of the fingers wide and resist pressure.
3. Ask the client to move the thumb toward the palm and then back to the neutral position.
4. Have the client grasp the nurse's hand, and note the strength of client's first and second fingers.

Level of Cognitive Ability: Applying
Client Needs: Health Promotion and Maintenance
Clinical Judgment/Cognitive Skills: Recognize Cues
Integrated Process: Clinical Judgment; Nursing Process/Assessment
Content Area: Health Assessment/Physical Exam: Neurologic
Health Problems: Adult Health: Musculoskeletal: Skeletal Injury
Priority Concepts: Clinical Judgment; Health Promotion

Answer: 2
Rationale: So that the nurse may assess the ulnar nerve status, the client is asked to spread all of the fingers wide and resist pressure. Weakness against pressure may indicate compromise of the ulnar nerve. Raising the forearm above the head assesses the flexion of the biceps and determines the status of the cutaneous nerve. Moving the thumb toward the palm and back describes the assessment of the status of the radial nerve. Having the client grasp the nurse's hand and assessing the strength of the first two fingers describes the assessment of the status of the medial nerve.
Test-Taking Strategy: Focus on the subject, assessing the status of the ulnar nerve. Recalling the location and function of this nerve will direct you to the correct answer.
Priority Nursing Tip: The ulnar nerve splits from the medial cord in the shoulder and descends along the medial aspect of the arm and along the forearm. It then enters the hand. The ulnar nerve is also responsible for the sensation that one feels when they "hit the funny bone," squashing the nerve.
Reference: Heuther, S., McCance, K., & Brashers, V. (2020). *Understanding pathophysiology* (7th ed., p. 317). Elsevier.

❖ **136.** A hospitalized client diagnosed with active pulmonary tuberculosis has been receiving multidrug therapy for the past month and is being prepared for discharge. Which finding indicates that respiratory isolation is no longer required and that medication therapy has been **effective**?
1. Stools are clay colored.
2. Sputum cultures are negative.
3. Tuberculin skin test is negative.
4. Nausea and vomiting have stopped.

Level of Cognitive Ability: Evaluating
Client Needs: Health Promotion and Maintenance
Clinical Judgment/Cognitive Skills: Evaluate Outcomes
Integrated Process: Clinical Judgment; Nursing Process/Evaluation
Content Area: Foundations of Care: Infection Control
Health Problems: Adult Health: Respiratory: Tuberculosis
Priority Concepts: Clinical Judgment; Infection

Answer: 2
Rationale: The primary laboratory test for pulmonary tuberculosis is a sputum culture. A negative culture indicates the effectiveness of treatment. Clay-colored stools, nausea, and vomiting are side effects of the medication that is used to treat tuberculosis; their presence or absence does not measure the therapeutic effectiveness of the medication. The tuberculin skin test is a screening tool rather than a diagnostic test for tuberculosis. Because the tuberculin skin test indicates exposure to the organism but not active disease, the test results will remain positive.
Test-Taking Strategy: Note the strategic word, *effective.* Remember that the absence of infectious organisms is a desired outcome in clients with communicable diseases. The sputum is the only laboratory test that will determine the absence of infectious organisms.
Priority Nursing Tip: Tuberculosis has an insidious onset, and many clients are not aware of signs/symptoms until the disease is well advanced.
Reference: Ignatavicius, D., et al. (2021). *Medical-surgical nursing: Concepts for interprofessional collaborative care* (10th ed., p. 578). Elsevier.

137. The nurse has conducted a class for pregnant clients diagnosed with diabetes mellitus about the signs/symptoms of potential complications. The nurse determines that the teaching was **effective** if a client makes which statement?

1. "I won't have any ultrasounds done because I am diabetic."
2. "I'm glad I don't have to worry about developing hypoglycemia while I am pregnant."
3. "I need to watch my weight for any sudden gains because I could develop what they call gestational hypertension."
4. "My insulin needs will decrease during the last 2 months because I will be using some of the baby's insulin supply."

Level of Cognitive Ability: Evaluating
Client Needs: Health Promotion and Maintenance
Clinical Judgment/Cognitive Skills: Evaluate Outcomes
Integrated Process: Clinical Judgment; Nursing Process/Evaluation
Content Area: Maternity: Antepartum
Health Problems: Maternity: Diabetes Mellitus
Priority Concepts: Glucose Regulation; Reproduction

Answer: 3
Rationale: A pregnant client with diabetes has a higher incidence of developing gestational hypertension than a pregnant client without diabetes does. Ultrasounds are done frequently during a diabetic pregnancy to check for congenital anomalies and to determine appropriate growth patterns. Hypoglycemia is a problem during pregnancy in the client diagnosed with diabetes mellitus and needs to be assessed throughout the pregnancy. Insulin needs will increase during the last trimester because of increased hormone levels that destroy circulating insulin.
Test-Taking Strategy: Note the strategic word, *effective*. Focus on the subject, a pregnant client diagnosed with diabetes mellitus. Ultrasounds will be done to monitor a pregnant client diagnosed with diabetes mellitus, and blood glucose levels will be monitored for the presence of hypoglycemia. From the remaining options, remember that insulin needs will increase during the last trimester of pregnancy. This will assist you in eliminating option 4.
Priority Nursing Tip: Oral hypoglycemics are not usually prescribed for use during pregnancy.
Reference: McKinney, E. S., et al. (2022). *Maternal child nursing* (6th ed., p. 561). Elsevier.

❖ **138.** A postpartum client recovering from disseminated intravascular coagulopathy is to be discharged on low dosages of an anticoagulant medication. What action would the nurse encourage the client to avoid?

1. Brushing the teeth
2. Taking acetylsalicylic acid (aspirin)
3. Walking long distances and climbing stairs
4. All activities because bruising injuries can occur

Level of Cognitive Ability: Applying
Client Needs: Health Promotion and Maintenance
Clinical Judgment/Cognitive Skills: Take Action
Integrated Process: Clinical Judgment; Nursing Process/Implementation
Content Area: Pharmacology: Cardiovascular: Anticoagulants
Health Problems: Maternity: Disseminated Intravascular Coagulation
Priority Concepts: Patient Education; Clotting

Answer: 2
Rationale: Aspirin is an antiplatelet medication and can interact with the anticoagulant medication and increase the clotting time beyond therapeutic ranges, so avoiding aspirin is a priority. The client does not need to avoid brushing the teeth but needs to be instructed to use a soft toothbrush. Walking and climbing stairs are acceptable activities. Not all activities need to be avoided.
Test-Taking Strategy: Note the subject, a client recovering from disseminated intravascular coagulopathy. Also, note the word *avoid* in the question. This word indicates the need to select the harmful activity for the client. Recalling that bleeding is an adverse effect of anticoagulants will direct you to the correct option.
Priority Nursing Tip: Disseminated intravascular coagulopathy is a maternal condition in which the clotting cascade is activated, resulting in the formation of clots in the microcirculation.
References: Lowdermilk, D., et al. (2020). *Maternity & women's health care* (12th ed., pp. 728–730). Elsevier; McKinney, E. S., et al. (2022). *Maternal child nursing* (6th ed., pp. 566, 1144). Elsevier.

139. The nurse teaches a client at risk for coronary artery disease about lifestyle changes needed to reduce known risks. The nurse determines that the client understands these necessary lifestyle changes if the client makes which statements? **Select all that apply.**
   ❑ 1. "I will attempt to stop smoking."
   ❑ 2. "I will be sure to include some exercise such as walking in my daily activities."
   ❑ 3. "I will work at losing some weight so that my weight is at normal range for my age."
   ❑ 4. "I will limit my sodium intake every day and avoid eating high-sodium foods such as hot dogs."
   ❑ 5. "I will schedule regular doctor appointments for physical examinations and monitoring my blood pressure."
   ❑ 6. "It is acceptable to eat red meat and cheese every day as I have been doing, as long as I cut down on the butter."

Level of Cognitive Ability: Evaluating
Client Needs: Health Promotion and Maintenance
Clinical Judgment/Cognitive Skills: Evaluate Outcomes
Integrated Process: Clinical Judgment; Nursing Process/Evaluation
Content Area: Adult Health: Cardiovascular
Health Problems: Adult Health: Cardiovascular: Coronary Artery Disease
Priority Concepts: Patient Education; Health Promotion

Answer: 2, 3, 4, 5
Rationale: Coronary artery disease affects the arteries that provide blood, oxygen, and nutrients to the myocardium. Modifiable risk factors include elevated serum cholesterol levels, cigarette smoking, hypertension, impaired glucose tolerance, obesity, physical inactivity, and stress. The client is instructed to stop smoking (not cut down), and the nurse would provide the client with resources to do so. The client is also instructed to maintain a normal weight and include physical activity in the daily schedule. The client needs to limit sodium intake and foods high in cholesterol, including red meat and cheese. The client must follow up with regular primary health care provider appointments for physical examinations and monitoring blood pressure.
Test-Taking Strategy: Focus on the subject, lifestyle changes to reduce the risk of coronary artery disease. Think about the pathophysiology associated with coronary artery disease. Read each option carefully and recall that coronary artery disease affects the arteries that provide blood, oxygen, and nutrients to the myocardium. This will assist in selecting the correct options.
Priority Nursing Tip: Modifiable risk factors for coronary artery disease are those that can be changed to reduce the risk (e.g., smoking, diet intake). Nonmodifiable risk factors for coronary artery disease are those that cannot be changed (e.g., age, race).
Reference: Ignatavicius, D., et al. (2021). *Medical-surgical nursing: Concepts for interprofessional collaborative care* (10th ed., pp. 700–701). Elsevier.

❖ **140.** What factors would the nurse consider for teaching a child about their disease and related health care measures? **Select all that apply.**
   ❑ 1. A child rarely forms misconceptions.
   ❑ 2. The older the child, the shorter the attention span.
   ❑ 3. A child's imagination may create greater fear than the truth.
   ❑ 4. A child may regress developmentally in a situation of illness.
   ❑ 5. It is not necessary to assess the child's knowledge before teaching.
   ❑ 6. A child may better manage uncomfortable information through role-playing.

Level of Cognitive Ability: Analyzing
Client Needs: Health Promotion and Maintenance
Clinical Judgment/Cognitive Skills: Generate Solutions
Integrated Process: Clinical Judgment; Nursing Process/Planning
Content Area: Foundations of Care: Communication
Health Problems: N/A
Priority Concepts: Development; Health Promotion

Answer: 3, 4, 6
Rationale: For children, the teaching-learning process may be fundamentally different from that used for adults, and the nurse needs to adjust the complexity and volume of information based on the child's age and cognitive level. The factors that need to be addressed when teaching children include the following: trust is essential to a therapeutic relationship; in general, the younger the child, the shorter the attention span; assessing the child's knowledge is important because children are exposed to various levels of information about health care; children form misconceptions easily, and a child's imagination may create greater fear than the truth; a child may regress developmentally in a situation of illness; and a child may better manage uncomfortable information through role-playing.
Test-Taking Strategy: Focus on the subject, factors to consider for teaching a child. Read each option carefully and think about the concepts of growth and development. This will assist in selecting the correct options.
Priority Nursing Tip: Many factors need to be considered when determining the best teaching method. One factor is age. At a younger age, people tend to be visual and hands-on learners, thus presenting charts and pictures will enhance learning. Adults typically like to have control over their learning; thus, it is best to include them in planning the process.
References: McKinney, E. S., et al. (2022) *Maternal child nursing* (6th ed., pp. 50–51). Elsevier; Potter, P., et al. (2021). *Fundamentals of nursing* (10th ed., p. 345). Elsevier.

141. The nurse is caring for a client diagnosed with end-stage renal disease. What areas are appropriate to assess to determine the client's wishes for end-of-life nursing care? **Select all that apply.**
- ❑ 1. Preferred place for death
- ❑ 2. Client expectations for nursing care
- ❑ 3. Financial responsibilities for the funeral
- ❑ 4. Where the funeral and burial will take place
- ❑ 5. Use of and the level of life-sustaining measures
- ❑ 6. Expectations regarding pain control and symptom management

Level of Cognitive Ability: Analyzing
Client Needs: Health Promotion and Maintenance
Clinical Judgment/Cognitive Skills: Prioritize Hypotheses
Integrated Process: Clinical Judgment; Nursing Process/Analysis
Content Area: Developmental Stages: End-of-Life
Health Problems: Adult Health: Renal and Urinary: Acute Kidney Injury and Chronic Kidney Disease
Priority Concepts: Clinical Judgment; Palliation

Answer: 1, 2, 5, 6
Rationale: The nurse must assess the client's wishes for end-of-life nursing care because these can influence how the nurse sets priorities for planning and implementing care. End-of-life assessment related to nursing care should include the preferred place for death, client expectations for nursing care, the use of and the level of life-sustaining measures, and expectations regarding pain control and symptom management. Financial responsibilities for the funeral and where the funeral and burial will take place are issues that the client may want to discuss, but they are unrelated to nursing care.
Test-Taking Strategy: Focus on the subject, end-of-life nursing care. Read each option and select those that relate to nursing care. Financial responsibilities for the funeral and where the funeral and burial will take place are unrelated to nursing care.
Priority Nursing Tip: Each client's end-of-life experience will be unique, and the nurse needs to plan care based on the client's wishes.
References: Ignatavicius, D., et al. (2021). *Medical-surgical nursing: Concepts for interprofessional collaborative care* (10th ed., pp. 1388–1389). Elsevier; Potter, P., et al. (2021). *Fundamentals of nursing* (10th ed., p. 750). Elsevier.

❖ **142.** The school nurse teaches an athletic coach how to prevent dehydration among athletes practicing in the hot weather. What is the **best** advice for the nurse to give to the coach?
1. Drink plenty of fluids before and after practice.
2. Have the athletes take a salt tablet before practice.
3. Reschedule practice for before school and after sunset.
4. Provide a fluid break every 30 minutes during practice.

Level of Cognitive Ability: Applying
Client Needs: Health Promotion and Maintenance
Clinical Judgment/Cognitive Skills: Generate Solutions
Integrated Process: Clinical Judgment; Nursing Process/Planning
Content Area: Foundations of Care: Fluids and Electrolytes
Health Problems: Adult Health: Cardiovascular: Hypovolemic Shock
Priority Concepts: Patient Education; Fluids and Electrolytes

Answer: 4
Rationale: Hot weather accelerates the body's loss of fluid and electrolytes during strenuous physical activity, so the nurse encourages the coach to schedule fluid breaks at 30-minute intervals so that the athletes can periodically rest and restore body fluids. Drinking fluid before and after practice is a reasonable suggestion; however, because the hot weather accelerates fluid and electrolyte losses, body fluids must be periodically replenished to maintain the fluid and electrolyte balance. Although a sodium load increases fluid retention, the nurse avoids suggesting salt tablets for the athletes because the nurse needs approval from each athlete's primary health care provider before recommending the salt. Rescheduling practice times is unrealistic.
Test-Taking Strategy: Focus on the subject, preventing dehydration. Note the strategic word, *best*; this indicates that each option could be a reasonable response for preventing dehydration. However, you must choose the option that is a better choice than the other three. Recall the principles of fluid and electrolyte balance and the causes of dehydration. Regularly scheduled fluid breaks every 30 minutes is the best answer because it is the option that addresses fluid and electrolyte balance directly, and it is also the most practical choice.
Priority Nursing Tip: Some causes of dehydration include decreased fluid intake, diaphoresis, vomiting, diarrhea, diabetic ketoacidosis, and extensive burns or other serious injuries.
Reference: Nix, S. (2022). *Williams' Basic nutrition and diet therapy* (16th ed., pp. 140–141, 290.). Elsevier.

143. The nurse instructs a client with coronary artery disease who is hospitalized about a low-fat diet. Which menu does the nurse provide for the client?
1. Shrimp, avocado, and tomato salad
2. Calf's liver, potato salad, and sherbet
3. Lean steak, mashed potatoes, and gravy
4. Turkey breast, boiled rice, and strawberries

Level of Cognitive Ability: Applying
Client Needs: Health Promotion and Maintenance
Clinical Judgment/Cognitive Skills: Take Action
Integrated Process: Nursing Process/Implementation
Content Area: Foundations of Care: Therapeutic Diets
Health Problems: Adult Health: Cardiovascular: Coronary Artery Disease
Priority Concepts: Patient Education; Nutrition

Answer: 4
Rationale: Turkey breast without the skin, boiled rice, and strawberries offer the client nourishing foods that are low in fat. Some sources of fat include meats, avocado, salad dressing, mayonnaise, butter, cheese, and bacon. The remaining options contain high-fat foods.
Test-Taking Strategy: Focus on the subject, a low-fat diet. Eliminate options 1 and 2 first because avocado and liver have a very high fat content. Potato salad usually contains mayonnaise, which is high in fat. Next, eliminate option 3 because meat is high in fat and mashed potatoes are not very palatable without butter or gravy, and both are high in fat. Option 4 does not contain high-fat foods.
Priority Nursing Tip: A low-fat diet is indicated for health problems such as obesity, atherosclerosis, diabetes mellitus, hyperlipidemia, hypertension, and myocardial infarction.
Reference: Nix, S. (2022). *Williams' Basic nutrition and diet therapy* (16th ed., pp. 38–39, 350–351). Elsevier.

❖ **144.** The camp nurse provides instructions regarding skin protection from the sun to the parents who are preparing their children for a camping adventure. Which statement by a parent indicates a **need for further teaching?**
1. "A protective sunscreen is best to prevent sunburn."
2. "My child won't need the sunscreen on cloudy, hazy days."
3. "I need to pack a hat, long-sleeved shirts, and long pants for my child to wear."
4. "My child needs to wear clothes that have a tightly woven material for greater protection from the sun's rays."

Level of Cognitive Ability: Evaluating
Client Needs: Health Promotion and Maintenance
Clinical Judgment/Cognitive Skills: Clinical Judgment; Evaluate Outcomes
Integrated Process: Teaching and Learning
Content Area: Pediatrics: Integumentary
Health Problems: Pediatric-Specific: Burns
Priority Concepts: Patient Education; Tissue Integrity

Answer: 2
Rationale: The sun's rays are as damaging to the skin on cloudy, hazy days as they are on sunny days. Sunscreens are recommended and need to be applied before exposure to the sun and reapplied frequently and liberally at least every 2 hours. A hat, long-sleeved shirt, and long pants need to be worn when out in the sun. Tightly woven materials provide greater protection from the sun's rays.
Test-Taking Strategy: Note the strategic words, *need for further teaching*. These words indicate a negative event query and ask you to select an option that is an incorrect statement. Eliminate options 1, 3, and 4 because these measures provide the greatest protection from the sun. Also recalling the concept that ultraviolet rays can be damaging regardless of cloudiness or haziness will assist in directing you to the correct option.
Priority Nursing Tip: To prevent skin damage from the sun's rays, the client needs to be instructed to avoid sun exposure between the hours of 1000 and 1600.
References: Ball, J., et al. (2019). *Seidel's Guide to physical examination; An interprofessional approach* (9th ed., p. 136). Elsevier; Hockenberry, M., Wilson, D., & Rodgers, C. (2019). *Wong's Nursing care of infants and children* (11th ed., p. 417). Elsevier.

145. A client has urinary calculi that are composed of uric acid, and the nurse teaches the client dietary measures to prevent the further development of the calculi. The nurse determines that the client understands the dietary measures if the client states that it is necessary to avoid consuming what food products?
1. Milk
2. Yogurt
3. Spinach, chocolate, and tea
4. Sardines, herring, and organ meats

Level of Cognitive Ability: Evaluating
Client Needs: Health Promotion and Maintenance
Clinical Judgment/Cognitive Skills: Evaluate Outcomes
Integrated Process: Clinical Judgment; Nursing Process/Evaluation
Content Area: Foundations of Care: Therapeutic Diets
Health Problems: Adult Health: Renal and Urinary: Calculi
Priority Concepts: Patient Education; Health Promotion

Answer: 4
Rationale: The client diagnosed with a uric acid stone needs to limit the intake of foods that are high in purines. Organ meats, sardines, herring, and other high-purine foods are eliminated from the diet. Foods with moderate levels of purines, such as red and white meats and some seafood, are also limited. Milk, yogurt, spinach, chocolate, and tea are recommended dietary changes to prevent calculi that are composed of calcium phosphate or calcium oxalate.
Test-Taking Strategy: Note the **subject**, a client with urinary calculi that are composed of uric acid. Note the word *avoid*, which asks you to select the incorrect food choice. Remembering that organ meats are high in purines will direct you to the correct option. Eliminate milk and yogurt as they are **comparable or alike** as both options belong to the dairy food group. Also note that the remaining options are **comparable or alike** in that they are foods that are avoided if the client has calcium phosphate or calcium oxalate calculi.
Priority Nursing Tip: Uric acid stones are usually caused by excess dietary purine or gout.
Reference: Ignatavicius, D., et al. (2021). *Medical-surgical nursing: Concepts for interprofessional collaborative care* (10th ed., pp. 1345, 1349). Elsevier.

❖ **146.** The nurse is teaching a birthing parent diagnosed with diabetes mellitus who delivered an infant who is large for gestational age (LGA) about the care of the infant. The nurse tells the birthing parent that infants who are LGA appear to be more mature because of their large size but that, in reality, these infants frequently need to be aroused to facilitate nutritional intake and attachment. Which statement by the birthing parent indicates the **need for further teaching** about the care of the infant?
1. "It's best to talk to babies when they are in a quiet, alert state."
2. "I will allow my baby to sleep through the night because rest is most important."
3. "I will breast-feed my baby every 2½ to 3 hours and will use arousal techniques."
4. "I will watch my baby closely because I know that babies who are LGA may not be as mature in their motor development."

Level of Cognitive Ability: Evaluating
Client Needs: Health Promotion and Maintenance
Clinical Judgment/Cognitive Skills: Evaluate Outcomes
Integrated Process: Clinical Judgment; Teaching and Learning
Content Area: Maternity: Newborn
Health Problems: Newborn: Preterm and Postterm Newborn
Priority Concepts: Patient Education; Development

Answer: 2
Rationale: Infants who are LGA tend to be more difficult to arouse and therefore must be aroused to facilitate nutritional intake and attachment opportunities. These infants also have problems maintaining a quiet, alert state. It is beneficial for the birthing parent to interact with the infant during this time to enhance and lengthen the quiet, alert state. Infants who are LGA need to be aroused for feedings, usually every 2 to 3 hours for breast-feeding. Although the infant is large, motor function is not usually as mature as it is in the term infant.
Test-Taking Strategy: Note the **strategic words**, *need for further teaching*. These words indicate a **negative event query** and ask you to select an option that is an incorrect statement. Focusing on the words *frequently need to be aroused* in the question will direct you to the correct option. The remaining options address observation and arousal.
Priority Nursing Tip: Monitor the newborn who is LGA for signs of hypoglycemia. Initiate feedings early to prevent the occurrence of hypoglycemia.
Reference: McKinney, E. S., et al. (2022). *Maternal child nursing* (6th ed., pp. 455, 643). Elsevier.

147. A client has been experiencing muscle weakness for a period of several months. The primary health care provider suspects polymyositis, and the client asks the nurse about the disorder. The nurse explains to the client that which occurs in this disorder?
1. Muscle fibers are inflamed.
2. Muscle fibers are thickened.
3. There is a decrease in elastic tissue.
4. There is an increase in fibrous tissue.

Level of Cognitive Ability: Applying
Client Needs: Health Promotion and Maintenance
Clinical Judgment/Cognitive Skills: Generate Solutions
Integrated Process: Nursing Process/Implementation
Content Area: Adult Health: Musculoskeletal
Health Problems: Adult Health: Musculoskeletal: Tissue or Ligament Injury
Priority Concepts: Patient Education; Inflammation

Answer: 1
Rationale: Polymyositis is a diffuse inflammatory disorder of skeletal (striated) muscle that is characterized by symmetrical weakness and atrophy. Increased fibrous tissue is seen in clients diagnosed with ankylosis. Thickened muscle fibers describe the opposite of what is noted with this disorder. Decreased elastic tissue, if it occurred in the aorta, would be noted in a client with Marfan's syndrome.
Test-Taking Strategy: Note the subject of the question, polymyositis. The ending, *-itis*, indicates inflammation. The only option that addresses inflammation is the correct one.
Priority Nursing Tip: Using medical terminology skills will assist you with determining what an unfamiliar condition presented in a test question means. For example, *poly-* means many; *-myo-* refers to muscle; and *-itis* indicates inflammation.
Reference: Harding M., et al. (2023). *Lewis's Medical-surgical nursing: Assessment and management of clinical problems* (12th ed., pp. 1723-1724). Elsevier.

❖ **148.** The nurse in an ambulatory clinic administers a tuberculin skin test to a client on a Monday. When would the nurse tell the client to return to the clinic to have the results read?
1. Thursday or Friday
2. The following Monday
3. Tuesday or Wednesday
4. Wednesday or Thursday

Level of Cognitive Ability: Applying
Client Needs: Health Promotion and Maintenance
Clinical Judgment/Cognitive Skills: Generate Solutions
Integrated Process: Nursing Process/Planning
Content Area: Foundations of Care: Diagnostic Tests
Health Problems: Adult Health: Respiratory: Tuberculosis
Priority Concepts: Health Promotion; Infection

Answer: 4
Rationale: The tuberculin skin test for tuberculosis is read in 48 to 72 hours; therefore, the client needs to return to the clinic on Wednesday or Thursday.
Test-Taking Strategy: Focus on the subject, the time frame for reading a tuberculin skin test after it is administered. Recalling that this test is read within 48 to 72 hours will direct you to the correct option.
Priority Nursing Tip: For a tuberculin skin test, once the result is positive, it will be positive in any future tests.
Reference: Pagana, K., Pagana, T., & Pagana, T. N. (2021). *Mosby's Diagnostic and laboratory test reference* (15th ed., pp. 904–905). Elsevier.

149. A client diagnosed with chronic obstructive pulmonary disease (COPD) is admitted to the hospital with an exacerbation of signs and symptoms. Which factor contributed **most** to the change in client status?
1. Decreased fat intake
2. Decreased fluid intake
3. Sleeping soundly during the night
4. Anxiety about the upcoming pulmonologist visit

Level of Cognitive Ability: Analyzing
Client Needs: Health Promotion and Maintenance
Clinical Judgment/Cognitive Skills: Recognize Cues
Integrated Process: Nursing Process/Assessment
Content Area: Adult Health: Respiratory
Health Problems: Adult Health: Respiratory: Chronic Obstructive Pulmonary Disease
Priority Concepts: Gas Exchange; Health Promotion

Answer: 2
Rationale: The client with exacerbation of COPD has ineffective coughing and excess sputum in the airways. The nurse assesses the client for contributing factors such as dehydration and a lack of knowledge of proper coughing techniques. The reduction of these factors helps limit exacerbations of the disease. Decreased fat intake, sleeping soundly, and anxiety related to scheduled pulmonologist visit are not directly associated with this change in condition.
Test-Taking Strategy: Note the strategic word, *most*. Also note the subject, exacerbation of COPD. This calls to mind the concept of sputum production and clearance. Evaluate each of the options in terms of the potential ability to inhibit sputum production or clearance. The fluid intake is the only factor that could affect the viscosity of secretions, thus affecting airway clearance.
Priority Nursing Tip: The client with COPD needs to be instructed to avoid environmental irritants such as smoke from fireplaces, pets, feather pillows, and aerosol sprays.
Reference: Lewis, S., et al. (2020). *Medical-surgical nursing: Assessment and management of clinical problems* (11th ed., pp. 564–565, 573). Elsevier.

150. A client diagnosed with acquired immunodeficiency syndrome (AIDS) gets recurrent *Candida* infections of the mouth (thrush). The nurse has given the client instructions to minimize the occurrence of thrush and determines that the client understands the instructions if which statement is made by the client?
1. "I should use a mouthwash at least once a week."
2. "I should use warm saline or water to rinse my mouth."
3. "I should brush my teeth and rinse my mouth once a day."
4. "Increasing the amount of red meat in my diet will keep this from recurring."

Level of Cognitive Ability: Evaluating
Client Needs: Health Promotion and Maintenance
Clinical Judgment/Cognitive Skills: Evaluate Outcomes
Integrated Process: Clinical Judgment; Nursing Process/Evaluation
Content Area: Adult Health: Immune
Health Problems: Adult Health: Immune: Immunodeficiency Syndrome
Priority Concepts: Immunity; Infection

Answer: 2
Rationale: When a client is in a state of immunosuppression or has decreased levels of some normal oral flora, an overgrowth of the normal flora *Candida* can occur. Careful routine mouth care is helpful to prevent the recurrence of *Candida* infections. The client should use a mouthwash that consists of warm saline or water. The time frames given for oral hygiene in options 1 and 3 are too infrequent. Red meat will not prevent thrush.
Test-Taking Strategy: Eliminate options 1 and 3 because they are comparable or alike and the time frames are too infrequent. From the remaining options, recalling that red meat is not likely to minimize the occurrence of thrush will direct you to the correct option.
Priority Nursing Tip: A *Candida* infection of the mucous membranes of the mouth appears as red and whitish patches.
Reference: Ignatavicius, D., et al. (2021). *Medical-surgical nursing: Concepts for interprofessional collaborative care* (10th ed., p. 332). Elsevier.

151. The nurse is teaching a client diagnosed with acquired immunodeficiency syndrome (AIDS) how to avoid foodborne illnesses. The nurse instructs the client to prevent acquiring infection from food by avoiding which item?
1. Raw oysters
2. Bottled water
3. Pasteurized milk
4. Products with sorbitol

Level of Cognitive Ability: Applying
Client Needs: Health Promotion and Maintenance
Clinical Judgment/Cognitive Skills: Take Action
Integrated Process: Teaching and Learning
Content Area: Adult Health: Immune
Health Problems: Adult Health: Immune: Immunodeficiency Syndrome
Priority Concepts: Patient Education; Immunity

Answer: 1
Rationale: The client who is at risk for immunosuppression is taught to avoid raw or undercooked seafood, meat, poultry, and eggs. The client needs to also avoid unpasteurized milk and dairy products. Fruits that can be peeled, as well as bottled beverages, are safe. The client may be taught to avoid sorbitol, but this is to diminish diarrhea and has nothing to do with foodborne infections.
Test-Taking Strategy: Focus on the subject, foodborne illness. Sorbitol can cause diarrhea, but it is unrelated to foodborne illness, so option 4 is eliminated first. Eliminate option 3 next because products that are pasteurized are free of microbes. From the remaining options, noting the word *raw* in option 1 will direct you to this option.
Priority Nursing Tip: Acquired immunodeficiency syndrome is considered to be a chronic illness. The disease has a long incubation period, sometimes 10 years or longer. Manifestations may not appear until late in the infection.
Reference: Nix, S. (2022). *Williams' Basic nutrition and diet therapy* (16th ed., pp. 221–222). Elsevier.

❖ 152. A client has a prescription for ketoconazole. Which instruction would the nurse teach the client to follow while taking this medication?
1. Avoid exposure to sunlight.
2. Limit alcohol to 2 ounces per day.
3. Take the medication with an antacid.
4. Take the medication on an empty stomach.

Level of Cognitive Ability: Applying
Client Needs: Health Promotion and Maintenance
Clinical Judgment/Cognitive Skills: Take Action
Integrated Process: Teaching and Learning
Content Area: Pharmacology: Immune: Antifungals
Health Problems: N/A
Priority Concepts: Patient Education; Safety

Answer: 1
Rationale: The client is taught that ketoconazole is an antifungal medication. The client should avoid exposure to sunlight because the medication increases photosensitivity. The client needs to avoid the concurrent use of alcohol because the medication is hepatotoxic. Antacids need to be avoided for 2 hours after it is taken because gastric acid is needed to activate the medication. This medication needs to be taken with food or milk.
Test-Taking Strategy: Focus on the subject, client instructions for ketoconazole. Use general guidelines related to medication administration to eliminate taking the medication with some alcohol and with an antacid. From the remaining options, it is necessary to know that the medication causes photosensitivity reaction and needs to be taken with food or milk.
Priority Nursing Tip: Ketoconazole, an antifungal medication, is hepatotoxic. Assess the client for a history of liver disorders and check the results of liver function blood tests.
Reference: Lewis, S., et al. (2020). *Medical-surgical nursing: Assessment and management of clinical problems* (11th ed., p. 410). Elsevier.

153. The nurse is planning to teach an adolescent client about sexuality. What would the nurse do **first**?
1. Inform the adolescent about the dangers of pregnancy.
2. Establish a relationship and determine prior knowledge.
3. Advise the adolescent to maintain sexual abstinence until marriage.
4. Provide written information about sexually transmitted infections.

Level of Cognitive Ability: Applying
Client Needs: Health Promotion and Maintenance
Clinical Judgment/Cognitive Skills: Generate Solutions
Integrated Process: Teaching and Learning
Content Area: Developmental Stages: Adolescent
Health Problems: N/A
Priority Concepts: Development; Sexuality

Answer: 2
Rationale: The first step in effective communication is establishing a relationship. By exploring the client's interest and prior knowledge, the nurse establishes rapport and assesses learning needs. The other options may or may not be later steps, depending on the data obtained.
Test-Taking Strategy: Note the strategic word, *first*. Use the steps of the nursing process, and select an assessment option. This will direct you to the correct option. When teaching, the nurse assesses motivation, interest, and level of knowledge before providing information.
Priority Nursing Tip: The nurse always needs to assess the client's readiness to learn before implementing a teaching plan.
Reference: McKinney, E. S., et al. (2022). *Maternal child nursing* (6th ed., pp. 159, 171). Elsevier.

❖ **154.** The nurse provides home care instructions to a client diagnosed with Cushing's syndrome. The nurse determines that the client understands the hospital discharge instructions if the client makes which statement?
1. "I need to eat foods low in potassium."
2. "I need to check the color of my stools."
3. "I need to check the temperature of my legs twice a day."
4. "I need to take aspirin rather than acetaminophen for a headache."

Level of Cognitive Ability: Evaluating
Client Needs: Health Promotion and Maintenance
Clinical Judgment/Cognitive Skills: Evaluate Outcomes
Integrated Process: Clinical Judgment; Nursing Process/ Evaluation
Content Area: Adult Health: Endocrine
Health Problems: Adult Health: Endocrine: Adrenal Disorders
Priority Concepts: Patient Education; Health Promotion

Answer: 2
Rationale: Cushing's syndrome results in an increased secretion of cortisol. Cortisol stimulates the secretion of gastric acid, and this can result in the development of peptic ulcers and gastrointestinal bleeding. The client needs to be encouraged to eat potassium-rich foods to correct the hypokalemia that occurs with this disorder. Cushing's syndrome does not affect temperature changes in the lower extremities. Aspirin can increase the risk for gastric bleeding and skin bruising.
Test-Taking Strategy: Focus on the subject, home care instructions for the client with Cushing's syndrome. Recalling the pathophysiology of this disorder and that cortisol stimulates the secretion of gastric acid will direct you to the correct option.
Priority Nursing Tip: Laboratory findings noted in Cushing's syndrome include hyperglycemia, hypernatremia, hypokalemia, and hypocalcemia.
Reference: Ignatavicius, D., et al. (2021). *Medical-surgical nursing: Concepts for interprofessional collaborative care* (10th ed., pp. 1242–1243, 1245). Elsevier.

155. A client diagnosed with heart failure and secondary hyperaldosteronism is started on spironolactone to manage this disorder. The nurse informs the client that the need for dosage adjustment may be necessary if which medication is also being taken?
1. Alprazolam
2. Warfarin sodium
3. Potassium chloride
4. Verapamil hydrochloride

Level of Cognitive Ability: Applying
Client Needs: Health Promotion and Maintenance
Clinical Judgment/Cognitive Skills: Take Action
Integrated Process: Clinical Judgment; Nursing Process/Implementation
Content Area: Adult Health: Cardiovascular
Health Problems: Adult Health: Cardiovascular: Heart Failure
Priority Concepts: Patient Education; Safety

Answer: 3
Rationale: Spironolactone is a potassium-sparing diuretic. If the client is also taking potassium chloride or another potassium supplement, the risk for hyperkalemia exists. Potassium doses need to be adjusted while the client is taking this medication. A dosage adjustment would not be necessary if the client was taking alprazolam, warfarin sodium, or verapamil hydrochloride.
Test-Taking Strategy: Focus on the subject, dosage adjustment in a client taking spironolactone. Recalling that spironolactone is a potassium-sparing diuretic will direct you to the correct option.
Priority Nursing Tip: Potassium-sparing diuretics act on the distal tubule to promote sodium and water excretion and potassium retention.
Reference: Lewis, S., et al. (2020). *Medical-surgical nursing: Assessment and management of clinical problems* (11th ed., pp. 745, 1168). Elsevier.

❖ **156.** The nurse is teaching health education classes to a group of expectant parents, and the topic is preventing cognitive impairment caused by congenital hypothyroidism. What would the nurse tell the parents is the **most effective** means of promoting early intervention?
1. Vitamin intake
2. Neonatal screening
3. Adequate protein intake
4. Limiting alcohol consumption

Level of Cognitive Ability: Applying
Client Needs: Health Promotion and Maintenance
Clinical Judgment/Cognitive Skills: Prioritize Hypotheses
Integrated Process: Teaching and Learning
Content Area: Maternity: Antepartum
Health Problems: Newborn: Hypothyroidism
Priority Concepts: Patient Education; Health Promotion

Answer: 2
Rationale: Congenital hypothyroidism is a common preventable cause of cognitive impairment. Neonatal screening is the only means of early diagnosis followed by intervention and the subsequent prevention of cognitive impairment. Newborn infants are screened for congenital hypothyroidism before discharge from the newborn nursery and before 7 days of life. Treatment is begun immediately, if necessary. Vitamin intake and adequate protein will not specifically prevent this disorder. Alcohol consumption during pregnancy needs to be restricted rather than just limited.
Test-Taking Strategy: Note the strategic words, *most effective*. Focus on the subject, promoting early identification. Vitamin intake, protein consumption, and alcohol restriction are measures to prevent all birth defects. In addition, note that neonatal screening is the umbrella option.
Priority Nursing Tip: With cognitive impairment, a child manifests below average intellectual functioning along with deficits in adaptive skills.
Reference: McKinney, E. S., et al. (2022) *Maternal child nursing* (6th ed., p. 1260). Elsevier.

157. The nurse is monitoring a client with type 1 diabetes mellitus and checks the laboratory result for the client's glycosylated hemoglobin drawn this morning. The nurse creates a teaching plan based on the understanding that this result indicates which finding?

Laboratory Results

Test and Results	Reference Range
HbA1c 10%	<6%

1. A normal value that indicates that the client is managing blood glucose control well
2. A value that does not offer information regarding the client's management of the disease
3. A low value that indicates that the client is not managing blood glucose control very well
4. A high value that indicates that the client is not managing blood glucose control very well

Level of Cognitive Ability: Analyzing
Client Needs: Health Promotion and Maintenance
Clinical Judgment/Cognitive Skills: Generate Solutions
Integrated Process: Clinical Judgment; Nursing Process/Planning
Content Area: Adult Health: Endocrine
Health Problems: Adult Health: Endocrine: Diabetes Mellitus
Priority Concepts: Patient Education; Glucose Regulation

Answer: 4
Rationale: Glycosylated hemoglobin is a measure of glucose control during the 6 to 8 weeks before the test. It is a reliable measure for determining the degree of glucose control in clients with diabetes over a period of time, and it is not influenced by dietary management 1 to 2 days before the test is done. The glycosylated hemoglobin level should be 6.0% or less for a client diagnosed with diabetes mellitus (based on individual physician recommendation), with elevated levels indicating poor glucose control.
Test-Taking Strategy: Focus on the subject, an elevated glycosylated hemoglobin level. Specific knowledge regarding the normal values for this test will direct you to the correct option. Remember that the level should be less than 6.0%.
Priority Nursing Tip: Hyperglycemia in a client with diabetes mellitus is usually the cause of an increase in the HbA1c (glycosylated hemoglobin) level.
Reference: Pagana, K., Pagana, T., & Pagana, T. N. (2021). *Mosby's Diagnostic and laboratory test reference* (15th ed., pp. 473–474). Elsevier.

❖ 158. The nurse is instructing a client diagnosed with type 1 diabetes mellitus about the management of hypoglycemic reactions. The nurse instructs the client that hypoglycemia **most likely** occurs during what time interval after insulin administration?
1. Peak
2. Onset
3. Duration
4. Anytime

Level of Cognitive Ability: Applying
Client Needs: Health Promotion and Maintenance
Clinical Judgment/Cognitive Skills: Take Action
Integrated Process: Teaching and Learning
Content Area: Adult Health: Endocrine
Health Problems: Adult Health: Endocrine: Diabetes Mellitus
Priority Concepts: Patient Education; Glucose Regulation

Answer: 1
Rationale: Insulin reactions are most likely to occur during the peak time after insulin administration, when the medication is at its maximum action. Peak action depends on the type of insulin, the amount administered, the injection site, and other factors.
Test-Taking Strategy: Note the strategic words, *most likely.* Focus on the subject, hypoglycemia. Remember that insulin is a hypoglycemic agent. The word *peak* means the highest point. Remembering this will assist with directing you to the correct option.
Priority Nursing Tip: Regular insulin peaks in 2 hours. NPH insulin peaks in 4 to 12 hours.
Reference: Ignatavicius, D., et al. (2021). *Medical-surgical nursing: Concepts for interprofessional collaborative care* (10th ed., pp. 1134–1135). Elsevier.

159. The nurse is caring for a client who is scheduled to have a thyroidectomy and provides instructions to the client about the surgical procedure. Which statement by the client indicates an understanding of the nurse's instructions?
1. "I will definitely have to continue taking antithyroid medication after this surgery."
2. "I need to place my hands behind my neck when I have to cough or change positions."
3. "I need to turn my head and neck front, back, and side to side every hour for the first 12 hours after surgery."
4. "I will immediately report to the emergency room if I experience tingling of my toes, fingers, and lips after surgery."

Level of Cognitive Ability: Evaluating
Client Needs: Health Promotion and Maintenance
Clinical Judgment/Cognitive Skills: Evaluate Outcomes
Integrated Process: Clinical Judgment; Nursing Process/Evaluation
Content Area: Adult Health: Endocrine
Health Problems: Adult Health: Endocrine: Thyroid Disorders
Priority Concepts: Patient Education; Safety

Answer: 2
Rationale: One way of reducing incisional tension is to teach the client how to support the neck when coughing or being repositioned. The removal of the thyroid does not mean that the client will be taking antithyroid medications postoperatively. The client is taught that, after thyroidectomy, tension needs to be avoided on the suture line because hemorrhage may develop. Likewise, during the postoperative period, the client needs to avoid any unnecessary movement of the neck; that is why sandbags and pillows are frequently used to support the head and neck. If a client experiences tingling in the fingers, toes, and lips, it is probably a result of injury to the parathyroid gland during surgery, resulting in hypocalcemia. These signs and symptoms need to be reported immediately.
Test-Taking Strategy: Focus on the subject, a client scheduled to have a thyroidectomy. Eliminate option 1 because of the wording stating that the medication would definitely be administered. Eliminate hourly head turning as this would place unusual strain on the surgical site. Eliminate the emergency room visit as the question asks about the surgical procedure and not potential discharge instructions.
Priority Nursing Tip: The nurse needs to ensure that a tracheostomy set, oxygen, and suction are at the bedside of a client after thyroidectomy.
Reference: Lewis, S., et al. (2020). *Medical-surgical nursing: Assessment and management of clinical problems* (11th ed., pp. 1154–1155). Elsevier.

❖ **160.** The nurse has been preparing a client diagnosed with chronic obstructive pulmonary disease (COPD) for discharge. Which statement by the client indicates the **need for further teaching** about nutrition?
1. "I will rest a few minutes before I eat."
2. "I will not eat as much cabbage as I once did."
3. "I will certainly try to drink 3 L of fluid every day."
4. "It's best to eat three large meals a day so that I will get all my nutrients."

Level of Cognitive Ability: Evaluating
Client Needs: Health Promotion and Maintenance
Clinical Judgment/Cognitive Skills: Evaluate Outcomes
Integrated Process: Clinical Judgment; Nursing Process/Evaluation
Content Area: Adult Health: Respiratory
Health Problems: Adult Health: Respiratory: Chronic Obstructive Pulmonary Disease
Priority Concepts: Patient Education; Gas Exchange

Answer: 4
Rationale: Large meals distend the abdomen and elevate the diaphragm, which may interfere with breathing for the client diagnosed with COPD. Resting before eating may decrease the fatigue that is often associated with COPD. Gas-forming foods may cause bloating, which interferes with normal diaphragmatic breathing. Adequate fluid intake helps liquefy pulmonary secretions.
Test-Taking Strategy: Note the strategic words, *need for further teaching.* These words indicate a negative event query and ask you to select an option that is an incorrect statement. Focusing on the client's diagnosis of COPD and recalling the activities that produce dyspnea will direct you to the correct option.
Priority Nursing Tip: The best diet for a client with COPD is to consume a high-calorie and high-protein diet with supplements.
Reference: Lewis, S., et al. (2020). *Medical-surgical nursing: Assessment and management of clinical problems* (11th ed., p. 572). Elsevier.

161. The nurse is preparing a client diagnosed with pneumonia for discharge. Which statement by the client would alert the nurse to the fact that the client **needs further teaching** before being discharged?

1. "I will take all of my antibiotics, even if I do feel 100% better."
2. "You can toss out that incentive spirometer as soon as I leave for home."
3. "I realize that it may be weeks before my usual sense of well-being returns."
4. "It is a good idea for me to take a nap every afternoon for the next couple of weeks."

Level of Cognitive Ability: Evaluating
Client Needs: Health Promotion and Maintenance
Clinical Judgment/Cognitive Skills: Evaluate Outcomes
Integrated Process: Clinical Judgment; Teaching and Learning
Content Area: Adult Health: Respiratory
Health Problems: Adult Health: Respiratory: Pneumonia
Priority Concepts: Patient Education; Gas Exchange

Answer: 2
Rationale: Deep breathing and coughing exercises and the use of incentive spirometry need to be practiced for 6 to 8 weeks after the client diagnosed with pneumonia is discharged from the hospital to keep the alveoli expanded and promote the removal of lung secretions. If the entire regimen of antibiotics is not taken, the client may suffer a relapse. The period of convalescence with pneumonia is often lengthy, and it may be weeks before the client feels a sense of well-being. Adequate rest is needed to maintain progress toward recovery.
Test-Taking Strategy: Note the strategic words, *needs further teaching.* These words indicate a negative event query and ask you to select an option that is an incorrect statement. Focusing on the client's diagnosis of pneumonia and recalling the need to promote the removal of lung secretions will direct you to the correct option.
Priority Nursing Tip: The client with pneumonia needs to be placed in a semi-Fowler's position to facilitate breathing and lung expansion.
Reference: Harding M., et al. (2023). *Lewis's Medical-surgical nursing: Assessment and management of clinical problems* (12th ed.). Elsevier. pp. 603-604.

❖ **162.** The nurse employed in a well-baby clinic is preparing to administer the scheduled recommended immunizations to a 2-month-old infant. After consultation with the pediatrician, the nurse would prepare to administer which vaccines at this time? **Select all that apply.**

❏ 1. Rotavirus (RV)
❏ 2. Pneumococcal virus (PCV)
❏ 3. Inactivated poliovirus (IPV)
❏ 4. Varicella; measles, mumps, and rubella (MMR)
❏ 5. *Haemophilus influenzae* type b conjugate (Hib)
❏ 6. Diphtheria and tetanus toxoids and acellular pertussis (DTaP)

Level of Cognitive Ability: Applying
Client Needs: Health Promotion and Maintenance
Clinical Judgment/Cognitive Skills: Generate Solutions
Integrated Process: Nursing Process/Planning
Content Area: Pediatrics: Infectious and Communicable Diseases
Health Problems: Pediatric-Specific: Immunizations
Priority Concepts: Development; Immunity

Answer: 1, 2, 3, 5, 6
Rationale: RV is administered at 2 months of age. PCV is administered at 2, 4, and 6 months of age and then between 12 and 15 months. IPV is administered at ages 2 and 4 months and then at age 4 to 6 years. Hib is administered at ages 2 and 4 months with a final dose administered at age 12 months or older. DTaP is administered at 2, 4, and 6 months of age; the fourth dose is administered as early as age 12 months, as long as 6 months have elapsed since the third dose. Varicella vaccine is administered at age 12 months or older. MMR is administered at age 12 to 18 months with the second dose at age 4 to 6 years.
Test-Taking Strategy: Note the subject, the recommended childhood immunization schedule. Note that the infant is 2 months of age, and remember that a 2-month-old infant is scheduled for RV, PCV, IPV, Hib, and DTaP.
Priority Nursing Tip: Immunization produces active acquired immunity.
Reference: Hockenberry, M., Wilson, D., & Rodgers, C. (2019). *Wong's Nursing care of infants and children* (11th ed., pp. 170–172). Elsevier.

163. The nurse makes a home care visit to a client diagnosed with Bell's palsy. Which statement by the client indicates a **need for further teaching?**
1. "I wear an eye patch at night."
2. "I am staying on a liquid diet."
3. "I wear dark glasses when I go out."
4. "I have been gently massaging my face."

Level of Cognitive Ability: Evaluating
Client Needs: Health Promotion and Maintenance
Clinical Judgment/Cognitive Skills: Evaluate Outcomes
Integrated Process: Clinical Judgment; Nursing Process/Evaluation
Content Area: Adult Health: Neurologic
Health Problems: Adult Health: Neurologic: Bell's Palsy
Priority Concepts: Patient Education; Intracranial Regulation

Answer: 2
Rationale: Bell's palsy is caused by a lower motor neuron lesion of the seventh cranial nerve that may result from infection, trauma, hemorrhage, meningitis, or tumor. It is not necessary for a client diagnosed with Bell's palsy to stay on a liquid diet. The client needs to be encouraged to chew on the unaffected side. Wearing an eye patch at night, dark glasses for daytime outings, and gently massaging the face identify accurate statements related to the management of Bell's palsy.
Test-Taking Strategy: Note the strategic words, *need for further teaching.* These words indicate a negative event query and ask you to select an option that is an incorrect statement. Recalling that Bell's palsy relates to the face will assist you in eliminating options 1, 3, and 4, which are appropriate interventions.
Priority Nursing Tip: Bell's palsy results in paralysis of one side of the face. Recovery usually occurs in a few weeks, without residual effects.
Reference: Harding M., et al. (2023). *Lewis's Medical-surgical nursing: Assessment and management of clinical problems* (12th ed., pp. p. 1616. Elsevier.

❖ **164.** The home care nurse is evaluating a client's understanding of the self-management of trigeminal neuralgia. Which client statement indicates that there is a **need for further teaching?**
1. "I need to chew on my good side."
2. "An analgesic will relieve my pain."
3. "I need to use warm mouthwash for oral hygiene."
4. "Taking my carbamazepine will help control my pain."

Level of Cognitive Ability: Evaluating
Client Needs: Health Promotion and Maintenance
Clinical Judgment/Cognitive Skills: Clinical Judgment; Evaluate Outcomes
Integrated Process: Teaching and Learning
Content Area: Adult Health: Neurologic
Health Problems: Adult Health: Neurologic: Trigeminal Neuralgia
Priority Concepts: Patient Education; Intracranial Regulation

Answer: 2
Rationale: Chronic irritation of cranial nerve V results in trigeminal neuralgia, and it is characterized by intermittent episodes of intense pain of sudden onset on the affected side of the face. The pain is rarely relieved by analgesics. It is recommended that clients chew on the unaffected side and use warm mouthwash for oral hygiene. Medications such as carbamazepine help control the pain of trigeminal neuralgia.
Test-Taking Strategy: Note the strategic words, *need for further teaching.* These words indicate a negative event query and ask you to select an option that is an incorrect statement. Recalling that trigeminal neuralgia is characterized by intense pain will direct you to the correct option.
Priority Nursing Tip: Situations that stimulate symptoms in the client with trigeminal neuralgia include cold, washing the face, chewing, or consuming food or fluids of extreme temperatures.
Reference: Lewis, S., et al. (2020). *Medical-surgical nursing: Assessment and management of clinical problems* (11th ed., p. 1422). Elsevier.

165. The nurse is caring for a client diagnosed with type 1 diabetes mellitus. Because the client is at risk for hypoglycemia, which instructions would the nurse teach the client to follow?
1. Keep glucose tablets handy.
2. Monitor the urine for acetone.
3. Report any feelings of drowsiness.
4. Omit the evening dose of NPH insulin if the client has been exercising.

Level of Cognitive Ability: Applying
Client Needs: Health Promotion and Maintenance
Clinical Judgment/Cognitive Skills: Generate Solutions
Integrated Process: Teaching and Learning
Content Area: Adult Health: Endocrine
Health Problems: Adult Health: Endocrine: Diabetes Mellitus
Priority Concepts: Patient Education; Glucose Regulation

Answer: 1
Rationale: Glucose tablets are taken if a hypoglycemic reaction occurs. Glucagon is also a medication that may be prescribed to be administered subcutaneously or intramuscularly if the client loses consciousness and is unable to take glucose by mouth. Glucagon releases glycogen stores and raises the blood glucose levels of clients with hypoglycemia. Family members can be taught to administer this medication and possibly to prevent an emergency department visit. Acetone in the urine may indicate hyperglycemia. Although signs/symptoms of hypoglycemia need to be taught to the client, drowsiness is not the initial and key sign of this complication. The nurse would not instruct a client to omit insulin.
Test-Taking Strategy: Focus on the **subject**, a client diagnosed with type 1 diabetes mellitus who is at risk for hypoglycemia. Eliminate option 4 first because the nurse would not instruct a client to omit insulin doses. Acetone in the urine and drowsiness can be eliminated next because they are not related to the **subject** of hypoglycemia.
Priority Nursing Tip: Hypoglycemia in the client with diabetes mellitus is caused by too much insulin or oral hypoglycemic agents, too little food, or excessive activity.
Reference: Lewis, S., et al. (2020). *Medical-surgical nursing: Assessment and management of clinical problems* (11th ed., pp. 1125–1126). Elsevier.

❖ **166.** The nurse is caring for a client with a precipitous labor. What information would the nurse provide to the client regarding this type of labor?
1. Induction may be necessary.
2. The onset of contractions is gradual.
3. The labor may last less than 3 hours.
4. A lengthy period of pushing may be necessary.

Level of Cognitive Ability: Applying
Client Needs: Health Promotion and Maintenance
Clinical Judgment/Cognitive Skills: Take Action
Integrated Process: Nursing Process/Implementation
Content Area: Maternity: Intrapartum
Health Problems: Maternity: Precipitous Labor and Delivery
Priority Concepts: Patient Education; Reproduction

Answer: 3
Rationale: Precipitous labor is defined as labor that lasts 3 hours or less for the entire labor and delivery. It usually has an abrupt rather than a gradual onset. Induction, particularly with an oxytocic agent, is contraindicated because of the enhanced stimulatory effects on the uterine muscle and an increased risk for fetal hypoxia.
Test-Taking Strategy: Focus on the **subject**, precipitous labor. The word *precipitous* will assist you with defining this condition. Note the relationship between this word and "less than 3 hours" in option 3.
Priority Nursing Tip: In the event of a precipitous labor, do not try to keep the fetus from being delivered.
Reference: McKinney, E. S., et al. (2022). *Maternal child nursing* (6th ed., p. 585). Elsevier.

167. The nurse is instructing a pregnant client regarding measures to prevent a recurrent episode of preterm labor. Which statement by the client indicates the **need for further teaching?**
1. "I will report any feeling of pelvic pressure."
2. "I will not engage in sexual intercourse at this time."
3. "I will adhere to the limitations in activity and stay off my feet."
4. "I will limit my fluid intake to three 8-ounce glasses of fluid per day."

Level of Cognitive Ability: Evaluating
Client Needs: Health Promotion and Maintenance
Clinical Judgment/Cognitive Skills: Evaluate Outcomes
Integrated Process: Clinical Judgment; Nursing Process/Evaluation
Content Area: Maternity: Antepartum
Health Problems: Maternity: Preterm Labor
Priority Concepts: Patient Education; Reproduction

Answer: 4
Rationale: Risks for preterm labor include dehydration. A client would not restrict fluids (except for those containing alcohol and caffeine). A sign of preterm labor may be pelvic pressure without the perception of a contraction. Mechanical stimulation of the cervix during intercourse can stimulate contractions. A decrease in activity and bed rest are often prescribed in an attempt to decrease pressure on the cervix and to increase uterine blood flow.
Test-Taking Strategy: Note the **strategic words,** *need for further teaching.* These words indicate a **negative event query** and ask you to select an option that is an incorrect statement. Focusing on the **subject** of the prevention of preterm labor will direct you to the correct option. Remember that it is generally not a good practice for the client to limit fluid intake to three 8-ounce glasses of fluid per day.
Priority Nursing Tip: Preterm labor occurs after the 20th week but before the 37th week of gestation.
Reference: McKinney, E. S., et al. (2022). *Maternal child nursing* (6th ed., pp. 587–588). Elsevier.

❖ **168.** The nurse has completed discharge teaching with the parents of a child diagnosed with glomerulonephritis. Which statement by the parents indicates a **need for further teaching?**
1. "We'll check our child's blood pressure every day."
2. "We'll test our child's urine for albumin every week."
3. "It'll be so good to have our child back in tap-dancing classes next week."
4. "We'll be sure that our child eats a lot of vegetables and does not add extra salt to food."

Level of Cognitive Ability: Evaluating
Client Needs: Health Promotion and Maintenance
Clinical Judgment/Cognitive Skills: Clinical Judgment; Evaluate Outcomes
Integrated Process: Teaching and Learning
Content Area: Pediatrics: Renal and Urinary
Health Problems: Pediatric-Specific: Urinary Tract Infection
Priority Concepts: Patient Education; Safety

Answer: 3
Rationale: Tap dancing classes 1 week after discharge would be unrealistic and involve a too rapid increase in activity. Glomerulonephritis results in destruction, inflammation, and sclerosis of the glomeruli of the kidneys. After discharge, parents can allow the child to return to their normal routine and activities, with adequate periods allowed for rest. Taking daily blood pressure, testing urine weekly for albumin, and restricting extra sodium are appropriate home care measures.
Test-Taking Strategy: Note the **strategic words,** *need for further teaching.* These words indicate a **negative event query** and ask you to select an option that is an incorrect statement. Select option 3 because tap dancing is an aggressive exercise.
Priority Nursing Tip: For the child with glomerulonephritis, foods high in potassium are restricted during periods of oliguria.
Reference: McKinney, E. S., et al. (2022) *Maternal child nursing* (6th ed., p. 1023). Elsevier.

169. The nurse is planning discharge teaching for the parents of a child who sustained a head injury and who is now receiving tapering doses of dexamethasone. The nurse plans to make which statement to the parents?
1. "This medication decreases the chance of infection."
2. "This medication will be discontinued after two doses."
3. "If your child's face becomes puffy, the medication dose needs to be increased."
4. "This medication is tapered to decrease the chance of recurring swelling in the brain."

Level of Cognitive Ability: Applying
Client Needs: Health Promotion and Maintenance
Clinical Judgment/Cognitive Skills: Generate Solutions
Integrated Process: Teaching and Learning
Content Area: Pharmacology: Endocrine: Corticosteroids
Health Problems: Pediatric-Specific: Head Injury
Priority Concepts: Patient Education; Safety

Answer: 4
Rationale: Dexamethasone sodium phosphate is a corticosteroid. The rebounding of cerebral edema is a side effect of dexamethasone sodium phosphate withdrawal if it is done abruptly. This medication decreases inflammation rather than infection. Facial edema is a common side effect that disappears when the medication is discontinued.
Test-Taking Strategy: Focus on the subject, a client taking dexamethasone sodium phosphate. Recall that this medication is a corticosteroid. Remember that tapering is required with corticosteroids to prevent a rebound effect as a result of adrenal insufficiency.
Priority Nursing Tip: Monitor the client receiving a corticosteroid for hypokalemia and hyperglycemia.
Reference: Hockenberry, M., Wilson, D., & Rodgers, C. (2019). *Wong's Nursing care of infants and children* (11th ed., pp. 153, 1123). Elsevier.

170. The nurse has implemented a plan of care for a client diagnosed with a cervical 5 (C5) spinal cord injury to promote health maintenance. Which client outcome indicates the **effectiveness** of the plan?
1. Maintenance of intact skin
2. Regaining of bladder and bowel control
3. Performance of activities of daily living independently
4. Independent transfer of self to and from the wheelchair

Level of Cognitive Ability: Evaluating
Client Needs: Health Promotion and Maintenance
Clinical Judgment/Cognitive Skills: Evaluate Outcomes
Integrated Process: Clinical Judgment; Nursing Process/Evaluation
Content Area: Adult Health: Neurologic
Health Problems: Adult Health: Neurologic: Spinal Cord Injury
Priority Concepts: Clinical Judgment; Intracranial Regulation

Answer: 1
Rationale: A C5 spinal cord injury results in quadriplegia with no sensation below the clavicle, including most of the arms and hands. The client maintains the partial movement of the shoulders and elbows. Maintaining intact skin is an outcome for spinal cord injury clients. The remaining options are inappropriate for this client.
Test-Taking Strategy: Note the strategic word, *effectiveness.* Focus on the subject, a client with a C5 spinal cord injury. Eliminate independent performance of daily activities and independent transfer to and from the wheelchair first because they are comparable or alike as both deal with independence in daily activities. From the remaining options, recalling the effects of a C5 spinal cord injury will assist you in eliminating regaining bowel and bladder function because it is unrealistic.
Priority Nursing Tip: The level of the spinal cord injury is assessed as the lowest spinal cord segment with intact motor and sensory function.
Reference: Lewis, S., et al. (2020). *Medical-surgical nursing: Assessment and management of clinical problems* (11th ed., pp. 1408–1409, 1418). Elsevier.

171. The home care nurse visits a child diagnosed with scarlet fever who is being treated with penicillin G potassium. The parent tells the nurse that the child has only voided a small amount of tea-colored urine since the previous day. The parent also reports that the child's appetite has decreased and that the child's face was swollen this morning. How would the nurse interpret these new signs/symptoms?

1. Nothing to be concerned about
2. Signs/symptoms of acute glomerulonephritis
3. Signs/symptoms of the normal progression of scarlet fever
4. Symptoms of an allergic reaction to penicillin G potassium

Level of Cognitive Ability: Analyzing
Client Needs: Health Promotion and Maintenance
Clinical Judgment/Cognitive Skills: Analyze Cues
Integrated Process: Clinical Judgment; Nursing Process/Analysis
Content Area: Pharmacology: Immune: Penicillins
Health Problems: Pediatric-Specific: Infectious/Communicable Diseases
Priority Concepts: Elimination; Infection

Answer: 2
Rationale: Scarlet fever is an infectious and communicable disease caused by group A beta-hemolytic streptococci. The signs/symptoms identified in the question indicate acute glomerulonephritis, indicative of nephrotoxicity. These signs/symptoms are not normal and should not be ignored. Although the child is receiving penicillin G potassium, these are not signs/symptoms of an allergic reaction.
Test-Taking Strategy: Eliminate option 1 and option 3 because these options are comparable or alike in that both reinforce normalcy. From the remaining options, recalling the complications of scarlet fever and the signs/symptoms of a medication reaction will direct you to the correct option.
Priority Nursing Tip: Scarlet fever is transmitted by direct contact with an infected person or droplet spread or indirectly by contact with contaminated articles or the ingestion of contaminated milk or other foods.
Reference: McKinney, E. S., et al. (2022). *Maternal child nursing* (6th ed., pp. 922, 1023). Elsevier.

❖ 172. A client who sustained a thoracic cord injury a year ago returns to the clinic for a follow-up visit, and the nurse notes a small reddened area on the coccyx. The client is not aware of the reddened area. After counseling the client to relieve pressure on the area by adhering to a turning schedule, which action by the nurse is **most appropriate?**

1. Teaching the client to feel for reddened areas
2. Asking a family member to assess the skin daily
3. Teaching the client to use a mirror for skin assessment
4. Scheduling the client to return to the clinic daily for a skin check

Level of Cognitive Ability: Applying
Client Needs: Health Promotion and Maintenance
Clinical Judgment/Cognitive Skills: Take Action
Integrated Process: Clinical Judgment; Nursing Process/Implementation
Content Area: Adult Health: Neurologic
Health Problems: Adult Health: Neurologic: Spinal Cord Injury
Priority Concepts: Patient Education; Tissue Integrity

Answer: 3
Rationale: The client needs to be encouraged to be as independent as possible. The most effective means of skin self-assessment for this client is with the use of a mirror. The redness cannot be felt. Asking a family member to assess the skin daily does not promote independence. It is unnecessary and unrealistic for the client to return to the clinic daily for a skin check.
Test-Taking Strategy: Note the strategic words, *most appropriate.* Recall that independence is vital to the rehabilitation of clients. Asking a family member to make a daily skin inspection or having the client return to the clinic daily for skin inspection involves others in performing a task that the client can do independently. Feeling for redness is an inaccurate assessment technique because redness cannot be felt. Teaching the client to use a mirror to assess skin integrity is the only option that addresses client self-assessment.
Priority Nursing Tip: Autonomic dysreflexia may occur with lesions or injuries above T6 and in cervical lesions.
Reference: Lewis, S., et al. (2020). *Medical-surgical nursing: Assessment and management of clinical problems* (11th ed., pp. 172, 1411–1412). Elsevier.

173. The nurse has given instructions to a client who is returning home after an arthroscopy of the knee. The nurse determines that the client understands the home care instructions if the client states the need to follow which instruction?

1. Resume strenuous exercise the following day.
2. Stay off the leg entirely for the rest of the day.
3. Refrain from eating food for the remainder of the day.
4. Report fever or site inflammation to the surgeon.

Level of Cognitive Ability: Evaluating
Client Needs: Health Promotion and Maintenance
Clinical Judgment/Cognitive Skills: Evaluate Outcomes
Integrated Process: Clinical Judgment; Nursing Process/Evaluation
Content Area: Foundations of Care: Diagnostic Tests
Health Problems: Adult Health: Musculoskeletal: Skeletal Injury
Priority Concepts: Patient Education; Health Promotion

Answer: 4
Rationale: After arthroscopy, signs/symptoms of infection need to be reported to the surgeon. The client is instructed to avoid strenuous exercise for at least a few days; however, the client can usually walk carefully on the leg after sensation has returned. The client may resume the usual diet.
Test-Taking Strategy: Focus on the subject, a client returning home after arthroscopy. Recalling that the procedure is invasive will direct you to reporting fever and signs of site inflammation. Additionally, the client is always taught which signs/symptoms of infection to report to the surgeon.
Priority Nursing Tip: An arthroscopy allows for an endoscopic examination of various joints and is done to diagnose and treat acute and chronic disorders of the joint.
Reference: Ignatavicius, D., et al. (2021). *Medical-surgical nursing: Concepts for interprofessional collaborative care* (10th ed., pp. 981–982). Elsevier.

❖ **174.** Allopurinol has been prescribed for a client to treat gouty arthritis. The nurse would tell the client to anticipate which prescription if an acute attack occurs?

1. Doubling the dose of the allopurinol
2. Stopping the allopurinol and taking acetylsalicylic acid (aspirin)
3. Stopping the allopurinol and taking a nonsteroidal antiinflammatory drug
4. Adding colchicine or a nonsteroidal antiinflammatory drug to the treatment plan

Level of Cognitive Ability: Applying
Client Needs: Health Promotion and Maintenance
Clinical Judgment/Cognitive Skills: Generate Solutions
Integrated Process: Teaching and Learning
Content Area: Pharmacology: Musculoskeletal: Antigout
Health Problems: Adult Health: Musculoskeletal: Gout
Priority Concepts: Patient Education; Pain

Answer: 4
Rationale: Allopurinol helps prevent an attack of gouty arthritis, but it does not relieve the pain. Therefore, another medication such as colchicine or a nonsteroidal antiinflammatory drug must be added if an acute attack occurs. Because acute attacks may occur more frequently early during the course of therapy with allopurinol, some primary health care providers recommend taking the two products concurrently during the first 3 to 6 months.
Test-Taking Strategy: Eliminate options 2 and 3 first because it is unlikely that medication will be stopped. From the remaining options, focus on the subject, gouty arthritis; recalling that an acute attack of gouty arthritis is painful will assist you with selecting option 4 because of the antiinflammatory action of the nonsteroidal antiinflammatory drug.
Priority Nursing Tip: Gout is a systemic disease in which urate crystals deposit in joints and other body tissues. Elevated uric acid levels can cause uric acid renal stones to form.
Reference: Lewis, S., et al. (2020). *Medical-surgical nursing: Assessment and management of clinical problems* (11th ed., pp. 1514–1515). Elsevier.

175. The nursing student is providing care to a preschooler diagnosed with an immunocompromised condition. The nursing instructor is reviewing with the nursing student a list of potential immunizations to be administered. The nursing instructor determines that the student understands the immunization schedule if the student identifies which as safe to administer to this child? **Select all that apply.**

- ❏ 1. OPV
- ❏ 2. MMR
- ❏ 3. DTaP
- ❏ 4. Varicella
- ❏ 5. Influenza
- ❏ 6. Meningococcal

Level of Cognitive Ability: Evaluating
Client Needs: Health Promotion and Maintenance
Clinical Judgment/Cognitive Skills: Evaluate Outcomes
Integrated Process: Teaching and Learning
Content Area: Pediatrics: Infectious and Communicable Diseases
Health Problems: Pediatric-Specific: Immunizations
Priority Concepts: Health Promotion; Immunity

Answer: 3, 5, 6
Rationale: DTaP, influenza, and meningococcal immunizations are recommended for clients who are immunocompromised. Either these vaccines provide passive immunity or the risk of complications from the potential illness outweigh the risk of the immunization. An individual who is immunocompromised, under ordinary circumstances, should not receive a live or attenuated vaccine. OPV, MMR, and varicella are all categorized as live or attenuated vaccines.
Test-Taking Strategy: Focus on the subject, immunizations that are safe to administer to the immunocompromised individual. Recognizing that this child should not typically receive a live or attenuated viral immunization will assist in eliminating OPV, MMR, and varicella.
Priority Nursing Tip: It is important for the nurse to store vaccines and to reconstitute the vaccine according to manufacturer's directions.
Reference: McKinney, E. S., et al. (2022). *Maternal child nursing* (6th ed., p. 77). Elsevier.

❖ **176.** A client with hypertension has received a prescription for lisinopril. The nurse teaches the client that which frequent side effect may occur?
1. Cough
2. Polyuria
3. Hypothermia
4. Hypertension

Level of Cognitive Ability: Applying
Client Needs: Health Promotion and Maintenance
Clinical Judgment/Cognitive Skills: Take Action
Integrated Process: Teaching and Learning
Content Area: Pharmacology: Cardiovascular: Angiotensin-Converting Enzyme (ACE) Inhibitors
Health Problems: Adult Health: Cardiovascular: Hypertension
Priority Concepts: Patient Education; Safety

Answer: 1
Rationale: Cough is a frequent side effect of therapy with any of the angiotensin-converting enzyme (ACE) inhibitors. Fever is an occasional side effect. Proteinuria is another common side effect, but polyuria is not. Hypertension is the reason to administer the medication rather than a side effect.
Test-Taking Strategy: Focus on the subject, a frequent side effect of lisinopril. Recalling that most ACE inhibitor medication names end in "-pril" and that ACE inhibitors are used to treat hypertension will assist you in eliminating option 4. From the remaining options, it is necessary to know that cough is a frequent side effect of these medications.
Priority Nursing Tip: Hypoglycemic reactions can occur in the client diagnosed with diabetes mellitus who is taking an ACE inhibitor.
Reference: Kizior, R., & Hodgson, B. (2023). *Saunders Nursing drug handbook 2023* (pp. 702–704). Elsevier.

177. The nurse has provided home-care instructions to a client who is taking lithium carbonate. Which client statement indicates that the client understands the prescribed regimen?
1. "I will restrict my water intake."
2. "I will make sure that my diet contains salt."
3. "I will keep my medication in the refrigerator."
4. "I will be careful to avoid eating foods high in potassium."

Level of Cognitive Ability: Evaluating
Client Needs: Health Promotion and Maintenance
Clinical Judgment/Cognitive Skills: Evaluate Outcomes
Integrated Process: Clinical Judgment; Nursing Process/Evaluation
Content Area: Pharmacology: Psychotherapeutics: Mood Stabilizers
Health Problems: Mental Health: Mood Disorders
Priority Concepts: Patient Education; Safety

Answer: 2
Rationale: Lithium is a mood stabilizer used to treat bipolar disorder. It replaces sodium ions in the cells and induces the excretion of sodium and potassium from the body. Client teaching includes the maintenance of sodium intake in the daily diet and increased fluid intake (at least 1 to 1½ L/day) during maintenance therapy. Lithium is stored at room temperature and protected from light and moisture.
Test-Taking Strategy: Focus on the subject, client teaching points for lithium carbonate. Recalling that lithium is a salt that replaces sodium ions and induces the excretion of sodium and potassium will direct you to the correct option.
Priority Nursing Tip: Blood samples to check serum lithium levels need to be drawn in the morning, 12 hours after the last dose was taken.
Reference: Varcarolis, E. & Fosbre, C. (2021). *Essentials of psychiatric mental health nursing: A communication approach to evidence-based care* (4th ed., pp. 237, 241). Elsevier.

❖ **178.** A client is given a prescription for an antipsychotic medication. The nurse instructs the client and family to report any signs/symptoms of pseudoparkinsonism and tells the family to monitor for effects that are indicative of this medication complication?
1. Tremors and hyperpyrexia
2. Motor restlessness and aphasia
3. Stooped posture and a shuffling gait
4. Muscle weakness and decreased salivation

Level of Cognitive Ability: Applying
Client Needs: Health Promotion and Maintenance
Clinical Judgment/Cognitive Skills: Recognize Cues
Integrated Process: Teaching and Learning
Content Area: Pharmacology: Psychotherapeutics: Antipsychotics
Health Problems: Mental Health: Schizophrenia
Priority Concepts: Patient Education; Safety

Answer: 3
Rationale: Pseudoparkinsonism is a common extrapyramidal side effect of antipsychotic medications. This condition is characterized by a stooped posture, a shuffling gait, a masklike facial appearance, drooling, tremors, and pill-rolling motions of the fingers. Hyperpyrexia is characteristic of the extrapyramidal side effect of neuroleptic malignant syndrome. Motor restlessness, aphasia, muscle weakness, and decreased salivation are not characteristic of pseudoparkinsonism.
Test-Taking Strategy: Focus on the subject, signs/symptoms of pseudoparkinsonism. Recalling the characteristics of Parkinson's disease will direct you to the correct option.
Priority Nursing Tip: Antipsychotic medications improve the thought processes and the behavior of the client with psychotic symptoms, especially clients with schizophrenia.
Reference: Varcarolis, E. & Fosbre, C. (2021). *Essentials of psychiatric mental health nursing: A communication approach to evidence-based care* (4th ed., p. 272). Elsevier.

179. A client who is taking tranylcypromine sulfate requests information about foods that are acceptable to eat while taking the medication. Which foods are safe to consume while taking this medication?
1. Yogurt
2. Raisins
3. Oranges
4. Smoked fish

Level of Cognitive Ability: Applying
Client Needs: Health Promotion and Maintenance
Clinical Judgment/Cognitive Skills: Generate Solutions
Integrated Process: Teaching and Learning
Content Area: Pharmacology: Psychotherapeutics: Monoamine Oxidase Inhibitors (MAOIs)
Health Problems: Mental Health: Mood Disorders
Priority Concepts: Patient Education; Safety

Answer: 3
Rationale: Tranylcypromine sulfate is classified as a MAOI; as such, tyramine-containing food need to be avoided. Oranges are permissible. Types of food to be avoided include, but are not limited to, yogurt, raisins, and smoked fish. Additionally, beer, wine, caffeinated beverages, pickled meats, yeast preparations, avocados, bananas, and plums are to be avoided.
Test-Taking Strategy: The food items in options 1, 2, and 4 are comparable or alike as they have high levels of tyramine. These are food items that are either processed or that contain some type of additive. The only natural food is oranges. Remember that, although bananas, avocados, and plums are natural foods, they are not permitted while taking an MAOI.
Priority Nursing Tip: Instruct the client taking an antipsychotic medication to report signs/symptoms of agranulocytosis, including sore throat, fever, and malaise.
Reference: Varcarolis, E. & Fosbre, C. (2021). *Essentials of psychiatric mental health nursing: A communication approach to evidence-based care* (4th ed., pp. 218, 220). Elsevier.

❖ **180.** The nurse is performing an assessment on a 3-year-old child with chicken pox. The child's parent tells the nurse that the child keeps scratching at night, and the nurse teaches the parent about measures that will prevent an alteration in skin integrity. Which statement by the parent indicates that teaching was **effective**?
1. "I need to place white gloves on my child's hands at night."
2. "I will apply generous amounts of a cortisone cream to prevent itching."
3. "I will give my child a glass of warm milk at bedtime to help my child sleep."
4. "I need to keep my child in a warm room at night so that the covers will not cause my child to scratch."

Level of Cognitive Ability: Evaluating
Client Needs: Health Promotion and Maintenance
Clinical Judgment/Cognitive Skills: Evaluate Outcomes
Integrated Process: Clinical Judgment; Nursing Process/Evaluation
Content Area: Pediatrics: Infectious and Communicable Diseases
Health Problems: Pediatric-Specific: Infectious/Communicable Diseases
Priority Concepts: Patient Education; Tissue Integrity

Answer: 1
Rationale: Gloves will keep the child from causing an alteration in skin integrity from scratching. Generous amounts of any topical cream can lead to medication toxicity. Warm milk will have no effect on itching. A warm room will increase the child's skin temperature and make the itching worse.
Test-Taking Strategy: Note the strategic word, *effective*. Note the subject, preventing an alteration in skin integrity in a 3-year-old child with chicken pox. Eliminate the warm room first because this action will promote itching. Consuming warm milk is eliminated next because it is unrelated to skin integrity. From the remaining options, the words *generous amounts* in option 2 provides you with a clue that this option is incorrect.
Priority Nursing Tip: Isolate high-risk children, such as children who have immunosuppressive disorders, from a child with a communicable disease.
Reference: Hockenberry, M., Wilson, D., & Rodgers, C. (2019). *Wong's Nursing care of infants and children* (11th ed., p. 180). Elsevier.

181. The nurse is providing instructions to a client with peptic ulcer disease about symptom management. Which statement by the client indicates that teaching was **effective?**
1. "I need to eat a snack at bedtime."
2. "I can take aspirin to relieve gastric pain."
3. "I need to take my antacid and famotidine at the same time."
4. "It is important that I eat slowly and chew my food thoroughly."

Level of Cognitive Ability: Evaluating
Client Needs: Health Promotion and Maintenance
Clinical Judgment/Cognitive Skills: Evaluate Outcomes
Integrated Process: Clinical Judgment; Nursing Process/Evaluation
Content Area: Adult Health: Gastrointestinal
Health Problems: Adult Health: Gastrointestinal: Peptic Ulcer Disease
Priority Concepts: Patient Education; Health Promotion

Answer: 4
Rationale: Eating slowly and chewing thoroughly helps prevent overdistention and reflux. Bedtime snacks are avoided because they can promote nighttime acid secretion. Acetaminophen is administered for routine pain relief during treatment. All nonsteroidal antiinflammatory drugs and aspirin are avoided. Antacids will interfere with the absorption of famotidine, a histamine-2 (H_2) receptor antagonist, and, therefore, should not be taken concurrently.
Test-Taking Strategy: Note the strategic word, *effective.* Focus on the subject, peptic ulcer disease and client teaching about the disorder. Use the concepts related to digestion to direct you to option 4.
Priority Nursing Tip: Famotidine is an H_2 receptor antagonist that suppresses the secretion of gastric acid, alleviates the symptoms of heartburn, and assists in preventing the complications associated with peptic ulcer disease.
Reference: Ignatavicius, D., et al. (2021). *Medical-surgical nursing: Concepts for interprofessional collaborative care* (10th ed., pp. 1101–1102). Elsevier.

❖ **182.** A client with a hiatal hernia asks the nurse about fluids that are safe to drink and that will not irritate the gastric mucosa. What fluid would the nurse tell the client to drink?
1. Apple juice
2. Orange juice
3. Tomato juice
4. Grapefruit juice

Level of Cognitive Ability: Applying
Client Needs: Health Promotion and Maintenance
Clinical Judgment/Cognitive Skills: Take Action
Integrated Process: Nursing Process/Implementation
Content Area: Foundations of Care: Therapeutic Diets
Health Problems: Adult Health: Gastrointestinal: Hernias
Priority Concepts: Nutrition; Tissue Integrity

Answer: 1
Rationale: Substances that are irritating to the client with hiatal hernia include tomato products and citrus fruits, which need to be avoided. Because caffeine stimulates gastric acid secretion, beverages that contain caffeine, such as coffee, tea, cola, and cocoa are also eliminated from the diet.
Test-Taking Strategy: Eliminate orange, tomato, and grapefruit juices because they are comparable or alike and are all citrus products. Additionally, apple juice is the least irritating to the stomach.
Priority Nursing Tip: With hiatal hernia, a portion of the stomach herniates through the diaphragm and into the thorax.
References: Ignatavicius, D., et al. (2021). *Medical-surgical nursing: Concepts for interprofessional collaborative care* (10th ed., p. 1081). Elsevier; Nix, S. (2022). *Williams' Basic nutrition and diet therapy* (16th ed., pp. 322, 527). Elsevier.

183. The nurse determines that the client with gastroesophageal reflux disease (GERD) **needs further teaching** regarding diet if which statement is made?
1. "I need to avoid coffee, tea, and chocolate."
2. "I should eat four to six small meals a day."
3. "It is important that I drink extra fluids during meals."
4. "I need to avoid snacking for 2 to 3 hours before bedtime."

Level of Cognitive Ability: Evaluating
Client Needs: Health Promotion and Maintenance
Clinical Judgment/Cognitive Skills: Evaluate Outcomes
Integrated Process: Clinical Judgment; Teaching and Learning
Content Area: Adult Health: Gastrointestinal
Health Problems: Adult Health: Gastrointestinal: Gastroesophageal Reflux Disease
Priority Concepts: Patient Education; Health Promotion

Answer: 3
Rationale: GERD is the backflow of gastric and duodenal contents into the esophagus. Fluids must be taken between meals rather than with meals to prevent the overdistention that leads to reflux. Coffee, tea, cola, and chocolate are eliminated from the diet because they decrease lower esophageal sphincter pressure and can potentiate reflux. Four to six smaller meals per day will help to prevent gastric overdistention. One of the primary factors in GERD is an incompetent lower esophageal sphincter. Adequate time needs to pass after snacking and before bedtime to decrease the risk for the reflux of gastric contents.
Test-Taking Strategy: Focus on the **strategic words**, *needs further teaching*. These words indicate a **negative event query** and the need to select the incorrect client statement. Think about the pathophysiology associated with this disorder to answer correctly. Eliminate options that indicate that the client has a proper understanding of the dietary management of GERD.
Priority Nursing Tip: Manifestations of GERD include heartburn, epigastric pain, dyspepsia, regurgitation, pain and difficulty with swallowing, and hypersalivation.
Reference: Nix, S. (2022). *Williams' Basic nutrition and diet therapy* (16th ed., p. 322). Elsevier.

❖ **184.** When preparing the client with a spinal cord injury who is experiencing bladder spasms and reflex incontinence for discharge to home, the nurse would provide which instruction to prevent the problem?
1. "Avoid caffeine in your diet."
2. "Take your temperature every day."
3. "Limit your fluid intake to 1000 mL/24 hours."
4. "Catheterize yourself every 2 hours as needed to prevent spasm."

Level of Cognitive Ability: Applying
Client Needs: Health Promotion and Maintenance
Clinical Judgment/Cognitive Skills: Generate Solutions
Integrated Process: Teaching and Learning
Content Area: Adult Health: Neurologic
Health Problems: Adult Health: Neurologic: Spinal Cord Injury
Priority Concepts: Patient Education; Elimination

Answer: 1
Rationale: Caffeine in the diet can contribute to bladder spasms and reflex incontinence; thus, it should be eliminated in the diet of the client with a spinal cord injury. The self-monitoring of the temperature is useful to detect infection, but it does nothing to alleviate bladder spasms. Limiting fluid intake does not prevent spasm, and it could place the client at further risk for urinary tract infection. Self-catheterization every 2 hours is too frequent and serves no useful purpose.
Test-Taking Strategy: Focus on the **subject**, preventive measures for bladder spasms and reflex incontinence. Eliminate options 3 and 4 first because they place the client at increased risk for urinary tract infection and are, therefore, not appropriate. From the remaining options, eliminate option 2 because this action would detect infection but does not deal with spasms and incontinence.
Priority Nursing Tip: For the client with a spinal cord injury, it is important for the nurse to institute measures to prevent urinary retention. Initiating a bladder control program and ensuring that the client maintains a fluid intake of 2000 mL/day are important measures.
Reference: Ignatavicius, D., et al. (2021). *Medical-surgical nursing: Concepts for interprofessional collaborative care* (10th ed., pp. 885, 1335). Elsevier.

❖ **185.** A client is diagnosed with organic erectile dysfunction, and the nurse is collecting subjective data from the client. After the assessment, the nurse explains to the client that which are causes of this disorder? **Select all that apply.**

- ❑ **1.** Stress
- ❑ **2.** Depression
- ❑ **3.** Hypertension
- ❑ **4.** Vascular disease
- ❑ **5.** Diabetes mellitus
- ❑ **6.** Alcohol consumption

Level of Cognitive Ability: Applying
Client Needs: Health Promotion and Maintenance
Clinical Judgment/Cognitive Skills: Take Action
Integrated Process: Teaching and Learning
Content Area: Adult Health: Reproductive
Health Problems: Adult Health: Reproductive: Menstruation Problems/Fertility/Infertility
Priority Concepts: Patient Education; Sexuality

Answer: 3, 4, 5, 6
Rationale: Erectile dysfunction is the inability to achieve or maintain an erection for sexual intercourse. Organic erectile dysfunction is a gradual deterioration of function; the person first notices diminishing firmness and a decrease in frequency of erections. Causes include inflammation of the prostate, urethra, or seminal vesicles; surgical procedures such as prostatectomy; pelvic fractures or lumbosacral injuries; vascular diseases, including hypertension; chronic neurologic conditions such as Parkinson's disease or multiple sclerosis; endocrine disorders such as diabetes mellitus or thyroid disorders; smoking and alcohol consumption; drugs; and poor overall health. Functional (not organic) erectile dysfunction usually has a psychological cause.
Test-Taking Strategy: Focus on the subject, cause of organic erectile dysfunction. Noting the word *organic* and recalling that these types of disorders have a physiologic cause will direct you to the correct options.
Priority Nursing Tip: Some factors that cause erectile dysfunction are modifiable, such as smoking and alcohol consumption. It is important for the nurse to inform the client of these modifiable factors and provide assistance in seeking necessary support services.
Reference: Lewis, S., et al. (2020). *Medical-surgical nursing: Assessment and management of clinical problems* (11th ed., p. 1273). Elsevier.

❖ **186.** Following a teaching session, the nurse determines that the client diagnosed with atherosclerosis understands dietary modifications to lower the risk of heart disease if which food selection is made?

1. Roast beef
2. Fresh cantaloupe
3. Broiled cheeseburger
4. Mashed potato with gravy

Level of Cognitive Ability: Evaluating
Client Needs: Health Promotion and Maintenance
Clinical Judgment/Cognitive Skills: Evaluate Outcomes
Integrated Process: Clinical Judgment; Nursing Process/Evaluation
Content Area: Foundations of Care: Therapeutic Diets
Health Problems: Adult Health: Cardiovascular: Coronary Artery Disease
Priority Concepts: Health Promotion; Nutrition

Answer: 2
Rationale: To lower the risk of heart disease, the diet needs to be low in saturated fat with the appropriate number of total calories. The client needs to eat less red meat (roast beef, cheeseburger) and eat more white meat with the skin removed. Dairy products used need to be low in fat, and foods with high amounts of empty calories (white gravy) need to be avoided.
Test-Taking Strategy: Focus on the subject, lowering the risk of heart disease. Use the fat content of the foods in the options as a guide to answering this question. Eliminate options 1 and 3 first because of the fat content of the described meats. From the remaining options, eliminate option 4 because only fresh fruits and vegetables are naturally low in fat.
Priority Nursing Tip: The nurse needs to stress to the client with coronary artery disease that the necessary dietary changes to prevent complications are not temporary and need to be maintained for life.
References: Lewis, S., et al. (2020). *Medical-surgical nursing: Assessment and management of clinical problems* (11th ed., pp. 703–705). Elsevier; Nix, S. (2022). *Williams' Basic nutrition and diet therapy* (16th ed., pp. 350–351). Elsevier.

187. A client being discharged to home after angioplasty via the right femoral groin has received the catheter insertion site discharge instructions from the nurse. Which client statement indicates that the client understands the instructions?
1. "Coolness or discoloration of the right foot is expected."
2. "I should expect a large area of bruising at the right groin."
3. "Temperature as high as 101° F (38.3° C) is not unusual a few days after the procedure."
4. "Mild discomfort in the right groin may occur, and acetaminophen should relieve the pain."

Level of Cognitive Ability: Evaluating
Client Needs: Health Promotion and Maintenance
Clinical Judgment/Cognitive Skills: Evaluate Outcomes
Integrated Process: Clinical Judgment; Nursing Process/Evaluation
Content Area: Adult Health: Cardiovascular
Health Problems: Adult Health: Cardiovascular: Coronary Artery Disease
Priority Concepts: Patient Education; Perfusion

Answer: 4
Rationale: The client may feel some mild discomfort at the catheter insertion site after angioplasty. This is usually relieved by analgesics such as acetaminophen. The client is taught to report to the primary health care provider any neurovascular changes to the affected leg; bleeding or bruising at the insertion site; and signs/symptoms of local infection, such as drainage at the site or increased temperature.
Test-Taking Strategy: Focus on the subject, client instructions after angioplasty. Knowing that bleeding and infection are complications of the procedure guides you in eliminating options 2 and 3. From the remaining options, eliminate option 1, knowing that neurovascular status should not be impaired by the procedure or by knowing that the area may be mildly uncomfortable.
Priority Nursing Tip: After angioplasty, the nurse needs to keep the client on bed rest and maintain the affected extremity in a straight position for 6 to 8 hours (or as prescribed).
Reference: Ignatavicius, D., et al. (2021). *Medical-surgical nursing: Concepts for interprofessional collaborative care* (10th ed., pp. 628–630). Elsevier.

188. The nurse is teaching dietary modifications to the client being treated for hypertension. The nurse would instruct the client to eat which snack foods? **Select all that apply.**
1. Raw carrots
2. Celery stalks
3. Frozen pizza
4. Cheese and crackers
5. Canned tomato soup

Level of Cognitive Ability: Applying
Client Needs: Health Promotion and Maintenance
Clinical Judgment/Cognitive Skills: Generate Solutions
Integrated Process: Teaching and Learning
Content Area: Foundations of Care: Therapeutic Diets
Health Problems: Adult Health: Cardiovascular: Hypertension
Priority Concepts: Patient Education; Nutrition

Answer: 1, 2
Rationale: Sodium needs to be avoided by the client with hypertension. Fresh fruits and vegetables such as carrots and celery are naturally lower in sodium. Hypertensive clients are also advised to keep fat intake to less than 30% of their total calories as part of prudent heart living. Each of the incorrect options contains high amounts of sodium, and frozen pizza and cheese and crackers are also likely to be higher in fat.
Test-Taking Strategy: Focus on the subject, the dietary modifications needed with hypertension. Eliminate frozen pizza, cheese and crackers, and canned tomato soup because they are comparable or alike as all are processed food items and have a high sodium value.
Priority Nursing Tip: A goal of treatment for the client with hypertension is to lower the blood pressure and prevent or lessen the extent of any organ damage.
Reference: Ignatavicius, D., et al. (2021). *Medical-surgical nursing: Concepts for interprofessional collaborative care* (10th ed., pp. 700–701). Elsevier.

189. The nurse teaches a client with hypertension to recognize the signs/symptoms that may occur during periods of elevated blood pressure. The nurse determines that the client has a **need for further teaching** if the client states that which sign/symptom is associated with this condition?
1. Epistaxis
2. Dizziness
3. Blurred vision
4. A feeling of fullness in the head

Level of Cognitive Ability: Evaluating
Client Needs: Health Promotion and Maintenance
Clinical Judgment/Cognitive Skills: Evaluate Outcomes
Integrated Process: Clinical Judgment; Nursing Process/Evaluation
Content Area: Adult Health: Cardiovascular
Health Problems: Adult Health: Cardiovascular: Hypertension
Priority Concepts: Patient Education; Perfusion

Answer: 4
Rationale: A feeling of fullness in the head is more likely associated with a sinus condition than hypertension. Cerebrovascular symptoms of hypertension include early morning headaches, occipital headaches, epistaxis, dizziness, blurred vision, lightheadedness, and vertigo. The client needs to be aware of these signs/symptoms and report them if they occur. The client needs to also be taught to self-monitor the blood pressure.
Test-Taking Strategy: Note the strategic words, *need for further teaching.* These words indicate a negative event query and ask you to select an option that is an incorrect sign or symptom. Focus on the subject, signs/symptoms of an elevated blood pressure. A feeling of fullness in the head is the vague option, whereas epistaxis, dizziness, and blurred vision are specific and related to hypertension.
Priority Nursing Tip: There is no known cause for primary (essential) hypertension. Secondary hypertension occurs as a result of other diseases or conditions.
Reference: Ignatavicius, D., et al. (2021). *Medical-surgical nursing: Concepts for interprofessional collaborative care* (10th ed., p. 705). Elsevier.

❖ 190. Which instruction would the nurse include in the teaching plan for a client taking iron supplements to correct iron-deficiency anemia?
1. Eat a low-fiber diet.
2. Limit the intake of fluids.
3. Limit the intake of meat, fish, and poultry.
4. Avoid taking the iron supplements with milk or antacids.

Level of Cognitive Ability: Applying
Client Needs: Health Promotion and Maintenance
Clinical Judgment/Cognitive Skills: Generate Solutions
Integrated Process: Teaching and Learning
Content Area: Foundations of Care: Therapeutic Diets
Health Problems: Adult Health: Hematologic: Anemias
Priority Concepts: Patient Education; Nutrition

Answer: 4
Rationale: The client needs to avoid taking the iron supplements with milk or antacids because these items decrease the absorption of iron. The client needs to also avoid taking the iron with food, if possible. Finally, the client needs to take in sufficient fiber and fluids to prevent constipation as a side effect of iron therapy. The client should increase the intake of natural sources of iron, such as meats, fish, and poultry.
Test-Taking Strategy: Focus on the subject, iron supplements. Eliminate a low-fiber diet and restricting fluids because constipation is a common side effect of iron therapy. Recalling that meat products contain iron helps you eliminate option 3 next. Remember that several medications have impaired absorption with milk products or antacids.
Priority Nursing Tip: Liquid iron preparations can stain the teeth. The client taking iron in the liquid form needs to be instructed to use a straw to take the medication and perform mouth care after taking the medication.
Reference: Lilley, L., Rainforth Collins, S., & Snyder J. (2020). *Pharmacology and the nursing process* (9th ed., pp. 846–847, 850). Elsevier.

Client Needs

191. A client with a colostomy reports a concern about appliance odor. The nurse recommends that the client use a deodorizing pouch and consume which deodorizing foods to decrease the odor?
1. Eggs
2. Yogurt
3. Cucumbers
4. Mushrooms

Level of Cognitive Ability: Applying
Client Needs: Health Promotion and Maintenance
Clinical Judgment/Cognitive Skills: Generate Solutions
Integrated Process: Teaching and Learning
Content Area: Adult Health: Gastrointestinal
Health Problems: Adult Health: Gastrointestinal: Nutrition/Malabsorption Problems
Priority Concepts: Patient Education; Elimination

Answer: 2
Rationale: Foods that help eliminate odor with a colostomy include yogurt, buttermilk, cranberry juice, and parsley. Foods that cause odor are many and include alcohol, beans, turnips, radishes, asparagus, onions, cucumbers, mushrooms, cabbage, eggs, and fish.
Test-Taking Strategy: Focus on the subject, deodorizing foods for a client with a colostomy. Remember that foods that cause gas in the client with normal gastrointestinal function also form gas in the gastrointestinal tract of the client with a colostomy. Use basic nutritional knowledge to eliminate eggs, cucumbers, and mushrooms.
Priority Nursing Tip: The normal color for the stoma of a colostomy is pink to bright red and shiny, indicating high vascularity.
Reference: Lewis, S., et al. (2020). *Medical-surgical nursing: Assessment and management of clinical problems* (11th ed., p. 956). Elsevier; https://www.ostomy.org.

❖ **192.** The nurse is demonstrating colostomy care to a client with a newly created colostomy. The nurse demonstrates the correct cutting of the appliance by making the circle how much larger than the client's stoma?
1. ⅛ inch
2. ¼ inch
3. ½ inch
4. 1 inch

Level of Cognitive Ability: Applying
Client Needs: Health Promotion and Maintenance
Clinical Judgment/Cognitive Skills: Take Action
Integrated Process: Teaching and Learning
Content Area: Skills: Elimination
Health Problems: Adult Health: Gastrointestinal: Nutrition/Malabsorption Problems
Priority Concepts: Patient Education; Elimination

Answer: 1
Rationale: The size of the opening for the appliance is generally cut ⅛ inch larger than the size of the client's stoma. This minimizes the amount of exposed skin but does not put pressure on the stoma. The larger sizes leave too much skin area exposed for irritation by gastrointestinal contents.
Test-Taking Strategy: Focus on the subject, colostomy care. Remember that the goal is to prevent stoma and skin irritation. Visualizing each of the appliance sizes in the options will direct you to the correct option.
Priority Nursing Tip: A pale pink colostomy stoma most likely indicates that the client has a low hemoglobin and hematocrit level.
Reference: Ignatavicius, D., et al. (2021). *Medical-surgical nursing: Concepts for interprofessional collaborative care* (10th ed., p. 1122). Elsevier.

193. The nurse teaches a client diagnosed with a spinal cord injury about measures to prevent autonomic hyperreflexia. Which statement by the client indicates the **need for further teaching?**
1. "It is best if I avoid tight clothing and lumpy bedclothes."
2. "I need to watch for headache, congestion, and flushed skin."
3. "Signs/symptoms I need to watch for include fever and chest pain."
4. "I need to pay close attention to how frequently my bowels move."

Level of Cognitive Ability: Evaluating
Client Needs: Health Promotion and Maintenance
Clinical Judgment/Cognitive Skills: Evaluate Outcomes
Integrated Process: Clinical Judgment; Nursing Process/Evaluation
Content Area: Adult Health: Neurologic
Health Problems: Adult Health: Neurologic: Spinal Cord Injury
Priority Concepts: Patient Education; Intracranial Regulation

Answer: 3
Rationale: Autonomic hyperreflexia generally occurs in a client with a spinal cord injury after the period of spinal shock resolves. It occurs with injuries above T6 and cervical injuries. Signs/symptoms of autonomic hyperreflexia include headache, congestion, flushed skin above the level of injury and cold skin below it, diaphoresis, nausea, and anxiety. Fever and chest pain are not associated with this condition.
Test-Taking Strategy: Note the strategic words, *need for further teaching.* These words indicate a negative event query and ask you to select an option that is an incorrect statement. Recalling the signs, symptoms, and causes of autonomic hyperreflexia will direct you to the correct option.
Priority Nursing Tip: Triggers of autonomic hyperreflexia include visceral stimulation from a distended bladder or an impacted rectum.
Reference: Ignatavicius, D., et al. (2021). *Medical-surgical nursing: Concepts for interprofessional collaborative care* (10th ed., p. 880). Elsevier.

❖ **194.** The nurse is discharging a client from the hospital who has a diagnosis of a thoracic 11 (T11) fracture with cord transection. The nurse has provided home care instructions to the client. Which action indicates the **need for further teaching** before discharge?
1. Client jokes about no longer needing to worry about birth control.
2. Client verbalizes about being careful to not eat as many dairy products.
3. Client verbalizes the need to eat meals at the same time every day.
4. Client agrees to wash the hands, perineum, and the catheter with soap and water before performing self-catheterization.

Level of Cognitive Ability: Evaluating
Client Needs: Health Promotion and Maintenance
Clinical Judgment/Cognitive Skills: Evaluate Outcomes
Integrated Process: Clinical Judgment; Nursing Process/Evaluation
Content Area: Adult Health: Neurologic
Health Problems: Adult Health: Neurologic: Spinal Cord Injury
Priority Concepts: Patient Education; Intracranial Regulation

Answer: 1
Rationale: Clients with spinal cord trauma remain fertile during their reproductive years, and contraception is necessary for those who are sexually active. However, oral contraceptives may increase the risk for thrombophlebitis. Clients with paralysis need to avoid dairy products to control the formation of urinary calculi. Meals should be eaten at the same time every day, and they need to include fiber and warm solid and liquid foods to promote and maintain the regular evacuation of the bowel. Clients who lack bladder control are taught to self-catheterize using clean technique.
Test-Taking Strategy: Note the strategic words, *need for further teaching.* These words indicate a negative event query and ask you to select an option that is an incorrect statement. Remember that the key aspects of dealing with a spinal cord injury client are nutrition and elimination. Not consuming as much dairy, eating meals at scheduled times, and implementing appropriate clean technique for catheterization address these areas.
Priority Nursing Tip: With complete transection of the cord, the spinal cord is severed completely, with total loss of sensation, movement, and reflex activity below the level of injury.
Reference: Ignatavicius, D., et al. (2021). *Medical-surgical nursing: Concepts for interprofessional collaborative care* (10th ed., pp. 886–887). Elsevier.

195. A client has been started on a monoamine oxidase inhibitor (MAOI). Which information would the nurse include when teaching the client about the medication?
1. This medication can cause severe drowsiness.
2. Client must avoid foods that contain tyramine.
3. The medication is associated with a high rate of abuse.
4. The medication will begin to alleviate symptoms of depression almost immediately.

Level of Cognitive Ability: Applying
Client Needs: Health Promotion and Maintenance
Clinical Judgment/Cognitive Skills: Generate Solutions
Integrated Process: Teaching and Learning
Content Area: Pharmacology: Psychotherapeutics: Monoamine Oxidase Inhibitors (MAOIs)
Health Problems: Mental Health: Mood Disorders
Priority Concepts: Patient Education; Safety

Answer: 2
Rationale: MAOIs are used to treat depression. Although MAOIs usually produce hypotension as a side effect, potentially lethal hypertension can occur if the client eats foods that contain tyramine. Such foods include aged cheeses, hot dogs, and beer, among others. The medication does not cause drowsiness, is not associated with a high rate of abuse, and does not act almost immediately.
Test-Taking Strategy: Focus on the subject, a client taking an MAOI. Recalling that MAOIs are associated with a food-medication interaction will direct you to the correct option.
Priority Nursing Tip: Instruct the client taking a MAOI to change positions slowly to prevent orthostatic hypotension.
Priority Concepts: Cognition; Health Promotion
Reference: Lilley, L., Rainforth Collins, S., & Snyder J. (2020). *Pharmacology and the nursing process* (9th ed., p. 257). Elsevier.

❖ 196. The nurse is creating a plan of care for an older client diagnosed with dementia. The nurse develops which realistic outcome for the client?
1. Client will function at the highest level of independence possible.
2. Client will be admitted to a nursing home to have the needs of activities of daily living met.
3. Client will complete all activities of daily living independently within a 1- to 1½-hour time frame.
4. The nursing staff will attend to all of client's activities of daily living needs during the hospital stay.

Level of Cognitive Ability: Creating
Client Needs: Health Promotion and Maintenance
Clinical Judgment/Cognitive Skills: Generate Solutions
Integrated Process: Clinical Judgment; Nursing Process/Planning
Content Area: Mental Health
Health Problems: Mental Health: Neurocognitive Impairment
Priority Concepts: Cognition; Health Promotion

Answer: 1
Rationale: All clients, regardless of age, need to be encouraged to perform at the highest level of independence possible. This contributes to the client's sense of control and well-being. Being admitted to a nursing home and having nursing staff perform all activities of daily living are not client-centered goals, and a 1- to 1½-hour time frame may not be realistic for an older client with dementia.
Test-Taking Strategy: Focus on the subject, a client diagnosed with dementia. Note the words *realistic outcome for the client*. Eliminate being admitted to the nursing home and having the nursing staff perform all activities of daily living first because they are not client-centered. From the remaining options, eliminate 1 to 1½ hours for completion of activities of daily living because of the unrealistic time frame.
Priority Nursing Tip: Providing a safe environment is the priority for a client with dementia.
Reference: Potter, P., et al. (2023). *Fundamentals of nursing* (11th ed., pp. 194–195). Elsevier.

197. Percussion is a physical assessment technique that is used to identify which findings? **Select all that apply.**
- ❑ 1. Fluid in body cavities
- ❑ 2. Borders of body organs
- ❑ 3. Consistency of body organs
- ❑ 4. Mobility of organs and other structures
- ❑ 5. Resilience and resistance of tissue and organs
- ❑ 6. Location, size, and density of an underlying structure

Level of Cognitive Ability: Applying
Client Needs: Health Promotion and Maintenance
Clinical Judgment/Cognitive Skills: Recognize Cues
Integrated Process: Clinical Judgment; Nursing Process/Assessment
Content Area: Health Assessment/Physical Exam: General Assessment Techniques
Health Problems: N/A
Priority Concepts: Clinical Judgment; Health Promotion

Answer: 1, 2, 3, 6
Rationale: Percussion involves tapping the body with the fingertips to evaluate the size, borders, and consistency of body organs and assess for fluid in body cavities. Through percussion, the location, size, and density of an underlying structure can be determined. Through palpation, assessment is done via the sense of touch. Measurements of specific physical signs, including resistance, resilience, roughness, texture, and mobility, can be made through palpation.
Test-Taking Strategy: Focus on the **subject**, percussion, and recall that percussion involves tapping the body with the fingertips. Visualize the effect of this assessment technique to determine what it evaluates.
Priority Nursing Tip: Physical assessment techniques include inspection, palpation, percussion, and auscultation.
References: Jarvis, C. (2020) *Physical examination and health assessment* (8th ed., pp. 113–114). Elsevier. Lewis, S., et al. (2020). *Medical-surgical nursing: Assessment and management of clinical problems* (11th ed., pp. 38, 465). Elsevier;

❖ **198.** A client is newly diagnosed with chronic obstructive pulmonary disease (COPD). The client returns home after a short hospitalization. The home care nurse would **most importantly** plan teaching strategies that are designed to do what?
1. Promote membership in support groups.
2. Encourage client to become a more active person.
3. Identify irritants in the home that interfere with breathing.
4. Improve oxygenation and minimize carbon dioxide retention.

Level of Cognitive Ability: Applying
Client Needs: Health Promotion and Maintenance
Clinical Judgment/Cognitive Skills: Generate Solutions
Integrated Process: Teaching and Learning
Content Area: Adult Health: Respiratory
Health Problems: Adult Health: Respiratory: Chronic Obstructive Pulmonary Disease
Priority Concepts: Gas Exchange; Safety

Answer: 4
Rationale: COPD is a disease state characterized by airflow obstruction. Improving oxygenation and minimizing carbon dioxide retention are the primary goals. The other options are interventions that will help with the achievement of this primary goal.
Test-Taking Strategy: Note the **strategic words**, *most importantly.* Use the ABCs—airway, breathing, and circulation—to direct you to the correct option.
Priority Nursing Tip: In COPD, progressive airflow limitation occurs. This is associated with an abnormal inflammatory response of the lungs that is not completely reversible.
Reference: Ignatavicius, D., et al. (2021). *Medical-surgical nursing: Concepts for interprofessional collaborative care* (10th ed., p. 550). Elsevier.

199. A client is being discharged from the hospital after a bronchoscopy that was performed a day earlier. After the discharge teaching, the client makes the following statements to the nurse. Which statement would the nurse identify as indicating a **need for further teaching?**
1. "I will stop smoking my cigarettes."
2. "I can expect to cough up bright red blood."
3. "I will get help immediately if I start having trouble breathing."
4. "I will use the throat lozenges as directed by my doctor until my sore throat goes away."

Level of Cognitive Ability: Evaluating
Client Needs: Health Promotion and Maintenance
Clinical Judgment/Cognitive Skills: Evaluate Outcomes
Integrated Process: Clinical Judgment; Nursing Process/Evaluation
Content Area: Foundations of Care: Diagnostic Tests
Health Problems: N/A
Priority Concepts: Patient Education; Gas Exchange

Answer: 2
Rationale: After bronchoscopy, expectorated secretions are inspected for hemoptysis, and if the client expectorates bright red blood, the primary health care provider is to be notified. The client needs to avoid smoking. The client needs to be observed for signs/symptoms of respiratory distress, including dyspnea, changes in respiratory rate, the use of accessory muscles, and changes in or absent lung sounds. A sore throat is common, and lozenges would be helpful to alleviate it.
Test-Taking Strategy: Note the strategic words, *need for further teaching*. These words indicate a negative event query and ask you to select an option that is an incorrect statement. Note the words *bright red* in option 2. Remember that bright red blood indicates active bleeding and that this needs to be reported to the primary health care provider immediately.
Priority Nursing Tip: After bronchoscopy, the nurse needs to maintain the client on nothing-by-mouth (NPO) status until the gag reflex returns.
Reference: Pagana, K., Pagana, T., & Pagana, T. N. (2021). *Mosby's Diagnostic and laboratory test reference* (15th ed., pp. 187–188). Elsevier.

❖ **200.** A client who is taking an antipsychotic medication is preparing for discharge. To facilitate health promotion for this client, what instruction would the nurse provide?
1. Avoid prolonged exposure to the sun.
2. Adhere to a strict tyramine-restricted diet.
3. Recognize the signs and symptoms of a relapse of depression.
4. Have therapeutic blood levels drawn because the medication has a narrow therapeutic range.

Level of Cognitive Ability: Applying
Client Needs: Health Promotion and Maintenance
Clinical Judgment/Cognitive Skills: Generate Solutions
Integrated Process: Teaching and Learning
Content Area: Pharmacology: Psychotherapeutics: Antipsychotics
Health Problems: Mental Health: Schizophrenia
Priority Concepts: Patient Education; Psychosis

Answer: 1
Rationale: Antipsychotic medications improve the thought processes and behaviors of a client with psychotic symptoms, especially a client with schizophrenia. Photosensitivity is a side effect of antipsychotic medications. Maintaining a strict tyramine-restricted diet is applicable to monoamine oxidase inhibitors (MAOIs). Antipsychotics are not used to treat depression. Lithium is a mood stabilizer that requires monitoring of medication blood levels.
Test-Taking Strategy: Focus on the subject, an antipsychotic medication to eliminate a relapse in depression. Eliminate a tyramine-restricted diet because this option relates to medications that are monoamine oxidase inhibitors. There is not a narrow range between therapeutic and toxic levels such as there is with lithium carbonate; therefore, drawing therapeutic blood levels can be eliminated.
Priority Nursing Tip: Monitor the client taking an antipsychotic medication for anticholinergic and extrapyramidal side effects.
Reference: Lewis, S., et al. (2020). *Medical-surgical nursing: Assessment and management of clinical problems* (11th ed., p. 410). Elsevier.

CHAPTER 9

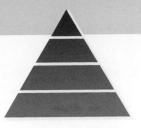

Psychosocial Integrity Practice Questions

1. A client with a diagnosis of schizophrenia is experiencing visual hallucinations. The nurse plans care based on the determination that this symptom is related to an alteration in brain function in which lobe of the cerebrum? **(Refer to the figure.)**

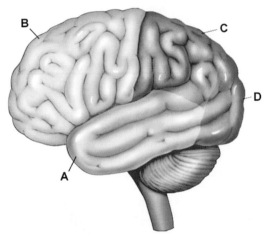

(From Patton, K. T., & Thibodeau, G. A. [2013]. *Anatomy & physiology* [8th ed.]. Mosby.)

1. A
2. B
3. C
4. D

Level of Cognitive Ability: Applying
Client Needs: Psychosocial Integrity
Clinical Judgment/Cognitive Skills: Generate Solutions
Integrated Process: Clinical Judgment: Nursing Process/Planning
Content Area: Mental Health
Health Problems: Mental Health: Schizophrenia
Priority Concepts: Clinical Judgment; Psychosis

Answer: 4
Rationale: Visual hallucinations indicate an alteration in brain function in the cerebrum. The occipital lobe is located in the back of the head, is primarily responsible for seeing and receiving information, and is responsible for visual hallucinations. The temporal lobe lies beneath the skull on both sides of the brain and is primarily responsible for hearing and receiving information via the ears. Symptoms indicating an alteration of function in the temporal lobe include auditory hallucinations, sensory aphasia, alterations in memory, and altered emotional responses. The frontal lobe is located in the anterior or front area of the brain and is primarily responsible for motor functions, higher thought processes such as decision-making, intellectual insight and judgment, and expression of emotion. Symptoms indicating an alteration of function in the frontal lobe include changes in affect, alteration in language production, alteration in motor function, impulsive behavior, and impaired decision-making. The parietal lobe lies beneath the skull at the back and top of the head and is primarily responsible for association and sensory perception. Symptoms indicating an alteration of function in the parietal lobe include alterations in sensory perceptions, difficulty with time concepts and calculating numbers, alteration in personal hygiene, and poor attention span.
Test-Taking Strategy: Focus on the subject, a client who is experiencing visual hallucinations. Use concepts related to anatomy and physiology of the brain to answer this question. Recalling the location of the occipital lobe and that this lobe is primarily responsible for seeing and receiving information via the eyes will assist in answering correctly.
Priority Nursing Tip: The client experiencing visual hallucinations is seeing things that are not there.
Reference: Varcarolis, E., & Fosbre, C. (2021). *Essentials of psychiatric mental health nursing: A communication approach to evidence-based care* (4th ed., p. 255). Elsevier.

2. A client with the diagnosis of acute pyelonephritis who is very shy and modest is scheduled for a voiding cystourethrogram. What about this procedure makes the nurse determine that this client would benefit from increased support and teaching about the procedure?
1. Radioactive material is inserted into the bladder.
2. Radiopaque contrast is injected into the bloodstream.
3. Client must void while the voiding process is filmed.
4. Client must lie on an x-ray table in a cold, barren room.

Level of Cognitive Ability: Applying
Client Needs: Psychosocial Integrity
Clinical Judgment/Cognitive Skills: Generate Solutions
Integrated Process: Nursing Process/Planning
Content Area: Foundations of Care: Diagnostic Tests
Health Problems: Mental Health: Anxiety
Priority Concepts: Clinical Judgment; Elimination

Answer: 3
Rationale: Having to void in the presence of others can be very embarrassing for clients, and it may actually interfere with the client's ability to void. The nurse teaches the client about the procedure to try to minimize stress from a lack of preparation and gives the client encouragement and emotional support. Screens may be used in the radiology department to try to provide an element of privacy during this procedure. The remaining options are incorrect and do not address the subject of support.
Test-Taking Strategy: Focus on the subject, a shy and modest client scheduled for a voiding cystourethrogram. Use your knowledge regarding this procedure. Noting the words *shy* and *modest* will direct you to the correct option.
Priority Nursing Tip: Pyelonephritis frequently follows untreated urinary tract infections and is associated with increased incidence of anemia, low birth weight, gestational hypertension, preterm labor and delivery, and premature rupture of the membranes.
Reference: Pagana, K., Pagana, T., & Pagana, T. N. (2021). *Mosby's Diagnostic and laboratory test reference* (15th ed., pp. 951–953). Elsevier.

3. A client with the diagnosis of mania emerges from the room topless while making sexual remarks and lewd gestures toward the staff and peers. Which action would the nurse take **first**?
1. Quietly approach client and escort to own room to get dressed.
2. Confront client on the inappropriateness of the behavior and offer client a time out.
3. Ask other clients to ignore the behavior; eventually client will return to their own room.
4. Approach client in the hallway and insist that client go to their own room immediately.

Level of Cognitive Ability: Applying
Client Needs: Psychosocial Integrity
Clinical Judgment/Cognitive Skills: Take Action
Integrated Process: Clinical Judgment; Nursing Process/Implementation
Content Area: Mental Health
Health Problems: Mental Health: Mood Disorders
Priority Concepts: Clinical Judgment; Mood and Affect

Answer: 1
Rationale: A person who is experiencing mania lacks insight and judgment, has poor impulse control, and is highly excitable. The nurse must take control without creating increased stress or anxiety for the client. Insisting that the client go to their own room may cause the nurse to be met with a great deal of resistance. Confronting the client and offering the client a consequence of time out may be meaningless to the client. Asking other clients to ignore the client is inappropriate. A quiet but firm approach while distracting the client (walking the client to their own room and helping the client to get dressed) achieves the goal of having the client dressed appropriately and preserving the client's psychosocial integrity.
Test-Taking Strategy: Note the strategic word, *first*. Focus on the subject, a client in a manic state. Recalling that the nurse must take control to protect the client will direct you to option 1.
Priority Nursing Tip: Bipolar disorder is characterized by episodes of mania and depression with periods of normal mood and activity in between. It is commonly treated with lithium carbonate, which can be toxic and requires regular monitoring of serum lithium levels.
Reference: Varcarolis, E., & Fosbre, C. (2021). *Essentials of psychiatric mental health nursing: A communication approach to evidence-based care* (4th ed., pp. 228, 236–237). Elsevier.

❖ **4.** After cardiac surgery to treat coronary artery disease, both the client and the family express anxiety regarding how to cope with the recovering process after discharge. Which available resource would the nurse plan to tell the client and family about to **best** address their concerns?

1. United Way
2. Client's local church
3. American Cancer Society Reach for Recovery
4. American Heart Association Mended Hearts Club

Level of Cognitive Ability: Applying
Client Needs: Psychosocial Integrity
Clinical Judgment/Cognitive Skills: Generate Solutions
Integrated Process: Nursing Process/Planning
Content Area: Adult Health: Cardiovascular
Health Problems: Mental Health: Anxiety
Priority Concepts: Anxiety; Patient Education

Answer: 4
Rationale: Most clients and families benefit from knowing that there are available resources to help them cope with the stress of self-care management at home. These can include telephone contact with the surgeon, cardiologist, and nurse; cardiac rehabilitation programs; and community support groups such as the American Heart Association Mended Hearts Club, which is a nationwide program with local chapters. The United Way provides a wide variety of services to people who may not otherwise be able to afford them. The library normally does not provide resources for coping with the recuperative process. The American Cancer Society Reach for Recovery helps those recovering after mastectomy.
Test-Taking Strategy: Note the strategic word, *best*. Focus on the subject, the available resource for the client who had cardiac surgery. Note that the options identify three organizations and a church. Noting that the client had cardiac surgery will direct you to option 4.
Priority Nursing Tip: Many hospitals sponsor health fairs, blood pressure screening, and risk factor modification programs. The Internet is a resource that can be used to locate such events.
Reference: Ignatavicius, D., et al. (2021). *Medical-surgical nursing: Concepts for interprofessional collaborative care* (10th ed., p. 774). Elsevier.

5. Which explanation by the nurse would **best** alleviate anxiety in a client with coronary artery disease about having a 12-lead electrocardiogram (ECG) diagnostic procedure?

1. "It's a simple test, but it's important to lie still during the procedure."
2. "It should only take about 20 minutes to complete the ECG tracing process."
3. "The ECG electrodes are painless and will record the electrical activity of your heart."
4. "The ECG can give the primary health care provider information about the status of your heart."

Level of Cognitive Ability: Applying
Client Needs: Psychosocial Integrity
Clinical Judgment/Cognitive Skills: Take Action
Integrated Process: Teaching and Learning
Content Area: Foundations of Care: Diagnostic Tests
Health Problems: Mental Health: Anxiety
Priority Concepts: Anxiety; Patient Education

Answer: 3
Rationale: The ECG uses painless electrodes that are applied to the chest and limbs. The procedure takes less than 5 minutes to complete, and it requires the client to lie still; therefore, option 2 is incorrect. The ECG measures the heart's electrical activity to determine rate, rhythm, and a variety of abnormalities. Options 1 and 4 are factual statements, but they are not stated to reduce anxiety.
Test-Taking Strategy: Focus on the subject, alleviating the client's anxiety about a 12-lead ECG, and noting the strategic word, *best*. Eliminate option 2 because it is inaccurate. Next, eliminate options 1 and 4 because they will not alleviate anxiety.
Priority Nursing Tip: An ECG is another noninvasive procedure that evaluates cardiac function and specifically examines structural and functional changes in the heart. The client must lie still, breathe normally, and refrain from talking during the test.
Reference: Ignatavicius, D., et al. (2021). *Medical-surgical nursing: Concepts for interprofessional collaborative care* (10th ed., pp. 638–639). Elsevier.

❖ **6.** The spouse of a client who is scheduled for the insertion of an implantable cardioverter-defibrillator (ICD) expresses anxiety about what would happen if the device discharges during physical contact. Which information is **most appropriate** for the nurse to provide to the spouse?
  1. Physical contact needs to be avoided whenever possible.
  2. The spouse would not feel or be harmed by the countershock.
  3. The shock would be felt, but it would not cause the spouse any harm.
  4. A warning device sounds before countershock, so there is time to move away.

Level of Cognitive Ability: Applying
Client Needs: Psychosocial Integrity
Clinical Judgment/Cognitive Skills: Take Action
Integrated Process: Teaching and Learning
Content Area: Adult Health: Cardiovascular
Health Problems: Mental Health: Anxiety
Priority Concepts: Anxiety; Patient Education

Answer: 3
Rationale: Clients and families are often fearful about the activation of the ICD. Their fears are about the device itself and also about the occurrence of life-threatening dysrhythmias that trigger its function. Family members need reassurance that, even if the device activates while they are touching the client, the level of the charge is not high enough to harm the family member, although it will be felt. The ICD emits a warning beep when the client is near magnetic fields, which could possibly deactivate it, but it does not beep before countershock.
Test-Taking Strategy: Note the strategic words, *most appropriate*. Focus on the subject, the spouse's anxiety about ICD, and use your knowledge of the function of the ICD to answer this question. This will direct you to the correct option. Remember that the shock would be felt, but it would not cause the spouse any harm.
Priority Nursing Tip: An ICD monitors cardiac rhythm and detects and terminates episodes of ventricular fibrillation and ventricular tachycardia.
Reference: Ignatavicius, D., et al. (2021). *Medical-surgical nursing: Concepts for interprofessional collaborative care* (10th ed., pp. 661–662). Elsevier.

7. An anxious client who is scheduled for permanent transvenous pacemaker insertion states to the nurse, "I know I need it, but I'm not sure this surgery is a great idea." Which nursing response would **best** help the nurse assess the client's preoperative concerns?
  1. "How does your family feel about the surgery?"
  2. "Has anyone taught you about the procedure yet?"
  3. "You sound extremely worried. Has anyone told you that the technology is really quite safe?"
  4. "You sound uncertain about the procedure. Can you tell me more about what has you concerned?"

Level of Cognitive Ability: Applying
Client Needs: Psychosocial Integrity
Clinical Judgment/Cognitive Skills: Generate Solutions
Integrated Process: Communication and Documentation
Content Area: Adult Health: Cardiovascular
Health Problems: Mental Health: Anxiety
Priority Concepts: Anxiety; Communication

Answer: 4
Rationale: Anxiety is common in the client with the need for pacemaker insertion. This can be related to a fear of life-threatening dysrhythmias or of the surgical procedure. Option 4 is the correct choice because it is open-ended and uses clarification as a communication technique to explore the client's concerns. Option 1 is not indicated because it asks about the family and deflects attention away from the client's concerns. Options 2 and 3 are closed-ended and are not exploratory.
Test-Taking Strategy: Note the strategic word, *best*. Use therapeutic communication techniques, focusing on the subject, addressing the client's preoperative concerns. Option 1 can be eliminated first because it addresses the family rather than the client. From the remaining options, the only option that addresses the client's concerns is option 4.
Priority Nursing Tip: A pacemaker is a temporary or permanent device that provides electrical stimulation and maintains the heart rate when the client's intrinsic pacemaker fails to provide a perfusing rhythm.
References: Ignatavicius, D., et al. (2021). *Medical-surgical nursing: Concepts for interprofessional collaborative care* (10th ed., pp. 648–649). Elsevier; Potter, P., et al. (2021). *Fundamentals of nursing* (10th ed., pp. 333–335). Elsevier.

8. A client with superficial varicose veins states to the nurse, "I hate these things. They're so ugly. I wish I could get them to go away." Which therapeutic response would be **most appropriate** for the nurse to make to the client?
1. "You should try sclerotherapy. It's great."
2. "What makes you so upset about having ugly varicose veins?"
3. "What have you been told about varicose veins and their management?"
4. "I understand how you feel, but you know, they really don't look all that bad."

Level of Cognitive Ability: Applying
Client Needs: Psychosocial Integrity
Clinical Judgment/Cognitive Skills: Take Action
Integrated Process: Communication and Documentation
Content Area: Adult Health: Cardiovascular
Health Problems: Mental Health: Coping
Priority Concepts: Anxiety; Communication

Answer: 3
Rationale: The client expressing distress about physical appearance has a risk for an altered body image. The nurse assesses the client's knowledge and self-management of the condition as a means of empowering the client and helping the client adapt to the body change. Options 1 and 4 are not therapeutic. Option 2 focuses only on the cosmetic aspect of varicose veins.
Test-Taking Strategy: Note the strategic words, *most appropriate.* Use therapeutic communication techniques. With questions that deal with client's feelings, select the option that facilitates the sharing of information and concerns by the client. The remaining options cut off or limit further comments by the client. Additionally, the correct option addresses assessment, which is the first step of the nursing process.
Priority Nursing Tip: Varicose veins occur from the weakening and dilation of vein walls and incompetence of the valves inside the veins. The client may feel pain in the legs with dull aching after standing, a feeling of fullness in the legs, and ankle edema.
References: Ignatavicius, D., et al. (2021). *Medical-surgical nursing: Concepts for interprofessional collaborative care* (10th ed., pp. 728–729). Elsevier; Potter, P., et al. (2021). *Fundamentals of nursing* (10th ed., pp. 333–335). Elsevier.

9. A client diagnosed with chronic kidney disease (CKD) has been told that hemodialysis will be required. The client becomes angry and states, "I'll never be the same now." Based on this information, which would the nurse identify as the client's **primary** concern?
1. Anxiety about the hemodialysis
2. Inability to think clearly because of the treatments needed
3. Potential for noncompliance because of concerns about the disease
4. Altered body image because of the physical changes that may occur

Level of Cognitive Ability: Analyzing
Client Needs: Psychosocial Integrity
Clinical Judgment/Cognitive Skills: Prioritize Hypotheses
Integrated Process: Clinical Judgment; Nursing Process/Analysis
Content Area: Adult Health: Renal and Urinary
Health Problems: Mental Health: Coping
Priority Concepts: Stress and Coping; Mood and Affect

Answer: 4
Rationale: A client with a renal disorder such as CKD may become angry in response to the permanence of the condition. Because of the physical changes and the change in lifestyle that may be required to manage a severe renal condition, the client may experience an altered body image. Anxiety is not appropriate because the client is exhibiting anger at this time. The client is not cognitively impaired, eliminating option 2, and is not stating a refusal to undergo therapy, so eliminate option 3.
Test-Taking Strategy: Note the strategic word, *primary.* Focus on the subject, an angry client who will have hemodialysis and states that they will never be the same. Note that the client's statement focuses on the self, which is consistent with altered body image.
Priority Nursing Tip: The client undergoing hemodialysis will either have a subclavian or femoral catheter for short-term or temporary use in acute kidney injury. This will be used until a fistula or graft is created and matures, which typically takes 6 weeks, or the short-term catheter may be required if the permanent fistula has failed because of infection or clotting.
References: Ignatavicius, D., et al. (2021). *Medical-surgical nursing: Concepts for interprofessional collaborative care* (10th ed., p. 1395). Elsevier; Potter, P., et al. (2021). *Fundamentals of nursing* (10th ed., pp. 77–78). Elsevier.

❖ **10.** A client with the diagnosis of hyperparathyroidism states to the nurse, "I can't stay on this diet. It is too difficult for me." Which therapeutic response by the nurse is **best** when intervening in this situation?
1. "Why do you think you find this diet plan difficult to adhere to?"
2. "It really isn't difficult to stick to this diet. Just avoid milk products."
3. "You are having a difficult time staying on this plan. Let's discuss this."
4. "It is very important that you stay on this diet to avoid forming renal calculi."

Level of Cognitive Ability: Applying
Client Needs: Psychosocial Integrity
Clinical Judgment/Cognitive Skills: Take Action
Integrated Process: Nursing Process/Implementation
Content Area: Foundations of Care: Therapeutic Diets
Health Problems: Mental Health: Coping
Priority Concepts: Communication; Nutrition

Answer: 3
Rationale: By paraphrasing the client's statement, the nurse can encourage the client to verbalize emotions. The nurse also sends feedback to the client that the message was understood. An open-ended statement or question such as this prompts a thorough response from the client. Option 1 requests information that the client may not be able to express. Option 2 devalues the client's feelings. Option 4 gives advice, which blocks communication.
Test-Taking Strategy: Note the strategic word, *best*. Use therapeutic communication techniques, and focus on the client's statement. Note that option 3 paraphrases the client's statement.
Priority Nursing Tip: After the nurse determines the cause of a client's difficulty in adhering to a prescribed diet, the nurse can develop a plan of care and refer the client to appropriate community support programs, such as nutritional programs.
References: Ignatavicius, D., et al. (2021). *Medical-surgical nursing: Concepts for interprofessional collaborative care* (10th ed., pp. 1262–1263). Elsevier; Potter, P., et al. (2021). *Fundamentals of nursing* (10th ed., pp. 333–335). Elsevier.

11. The nurse is caring for a client with a new diagnosis of type 1 diabetes mellitus who is very anxious. The nurse recognizes that which teaching plan component is **most important initially**?
1. Knowledge of the diabetic diet
2. Understanding of the diagnosis
3. Monitoring of blood glucose levels
4. Correct technique for administering insulin

Level of Cognitive Ability: Applying
Client Needs: Psychosocial Integrity
Clinical Judgment/Cognitive Skills: Prioritize Hypotheses
Integrated Process: Clinical Judgment; Teaching and Learning
Content Area: Adult Health: Endocrine
Health Problems: Mental Health: Anxiety
Priority Concepts: Patient Education; Glucose Regulation

Answer: 2
Rationale: Before educating about a disease process, it is important that the client understands the components of the disease process. After this teaching, the actual components of diet, blood glucose testing, and insulin injections can be taught.
Test-Taking Strategy: Note the strategic words, *most important* and *initially*. All of the options may be appropriate to assess, but note that options 1, 3, and 4 relate to specific components of the teaching. Option 2 is the umbrella option, and, considering the principles of teaching and learning, this aspect needs to be assessed before the implementation of teaching.
Priority Nursing Tip: The management of diabetes mellitus is complicated and involves considerable client involvement and education, so it is important for the nurse to ensure that the client understands the disease process.
Reference: Ignatavicius, D., et al. (2021). *Medical-surgical nursing: Concepts for interprofessional collaborative care* (10th ed., pp. 1296, 1298). Elsevier.

❖ **12.** A client with a new diagnosis of type 1 diabetes mellitus has been seen for 3 consecutive days in the emergency department with hyperglycemia. During the assessment, the client states to the nurse, "I'm sorry to keep bothering you every day, but I just can't give myself those awful shots." Which is the **most appropriate** therapeutic response by the nurse?
1. "I couldn't give myself a shot either."
2. "You must learn to give yourself the shots."
3. "Let me see if we can change your medication."
4. "Have you had instructions on injecting yourself?"

Level of Cognitive Ability: Applying
Client Needs: Psychosocial Integrity
Clinical Judgment/Cognitive Skills: Take Action
Integrated Process: Communication and Documentation
Content Area: Adult Health: Endocrine
Health Problems: Mental Health: Coping
Priority Concepts: Anxiety; Glucose Regulation

Answer: 4
Rationale: It is important to determine and deal with a client's underlying fear of self-injection. The nurse would determine whether a knowledge deficit exists. Positive reinforcement needs to occur rather than focusing on negative behaviors. Demanding that the client perform a behavior or skill is inappropriate. The nurse would not offer a change in regimen that cannot be accomplished.
Test-Taking Strategy: Note the strategic words, *most appropriate*. Use therapeutic communication techniques. Options 1, 2, and 3 are not therapeutic. In addition, option 3 may provide false reassurance regarding a potential change in medications.
Priority Nursing Tip: Common sites for the injection of insulin include the upper arm, abdomen, thighs, lower back, and buttocks.
References: Ignatavicius, D., et al. (2021). *Medical-surgical nursing: Concepts for interprofessional collaborative care* (10th ed., p. 1279). Elsevier; Potter, P., et al. (2021). *Fundamentals of nursing* (10th ed., pp. 333–335). Elsevier.

13. The nurse requests that a client with a diagnosis of diabetes mellitus ask family members to attend an educational conference about the administration of insulin. The client questions why they need to be included, as "it is not their disease." Which statement is **best** for the nurse to respond?
1. "Family members are at risk of developing diabetes."
2. "Family members can take you to your appointments."
3. "Nurses will need someone to call and check on a client's progress."
4. "Families often work together toward the successful management of diabetes."

Level of Cognitive Ability: Applying
Client Needs: Psychosocial Integrity
Clinical Judgment/Cognitive Skills: Take Action
Integrated Process: Communication and Documentation
Content Area: Adult Health: Endocrine
Health Problems: Mental Health: Coping
Priority Concepts: Communication; Glucose Regulation

Answer: 4
Rationale: Families and significant others may be included in diabetes education to assist with adjustments of the diabetic regimen. Having positive family members involved will be a support to the client in assuming independent care. Although the other options are not incorrect, they do not reinforce the importance of family involvement in the client's care.
Test-Taking Strategy: Note the strategic word, *best*. Use of therapeutic communication techniques will promote independence in coping with a chronic illness. None of the remaining options promote independence.
Priority Nursing Tip: Some chronic complications of diabetes mellitus include diabetic retinopathy, diabetic nephropathy, and diabetic neuropathy.
References: Ignatavicius, D., et al. (2021). *Medical-surgical nursing: Concepts for interprofessional collaborative care* (10th ed., pp. 1295–1296). Elsevier; Potter, P., et al. (2021). *Fundamentals of nursing.* (10th ed., pp. 333–335) Elsevier.

❖ **14.** A client has recently been diagnosed with polycystic kidney disease. The nurse has a series of discussions with the client that are intended to help the client cope with the disorder. Which would the nurse plan to include as part of one of these discussions?
1. Ongoing fluid restriction
2. The need for genetic counseling
3. The risk of hypotensive episodes
4. Depression regarding massive edema

Level of Cognitive Ability: Applying
Client Needs: Psychosocial Integrity
Clinical Judgment/Cognitive Skills: Generate Solutions
Integrated Process: Clinical Judgment; Nursing Process/Planning
Content Area: Adult Health: Renal and Urinary
Health Problems: Mental Health: Coping
Priority Concepts: Patient Education; Elimination

Answer: 2
Rationale: Adult polycystic kidney disease is a hereditary disorder that is inherited as an autosomal-dominant trait. Because of this, the client and the extended family need genetic counseling. Ongoing fluid restriction is unnecessary. The client is likely to have hypertension rather than hypotension. Massive edema is not part of the clinical picture of this disorder.
Test-Taking Strategy: Focus on the subject, polycystic kidney disease. Use knowledge about the characteristics of this disease. This disease is a hereditary disease that does not have a need for fluid restriction or conditions related to blood pressure.
Priority Nursing Tip: In polycystic kidney disease, a cystic formation and hypertrophy of the kidneys leads to cystic rupture, infection, formation of scar tissue, and damaged nephrons. There is no specific treatment to arrest the progress of the destructive cysts.
Reference: Lewis, S., et al. (2020). *Medical-surgical nursing: Assessment and management of clinical problems* (11th ed., 1041–1042). Elsevier.

15. The nurse is admitting a client who is to undergo ureterolithotomy. Which would the nurse assess in order to determine if the client is ready for surgery? **Select all that apply.**
❑ 1. The need for a visit from a support group
❑ 2. The knowledge of postoperative activities
❑ 3. An understanding of the surgical procedure
❑ 4. Expected outcomes of the surgical procedure
❑ 5. Feelings or anxieties about the surgical procedure

Level of Cognitive Ability: Analyzing
Client Needs: Psychosocial Integrity
Clinical Judgment/Cognitive Skills: Recognize Cues
Integrated Process: Clinical Judgment; Nursing Process/Assessment
Content Area: Adult Health: Renal and Urinary
Health Problems: Adult Health: Renal and Urinary: Strictures
Priority Concepts: Caregiving; Elimination

Answer: 2, 3, 4, 5
Rationale: Ureterolithotomy is the removal of a calculus from the ureter using either a flank or abdominal incision. The client needs to have an understanding of the same items as are required for any surgery, including knowledge of the procedures, the expected outcome, the postoperative routines, and any expected discomfort. The client needs to also be assessed for any concerns or anxieties before surgery. Because no urinary diversion is created during this procedure, the client has no need for a visit from a member of a support group.
Test-Taking Strategy: Focus on the subject, the client's readiness for surgery. This will assist in directing you to the correct options.
Priority Nursing Tip: Problems resulting from urinary calculi are pain, obstruction, tissue trauma, secondary hemorrhage, and infection. A stone analysis will be done after passage to determine the type of stone and assist in determining treatment.
Reference: Ignatavicius, D., et al. (2021). *Medical-surgical nursing: Concepts for interprofessional collaborative care* (10th ed., pp. 1348–1349). Elsevier.

❖ **16.** The spouse of a dying client states to the nurse, "I don't think I can come anymore and watch my spouse die. It's chewing me up too much!" Which is the **most** therapeutic response the nurse would make to the spouse?
1. "It's hard to watch someone you love die. You've been here with your spouse every day. Are you taking any time for yourself?"
2. "Focus on your spouse's pain rather than yours. I know it's hard, but this isn't about what's happening to you, you know."
3. "I know it's hard for you, but your spouse would know if you're not there, and you would feel so very guilty all of the rest of your days."
4. "I think you're making the right decision. Your spouse feels your love. You don't have to come every day. I'll take care of your spouse for you."

Level of Cognitive Ability: Applying
Client Needs: Psychosocial Integrity
Clinical Judgment/Cognitive Skills: Take Action
Integrated Process: Communication and Documentation
Content Area: Developmental Stages: End-of-Life Care
Health Problems: Mental Health: Coping
Priority Concepts: Caregiving; Communication

Answer: 1
Rationale: The most therapeutic response is the one that is empathetic and that reflects the nurse's understanding of the client's, or in this case, the spouse's, stress and emotional pain. In the correct option, the nurse suggests that the client take time for self. Option 2 is an example of a nontherapeutic and judgmental attitude that places blame. Option 3 makes statements that the nurse cannot know are true (the client may not, in fact, know if the spouse visits), and it predicts feelings of guilt, which is inappropriate. Option 4 fosters dependency and gives advice, which is nontherapeutic.
Test-Taking Strategy: Note the strategic word, *most.* Use therapeutic communication techniques to answer the question. The correct option is the only option that is therapeutic and that addresses the spouse's feelings.
Priority Nursing Tip: Respite care provides support to the caregiver(s) of the client requiring long-term care. This allows family members and significant others involved in the client's care time to care for themselves.
Reference: Potter, P., et al. (2021). *Fundamentals of nursing* (10th ed., pp. 333–335, 743). Elsevier.

17. While in the dining area, an adult client at the retirement center yells, "This turkey is dry and cold! I can't stand the food here!" Which is the **best** response by the nurse to the client's behavior?
1. "Now look what you've done! You're ruining this meal for the whole community. Aren't you ashamed of yourself?"
2. "I think you had better return to your apartment now. I'll make arrangements for a new meal to be served to you there."
3. "Let me get you another serving that is more to your liking. Would you like to see the chef and select your own serving?"
4. "One of the things that was agreed upon was that anyone who did not use appropriate behavior would be asked to leave the dining room. Please leave now."

Level of Cognitive Ability: Applying
Client Needs: Psychosocial Integrity
Clinical Judgment/Cognitive Skills: Take Action
Integrated Process: Communication and Documentation
Content Area: Foundations of Care: Communication
Health Problems: Mental Health: Violence
Priority Concepts: Communication; Professional Identity

Answer: 3
Rationale: Asking the client to accompany the nurse to the kitchen respects the client's need for control, removes the angry client from the dining room, and may offer the nurse an opportunity to assess what is happening with the client. Agency procedure needs to be followed regarding those who are allowed access to the facility kitchen. Option 1 is angry, aggressive, and nontherapeutic. Option 2 could provoke a regressive struggle between the nurse and the client and cause more anger in the client. In option 4, the nurse is authoritative, and it would not be appropriate to ask the client to leave. This action may set up an aggressive struggle between the nurse and the client.
Test-Taking Strategy: Note the strategic word, *best.* Use therapeutic communication techniques and your knowledge about the care of an angry client. Option 3 is the only option that addresses the client's angry feelings, and it also provides the nurse with an opportunity to further assess the client.
Priority Nursing Tip: The aging client may experience a sense of loss of control, particularly if the client has been moved from their own home into a care facility. The nurse needs to allow the client to exercise as much control as possible through decision-making and other means.
Reference: Varcarolis, E., & Fosbre, C. (2021). *Essentials of psychiatric mental health nursing: A communication approach to evidence-based care* (4th ed., pp. 93–95). Elsevier.

❖ **18.** When the home care nurse arrives, the client with a diagnosis of emphysema is smoking. Which statement by the nurse would be **most** therapeutic?

1. "Well, I can see you never got to the stop smoking clinic."
2. "Now that your secret is out, may we decide what you are going to do?"
3. "Did you explore the stop smoking program at the senior citizens center?"
4. "I wonder if you realize that by smoking you are slowly killing yourself."

Level of Cognitive Ability: Applying
Client Needs: Psychosocial Integrity
Clinical Judgment/Cognitive Skills: Take Action
Integrated Process: Communication and Documentation
Content Area: Adult Health: Respiratory
Health Problems: Mental Health: Addictions
Priority Concepts: Communication; Gas Exchange

Answer: 3
Rationale: Clients with emphysema must avoid smoking and all airborne irritants. The nurse who observes a maladaptive behavior in a client would not make judgmental comments and would instead explore an adaptive strategy with the client without being overly controlling. This will place the decision-making in the client's hands and provide an avenue for the client to share what may be expressions of frustration about an inability to stop what is essentially a physiologic addiction. Option 1 is an intrusive use of sarcastic humor that is degrading to the client. Option 2 is a disciplinary remark and places a barrier between the nurse and the client within the therapeutic relationship. In option 4, the nurse preaches and is judgmental.
Test-Taking Strategy: Note the strategic word, *most*. Use therapeutic communication techniques. Option 3 recognizes and addresses the client's behavior and explores an avenue for dealing with the behavior.
Priority Nursing Tip: Emphysema occurs when there is abnormal permanent enlargement of air spaces distal to the terminal bronchioles, with destruction of alveolar walls without obvious fibrosis.
References: Ignatavicius, D., et al. (2021). *Medical-surgical nursing: Concepts for interprofessional collaborative care* (10th ed., p.544). Elsevier; Potter, P., et al. (2021). *Fundamentals of nursing* (10th ed., pp. 333–335). Elsevier.

19. A client is to have arterial blood gases drawn. While the nurse is performing Allen's test, the client states to the nurse, "What are you doing? No one else has done that!" Which response to the client is **most** therapeutic?

1. "I assure you that I am doing the correct procedure. I cannot account for what others do."
2. "This step is crucial to safe blood withdrawal. I would not let anyone take my blood until they did this."
3. "Oh? You have questions about this? You need to insist that they all do this procedure before drawing up your blood."
4. "This is a routine precautionary step that simply makes certain your circulation is intact before a blood sample is obtained."

Level of Cognitive Ability: Applying
Client Needs: Psychosocial Integrity
Clinical Judgment/Cognitive Skills: Take Action
Integrated Process: Communication and Documentation
Content Area: Foundations of Care: Diagnostic Tests
Health Problems: Mental Health: Anxiety
Priority Concepts: Patient Education; Safety

Answer: 4
Rationale: Allen's test is performed to assess collateral circulation in the hand before drawing a radial artery blood specimen. The therapeutic response provides information to the client. Option 1 is defensive and nontherapeutic in that it offers false reassurance. Option 2 identifies client advocacy, but it is overly controlling and aggressive, and undermines treatment. Option 3 is aggressive, controlling, and nontherapeutic in its disapproving stance.
Test-Taking Strategy: Note the strategic word, *most*. Use therapeutic communication techniques. Option 4 addresses the subject, explaining an Allen's test to a questioning client, and provides information to the client in an appropriate manner.
Priority Nursing Tip: Before an arterial blood gas (ABG) is drawn, the client needs to rest for 30 minutes to ensure accurate measurement of body oxygenation. If the client is wearing oxygen, it would not be turned off unless the ABG sample is prescribed to be drawn with the client breathing room air.
References: Pagana, K., Pagana, T., & Pagana, T. N. (2021). *Mosby's Diagnostic and laboratory test reference* (15th ed., p. 109). Elsevier; Potter, P., et al. (2021). *Fundamentals of nursing* (10th ed., pp. 333–335). Elsevier.

❖ **20.** A client reports having difficulty concentrating and is having outbursts of anger, as well as feeling "keyed up" all the time. The client reveals that the behaviors began soon after witnessing the murder of a good friend. The nurse would suspect which stressor before communicating with the client?
1. Social phobia
2. Panic disorder
3. Post-traumatic stress disorder (PTSD)
4. Obsessive-compulsive disorder (OCD)

Level of Cognitive Ability: Analyzing
Client Needs: Psychosocial Integrity
Clinical Judgment/Cognitive Skills: Analyze Cues
Integrated Process: Clinical Judgment; Nursing Process/Analysis
Content Area: Mental Health
Health Problems: Mental Health: Post-Traumatic Stress Disorder
Priority Concepts: Anxiety; Stress

Answer: 3
Rationale: PTSD is a response to an event that would be markedly distressing to almost anyone. Characteristic symptoms include a sustained level of anxiety, difficulty sleeping, irritability, difficulty concentrating, and outbursts of anger. Panic disorders and social phobia are characterized by a specific fear of an object or situation. OCD involves some repetitive thoughts or behaviors.
Test-Taking Strategy: Focus on the data in the question. Eliminate options 1 and 2 first because they are comparable or alike. From the remaining options, recalling that OCD relates to a repetitive thought or behavior will direct you to the correct option.
Priority Nursing Tip: Common stressors that can result in PTSD include a natural disaster; terrorist attack; combat experiences; accidents; rape; crime or violence; sexual, physical, and emotional abuse; and reexperiencing the event as flashbacks.
Reference: Varcarolis, E., & Fosbre, C. (2021). *Essentials of psychiatric mental health nursing: A communication approach to evidence-based care* (4th ed., pp. 121–123). Elsevier.

21. A client states to the nurse, "I can't get any help with my care! I call and call, but the nurses never answer my light. Last night one of them told me they had other clients besides me! I'm very sick, but the nurses don't care!" Which statement would the nurse plan to make to address the client's **primary** concern?
1. "I think you are being very impatient. The nurses come as quickly as they can."
2. "I can hear your anger. That nurse had no right to speak to you that way. I will report her."
3. "You poor thing! I'm so sorry this happened to you. That nurse needs to be reprimanded immediately."
4. "It's hard to be in bed and to have to ask for help. You feel that the nurses do not seem to care?"

Level of Cognitive Ability: Applying
Client Needs: Psychosocial Integrity
Clinical Judgment/Cognitive Skills: Generate Solutions
Integrated Process: Clinical Judgment; Nursing Process/Planning
Content Area: Foundations of Care: Communication
Health Problems: Mental Health: Coping
Priority Concepts: Communication; Professional Identity

Answer: 4
Rationale: *Empathy* is a term that describes the nurse's capacity to enter into the life of another person and to perceive how the client is feeling and what meaning this has for the client. In option 4, the nurse displays empathy and shares perceptions. The sharing of perceptions asks the client to validate the nurse's understanding of what the client is feeling and thinking. It opens the door for the client to share concerns, fears, and anxieties. In option 1, the nurse is assertive and also defends the nursing staff. In option 2, the nurse expresses the client's frustration by labeling the client's feelings as angry and disapproving of the nursing staff. This is splitting, and it is nontherapeutic. Option 3 is a social response, and it is demeaning to the client.
Test-Taking Strategy: Note the strategic word, *primary.* Use therapeutic communication techniques. Focus on the client's statement in the question. Note the relationship between the client's statement and option 4. In addition, in this option, the nurse validates the client's feelings.
Priority Nursing Tip: The nurse would encourage the client to share thoughts and feelings. This will assist to uncover other feelings, anxieties, or fears the client is having.
Reference: Varcarolis, E., & Fosbre, C. (2021). *Essentials of psychiatric mental health nursing: A communication approach to evidence-based care* (4th ed., pp. 93–95, 113). Elsevier.

Client Needs

❖ **22.** A client has a newly applied long leg cast to stabilize a right proximal fractured tibia. During rounds at night, the nurse finds the client restless, withdrawn, and unusually quiet. Which nursing statement would be **most appropriate**?
1. "Are you uncomfortable?"
2. "Tell me what you are feeling."
3. "You'll feel better in the morning."
4. "I'll get your pain medication right away."

Level of Cognitive Ability: Applying
Client Needs: Psychosocial Integrity
Clinical Judgment/Cognitive Skills: Generate Solutions
Integrated Process: Communication and Documentation
Content Area: Foundations of Care: Communication
Health Problems: Mental Health: Coping
Priority Concepts: Communication; Culture

Answer: 2
Rationale: Option 2 is open-ended and makes no assumptions about the client's psychological or emotional state. Option 1 is incorrect because, for some clients, stoicism is valued, so the client may deny any pain when asked. False reassurance is never therapeutic, which makes option 3 incorrect. Option 4 is incorrect because an assessment is necessary before administering medication for pain.
Test-Taking Strategy: Note the strategic words, *most appropriate*. Use therapeutic communication techniques. Recalling that the client's feelings are the priority will direct you to the correct option.
Priority Nursing Tip: The nurse must be aware of different types of client reactions to pain.
Reference: Varcarolis, E., & Fosbre, C. (2021). *Essentials of psychiatric mental health nursing: A communication approach to evidence-based care* (4th ed., pp. 93–95). Elsevier.

23. A client diagnosed with moderate dementia is prescribed oral anticoagulant therapy while hospitalized. The nurse identifies which discharge scenario as being the **best** support system for successful anticoagulant therapy monitoring?
1. Client has a home health aide coming to the house for 9 weeks.
2. Client was going to stay with a family member in the family member's home indefinitely.
3. Client was going to have blood work drawn in the home by a local laboratory.
4. Client has a good friend living next door who would take the client to the doctor.

Level of Cognitive Ability: Analyzing
Client Needs: Psychosocial Integrity
Clinical Judgment/Cognitive Skills: Generate Solutions
Integrated Process: Nursing Process/Planning
Content Area: Pharmacology: Cardiovascular: Anticoagulants
Health Problems: Mental Health: Neurocognitive Impairment
Priority Concepts: Family Dynamics; Health Promotion

Answer: 2
Rationale: The client taking anticoagulant therapy needs to be informed about the medication, its purpose, and the necessity of taking the proper dose at the specified times. If the client is unwilling or unable to comply with the medication regimen, the continuance of the regimen needs to be questioned. Option 2 provides a direct support system. Clients may need support systems in place to enhance compliance with therapy. Option 1 facilitates reminding the client to take the medication, option 3 facilitates blood work only, and option 4 facilitates medical care.
Test-Taking Strategy: Note the strategic word, *best*. Note the subject, the best support system for a client on oral anticoagulant therapy. Note that option 2 is the only option that indicates direct support for the client.
Priority Nursing Tip: Anticoagulants are administered when there is evidence of or likelihood of clot formation. Such situations include myocardial infarction, unstable angina, atrial fibrillation, deep vein thrombosis, pulmonary embolism, and the presence of mechanical heart valves.
Reference: Ignatavicius, D., et al. (2021). *Medical-surgical nursing: Concepts for interprofessional collaborative care* (10th ed., pp. 724, 852–853). Elsevier.

24. A client who has undergone successful femoral-popliteal bypass grafting of the leg states to the nurse, "I hope everything goes well after this and that I don't lose my leg. I'm so afraid that I'll have gone through this for nothing." Which **most** therapeutic response would the nurse make to the client?
1. "I can understand what you mean. I'd be nervous too if I were in your shoes."
2. "This surgery is so successful that I wouldn't be concerned at all if I were you."
3. "Complications are possible, but you have a good deal of control if you make the lifestyle adjustments we talked about."
4. "Stress isn't helpful for you. You should probably just try to relax. You shouldn't worry unless something actually happens."

Level of Cognitive Ability: Applying
Client Needs: Psychosocial Integrity
Clinical Judgment/Cognitive Skills: Generate Solutions
Integrated Process: Communication and Documentation
Content Area: Adult Health: Cardiovascular
Health Problems: Mental Health: Coping
Priority Concepts: Communication; Perfusion

Answer: 3
Rationale: Clients frequently fear that they will ultimately lose a limb or become debilitated in some other way. Option 3 acknowledges the client's concerns and empowers the client to improve their health, which will ultimately reduce concern about the risk of complications. Option 1 feeds into the client's anxiety and is not therapeutic. Option 2 gives false reassurance. Option 4 is meant to be reassuring, but it offers no suggestions to empower the client.
Test-Taking Strategy: Note the strategic word, *most.* Use therapeutic communication techniques. Option 3 is the only option that acknowledges the client's concerns and addresses the client's control over the situation.
Priority Nursing Tip: The client undergoing femoral-popliteal bypass grafting who is returning home needs to progressively return to their normal routine. Additionally, the client needs to limit pushing or pulling objects for 6 weeks; maintain incision care and report signs of redness, swelling, or discharge; avoid crossing the legs; use prescribed medications; and maintain the prescribed therapeutic diet.
References: Lewis, S., et al. (2020). *Medical-surgical nursing: Assessment and management of clinical problems* (11th ed., pp. 803–804). Elsevier; Potter, P., et al. (2021). *Fundamentals of nursing* (10th ed., pp. 333–335). Elsevier.

25. A client is about to undergo a pericardiocentesis to help manage rapidly accumulating pericardial effusion. What is the **best** plan for the nurse to implement to alleviate the client's apprehension?
1. Suggesting client watch television during the procedure as a distraction
2. Talking to client from the foot of the bed and assisting with the procedure
3. Staying beside client to give information and encouragement during the procedure
4. Assuring client that, even though there are other clients needing care, client's needs are most important

Level of Cognitive Ability: Applying
Client Needs: Psychosocial Integrity
Clinical Judgment/Cognitive Skills: Generate Solutions
Integrated Process: Nursing Process/Planning
Content Area: Adult Health: Cardiovascular
Health Problems: Mental Health: Coping
Priority Concepts: Anxiety; Communication

Answer: 3
Rationale: Clients who develop sudden complications are in situational crisis and need therapeutic intervention. Staying with the client and giving information and encouragement is part of building and maintaining trust in the nurse–client relationship. Options 1 and 4 distance the nurse from the client psychosocially. The nurse would ask another caregiver to be available to assist with the procedure.
Test-Taking Strategy: Note the strategic word, *best.* Use therapeutic communication techniques. Option 3 is the only option that provides direct contact with and assistance to the client.
Priority Nursing Tip: A pericardiocentesis involves aspiration of fluid from the pericardium. It is generally done with the guidance of ultrasound so as to minimize complications.
References: Ignatavicius, D., et al. (2021). *Medical-surgical nursing: Concepts for interprofessional collaborative care* (10th ed., pp. 690–691). Elsevier; Potter, P., et al. (2021). *Fundamentals of nursing* (10th ed., pp. 333–335). Elsevier.

❖ **26.** The nurse has created a teaching plan for a client prescribed spironolactone. On which psychosocial side effect of the medication would the nurse base the teaching plan?
1. Edema
2. Hair loss
3. Weight loss
4. Decreased libido

Level of Cognitive Ability: Applying
Client Needs: Psychosocial Integrity
Clinical Judgment/Cognitive Skills: Generate Solutions
Integrated Process: Nursing Process/Planning
Content Area: Pharmacology: Cardiovascular: Diuretics
Health Problems: Mental Health: Coping
Priority Concepts: Patient Education; Fluids and Electrolytes

Answer: 4
Rationale: The nurse needs to be aware of the fact that the client taking spironolactone, a potassium-sparing diuretic, may experience body image changes that result from a threatened sexual identity. These are related to decreased libido, gynecomastia in biologically born males, and hirsutism in biologically born females. Edema, weight loss, and hair loss are not specifically associated with the use of this medication.
Test-Taking Strategy: Recall your knowledge regarding the side effects of spironolactone. Eliminate options 2 and 3 because they are comparable or alike options. From the remaining options, focusing on the word "psychosocial" in the question will direct you to the correct option.
Priority Nursing Tip: Spironolactone is a potassium-sparing diuretic. A primary concern with administering potassium-sparing diuretics is hyperkalemia.
Reference: Kizior, R., & Hodgson, B. (2022). *Saunders nursing drug handbook 2022* (p. 1099). Elsevier.

27. The nurse is caring for a client who is recovering from an episode of autonomic hyperreflexia. Which statement would the nurse make to the client to **most** encourage therapeutic communication?
1. "How could your home care nurse let this happen?"
2. "Now that this problem is taken care of, I'm sure you'll be fine."
3. "I have some time if you would like to talk about what happened to you."
4. "I'm sure you now understand the importance of preventing this from occurring."

Level of Cognitive Ability: Applying
Client Needs: Psychosocial Integrity
Clinical Judgment/Cognitive Skills: Take Action
Integrated Process: Communication and Documentation
Content Area: Adult Health: Neurologic
Health Problems: Adult Health: Neurologic: Spinal Cord Injury
Priority Concepts: Communication; Stress

Answer: 3
Rationale: Option 3 encourages the client to discuss their feelings. Options 1 and 4 show disapproval, and option 2 provides false reassurance; these are nontherapeutic techniques.
Test-Taking Strategy: Note the strategic word, *most.* Use therapeutic communication techniques to identify the correct answer. Remembering to always address the client's concerns and feelings first will direct you to the correct option.
Priority Nursing Tip: Autonomic dysreflexia occurs with spinal cord lesions or injuries above T6. If autonomic dysreflexia occurs, immediately place the client in high-Fowler's position.
References: Ignatavicius, D., et al. (2021). *Medical-surgical nursing: Concepts for interprofessional collaborative care* (10th ed., p. 882). Elsevier; Potter, P., et al. (2021). *Fundamentals of nursing* (10th ed., pp. 333–335). Elsevier.

28. While the nurse is assisting with bathing, the client who has sustained a spinal cord injury states, "I can't do this. I wish I were dead." Which therapeutic response would the nurse make to encourage communication?
1. "Why do you say that?"
2. "You wish you were dead?"
3. "Would you prefer a shower instead?"
4. "Are you frustrated with your limitations?"

Level of Cognitive Ability: Applying
Client Needs: Psychosocial Integrity
Clinical Judgment/Cognitive Skills: Generate Solutions
Integrated Process: Communication and Documentation
Content Area: Adult Health: Neurologic
Health Problems: Mental Health: Coping
Priority Concepts: Communication; Stress and Coping

Answer: 2
Rationale: Clarifying is a therapeutic technique that involves restating what was said to obtain additional information. By asking "why" in option 1, the nurse puts the client on the defensive. Option 3 changes the subject. In option 4, the nurse presumes limitations.
Test-Taking Strategy: Use therapeutic communication techniques. Remember to focus on the client's feelings. Option 2 involves clarifying and restating, and it is the only option that will encourage the client to verbalize feelings and concerns.
Priority Nursing Tip: Trauma to the spinal cord causes partial or complete disruption of the nerve tracts and neurons. Loss of motor function, sensation, reflex activity, and bowel and bladder control may result; therefore, the client is likely to feel a sense of loss of control.
References: Ignatavicius, D., et al. (2021). *Medical-surgical nursing: Concepts for interprofessional collaborative care* (10th ed., p. 877). Elsevier; Potter, P., et al. (2021). *Fundamentals of nursing* (10th ed., pp. 333–335). Elsevier.

29. Family members of a client who attempted suicide are tearful. Which statement by the nurse would be **most** helpful in the management of their concerns?
1. "I'll check on when you will be able to see your loved one."
2. "Believe me when I say that everything possible is being done."
3. "Don't worry. You have absolutely nothing to feel guilty about."
4. "I certainly can see that you are terribly worried about your loved one."

Level of Cognitive Ability: Applying
Client Needs: Psychosocial Integrity
Clinical Judgment/Cognitive Skills: Take Action
Integrated Process: Caring
Content Area: Foundations of Care: Communication
Health Problems: Mental Health: Suicide
Priority Concepts: Communication; Family Dynamics

Answer: 4
Rationale: Option 4 addresses the family's feelings and displays empathy. Options 1, 2, and 3 are communication blocks. Option 1 focuses on an important issue at an inappropriate time. Option 2 uses clichés and false reassurance. Option 3 labels the family's behavior without their validation.
Test-Taking Strategy: Note the strategic word, *most*. Use therapeutic communication techniques. Option 4 involves clarifying, and it is the only option that will encourage the family to verbalize feelings and concerns.
Priority Nursing Tip: All suicide behavior is serious regardless of the intent. Suicide ideation requires constant attention and typically one-on-one observation. The client at risk must be placed on suicide precautions.
Reference: Varcarolis, E., & Fosbre, C. (2021). *Essentials of psychiatric mental health nursing: A communication approach to evidence-based care* (4th ed., pp. 93–95, 372). Elsevier.

❖ **30.** The nurse is caring for an 11-year-old child who has been physically abused. Which therapeutic action would the nurse include in the plan of care?
1. Encouraging the child to confront the abuser
2. Providing a care environment that fosters trust
3. Teaching the child to make wise choices when faced with possible abuse
4. Reinforcing for the child that not all adults are capable of abusing children

Level of Cognitive Ability: Applying
Client Needs: Psychosocial Integrity
Clinical Judgment/Cognitive Skills: Generate Solutions
Integrated Process: Clinical Judgment; Caring
Content Area: Mental Health
Health Problems: Mental Health: Abuse/Neglect
Priority Concepts: Interpersonal Violence; Safety

Answer: 2
Rationale: The abused child usually requires long-term therapeutic support. The environment provided during the child's healing must include one in which trust and empathy are modeled and provided for the child. Option 2 is therapeutic because it provides the child with a nurturing and supportive environment in which to begin the healing process. Option 1 reinforces fear, which would not be encouraged. Options 3 and 4 ask the child to behave or assume beliefs with a maturity beyond that which would be expected of an 11-year-old child.
Test-Taking Strategy: Use therapeutic communication techniques. Option 2 is the only option that provides support to the child.
Priority Nursing Tip: Nurses are legally required to report all cases of suspected child abuse to the appropriate local or state agency. Documentation of information related to the suspected abuse needs to be done in an objective manner.
Reference: Varcarolis, E., & Fosbre, C. (2021). *Essentials of psychiatric mental health nursing: A communication approach to evidence-based care* (4th ed., pp. 93–95, 343). Elsevier.

31. Which psychosocial factor obtained during an assessment of an older client places the client **most** at risk for abuse?
1. Client resides in an apartment in a low-income neighborhood.
2. Client shows several signs and symptoms of clinical depression.
3. Client is completely dependent on family members for both food and medicine.
4. Client has been diagnosed with and is being treated for several chronic illnesses.

Level of Cognitive Ability: Analyzing
Client Needs: Psychosocial Integrity
Clinical Judgment/Cognitive Skills: Recognize Cues
Integrated Process: Clinical Judgment; Nursing Process/Assessment
Content Area: Health Assessment/Physical Exam: Health History
Health Problems: Mental Health: Abuse/Neglect
Priority Concepts: Development; Interpersonal Violence

Answer: 3
Rationale: Elder abuse is sometimes the result of frustrated adult children who find themselves caring for dependent parents. Increasing demands by parents for care and financial support can cause resentment and a feeling of being burdened. The issues of abuse are not bound to socioeconomic status (option 1). Option 2 relates to depression rather than the risk for abuse. Option 4 relates to a physical factor rather than a psychosocial factor.
Test-Taking Strategy: Note the strategic word, *most*. Then note the words *psychosocial factor*, and focus on the subject, the risk for elder abuse. Noting the words *completely dependent* in option 3 will direct you to this option.
Priority Nursing Tip: Factors that contribute to elder abuse and neglect include long-standing family violence, caregiver stress, and the individual's increasing dependence on others. The interaction between the older adult and caregiver can provide important clues about the relationship.
Reference: Varcarolis, E., & Fosbre, C. (2021). *Essentials of psychiatric mental health nursing: A communication approach to evidence-based care* (4th ed., pp. 351–352). Elsevier.

❖ **32.** The nurse is caring for a dying client who states, "Will you be the executor of my will?" How would the nurse **best** respond to this client?

1. "I must decline your offer because I am your nurse."
2. "I will carry out your will according to your wishes."
3. "It is an honor to be named the executor of your will."
4. "Tell me more so that I can understand your thinking."

Level of Cognitive Ability: Applying
Client Needs: Psychosocial Integrity
Clinical Judgment/Cognitive Skills: Take Action
Integrated Process: Nursing Process/Implementation
Content Area: Leadership/Management: Ethical/Legal
Health Problems: Mental Health: Grief/Loss
Priority Concepts: Ethics; Health Care Law

Answer: 4
Rationale: The client's question reflects their thoughts about the will and how to obtain an executor, but the question does not reveal why the client is asking the nurse to be executor, and it also does not address other important information. In option 4, the nurse seeks clarification while acknowledging the client's statement. Most agencies do not allow the nurse to be the executor of a client's will (option 3). The other options fail to regard the potential consequences, think critically, or explore the client's motivation and needs.
Test-Taking Strategy: Note the strategic word, *best*. Use therapeutic communication techniques. Option 4 is the only option that addresses the client's thoughts and feelings.
Priority Nursing Tip: A living will is one example of the execution of the Patient's Bill of Rights (Patient Care Partnership), which reflects acknowledgment of a client's right to participate in their health care with an emphasis on client autonomy.
Reference: Potter, P., et al. (2021). *Fundamentals of nursing* (10th ed., pp. 310, 333–335). Elsevier.

33. A client experiencing urticaria (hives) and pruritus states to the nurse, "What am I going to do? I'm getting married next week, and I'll probably be covered in this rash and itching like crazy." Which statement made by the nurse is the **most** therapeutic?

1. "You're troubled that this will extend into your wedding?"
2. "It's probably just due to prewedding jitters. You'll be fine."
3. "The antihistamine will help a great deal, just you wait and see."
4. "Do you think this would really be something that could ruin your wedding?"

Level of Cognitive Ability: Applying
Client Needs: Psychosocial Integrity
Clinical Judgment/Cognitive Skills: Take Action
Integrated Process: Communication and Documentation
Content Area: Foundations of Care: Communication
Health Problems: Mental Health: Coping
Priority Concepts: Anxiety; Communication

Answer: 1
Rationale: The therapeutic communication technique that the nurse uses in option 1 is reflection. In option 2, the nurse minimizes the client's anxiety and fears. In option 3, the nurse talks about antihistamines and asks the client to "wait and see." This is nontherapeutic because the nurse is making promises that may not be kept. In addition, the response is closed-ended and shuts off the client's expression of feelings. In option 4, the nurse responds without sensitivity.
Test-Taking Strategy: Note the strategic word, *most*. Use therapeutic communication techniques. Options 2, 3, and 4 are nontherapeutic responses. Option 1 addresses the client's feelings.
Priority Nursing Tip: Antihistamines are used to treat the common cold, rhinitis, nausea and vomiting, motion sickness, and urticaria and as a sleep aid. These medications can cause central nervous system depression if taken with alcohol, opioids, hypnotics, and barbiturates.
References: Ignatavicius, D., et al. (2021). *Medical-surgical nursing: Concepts for interprofessional collaborative care* (10th ed., p. 448). Elsevier; Potter, P., et al. (2021). *Fundamentals of nursing* (10th ed., pp. 333-–335). Elsevier.

❖ **34.** Which statement made by a client who has experienced a spinal cord injury resulting in chronic immobility issues warrants **immediate** follow-up by the nurse to ensure client safety?
1. "I'm so angry that this happened to me."
2. "I really don't want to live my life like this."
3. "I'm definitely not looking forward to going home."
4. "I don't know if I can make all these major adjustments to my life."

Level of Cognitive Ability: Analyzing
Client Needs: Psychosocial Integrity
Clinical Judgment/Cognitive Skills: Recognize Cues
Integrated Process: Clinical Judgment; Nursing Process/Assessment
Content Area: Adult Health: Neurologic
Health Problems: Mental Health: Coping
Priority Concepts: Mood and Affect; Functional Ability

Answer: 2
Rationale: It is important to allow the client with a spinal cord injury to verbalize their feelings. If the client indicates a desire to discuss their feelings, the nurse would respond therapeutically. Expressions of hopelessness or despair require immediate attention because they can indicate that the client is harboring suicidal ideations. Although the remaining statements require follow-up, they lack that serious component of despair and/or hopelessness.
Test-Taking Strategy: Focus on the subject, the client statement that *warrants follow-up*. Note the strategic word, *immediate*. Recognize that depression is a common factor among such clients and can lead to thoughts of suicide.
Priority Nursing Tip: Autonomic dysreflexia is a concern for the client with a spinal cord injury. Autonomic dysreflexia occurs with spinal lesions or injury above T6. Severe hypertension occurs in autonomic dysreflexia; therefore, immediately place the client in the high-Fowler's position and eliminate the noxious stimuli causing the problem.
Reference: Ignatavicius, D., et al. (2021). *Medical-surgical nursing: Concepts for interprofessional collaborative care* (10th ed., pp. 885–886). Elsevier.

35. The nurse is caring for a client with a diagnosis of a mild cerebral bleed resulting from a small cerebral aneurysm rupture. The client reports feeling anxious and restless about family visiting soon. Which comment by the client would assist the nurse in identifying the reason for the anxiety?
1. "My child came to visit me yesterday."
2. "At least I can speak and answer questions."
3. "I have a problem turning my neck to the side."
4. "Look at me, I can no longer be the head of my family."

Level of Cognitive Ability: Analyzing
Client Needs: Psychosocial Integrity
Clinical Judgment/Cognitive Skills: Recognize Cues
Integrated Process: Clinical Judgment; Nursing Process/Assessment
Content Area: Adult Health: Neurologic
Health Problems: Mental Health: Anxiety
Priority Concepts: Anxiety; Intracranial Regulation

Answer: 4
Rationale: With a mild bleed from a cerebral aneurysm rupture the client usually remains alert but has nuchal rigidity with possible neurologic deficits, depending on the area of the bleed. Because these clients remain alert, they are acutely aware of the neurologic deficits and frequently have some degree of body image disturbance. Option 4 alludes to the client's self-perception about not being able to be the head of the family now. The remaining client statements are unrelated to anxiety and restlessness.
Test-Taking Strategy: Focus on the subject, the client is feeling restless and anxious, and note the words *about family visiting soon*. Using your knowledge of the effects of this disorder and focusing on the client's behavior will direct you to option 4.
Priority Nursing Tip: For the client with a cerebral aneurysm, bed rest is usually maintained with the head of the bed elevated 30 to 45 degrees to prevent pressure on the aneurysm site that can lead to rupture.
References: Heuther, S., McCance, K., & Brashers, V. (2020). *Understanding pathophysiology* (7th ed., pp. 596–597). Elsevier; Potter, P., et al. (2021). *Fundamentals of nursing* (10th ed., pp. 333–335). Elsevier.

❖ **36.** When planning the care of the client diagnosed with thromboangiitis obliterans (Buerger's disease), the nurse incorporates information on which support service to **best** help the client cope with the lifestyle changes that are needed to control the disease process?
1. Pain management clinic
2. Smoking cessation program
3. Consultation with a dietician
4. Referral to a medical social worker

Level of Cognitive Ability: Applying
Client Needs: Psychosocial Integrity
Clinical Judgment/Cognitive Skills: Generate Solutions
Integrated Process: Nursing Process/Planning
Content Area: Adult Health: Cardiovascular
Health Problems: Mental Health: Coping
Priority Concepts: Health Promotion; Stress and Coping

Answer: 2
Rationale: Smoking is highly detrimental to the client with Buerger's disease, and clients are recommended to stop completely. Because smoking is a form of chemical dependency, referral to a smoking cessation program may be helpful for many clients. For many clients, symptoms are relieved or alleviated when smoking stops. None of the remaining options are directly related to the physiology associated with this condition.
Test-Taking Strategy: Note the strategic word, *best*. Focus on the subject, Buerger's disease. Recalling that the treatment goals are the same as for peripheral vascular disease will direct you to the correct option.
Priority Nursing Tip: Buerger's disease is an occlusive disease of the median and small arteries and veins. The distal upper and lower limbs are affected most commonly.
Reference: Ignatavicius, D., et al. (2021). *Medical-surgical nursing: Concepts for interprofessional collaborative care* (10th ed., p. 720). Elsevier.

37. While assessing a 14-year-old child, the nurse notes bruises and cigarette burns on the child's chest and rope burns on the buttocks. The child states, "I'm afraid to go home because my stepparent will be angry with me for telling you what happened." The nurse would make which therapeutic response to the child?
1. "You can't go back there with that parent. How do you think your other parent will react?"
2. "You must know that your presence in the house will only irritate your stepparent more."
3. "I am sorry that this has happened to you, but you will be safe here until plans can be made."
4. "Let's keep this between you, me, and the primary health care provider until we formulate further plans to assist you."

Level of Cognitive Ability: Applying
Client Needs: Psychosocial Integrity
Clinical Judgment/Cognitive Skills: Take Action
Integrated Process: Caring
Content Area: Mental Health
Health Problems: Mental Health: Abuse/Neglect
Priority Concepts: Interpersonal Violence; Safety

Answer: 3
Rationale: A child who has been physically and sexually abused needs to be admitted to the hospital. This will provide time for a more comprehensive evaluation while protecting the child from further abuse. The correct option also provides an empathic statement that supports the child to appropriately perceive self as the victim while assuring the child of protection from abuse. In option 1, the nurse does not respond with a calm and reassuring communication style or maintain a professional attitude. Option 2, which holds an innuendo, appears to accuse the victim of teasing the stepparent and is thus incorrect; it is also judgmental, controlling, and demeaning. The nurse's suggestion in option 4 is not only incorrect but also passive in its stance.
Test-Taking Strategy: Use therapeutic communication techniques and your knowledge of the care of the child who has been physically abused. Recalling that the priority is the safety of the victim will direct you to option 3.
Priority Nursing Tip: Ensuring a safe environment is the priority for a child who is a victim of abuse.
Reference: Varcarolis, E., & Fosbre, C. (2021). *Essentials of psychiatric mental health nursing: A communication approach to evidence-based care* (4th ed., pp. 333–335, 344). Elsevier.

❖ **38.** While providing care to a 12-year-old client, the nurse notes small round burn scars on the client's arms and legs, bruising on the buttocks, and tenderness of the right jaw. The client is anxious, has poor eye contact, and denies being injured at home when the nurse asks questions. Based on these observations, the nurse suspects victimization. Which is the **next priority** question the nurse would therapeutically ask the client in providing a safe environment for the client?

1. "Are you sure your parents didn't do this?"
2. "You need to tell me now, or I'll call security. Who did this to you?"
3. "Is someone bullying you at school, or at home, or in your neighborhood?"
4. "I can see this is difficult for you to talk about. You are safe here, but I need to ask you, who hurt you like this?"

Level of Cognitive Ability: Applying
Client Needs: Psychosocial Integrity
Clinical Judgment/Cognitive Skills: Take Action
Integrated Process: Clinical Judgment; Nursing Process/Implementation
Content Area: Mental Health
Health Problems: Mental Health: Abuse/Neglect
Priority Concepts: Interpersonal Violence; Safety

Answer: 4
Rationale: Based on the nurse's assessment data, the suspect of victimization needs to be analyzed to determine how the client received the old and new injuries. Option 4 offers the therapeutic approach for obtaining information using an open-ended question. It is important to determine if the injuries resulted from a family member or someone else outside the home. There are many forms of abuse besides physical abuse to consider, such as sexual, emotional, and psychological abuse. Identifying the victimizer is important to stop the abuse and avoid further injuries. Safety is a priority concern for the client while in the care of the nurse and then after discharge from care. Option 1 implies that the nurse is challenging if the client is telling the truth. Option 2 could be perceived as demanding and a threat to the client to answer the question. Option 3 focuses on outside the family, but there is not enough information given in the question to determine whether a family member is not suspected.
Test-Taking Strategy: Note the strategic words, *next* and *priority*. Focus on the subject, suspect injuries from victimization. Use therapeutic communication techniques to further analyze the client's situation.
Priority Nursing Tip: Nurses are legally required to report all cases of suspected child abuse to the appropriate local or state agency. A safe environment must be provided for the victim.
Reference: Varcarolis, E., & Fosbre, C. (2021). *Essentials of psychiatric mental health nursing: A communication approach to evidence-based care* (4th ed., p. 344). Elsevier.

39. A client with arterial leg ulcers tells the nurse, "I'm so discouraged. I have had this pain for more than a year now. The pain never seems to go away. I can't do anything, and I feel as though I'll never get better." The nurse determines that which is the **priority** client concern?

1. Fatigue
2. Uneasiness
3. Chronic pain
4. An acute illness

Level of Cognitive Ability: Analyzing
Client Needs: Psychosocial Integrity
Clinical Judgment/Cognitive Skills: Prioritize Hypotheses
Integrated Process: Clinical Judgment; Nursing Process/Analysis
Content Area: Adult Health: Cardiovascular
Health Problems: Adult Health: Cardiovascular: Vascular Disorders
Priority Concepts: Mood and Affect; Pain

Answer: 3
Rationale: The major focus of the client's complaint is the experience of pain. Pain that has a duration of more than 3 months is defined as chronic pain and does not indicate an acute illness. There are no data in the question that indicate fatigue or uneasiness.
Test-Taking Strategy: Note the strategic word, *priority*. Focusing on the words *pain for more than a year now* will direct you to the correct option.
Priority Nursing Tip: The client with nonhealing arterial ulcerations needs to monitor the site and report signs of infection. These signs include redness, edema, and warmth at the affected area. In addition, an elevated temperature and change in vital signs may be signs of infection and need to be reported.
Reference: Ignatavicius, D., et al. (2021). *Medical-surgical nursing: Concepts for interprofessional collaborative care* (10th ed., pp. 46, 72). Elsevier.

❖ **40.** A client with a diagnosis of valvular heart disease is being considered for mechanical valve replacement. Which circumstance is **essential** to assess before the surgery is performed?
1. The physical demands of client's lifestyle
2. The ability to comply with anticoagulant therapy for life
3. The ability to participate in a cardiac rehabilitation program
4. The likelihood of the client experiencing body image problems

Level of Cognitive Ability: Analyzing
Client Needs: Psychosocial Integrity
Clinical Judgment/Cognitive Skills: Prioritize Hypotheses
Integrated Process: Nursing Process/Assessment
Content Area: Adult Health: Cardiovascular
Health Problems: Adult Health: Cardiovascular: Inflammatory/Infections/Structural Problems
Priority Concepts: Adherence; Perfusion

Answer: 2
Rationale: Mechanical valves carry the associated risk of thromboemboli, which require long-term anticoagulation with warfarin sodium. No data in the question indicate that physical demands exist in the client's lifestyle. Not all clients who undergo cardiac surgery require cardiac rehabilitation. Body image problems are important but not critical.
Test-Taking Strategy: Focus on the strategic word, *essential*. Recalling that mechanical valves are thrombogenic will direct you to the correct option.
Priority Nursing Tip: A priority concern when the client is taking an anticoagulant is bleeding.
Reference: Ignatavicius, D., et al. (2021). *Medical-surgical nursing: Concepts for interprofessional collaborative care* (10th ed., pp. 685–686). Elsevier.

41. A client who has a history of depression has been prescribed a beta-adrenergic blocking agent for the management of angina pectoris. Which consideration is **most important** when the nurse plans to counsel this client about the effects of this medication?
1. Risk of tachycardia
2. Probability of fatigue
3. High incidence of hypoglycemia
4. Possible exacerbation of depression

Level of Cognitive Ability: Analyzing
Client Needs: Psychosocial Integrity
Clinical Judgment/Cognitive Skills: Generate Solutions
Integrated Process: Clinical Judgment; Nursing Process/Planning
Content Area: Pharmacology: Cardiovascular: Beta Blockers
Health Problems: Mental Health: Mood Disorders
Priority Concepts: Clinical Judgment; Mood and Affect

Answer: 4
Rationale: Clients with depression or a history of depression have experienced an exacerbation of depression after beginning therapy with beta-adrenergic blocking agents. These clients need to be monitored carefully if these agents are prescribed. The medication would cause bradycardia rather than tachycardia. Fatigue is a possible side effect, but it is not the most important item. Hypoglycemia is a sign that is masked with beta blockers.
Test-Taking Strategy: Note the strategic words, *most important*. Focus on the subject, the effects of a beta-adrenergic blocking agent. Note the word *depression* in the question to direct you to the correct option. Clients with depression or a history of depression have experienced an exacerbation of depression after beginning therapy with beta-adrenergic blocking agents. These clients need to be monitored carefully if these agents are prescribed.
Priority Nursing Tip: The goal of treatment for angina is to provide relief of the acute attack, correct the imbalance between myocardial oxygen supply and demand, and prevent the progression of the disease and further attacks to reduce the risk of myocardial infarction.
Reference: Lilley, L., Rainforth Collins, S., & Snyder J. (2023). *Pharmacology and the nursing process* (10th ed.). St. Louis: Elsevier. p. 308.

❖ **42.** The nurse is caring for a client with a diagnosis of terminal cancer of the throat. The family tells the nurse that they have spoken to the primary health care provider regarding taking their loved one home. The nurse plans to coordinate discharge planning. Which service would be **most** supportive to the client and the family?
1. Hospice care
2. The American Cancer Society
3. The American Lung Association
4. Local religious and social organizations

Level of Cognitive Ability: Applying
Client Needs: Psychosocial Integrity
Clinical Judgment/Cognitive Skills: Generate Solutions
Integrated Process: Nursing Process/Planning
Content Area: Adult Health: Oncology
Health Problems: Mental Health: Coping
Priority Concepts: Caregiving; Palliative Care

Answer: 1
Rationale: Hospice care provides an environment that emphasizes caring rather than curing; the emphasis is on palliative care. One of the major goals of hospice care is that clients be free of pain and other symptoms that do not allow them to maintain a quality life. An interdisciplinary approach is used. Although the remaining options may be helpful, they are not the most supportive of the options provided.
Test-Taking Strategy: Note the strategic word, *most*. Knowledge regarding the goals and services provided by hospice care will assist you with answering the question. Think about what each support service presented in the options will provide for meeting this client's needs. This will assist with directing you to the correct option.
Priority Nursing Tip: With hospice care the client and the family are the focus of nursing care, and the goal is to relieve pain and facilitate an optimal quality of life.
Reference: Ignatavicius, D., et al. (2021). *Medical-surgical nursing: Concepts for interprofessional collaborative care* (10th ed., pp. 137–139). Elsevier.

43. The home care nurse is caring for an anxious client with lung cancer with acute cancer pain. Which is the **most appropriate** way to assess the client's pain?
1. Client's pain rating
2. Nurse's impression of client's pain
3. Verbal and nonverbal clues from client
4. Pain relief after appropriate nursing intervention

Level of Cognitive Ability: Applying
Client Needs: Psychosocial Integrity
Clinical Judgment/Cognitive Skills: Recognize Cues
Integrated Process: Nursing Process/Assessment
Content Area: Adult Health: Oncology
Health Problems: Mental Health: Anxiety
Priority Concepts: Clinical Judgment; Pain

Answer: 1
Rationale: The client's perception of pain is the hallmark of pain assessment. Usually noted by the client's rating on a scale of 1 to 10, the assessment is documented and followed with appropriate medical and nursing interventions. The nurse's impression and the verbal and nonverbal clues are subjective data. Pain relief after intervention is appropriate but relates to evaluation.
Test-Taking Strategy: Note the strategic words, *most appropriate*. Using the steps of the nursing process, note that the correct option addresses the client directly.
Priority Nursing Tip: The nurse must assess the client's pain; pain is what the client describes or says that it is. The nurse must not undermedicate the client with cancer who is in pain.
Reference: Ignatavicius, D., et al. (2021). *Medical-surgical nursing: Concepts for interprofessional collaborative care* (10th ed., p. 79). Elsevier.

❖ **44.** A prenatal client has been told during a primary health care provider office visit that testing is positive for human immunodeficiency virus (HIV). The client cried and was significantly distressed regarding this news. Which client concern would this assessment data **best** support?

1. Pain
2. Nonadherence
3. Anticipatory grieving
4. High risk for infection

Level of Cognitive Ability: Analyzing
Client Needs: Psychosocial Integrity
Clinical Judgment/Cognitive Skills: Prioritize Hypotheses
Integrated Process: Clinical Judgment; Nursing Process/Analysis
Content Area: Maternity: Antepartum
Health Problems: Mental Health: Coping
Priority Concepts: Stress and Coping; Immunity

Answer: 3
Rationale: A life-threatening diagnosis such as HIV will stimulate the anticipatory grief response. Anticipatory grief occurs when the client, family, and loved ones know that the client will die. The prenatal client with HIV is forced to make important changes in their life, frequently resulting in grief related to lost future dreams and diminished self-esteem as a result of an inability to achieve life goals. Although the remaining options may be appropriate problem statements, they do not address the information given in the question.
Test-Taking Strategy: Note the strategic word, *best*. Focus on the data in the question. A client who is distressed and crying is supporting data for the problem statement of anticipatory grieving.
Priority Nursing Tip: During the prenatal period, the primary health care providers must focus on preventing opportunistic infections in the client with HIV. Procedures that increase the risk of perinatal transmission, such as amniocentesis and fetal scalp sampling, need to be avoided.
Reference: McKinney, E. S., et al. (2022). *Maternal child nursing* (6th ed., pp. 519, 573–574). Elsevier.

45. The nurse is assessing a client's suicide potential. Which question is **most important** for the nurse to ask the client?

1. "Why do you want to hurt yourself?"
2. "Do you have a plan to hurt yourself?"
3. "Has anyone in your family committed suicide?"
4. "Can you describe how you are feeling right now?"

Level of Cognitive Ability: Analyzing
Client Needs: Psychosocial Integrity
Clinical Judgment/Cognitive Skills: Recognize Cues
Integrated Process: Clinical Judgment; Nursing Process/Assessment
Content Area: Mental Health
Health Problems: Mental Health: Suicide
Priority Concepts: Mood and Affect; Safety

Answer: 2
Rationale: When assessing for suicide risk, the nurse must evaluate whether the client has a suicide plan. Clients who have a definitive plan pose a greater risk for suicide. Options 3 and 4 may also be questions that the nurse would ask, but they are not the most important. The nurse avoids the use of the word *why* when communicating with a client. The use of this word may place the client on the defensive; additionally, the client may not even know the reason for wanting to hurt self.
Test-Taking Strategy: Note the strategic words, *most important*. Recalling the importance of assessing for a suicide plan will direct you to the correct option.
Priority Nursing Tip: The client who has a plan to commit suicide must be placed on suicide precautions.
Reference: Varcarolis, E., & Fosbre, C. (2021). *Essentials of psychiatric mental health nursing: A communication approach to evidence-based care* (4th ed., pp. 370, 372). Elsevier.

❖ **46.** The nurse is caring for a client who is receiving electroconvulsive therapy (ECT) for a diagnosis of major depressive disorder. Which assessment findings would the nurse identify as expected short-term side effects of ECT that do not require notifying the primary health care provider? **Select all that apply.**
- ❑ 1. Confusion
- ❑ 2. Memory loss
- ❑ 3. Hypertension
- ❑ 4. Disorientation
- ❑ 5. Heart palpitations

Level of Cognitive Ability: Analyzing
Client Needs: Psychosocial Integrity
Clinical Judgment/Cognitive Skills: Recognize Cues
Integrated Process: Nursing Process/Assessment
Content Area: Mental Health
Health Problems: Mental Health: Mood Disorders
Priority Concepts: Clinical Judgment; Mood and Affect

Answer: 1, 2, 4
Rationale: The major expected side effects of ECT are confusion, disorientation, and memory loss. A change in blood pressure or presence of heart palpitations would not be anticipated side effects and would be causes for concern. If hypertension or presence of heart palpitations occurred after ECT, the primary health care provider needs to be notified.
Test-Taking Strategy: Focus on the subject, expected side effects of ECT. Recall that the side effects of ECT do not include cardiovascular changes.
Priority Nursing Tip: Electroconvulsive therapy may be used to treat depression. It consists of inducing a seizure by passing an electrical current through electrodes attached to the temples. It is not always effective in clients with dysthymic depression, depression and personality disorders, drug dependence, or depression secondary to situational or social difficulties.
Reference: Varcarolis, E., & Fosbre, C. (2021). *Essentials of psychiatric mental health nursing: A communication approach to evidence-based care* (4th ed., pp. 25, 221). Elsevier.

47. During the admission assessment of a client with a history of alcohol abuse for diagnosis of ruptured esophageal varices, the client says, "I deserve this. I brought it on myself." Which response is **most** therapeutic for the nurse to make to the client?
1. "Would you like to talk to the chaplain?"
2. "Is there some reason you feel you deserve this?"
3. "Not all esophageal varices are caused by alcohol."
4. "That is something to think about when you leave the hospital."

Level of Cognitive Ability: Applying
Client Needs: Psychosocial Integrity
Clinical Judgment/Cognitive Skills: Take Action
Integrated Process: Communication and Documentation
Content Area: Adult Health: Gastrointestinal
Health Problems: Mental Health: Addictions
Priority Concepts: Caregiving; Communication

Answer: 2
Rationale: Ruptured esophageal varices are often a complication of cirrhosis of the liver, and the most common type of cirrhosis is caused by chronic alcohol abuse. It is important to obtain an accurate history regarding the client's alcohol intake. If the client is ashamed or embarrassed, the client may not respond accurately. Option 2 is open-ended and allows the client to discuss their feelings about drinking. Option 1 blocks the nurse–client communication process. Options 3 and 4 are somewhat judgmental.
Test-Taking Strategy: Note the strategic word, *most*. Use therapeutic communication techniques to direct you to the correct option. Remember that the client's feelings need to be addressed first.
Priority Nursing Tip: Rupture and resultant hemorrhage of the esophageal varices is primary concerns because this is a life-threatening situation.
References: Ignatavicius, D., et al. (2021). *Medical-surgical nursing: Concepts for interprofessional collaborative care* (10th ed., pp. 1156-1157). Elsevier; Potter, P., et al. (2021). *Fundamentals of nursing* (10th ed., pp. 333–335). Elsevier.

48. The nurse is performing a neurologic assessment on a client with a diagnosis of dementia and assessing the function of the frontal lobe of the brain. Which would the nurse assess to yield the **best** information about this area of functioning?
1. Eye movements
2. Feelings or emotions
3. Level of consciousness
4. Insight, judgment, and planning

Level of Cognitive Ability: Applying
Client Needs: Psychosocial Integrity
Clinical Judgment/Cognitive Skills: Recognize Cues
Integrated Process: Nursing Process/Assessment
Content Area: Adult Health: Neurologic
Health Problems: Mental Health: Neurocognitive Impairment
Priority Concepts: Clinical Judgment; Cognition

Answer: 4
Rationale: Insight, judgment, and planning are part of the function of the frontal lobe. Eye movements are under the control of cranial nerves III, IV, and VI. Feelings and emotions are part of the role of the limbic system. The level of consciousness is controlled by the reticular activating system.
Test-Taking Strategy: Focus on the subject, the frontal lobe of the brain. Note the strategic word, *best*. Recalling the location of the frontal lobe and that this lobe is primarily responsible for insight and reasoning will assist in answering correctly.
Priority Nursing Tip: A common type of dementia is Alzheimer's disease. Dementia results in a self-care deficit. Long-term and short-term memory loss occur, with impairment in judgment, abstract thinking, problem-solving ability, and behavior.
Reference: Ignatavicius, D., et al. (2021). *Medical-surgical nursing: Concepts for interprofessional collaborative care* (10th ed., p. 826). Elsevier.

49. The client who is dying states to the nurse, "I hope I am worthy of heaven." Which intervention would the nurse implement **first** after determining that this client is experiencing fear?
1. Help client express fears.
2. Assess the nature of client's fears.
3. Help client identify coping mechanisms that were successful in the past.
4. Document verbal and nonverbal expressions of fear and other significant data.

Level of Cognitive Ability: Applying
Client Needs: Psychosocial Integrity
Clinical Judgment/Cognitive Skills: Take Action
Integrated Process: Nursing Process/Implementation
Content Area: Developmental Stages: End-of-Life Care
Health Problems: Mental Health: Coping
Priority Concepts: Anxiety; Palliative Care

Answer: 2
Rationale: Fear can range from a paralyzing, overwhelming feeling to a mild concern. Therefore, the nurse would first assess the nature of the client's fears to know how best to help the client. Next, the nurse would help the client express their fears. The client's fears may not be limited to the fear of dying, and the nurse needs this information to help the client. Once the nurse is aware of the client's fears, the methods that the client used to cope with fear in the past are identified. From the interventions listed, the nurse would document verbal and nonverbal expressions of fear and any other significant data as a final intervention.
Test-Taking Strategy: Note the strategic word, *first.* Use the steps of the nursing process to assist you with determining the order of priority of the nursing interventions. An assessment of the client's fear would be the first intervention.
Priority Nursing Tip: The nurse needs to avoid repeated, unnecessary assessments on a dying client. Assessment needs to be limited to obtaining essential data.
Reference: Lewis, S., et al. (2020). *Medical-surgical nursing: Assessment and management of clinical problems* (11th ed., pp. 136–137). Elsevier.

Client Needs

❖ 50. Fluoxetine hydrochloride is prescribed for a client with a diagnosis of depression. The nurse provides instructions to the client regarding the administration of the medication. Which statement by the client indicates an understanding about administration of the medication?
1. "I need to take the medication with my evening meal."
2. "I need to take the medication at noon with an antacid."
3. "I need to take the medication in the morning when I first arise."
4. "I need to take the medication right before bedtime with a snack."

Level of Cognitive Ability: Evaluating
Client Needs: Psychosocial Integrity
Clinical Judgment/Cognitive Skills: Evaluate Outcomes
Integrated Process: Nursing Process/Evaluation
Content Area: Pharmacology: Psychiatric: Selective Serotonin Reuptake Inhibitors (SSRIs)
Health Problems: Mental Health: Mood Disorders
Priority Concepts: Patient Education; Safety

Answer: 3
Rationale: Fluoxetine hydrochloride is an antidepressant and is administered in the early morning without consideration of meals. The remaining options present either incorrect times or incorrect conditions to take this medication.
Test-Taking Strategy: Eliminate options that are comparable or alike, and indicate taking the medication with an antacid or food.
Priority Nursing Tip: For the depressed client, the nurse would assess for homicidal and suicidal ideation and provide safety from suicidal actions. Additional interventions would be to assist with activities of daily living, remind the client of times when they felt better and were successful, and spend time with the client to communicate the client's value.
Reference: Burchum, J., & Rosenthal, L. (2022). *Lehne's Pharmacology for nursing care* (11th ed., pp. 368–369). Elsevier.

51. A parent brings their previously continent 6-year-old child to the pediatric clinic because the child has resumed bedwetting. The nurse assesses the home environment and discovers that there is a new baby at home. Which **best** describes for the parent the defense mechanism the child is using?
1. Regression
2. Repression
3. Identification
4. Rationalization

Level of Cognitive Ability: Analyzing
Client Needs: Psychosocial Integrity
Clinical Judgment/Cognitive Skills: Analyze Cues
Integrated Process: Nursing Process/Analysis
Content Area: Pediatrics: Renal and Urinary
Health Problems: Mental Health: Coping
Priority Concepts: Patient Education; Stress and Coping

Answer: 1
Rationale: The defense mechanism of regression is characterized by returning to an earlier form of expressing an impulse. Option 2 is characterized by blocking a wish or desire from conscious expression. Option 3 occurs when a person models behavior after someone else. Option 4 occurs when a person unconsciously falsifies an experience by giving a "rational" explanation.
Test-Taking Strategy: Note the strategic word, *best*. Focus on the subject, the defense mechanism the child is using. Noting the words *resumed bedwetting* will direct you to the correct option.
Priority Nursing Tip: A defense mechanism is a coping mechanism used in an effort to protect the individual from feelings of anxiety. As anxiety increases and becomes overwhelming, the individual copes by using defense mechanisms to protect the ego and decrease anxiety.
Reference: McKinney, E. S., et al. (2022). *Maternal child nursing* (6th ed., pp. 69–70, 127) Elsevier.

52. The nurse is obtaining a health history from an adolescent. Which statement by the adolescent indicates a **need for follow-up** assessment and intervention?
1. "When I get stressed out about school, I just like to be alone."
2. "I find myself very moody. I'm happy one minute and crying the next."
3. "I don't eat any fatty foods, and I've already lost 8 pounds in 2 weeks."
4. "I can't seem to wake up in the morning. I would sleep until noon if I could."

Level of Cognitive Ability: Evaluating
Client Needs: Psychosocial Integrity
Clinical Judgment/Cognitive Skills: Evaluate Outcomes
Integrated Process: Nursing Process/Evaluation
Content Area: Developmental Stages: Adolescent
Health Problems: Mental Health: Eating Disorders
Priority Concepts: Development; Nutrition

Answer: 3
Rationale: During the adolescent period, there is a heightened awareness of body image and peer pressure to go on excessively restrictive diets. The extreme limitation of omitting all fat in the diet and losing weight during a time of growth suggests inadequate nutrition and a possible eating disorder. The remaining options are normal behaviors or feelings that occur during adolescence.
Test-Taking Strategy: Note the strategic words, *need for follow-up.* These words indicate a negative event query and ask you to select the option that identifies a statement made by the adolescent that is of concern. Eliminate options that suggest normal behaviors or feelings demonstrated during adolescence. The correct option indicates a problem or abnormality.
Priority Nursing Tip: The nurse must remember that the adolescent may be preoccupied with body image and needs to encourage and support independence. Additionally, the nurse needs to provide privacy during examination and engage in conversation about the adolescent's interests.
Reference: McKinney, E. S., et al. (2022). *Maternal child nursing* (6th ed., pp. 165–166). Elsevier.

53. The nurse is caring for a client who has been diagnosed with bipolar disorder and is in a manic state. The nurse determines that which group of foods would be **best** for this client?
1. Beef stew, fruit salad, tea
2. Cheeseburger, banana, milk
3. Macaroni and cheese, apple, milk
4. Scrambled eggs, orange juice, coffee

Level of Cognitive Ability: Applying
Client Needs: Psychosocial Integrity
Clinical Judgment/Cognitive Skills: Generate Solutions
Integrated Process: Nursing Process/Planning
Content Area: Mental Health
Health Problems: Mental Health: Mood Disorders
Priority Concepts: Mood and Affect; Nutrition

Answer: 2
Rationale: The client in a manic state often has inadequate food and fluid intake as a result of physical agitation. Foods that the client can eat "on the run" are best because the client is too active to sit at meals and use utensils. Additionally, clients in a manic state should not have any products that contain caffeine.
Test-Taking Strategy: Note the strategic word, *best.* Focus on the words *manic state.* Note that the remaining options are comparable or alike in that the client needs to sit to eat some of these food items. Remember the concept of "finger foods" with regard to the client with mania.
Priority Nursing Tip: For the client in a manic state, the nurse needs to maintain safety for the client, others, and self. The nurse needs to maintain large personal space, use a nonaggressive posture, a calm approach, and communicate with a calm, clear tone of voice.
Reference: Varcarolis, E., & Fosbre, C. (2021). *Essentials of psychiatric mental health nursing: A communication approach to evidence-based care* (4th ed., p. 238). Elsevier.

❖ **54.** The nurse is caring for a child who is a victim of abuse and has determined that the child uses repression to cope with past life experiences. Which activity would the nurse implement as part of the nursing care plan?
1. Encourage the child to use therapeutic play to act out past experiences.
2. Tell the child to let the past go and concentrate on the present and future.
3. Place the child on medications that will help the child forget the incidents.
4. Have the child talk about the abuse in detail during the first therapy session.

Level of Cognitive Ability: Applying
Client Needs: Psychosocial Integrity
Clinical Judgment/Cognitive Skills: Generate Solutions
Integrated Process: Clinical Judgment; Nursing Process/Planning
Content Area: Mental Health
Health Problems: Mental Health: Coping
Priority Concepts: Stress and Coping; Interpersonal Violence

Answer: 1
Rationale: Therapeutic play is used to reduce the trauma of illness and hospitalizations. It is a nonthreatening avenue through which the child can use artwork, dolls, or puppets to act out frightening life experiences. Option 3 would be extremely threatening to the child and nontherapeutic. Options 2 and 4 devalue the child and force the child to further repress harmful past experiences rather than facing them and moving on.
Test-Taking Strategy: Use therapeutic communication techniques to eliminate options 2 and 4. From the remaining options, note the relationship of the words *past life experiences* in the question and *past experiences* in the correct option.
Priority Nursing Tip: Repression is the unconscious process in which the client blocks undesirable and unacceptable thoughts from conscious expression.
Reference: Varcarolis, E., & Fosbre, C. (2021). *Essentials of psychiatric mental health nursing: A communication approach to evidence-based care* (4th ed., pp. 93–95, 138). Elsevier.

55. An older client is brought to the emergency department by a family member with whom the client lives. The nurse observes that the client has poor hygiene, contractures, and pressure ulcers on the sacrum, the scapula, and the heels. Based on the nurse's assessment data, the client is suspected of which form of victimization?
1. Sexual abuse
2. Physical abuse
3. Emotional abuse
4. Psychological abuse

Level of Cognitive Ability: Analyzing
Client Needs: Psychosocial Integrity
Clinical Judgment/Cognitive Skills: Analyze Cues
Integrated Process: Nursing Process/Analysis
Content Area: Mental Health
Health Problems: Mental Health: Abuse/Neglect
Priority Concepts: Clinical Judgment; Interpersonal Violence

Answer: 2
Rationale: Victimization in a family can take many forms. When analyzing a specific client situation, the nurse must understand which form of abuse is being considered. Physical abuse can take the form of battering (hitting, slapping, striking), or it can be more subtle, such as neglect (the failure to meet basic needs). Sexual abuse can involve unwanted sexual remarks, sexual advances, and physical sexual acts. Emotional and psychological abuse can involve inflicting verbal statements that cause mental anguish or alienation of the victim.
Test-Taking Strategy: Note the subject, the form of victimization. Focus on the words that relate to physical abuse in the question such as the description of the client. The correct option is the only choice that fits the description in the question.
Priority Nursing Tip: Victims of abuse are often isolated socially by their abusers.
Reference: Varcarolis, E., & Fosbre, C. (2021). *Essentials of psychiatric mental health nursing: A communication approach to evidence-based care* (4th ed., pp. 351–352). Elsevier.

❖ **56.** A client diagnosed with schizophrenia is admitted to the inpatient mental health unit. The client states, "I am Elizabeth, the Queen of England." Which would the nurse recognize this client's statement is indicating?
1. Visual illusion
2. Loose association
3. Grandeur delusion
4. Auditory hallucination

Level of Cognitive Ability: Analyzing
Client Needs: Psychosocial Integrity
Clinical Judgment/Cognitive Skills: Analyze Cues
Integrated Process: Nursing Process/Analysis
Content Area: Mental Health
Health Problems: Mental Health: Schizophrenia
Priority Concepts: Clinical Judgment; Psychosis

Answer: 3
Rationale: A delusion is an important personal belief that is almost certainly not true and that resists modification. An illusion is a misperception or misinterpretation of externally real stimuli. Loose association is thinking that is characterized by speech in which ideas that are unrelated shift from one subject to another. A hallucination is a false perception.
Test-Taking Strategy: Note the subject, what the client's statement indicates. Focus on the word *queen* in the question. Making a reference to being a queen is a grandiose assumption.
Priority Nursing Tip: In delusions of grandeur, the client attaches special significance to self in relation to others or the universe and has an exaggerated sense of self that has no basis in reality.
Reference: Varcarolis, E., & Fosbre, C. (2021). *Essentials of psychiatric mental health nursing: A communication approach to evidence-based care* (4th ed., p. 254). Elsevier.

57. A client who has been newly admitted to the mental health unit with a diagnosis of bipolar disorder is trying to organize a dance with the other clients on the unit. The nurse would encourage which action to decrease stimulation?
1. Seek assistance from other staff members.
2. Engage the help of other clients on the unit to accomplish the task.
3. Stop the planning and firmly tell client that this task is inappropriate.
4. Postpone organizing the dance and engage client in a writing activity.

Level of Cognitive Ability: Applying
Client Needs: Psychosocial Integrity
Clinical Judgment/Cognitive Skills: Take Action
Integrated Process: Nursing Process/Implementation
Content Area: Mental Health
Health Problems: Mental Health: Mood Disorders
Priority Concepts: Clinical Judgment; Psychosis

Answer: 4
Rationale: Because the client with bipolar disorder is easily stimulated by the environment, sedentary activities are the best outlets for energy release. Most bipolar clients enjoy writing, so the writing task is appropriate. An activity such as planning a dance may be appropriate at some point, but not for the newly admitted client who is likely to have impaired judgment and a short attention span. Options 1 and 2 encourage planning the activity and therefore increase client stimulation. Option 3 could result in an angry outburst by the client.
Test-Taking Strategy: Focus on the subject, the activity that will decrease stimulation. Options 1 and 2 encourage activity and need to be eliminated. Option 3 tells the client that the activity is inappropriate, and this could result in an angry outburst by the client. The correct option is the only choice that limits activity.
Priority Nursing Tip: Bipolar disorder is commonly treated with lithium carbonate. This medication can result in toxicity and requires regular monitoring of serum lithium levels.
Reference: Varcarolis, E., & Fosbre, C. (2021). *Essentials of psychiatric mental health nursing: A communication approach to evidence-based care* (4th ed., p. 236.). Elsevier.

❖ **58.** A client diagnosed with an obsessive-compulsive disorder spends many hours during the day and night washing hands. The nurse would **initially** allow the client to continue this behavior because it has what therapeutic effect for the client?
1. Relieves client's anxiety
2. Decreases the chance of infection
3. Gives client a feeling of self-control
4. Increases client's sense of self-esteem

Level of Cognitive Ability: Applying
Client Needs: Psychosocial Integrity
Clinical Judgment/Cognitive Skills: Generate Solutions
Integrated Process: Nursing Process/Planning
Content Area: Mental Health
Health Problems: Mental Health: Obsessive Compulsive Disorders
Priority Concepts: Anxiety; Clinical Judgment

Answer: 1
Rationale: The compulsive act provides immediate relief from anxiety and is used to cope with stress, conflict, or pain. Options 2 and 3 are also incorrect interpretations of the client's need to perform this behavior. Although the client may feel the need to increase self-esteem, that is not the primary goal of this behavior.
Test-Taking Strategy: Focusing on the strategic word, *initially*, and recalling the effect of compulsive acts will direct you to the correct option.
Priority Nursing Tip: For the client with obsessive-compulsive disorder, the nurse would ensure that basic needs are met, such as food, rest, and grooming. Also, the nurse would help the client identify situations that precipitate compulsive behavior and encourage the client to verbalize thoughts and feelings when these situations arise.
Reference: Varcarolis, E., & Fosbre, C. (2021). *Essentials of psychiatric mental health nursing: A communication approach to evidence-based care* (4th ed., pp. 143–144). Elsevier.

59. An adolescent is preparing to return home after psychiatric hospitalization for a suicide attempt. Which actions would be **most effective** to support family processes when the client returns home? **Select all that apply.**
1. Make a video of the ride home in the car.
2. Identify the family's strengths and weaknesses.
3. Ask that the parent's boyfriend move out of the home.
4. Provide and offer the family appropriate options and resources.
5. Encourage communication and the sharing of feelings among the family members.

Level of Cognitive Ability: Applying
Client Needs: Psychosocial Integrity
Clinical Judgment/Cognitive Skills: Generate Solutions
Integrated Process: Clinical Judgment/Nursing Process/Planning
Content Area: Mental Health
Health Problems: Mental Health: Suicide
Priority Concepts: Mood and Affect; Safety

Answer: 2, 4, 5
Rationale: After the crisis time of a family member's suicide attempt, safety for the recovering individual is a priority. Families can provide support and encouragement in a caring home environment. Options 2, 4, and 5 offer helpful ways to enhance the family processes. Options 1 and 3 are clearly the least effective options because there is no information in the question that indicates that these actions are relative to the suicide attempt.
Test-Taking Strategy: Note the strategic words, *most effective*. Focus on the data in the question, and note that options 2, 4, and 5 identify positive measures.
Priority Nursing Tip: High-risk groups for suicide include clients with a history of previous suicide attempts, family history of suicide attempts, adolescents, older adults, disabled or terminally ill clients, clients with personality disorders, clients with organic brain syndrome or dementia, depressed or psychotic clients, and substance abusers.
Reference: Varcarolis, E., & Fosbre, C. (2021). *Essentials of psychiatric mental health nursing: A communication approach to evidence-based care* (4th ed., pp. 368, 373). Elsevier.

❖ **60.** An 11-year-old child scheduled for a diagnostic procedure is anxious about having an intravenous line inserted and receiving an intramuscular injection. Which form of communication would the nurse use in preparing the child for the procedure?
1. Reassuring the child by introducing the equipment used
2. Teaching the parents so that they can explain everything to the child
3. Telling the child not to worry because the doctors take care of everything
4. Using pictures, concrete words, and demonstrations to describe what will happen

Level of Cognitive Ability: Applying
Client Needs: Psychosocial Integrity
Clinical Judgment/Cognitive Skills: Generate Solutions
Integrated Process: Clinical Judgment/Nursing Process/Planning
Content Area: Foundations of Care: Communication
Health Problems: Mental Health: Anxiety
Priority Concepts: Communication; Development

Answer: 4
Rationale: The school-age child understands best with visual aids and concrete language. Option 1 does not fully address the child's concerns. Option 2 inappropriately delegates the responsibility for teaching to the parents. Option 3 is not therapeutic.
Test-Taking Strategy: Use therapeutic communication techniques. Option 1 doesn't fully address the issue. In option 2, a nursing responsibility is inappropriately delegated to parents, and option 3 is nontherapeutic.
Priority Nursing Tip: For the school-age child, the nurse would provide reassurance to help in alleviating fears and anxieties. In addition to using pictures, concrete words, and demonstrations to describe what will happen, the nurse can use medical play techniques.
Reference: McKinney, E. S., et al. (2022) *Maternal child nursing* (6th ed., p. 54). Elsevier.

61. The nurse observes an anxious client blocking the hallway, walking three steps forward and then two steps backward. Other clients are agitated and trying to get past the client. How would the nurse intervene?
1. Stand alongside client and say, "You're very anxious today."
2. Attempt to stop the behavior and say, "You're going to get exhausted."
3. Take client to the lounge and say, "Relax and watch television now."
4. Walk alongside client and say, "You're not going anywhere very fast doing this."

Level of Cognitive Ability: Applying
Client Needs: Psychosocial Integrity
Clinical Judgment/Cognitive Skills: Take Action
Integrated Process: Clinical Judgment/Nursing Process/Implementation
Content Area: Mental Health
Health Problems: Mental Health: Anxiety
Priority Concepts: Anxiety; Communication

Answer: 1
Rationale: An important consideration when alleviating anxiety is to assist the client with recognizing the behavior. Options 2 and 3 do not address the increased anxiety and the need to control the underlying behavior, and they may even escalate the behavior. Option 4 does not raise the client to a functioning level.
Test-Taking Strategy: Focus on the subject, dealing with a client who is anxious. Note the word *anxious* in the question and in the correct option. Remember that it is important to assist the client with recognizing their own behavior.
Priority Nursing Tip: Cognitive therapy is one treatment modality for anxiety. This therapy involves an active, directive, time-limited, structured approach and is based on the principle that how an individual feels and behaves is determined by how the individual thinks about the world and their place in it.
Reference: Varcarolis, E., & Fosbre, C. (2021). *Essentials of psychiatric mental health nursing: A communication approach to evidence-based care* (4th ed., pp. 141, 145). Elsevier.

❖ **62.** The nurse is assisting with providing a form of psychotherapy in which the client acts out situations that are of emotional significance. Based on this assessment data, which form of therapy would the nurse expect the primary health care provider has prescribed?
1. Psychodrama
2. Reality therapy
3. Psychoanalytic therapy
4. Short-term dynamic psychotherapy

Level of Cognitive Ability: Applying
Client Needs: Psychosocial Integrity
Clinical Judgment/Cognitive Skills: Generate Solutions
Integrated Process: Clinical Judgment/Nursing Process/Planning
Content Area: Mental Health
Health Problems: Mental Health: Coping
Priority Concepts: Stress and Coping; Psychosis

Answer: 1
Rationale: Psychodrama involves the enactment of emotionally charged situations. Reality therapy is used for individuals with cognitive impairment. Both short-term dynamic psychotherapy and psychoanalytic therapy depend on techniques that are drawn from psychoanalysis.
Test-Taking Strategy: Focus on the **subject**, the specific form of psychotherapy. Note the words *the client acts out situations*. These words will assist you by providing you with the definition of psychodrama.
Priority Nursing Tip: Psychotherapy consists of three levels: supportive therapy, reeducative therapy, and reconstructive therapy. These modalities use a therapeutic relationship to modify the client's feelings, attitudes, and behaviors.
Reference: Varcarolis, E., & Fosbre, C. (2021). *Essentials of psychiatric mental health nursing: A communication approach to evidence-based care* (4th ed., p. 126). Elsevier.

63. A client with the diagnosis of mania is placed in a seclusion room after an outburst of violent behavior that involved a physical assault on another client. Which intervention would the nurse include in the plan of care before seclusion?
1. Ask client if they understand why the seclusion is necessary.
2. Remain silent because verbal interaction would be too stimulating.
3. Tell client that they will be allowed to come out when they can behave.
4. Inform client that they are being secluded to help regain self-control.

Level of Cognitive Ability: Applying
Client Needs: Psychosocial Integrity
Clinical Judgment/Cognitive Skills: Generate Solutions
Integrated Process: Clinical Judgment/Nursing Process/Planning
Content Area: Mental Health
Health Problems: Mental Health: Mood Disorders
Priority Concepts: Mood and Affect; Safety

Answer: 4
Rationale: Seclusion is a process in which a client is placed alone in a specially designed room for protection and close supervision. This client is removed to a nonstimulating environment as a result of their behavior. Options 1, 2, and 3 are nontherapeutic actions. Additionally, option 3 implies punishment. It is best to directly inform the client of the purpose of the seclusion.
Test-Taking Strategy: Focus on the **subject**, care to the client in seclusion. Also, use **therapeutic communication techniques**. Select the option that presents reality most clearly to the client. Option 4 is the only option that provides a clear and direct purpose of the seclusion.
Priority Nursing Tip: While in seclusion, the client is monitored continuously and must be protected from all sources of harm.
Reference: Varcarolis, E., & Fosbre, C. (2021). *Essentials of psychiatric mental health nursing: A communication approach to evidence-based care* (4th ed., pp. 93–95, 383). Elsevier.

64. A client diagnosed with angina pectoris is extremely anxious after being hospitalized. Which would the nurse do to minimize the client's anxiety?
1. Provide care choices to client.
2. Keep the door open and the hallway lights on at night.
3. Encourage client to limit visitors to as few as possible.
4. Arrange for client to share a room with a cognitively alert client.

Level of Cognitive Ability: Applying
Client Needs: Psychosocial Integrity
Clinical Judgment/Cognitive Skills: Take Action
Integrated Process: Clinical Judgment/Nursing Process/Implementation
Content Area: Adult Health: Cardiovascular
Health Problems: Mental Health: Anxiety
Priority Concepts: Anxiety; Caregiving

Answer: 1
Rationale: General interventions to minimize anxiety in the hospitalized client include providing information, social support, and control over choices related to care, as well as acknowledging the client's feelings. Leaving the door open with the hallway lights on may keep the client oriented, but these actions may interfere with sleep and increase anxiety. Limiting visitors reduces social support. The sharing of a room may not necessarily meet the client's needs.
Test-Taking Strategy: Focus on the subject, minimizing anxiety. Thinking about each option and how it may either increase or minimize anxiety will direct you to the correct option.
Priority Nursing Tip: Angina pectoris is chest pain resulting from myocardial ischemia caused by inadequate myocardial blood and oxygen supply. In addition to anxiety, the client with angina may experience dyspnea, pallor, sweating, palpitations and tachycardia, dizziness and faintness, hypertension, or digestive disturbances.
Reference: Lewis, S., et al. (2020). *Medical-surgical nursing: Assessment and management of clinical problems* (11th ed., pp. 726–727, 1535). Elsevier.

65. A client diagnosed with catatonic schizophrenia demonstrates severe withdrawal by lying on the bed with the body pulled into a fetal position. Which action by the nurse is **most appropriate** to increase interpersonal communication?
1. Ask client direct questions to encourage talking.
2. Leave client alone and intermittently check on client.
3. Sit beside client in silence and occasionally ask open-ended questions.
4. Take client into the dayroom with the other clients to encourage interaction.

Level of Cognitive Ability: Applying
Client Needs: Psychosocial Integrity
Clinical Judgment/Cognitive Skills: Take Action
Integrated Process: Clinical Judgment/Nursing Process/Implementation
Content Area: Mental Health
Health Problems: Mental Health: Schizophrenia
Priority Concepts: Caregiving; Psychosis

Answer: 3
Rationale: Clients who are withdrawn may be immobile and mute, and they require consistent, repeated approaches. Intervention includes the establishment of interpersonal contact. The nurse facilitates communication with the client by sitting in silence, asking open-ended questions, and pausing to provide opportunities for the client to respond. Asking this client direct questions is not therapeutic. The client is not to be left alone. This client is not capable of interaction in the dayroom.
Test-Taking Strategy: Note the strategic words, *most appropriate*. Focus on the subject, increasing interpersonal communication. Eliminate option 2 because the nurse would not leave the client alone. Option 4 relies on other clients to care for this client; this is inappropriate and it should be eliminated next. From the remaining options, recall that asking direct questions to this client would not be therapeutic.
Priority Nursing Tip: Catatonic posturing occurs when the client holds bizarre positions for long periods of time. Medications used to treat schizophrenia have reduced the likelihood of catatonic posturing occurring.
Reference: Varcarolis, E., & Fosbre, C. (2021). *Essentials of psychiatric mental health nursing: A communication approach to evidence-based care* (4th ed., p. 257). Elsevier.

❖ **66.** The nurse is interviewing a client being admitted to the mental health inpatient unit who was involved in a fire 2 months ago. The client is reporting insomnia, difficulty concentrating, nervousness, hypervigilance, and frequently thinking about fires. The nurse would recognize these complaints to be indications of which disorder?

1. Phobia
2. Dissociative disorder
3. Obsessive-compulsive disorder
4. Post-traumatic stress disorder (PTSD)

Level of Cognitive Ability: Analyzing
Client Needs: Psychosocial Integrity
Clinical Judgment/Cognitive Skills: Analyze Cues
Integrated Process: Clinical Judgment/Nursing Process/Analysis
Content Area: Mental Health
Health Problems: Mental Health: Post-Traumatic Stress Disorder
Priority Concepts: Clinical Judgment; Psychosis

Answer: 4
Rationale: PTSD is precipitated by events that are overwhelming, unpredictable, and sometimes life-threatening. Typical symptoms of PTSD include difficulty concentrating, sleep disturbances, intrusive recollections of the traumatic event, hypervigilance, and anxiety. These symptoms are not characteristic of the disorders noted in options 1, 2, and 3.
Test-Taking Strategy: Note the subject, the disorder that the client is experiencing. Focus on the words *fire* and *disorder* in the question regarding the client's complaints. Recalling that having flashbacks of traumatic events is a common symptom of PTSD will direct you to the correct option.
Priority Nursing Tip: Assist the client with PTSD to develop adaptive coping mechanisms and to use relaxation techniques.
Reference: Foster, K., et al. (2021). *Mental health in nursing, theory and practice for clinical settings* (5th ed., pp. 163, 167–168). Elsevier.

67. A 16-year-old client diagnosed with Crohn's disease is hospitalized. Which statement by the client would alert the nurse to a potential developmental problem?

1. "I'd like my hair washed before my friends get here."
2. "Is it okay if I have a couple of friends in to visit me this evening?"
3. "Please tell my friends not to visit, since I'll see them back at school next week."
4. "When my friends get here, I would like to play some computer games with them."

Level of Cognitive Ability: Analyzing
Client Needs: Psychosocial Integrity
Clinical Judgment/Cognitive Skills: Analyze Cues
Integrated Process: Clinical Judgment/Nursing Process/Analysis
Content Area: Developmental Stages: Adolescent
Health Problems: Mental Health: Coping
Priority Concepts: Clinical Judgment; Development

Answer: 3
Rationale: Adolescents who withdraw from peers into isolation struggle with developing identity, so option 3 would cause the nurse to be concerned. It is appropriate for the client to ask for hygiene measures to be attended to before the peer group arrives. Option 2 indicates that the client is eager for companionship. Adolescents often develop special interests within their groups that may help them maximize certain skills, such as with computers.
Test-Taking Strategy: Eliminate the options that are comparable or alike, and indicate that the client is anticipating the arrival of a peer group, which is appropriate. The correct option indicates that the client may be withdrawing from appropriate relationships.
Priority Nursing Tip: For the hospitalized adolescent, separation from friends is a source of anxiety. Additionally, adolescents are not sure whether they want their parents with them when they are hospitalized.
Reference: McKinney, E. S., et al. (2022). *Maternal child nursing* (6th ed., pp. 793, 986–987). Elsevier.

❖ **68.** The nurse obtains an electrocardiogram (ECG) rhythm strip for an adult client who is anxious about the results. The ECG shows that the heart rate is 90 beats/min. Which statement would the nurse make to the client to relieve anxiety?

1. The rate is normal.
2. There is no need to worry.
3. A slower heart rate is preferred.
4. Medication specific to the problem will be prescribed.

Level of Cognitive Ability: Applying
Client Needs: Psychosocial Integrity
Clinical Judgment/Cognitive Skills: Take Action
Integrated Process: Clinical Judgment/Nursing Process/Implementation
Content Area: Adult Health: Cardiovascular
Health Problems: Mental Health: Coping
Priority Concepts: Anxiety; Clinical Judgment

Answer: 1
Rationale: A normal adult resting pulse rate ranges between 60 and 100 beats/min; therefore, the rate is normal. The nurse would not tell a client not to worry. Options 3 and 4 indicate that the ECG is abnormal.
Test-Taking Strategy: Recall knowledge of the basic range of pulse rates for an adult. Option 2 is not therapeutic because telling the client not to worry is an inappropriate action. Eliminate options 3 and 4 because they are comparable or alike and indicate that a problem exists.
Priority Nursing Tip: Obtaining a baseline measurement of the client's vital signs will allow the nurse to determine any changes. The nurse can also measure the client's pulse rate and blood pressure in sitting, standing, and lying positions and compare the readings.
References: Pagana, K., Pagana, T., & Pagana, T. N. (2021). *Mosby's Diagnostic and laboratory test reference* (15th ed., pp. 352-353). Elsevier; Potter, P., et al. (2021). *Fundamentals of nursing* (10th ed., p. 468). Elsevier.

69. Which behavior is a sign of depression that a client could exhibit when recovering from a myocardial infarction?

1. Reports insomnia at night
2. Consumes 25% of meals and shows little interest when doing client teaching
3. Ignores activity restrictions and does not report the experience of chest pain with activity
4. Expresses apprehension about leaving the hospital and requests that someone stay in the room at night

Level of Cognitive Ability: Analyzing
Client Needs: Psychosocial Integrity
Clinical Judgment/Cognitive Skills: Recognize Cues
Integrated Process: Clinical Judgment/Nursing Process/Assessment
Content Area: Adult Health: Cardiovascular
Health Problems: Mental Health: Mood Disorders
Priority Concepts: Clinical Judgment; Mood and Affect

Answer: 2
Rationale: Signs of depression include withdrawal, lack of interest, crying, anorexia, and apathy. Insomnia may be a sign of anxiety or fear. Ignoring symptoms and activity restrictions are signs of denial. Apprehension is a sign of anxiety.
Test-Taking Strategy: Focus on the subject, sign of depression. Recalling that anorexia and a lack of interest are associated with depression will direct you to the correct option.
Priority Nursing Tip: The nurse would monitor a depressed client closely for signs of suicidal ideation. If the client presents with increased energy, monitor closely because it could mean the client now has the energy to perform the suicide act.
Reference: Ignatavicius, D., et al. (2021). *Medical-surgical nursing: Concepts for interprofessional collaborative care* (10th ed., p. 772). Elsevier.

❖ **70.** A client who recently had a gastrostomy feeding tube inserted refuses to participate in the plan of care, will not make eye contact, and does not speak to family or visitors. Which type of coping mechanism would the nurse assess the client is using?
1. Denial
2. Distancing
3. Regression
4. Suppression

Level of Cognitive Ability: Analyzing
Client Needs: Psychosocial Integrity
Clinical Judgment/Cognitive Skills: Analyze Cues
Integrated Process: Clinical Judgment/Nursing Process/Assessment
Content Area: Mental Health
Health Problems: Mental Health: Coping
Priority Concepts: Anxiety; Stress and Coping

Answer: 2
Rationale: Distancing is an unwillingness or inability to discuss events. The behaviors described are not associated with any of the other options.
Test-Taking Strategy: Note the subject, the type of coping mechanism that the client is using. Focus on the words *will not make eye contact,* and *does not speak to family or visitors* in the question. Noting the client's behavior will direct you to the correct option.
Priority Nursing Tip: Coping mechanisms are methods used to decrease anxiety. The use of a coping mechanism can be conscious, unconscious, constructive, destructive, task oriented in relation to direct problem-solving, or defense oriented and regulating in response to protect oneself.
Reference: Potter, P., et al. (2021). *Fundamentals of nursing* (10th ed., p. 763). Elsevier; https://en.wikipedia.org/wiki/Distancing_(psychology).

71. The nurse is reviewing the preoperative teaching plan for a client who is anxious about a scheduled radical neck dissection for laryngeal cancer. Which part of the nursing care plan would the nurse **initially** focus on?
1. The financial status of client
2. Postoperative communication techniques
3. Information given to client by the surgeon
4. Client's support systems and coping behaviors

Level of Cognitive Ability: Applying
Client Needs: Psychosocial Integrity
Clinical Judgment/Cognitive Skills: Prioritize Hypotheses
Integrated Process: Clinical Judgment/Nursing Process/Planning
Content Area: Adult Health: Oncology
Health Problems: Mental Health: Anxiety
Priority Concepts: Patient Education; Clinical Judgment

Answer: 3
Rationale: The first step in client teaching is establishing what the client already knows. This allows the nurse not only to correct any misinformation, especially in an anxious client, but also to determine the starting point for teaching and to implement the education at the client's level. Although the remaining options may be components of the plan, they are not the initial focus.
Test-Taking Strategy: Note the strategic word, *initially.* Remember that determining what the client already knows provides a starting point for teaching.
Priority Nursing Tip: Because of the potential for edema formation, airway patency is always a priority concern for any client who underwent surgery in the neck area.
Reference: Lewis, S., et al. (2020). *Medical-surgical nursing: Assessment and management of clinical problems* (11th ed., pp. 493, 498). Elsevier.

❖ **72.** The community health nurse is conducting an awareness workshop on adolescent suicide. Which circumstances would the nurse discuss as risk factors? **Select all that apply.**
- ❑ 1. Family violence
- ❑ 2. Use of alcohol or drugs
- ❑ 3. Strong peer relationships
- ❑ 4. Family history of depression
- ❑ 5. Adequate family financial resources

Level of Cognitive Ability: Applying
Client Needs: Psychosocial Integrity
Clinical Judgment/Cognitive Skills: Recognize Cues
Integrated Process: Clinical Judgment/Nursing Process/Assessment
Content Area: Mental Health
Health Problems: Mental Health: Suicide
Priority Concepts: Development; Mood and Affect

Answer: 1, 2, 4
Rationale: Risk factors for suicide among adolescents are depression; a family history of mental health disorders, especially depression and suicide; previous attempts at suicide; family violence or abuse; substance abuse; poor school performance; feelings of worthlessness or hopelessness; and homosexuality.
Test-Taking Strategy: Focus on the subject, the risk factors for suicide. Noting the words *strong* in option 3 and *adequate* in option 5 will assist in eliminating these options as risk factors.
Priority Nursing Tip: The client who is at suicide risk and is taking an antidepressant must be monitored closely, especially during the period in which the medication begins to take effect, which is in about 4 to 6 weeks. The client experiences an unusual burst of energy once the medication begins to take effect, which may further motivate the client to carry out the suicide plan.
Reference: Varcarolis, E., & Fosbre, C. (2021). *Essentials of psychiatric mental health nursing: A communication approach to evidence-based care* (4th ed., p. 368). Elsevier.

73. A preschool child is placed in traction for a femur fracture. The child has started being incontinent during the day, even though the child has been toilet trained for a year. The parent is very upset about the situation. The nurse explains to the parent that this behavior is recognized as which psychosocial adaptation?
1. A body image disturbance
2. Attention-seeking behavior
3. Opposition to authority figures
4. Regressing to earlier developmental behavior

Level of Cognitive Ability: Applying
Client Needs: Psychosocial Integrity
Clinical Judgment/Cognitive Skills: Analyze Cues
Integrated Process: Clinical Judgment/Nursing Process/Analysis
Content Area: Developmental Stages: Preschool
Health Problems: Mental Health: Coping
Priority Concepts: Stress and Coping; Development

Answer: 4
Rationale: The monotony of immobilization can lead to sluggish intellectual and psychomotor responses. Regressive behaviors are not uncommon in immobilized young children, and they usually do not require professional intervention. Body image may or may not be affected by long-term immobilization, but it does not relate to the information presented in the question. The remaining options are not relevant to the described situation.
Test-Taking Strategy: Focus on the subject, the behavior and psychosocial adaptation of the preschooler. This will eliminate option 1. From the remaining options, recalling that regression is a normal psychologic response to immobilization will direct you to option 4.
Priority Nursing Tip: The nurse needs to plan care for the hospitalized preschooler, recalling that the hospitalized preschooler may be quietly withdrawn and uninterested in the environment, become uncooperative by refusing to eat or take medication, and repeatedly ask when the parents will be visiting.
Reference: McKinney, E. S., et al. (2022). *Maternal child nursing* (6th ed., pp. 69–70, 792). Elsevier.

Client Needs

❖ **74.** The nurse is assessing a client to determine the client's adjustment to presbycusis. Which indicates successful adaptation by the client to this problem?
   1. Proper use of a hearing aid
   2. Denial of a hearing impairment
   3. Withdrawal from social activities
   4. Reluctance to answer the telephone

Level of Cognitive Ability: Evaluating
Client Needs: Psychosocial Integrity
Clinical Judgment/Cognitive Skills: Evaluate Outcomes
Integrated Process: Clinical Judgment/Nursing Process/Evaluation
Content Area: Adult Health: Ear
Health Problems: Mental Health: Coping
Priority Concepts: Clinical Judgment; Sensory Perception

Answer: 1
Rationale: Presbycusis occurs as part of the aging process; it is a progressive sensorineural hearing loss. Clients show adequate adaptation by obtaining and regularly using a hearing aid. Some clients may not adapt well to the impairment, denying its presence. Others withdraw from social interactions and contact with others, embarrassed by the problem and the need to wear a hearing aid.
Test-Taking Strategy: Focus on the subject, successful adaptation to the problem. A review of each of the options shows that the only option with positive wording is option 1. The incorrect options indicate a need for further adaptation.
Priority Nursing Tip: Presbycusis is a gradual nerve degeneration associated with aging; it leads to degeneration or atrophy of the ganglion cells in the cochlea and a loss of elasticity of the basilar membranes.
Reference: Lewis, S., et al. (2020). *Medical-surgical nursing: Assessment and management of clinical problems* (11th ed., pp. 378, 392). Elsevier.

75. The nurse is preparing to implement suicide precautions for a suicidal client. Which nursing interventions are included with regard to these precautions? **Select all that apply.**
   ❏ 1. Maintain arm's length distance with client at all times.
   ❏ 2. Ensure that meal trays contain no glass or metal silverware.
   ❏ 3. Carefully watch client swallow each dose of medication.
   ❏ 4. Conduct one-on-one nursing observation and interaction 24 hours a day.
   ❏ 5. Document client's mood, verbatim statements, and behaviors every 15 to 30 minutes per protocol.
   ❏ 6. Allow client to totally cover self with the bedcovers during sleep at night as long as the nurse is present.

Level of Cognitive Ability: Applying
Client Needs: Psychosocial Integrity
Clinical Judgment/Cognitive Skills: Take Action
Integrated Process: Clinical Judgment/Nursing Process/Implementation
Content Area: Mental Health
Health Problems: Mental Health: Suicide
Priority Concepts: Mood and Affect; Safety

Answer: 1, 2, 3, 4, 5
Rationale: Suicide precautions involve constant observation of the client by the nursing staff. This intense attention from the nurse provides for safety and also allows for constant reassessment of risk. Suicide precautions include maintaining arm's length distance with the client at all times; ensuring that meal trays contain no glass or metal silverware; carefully watching the client swallow each dose of medication; conducting one-on-one nursing observation and interaction 24 hours a day and explaining to the client the procedures involved with suicide precautions; and documenting client's mood, verbatim statements, and behaviors every 15 to 30 minutes per protocol. During observation when the client is sleeping, the client's hands need to always be in view and not under the bedcovers.
Test-Taking Strategy: Focus on the subject, suicide precautions. Read each option carefully, keeping safety in mind. The only option that presents a risk is option 6, allowing the client to totally cover self with the bedcovers during sleep at night. Remember that the client's hands need to always be in view.
Priority Nursing Tip: If a client is known to be at risk for suicide, the client must be monitored closely. A staff member must be within arm's length of this client, and any potentially dangerous objects must be removed from the client's environment and living space.
Reference: Varcarolis, E., & Fosbre, C. (2021). *Essentials of psychiatric mental health nursing: A communication approach to evidence-based care* (4th ed., p. 372). Elsevier.

❖ **76.** A client diagnosed with a severe ulcer of the right foot is told that a right leg amputation may be necessary. Which signs or client behaviors indicative of anticipatory grief would the nurse monitor the client for? **Select all that apply.**
- ❑ **1.** Stating a fear of the future and unknown
- ❑ **2.** Engaging in periods of weeping or raging
- ❑ **3.** Expressing anger at the medical professionals
- ❑ **4.** Expressing a feeling of unreality and disbelief
- ❑ **5.** Expressing a desire to run away from the situation
- ❑ **6.** Stating that the client knows all that is needed to know about the condition

Level of Cognitive Ability: Analyzing
Client Needs: Psychosocial Integrity
Clinical Judgment/Cognitive Skills: Recognize Cues
Integrated Process: Clinical Judgment/Nursing Process/Assessment
Content Area: Mental Health
Health Problems: Mental Health: Grief/Loss
Priority Concepts: Clinical Judgment; Stress and Coping

Answer: 1, 2, 3, 4, 5
Rationale: Anticipatory grief refers to the intellectual and emotional responses and behaviors by which individuals, families, or communities work through the process of modifying self-concept based on the perception of potential loss. Signs of anticipatory grief include fears of the future and the unknown, periods of weeping or raging, anger at medical professionals, a feeling of unreality and disbelief, a desire to run away from the situation, feelings of emptiness or of being lost, a sense of being numb and fatigued, a need to oversee every detail of care, pronounced clinging to or dependency on other family members, and fear of going crazy. A statement by the client that the client knows all the client needs to know about the condition is not a sign of anticipatory grieving; it may indicate another client problem such as avoidance or fear.
Test-Taking Strategy: Focus on the subject, the signs/client behaviors of anticipatory grief. Recall that anticipatory grief involves the intellectual and emotional responses and behaviors by which an individual works through the process of modifying self-concept based on the perception of potential loss. Read each option, keeping the subject of the question and the definition of anticipatory grief in mind to assist in answering correctly.
Priority Nursing Tip: The stages of the grief process include denial, bargaining, anger, depression, and acceptance. These stages can be experienced in any order and at any time during the grieving process.
Reference: Potter, P., et al. (2021). *Fundamentals of nursing* (10th ed., pp. 742–743). Elsevier; Varcarolis, E., & Fosbre, C. (2021). *Essentials of psychiatric mental health nursing: A communication approach to evidence-based care* (4th ed., p. 393). Elsevier.

77. The nurse manager is discussing seclusion procedures for clients with a mental health disorder with the nursing staff. Under which circumstances is seclusion contraindicated? **Select all that apply.**
- ❑ **1.** Client has severe dementia.
- ❑ **2.** Client requests to be secluded.
- ❑ **3.** Client experienced a severe drug overdose.
- ❑ **4.** Client presents a clear and present danger to self or others.
- ❑ **5.** Client has been legally detained for involuntary treatment and is thought to pose an escape risk.
- ❑ **6.** Staffing ratios are not sufficient to provide an involuntarily committed client with sufficient supervision.

Level of Cognitive Ability: Applying
Client Needs: Psychosocial Integrity
Clinical Judgment/Cognitive Skills: Recognize Cues
Integrated Process: Clinical Judgment/Nursing Process/Assessment
Content Area: Mental Health
Health Problems: Mental Health: Abuse/Neglect
Priority Concepts: Health Care Law; Safety

Answer: 1, 3, 6
Rationale: Seclusion is the confinement of a client to a room in which the client is prevented from leaving. General contraindications to seclusion include extremely unstable medical or mental health conditions; delirium or dementia leading to inability to tolerate decreased stimulation; severe suicidal tendencies; severe drug reactions or overdoses or the need for close monitoring of drug doses; and desire for punishment of the client or convenience of the staff. Seclusion may be used for the following circumstances: the client presents a clear and present danger to self or others, the client has been legally detained for involuntary treatment and is thought to pose an escape risk, and the client requests to be secluded.
Test-Taking Strategy: Focus on the subject, contraindications to seclusion. Noting the word *severe* in options 1 and 3 will assist in selecting these options. Noting that option 6 indicates that seclusion is needed for the convenience of the nursing staff will assist in selecting this option.
Priority Nursing Tip: Seclusion is used most commonly when a client presents a risk to self or other people in the area. The client must be monitored continuously while in seclusion to ensure client safety. A liability issue is present if a client is secluded without reasonable grounds for seclusion.
Reference: Varcarolis, E., & Fosbre, C. (2021). *Essentials of psychiatric mental health nursing: A communication approach to evidence-based care* (4th ed., p. 67). Elsevier.

❖ **78.** During an office visit, a prenatal client diagnosed with mitral stenosis states being under a lot of stress lately. During the examination, the client questions the nurse about the assessment and behaves anxiously. Which is the appropriate nursing action at this time?
1. Tell client not to worry.
2. Refer client to a counselor.
3. Assume that client's anxiety will lessen when the assessment is finished.
4. Explain the purpose of the nurse's actions and answer client's questions.

Level of Cognitive Ability: Applying
Client Needs: Psychosocial Integrity
Clinical Judgment/Cognitive Skills: Take Action
Integrated Process: Clinical Judgment/Nursing Process/Implementation
Content Area: Maternity: Antepartum
Health Problems: Mental Health: Coping
Priority Concepts: Clinical Judgment; Communication

Answer: 4
Rationale: In the prenatal client with cardiac issues, stress needs to be reduced as much as possible. The client needs to be provided with honest and informed answers to questions to help alleviate unnecessary fears and emotional stress. Explaining the purpose of nursing actions will assist with decreasing the stress level of the client. The remaining options are nontherapeutic because they neglect to deal with the client's concerns.
Test-Taking Strategy: Use therapeutic communication techniques to answer the question. The client's concerns and feelings would always be addressed, and the correct option is the only choice that does this.
Priority Nursing Tip: In mitral stenosis, valvular tissue thickens and narrows the valve opening, preventing blood flow through the heart. If the client requires a valve replacement, the nurse needs to inform the client that thromboembolism is a problem after valve replacement with a mechanical prosthetic valve, and lifetime anticoagulant therapy is required.
Reference: McKinney, E. S., et al. (2022). *Maternal child nursing* (6th ed., pp. 27, 565–566). Elsevier.

79. A postpartum client with a diagnosis of gestational diabetes is scheduled for discharge. During the discharge teaching, the anxious client asks the nurse, "Do I have to worry about this diabetes anymore?" Which is the **most appropriate** response by the nurse?
1. "Your blood glucose level is within normal limits now, so you will be all right."
2. "You will have to worry about the diabetes only if you become pregnant again."
3. "You will be at risk for developing gestational diabetes with your next pregnancy and also for developing diabetes mellitus."
4. "When you have gestational diabetes, you have diabetes forever, and you must be treated with medication for the rest of your life."

Level of Cognitive Ability: Applying
Client Needs: Psychosocial Integrity
Clinical Judgment/Cognitive Skills: Take Action
Integrated Process: Clinical Judgment/Nursing Process/Implementation
Content Area: Maternity: Postpartum
Health Problems: Mental Health: Anxiety
Priority Concepts: Glucose Regulation; Reproduction

Answer: 3
Rationale: The client is at risk for developing gestational diabetes with each pregnancy. The client also has an increased risk for developing diabetes mellitus and needs to comply with follow-up assessments. The client also needs to be taught techniques to lower the risk for developing diabetes mellitus, such as weight control. The diagnosis of gestational diabetes mellitus indicates that this client has an increased risk for developing diabetes mellitus; however, with proper care, it may not develop.
Test-Taking Strategy: Note the strategic words, *most appropriate.* Note the subject, the long-term effect of gestational diabetes. In addition, use therapeutic communication techniques to answer the question and direct you to the correct option.
Priority Nursing Tip: Pregnant clients should be screened for gestational diabetes between 24 and 28 weeks of pregnancy. Insulin, rather than oral hypoglycemic agents, is prescribed for use during pregnancy.
Reference: McKinney, E. S., et al. (2022). *Maternal child nursing* (6th ed., pp. 27, 560). Elsevier.

❖ **80.** The nurse is performing an assessment on a 16-year-old client who has been diagnosed with anorexia nervosa. Which statement by the client would the nurse identify as a **priority** requiring a **need for further teaching?**
  1. "I check my weight every day without fail."
  2. "I exercise 3 to 4 hours every day to keep my slim figure."
  3. "I've been told that I am 10% below my ideal body weight."
  4. "My best friend was in the hospital with this disorder a year ago."

Level of Cognitive Ability: Evaluating
Client Needs: Psychosocial Integrity
Clinical Judgment/Cognitive Skills: Evaluate Outcomes
Integrated Process: Clinical Judgment/Nursing Process/Evaluation
Content Area: Mental Health
Health Problems: Mental Health: Eating Disorders
Priority Concepts: Clinical Judgment; Nutrition

Answer: 2
Rationale: Exercising 3 to 4 hours every day is excessive physical activity and unrealistic for a 16-year-old. The nurse needs to further assess this statement immediately to find out why the client feels the need to exercise this much to maintain their figure. It is not considered abnormal to check the weight every day; many clients with anorexia nervosa check their weight close to 20 times a day. A weight that exceeds 15% below the ideal weight is significant for clients with anorexia nervosa. Although it is unfortunate that the client's best friend had this disorder, this is not considered a major threat to this client's physical well-being.
Test-Taking Strategy: Note the strategic words, *priority* and *need for further teaching*. The words *need for further teaching* indicate a negative event query and ask you to select the option that identifies a concern. Eliminate options 3 and 4 first because these client statements are not significant or abnormal. From the remaining options, knowledge regarding the manifestations associated with anorexia nervosa will direct you to the correct option.
Priority Nursing Tip: The onset of anorexia nervosa is often associated with a stressful life event. The client intensely fears obesity, body image is distorted, and the client has a disturbed self-concept.
Reference: Varcarolis, E., & Fosbre, C. (2021). *Essentials of psychiatric mental health nursing: A communication approach to evidence-based care* (4th ed., pp. 186–187). Elsevier.

81. A client is demonstrating confusion as a result of a prolonged length of hospital stay requiring bed rest. The client receives a prescription for progressive ambulation as tolerated. Which is the **best** nursing intervention to use to implement the prescription?
  1. Ambulate to client's bathroom 3 times a day.
  2. Ambulate in the room for short distances frequently.
  3. Ambulate in the hall progressively 3 times a day.
  4. Assist with range-of-motion exercises 3 times a day.

Level of Cognitive Ability: Applying
Client Needs: Psychosocial Integrity
Clinical Judgment/Cognitive Skills: Generate Solutions
Integrated Process: Clinical Judgment/Nursing Process/Planning
Content Area: Skills: Activity/Mobility
Health Problems: Mental Health: Neurocognitive Impairment
Priority Concepts: Clinical Judgment; Sensory Perception

Answer: 3
Rationale: The cause of the client's confusion is bed rest and decreased sensory stimulation from a prolonged length of stay; therefore, the best intervention is to ambulate the client in the hall to increase sensory stimulation. Hopefully the stimulation can help decrease the confusion. Options 1 and 2 do not address the client's need for sensory stimulation. The nurse performs option 4 in preparation for ambulation while the client is on bed rest.
Test-Taking Strategy: Note the strategic word, *best*. Focus on the subject, client confusion as a result of bed rest and a prolonged length of hospital stay. Eliminate option 4 first because this action should have been performed in preparation for ambulation. Next eliminate options 1 and 2 because they are comparable or alike in that they both address ambulating the client in the hospital room.
Priority Nursing Tip: Special senses changes that may occur as a result of decreased sensory stimulation and aging include decreased visual acuity, decreased accommodation in the eyes, decreased peripheral vision and increased sensitivity to glare, presbyopia and cataract formation, possible loss of hearing ability, inability to discern taste of food, decreased sense of smell, changes in touch sensation, and decreased pain awareness.
Reference: Potter, P., et al. (2021). *Fundamentals of nursing* (10th ed., pp. 823, 835). Elsevier.

❖ **82.** The nurse is caring for an older client who has been placed in Buck's extension traction after a hip fracture. During the assessment of the client, the nurse notes that the client is disoriented. Which is the **most appropriate** nursing intervention for this client?
   1. Apply restraints to client.
   2. Ask the family to stay with client.
   3. Ask the laboratory to perform electrolyte studies.
   4. Reorient client to time, place, and person frequently.

Level of Cognitive Ability: Applying
Client Needs: Psychosocial Integrity
Clinical Judgment/Cognitive Skills: Take Action
Integrated Process: Clinical Judgment/Nursing Process/Implementation
Content Area: Adult Health: Musculoskeletal
Health Problems: Mental Health: Neurocognitive Impairment
Priority Concepts: Clinical Judgment; Cognition

***Answer:* 4**
Rationale: An inactive older person may become disoriented as a result of a lack of sensory stimulation. The appropriate nursing intervention would be to frequently reorient the client and place objects such as a clock and a calendar in the client's room to maintain orientation. Restraints may cause further disorientation and would not be applied unless specifically prescribed. Agency policies and procedures need to be followed before the application of restraints. The family can assist with the orientation of the client, but it is not appropriate to ask the family to stay with the client. It is not within the scope of nursing practice to prescribe laboratory studies.
Test-Taking Strategy: Note the strategic words, *most appropriate*. Focus on the subject, the appropriate intervention for the client who is disoriented. Eliminate option 3 first because it is not within the realm of nursing practice to prescribe laboratory studies. Next eliminate option 1 because restraints may add to the disorientation that the client is experiencing. It is not appropriate to place the responsibility of the client on the family, so option 2 should be eliminated. In addition, note the relationship between the words *disoriented* in the question and *reorient* in option 4.
Priority Nursing Tip: The nurse would ask the family of a client who is disoriented to bring items from home, such as family photographs for placement at the client's bedside.
Reference: Ignatavicius, D., et al. (2021). *Medical-surgical nursing: Concepts for interprofessional collaborative care* (10th ed., pp. 848, 1037, 1044). Elsevier.

83. An 8-year-old is admitted to the hospital after being sexually abused by an adult family member. The child is withdrawn and appears frightened. Which describes the **best** plan for the **initial** nursing encounter to convey concern and support?
   1. Introduce self and explain to the child that they are safe now here in the hospital.
   2. Introduce self and tell the child that you would like to sit with the child for a little while.
   3. Introduce self and then ask the child to express how they feel about the events leading up to this hospital admission.
   4. Introduce self, explain your role, and ask the child to act out the sexual encounter with the abuser with the use of art therapy.

Level of Cognitive Ability: Applying
Client Needs: Psychosocial Integrity
Clinical Judgment/Cognitive Skills: Generate Solutions
Integrated Process: Clinical Judgment/Nursing Process/Caring
Content Area: Mental Health
Health Problems: Mental Health: Abuse/Neglect
Priority Concepts: Caregiving; Interpersonal Violence

***Answer:* 2**
Rationale: Victims of sexual abuse may exhibit fear and anxiety regarding what has just occurred. In addition, they may fear that the abuse could be repeated. When initiating contact with a child victim of sexual abuse who demonstrates a fear of others, the nurse must convey a willingness to spend time and move slowly to initiate activities that may be perceived as threatening. After a rapport is established, the nurse may explore the child's feelings or use various therapeutic modalities to encourage the recounting of the sexual encounter. Option 2 conveys a plan for an initial encounter that establishes trust by sitting with the child in a nonthreatening atmosphere. Option 1 does not convey concern and support by the nurse. Options 3 and 4 may be implemented after trust and rapport are established.
Test-Taking Strategy: Note the strategic words, *best* and *initial*. Use therapeutic communication techniques. Recalling that rapport needs to be established first will direct you to the correct option.
Priority Nursing Tip: Sexual abuse can involve incest, molestation, exhibitionism, use of pornography, prostitution, or pedophilia; the findings associated with sexual abuse may not be easily apparent in the child.
Reference: McKinney, E. S., et al. (2022). *Maternal child nursing* (6th ed., pp. 723, 1342). Elsevier.

❖ **84.** A victim of a sexual assault is being seen in the crisis center for a third visit. The victim states that, although the rape occurred nearly 2 months ago, it still feels "as though the rape just happened yesterday." Which statement is **most appropriate** for the nurse to use as a response?

1. "In reality, the rape did not just occur. It has been over 2 months now."
2. "What can you do to alleviate some of your fears about being assaulted again?"
3. "In time, our goal will be to help you move on from these strong feelings about your rape."
4. "Tell me more about those aspects of the rape that cause you to feel like the rape just occurred."

Level of Cognitive Ability: Applying
Client Needs: Psychosocial Integrity
Clinical Judgment/Cognitive Skills: Take Action
Integrated Process: Clinical Judgment/Nursing Process/Implementation
Content Area: Mental Health
Health Problems: Mental Health: Coping
Priority Concepts: Communication; Interpersonal Violence

Answer: 4
Rationale: Option 4 allows for the client to express ideas and feelings more fully and portrays an unhurried, nonjudgmental, supportive attitude. Clients need to be reassured that their feelings are normal and that they may freely express their concerns in a safe care environment. Although option 1 is true, it immediately blocks communication. Option 2 places the problem-solving totally on the client. Option 3 places the client's feelings on hold.
Test-Taking Strategy: Note the strategic words, *most appropriate*. Use therapeutic communication techniques. Option 4 specifically addresses the client's feelings and concerns. Remember to always address the client's feelings first.
Priority Nursing Tip: For the client who is a victim of rape, rape trauma syndrome may occur. The client may experience sleep disturbances; nightmares; loss of appetite; fears; anxiety; phobias; suspicion; a decrease in activities and motivation; disruptions in relationships with the partner, family, or friends; self-blame, guilt, and shame; lowered self-esteem; feelings of worthlessness; and somatic complaints.
Reference: Varcarolis, E., & Fosbre, C. (2021). *Essentials of psychiatric mental health nursing: A communication approach to evidence-based care.* (4th ed., pp. 93–95, 360). Elsevier.

85. Which instruction would the nurse give the staff when formulating the plan of care for a client diagnosed with paranoid personality disorder?

1. Have client sign a release of information form.
2. Avoid laughing or whispering in front of client.
3. Increase the socialization of client with unit peers.
4. Begin educating client about available social supports.

Level of Cognitive Ability: Applying
Client Needs: Psychosocial Integrity
Clinical Judgment/Cognitive Skills: Generate Solutions
Integrated Process: Clinical Judgment/Nursing Process/Planning
Content Area: Mental Health
Health Problems: Mental Health: Personality Disorders
Priority Concepts: Caregiving; Psychosis

Answer: 2
Rationale: A client experiencing paranoia is distrustful and suspicious of others. The health care team needs to establish rapport and trust with the client. Laughing or whispering in front of the client would increase the client's paranoia. The remaining options ask the client to trust on a multitude of levels. These options are too intrusive for a client who is paranoid.
Test-Taking Strategy: Focus on the subject, the plan of care for a client diagnosed with paranoia. Recalling that the client with paranoia is distrustful and suspicious of others will direct you to the correct option.
Priority Nursing Tip: The client diagnosed with a paranoid disorder has a concrete, pervasive delusional system characterized by persecutory and grandiose beliefs. The client is often viewed by others as hostile, stubborn, and defensive, and the client commonly exhibits suspiciousness and mistrust of others.
Reference: Varcarolis, E., & Fosbre, C. (2021). *Essentials of psychiatric mental health nursing: A communication approach to evidence-based care* (4th ed., pp. 170, 175). Elsevier.

❖ **86.** The nurse is assessing a client who was just admitted to the psychiatric unit. The client says, "You won't have to worry about me much longer." Which meaning would the nurse interpret from this statement?
1. An intention of suicide
2. An expression of depression
3. An intention of self-mutilation
4. An expression of hopelessness

Level of Cognitive Ability: Analyzing
Client Needs: Psychosocial Integrity
Clinical Judgment/Cognitive Skills: Analyze Cues
Integrated Process: Clinical Judgment/Nursing Process/Analysis
Content Area: Mental Health
Health Problems: Mental Health: Suicide
Priority Concepts: Clinical Judgment; Safety

Answer: 1
Rationale: A client who is at risk for suicide who says, "You won't have to worry about me much longer," is making an expression of a suicidal intent. Although depression, self-mutilation, and hopelessness may relate to violence to oneself, the statement that they will not be around is a direct comment about the act of suicide.
Test-Taking Strategy: Focus on the subject, interpreting the client's statement. Noting the words, *You won't have to worry about me much longer*, will direct you to the correct option.
Priority Nursing Tip: All suicide behavior is extremely serious regardless of the intent. Suicide ideation requires constant attention and, typically, one-on-one observation. The client with a suicide plan must be placed on suicide precautions.
Reference: Varcarolis, E., & Fosbre, C. (2021). *Essentials of psychiatric mental health nursing: A communication approach to evidence-based care* (4th ed., pp. 369–370). Elsevier.

87. The nurse notes that an assigned client is lying tense in bed and staring at the cardiac monitor. The client states, "There sure are a lot of wires around there. I sure hope we don't get hit by lightning." Which is the **most appropriate** nursing response?
1. "Your family can stay tonight if they wish."
2. "Would you like a mild sedative to help you relax?"
3. "The hospital is well equipped to shield a lightning strike."
4. "Yes, all the wires must be scary. Let's talk about the cardiac monitor."

Level of Cognitive Ability: Applying
Client Needs: Psychosocial Integrity
Clinical Judgment/Cognitive Skills: Take Action
Integrated Process: Clinical Judgment/Nursing Process/Implementation
Content Area: Adult Health: Cardiovascular
Health Problems: Mental Health: Coping
Priority Concepts: Anxiety; Communication

Answer: 4
Rationale: The nurse would initially validate the client's concern and then assess the client's knowledge regarding the cardiac monitor. This gives the nurse an opportunity to provide the client education if necessary. None of the remaining options address the client's concern. In addition, pharmacologic interventions would be considered only if necessary.
Test-Taking Strategy: Note the strategic words, *most appropriate*. Use therapeutic communication techniques. Remember to address the client's feelings first. The correct option is the only option that addresses the client's feelings.
Priority Nursing Tip: The client needs to be oriented to the room upon admission to the hospital. Any medical equipment should be explained, and explanations need to be repeated for the client if necessary. Decreasing sensory stimulation will allow the client to rest, which is important for the process of recovery.
References: Lewis, S., et al. (2020). *Medical-surgical nursing: Assessment and management of clinical problems* (11th ed., p. 669). Elsevier; Potter, P., et al. (2021). *Fundamentals of nursing.* (10th ed., pp. 333–335). Elsevier.

❖ **88.** A young adult client diagnosed with a spinal cord injury tells the nurse, "It's so depressing that I'll never get to have sex again." Which is the realistic reply for the nurse to make to the client?

1. "It must feel horrible to know you can never have sex again."
2. "It's still possible to have a sexual relationship, but it will be different."
3. "You're young, so you'll adapt to this more easily than if you were older."
4. "Because of body reflexes, sexual functioning will be no different than before."

Level of Cognitive Ability: Applying
Client Needs: Psychosocial Integrity
Clinical Judgment/Cognitive Skills: Take Action
Integrated Process: Clinical Judgment/Nursing Process/Implementation
Content Area: Adult Health: Neurologic
Health Problems: Mental Health: Coping
Priority Concepts: Functional Ability; Sexuality

Answer: 2
Rationale: It is possible to have a sexual relationship after a spinal cord injury, but it is different from what the client will have experienced before the injury. Those who have a penis may experience reflex erections, although they may not ejaculate. Those with vaginas can have adductor spasm. Sexual counseling may help the client adapt to changes in sexuality after a spinal cord injury.
Test-Taking Strategy: Use knowledge regarding the effects of a spinal cord injury and therapeutic communication techniques in chronic conditions to answer correctly. The correct option addresses the subject, sexual relationships after spinal cord injury; it is accurate and is a therapeutic response.
Priority Nursing Tip: The complications associated with a spinal cord injury depend on the level of the injury. One complication is autonomic dysreflexia. Autonomic dysreflexia occurs with spinal lesions above the level of T6.
References: Ignatavicius, D., et al. (2021). *Medical-surgical nursing: Concepts for interprofessional collaborative care* (10th ed., p. 885). Elsevier; Potter, P., et al. (2021). *Fundamentals of nursing* (10th ed., pp. 333–335). Elsevier.

89. A family member of a client diagnosed with a brain tumor states that they are feeling distraught and guilty for not encouraging the client to seek medical evaluation earlier. Which information would the nurse incorporate when formulating a response to the family member's statement?

1. A brain tumor presents with few sights/symptoms.
2. It is true that brain tumors are easily recognizable.
3. Brain tumors are never detected until very late in their course.
4. The signs/symptoms of a brain tumor may be easily attributed to another cause.

Level of Cognitive Ability: Applying
Client Needs: Psychosocial Integrity
Clinical Judgment/Cognitive Skills: Generate Solutions
Integrated Process: Clinical Judgment/Nursing Process/Caring
Content Area: Adult Health: Neurologic
Health Problems: Mental Health: Coping
Priority Concepts: Communication; Stress and Coping

Answer: 4
Rationale: Signs and symptoms of a brain tumor vary depending on location, and they may easily be attributed to another cause. Symptoms include headache, vomiting, visual disturbances, and changes in intellectual abilities or personality. Seizures occur in some clients. These symptoms can be easily attributed to other causes. The family requires support to assist them during the normal grieving process. Options 1, 2, and 3 are inaccurate statements.
Test-Taking Strategy: Eliminate option 3 first because it contains the closed-ended word "never." From the remaining options, recall that the tumor does present with signs/symptoms, but it is not always easily diagnosed since the symptoms of a brain tumor may be easily attributed to another cause. Also note the word *may* in the correct option.
Priority Nursing Tip: The brain is a common site of metastasis for cancers that originate in the lungs and the breast. Tumors that originate in the brain primarily affect the central nervous system and its associated functions.
Reference: Ignatavicius, D., et al. (2021). *Medical-surgical nursing: Concepts for interprofessional collaborative care* (10th ed., p. 922). Elsevier.

90. A client has a hip fracture repair with a prosthetic implant placed. On the day after the implant, the nurse finds the client surrounded by papers from the client's briefcase and planning a phone meeting. The nurse plans to discuss activities with the client and would base the discussion on which information?
1. Rest is an essential component of bone healing.
2. Setting limits on a client's behavior is a mandated nursing role.
3. Not keeping up with the job will increase client's stress level.
4. Involvement in the job will keep client from becoming bored.

Level of Cognitive Ability: Applying
Client Needs: Psychosocial Integrity
Clinical Judgment/Cognitive Skills: Generate Solutions
Integrated Process: Clinical Judgment/Nursing Process/Planning
Content Area: Adult Health: Musculoskeletal
Health Problems: Mental Health: Coping
Priority Concepts: Clinical Judgment; Mobility

Answer: 1
Rationale: Rest is an essential component of bone healing. Nurses can help clients understand the importance of rest and find ways to balance work demands to promote healing. Stress needs to be kept to a minimum to promote bone healing. Nurses cannot demand these changes, but they need to encourage clients to choose them. Setting limits on a client's behavior is not a mandated nursing role. It may relieve stress to do work; however, during the immediate period after the implant, it may not be therapeutic.
Test-Taking Strategy: Eliminate options 3 and 4 because they are comparable or alike in that they both relate to the client's job. From the remaining options, note that option 1 is the umbrella option, and it addresses rest after hip fracture repair with a prosthetic implant.
Priority Nursing Tip: Although rare, a fat embolism can occur as a result of a bone fracture. A fat embolism originates in the bone marrow and occurs when a fat globule is released into the bloodstream. If the nurse suspects this, the nurse must notify the primary health care provider immediately.
Reference: Ignatavicius, D., et al. (2021). *Medical-surgical nursing: Concepts for interprofessional collaborative care* (10th ed., pp. 1032, 1044). Elsevier.

91. A charge nurse observes an unlicensed assistive personnel (UAP) talking in an unusually loud voice to a client with schizophrenia experiencing delirium. Which **priority** action would the charge nurse take?
1. Enter the room and inform client that everything is all right.
2. Speak to the UAP immediately while in client's room to solve the problem.
3. Ensure client's safety, calmly ask the UAP to step outside the room, and inform the UAP that their voice was unusually loud.
4. Explain to the UAP that speaking so loudly is tolerated only if client is talking loudly and the UAP needs to get client's attention.

Level of Cognitive Ability: Applying
Client Needs: Psychosocial Integrity
Clinical Judgment/Cognitive Skills: Take Action
Integrated Process: Clinical Judgment/Nursing Process/Implementation
Content Area: Leadership/Management: Delegating/Supervising
Health Problems: Mental Health: Schizophrenia
Priority Concepts: Communication; Leadership

Answer: 3
Rationale: The nurse must ascertain that the client is safe and then discuss the matter with the UAP in an area away from the hearing of the client. If the client hears the conversation, the client may become more confused or agitated. The remaining options are incorrect actions for this situation.
Test-Taking Strategy: Note the strategic word, *priority*. Focus on the subject, the action that the charge nurse should take. Use therapeutic communication techniques to answer correctly. Also note that the correct option addresses client safety.
Priority Nursing Tip: Methods that can be used to enhance communication include using written words if the client is able to see, read, and write; providing plenty of light in the room; getting the attention of the client before beginning to speak; facing the client when speaking; and talking in a room without distracting noises.
Reference: Varcarolis, E., & Fosbre, C. (2021). *Essentials of psychiatric mental health nursing: A communication approach to evidence-based care* (4th ed., p. 284). Elsevier.

92. A teenager diagnosed with celiac disease arrives at the emergency department reporting profuse, watery diarrhea after a pizza party the night before. The client states, "I don't want to be different from my friends." Which client concern would the nurse focus on when planning a response to the client?
1. Diarrhea
2. Low self-esteem
3. Deficient fluid volume
4. Increased inflammation

Level of Cognitive Ability: Analyzing
Client Needs: Psychosocial Integrity
Clinical Judgment/Cognitive Skills: Generate Solutions
Integrated Process: Clinical Judgment/Nursing Process/Planning
Content Area: Mental Health
Health Problems: Mental Health: Coping
Priority Concepts: Communication; Coping

Answer: 2
Rationale: The client expresses concern about being different from friends. Celiac crisis is a medical diagnosis that often involves diarrhea. Although the question states that the client has profuse, watery diarrhea, no data identify an actual deficient fluid volume or increased inflammation.
Test-Taking Strategy: Focus on the subject of a client feeling different. Focus on the client's statement and note the relationship of the statement and the correct option. Also note that the incorrect options are comparable or alike and identify physiologic problems.
Priority Nursing Tip: The client with celiac disease has intolerance to gluten, the protein component of wheat, barley, rye, and oats. Consuming products containing these components results in the accumulation of the amino acid glutamine, which is toxic to the intestinal mucosal cells.
Reference: McKinney, E. S., et al. (2022). *Maternal child nursing* (6th ed., pp. 996–997). Elsevier.

93. The nurse develops a plan of care for a 1-month-old infant diagnosed with intussusception. Which nursing measure would be **most effective** to provide psychosocial support for the parent–child relationship?
1. Provide educational materials.
2. Encourage the parents to room-in with their infant.
3. Initiate home nutritional support as early as possible.
4. Encourage the parents to go home and get some sleep.

Level of Cognitive Ability: Applying
Client Needs: Psychosocial Integrity
Clinical Judgment/Cognitive Skills: Generate Solutions
Integrated Process: Clinical Judgment/Nursing Process/Planning
Content Area: Pediatrics: Gastrointestinal
Health Problems: Pediatric-Specific: Intussusception
Priority Concepts: Anxiety; Development

Answer: 2
Rationale: Rooming-in is effective for reducing separation anxiety and preserving the parent–child relationship. Educational materials may be beneficial, but they will not provide psychosocial support for the parent–child relationship. Home nutritional support is not usually necessary in the situation described. Parents are under stress when a child is ill and hospitalized, and telling a parent to go home and sleep will not relieve this stress.
Test-Taking Strategy: Note the strategic words, *most effective*. Focus on the words *parent–child relationship*. The only choice that addresses the parent–child relationship is the correct option.
Priority Nursing Tip: Intussusception occurs when one portion of the bowel telescopes into another portion of the bowel and results in obstruction to the passage of intestinal contents. The nurse must monitor for signs and symptoms of obstruction, perforation, and shock, including fever, increased heart rate, changes in level of consciousness or blood pressure, and respiratory distress.
Reference: McKinney, E. S., et al. (2022). *Maternal child nursing* (6th ed., p. 789). Elsevier.

❖ **94.** Which comment made by the parents of an infant with a penis who will have a surgical repair of a hernia indicates a **need for further teaching** by the nurse?
1. "I understand that surgery will repair the hernia."
2. "I don't know if my child will be able to have a child when grown up."
3. "The day nurse told me to give my child sponge baths for a few days after surgery."
4. "I'll need to buy extra diapers because we need to change them frequently now."

Level of Cognitive Ability: Evaluating
Client Needs: Psychosocial Integrity
Clinical Judgment/Cognitive Skills: Evaluate Outcomes
Integrated Process: Clinical Judgment/Nursing Process/Evaluation
Content Area: Pediatrics: Gastrointestinal
Health Problems: Mental Health: Anxiety
Priority Concepts: Anxiety; Patient Education

Answer: **2**
Rationale: The anatomic location of a hernia frequently causes more psychological concern to the parents than does the actual condition or treatment. The remaining options all indicate accurate understanding associated with the surgery. The correct option is an incorrect comment requiring follow-up.
Test-Taking Strategy: Focus on the strategic words, *need for further teaching.* These words indicate a negative event query and the need to select the incorrect statement. Options 1, 3, and 4 do not require follow-up, whereas option 2 reflects parental fear and identifies a need for further assessment.
Priority Nursing Tip: A hernia occurs as a result of a weakened muscle wall. After surgical repair, the child or parents of a child who underwent repair need to be informed about the importance of allowing the site to heal.
Reference: McKinney, E. S., et al. (2022). *Maternal child nursing* (6th ed., p. 973). Elsevier.

95. The nurse is leading a crisis intervention group comprising high school students who have experienced the recent death of a classmate who committed suicide. The students are experiencing disbelief as they review the details of the suicide. Which would be the **initial** therapeutic action by the nurse?
1. Ask how the students recovered from a death event in the past.
2. Reinforce the students' ability to work through this death event.
3. Inquire about the students' perception of their classmate's suicide.
4. Reinforce the students' sense of growth through this death experience.

Level of Cognitive Ability: Applying
Client Needs: Psychosocial Integrity
Clinical Judgment/Cognitive Skills: Take Action
Integrated Process: Clinical Judgment/Nursing Process/Implementation
Content Area: Mental Health
Health Problems: Mental Health: Suicide
Priority Concepts: Communication; Coping

Answer: **3**
Rationale: It is essential to determine the students' views. Inquiring about the students' perception of the suicide will specifically identify the appraisal of the suicide and the meaning of the perception. Although option 1 is exploratory, it does not address the "here-and-now" appraisal in terms of the classmate's suicide. Although the nurse is interested in how students have coped in the past, this inquiry would not be the most immediate assessment. Options 2 and 4 are attempts to foster students' self-esteem. Such an approach is premature at this point.
Test-Taking Strategy: Note the strategic word, *initial.* Use the steps of the nursing process to eliminate options 2 and 4. Options 2 and 4 are also comparable or alike in that they are attempts to foster students' self-esteem. From the remaining options, consider the subject of the question, high school students who recently lost a classmate to suicide, and select the option that deals with the here and now. The nurse must first determine the students' perception and appraisal of the stressful event.
Priority Nursing Tip: The nurse's role in the grief and loss process includes communicating with those involved in the crisis. The nurse must consider the client's culture, religion, family structure, individual life experiences, coping skills, and support systems.
Reference: Varcarolis, E., & Fosbre, C. (2021). *Essentials of psychiatric mental health nursing: A communication approach to evidence-based care* (4th ed., pp. 368, 373–374). Elsevier.

❖ **96.** A hospitalized client has participated in substance abuse therapy group sessions. Which statement by the client would **best** indicate that the client has assimilated session topics, understood coping response styles, and processed information effectively for self-use?

1. "I'll keep all my appointments, and I'll do everything I'm supposed to. That way nothing will go wrong."
2. "I know I'm ready to be discharged. I feel like I'll have no problem saying no and leaving a group of friends if they are drinking."
3. "This group has really helped a lot. I know that it will be different when I go home. But I'm sure that my family and friends will all help me like the people in this group have. They'll all help me, I know they will. They won't let me go back to old ways."
4. "I'm looking forward to leaving here, but I know that I will miss all of you. So, I'm happy, and I'm sad. I'm excited, and I'm scared. I know that I have to work hard to be strong and that everyone isn't going to be as helpful as you all have been. I know it isn't going to be easy, but I'm going to try as hard as I can."

Level of Cognitive Ability: Evaluating
Client Needs: Psychosocial Integrity
Clinical Judgment/Cognitive Skills: Evaluate Outcomes
Integrated Process: Clinical Judgment/Nursing Process/Evaluation
Content Area: Mental Health
Health Problems: Mental Health: Addictions
Priority Concepts: Addiction; Coping

Answer: 4
Rationale: In option 4, the client is expressing real concern and ambivalence about discharge from the hospital. The client demonstrates an ability to perceive reality in the appraisal regarding the lifestyle changes that will have to be initiated, as well as the fact that the client will have to work hard and develop new friends and meeting places. With the defense mechanism of denial, the person denies reality. There can be varying degrees of this denial. In option 1 the client is concrete and procedure oriented; again, the client verbalizes denial. Option 2 identifies denial. In option 3 the client is relying heavily on others, and the client's locus of control is external.
Test-Taking Strategy: Note the strategic word, *best.* Select the option that identifies the most realistic client verbalization. Recalling that a person in denial is unable to face reality will assist you with eliminating the remaining options.
Priority Nursing Tip: A defense mechanism is a coping device used in an effort to protect the individual from feelings of anxiety. As anxiety increases and becomes overwhelming, the individual copes by using defense mechanisms to protect the ego and decrease anxiety.
Reference: Varcarolis, E., & Fosbre, C. (2021). *Essentials of psychiatric mental health nursing: A communication approach to evidence-based care* (4th ed., pp. 325–326). Elsevier.

97. A client recovering from a diagnosed head injury becomes anxious at times. Which nursing action is **most appropriate** when attempting to calm this client?

1. Assign client a new task to master.
2. Turn on the television to a musical program.
3. Make client aware that the behavior is undesirable.
4. Talk about the family pictures on display in client's room.

Level of Cognitive Ability: Applying
Client Needs: Psychosocial Integrity
Clinical Judgment/Cognitive Skills: Take Action
Integrated Process: Clinical Judgment/Nursing Process/Implementation
Content Area: Adult Health: Neurologic
Health Problems: Mental Health: Anxiety
Priority Concepts: Anxiety; Intracranial Regulation

Answer: 4
Rationale: Providing familiar objects will decrease anxiety. Decreasing environmental stimuli also aids in reducing agitation for the head-injured client. Option 1 does not simplify the environment because a new task may be frustrating. Option 2 increases stimuli. In option 3 the nurse uses negative reinforcement to help the client adjust.
Test-Taking Strategy: Note the strategic words, *most appropriate.* Focus on the subject, the measure that will calm a client who is agitated. Identify those options that may increase stimuli, agitation, and frustration. This will assist you with eliminating the remaining options.
Priority Nursing Tip: For the client with a head injury, the nurse would monitor for cerebrospinal fluid (CSF) drainage, such as from the nose. CSF can be distinguished from other fluids by the presence of concentric rings (yellowish stain surrounded by bloody fluid) when the fluid is placed on a white sterile background, such as a gauze pad. CSF also tests positive for glucose when tested using a strip test.
Reference: Ignatavicius, D., et al. (2021). *Medical-surgical nursing: Concepts for interprofessional collaborative care* (10th ed., p. 921). Elsevier.

❖ **98.** A client recovering from a stroke has become irritable and angry regarding self-limitations. Which is the **best** nursing approach to help the client regain motivation to keep trying to succeed as capable?
1. Ignore the behavior, knowing client is grieving.
2. Allow longer and more frequent visitation by the spouse.
3. Use supportive statements to correct client's behavior.
4. Stress that the nurses are experienced and know how client feels.

Level of Cognitive Ability: Applying
Client Needs: Psychosocial Integrity
Clinical Judgment/Cognitive Skills: Generate Solutions
Integrated Process: Clinical Judgment/Nursing Process/Planning
Content Area: Adult Health: Neurologic
Health Problems: Mental Health: Coping
Priority Concepts: Stress and Coping; Intracranial Regulation

Answer: 3
Rationale: Clients who have experienced a stroke have many and varied needs. It is also important to support and praise the client for accomplishments. The client may need their behavior pointed out so that correction can take place, and the client's behavior should not be ignored. Spouses of a stroke client are often grieving; therefore, more visitations may not be helpful. Additionally, short visits are often encouraged. Stating that the nurse knows how the client feels is inappropriate.
Test-Taking Strategy: Note the strategic word, *best*. Use therapeutic communication techniques to eliminate options 1 and 4. From the remaining choices, option 3 is the only one that addresses the client's behavior described in the question.
Priority Nursing Tip: For the client at risk for increased intracranial pressure, the nurse would ensure that the client avoids extreme hip and neck flexion; extreme hip flexion may increase intrathoracic pressure, whereas extreme neck flexion prohibits venous drainage from the brain.
References: Ignatavicius, D., et al. (2021). *Medical-surgical nursing: Concepts for interprofessional collaborative care* (10th ed., pp. 910–911). Elsevier; Potter, P., et al. (2021). *Fundamentals of nursing* (10th ed., pp. 333–335). Elsevier.

99. An older client is admitted to the hospital with a fractured hip and is experiencing periods of confusion. The nurse develops a plan of care and would identify which psychosocial outcome as having the greatest impact on improving the client's cognitive abilities?
1. Improved sleep patterns
2. Reduced family fears and anxiety
3. Meeting self-care needs independently
4. Increased ability to concentrate and participate in care

Level of Cognitive Ability: Applying
Client Needs: Psychosocial Integrity
Clinical Judgment/Cognitive Skills: Generate Solutions
Integrated Process: Clinical Judgment/Nursing Process/Planning
Content Area: Foundations of Care: Communication
Health Problems: Mental Health: Neurocognitive Impairment
Priority Concepts: Clinical Judgment; Cognition

Answer: 4
Rationale: The client needs to be able to concentrate and participate in own care. When the client is able to do that, the nurse can work with the client to achieve the other outcomes. Options 1 and 3 address physiologic needs rather than psychosocial outcomes. Option 2 is a secondary need and does not address the client.
Test-Taking Strategy: Focus on the subject, psychosocial outcome, and that the client is confused. Select the option that will have the greatest impact on the client's ability to function psychosocially. Option 2 can be eliminated because it does not address the client. Options 1 and 3 address physiologic rather than psychosocial needs.
Priority Nursing Tip: For the client who has experienced a hip fracture, the nurse must maintain the leg and hip in proper alignment and prevent internal or external rotation, as well as extreme hip flexion.
Reference: Ignatavicius, D., et al. (2021). *Medical-surgical nursing: Concepts for interprofessional collaborative care* (10th ed., p. 1034). Elsevier.

❖ 100. The nurse is caring for a terminally ill woman who is in the terminal stage of diagnosed breast cancer. The nurse would know which client behavior is characteristic of anticipatory grieving?
1. Discusses thoughts and feelings related to loss
2. Has prolonged emotional reactions and outbursts
3. Verbalizes unrealistic goals and plans for the future
4. Ignores untreated medical conditions that require treatment

Level of Cognitive Ability: Analyzing
Client Needs: Psychosocial Integrity
Clinical Judgment/Cognitive Skills: Analyze Cues
Integrated Process: Clinical Judgment/Nursing Process/Analysis
Content Area: Developmental Stages: End-of-Life
Health Problems: Mental Health: Grief/Loss
Priority Concepts: Clinical Judgment; Coping

Answer: 1
Rationale: The nurse can determine the client's stage of anticipatory grief by observing the client's behavior. The remaining options are examples of dysfunctional grieving.
Test-Taking Strategy: Focus on the subject, anticipatory grieving. Note that the remaining options are comparable or alike, and indicate dysfunctional grieving. Also noting the words *prolonged, unrealistic,* and *ignores* in these options will assist you in eliminating them.
Priority Nursing Tip: The nurse's role in the grief and loss process includes communicating with the client, family members, and significant others.
Reference: Lewis, S., et al. (2020). *Medical-surgical nursing: Assessment and management of clinical problems* (11th ed., pp. 131, 1206). Elsevier.

101. The nurse determines that a client is beginning to experience shock and hemorrhage as a result of a partial inversion of the uterus. The client asks in an apprehensive voice, "What is happening to me? I feel so funny, and I know I'm bleeding. Am I dying?" Which typical response is the client experiencing during this medical emergency?
1. Panic as a result of shock
2. Anticipatory grieving related to the fear of dying
3. Depression related to postpartum hormonal changes
4. Fear and anxiety related to unexpected and unknown changes

Level of Cognitive Ability: Analyzing
Client Needs: Psychosocial Integrity
Clinical Judgment/Cognitive Skills: Analyze Cues
Integrated Process: Clinical Judgment/Nursing Process/Analysis
Content Area: Complex Care: Shock
Health Problems: Mental Health: Anxiety
Priority Concepts: Caregiving; Clinical Judgment

Answer: 4
Rationale: Feelings of loss of control are common causes of anxiety, and the unknown is the most common cause of fear. Apprehension and feelings of impending doom are also associated with shock, but the information in the question does not suggest panic at this point. Anticipatory grieving occurs when there is knowledge of the impending loss, but it is not associated with a sudden situational crisis such as this one. It is far too early for the onset of postpartum depression.
Test-Taking Strategy: Note the subject, the response that the client is experiencing. Focus on the words *I feel so funny* in the question and *unexpected and unknown changes* in option 4.
Priority Nursing Tip: For the postpartum client experiencing uterine atony, the nurse would massage the fundus, taking care not to overmassage. If the client is hemorrhaging, the nurse would remain with the client and ask another nurse to contact the primary health care provider.
Reference: McKinney, E. S., et al. (2022). *Maternal child nursing* (6th ed., pp. 604, 610). Elsevier.

❖ **102.** A perinatal home care nurse has just assessed the fetal status of a client with a diagnosis of partial placental abruption at 20 weeks' gestation. The client is experiencing new bleeding and reports less fetal movement. The nurse informs the client that the obstetrician will be contacted for possible hospital admission. The client begins to cry quietly while holding the abdomen with the hands. The client murmurs, "No, no, you can't go, my little baby." The nurse would recognize the client's behavior as an indication of which psychosocial reaction?
1. Fear of hospitalization
2. Fear of loss and the death of the fetus
3. Grief due to potential loss of the fetus
4. Cognitive confusion as a result of shock

Level of Cognitive Ability: Analyzing
Client Needs: Psychosocial Integrity
Clinical Judgment/Cognitive Skills: Analyze Cues
Integrated Process: Clinical Judgment/Nursing Process/Analysis
Content Area: Maternity: Intrapartum
Health Problems: Mental Health: Grief/Loss
Priority Concepts: Stress and Coping; Reproduction

Answer: 3
Rationale: Grief occurs when a client has knowledge of an impending loss, such as when signs of fetal distress accelerate. The first stages of grieving may be characterized by shock; emotional numbness; disbelief; and strong emotions such as tears, screaming, or anger. The remaining options are not focused on the client's expressed concerns.
Test-Taking Strategy: Focus on the subject, the client's psychosocial reaction. Options 1 and 4 can be eliminated because there is no indication of pain or confusion. Although options 2 and 3 are somewhat similar, one suggests a fetal death and the other a potential loss. There is no indication of fetal death. The client perceives this as a potential loss. With this knowledge, option 3 is the only correct answer.
Priority Nursing Tip: In placenta abruptio, there is dark red vaginal bleeding, uterine pain or tenderness or both, and uterine rigidity. In placenta previa, there is painless, bright red vaginal bleeding, and the uterus is soft, relaxed, and nontender.
Reference: McKinney, E. S., et al. (2022) *Maternal child nursing* (6th ed., pp. 537, 540–541). Elsevier.

103. A postoperative client has been vomiting and has absent bowel sounds, and paralytic ileus has been diagnosed. The physician prescribes the insertion of a nasogastric tube. The nurse explains the purpose of the tube and the insertion procedure to the client. The client says to the nurse, "I'm not sure I can take any more of this treatment." Which therapeutic response would the nurse make to the client?
1. "Let's just put the tube down so that you can get well."
2. "If you don't have this tube put down, you will just continue to vomit."
3. "You are feeling tired and frustrated with your recovery from surgery?"
4. "It is your right to refuse any treatment. I'll notify the primary physician."

Level of Cognitive Ability: Applying
Client Needs: Psychosocial Integrity
Clinical Judgment/Cognitive Skills: Take Action
Integrated Process: Caring
Content Area: Foundations of Care: Communication
Health Problems: Mental Health: Coping
Priority Concepts: Communication; Professional Identity

Answer: 3
Rationale: In option 3, the nurse uses empathy. Empathy, comprehending, and sharing a client's frame of reference are important components of the nurse–client relationship. This assists clients with expressing and exploring feelings, which can lead to problem-solving. The other options are examples of barriers to effective communication, including option 1, which is stereotyping; option 2, which is defensiveness; and option 4, which is showing disapproval.
Test-Taking Strategy: Use therapeutic communication techniques. Option 3 is an open-ended question and a communication tool; it also focuses on the client's feelings.
Priority Nursing Tip: In the postoperative period, vomiting, abdominal distention, and the absence of bowel sounds may be signs of paralytic ileus.
Reference: Potter, P., et al. (2021). *Fundamentals of nursing* (10th ed., pp. 333–335, 1224). Elsevier.

❖ **104.** The nurse implements which de-escalation techniques with a client who is extremely angry and exhibiting increasingly agitated behavior? **Select all that apply.**
- ❑ 1. Avoid verbal struggles.
- ❑ 2. Provide clear options to client.
- ❑ 3. Use therapeutic touch on client's shoulder.
- ❑ 4. Maintain both client's self-esteem and dignity.
- ❑ 5. Establish what client considers to be their own needs.
- ❑ 6. Use a firm and assertive tone of voice when speaking to client.

Level of Cognitive Ability: Applying
Client Needs: Psychosocial Integrity
Clinical Judgment/Cognitive Skills: Take Action
Integrated Process: Clinical Judgment/Nursing Process/Implementation
Content Area: Mental Health
Health Problems: Mental Health: Violence
Priority Concepts: Interpersonal Violence; Safety

Answer: 1, 2, 4, 5
Rationale: When the client is angry and exhibits increasingly agitated behavior, the nurse would employ de-escalation techniques to prevent client violence and assaultive behaviors. These techniques include assessing the situation, using a calm and clear tone of voice when communicating with the client, remaining calm, avoiding verbal struggles, presenting clear options to the client, and maintaining the client's self-esteem and dignity. The nurse would establish what the client considers to be their own need and maintain a large personal space (touching the client could increase agitation).
Test-Taking Strategy: Focus on the subject, de-escalation techniques. In selecting the correct answers, determine if the technique would calm or further agitate the client. Remember the need to maintain a calm approach and a large distance from the client.
Priority Nursing Tip: When using de-escalation techniques, the nurse needs to remain calm and centered. The nurse would encourage the client to use slow breathing, which will help in successful de-escalation.
Reference: Varcarolis, E., & Fosbre, C. (2021). *Essentials of psychiatric mental health nursing: A communication approach to evidence-based care* (4th ed., p. 381). Elsevier.

105. A client who is receiving total parenteral nutrition (TPN) tells the nurse, "I'm not sure that I want to receive an infusion of lipids because it could make me obese." Which **initial** action would the nurse take?
1. Inquire how illness affects client's self-concept.
2. Ask the provider to discuss the benefits of intralipids.
3. State that intralipids supply essential fatty acids for life.
4. Explain how intralipids replace dietary sources of lipids.

Level of Cognitive Ability: Applying
Client Needs: Psychosocial Integrity
Clinical Judgment/Cognitive Skills: Take Action
Integrated Process: Clinical Judgment/Nursing Process/Implementation
Content Area: Foundations of Care: Communication
Health Problems: Mental Health: Coping
Priority Concepts: Caregiving; Nutrition

Answer: 1
Rationale: A client who receives TPN is at risk for developing an essential fatty acid deficiency; however, this client's comment requires more than a simple informational response initially. Thus, the nurse responds with option 1 to assist the client with self-expression and to deal with aspects of illness and treatment. Option 2 delays client self-expression and devalues the client's feelings. Options 3 and 4 provide information only.
Test-Taking Strategy: Note the strategic word, *initial*. This should cue you to use therapeutic communication techniques to focus on the client's feelings because the client's feelings must be assessed before the nurse can provide comprehensive information and adapt the information accordingly. Option 1 is the only choice that addresses the client's feelings.
Priority Nursing Tip: Total parenteral nutrition is the least desirable form of nutrition and is used when there is no other nutritional alternative. Other forms of administering nutrition such as oral or via a gastrointestinal tube are initiated first.
Reference: Potter, P., et al. (2021). *Fundamentals of nursing* (10th ed., pp. 333–335, 999). Elsevier.

❖ **106.** A client has been diagnosed with terminal cancer and is using opioid analgesics for pain relief. Which action by the home care nurse would **best** allay the client's anxiety about becoming addicted to the pain medication?
1. Encouraging client to hold off as long as possible between doses of pain medication
2. Encouraging client to take lower doses of medications even though the pain is not well controlled
3. Explaining to client that the fears are justified but would be of no concern during the final stages of care
4. Explaining to client that addiction rarely occurs in individuals who are taking medication appropriately to relieve pain

Level of Cognitive Ability: Applying
Client Needs: Psychosocial Integrity
Clinical Judgment/Cognitive Skills: Take Action
Integrated Process: Clinical Judgment/Nursing Process/Implementation
Content Area: Pharmacology: Pain: Opioid Analgesics
Health Problems: Mental Health: Anxiety
Priority Concepts: Caregiving; Pain

Answer: 4
Rationale: Clients who are on opioid analgesics often have well-founded fears about addiction, even in the face of pain. The nurse has the responsibility to provide correct information about the likelihood of addiction while still maintaining adequate pain control. Addiction is rare for individuals who are taking medication to relieve pain. Allowing the client to be in pain, as in options 1 and 2, is not acceptable nursing practice. Option 3 is only partially correct in that it acknowledges the client's fear.
Test-Taking Strategy: Note the strategic word, *best*. Options 1 and 2 are comparable or alike options and would be eliminated because both are related to medication dosage. Focusing on the words *allay the client's anxiety* will also assist in selecting the best answer.
Priority Nursing Tip: The nurse needs to continually assess the client with terminal cancer for signs of pain. The nurse needs to ensure that measures to reduce and eliminate the pain are effective.
Reference: Ignatavicius, D., et al. (2021). *Medical-surgical nursing: Concepts for interprofessional collaborative care* (10th ed., pp. 86, 89–90). Elsevier.

107. A client recovering from pneumonia is very anxious about receiving chest physiotherapy (CPT) for the first time at home. When planning for the client's care, which concept about CPT would the home care nurse use to reassure the client?
1. CPT will help client cough more often.
2. There are no risks associated with this procedure.
3. CPT will resolve all of client's respiratory symptoms.
4. CPT will assist with mobilizing secretions to enhance more effective breathing.

Level of Cognitive Ability: Applying
Client Needs: Psychosocial Integrity
Clinical Judgment/Cognitive Skills: Generate Solutions
Integrated Process: Clinical Judgment/Nursing Process/Planning
Content Area: Adult Health: Respiratory
Health Problems: Mental Health: Anxiety
Priority Concepts: Client Education; Gas Exchange

Answer: 4
Rationale: CPT is an intervention to assist with mobilizing and clearing secretions to enhance more effective breathing. CPT will assist the client with coughing if the secretions have been mobilized and the cough stimulus is present. There are risks associated with CPT, including cardiac, gastrointestinal, neurologic, and pulmonary effects. It will not resolve all of the client's respiratory symptoms.
Test-Taking Strategy: Eliminate options 2 and 3 because they contain the closed-ended words "no" and "all." Option 4 is the umbrella option and contains most of the purposes of CPT.
Priority Nursing Tip: Contraindications for chest physiotherapy include unstable vital signs, increased intracranial pressure, bronchospasm, history of pathologic fractures, rib fractures, and chest incisions.
References: Ignatavicius, D., et al. (2021). *Medical-surgical nursing: Concepts for interprofessional collaborative care* (10th ed., p. 552). Elsevier; Potter, P., et al. (2021). *Fundamentals of nursing* (10th ed., p. 933). Elsevier.

❖ **108.** A client diagnosed with cardiomyopathy stops eating, takes long naps, and turns away from the nurse when the nurse talks to the client. The nurse would make which interpretation about this behavior?
1. Client is depressed.
2. Client is noncompliant.
3. Client has intractable pain.
4. Client is unable to tolerate activity.

Level of Cognitive Ability: Analyzing
Client Needs: Psychosocial Integrity
Clinical Judgment/Cognitive Skills: Analyze Cues
Integrated Process: Clinical Judgment/Nursing Process/Analysis
Content Area: Mental Health
Health Problems: Mental Health: Mood Disorders
Priority Concepts: Clinical Judgment; Mood and Affect

Answer: 1
Rationale: Depression is a common problem related to clients who have long-term and debilitating illnesses. None of the remaining options are related to the symptoms present in the question and therefore are not appropriate interpretations.
Test-Taking Strategy: Note the subject, interpretation of the client's behavior. Focus on the words *stops eating, takes long naps,* and *turns away from the nurse* in the question. On the basis of the data presented, the only appropriate interpretation is depression.
Priority Nursing Tip: Cardiomyopathy is a subacute or chronic disorder of the heart muscle. Treatment is palliative, not curative. The client needs assistance with numerous required lifestyle changes and has a shortened life span.
Reference: Lewis, S., et al. (2020). *Medical-surgical nursing: Assessment and management of clinical problems* (11th ed., pp. 727, 794). Elsevier.

109. The nurse is caring for a pregnant client who has been hospitalized for the stabilization of diabetes mellitus. The client tells the nurse that their spouse is caring for their 2-year-old child. Which short-term psychosocial outcome would the nurse develop for the client?
1. Be alert to the risks of early labor and birth.
2. Protect client from injuries that can result from seizures.
3. Teach client and family about diabetes and its implications.
4. Provide emotional support and education about interrupted family processes.

Level of Cognitive Ability: Analyzing
Client Needs: Psychosocial Integrity
Clinical Judgment/Cognitive Skills: Generate Solutions
Integrated Process: Clinical Judgment/Nursing Process/Planning
Content Area: Maternity: Antepartum
Health Problems: Mental Health: Coping
Priority Concepts: Glucose Regulation; Health Promotion

Answer: 4
Rationale: The short-term psychosocial well-being of the family is at risk as a result of the hospitalization of the client. Options 1 and 2 are unrelated to diabetes mellitus and are more related to gestational hypertension. Teaching about diabetes mellitus is a long-term goal related to diabetes.
Test-Taking Strategy: Eliminate options 1 and 2 because they are unrelated to diabetes mellitus. Next, note the words *short-term psychosocial outcome,* and focus on the data in the question to direct you to option 4. In addition, the incorrect options are comparable or alike in that they are all physiologic outcomes.
Priority Nursing Tip: The pregnant client will need to use insulin to control the blood glucose levels.
Reference: McKinney, E. S., et al. (2022). *Maternal child nursing* (6th ed., pp. 561–563). Elsevier.

❖ **110.** An anxious new parent is trying to decide whether to have the newborn baby circumcised. The nurse would make which statement to assist the parent with making the decision?
1. "Discuss the procedure with the other members of your family."
2. "You know, they say it prevents cancer and sexually transmitted infections, so I would definitely have my baby circumcised."
3. "Circumcision is a difficult decision, but your primary health care provider is the best, and it's better to get it done now than later."
4. "Circumcision is a difficult decision. Here, read this information pamphlet that discusses the pros and cons, and we will discuss any concerns and questions that you have after you read it."

Level of Cognitive Ability: Applying
Client Needs: Psychosocial Integrity
Clinical Judgment/Cognitive Skills: Take Action
Integrated Process: Communication and Documentation
Content Area: Maternity: Newborn
Health Problems: Mental Health: Anxiety
Priority Concepts: Patient Education; Communication

Answer: 4
Rationale: Informed decision-making is the strategic point when answering this question. The nurse would provide educational materials and answer questions pertaining to the education of the parent. Providing written information to the parent will give the parent the information needed to make an educated and informed decision. The nurse's personal thoughts and feelings should not be part of the educational process. The remaining options are not well focused on answering the parent's concerns.
Test-Taking Strategy: Use therapeutic communication techniques. The remaining options are communication blocks because the nurse is providing a personal opinion to the client.
Priority Nursing Tip: The nurse needs to instruct the parent of a newborn who has been circumcised to monitor urine output and for signs of urinary retention.
Reference: McKinney, E. S., et al. (2022). *Maternal child nursing* (6th ed., pp. 52, 477–478). Elsevier.

111. The nurse is planning care for a client who is experiencing anxiety after a myocardial infarction. Which **priority** nursing intervention would be included in the plan of care?
1. Answer questions with factual information.
2. Provide detailed explanations of all procedures.
3. Encourage family involvement during the acute phase.
4. Administer an antianxiety medication to promote relaxation.

Level of Cognitive Ability: Applying
Client Needs: Psychosocial Integrity
Clinical Judgment/Cognitive Skills: Generate Solutions
Integrated Process: Clinical Judgment/Nursing Process/Planning
Content Area: Adult Health: Cardiovascular
Health Problems: Mental Health: Coping
Priority Concepts: Anxiety; Communication

Answer: 1
Rationale: Accurate information reduces fear, strengthens the nurse–client relationship, and assists the client with dealing realistically with the situation. Providing detailed information may increase the client's anxiety. Information needs to be provided simply and clearly. Encouraging family involvement may or may not be helpful. Medication should not be used unless necessary.
Test-Taking Strategy: Note the strategic word, *priority,* and the word *anxiety* in the question. Eliminate option 2 first because of the word *detailed.* Eliminate option 4 next because medication would not be the first intervention to alleviate anxiety; however, it may be necessary if other strategies are not effective. From the remaining options, eliminate option 3 because limiting family involvement does not reduce anxiety in all situations.
Priority Nursing Tip: Myocardial infarction causes ischemia to the heart muscle. Ischemia can lead to necrosis of the myocardial tissue if blood flow is not restored.
Reference: Ignatavicius, D., et al. (2021). *Medical-surgical nursing: Concepts for interprofessional collaborative care* (10th ed., pp. 772, 774). Elsevier.

❖ **112.** A client recovering from an acute myocardial infarction will be discharged in 1 day. Which client action on the evening before discharge suggests that the client is in the denial about the medical condition?
1. Requests a sedative for sleep at 2200
2. Expresses a hesitancy to leave the hospital
3. Consumes 25% of foods and fluids given for supper
4. Walks up and down three flights of stairs unsupervised

Level of Cognitive Ability: Analyzing
Client Needs: Psychosocial Integrity
Clinical Judgment/Cognitive Skills: Analyze Cues
Integrated Process: Clinical Judgment/Nursing Process/Analysis
Content Area: Adult Health: Cardiovascular
Health Problems: Mental Health: Coping
Priority Concepts: Clinical Judgment; Stress and Coping

Answer: 4
Rationale: Ignoring activity limitations and avoiding lifestyle changes are signs of the denial stage. Walking three flights of stairs should be a supervised activity during this phase of the recovery process. Option 1 is an appropriate client action on the evening before discharge. Option 2 may be a manifestation of anxiety or fear rather than denial. Option 3 is a manifestation of depression rather than denial.
Test-Taking Strategy: Focus on the subject, the client action that indicates denial. Option 4 is the only option that identifies denial. Option 1 is an appropriate client request. Option 2 identifies anxiety or fear. Option 3 identifies depression.
Priority Nursing Tip: Pain relief increases oxygen supply to the myocardium; the nurse should administer morphine sulfate as prescribed as a priority in managing pain in the client having a myocardial infarction.
Reference: Ignatavicius, D., et al. (2021). *Medical-surgical nursing: Concepts for interprofessional collaborative care* (10th ed., pp. 626, 772–773). Elsevier.

113. The nurse is caring for a client diagnosed with Hodgkin's disease who will be receiving radiation and chemotherapy. Which statement by the client indicates a positive coping mechanism to be used during these treatments?
1. "I won't leave the house bald."
2. "Losing my hair won't bother me."
3. "I will be one of the few who doesn't lose my hair."
4. "I have selected a wig, even though I will miss my own hair."

Level of Cognitive Ability: Evaluating
Client Needs: Psychosocial Integrity
Clinical Judgment/Cognitive Skills: Evaluate Outcomes
Integrated Process: Clinical Judgment/Nursing Process/Evaluation
Content Area: Adult Health: Oncology
Health Problems: Mental Health: Coping
Priority Concepts: Self-Management; Stress and Coping

Answer: 4
Rationale: A combination of radiation and chemotherapy often causes alopecia. To make use of positive coping mechanisms, the client must identify personal feelings and positive interventions to deal with side effects. None of the remaining options are positive coping mechanisms.
Test-Taking Strategy: Focus on the subject, a positive coping mechanism. The remaining options all involve avoidance and denial. Option 4 is the only choice that addresses a positive coping mechanism.
Priority Nursing Tip: A coping mechanism involves any effort to decrease anxiety.
Reference: Ignatavicius, D., et al. (2021). *Medical-surgical nursing: Concepts for interprofessional collaborative care* (10th ed., pp. 391, 812). Elsevier.

❖ **114.** A client diagnosed with diabetic ketoacidosis (DKA) is admitted to the hospital. The client's adult child says to the nurse, "My other parent died last month, and now this. I've been trying to follow all of the instructions the doctor gave me, but what have I done wrong?" Which therapeutic response would the nurse make to the client's adult child?

1. "Tell me what you think you did wrong."
2. "Maybe we can keep your parent in the hospital for a while longer to give you a rest."
3. "You should talk to the social worker about getting you someone at home who has more experience managing the care of a client with diabetes."
4. "An emotional stress such as your parent's death can trigger DKA in a client with diabetes, even though the prescribed regimen is being followed."

Level of Cognitive Ability: Applying
Client Needs: Psychosocial Integrity
Clinical Judgment/Cognitive Skills: Take Action
Integrated Process: Clinical Judgment/Nursing Process/Implementation
Content Area: Foundations of Care: Communication
Health Problems: Mental Health: Coping
Priority Concepts: Communication; Glucose Regulation

Answer: 4
Rationale: Environment, infection, or an emotional stressor can initiate the physiologic mechanism of DKA. Options 1 and 3 substantiate the adult child's feelings of guilt and incompetence. Option 2 is not a cost-effective intervention.
Test-Taking Strategy: Identify the option that focuses on therapeutic communication techniques. Eliminate option 2 first because this option is not cost effective. Options 1 and 3 devalue the client and block therapeutic communication, so they are eliminated next.
Priority Nursing Tip: Diabetic ketoacidosis is a life-threatening complication of diabetes mellitus that develops when a severe insulin deficiency occurs. Hyperglycemia progresses to ketoacidosis over a period of several hours to days. DKA occurs in clients with type 1 diabetes mellitus, persons with undiagnosed diabetes, and persons who stop prescribed treatment for diabetes.
References: Ignatavicius, D., et al. (2021). *Medical-surgical nursing: Concepts for interprofessional collaborative care* (10th ed., p. 1269). Elsevier; Potter, P., et al. (2021). *Fundamentals of nursing* (10th ed., pp. 333–335). Elsevier.

115. The nurse has been working with a victim of rape in an outpatient setting for the past 4 weeks. The nurse would recognize that which of the following is an unrealistic short-term goal for the client?

1. Client will verbalize feelings about the rape event.
2. Client will resolve feelings of fear and anxiety related to the rape trauma.
3. Client will experience physical healing of the wounds that were incurred during the rape.
4. Client will participate in the treatment plan by following through with treatment options.

Level of Cognitive Ability: Understanding
Client Needs: Psychosocial Integrity
Clinical Judgment/Cognitive Skills: Generate Solutions
Integrated Process: Clinical Judgment/Nursing Process/Planning
Content Area: Mental Health
Health Problems: Mental Health: Coping
Priority Concepts: Stress and Coping; Interpersonal Violence

Answer: 2
Rationale: Short-term goals include the beginning stages of dealing with the rape trauma. Clients will initially be expected to keep appointments, participate in care, start to explore feelings, and begin to heal the physical wounds that were inflicted at the time of the rape. The resolution of feelings of anxiety and fear is a long-term goal.
Test-Taking Strategy: Focus on the subject, an unrealistic short-term goal for a rape victim. Consider each option and the reality of it being achieved in the short-term. Note the word *resolve* in option 2. This word will provide you with the clue that this option is a long-term goal.
Priority Nursing Tip: For the client who is a victim of rape, rape trauma syndrome may occur. The client may experience sleep disturbances; nightmares; loss of appetite; fears; anxiety; phobias; suspicion; a decrease in activities and motivation; disruptions in relationships with partner, family, or friends; self-blame; guilt and shame; lowered self-esteem; feelings of worthlessness; and somatic complaints.
Reference: Varcarolis, E., & Fosbre, C. (2021). *Essentials of psychiatric mental health nursing: A communication approach to evidence-based care* (4th ed., p. 360). Elsevier.

❖ **116.** A client is admitted to a surgical unit with a diagnosis of cancer. The client is scheduled for surgery in the morning. When the nurse enters the room and begins the surgical preparation, the client states, "I'm not having surgery. You must have the wrong person! My test results were negative. I'll be going home tomorrow." The nurse recognizes the client's statement as indicative of which defense mechanism?
1. Denial
2. Psychosis
3. Delusions
4. Displacement

Level of Cognitive Ability: Understanding
Client Needs: Psychosocial Integrity
Clinical Judgment/Cognitive Skills: Analyze Cues
Integrated Process: Clinical Judgment/Nursing Process/Analysis
Content Area: Foundations of Care: Communication
Health Problems: Mental Health: Coping
Priority Concepts: Coping; Self-Management

Answer: 1
Rationale: By definition, ego defense mechanisms are operations outside of a person's awareness that the ego calls into play to protect against anxiety. Denial is the defense mechanism that blocks out painful or anxiety-inducing events or feelings. In this case, the client cannot deal with the upcoming surgery for cancer and therefore denies the illness. Psychosis and delusions are not defense mechanisms. Displacement is the discharging of pent-up feelings on people who are less dangerous than those who initially aroused the feelings.
Test-Taking Strategy: Focus on the subject, ego defense mechanism. Options 2 and 3 are eliminated first because these are not ego defense mechanisms. From the remaining options, focus on the client's statement to direct you to option 1.
Priority Nursing Tip: For the client using defense mechanisms, the nurse would assist the client to identify the source of anxiety and explore methods to reduce anxiety.
Reference: Potter, P., et al. (2021). *Fundamentals of nursing* (10th ed., p. 348). Elsevier.

117. A community health nurse working in an industrial setting has received a memo indicating that a large number of employees will be laid off during the next 2 weeks. An analysis of previous layoffs suggested that workers experienced role crises, indecision, and depression. Using this information, which actions would the nurse implement to begin assisting employees?
1. Help the workers acquire unemployment benefits to avoid a gap in income.
2. Reduce the staff in the occupational health department of the industrial setting.
3. Notify insurance carriers of the upcoming event to assist with potential health care alterations.
4. Identify referral, counseling, and vocational rehabilitative services for the employees being laid off.

Level of Cognitive Ability: Applying
Client Needs: Psychosocial Integrity
Clinical Judgment/Cognitive Skills: Take Action
Integrated Process: Clinical Judgment/Nursing Process/Implementation
Content Area: Leadership/Management: Prioritizing
Health Problems: Mental Health: Crisis
Priority Concepts: Leadership: Stress and Coping

Answer: 4
Rationale: In preparation for this crisis, the nurse would identify the services that are available to the employees. These resources will provide immediate avenues for assistance when the layoff occurs. Additional information about the industrial setting is needed to determine whether options 1, 2, and 3 are necessary or possible.
Test-Taking Strategy: Use the steps of the nursing process to direct you to the correct option. This option refers to the assessment of resources and services for employees.
Priority Nursing Tip: One role of the community health nurse is to perform a needs assessment for the individuals with whom the nurse is working. The needs assessment is important to identify the potential underlying factors that may play a role in the client's ability to function normally.
Reference: Varcarolis, E., & Fosbre, C. (2021). *Essentials of psychiatric mental health nursing: A communication approach to evidence-based care* (4th ed., pp. 333, 335). Elsevier.

❖ **118.** A primigravida client who came to the clinic has been diagnosed with a urinary tract infection. The client repeatedly verbalizes concern regarding the safety of the fetus. Which would the nurse address **first**?
1. Maternal and infant safety
2. Obtaining a sedative prescription
3. Instructions regarding improved hygiene
4. Instructions regarding medication compliance

Level of Cognitive Ability: Applying
Client Needs: Psychosocial Integrity
Clinical Judgment/Cognitive Skills: Generate Solutions
Integrated Process: Clinical Judgment/Nursing Process/Planning
Content Area: Maternity: Antepartum
Health Problems: Maternity: Infection/Inflammation
Priority Concepts: Anxiety; Infection

Answer: 1
Rationale: The primary concern of this client is the safety of the fetus rather than concern about self. The priority for the nurse to address at this time is the issues regarding safety. The remaining options lack this priority.
Test-Taking Strategy: Note the strategic word, *first.* Eliminate option 2 because it is out of the nursing scope of practice. Focusing on the data in the question and noting the words *verbalizes concern* will direct you to the correct option.
Priority Nursing Tip: Some of the predisposing conditions for urinary tract infection in a pregnant client include a history of urinary tract infections, sickle cell trait, poor hygiene, anemia, and diabetes mellitus.
Reference: McKinney, E. S., et al. (2022). *Maternal child nursing* (6th ed., pp. 569, 571). Elsevier.

119. The nurse is planning interventions for counseling a pregnant client diagnosed with sickle cell anemia. Which would be the **most important** psychosocial intervention at this time?
1. Help client identify concerns.
2. Avoid discussing the details of the disease.
3. Allow client to be alone if client is crying.
4. Encourage family and friends to visit client frequently.

Level of Cognitive Ability: Applying
Client Needs: Psychosocial Integrity
Clinical Judgment/Cognitive Skills: Generate Solutions
Integrated Process: Clinical Judgment/Nursing Process/Planning
Content Area: Maternity: Antepartum
Health Problems: Mental Health: Coping
Priority Concepts: Caregiving; Coping

Answer: 1
Rationale: One of the most important nursing roles is providing emotional support to the client and family during the counseling process. Option 2, like option 4, is nontherapeutic. Option 3 is only appropriate if the client requests to be alone; if this is not requested, the nurse is abandoning the client in a time of need. Option 4 overwhelms the client with information while the client is trying to cope with the news of the disease.
Test-Taking Strategy: Note the strategic words, *most important.* Eliminate option 2 because of the closed-ended word "avoid." Additionally, this action is nontherapeutic. From the remaining options, remember that the client's feelings are the priority, and an extremely important role of the nurse is to provide emotional support.
Priority Nursing Tip: Situations that precipitate sickling in sickle cell anemia include fever, dehydration, and emotional or physical stress. Any condition that increases the need for oxygen or alters the transport of oxygen can result in sickle cell crisis.
Reference: McKinney, E. S., et al. (2022). *Maternal child nursing* (6th ed., p. 568). Elsevier.

❖ **120.** A neonatal intensive care nurse is caring for a newborn with a suspected diagnosis of erythroblastosis fetalis. Which therapeutic statement would the nurse make to the parents at this time?
  1. "Your infant is very sick. The next 24 hours are the most crucial."
  2. "This is a common neonatal problem, so the prognosis is very good."
  3. "You have reason to worry, but we have everything needed to care for your baby right here in this hospital."
  4. "You must have many concerns. Please ask me any questions that you have so that I can explain your infant's care."

Level of Cognitive Ability: Applying
Client Needs: Psychosocial Integrity
Clinical Judgment/Cognitive Skills: Take Action
Integrated Process: Clinical Judgment/Nursing Process/Implementation
Content Area: Maternity: Newborn
Health Problems: Mental Health: Anxiety
Priority Concepts: Communication; Stress and Coping

Answer: 4
Rationale: Parental anxiety is expected in relation to the care of the infant with erythroblastosis fetalis. This anxiety is caused by a lack of knowledge regarding the disease process, treatments, and expected outcomes. Parents need to be encouraged to verbalize concerns and participate in the care as appropriate. The nurse would not tell the parents to be or to not be concerned. Option 1 will produce anxiety in the parents. The remaining options lack that focus.
Test-Taking Strategy: Use therapeutic communication techniques. Eliminate options 2 and 3 because they are comparable or alike and are blocks to communication. Eliminate option 1 because it will produce anxiety in the parents. Remember to address the clients' feelings and concerns. The correct option is the only choice that encourages communication.
Priority Nursing Tip: Erythroblastosis fetalis is the destruction of red blood cells that results from an antigen–antibody reaction. The nurse would administer Rho(D) immune globulin (RhoGAM) to the birthing parent during the first 72 hours after delivery if the Rh-negative birthing parent delivers an Rh-positive fetus but remains unsensitized.
Reference: McKinney, E. S., et al. (2022). *Maternal child nursing* (6th ed., pp. 50–51, 649). Elsevier.

121. The nurse is preparing a plan of care for a client demonstrating mania. Which interventions would be included in the plan of care? **Select all that apply.**
  ❑ 1. Place client in seclusion.
  ❑ 2. Ignore any client complaints.
  ❑ 3. Use a firm and calm approach.
  ❑ 4. Use short and concise explanations and statements.
  ❑ 5. Remain neutral and avoid power struggles and value judgments.
  ❑ 6. Firmly redirect energy into more appropriate and constructive channels.

Level of Cognitive Ability: Applying
Client Needs: Psychosocial Integrity
Clinical Judgment/Cognitive Skills: Generate Solutions
Integrated Process: Clinical Judgment/Nursing Process/Planning
Content Area: Mental Health
Health Problems: Mental Health: Mood Disorders
Priority Concepts: Mood and Affect; Psychosis

Answer: 3, 4, 5, 6
Rationale: A client with mania will be extremely restless, disorganized, and chaotic. Grandiose plans are extremely out of touch with reality, and judgment is poor. Interventions for the client in acute mania include using a firm and calm approach to provide structure and control, using short and concise explanations or statements because of the client's short attention span, remaining neutral and avoiding power struggles and value judgments, being consistent in approach and expectations, having frequent staff meetings to plan consistent approaches and to set agreed-on limits to avoid manipulation by the client, hearing and acting on legitimate client complaints, and redirecting energy into more appropriate and constructive channels.
Test-Taking Strategy: Focus on the subject, a client with mania. Read each option and think about the manifestations that occur in the client with mania and how the intervention may or may not assist the client. Eliminate option 1 because of the word *seclusion* and option 2 because of the word *ignore.*
Priority Nursing Tip: Clients experiencing mania may also experience a disruption in their sleep pattern. Special considerations in room assignment need to be made for the client experiencing mania. Ideally these clients should be in a private room so as not to disturb other clients and to decrease sensory stimulation.
Reference: Varcarolis, E., & Fosbre, C. (2021). *Essentials of psychiatric mental health nursing: A communication approach to evidence-based care* (4th ed., p. 237). Elsevier.

❖ **122.** The nurse is planning care for a client with an intrauterine fetal demise. Which are appropriate goals for this client? **Select all that apply.**
  ❑ 1. Client's grieving process will be limited to 6 months.
  ❑ 2. Client and family will discuss plans for going home without the infant.
  ❑ 3. Client and family will express their grief about the loss of their desired infant.
  ❑ 4. Client will recognize that thoughts of worthlessness and suicide are normal after a loss.
  ❑ 5. Client and family will contact their pastor or grief counselor for support after discharge.

Level of Cognitive Ability: Applying
Client Needs: Psychosocial Integrity
Clinical Judgment/Cognitive Skills: Generate Solutions
Integrated Process: Clinical Judgment/Nursing Process/Planning
Content Area: Maternity: Postpartum
Health Problems: Mental Health: Grief/Loss
Priority Concepts: Caregiving; Stress and Coping

Answer: 2, 3, 5
Rationale: It is important for the nurse to assess whether the client is undergoing the normal grieving process. Options 2, 3, and 5 are appropriate goals. Signs that are causes for concern and that are not part of the normal grieving process include thoughts of worthlessness and suicide and limiting the grieving process to a short amount of time.
Test-Taking Strategy: Focus on the subject, appropriate goals. These words will direct you to options 2, 3, and 5. Options 1 and 4 are inappropriate because thoughts of worthlessness and suicide and limiting the grieving process to a short amount of time are causes for concern.
Priority Nursing Tip: For the client with intrauterine fetal demise, there is a risk for disseminated intravascular coagulation (DIC).
Reference: McKinney, E. S., et al. (2022). *Maternal child nursing* (6th ed., pp. 520–522). Elsevier.

123. A client diagnosed with severe preeclampsia is admitted to the hospital. The client is a student at a local college and insists on continuing studies while in the hospital, despite being instructed to rest. The client studies approximately 10 hours a day and has numerous visits from fellow students, family, and friends. Which intervention would the nurse use to **best** assist the client with promoting rest?
  1. Ask client why they are not complying with the prescription for bed rest.
  2. Develop a routine with client to balance studies and rest needs.
  3. Include a significant other in helping client understand the need for bed rest.
  4. Instruct client that the health of the baby is more important than studies at this time.

Level of Cognitive Ability: Applying
Client Needs: Psychosocial Integrity
Clinical Judgment/Cognitive Skills: Generate Solutions
Integrated Process: Clinical Judgment; Nursing Process/Planning
Content Area: Maternity: Antepartum
Health Problems: Maternity: Gestational Hypertension/Preeclampsia and Eclampsia
Priority Concepts: Caregiving; Reproduction

Answer: 2
Rationale: Option 2 involves the client in the decision-making process. In options 1 and 4 the nurse is judging the client's choices and asking probing questions; this will cause a breakdown in communication. Option 3 persuades the client's significant other to disagree with the client's actions. This could cause problems with the relationship between the client and the significant other, and it could also cause conflict in the client's communication with the health care workers.
Test-Taking Strategy: Note the strategic word, *best*. Focus on the subject, assisting the client with promoting rest. The remaining options are blocks to both communication and a therapeutic nurse–client relationship. The correct option is the most thorough nursing action because it addresses both rest and studies and involves the client in the decision-making process.
Priority Nursing Tip: Signs of preeclampsia are hypertension, generalized edema, and proteinuria.
Reference: McKinney, E. S., et al. (2022). *Maternal child nursing* (6th ed., pp. 544–545). Elsevier.

❖ **124.** A pregnant client is newly diagnosed with gestational diabetes. The client cries when receiving this information and keeps repeating, "What have I done to cause this? If only I could live my life over." Considering this statement, which concern would the nurse identify for the client?

1. Injury to the fetus because of maternal distress
2. Low self-esteem because of pregnancy complications
3. Lack of understanding about diabetic self-care during pregnancy
4. Poorly perceived body image caused by complications of pregnancy

Level of Cognitive Ability: Analyzing
Client Needs: Psychosocial Integrity
Clinical Judgment/Cognitive Skills: Analyze Cues
Integrated Process: Clinical Judgment/Nursing Process/Analysis
Content Area: Maternity: Antepartum
Health Problems: Mental Health: Coping
Priority Concepts: Stress and Coping; Reproduction

Answer: 2
Rationale: The client is putting the blame for the diabetes on self, thus lowering self-esteem. The client is expressing fear and grief. There are no data in the question to support the problems in options 1 and 4. Client lack of understanding is important to consider but not at this time because the client will not be able to comprehend information in the client's current state.
Test-Taking Strategy: Focus on the subject, the appropriate problem for the client situation described in the question. Note the words *what have I done.* The remaining options do not address the concerns the client is having.
Priority Nursing Tip: Gestational diabetes occurs in pregnancy in clients not previously diagnosed as diabetic and occurs when the pancreas cannot respond to the demand for more insulin.
Reference: McKinney, E. S., et al. (2022). *Maternal child nursing* (6th ed., pp. 561–563). Elsevier.

125. A client states to the nurse, "I'm going to die, and I wish my family would stop hoping for a cure! I get so angry when they carry on like this! After all, I'm the one who's dying." Which therapeutic response would the nurse make to the client?

1. "Have you shared your feelings with your family?"
2. "I think we should talk more about your anger at your family."
3. "You're feeling angry that your family continues to hope for you to be cured?"
4. "Well, it sounds like you're being pretty pessimistic. After all, years ago people died of pneumonia."

Level of Cognitive Ability: Applying
Client Needs: Psychosocial Integrity
Clinical Judgment/Cognitive Skills: Take Action
Integrated Process: Clinical Judgment Caring
Content Area: Developmental Stages: End-of-Life
Health Problems: Mental Health: Coping
Priority Concepts: Communication; Coping

Answer: 3
Rationale: Reflection is the therapeutic communication technique that redirects the client's feelings back at the client to validate what the client is saying. Option 3 uses the therapeutic technique of reflection. In option 1, the nurse is attempting to assess the client's ability to openly discuss feelings with family members. In option 2, the nurse attempts to use focusing, but the attempt to discuss central issues seems premature. In option 4, the nurse makes a judgment, and this is not therapeutic in the one-to-one relationship. Although this is an appropriate assessment for this client, the timing is somewhat premature, and it closes off the facilitation of the client's feelings.
Test-Taking Strategy: Use therapeutic communication techniques to answer the question. The correct option is the only choice that uses a therapeutic technique. Also, note the word *angry* in the question and the correct option.
Priority Nursing Tip: Successful communication includes appropriateness, efficiency, flexibility, and feedback. Communication also needs to be goal-directed within a professional framework.
Reference: Potter, P., et al. (2021). *Fundamentals of nursing* (10th ed., pp. 198, 333–335). Elsevier.

❖ **126.** The nurse is caring for a client who says, "I don't want to talk with you because you're only the nurse. I'll wait for my doctor." Which statement would the nurse say in response to the client?

1. "I'm saddened by the way you dismissed me."
2. "I understand. So should I call your primary health care provider?"
3. "Your primary health care provider directs me in your nursing care."
4. "So then, you would prefer to speak with your primary health care provider?"

Level of Cognitive Ability: Applying
Client Needs: Psychosocial Integrity
Clinical Judgment/Cognitive Skills: Take Action
Integrated Process: Clinical Judgment/Nursing Process/Implementation
Content Area: Foundations of Care: Communication
Health Problems: N/A
Priority Concepts: Communication; Professional Identity

Answer: 2
Rationale: The nurse uses techniques of therapeutic communication to reflect the client's statement (option 2), redirect feelings back to the client for validation, and focus on the client's desire to talk with the doctor. Options 1 and 3 are nontherapeutic responses and are defensive responses. Option 4 reinforces the client's behavior and does not encourage client expression of feelings.
Test-Taking Strategy: Use therapeutic communication techniques. The correct option is the only therapeutic response. This response focuses on the client's concern and reflects back the statement made by the client.
Priority Nursing Tip: Communication includes both verbal and nonverbal expression. Anxiety on the part of the nurse or client may impede communication.
Reference: Potter, P., et al. (2021). *Fundamentals of nursing* (10th ed., pp. 333–335). Elsevier.

127. A client awaiting surgery for the removal of a pancreatic mass shares with the nurse concerns about not waking up after receiving the anesthesia. Which therapeutic response is **most appropriate** for the nurse to make to the client?

1. "This is a very common concern."
2. "Tell me what makes you feel concerned about the anesthesia."
3. "I had surgery a year ago and was afraid of the same thing. I did just fine."
4. "You have the best anesthesiologist in this hospital. There is no need to be scared."

Level of Cognitive Ability: Applying
Client Needs: Psychosocial Integrity
Clinical Judgment/Cognitive Skills: Take Action
Integrated Process: Clinical Judgment/Nursing Process/Implementation
Content Area: Foundations of Care: Communication
Health Problems: Mental Health: Coping
Priority Concepts: Anxiety; Communication

Answer: 2
Rationale: This client is concerned about surgery and is expressing fear about the anesthesia. The therapeutic response to the client is the one that encourages the client to express their concerns. Option 1 is a stereotypical response. Option 3 avoids the client's concern and focuses on the nurse's personal experience. Option 4 also avoids the client's concern.
Test-Taking Strategy: Note the strategic words, *most appropriate*. Use therapeutic communication techniques, and focus on the client's feelings. The only response that addresses the client's feelings is the correct option.
Priority Nursing Tip: The nurse must keep the client who is undergoing surgery and has received preoperative medications in bed. The call bell needs to be placed next to the client, and the client needs to be instructed not to get out of bed and to call for assistance if needed.
Reference: Potter, P., et al. (2021). *Fundamentals of nursing* (10th ed., pp. 333–335). Elsevier.

❖ **128.** A community health nurse visits a recently widowed retired military client. When the nurse visits, the ordinarily immaculate house is in chaos, and the client is disheveled and has an alcohol type of odor on their breath. Which therapeutic statement would the nurse make to the client?
1. "I can see this isn't a good time to visit."
2. "You seem to be having a very troubling time."
3. "Do you think your spouse would want you to behave like this?"
4. "What are you doing? How much are you drinking and for how long?"

Level of Cognitive Ability: Applying
Client Needs: Psychosocial Integrity
Clinical Judgment/Cognitive Skills: Take Action
Integrated Process: Clinical Judgment; Nursing Process/Implementation
Content Area: Foundations of Care: Communication
Health Problems: Mental Health: Coping
Priority Concepts: Communication; Coping

Answer: 2
Rationale: The therapeutic statement is the one that helps the client explore the situation and express feelings. Reflection, by telling the client that the nurse realizes this is a troubled or difficult time, is empathic, and it will assist the client with beginning to ventilate their feelings. Option 1 uses humor to avoid therapeutic intimacy and effective problem-solving. Option 3 uses admonishment and tries to shame the client, which is not therapeutic or professional. This social communication belittles the client, will likely cause anger, and may evoke "acting out" by the client. Option 4 uses social communication.
Test-Taking Strategy: Use therapeutic communication techniques. Remember to focus on the client's behavior and feelings. This will direct you to the correct option.
Priority Nursing Tip: Therapeutic communication techniques should always be used when communicating with the client, family, or significant other.
Reference: Varcarolis, E., & Fosbre, C. (2021). *Essentials of psychiatric mental health nursing: A communication approach to evidence-based care* (4th ed., pp. 93–95). Elsevier.

129. A client states to the nurse, "I don't do anything right. I'm such a loser." Which therapeutic statement would the nurse make to the client?
1. "You don't do anything right?"
2. "You do things right all the time."
3. "Can we identify things you do right?"
4. "You are not a loser, you are depressed."

Level of Cognitive Ability: Applying
Client Needs: Psychosocial Integrity
Clinical Judgment/Cognitive Skills: Take Action
Integrated Process: Communication and Documentation
Content Area: Foundations of Care: Communication
Health Problems: Mental Health: Crisis
Priority Concepts: Communication; Coping

Answer: 1
Rationale: Option 1 provides the client with the opportunity to verbalize. With this statement, the nurse can learn more about what the client really means by the statement. The remaining options are closed statements and do not encourage the client to explore further.
Test-Taking Strategy: Use therapeutic communication techniques. The correct option repeats the client's statement and encourages further communication.
Priority Nursing Tip: Nontherapeutic communication techniques block the communication process and should never be used by the nurse in the communication process.
Reference: Varcarolis, E., & Fosbre, C. (2021). *Essentials of psychiatric mental health nursing: A communication approach to evidence-based care* (4th ed., pp. 93–95). Elsevier.

❖ **130.** A client who is experiencing suicidal thoughts shares with the nurse, "I was awake most of the night. It just doesn't seem worth it anymore. Why not just end it all?" Which response would the nurse make to **best** further assess the client?
1. "Did you sleep at all last night?"
2. "Tell me what you mean by that."
3. "I know you have had a stressful night."
4. "I'm sure that your family is worried about you."

Level of Cognitive Ability: Applying
Client Needs: Psychosocial Integrity
Clinical Judgment/Cognitive Skills: Take Action
Integrated Process: Clinical Judgment/Nursing Process/Implementation
Content Area: Mental Health
Health Problems: Mental Health: Suicide
Priority Concepts: Communication; Safety

Answer: 2
Rationale: Option 2 allows the client the opportunity to tell the nurse more about what their current thoughts are. Option 1 changes the subject and may block communication. Although option 3 offers empathy to the client, it does not further assess the client. Option 4 is false reassurance and may block communication.
Test-Taking Strategy: Note the strategic word, *best*, followed by the words *further assess*. Use the steps of the nursing process and therapeutic communication techniques to select the correct option. Options 3 and 4 can be eliminated first because they do not reflect assessment. Both options 1 and 2 relate to assessment, but option 2 is directly related to the subject of the question, suicide, and is the most therapeutic.
Priority Nursing Tip: The nurse should develop a safety plan with the suicidal client that provides a written list of coping strategies and sources of support.
Reference: Varcarolis, E., & Fosbre, C. (2021). *Essentials of psychiatric mental health nursing: A communication approach to evidence-based care* (4th ed., pp. 93–95, 369). Elsevier.

131. A client states to the nurse, "I am afraid that my child might have another febrile seizure." Which therapeutic statement is **best** for the nurse to make to the client?
1. "Tell me what frightens you the most about seizures."
2. "Tylenol can prevent another seizure from occurring."
3. "Most children will never experience a second seizure."
4. "Why worry about something that you cannot control?"

Level of Cognitive Ability: Applying
Client Needs: Psychosocial Integrity
Clinical Judgment/Cognitive Skills: Take Action
Integrated Process: Clinical Judgment/Nursing Process/Implementation
Content Area: Pediatrics: Neurologic
Health Problems: Mental Health: Anxiety
Priority Concepts: Communication; Stress and Coping

Answer: 1
Rationale: Option 1 is the only response that is an open-ended statement and that provides the client with an opportunity to express feelings. Options 2 and 3 are incorrect because the nurse is giving false reassurance that a seizure will not recur or that it can be prevented in this child. Option 4 is incorrect because it blocks communication by giving a flippant response to an expressed fear.
Test-Taking Strategy: Note the strategic word, *best*, and use therapeutic communication techniques to identify the correct answer. The remaining options all violate the principles of therapeutic communication and actually block communication.
Priority Nursing Tip: For the client experiencing a seizure, the nurse needs to ensure airway patency, have suction equipment and oxygen available, time the seizure episode, place a pillow or folded blanket under the client's head, loosen restrictive clothing, remove eyeglasses if present, and clear the area of any hazardous objects.
Reference: McKinney, E. S., et al. (2022). *Maternal child nursing* (6th ed., pp. 59–60, 1306). Elsevier.

❖ **132.** A client has just given birth to a newborn who has a cleft lip and palate. When planning to talk with the client, the nurse recognizes that the client needs to **first** work through which emotion before bonding can occur?
1. Guilt
2. Grief
3. Anger
4. Depression

Level of Cognitive Ability: Understanding
Client Needs: Psychosocial Integrity
Clinical Judgment/Cognitive Skills: Generate Solutions
Integrated Process: Clinical Judgment/Nursing Process/Planning
Content Area: Maternity: Postpartum
Health Problems: Mental Health: Grief/Loss
Priority Concepts: Caregiving; Coping

Answer: 2
Rationale: The nurse needs to recognize that a birthing parent will go through the grief process after giving birth to a child with a birth defect. After the grief process, the birthing parent can begin to focus on bonding with the infant. The remaining options are incorrect because they are each only one component of the grief process.
Test-Taking Strategy: Note the strategic word, *first.* Eliminate options that are incorrect because they are each only one component of the grief process.
Priority Nursing Tip: The nurse's role in the grief and loss process includes communicating with the client and family members. The nurse must consider the client's culture, religion, family structure, individual life experiences, coping skills, and support systems.
Reference: McKinney, E. S., et al. (2022). *Maternal child nursing* (6th ed., pp. 808–809, 969). Elsevier.

133. An infant has been diagnosed with acute chalasia. During the nursing history, the parent tells the nurse, "I am concerned that I am somehow causing my infant to vomit after feeding." Considering this statement, which concern would the nurse identify for the parent?
1. An unrealistic expectation of self
2. Denial that chalasia is a physiologic defect
3. Lack of understanding about feeding an infant with chalasia
4. Anxiety about the need for hospitalization of the infant for chalasia

Level of Cognitive Ability: Understanding
Client Needs: Psychosocial Integrity
Clinical Judgment/Cognitive Skills: Analyze Cues
Integrated Process: Clinical Judgment/Nursing Process/Analysis
Content Area: Pediatrics: Gastrointestinal
Health Problems: Mental Health: Anxiety
Priority Concepts: Family Dynamics; Stress and Coping

Answer: 1
Rationale: The infant is vomiting because of a physiologic problem that is not caused by the parent. The misconception that the parent is responsible for the problem is an unrealistic expectation of self and may result in the parent having a decreased perception of the ability to adequately parent the child. The nurse needs to assist the parent with understanding that the parent is not responsible for the child's condition. There are no data in the question to support that the parent is experiencing denial that chalasia is a physiologic defect. There are insufficient data to support that the parent lacks understanding on feeding techniques for a child with chalasia. The parent's statement does not reflect symptoms of anxiety regarding the child's hospitalization. The parent states a concern regarding own behavior.
Test-Taking Strategy: Focus on the subject, that the parent is blaming self for the child's health problem. The only option that relates to this subject is option 1.
Priority Nursing Tip: Chalasia occurs when there is an abnormal relaxation of a body orifice, such as the cardiac sphincter. This disorder is commonly associated with gastroesophageal reflux disease (GERD).
Reference: Hockenberry, M., Wilson, D., & Rodgers, C. (2019). *Wong's Nursing care of infants and children* (11th ed., p. 847). Elsevier.

❖ **134.** A client who experienced a myocardial infarction (MI) 4 days ago refuses to dangle at the bedside, saying, "If my doctor tells me to do it, I will. Otherwise, I won't." Which behavior would the nurse determine that the client is displaying?
1. Anger
2. Denial
3. Depression
4. Dependency

Level of Cognitive Ability: Understanding
Client Needs: Psychosocial Integrity
Clinical Judgment/Cognitive Skills: Analyze Cues
Integrated Process: Clinical Judgment; Nursing Process/Analysis
Content Area: Adult Health: Cardiovascular
Health Problems: Mental Health: Coping
Priority Concepts: Stress and Coping; Perfusion

Answer: 4
Rationale: Clients may experience numerous emotional and behavioral responses after an MI. Dependency is one response that may be manifested by the client's refusal to perform any tasks or activities unless specifically approved by the primary health care provider. Although the client's statement may express anger to some degree, it most specifically addresses dependency. There are no data in the question to support denial or depression.
Test-Taking Strategy: Focus on the subject of a client who refuses to perform tasks after an MI. Begin by eliminating options 2 and 3 because the client is not exhibiting signs of denial or depression. From the remaining options, focus on the client's statement to direct you to option 4.
Priority Nursing Tip: Dependency is evident when the client who sustained an MI is refusing to perform activities unless approved by the primary health care provider; this behavior reflects fear of causing another MI. The client also prefers to be monitored by electrocardiogram (ECG) at all times and is hesitant to leave the cardiac nursing unit or the hospital.
Reference: Lewis, S., et al. (2020). *Medical-surgical nursing: Assessment and management of clinical problems* (11th ed., p. 727). Elsevier.

135. The nurse is assessing a client who was admitted to the hospital with a diagnosis of urinary calculi. The client received 4 mg of morphine sulfate approximately 2 hours previously. The client states to the nurse, "I'm scared to death that it'll come back." Based on these statements, which concern would the nurse identify for this client at this time?
1. Fear of dying
2. Lack of understanding about the disease process
3. Anxiety about the anticipation of recurrent severe pain
4. Retention of urine from the obstruction of the urinary tract by calculi

Level of Cognitive Ability: Understanding
Client Needs: Psychosocial Integrity
Clinical Judgment/Cognitive Skills: Analyze Cues
Integrated Process: Clinical Judgment; Nursing Process/Analysis
Content Area: Adult Health: Renal and Urinary
Health Problems: Mental Health: Anxiety
Priority Concepts: Anxiety; Clinical Judgment

Answer: 3
Rationale: The client stated, "I'm scared to death that it'll come back." The anticipation of the recurring pain produces anxiety and threatens the client's psychological integrity. There is no evidence that the client has a calculus in the right ureter. There is also no evidence that the client has lack of knowledge or urinary retention.
Test-Taking Strategy: Focus on the subject, the appropriate client problem based on the client's statement. Note the words *I'm scared to death that it'll come back,* and note the relationship of these words to option 3.
Priority Nursing Tip: Problems resulting from urinary calculi are pain, obstruction, tissue trauma, secondary hemorrhage, and infection.
Reference: Ignatavicius, D., et al. (2021). *Medical-surgical nursing: Concepts for interprofessional collaborative care* (10th ed., pp. 1345, 1349). Elsevier.

❖ **136.** The nurse is observing the parents at the bedside of their small-for-gestational-age (SGA) infant, who was born at 27 weeks' gestation. The infant's parent states, "My baby is so tiny and fragile. I'll never be able to hold my baby with all those tubes." Considering this statement, which concern would the nurse identify for the parent?

1. Impaired adjustment
2. Trouble with family coping
3. Potential for compromised parenting
4. Difficulty understanding health concerns

Level of Cognitive Ability: Understanding
Client Needs: Psychosocial Integrity
Clinical Judgment/Cognitive Skills: Analyze Cues
Integrated Process: Clinical Judgment/Nursing Process/Analysis
Content Area: Maternity: Postpartum
Health Problems: Mental Health: Coping
Priority Concepts: Stress and Coping; Family Dynamics

Answer: 3
Rationale: Parents of a high-risk neonate, such as a preterm infant who is SGA, are at risk for compromised parenting. Parent–infant bonding is affected if the infant does not exhibit normal newborn characteristics. Option 1 involves the nonacceptance of a health status change or an inability to solve a problem or set a goal. Option 2 involves the identification of trouble with family coping. Option 4 addresses the condition's characteristics.
Test-Taking Strategy: Focus on the subject, the appropriate client problem based on the client's statement. Eliminate option 4 first because this is not a role of the parent and is a nursing function. Note the words *"I'll never be able to hold my baby."* This will assist with directing you to compromised parenting.
Priority Nursing Tip: For the infant who is SGA, the nurse must maintain airway patency and cardiopulmonary function and maintain the infant's body temperature.
Reference: Hockenberry, M., Wilson, D., & Rodgers, C. (2019). *Wong's Nursing care of infants and children* (11th ed., pp. 81–82, 272). Elsevier.

137. A client has just delivered by the vaginal route an infant who is large for gestational age (LGA). The client verbalizes concern regarding the infant's facial bruising and causing pain to the site if touched. Which therapeutic statement would the nurse make to alleviate the client's concerns?

1. "I can show you how to gently stroke the face and not cause pain."
2. "It is a normal finding in large babies and nothing to be concerned about."
3. "The bruising is caused by polycythemia, which usually leads to jaundice."
4. "Because the bruising is painful, it is advisable that you do not touch the baby's face."

Level of Cognitive Ability: Applying
Client Needs: Psychosocial Integrity
Clinical Judgment/Cognitive Skills: Take Action
Integrated Process: Clinical Judgment; Nursing Process/Implementation
Content Area: Maternity: Postpartum
Health Problems: Mental Health: Anxiety
Priority Concepts: Communication; Stress and Coping

Answer: 1
Rationale: The parent of an infant who is LGA and has facial bruising may be reluctant to interact with the infant because of concern about causing additional pain to the infant. Touching the infant gently with the fingertips should be encouraged. The bruising is temporary. Option 2 does not address the parent's verbalized concerns. The infant who is LGA may have polycythemia, which can contribute to bruising, but the bruising is not actually caused by the polycythemia. Option 4 advises the parent not to touch the baby's face because the bruising is painful, but touch is an important component of the attachment process.
Test-Taking Strategy: Note the subject, causing pain to infant's facial bruising if touched and alleviating the client's concern. Eliminate options 2 and 3 first, which do not specifically address the subject of touch. From the remaining options, note the relationship of the word *touch* in the question and the word *stroke* in the correct option.
Priority Nursing Tip: For the infant who is LGA, the nurse needs to monitor vital signs, monitor blood glucose levels and for signs of hypoglycemia, and initiate early feedings.
Reference: McKinney, E. S., et al. (2022). *Maternal child nursing* (6th ed., pp. 52, 643–644). Elsevier.

❖ **138.** A client diagnosed with myasthenia gravis is ready to return home. The client confides about being concerned that the partner will no longer find the client physically attractive. Which client-focused action would the nurse encourage in the plan of care?

1. Attend a support group.
2. Cease dwelling on the negative.
3. Reach out for help to face this fear.
4. Share feelings with the partner.

Level of Cognitive Ability: Applying
Client Needs: Psychosocial Integrity
Clinical Judgment/Cognitive Skills: Generate Solutions
Integrated Process: Clinical Judgment/Nursing Process/Planning
Content Area: Adult Health: Neurologic
Health Problems: Mental Health: Anxiety
Priority Concepts: Stress and Coping; Sexuality

Answer: 4
Rationale: Talking to the client about sharing feelings with the partner directly addresses the subject of the question. Encouraging the client to start a support group will not address the client's immediate and individual concerns. Options 2 and 3 are blocks to communication and avoid the client's concern.
Test-Taking Strategy: Focus on the subject, the concerns of a client with myasthenia gravis, and use therapeutic communication techniques. Only the correct option addresses the client's immediate concern. Remember to address the client's feelings and concerns first.
Priority Nursing Tip: Myasthenia gravis is a neuromuscular disease characterized by considerable weakness and abnormal fatigue of the voluntary muscles. A defect in the transmission of nerve impulses at the myoneural junction occurs.
References: Lewis, S., et al. (2020). *Medical-surgical nursing: Assessment and management of clinical problems* (11th ed., pp. 1377–1378). Elsevier; Potter, P., et al. (2021). *Fundamentals of nursing* (10th ed., pp. 333–335). Elsevier.

139. A 9-year-old child is hospitalized in traction for 2 months after a car accident. Which intervention would the nurse plan to use to **best** promote psychosocial development?

1. Providing a music player
2. Tutoring to keep the child up with schoolwork
3. Providing a phone for calling family and friends
4. Placing computer games, a television, and videos at the bedside

Level of Cognitive Ability: Applying
Client Needs: Psychosocial Integrity
Clinical Judgment/Cognitive Skills: Generate Solutions
Integrated Process: Clinical Judgment/Nursing Process/Planning
Content Area: Pediatrics: Musculoskeletal
Health Problems: Pediatric-Specific: Fractures
Priority Concepts: Development; Health Promotion

Answer: 2
Rationale: The developmental task of the school-age child is industry versus inferiority. The child achieves success by mastering skills and knowledge. Maintaining schoolwork provides for accomplishment and prevents feelings of inferiority that may be caused by lagging behind the rest of the class. The other options provide diversion and are of lesser importance for a child of this age.
Test-Taking Strategy: Note the strategic word, *best*. Note the words *psychosocial development* in the question. Note the age of the child, and determine the developmental task for this child. Eliminate those options that address social and diversional issues, whereas the correct option specifically addresses psychosocial development.
Priority Nursing Tip: For the school-age child, the nurse should use photographs, books, dolls, and videos to explain medical procedures.
Reference: McKinney, E. S., et al. (2022). *Maternal child nursing* (6th ed., p. 793). Elsevier.

❖ **140.** A client who is in halo traction states to the visiting nurse, "I can't get used to this contraption. I can't see properly on the side, and I keep misjudging where everything is." Which therapeutic response would the nurse make to the client?

1. "If I were you, I would have had the surgery rather than suffer like this."
2. "No one ever gets used to that thing! It's horrible. Many of our sports people who are in it complain vigorously."
3. "Halo traction involves many difficult adjustments. Practice scanning with your eyes after standing up and before you move around."
4. "Why do you feel like this when you could have died from a broken neck? This is the way it is for several months. You need to be more accepting, don't you think?"

Level of Cognitive Ability: Applying
Client Needs: Psychosocial Integrity
Clinical Judgment/Cognitive Skills: Take Action
Integrated Process: Clinical Judgment/Nursing Process/Implementation
Content Area: Adult Health: Musculoskeletal
Health Problems: Mental Health: Coping
Priority Concepts: Communication; Stress and Coping

Answer: 3
Rationale: In option 3, the nurse employs empathy and reflection. The nurse then offers a strategy for problem-solving, which helps increase the peripheral vision of the client in halo traction. In option 1, the nurse undermines the client's faith in the medical treatment being employed by giving advice that is insensitive and unprofessional. In option 2, the nurse provides a social response that contains emotionally charged language that could increase the client's anxiety. In option 4, the nurse uses excessive questioning and gives advice, which is nontherapeutic.
Test-Taking Strategy: Seek the option that represents a therapeutic communication technique. Focus on the client's statement, and note that option 3 is the only statement that addresses the client's concern.
Priority Nursing Tip: Halo traction involves the insertion of pins or screws into the client's skull and application of a circular fixation device and halo jacket or cast; it is used to immobilize the cervical spine. The nurse would instruct the client to notify the primary health care provider if the halo vest or ring bolts loosen.
References: Ignatavicius, D., et al. (2021). *Medical-surgical nursing: Concepts for interprofessional collaborative care* (10th ed., p. 883). Elsevier; Potter, P., et al. (2021). *Fundamentals of nursing* (10th ed., pp. 333–335). Elsevier.

141. An older client has been admitted to the hospital diagnosed with a hip fracture. The nurse prepares a plan of care for the client and identifies desired outcomes related to surgery and impaired physical mobility. Which statement by the client supports a positive adjustment to the surgery and impairment in mobility?

1. "Hurry up and go away. I want to be alone."
2. "What took you so long? I called for you 30 minutes ago."
3. "I wish you nurses would leave me alone! You are all telling me what to do!"
4. "I am a little nervous and find it difficult to concentrate since the surgeon talked with me about the surgery tomorrow."

Level of Cognitive Ability: Evaluating
Client Needs: Psychosocial Integrity
Clinical Judgment/Cognitive Skills: Evaluate Outcomes
Integrated Process: Clinical Judgment/Nursing Process/Evaluation
Content Area: Foundations of Care: Communication
Health Problems: Mental Health: Anxiety
Priority Concepts: Anxiety; Mobility

Answer: 4
Rationale: Option 4 reflects an individual with moderate anxiety caused by a difficulty to concentrate. It most appropriately supports a positive adjustment. Option 1 demonstrates withdrawal behavior. Option 2 is a demanding response. Option 3 demonstrates acting out by the client. Demanding, acting out, and withdrawn clients have not coped with or adjusted to the injury or disease.
Test-Taking Strategy: Focus on the subject, positive adjustment to surgery and impairment in mobility. This will help you eliminate the incorrect options. Remember that age and impaired mobility in combination with medications often contribute to anxiety and difficulty concentrating.
Priority Nursing Tip: Common fears before surgery include fear of death, fear of pain and discomfort, fear of mutilation or alteration in body image, fear of anesthesia, and fear of disruption of life functioning or patterns.
Reference: Ignatavicius, D., et al. (2021). *Medical-surgical nursing: Concepts for interprofessional collaborative care* (10th ed., pp. 1034, 1042). Elsevier.

❖ **142.** A client who is quadriplegic frequently makes lewd sexual suggestions and uses profanity. The nurse concludes that the client is inappropriately using displacement. Which concern would the nurse identify as being appropriate for this client?
1. Disuse syndrome
2. Lack of coping skills
3. Negative body image
4. Lack of awareness of surroundings

Level of Cognitive Ability: Understanding
Client Needs: Psychosocial Integrity
Clinical Judgment/Cognitive Skills: Analyze Cues
Integrated Process: Clinical Judgment/Nursing Process/Analysis
Content Area: Mental Health
Health Problems: Mental Health: Coping
Priority Concepts: Clinical Judgment; Coping

Answer: 2
Rationale: Lack of coping skills is evident when the client demonstrates an impaired ability to adapt to meeting life's demands and roles. This client is displacing feelings onto the environment instead of using them in a constructive fashion. Option 3 may be appropriate, but it has nothing to do with the displacement that the client is currently using. Options 1 and 4 have no relation to this situation.
Test-Taking Strategy: Note that the question addresses the subject of the defense mechanism of displacement. Focus on the information in the subject and remember that the use of displacement indicates lack of coping skills. This will direct you to the correct option.
Priority Nursing Tip: When the person is using displacement as a defense mechanism, the person's feelings toward one person are directed to another who is less threatening to satisfy an impulse with a substitute object.
Reference: Varcarolis, E., & Fosbre, C. (2021). *Essentials of psychiatric mental health nursing: A communication approach to evidence-based care* (4th ed., p. 138). Elsevier.

143. The nurse in the newborn nursery is caring for a preterm infant. Which is the **best** method the nurse can implement to assist the parents with developing attachment behaviors?
1. Support visits by family and friends.
2. Encourage the parents to touch and speak to their infant.
3. Report only positive qualities and progress to the parents.
4. Provide information regarding infant development and stimulation.

Level of Cognitive Ability: Applying
Client Needs: Psychosocial Integrity
Clinical Judgment/Cognitive Skills: Take Action
Integrated Process: Clinical Judgment/Nursing Process/Implementation
Content Area: Maternity: Newborn
Health Problems: Newborn: Preterm and Postterm Newborn
Priority Concepts: Caregiving; Family Dynamics

Answer: 2
Rationale: Parents' involvement through touch and voice establishes and initiates the bonding process in the parent–infant relationship. Their active participation builds their confidence and supports the parenting role. Family visits will not encourage parental attachments. Providing information and emphasizing only positives are not incorrect actions, but they do not relate to the attachment process.
Test-Taking Strategy: Note the strategic word, best. Focus on the subject, attachment behaviors. The only option that addresses attachment behaviors is the correct option.
Priority Nursing Tip: The primary concern for preterm infants is immaturity of all body systems.
Reference: McKinney, E. S., et al. (2022). *Maternal child nursing* (6th ed., pp. 423–424). Elsevier.

❖ **144.** A 16-year-old client diagnosed with diabetes is admitted for hyperglycemia. The client states, "I'm fed up with having my life ruled by diets, doctors' prescriptions, and machines!" Based on this assessment data, which is the **priority** client concern?
1. A chronic illness
2. A personal crisis
3. Feelings of loss of control
4. Lack of understanding about nutrition

Level of Cognitive Ability: Analyzing
Client Needs: Psychosocial Integrity
Clinical Judgment/Cognitive Skills: Analyze Cues
Integrated Process: Clinical Judgment/Nursing Process/Analysis
Content Area: Developmental Stages: Adolescent
Health Problems: Mental Health: Coping
Priority Concepts: Adherence; Development

Answer: 3
Rationale: The client is an adolescent. Adolescents strive for identity and independence, and the situation describes a common fear of loss of control. Therefore, the priority problem relates to these feelings of loss of control. Although the client has a chronic illness and may be experiencing a personal crisis, the client's statement focuses on loss of control. There is no information in the question that indicates a lack of knowledge.
Test-Taking Strategy: Note the strategic word, *priority.* Focus on the data in the question and the client's statement to direct you to the correct option.
Priority Nursing Tip: The adolescent may be preoccupied with body image, and the nurse would encourage and support independence.
Reference: McKinney, E. S., et al. (2022). *Maternal child nursing* (6th ed., pp. 1274–1275). Elsevier.

145. The client angrily tells the nurse that the primary health care provider (PHCP) purposefully provided incorrect information. Which responses by the nurse to the client support therapeutic communication? **Select all that apply.**
☐ 1. "I'm certain that the PHCP would not lie to you."
☐ 2. "I'm not sure what you mean by that statement."
☐ 3. "Can you describe the information that you are referring to?"
☐ 4. "Do you think it would be helpful to talk to your doctor about this?"
☐ 5. "You can check the information on lots of websites on the Internet."

Level of Cognitive Ability: Applying
Client Needs: Psychosocial Integrity
Clinical Judgment/Cognitive Skills: Take Action
Integrated Process: Communication and Documentation
Content Area: Foundations of Care: Communication
Health Problems: N/A
Priority Concepts: Communication; Professional Identity

Answer: 2, 3, 4
Rationale: Options 2 and 3 attempt to clarify the information to which the client is referring. Option 4 attempts to explore whether the client is comfortable talking to the PHCP about this issue and encourages direct confrontation. Options 1 and 5 hinder communication by disagreeing with the client and referring the client to the internet instead of the PHCP for clarification. This technique could make the client defensive and block further communication.
Test-Taking Strategy: Focus on the subject, the response that would support communication. Disagreeing with or challenging a client's response will hinder or block therapeutic communication.
Priority Nursing Tip: Agreeing or disagreeing with the client is a nontherapeutic communication technique.
Reference: Potter, P., et al. (2021). *Fundamentals of nursing* (10th ed., pp. 333–335). Elsevier.

❖ **146.** A client with a diagnosis of depression states to the nurse, "I should have died. I've always been a failure." Which therapeutic response would the nurse make to the client?
1. "You don't see anything positive?"
2. "You still have a great deal to live for."
3. "Feeling like a failure is part of your illness."
4. "You've been feeling like a failure for some time now?"

Level of Cognitive Ability: Applying
Client Needs: Psychosocial Integrity
Clinical Judgment/Cognitive Skills: Take Action
Integrated Process: Communication and Documentation
Content Area: Mental Health
Health Problems: Mental Health: Mood Disorders
Priority Concepts: Communication; Mood and Affect

Answer: 4
Rationale: Responding to the feelings expressed by a client is an effective therapeutic communication technique. The correct option is an example of the use of restating. Options 1, 2, and 3 block communication because they minimize the client's experience and do not facilitate the exploration of the client's expressed feelings.
Test-Taking Strategy: Use therapeutic communication techniques to answer this question. Remember to address the client's feelings and concerns. The correct option is the only option that is stated in the form of a question and that is open-ended, thus encouraging the verbalization of feelings.
Priority Nursing Tip: Any client with depression needs to be carefully assessed for a risk for suicide.
Reference: Varcarolis, E., & Fosbre, C. (2021). *Essentials of psychiatric mental health nursing: A communication approach to evidence-based care* (4th ed., pp. 93–95). Elsevier.

147. Two months after a right mastectomy for breast cancer, a client comes to the office for a follow-up appointment. After being diagnosed with cancer in the right breast, the client was told that the risk for cancer in the left breast existed. When asked about breast self-examination (BSE) practices since the surgery, the client replied, "I don't need to do that anymore." The nurse interprets this response to be using which coping mechanism?
1. Denial
2. Grief and mourning
3. Change in body image
4. Change in role pattern

Level of Cognitive Ability: Analyzing
Client Needs: Psychosocial Integrity
Clinical Judgment/Cognitive Skills: Analyze Cues
Integrated Process: Clinical Judgment/Nursing Process/Analysis
Content Area: Health Assessment/Physical Exam: Breasts
Health Problems: Mental Health: Coping
Priority Concepts: Adherence: Stress and Coping

Answer: 1
Rationale: The coping strategy of denying or minimizing a health problem can produce health situations that may be life-threatening. Denial can lead to an avoidance of self-care measures, such as taking medications or performing a BSE. None of the remaining options are coping mechanism.
Test-Taking Strategy: Focus on the subject, the coping mechanism that the client is using. Note the words *I don't need to do that anymore*. Eliminate options that are not directly related to the client's statement.
Priority Nursing Tip: Denial is the disowning of consciously intolerable thoughts and impulses.
Reference: Potter, P., et al. (2021). *Fundamentals of nursing* (10th ed., p. 348). Elsevier.

❖ **148.** In the plan of care of the client in the terminal stages of diagnosed cancer, one of the goals is that the client verbalizes acceptance of impending death. Which client statement indicates to the nurse that this goal has been reached?
   1. "I just want to live until my 100th birthday."
   2. "I would like to have my family here when I die."
   3. "I'll be ready to die when my children finish school."
   4. "I want to go to my child's wedding. Then I'll be ready to die."

Level of Cognitive Ability: Evaluating
Client Needs: Psychosocial Integrity
Clinical Judgment/Cognitive Skills: Evaluate Outcomes
Integrated Process: Clinical Judgment/Nursing Process/Evaluation
Content Area: Developmental Stages: End-of-Life
Health Problems: Mental Health: Coping
Priority Concepts: Caregiving; Coping

Answer: 2
Rationale: Acceptance is often characterized by plans for death. Often the client wants loved ones nearby. The remaining options all reflect the bargaining stage of coping during which the client tries to negotiate with their higher power or fate.
Test-Taking Strategy: Note that options 1, 3, and 4 are comparable or alike. These options all demonstrate negotiating for something else to happen before death occurs. The correct option is different, and it is the option that reflects acceptance.
Priority Nursing Tip: Outcomes related to care during illness and the dying experience should be based on the client's wishes.
Reference: Potter, P., et al. (2021). *Fundamentals of nursing* (10th ed., p. 348). Elsevier.

149. The nurse is caring for a client diagnosed with colon cancer who is receiving an antimetabolite for chemotherapy. Which self-care measures to better cope with side effects would the nurse plan to discuss with the client? **Select all that apply.**
   ❑ 1. The significance of wearing cotton gloves
   ❑ 2. The importance of rinsing the mouth after eating
   ❑ 3. The use of cosmetics to hide drug-induced rashes
   ❑ 4. The use of wigs, which are often covered by insurance
   ❑ 5. Proper dental hygiene with the use of a foam toothbrush

Level of Cognitive Ability: Applying
Client Needs: Psychosocial Integrity
Clinical Judgment/Cognitive Skills: Generate Solutions
Integrated Process: Clinical Judgment/Nursing Process/Planning
Content Area: Pharmacology: Oncology: Antimetabolites
Health Problems: Mental Health: Coping
Priority Concepts: Coping; Patient Teaching

Answer: 2, 3, 4, 5
Rationale: Antimetabolites are effective chemotherapeutic agents and include folic acid, pyrimidine, or purine analogues. There are many common side effects from chemotherapy that can cause the client physical and psychological distress. Options 2, 3, 4, and 5 are self-care activities the nurse can discuss with the client to help reduce this distress and minimize their impact on body changes while receiving chemotherapy. Option 1 is unrelated to client care when receiving chemotherapy.
Test-Taking Strategy: Focus on the subject of self-care measures while receiving chemotherapy. Recalling that cotton gloves are not relative to side effects of chemotherapy will direct you to the correct option.
Priority Nursing Tip: The nurse needs to provide the client with information about obtaining a wig, special skin products, foam toothbrush, cosmetics, and other personal care items. The nurse would also inform the client about how the body recovers after chemotherapy, such as hair growing back, but may be a different color and texture.
Reference: Lewis, S., et al. (2020). *Medical-surgical nursing: Assessment and management of clinical problems* (11th ed., p. 244). Elsevier.

❖ **150.** A client diagnosed with hyperaldosteronism has developed kidney failure and states to the nurse, "This means that I will die very soon." Which is the **most appropriate** therapeutic response for the nurse to make to the client?
1. "You will do just fine."
2. "What are you thinking about?"
3. "You sound discouraged today."
4. "I read that death is a beautiful experience."

Level of Cognitive Ability: Applying
Client Needs: Psychosocial Integrity
Clinical Judgment/Cognitive Skills: Take Action
Integrated Process: Clinical Judgment/Nursing Process/Implementation
Content Area: Foundations of Care: Communication
Health Problems: Mental Health: Coping
Priority Concepts: Communication; Coping

Answer: 3
Rationale: Option 3 uses the therapeutic communication technique of reflection, and it both clarifies and encourages the further expression of the client's feelings. Options 1 and 4 deny the client's concerns and provide false reassurance. Option 2 requests an explanation and does not encourage the expression of feelings.
Test-Taking Strategy: Note the strategic words, *most appropriate.* Use therapeutic communication techniques. Note that option 3 facilitates the client's expression of feelings. Remember to focus on the client's feelings.
Priority Nursing Tip: The signs and symptoms of acute kidney injury are primarily caused by the retention of nitrogenous wastes, the retention of fluids, and the inability of the kidneys to regulate electrolytes. Kidney failure affects all major body systems and may require dialysis to maintain life.
References: Ignatavicius, D., et al. (2021). *Medical-surgical nursing: Concepts for interprofessional collaborative care* (10th ed., p. 1246). Elsevier; Potter, P., et al. (2021). *Fundamentals of nursing* (10th ed., pp. 333–335). Elsevier.

151. A client diagnosed with diabetes mellitus has expressed frustration with learning the diabetic regimen and insulin administration. Which would be the **initial** action by the home care nurse?
1. Attempt to identify the cause of the frustration.
2. Call the primary health care provider to discuss client's problem.
3. Offer to administer the insulin on a daily basis until client is ready to learn.
4. Continue with teaching, knowing that client will overcome any frustrations.

Level of Cognitive Ability: Applying
Client Needs: Psychosocial Integrity
Clinical Judgment/Cognitive Skills: Take Action
Integrated Process: Clinical Judgment/Nursing Process/Implementation
Content Area: Foundations of Care: Communication
Health Problems: Mental Health: Anxiety
Priority Concepts: Client Education; Anxiety

Answer: 1
Rationale: The home care nurse must determine what is causing the client's frustration. The issue needs to be addressed by the nurse before involving the provider. Administering the insulin provides only a short-term solution. Continuing to teach may only further block the learning process.
Test-Taking Strategy: Note the strategic word, *initial,* as you select your answer. Use the steps of the nursing process. Assessment is the first step. The remaining options represent the implementation phase of the nursing process. The only assessment option is the correct option.
Priority Nursing Tip: The nurse needs to assist the client in making the necessary lifestyle adjustments to manage diabetes mellitus.
Reference: Ignatavicius, D., et al. (2021). *Medical-surgical nursing: Concepts for interprofessional collaborative care* (10th ed., pp. 1295–1296). Elsevier.

❖ **152.** A client diagnosed with cancer is placed on permanent total parenteral nutrition as a means of providing nutrition. Which is the rationale for the nurse to include psychosocial support when planning care for this client?
1. Death is imminent.
2. Client will need to adjust to the idea of living without eating by the usual route.
3. Total parenteral nutrition requires disfiguring surgery for permanent port implantation.
4. Nausea and vomiting occur regularly with this type of treatment and will prevent client from participating in social activity.

Level of Cognitive Ability: Applying
Client Needs: Psychosocial Integrity
Clinical Judgment/Cognitive Skills: Generate Solutions
Integrated Process: Clinical Judgment/Nursing Process/Planning
Content Area: Skills: Nutrition
Health Problems: Mental Health: Coping
Priority Concepts: Stress and Coping; Nutrition

Answer: 2
Rationale: Permanent total parenteral nutrition is indicated for clients who can no longer absorb nutrients via the enteral route. These clients will no longer take nutrition orally. The remaining options are inaccurate. There is no indication in the question that death is imminent. Permanent port implantation is not disfiguring. Total parenteral nutrition does not cause nausea and vomiting.
Test-Taking Strategy: Focus on the subject, psychosocial support for the client receiving total parenteral nutrition. Note the words *permanent* and *as a means of providing nutrition* in the question, and note the relationship between these words and option 2. Option 2 states *living without eating by the usual route.* Also, knowledge regarding total parenteral nutrition therapy will assist you with eliminating the incorrect options.
Priority Nursing Tip: Total parenteral nutrition is the administration of a nutritionally complete formula through a central or peripheral intravenous catheter.
Reference: Lewis, S., et al. (2020). *Medical-surgical nursing: Assessment and management of clinical problems* (11th ed., p. 865). Elsevier.

153. A client who is to be discharged to home with a temporary colostomy states to the nurse, "I know I've changed this thing once, but I just don't know how I'll do it by myself when I'm home alone. Can't I stay here until the surgeon puts it back?" Which therapeutic response would the nurse make to **best** deal with the client's concerns?
1. "This is only temporary, but with your level of anxiety you need to hire a nurse companion until your surgery."
2. "So you're saying that, although you've practiced changing your colostomy bag once, you don't feel comfortable on your own yet?"
3. "Well, your insurance will not pay for a longer stay just to practice changing your colostomy, so you'll have to fight it out with them."
4. "Going home to care for yourself still feels pretty overwhelming? I will schedule you for home visits until you're feeling more comfortable."

Level of Cognitive Ability: Applying
Client Needs: Psychosocial Integrity
Clinical Judgment/Cognitive Skills: Take Action
Integrated Process: Clinical Judgment/Nursing Process/Implementation
Content Area: Foundations of Care: Communication
Health Problems: Mental Health: Anxiety
Priority Concepts: Anxiety; Communication

Answer: 4
Rationale: The client is expressing feelings of fear and helplessness. Option 4 assists with meeting this client's needs. Option 1 provides information that the client already knows and then problem-solves by using a client-centered action, which would probably overwhelm the client. Option 2 is restating, but this response could cause the client to feel more helpless because the client's fears are reflected back to the client. Option 3 provides what is probably accurate information, but the words *just to practice* can be interpreted by the client as belittling.
Test-Taking Strategy: Note the strategic word, best. Use therapeutic communication techniques, and focus on the subject of the question, fear of being discharged home without help. This will eliminate options 1 and 3. From the remaining options, remember the subject of the question, and address the client's feelings and concerns. Option 2 is restating, but this intervention could cause the client to feel more helpless. Option 4 addresses the client's fear and dependency (helplessness) needs.
Priority Nursing Tip: For the client with a colostomy, the nurse needs to monitor stoma color. A dark blue, purple, or black stoma indicates compromised circulation, requiring primary health care provider notification.
References: Ignatavicius, D., et al. (2021). *Medical-surgical nursing: Concepts for interprofessional collaborative care* (10th ed., p. 1123). Elsevier; Potter, P., et al. (2021). *Fundamentals of nursing* (10th ed., pp. 333–335). Elsevier.

❖ **154.** The parents of a newborn infant diagnosed with congenital hypothyroidism and Down syndrome tell the nurse how despondent they are that their child was born with these problems. They had many plans for a normal child, and now these will need to be adjusted. On the basis of these statements, the nurse identifies which concern for the parents?
1. Inability to cope with change
2. Anger about lost opportunities
3. Trouble adjusting to a child born with medical issues
4. Depression associated with the birth of a child with defects

Level of Cognitive Ability: Analyzing
Client Needs: Psychosocial Integrity
Clinical Judgment/Cognitive Skills: Analyze Cues
Integrated Process: Clinical Judgment; Nursing Process/Analysis
Content Area: Maternity: Newborn
Health Problems: Mental Health: Coping
Priority Concepts: Stress and Coping; Mood and Affect

Answer: 4
Rationale: Depression is a normal part of the grieving process. It is a reaction to practical implications related to loss. Although the parents may have trouble adjusting and have anger, the best answer is to address their depression and sadness. The grief process includes intellectual and emotional responses and behaviors by which individuals and families work through the process of modifying their self-concepts on the basis of the perception of potential loss. Characteristics include expressions of sorrow and distress at the potential loss.
Test-Taking Strategy: Focus on the subject, the appropriate problem based on the parent's statement. Noting the words *how despondent they are* will lead you to the answer regarding depression.
Priority Nursing Tip: Down syndrome is a congenital condition that results in moderate to severe retardation and has been linked to an extra G chromosome, chromosome 21 (trisomy 21).
Reference: McKinney, E. S., et al. (2022). *Maternal child nursing* (6th ed., pp. 805, 1258–1260). Elsevier.

155. The nurse is caring for a client who has been diagnosed with schizophrenia. The client is unable to speak, although there is no known pathologic dysfunction. Based on this information, the nurse determines that the client is experiencing which type of dysfunctional communication?
1. Mutism
2. Verbigeration
3. Pressured speech
4. Poverty of speech

Level of Cognitive Ability: Analyzing
Client Needs: Psychosocial Integrity
Clinical Judgment/Cognitive Skills: Analyze Cues
Integrated Process: Clinical Judgment/Nursing Process/Analysis
Content Area: Mental Health
Health Problems: Mental Health: Schizophrenia
Priority Concepts: Communication; Psychosis

Answer: 1
Rationale: Mutism is the absence of verbal speech. The client does not communicate verbally despite an intact physical and structural ability to speak. Verbigeration is the purposeless repetition of words or phrases. Pressured speech refers to a rapidity of speech that reflects the client's racing thoughts. Poverty of speech involves diminished amounts of speech or monotonic replies.
Test-Taking Strategy: Focus on the subject, an inability to speak. This will assist you with eliminating options 2 and 3. From the remaining options, recalling that poverty of speech indicates a diminished amount of speech will assist you with eliminating option 4.
Priority Nursing Tip: Clients with schizophrenia may experience hallucinations. For a client with hallucinations, safety is the first priority; the nurse needs to ensure that the client does not have an auditory command telling the client to harm self or others.
Reference: Varcarolis, E., & Fosbre, C. (2021). *Essentials of psychiatric mental health nursing: A communication approach to evidence-based care* (4th ed., p. 260). Elsevier.

❖ **156.** A client diagnosed with schizophrenia states to the nurse, "I am a spy for the FBI. I am an eye, an eye in the sky." Based on this information, the nurse knows that the client is exhibiting which abnormal thought process?
1. Echolalia
2. Word salad
3. Clang associations
4. Loosened associations

Level of Cognitive Ability: Understanding
Client Needs: Psychosocial Integrity
Clinical Judgment/Cognitive Skills: Analyze Cues
Integrated Process: Clinical Judgment/Nursing Process/Analysis
Content Area: Mental Health
Health Problems: Mental Health: Schizophrenia
Priority Concepts: Communication; Psychosis

Answer: 3
Rationale: The repetition of words or phrases that are similar in sound and in no other way (rhyming) is one altered thought and language pattern seen in clients with schizophrenia. Clang associations often take the form of rhyming. Echolalia is the involuntary parrotlike repetition of words spoken by others. Word salad is the use of words with no apparent meaning attached to them or to their relationship to one another. Loosened associations occur when the individual speaks with frequent changes of subject and when the content is only obliquely related.
Test-Taking Strategy: Focus on the subject, the abnormal thought process that the client is experiencing. Also, note the client's statement. Recalling that clang associations often take the form of rhyming will direct you to the correct option.
Priority Nursing Tip: Abnormal thought processes displayed by the mentally ill client occur as a result of the psychiatric disorder.
Reference: Varcarolis, E., & Fosbre, C. (2021). *Essentials of psychiatric mental health nursing: A communication approach to evidence-based care* (4th ed., p. 260). Elsevier.

157. The nurse is planning the hospital discharge of a young client who has been newly diagnosed with type 1 diabetes mellitus. The client expresses concern about self-administering insulin while in school with other students around. Which statement by the nurse **best** addresses the client's need for support at this time?
1. "Oh, don't worry about that! You'll do fine!"
2. "You could leave school early and take your insulin at home."
3. "You shouldn't be embarrassed by your diabetes. Lots of people have this disease."
4. "Ask the school nurse about identifying a private area for you to use for injections."

Level of Cognitive Ability: Applying
Client Needs: Psychosocial Integrity
Clinical Judgment/Cognitive Skills: Take Action
Integrated Process: Clinical Judgment/Nursing Process/Implementation
Content Area: Pediatrics: Metabolic/Endocrine
Health Problems: Mental Health: Anxiety
Priority Concepts: Stress and Coping; Glucose Regulation

Answer: 4
Rationale: When planning this client's role transition, the nurse functions in the role of a problem-solver by assisting the client with adapting to their illness. In option 4, the nurse offers information that addresses the client's need and that promotes or assists the client with reaching a decision that optimizes a sense of well-being. Options 1 and 3 are inappropriate statements and blocks to communication. Option 2 requires a change in lifestyle.
Test-Taking Strategy: Note the strategic word, *best*. Use therapeutic communication techniques, and focus on the subject, a concern about self-administering insulin while in school. Options 1 and 3 are comparable or alike because they are nontherapeutic, so eliminate those options first. From the remaining options, select option 4 because it promotes the client's ability to continue the present lifestyle, whereas option 2 requires a change in lifestyle.
Priority Nursing Tip: Schools vary with regard to the availability of nursing services. The parents of a child with diabetes mellitus will need to work with school administration to determine appropriate staff and resources to ensure proper administration of insulin for their child as needed.
Reference: McKinney, E. S., et al. (2022). *Maternal child nursing* (6th ed., pp. 159, 1274–1275). Elsevier.

❖ **158.** The nurse is preparing a client for a parathyroidectomy when the client states, "I guess I'll have to wear a scarf after this surgery." Considering this statement, which concern would the nurse address?
   1. Denial that the surgery is necessary
   2. Trouble coping with the need for surgery
   3. Issues with potential changes to body image
   4. Anxiety about postsurgical altered function

Level of Cognitive Ability: Applying
Client Needs: Psychosocial Integrity
Clinical Judgment/Cognitive Skills: Generate Solutions
Integrated Process: Clinical Judgment/Nursing Process/Planning
Content Area: Adult Health: Endocrine
Health Problems: Mental Health: Coping
Priority Concepts: Clinical Judgment; Coping

Answer: 3
Rationale: The client's statement reflects a psychosocial concern regarding their appearance after surgery, so option 3 is the correct option. The remaining options identify unsuitable problems that are not supported by the provided client data.
Test-Taking Strategy: Note the subject, the client is expressing a concern about a possible scar. With this in mind, eliminate option 4 because the client is not demonstrating anxious behavior. Next, option 1 can be eliminated because denial is a way of avoiding concerns. Eliminate option 2 because the client expresses a realistic method of coping with a surgical scar.
Priority Nursing Tip: The appearance of the incision after parathyroidectomy may be distressing to the client. The nurse needs to reassure the client that the scar will fade in color and decrease in size over time.
Reference: Ignatavicius, D., et al. (2021). *Medical-surgical nursing: Concepts for interprofessional collaborative care* (10th ed., pp. 1259, 1262–1263). Elsevier.

159. The significant other of a client diagnosed with Graves' disease expresses concern regarding the client's bursts of temper, nervousness, and an inability to concentrate on even trivial tasks. On the basis of this information, the nurse would identify which concern for the client?
   1. Grief
   2. Socialization issues
   3. Issues related to sensory perception
   4. Trouble with coping with a disease process

Level of Cognitive Ability: Understanding
Client Needs: Psychosocial Integrity
Clinical Judgment/Cognitive Skills: Analyze Cues
Integrated Process: Clinical Judgment/Nursing Process/Analysis
Content Area: Adult Health: Endocrine
Health Problems: Mental Health: Coping
Priority Concepts: Clinical Judgment; Coping

Answer: 4
Rationale: A client with Graves' disease may become irritable, nervous, or depressed. The signs and symptoms in the question support option 4. The information in the question does not support the remaining options.
Test-Taking Strategy: Focus on the subject, the appropriate client problem based on the client's behavior. Note the behaviors of bursts of temper, nervousness, and an inability to concentrate on even trivial tasks in the question. This will direct you to the correct option.
Priority Nursing Tip: Graves' disease causes an enlarged thyroid gland, also known as *goiter*. The client may experience palpitations, cardiac dysrhythmias, protruding eyeballs, hypertension, heat intolerance, diaphoresis, weight loss, and diarrhea. Smooth, soft skin and hair; nervousness and fine tremors; and personality changes may also be noted in the client with Graves' disease.
Reference: Ignatavicius, D., et al. (2021). *Medical-surgical nursing: Concepts for interprofessional collaborative care* (10th ed., pp. 1255–1256). Elsevier.

❖ **160.** A client who was admitted for the treatment of thyroid storm (hyperthyroidism) is preparing for discharge. The client is anxious about the illness and is, at times, emotionally labile. Which action is **most appropriate** for the nurse to implement at this time?
  1. Assist client with identifying coping skills, support systems, and potential stressors.
  2. Avoid teaching client anything about the disease until the client is emotionally stable.
  3. Reassure client that everything will usually be fine after returning to one's home and family.
  4. Explain that one must be able to control one's behavior before being discharged to home.

Level of Cognitive Ability: Applying
Client Needs: Psychosocial Integrity
Clinical Judgment/Cognitive Skills: Take Action
Integrated Process: Clinical Judgment/Nursing Process/Implementation
Content Area: Adult Health: Endocrine
Health Problems: Mental Health: Anxiety
Priority Concepts: Anxiety; Stress and Coping

Answer: 1
Rationale: It is normal for clients who experience thyroid storm (hyperthyroidism) to continue to be anxious and emotionally labile at the time of discharge. The best intervention is to help the client cope with these changes in behavior and to anticipate potential stressors so that symptoms will not be as severe. Options 2 and 3 block communication by either avoiding the issue or providing false reassurance. The confrontation described in option 4 will only heighten the client's anxiety.
Test-Taking Strategy: Note the strategic words, *most appropriate.* Use therapeutic communication techniques. Eliminate options 2 and 3 because they are blocks to communication. From the remaining options, note the words *anxious about the illness.* Eliminate option 4 because it will heighten the client's anxiety.
Priority Nursing Tip: Thyroid storm occurs in a client with uncontrollable hyperthyroidism. It can be caused by manipulation of the thyroid gland during surgery and the release of thyroid hormone into the bloodstream; it also can occur from severe infection and stress.
References: Ignatavicius, D., et al. (2021). *Medical-surgical nursing: Concepts for interprofessional collaborative care* (10th ed., p. 1260). Elsevier; Potter, P., et al. (2021). *Fundamentals of nursing* (10th ed., pp. 333–335). Elsevier.

161. The nurse is caring for a client who has been admitted to the hospital for the insertion of a subclavian central venous catheter (CVC). The client is anxious because their employment position requires frequently working with the public. With this assessment data, which client concern would be the **priority** when managing care?
  1. Poor self-care
  2. Body image insecurity
  3. Neck range-of-motion restrictions
  4. Uncontrolled pain related to the CVC

Level of Cognitive Ability: Analyzing
Client Needs: Psychosocial Integrity
Clinical Judgment/Cognitive Skills: Prioritize Hypotheses
Integrated Process: Clinical Judgment/Nursing Process/Planning
Content Area: Leadership/Management: Management of Care
Health Problems: Mental Health: Coping
Priority Concepts: Stress and Coping; Functional Ability

Answer: 2
Rationale: Psychosocial assessment includes client data related to psychological and social issues. The CVC can create socially awkward situations and impair the client's security in body image. The client data presented do not support assessing the client for poor self-care. Although pain and neck range of motion are valid issues for this client, options 3 and 4 are physiologic issues and do not relate to the concerns of the client.
Test-Taking Strategy: Note the strategic word, *priority,* and the subject, subclavian CVC. The client data presented do not support poor self-care. Pain and restricted neck movements are physical concerns. Also, note that the client is concerned because the client is in a professional job working with the public to assist in answering correctly.
Priority Nursing Tip: For central line insertion, tubing change, and line removal, place the client in Trendelenburg or in the supine position if not contraindicated. Instruct the client to perform the Valsalva maneuver to increase pressure in the central veins when the intravenous system is open, such as during tubing changes.
Reference: Lewis, S., et al. (2020). *Medical-surgical nursing: Assessment and management of clinical problems* (11th ed., pp. 292–293, 301). Elsevier.

❖ **162.** A 12-year-old client is seen in the health care clinic. During the assessment, which finding would suggest to the nurse that the client is experiencing a disruption in the development of self-concept?
1. The child has many friends.
2. The child has a part-time babysitting job.
3. The child has an intimate relationship with a significant other.
4. The child enjoys playing chess and mastering new skills with this game.

Level of Cognitive Ability: Analyzing
Client Needs: Psychosocial Integrity
Clinical Judgment/Cognitive Skills: Recognize Cues
Integrated Process: Clinical Judgment/Nursing Process/Assessment
Content Area: Developmental Stages: Adolescent
Health Problems: Mental Health: Coping
Priority Concepts: Development; Health Promotion

Answer: 3
Rationale: The formation of an intimate relationship would not be expected until young adulthood. Friends are important and appropriate for members of this age-group. A sense of industry is appropriate for this age-group, and it may be exhibited by the child having a part-time job. The increase in self-esteem associated with skill mastery is an important part of development for the school-age child.
Test-Taking Strategy: Note the subject, that the child is experiencing disruption in the development of self-concept. Focus on normal growth and development. Noting the age of the child in the question will assist you with eliminating the remaining options.
Priority Nursing Tip: The school-age child is usually highly social, independent, and involved with activities.
Reference: Hockenberry, M., Wilson, D., & Rodgers, C. (2019). *Wong's Nursing care of infants and children* (11th ed., pp. 470, 472–473). Elsevier.

163. A client who has been newly diagnosed with tuberculosis (TB) is hospitalized and will be on respiratory isolation for at least 2 weeks. Which intervention is **most appropriate** in planning to prevent psychosocial distress in the client?
1. Noting whether client has visitors
2. Instructing all staff members to not touch client
3. Giving client a roommate with TB who persistently tries to talk
4. Removing the calendar and clock in the room so that client will not obsess about time

Level of Cognitive Ability: Applying
Client Needs: Psychosocial Integrity
Clinical Judgment/Cognitive Skills: Generate Solutions
Integrated Process: Clinical Judgment/Nursing Process/Planning
Content Area: Adult Health: Respiratory
Health Problems: Adult Health: Respiratory: Tuberculosis
Priority Concepts: Stress and Coping; Infection

Answer: 1
Rationale: The nurse needs to note whether the client has visitors and social contacts because the presence of others can offer positive stimulation. Touch may be important to help the client feel socially acceptable. A roommate who insists on talking could create sensory overload. In addition, the client on respiratory isolation needs to be in a private room. The calendar and clock are needed to promote orientation to time.
Test-Taking Strategy: Note the strategic words, *most appropriate.* Focus on the subject, the intervention to prevent psychosocial distress in the client with TB. Eliminate option 3 first because the client needs to be in a private room. From the remaining options, noting that the client will be on respiratory isolation for at least 2 weeks and recalling the basic principles related to sensory overload will direct you to option 1.
Priority Nursing Tip: An individual who has received a bacillus Calmette-Guérin vaccine will have a positive tuberculin skin test result and should be evaluated for TB with a chest x-ray.
Reference: Ignatavicius, D., et al. (2021). *Medical-surgical nursing: Concepts for interprofessional collaborative care* (10th ed., pp. 550, 577). Elsevier.

❖ **164.** The nurse is interviewing a client diagnosed with chronic obstructive pulmonary disease (COPD) who has a respiratory rate of 35 breaths/min and who is experiencing extreme dyspnea. On the basis of the nurse's observations, which is the appropriate client concern?
1. Lack of knowledge about COPD
2. Difficulty coping related with a situational crisis
3. Negative self-image because of neurologic deficit
4. Restricted verbal communication because of a physical barrier

Level of Cognitive Ability: Analyzing
Client Needs: Psychosocial Integrity
Clinical Judgment/Cognitive Skills: Analyze Cues
Integrated Process: Clinical Judgment/Nursing Process/Analysis
Content Area: Adult Health: Respiratory
Health Problems: Mental Health: Coping
Priority Concepts: Communication; Gas Exchange

Answer: 4
Rationale: A client with COPD may suffer physical or psychological alterations that impair communication. To speak spontaneously and clearly, a person must have an intact respiratory system. Extreme dyspnea is a physical alteration that affects speech. There are no data in the question that support the remaining options.
Test-Taking Strategy: Focus on the subject, that the client is experiencing extreme dyspnea during an interview. Based on this, option 4 is the only option that addresses this subject.
Priority Nursing Tip: For the client with COPD, the nurse would not change the oxygen flow rate without a health care provider's prescription. Low concentration of oxygen may be prescribed because the stimulus to breathe is a low arterial Po_2 instead of an increased Pco_2.
Reference: Ignatavicius, D., et al. (2021). *Medical-surgical nursing: Concepts for interprofessional collaborative care* (10th ed., pp. 545, 547–548, 550). Elsevier.

165. While intoxicated, a client received a severe full-thickness burn to the left leg. After an unsuccessful response to treatment, an amputation is required. After signing the informed consent form, the nurse observes that the client appears withdrawn. Which action would the nurse implement at this time?
1. Let client have some time alone to grieve about the future loss of the limb.
2. Teach client that the injury was a result of alcohol abuse, and suggest counseling.
3. Communicate with client in a manner that reflects that client appears to be upset.
4. Inform the primary health care provider of client's behavior, and request medication to assist with coping.

Level of Cognitive Ability: Applying
Client Needs: Psychosocial Integrity
Clinical Judgment/Cognitive Skills: Take Action
Integrated Process: Clinical Judgment/Nursing Process/Implementation
Content Area: Adult Health: Integumentary
Health Problems: Mental Health: Coping
Priority Concepts: Communication; Stress and Coping

Answer: 3
Rationale: Reflection statements tend to elicit a deeper awareness of feelings. A well-timed reflection can reveal an emotion that has escaped the client's notice. Additionally, option 3 validates the perception that the client is upset. Options 1 and 4 address interventions before assessing the situation. Option 2 is inappropriate and a block to communication.
Test-Taking Strategy: Use therapeutic communication techniques. Focus on the client's feelings, and select the option that encourages the client to express feelings and to talk more. This will direct you to the correct option.
Priority Nursing Tip: For the client undergoing amputation, the nurse should encourage verbalization regarding loss of the body part and assist the client to identify coping mechanisms to deal with the loss.
References: Ignatavicius, D., et al. (2021). *Medical-surgical nursing: Concepts for interprofessional collaborative care* (10th ed., p. 1050). Elsevier; Potter, P., et al. (2021). *Fundamentals of nursing* (10th ed., pp. 333–335). Elsevier.

❖ **166.** The nurse is caring for a client diagnosed with left-sided Bell's palsy. Which statement by the client shows a **need for further teaching** by the nurse?
1. "My left eye is tearing a lot."
2. "I have trouble closing my left eyelid."
3. "I don't know how I'll live with this stroke."
4. "I can't feel anything on the left side of my face."

Level of Cognitive Ability: Evaluating
Client Needs: Psychosocial Integrity
Clinical Judgment/Cognitive Skills: Evaluate Outcomes
Integrated Process: Clinical Judgment/Nursing Process/Evaluation
Content Area: Adult Health: Neurologic
Health Problems: Mental Health: Anxiety
Priority Concepts: Patient Education; Anxiety

Answer: 3
Rationale: Bell's palsy is an inflammatory condition that involves the facial nerve (cranial nerve VII). Although it results in facial paralysis, it is not the same as a stroke. Many clients fear that they have had a stroke when the symptoms of Bell's palsy appear, and they commonly believe that the paralysis is permanent. Symptoms resolve, although it may take several weeks. The remaining options are expected assessment findings of the client with Bell's palsy.
Test-Taking Strategy: Note the strategic words, *need for further teaching.* These words indicate a negative event query and ask you to select an option that is an incorrect client statement. Recalling that this disorder is a temporary condition will direct you to the correct option, which identifies an inaccurate understanding of the disorder and thus requires further exploration.
Priority Nursing Tip: Bell's palsy is characterized by the inability to raise the eyebrows, frown, smile, close the eyelids, or puff out the cheeks.
Reference: Lewis, S., et al. (2020). *Medical-surgical nursing: Assessment and management of clinical problems* (11th ed., p. 1424). Elsevier.

167. A client has a scheduled office visit due to a new diagnosis of diabetes mellitus. The client tells the nurse they are anxious about self-administering insulin and so have trouble maintaining proper health. Which teaching/learning strategy would the nurse **initially** plan to implement?
1. Teach a family member to give client the insulin.
2. Leave a list of instructions at the bedside for practicing the insulin injections.
3. Insert the needle, and have client push in the plunger and remove the needle.
4. Give the injection until client feels sufficiently confident to perform it alone.

Level of Cognitive Ability: Applying
Client Needs: Psychosocial Integrity
Clinical Judgment/Cognitive Skills: Generate Solutions
Integrated Process: Clinical Judgment/Nursing Process/Planning
Content Area: Adult Health: Endocrine
Health Problems: Mental Health: Anxiety
Priority Concepts: Anxiety; Patient Education

Answer: 3
Rationale: Some clients find it difficult to insert a needle into their own skin. For these clients, the nurse might assist by selecting the site and inserting the needle. Then, as a first step in self-injection, the client can push in the plunger and remove the needle. The remaining options place the client in a dependent role.
Test-Taking Strategy: Note the strategic word, *initially.* Focus on the subject, anxiety regarding the self-administration of insulin. The correct option allows the client to participate in this activity. Eliminate options that place the client in a dependent position. Also note that the correct option addresses the subject of self-administration.
Priority Nursing Tip: Insulin injected into the abdomen may absorb more evenly and rapidly than at other sites.
Reference: Lewis, S., et al. (2020). *Medical-surgical nursing: Assessment and management of clinical problems* (11th ed., p. 1116). Elsevier.

❖ **168.** A client who is in labor has human immunodeficiency virus (HIV) and anxiously states to the nurse, "I know I will have a sick-looking baby." Which appropriate therapeutic response would the nurse make?
1. "You are very sick, but your baby may not be."
2. "All babies are beautiful. I am sure your baby will be, too."
3. "You have concerns about how HIV will affect your baby?"
4. "There is no reason to worry. Our neonatal unit offers the latest treatments available."

Level of Cognitive Ability: Applying
Client Needs: Psychosocial Integrity
Clinical Judgment/Cognitive Skills: Take Action
Integrated Process: Communication and Documentation
Content Area: Maternity: Intrapartum
Health Problems: Mental Health: Anxiety
Priority Concepts: Communication; Anxiety

Answer: 3
Rationale: Option 3 is the most therapeutic response, and it will elicit the best information. It addresses the therapeutic communication technique of paraphrasing. Option 3 also is an open-ended response that will provide an opportunity for the client to verbalize concerns. Parents need to know that their baby will not look sick from HIV at birth and that there may be a period of uncertainty before it is known whether the baby has acquired the infection. Options 1 and 2 provide false reassurances. The client should not be told that there is no reason to worry.
Test-Taking Strategy: Use therapeutic communication techniques. Remember to address the client's feelings and concerns. This will direct you to the correct option.
Priority Nursing Tip: Infants at risk for HIV infection need to receive all recommended immunizations at the regular schedule; however, no live vaccines should be administered.
Reference: McKinney, E. S., et al. (2022). *Maternal child nursing* (6th ed., pp. 26–27, 944). Elsevier.

169. A client who is scheduled for an abdominal peritoneoscopy asks the home care nurse, "The surgeon told me to restrict food and liquids for at least 8 hours before this procedure and to use a Fleet enema 4 hours before entering the hospital. Do people ever get into trouble after this procedure?" Which is the **most appropriate** therapeutic response the nurse would make to the client?
1. "Any invasive procedure brings risk with it. You need to report any shoulder pain immediately."
2. "You seem to understand the preparation very well. Are you having any concerns about the procedure?"
3. "Trouble? There is never any trouble with this procedure. That's why the surgeon will use local anesthesia."
4. "There are relatively few problems, especially if you are having local anesthesia, but vaginal bleeding needs to be reported immediately."

Level of Cognitive Ability: Applying
Client Needs: Psychosocial Integrity
Clinical Judgment/Cognitive Skills: Take Action
Integrated Process: Clinical Judgment/Nursing Process/ Implementation
Content Area: Skills: Perioperative Care
Health Problems: Mental Health: Anxiety
Priority Concepts: Clinical Judgment; Communication

Answer: 2
Rationale: Abdominal peritoneoscopy is performed to directly visualize the liver, gallbladder, spleen, and stomach after the insufflation of nitrous oxide. During the procedure, a rigid laparoscope is inserted through a small incision in the abdomen. A microscope in the endoscope allows for the visualization of the organs and provides a way to collect a specimen for biopsy or remove small tumors. The appropriate response is the one that facilitates the expression of the client's feelings. Option 1 may increase the client's anxiety. In option 3, the nurse states that no problems are associated with this procedure; this is closed-ended and is incorrect. Although option 4 contains accurate information, the word *immediately* can increase the client's anxiety.
Test-Taking Strategy: Note the strategic words, *most appropriate*. Use therapeutic communication techniques to identify the client's feelings and concerns. The correct option is the appropriate response because it provides an opportunity for the client to verbalize concerns.
Priority Nursing Tip: After endoscopic procedures in which the throat is sprayed with an anesthetic, the nurse needs to monitor for the return of a gag reflex before giving the client any oral substance. If the gag reflex has not returned and food or fluids are administered, the client could aspirate.
References: Lewis, S., et al. (2020). *Medical-surgical nursing: Assessment and management of clinical problems* (11th ed., p. 843). Elsevier; Potter, P., et al. (2021). *Fundamentals of nursing.* (10th ed., pp. 333–335). Elsevier.

❖ **170.** The nurse is caring for a client during a precipitous labor. The nurse would anticipate that the client will require care for which emotional need?
1. Support in maintaining a sense of control
2. Less pain and anxiety than with a normal labor
3. A sense of satisfaction regarding the quick labor
4. Fewer fears regarding the effect of labor on the newborn infant

Level of Cognitive Ability: Analyzing
Client Needs: Psychosocial Integrity
Clinical Judgment/Cognitive Skills: Generate Solutions
Integrated Process: Clinical Judgment/Nursing Process/Planning
Content Area: Maternity: Intrapartum
Health Problems: Mental Health: Anxiety
Priority Concepts: Clinical Judgment; Reproduction

Answer: 1
Rationale: The client experiencing a precipitous labor may have more difficulty maintaining control because of the abrupt onset and quick progression of the labor. This may be very different from previous labor experiences; therefore, the client needs support from the nurse to understand and adapt to the rapid progression. The contractions often increase in intensity very quickly, which adds to the client's pain, anxiety, and lack of control. The client may also have an increased amount of concern about the effect of the labor on the newborn infant. A lack of control over the situation in combination with increased pain and anxiety can result in a decreased level of satisfaction with the labor and delivery experience.
Test-Taking Strategy: Focus on the subject, precipitous labor, and the client's reaction to this type of labor in selecting the correct option. Thinking about the definition and characteristics of a precipitous labor will direct you to the correct option.
Priority Nursing Tip: A precipitous labor is a labor lasting less than 3 hours.
Reference: McKinney, E. S., et al. (2022). *Maternal child nursing* (6th ed., pp. 585–586). Elsevier.

171. The nurse is planning care for a client who presents in active labor with a history of a previous cesarean delivery. The client complains of a "tearing" sensation in the lower abdomen. The client is upset, and expresses concern for the safety of the baby. Which therapeutic response to the client would the nurse make?
1. "Try not to worry, you and your baby are in good hands."
2. "I can understand that you are fearful. We are doing everything possible for your baby."
3. "I don't have time to answer questions now, but I'll plan for us to have time to talk later."
4. "I understand your concerns. I'll let your primary health care provider know you need to talk."

Level of Cognitive Ability: Applying
Client Needs: Psychosocial Integrity
Clinical Judgment/Cognitive Skills: Take Action
Integrated Process: Clinical Judgment/Nursing Process/Implementation
Content Area: Maternity: Intrapartum
Health Problems: Mental Health: Coping
Priority Concepts: Reproduction; Stress and Coping

Answer: 2
Rationale: Clients have a concern for the safety of their baby during labor and delivery, especially when a problem arises. Empathy and a calm attitude with realistic reassurances are important aspects of client care. Dismissing or ignoring the client's concerns can lead to increased fear and a lack of cooperation. Option 1 uses a cliché and provides false reassurance. Options 3 and 4 place the client's feelings on hold.
Test-Taking Strategy: Use therapeutic communication techniques. Eliminate options 3 and 4 because they place the client's feelings on hold. Next eliminate option 1 because the client should not be told to not worry.
Priority Nursing Tip: Breathing techniques can be used to enhance relaxation for the pregnant client. They also provide a focus for the client during contractions and can interfere with pain sensory transmission.
Reference: McKinney, E. S., et al. (2022). *Maternal child nursing* (6th ed., pp. 26–27, 321). Elsevier.

❖ **172.** A newborn infant is diagnosed with an undescended testicle (cryptorchidism), and these findings are shared with the parents. The parents ask questions about the condition. The nurse would respond to the parents that which condition can occur and have a psychosocial impact if the undescended testicle is not corrected?
1. Atrophy
2. Infertility
3. Malignancy
4. Feminization

Level of Cognitive Ability: Applying
Client Needs: Psychosocial Integrity
Clinical Judgment/Cognitive Skills: Take Action
Integrated Process: Clinical Judgment/Nursing Process/Implementation
Content Area: Maternity: Newborn
Health Problems: Mental Health: Coping
Priority Concepts: Patient Education; Reproduction

Answer: 2
Rationale: Infertility can occur with this condition because proper function of the testes in producing fertile sperm depends on a temperature of less than 98.6° F (37.0° C). The psychological effects of an "empty scrotum" could affect the client's perception of self and the ability to reproduce. Options 1 and 3 are possible physical consequences of a failure to treat cryptorchidism rather than psychosocial consequences. Because all of the hormones that are responsible for secondary sex characteristics continue to be secreted directly into the bloodstream, option 4 is not correct.
Test-Taking Strategy: Focusing on the subject, the psychosocial impact of an undescended testicle (cryptorchidism) will assist you with eliminating options 1 and 3. From the remaining options, it is necessary to know that infertility can occur if the condition is not corrected.
Priority Nursing Tip: Cryptorchidism is a condition in which one or both testes fail to descend through the inguinal canal into the scrotal sac.
Reference: McKinney, E. S., et al. (2022). *Maternal child nursing* (6th ed., pp. 1017–1018). Elsevier.

173. The birthing parent of a newborn diagnosed with hydrocephalus is concerned about the complication of mental retardation. The parent states to the nurse, "I'm not sure if I can care for my baby at home." Which therapeutic response would the nurse make to the parent?
1. "All babies have individual needs."
2. "Parents instinctively know what is best for their babies."
3. "You have concerns about your baby's condition and care?"
4. "There is no reason to worry. You have a good pediatrician."

Level of Cognitive Ability: Applying
Client Needs: Psychosocial Integrity
Clinical Judgment/Cognitive Skills: Take Action
Integrated Process: Clinical Judgment/Nursing Process/Implementation
Content Area: Maternity: Newborn
Health Problems: Mental Health: Coping
Priority Concepts: Communication; Stress and Coping

Answer: 3
Rationale: Paraphrasing is restating the parent's message in the nurse's own words. Option 3 demonstrates the therapeutic technique of paraphrasing. In option 1 the nurse is minimizing the social needs involved with the baby's diagnosis, which is harmful for the nurse–parent relationship. In options 2 and 4, the nurse is offering false reassurance, and these types of responses will block communication.
Test-Taking Strategy: Use therapeutic communication techniques to answer the question. The correct option is the only therapeutic response, and it demonstrates paraphrasing. This is the only option that will provide the client with an opportunity to verbalize concerns.
Priority Nursing Tip: Hydrocephalus results in head enlargement and increased intracranial pressure due to an abnormal buildup of fluid in the ventricles of the brain.
Reference: McKinney, E. S., et al. (2022). *Maternal child nursing* (6th ed., pp. 59, 1296–1297). Elsevier.

Client Needs

❖ **174.** A preschooler has just been diagnosed with impetigo. The child's parent tells the nurse, "But my children take baths every day." Which therapeutic response would the nurse make to the parent?
1. "You are concerned about how your child got impetigo?"
2. "There is no need to worry. We will not tell your day care provider why your child is absent."
3. "Not only do you have to do a better job of keeping your children clean, you must also wash your hands more frequently."
4. "You should have seen the doctor before the wound became infected, and then you would not have had to worry about the child having impetigo."

Level of Cognitive Ability: Applying
Client Needs: Psychosocial Integrity
Clinical Judgment/Cognitive Skills: Take Action
Integrated Process: Clinical Judgment/Nursing Process/Implementation
Content Area: Pediatrics: Infectious and Communicable Diseases
Health Problems: Mental Health: Anxiety
Priority Concepts: Communication; Tissue Integrity

Answer: 1
Rationale: By paraphrasing what the parent tells the nurse, the nurse is addressing the parent's concerns. Option 1 demonstrates the therapeutic technique of paraphrasing. The remaining options are blocks to communication because they make the parent feel guilty for the child's illness.
Test-Taking Strategy: Use therapeutic communication techniques to answer the question. Option 1 is the only therapeutic technique, and it demonstrates paraphrasing. This is the only option that will provide the client with an opportunity to verbalize concerns. Eliminate options that are blocks to communication.
Priority Nursing Tip: A child with an integumentary disorder needs to be monitored for signs of a skin infection or a systemic infection.
Reference: McKinney, E. S., et al. (2022). *Maternal child nursing* (6th ed., pp. 50, 1187–1188). Elsevier.

175. The nurse is preparing to care for a child with anemia from a culture that is different from the nurse's. Which is the **best** way to address the cultural needs of the child and family when the child is admitted to the health care facility?
1. Address only those issues that directly affect the nurse's care of the child.
2. Ask questions, and explain to the family why the questions are being asked.
3. Explain that cultural practices need to be discontinued during hospitalization.
4. Ignore cultural needs because they are not important to health care professionals.

Level of Cognitive Ability: Applying
Client Needs: Psychosocial Integrity
Clinical Judgment/Cognitive Skills: Generate Solutions
Integrated Process: Clinical Judgment/Nursing Process/Caring
Content Area: Foundations of Care: Spirituality, Culture, and Ethnicity
Health Problems: Pediatric-Specific: Anemias
Priority Concepts: Culture; Communication

Answer: 2
Rationale: When caring for individuals from a different culture, ask questions about their specific cultural needs and means of treatment. An understanding of the family's beliefs and health practices is essential to successful interventions for that particular family. Eliminate the options that ignore the cultural beliefs and values of the client.
Test-Taking Strategy: Note the strategic word, *best*. Focus on the subject, cultural needs. Eliminate options that are judgmental. In addition, these options are comparable or alike in that they ignore the cultural practices and values of the client.
Priority Nursing Tip: When caring for a client from a different culture, the nurse needs to treat the client with respect and appreciate the differences and diversity of beliefs about health, illness, and treatment modalities.
Reference: McKinney, E. S., et al. (2022). *Maternal child nursing* (6th ed., pp. 39, 1125). Elsevier.

❖ **176.** A client with a T1 spinal cord injury has just learned that the cord was completely severed. The client says, "I'm no good to anyone. I might as well be dead." Which **most** therapeutic response would the nurse make to the client?
   1. "You're not a useless person at all."
   2. "I'll ask the psychologist to see you about this."
   3. "You appear to be feeling troubled about things."
   4. "It makes me uncomfortable when you talk this way."

Level of Cognitive Ability: Applying
Client Needs: Psychosocial Integrity
Clinical Judgment/Cognitive Skills: Take Action
Integrated Process: Communication and Documentation
Content Area: Adult Health: Neurologic
Health Problems: Mental Health: Coping
Priority Concepts: Communication; Stress and Coping

Answer: 3
Rationale: Restating and reflecting keep the lines of communication open and encourage the client to expand on current feelings of unworthiness and loss that require exploration. The nurse can block communication by showing discomfort and disapproval or postponing the discussion of issues. Grief is a common reaction to a loss of function. The nurse facilitates grieving through open communication.
Test-Taking Strategy: Note the strategic word, *most*. Use therapeutic communication techniques. Eliminate options that block communication. The correct option identifies the therapeutic communication technique of restating and reflecting.
Priority Nursing Tip: Trauma to the spinal cord causes partial or complete disruption of the nerve tracts and neurons.
References: Ignatavicius, D., et al. (2021). *Medical-surgical nursing: Concepts for interprofessional collaborative care* (10th ed., pp. 828, 877). Elsevier; Potter, P., et al. (2021). *Fundamentals of nursing* (10th ed., pp. 333–335). Elsevier.

177. The nurse enters the room of a client who has been diagnosed having a myocardial infarction (MI) and finds the client quietly crying. After determining that there is no physiologic reason for the client's distress, how would the nurse **best** respond?
   1. "Do you want me to call your children?"
   2. "Can you tell me a little about what has you so upset?"
   3. "Try not to be so upset. Psychological stress is bad for your heart."
   4. "I understand how you feel. I'd cry, too, if I had a major heart attack."

Level of Cognitive Ability: Applying
Client Needs: Psychosocial Integrity
Clinical Judgment/Cognitive Skills: Take Action
Integrated Process: Communication and Documentation
Content Area: Adult Health: Cardiovascular
Health Problems: Mental Health: Coping
Priority Concepts: Stress and Coping; Communication

Answer: 2
Rationale: Clients with MI often have anxiety or fear. The nurse allows the client to express concerns by showing genuine interest and concern and facilitating communication using therapeutic communication techniques. The correct option provides the client with an opportunity to express concerns. The remaining options do not address the client's feelings or promote client verbalization.
Test-Taking Strategy: Note the strategic word, *best*. Use therapeutic communication techniques that have an exploratory approach because the question does not identify why the client is upset. This technique helps you eliminate each of the incorrect options.
Priority Nursing Tip: Cardiac rehabilitation is the process of actively assisting the client with cardiac disease to achieve and maintain a vital and productive life within the limitations of the heart disease.
References: Ignatavicius, D., et al. (2021). *Medical-surgical nursing: Concepts for interprofessional collaborative care* (10th ed., p. 621). Elsevier; Potter, P., et al. (2021). *Fundamentals of nursing* (10th ed., pp. 333–335). Elsevier.

❖ **178.** A client diagnosed with a recent complete T4 spinal cord transection tells the nurse about looking forward to walking again as soon as the spinal shock resolves. Which statement provides the **most** accurate basis for planning a response to the client?

1. Client is projecting by insisting that walking is the rehabilitation goal.
2. To speed acceptance, client needs reinforcement that client will not walk again.
3. Denial can be protective while client deals with the anxiety created by the new disability.
4. Client needs to move through the grieving process rapidly to benefit from rehabilitation.

Level of Cognitive Ability: Applying
Client Needs: Psychosocial Integrity
Clinical Judgment/Cognitive Skills: Generate Solutions
Integrated Process: Clinical Judgment/Nursing Process/Planning
Content Area: Adult Health: Neurologic
Health Problems: Mental Health: Coping
Priority Concepts: Caregiving; Coping

Answer: 3
Rationale: During the adjustment period that occurs the first few weeks after a spinal cord injury, clients may use denial as a defense mechanism. Denial may decrease anxiety temporarily, and it is a normal part of grieving. After the spinal shock resolves, the prolonged or excessive use of denial may impair rehabilitation. However, rehabilitation programs include psychological counseling to deal with denial and grief.
Test-Taking Strategy: Note the strategic word, *most*. Focus on the subject, the physiologic effects of a T4 spinal cord injury. The words *walking is the rehabilitation goal*, *speed acceptance*, and *move through the grieving process rapidly* are indicators that these are incorrect options. Also, focus on the client's statement, which is an indication of denial, to direct you to option 3.
Priority Nursing Tip: In spinal shock, a sudden depression of reflex activity in the spinal cord occurs below the level of injury (areflexia).
References: Ignatavicius, D., et al. (2021). *Medical-surgical nursing: Concepts for interprofessional collaborative care* (10th ed., p. 828). Elsevier; Potter, P., et al. (2021). *Fundamentals of nursing* (10th ed., p. 348). Elsevier.

179. The nurse is developing a plan of care for a client scheduled for an above-the-knee leg amputation. Which action would the nurse include in the plan of care when addressing the psychosocial needs of the client?

1. Explain to client that open grieving is abnormal.
2. Encourage client to express feelings about body changes.
3. Advise client to seek psychological treatment after surgery.
4. Discourage sharing with others who have had similar experiences.

Level of Cognitive Ability: Applying
Client Needs: Psychosocial Integrity
Clinical Judgment/Cognitive Skills: Generate Solutions
Integrated Process: Clinical Judgment/Nursing Process/Planning
Content Area: Adult Health: Musculoskeletal
Health Problems: Mental Health: Coping
Priority Concepts: Caregiving; Stress and Coping

Answer: 2
Rationale: Surgical incisions or the loss of a body part can alter a client's body image. The onset of problems coping with these changes may occur during the immediate or extended postoperative stage. Nursing interventions primarily involve providing psychological support. The nurse should encourage the client to express how they feel about these postoperative changes that will affect their life. Option 1 is an incorrect statement because open grieving is normal. The nurse is giving advice in option 3, and option 4 indicates disapproval.
Test-Taking Strategy: Focus on the subject, the psychosocial needs of the client undergoing amputation. Also, use therapeutic communication techniques. Remember to always focus on the client's feelings first. This will direct you to option 2.
Priority Nursing Tip: After amputation, avoid elevating the residual limb on a pillow to prevent hip flexion contractures.
References: Ignatavicius, D., et al. (2021). *Medical-surgical nursing: Concepts for interprofessional collaborative care* (10th ed.; pp. 1046, 1050). Elsevier; Potter, P., et al. (2021). *Fundamentals of nursing* (10th ed., pp. 333–335). Elsevier.

❖ **180.** A client diagnosed with pulmonary edema exhibits severe anxiety. The nurse is preparing to carry out a prescribed treatment. Which intervention would the nurse use to meet the needs of the client in a holistic manner?
1. Ask a family member to stay with client during the procedure.
2. Give client the call bell, and encourage its use if client feels worse.
3. Leave client alone only to gather the required equipment and medications.
4. Stay with client, and ask another nurse to gather needed equipment and supplies.

Level of Cognitive Ability: Applying
Client Needs: Psychosocial Integrity
Clinical Judgment/Cognitive Skills: Take Action
Integrated Process: Clinical Judgment/Nursing Process/Implementation
Content Area: Adult Health: Cardiovascular
Health Problems: Mental Health: Anxiety
Priority Concepts: Anxiety; Caregiving

Answer: 4
Rationale: Pulmonary edema is accompanied by extreme fear and anxiety. Because the client typically experiences a sense of impending doom, the nurse would remain with the client as much as possible. Family members can emotionally support the client, but they are not able to respond to physiologic needs and symptoms. In fact, they are typically in psychological distress themselves. Options 2 and 3 do not provide for the psychological needs of the client in distress.
Test-Taking Strategy: Focus on the subject, a client with pulmonary edema who exhibits severe anxiety. Identify the word *holistic*. This word guides you to consider both the physical and emotional well-being of the client. The correct option is the only choice that addresses both needs.
Priority Nursing Tip: If pulmonary edema occurs, the nurse would place the client in a high-Fowler's position; administer oxygen; assess the client quickly, including lung sounds; ensure that an intravenous access device is in place; prepare for the administration of a diuretic and morphine sulfate and insertion of a Foley catheter; prepare for intubation and ventilator support, if required; and document the event, actions taken, and the client's response.
Reference: Ignatavicius, D., et al. (2021). *Medical-surgical nursing: Concepts for interprofessional collaborative care* (10th ed., pp. 592, 678). Elsevier.

181. The family of a client diagnosed with a myocardial infarction complicated by cardiogenic shock is visibly anxious and upset about the client's condition. Which would the nurse plan to implement to provide support to the family?
1. Offer them coffee and other beverages on a regular basis.
2. Insist that they go home to sleep at night to keep up their own strength.
3. Ask the hospital chaplain to sit with them until client's condition stabilizes.
4. Provide flexible visiting times according to client's condition and family needs.

Level of Cognitive Ability: Applying
Client Needs: Psychosocial Integrity
Clinical Judgment/Cognitive Skills: Generate Solutions
Integrated Process: Clinical Judgment/Nursing Process/Planning
Content Area: Adult Health: Cardiovascular
Health Problems: Mental Health: Anxiety
Priority Concepts: Anxiety; Stress and Coping

Answer: 4
Rationale: The use of flexible visiting hours meets the needs of both the client and family for reducing the anxiety levels of both. Offering the family beverages does not provide support. Insisting that the family go home is nontherapeutic. Although the chaplain may provide support, it is unrealistic for the chaplain to stay until the client stabilizes.
Test-Taking Strategy: Note the subject, the method of providing support to a client's anxious family. Options 2 and 3 may or may not be helpful, depending on the client and family situation. Coffee and beverages, although probably helpful to many, do not provide support.
Priority Nursing Tip: Cardiogenic shock is failure of the heart to pump adequately, thereby reducing cardiac output and compromising tissue perfusion.
Reference: Lewis, S., et al. (2020). *Medical-surgical nursing: Assessment and management of clinical problems* (11th ed., pp. 1580, 1583). Elsevier.

❖ **182.** A client having premature ventricular contractions (PVCs) states to the nurse, "I'm so afraid that something bad will happen." Which action by the nurse provides the **most immediate** help to the client?
1. Telephoning client's family
2. Using a television to distract client
3. Having a staff member stay with client
4. Giving reassurance that nothing will happen to client

Level of Cognitive Ability: Applying
Client Needs: Psychosocial Integrity
Clinical Judgment/Cognitive Skills: Take Action
Integrated Process: Clinical Judgment/Nursing Process/Implementation
Content Area: Adult Health: Cardiovascular
Health Problems: Mental Health: Coping
Priority Concepts: Anxiety; Stress and Coping

Answer: 3
Rationale: When a client experiences fear, the nurse can provide a calm, safe environment by offering appropriate reassurance, using therapeutic touch, and having someone remain with the client as much as possible. Options 1 and 2 do not address the client's fear, and option 4 provides false reassurance.
Test-Taking Strategy: Note the strategic words, *most immediate*, in selecting the correct option. Options 1 and 2 are comparable or alike options because they do not address the immediate concern of fear. Next, focusing on the strategic words will direct you to the correct option.
Priority Nursing Tip: For the client experiencing PVCs, notify the primary health care provider if the client complains of chest pain or if the PVCs increase in frequency, are multifocal, occur on the T wave (R on T), or occur in runs of ventricular tachycardia.
Reference: Lewis, S., et al. (2020). *Medical-surgical nursing: Assessment and management of clinical problems* (11th ed., pp. 726, 766–767). Elsevier.

183. A client diagnosed with Raynaud's disease tells the nurse that they have a stressful job and do not handle stressful situations well. Which life change would the nurse suggest the client consider to help alleviate stress?
1. Change to a less stressful job.
2. Seek help from a psychologist.
3. Consider a stress management program.
4. Use earplugs to minimize environmental noise.

Level of Cognitive Ability: Applying
Client Needs: Psychosocial Integrity
Clinical Judgment/Cognitive Skills: Take Action
Integrated Process: Clinical Judgment/Nursing Process/Implementation
Content Area: Adult Health: Cardiovascular
Health Problems: Mental Health: Anxiety
Priority Concepts: Stress and Coping; Patient Education

Answer: 3
Rationale: Stress can trigger the vasospasm that occurs with Raynaud's disease, so referral to a stress management program or the use of biofeedback training may be helpful. Option 1 is unrealistic. Option 2 is not necessarily required at this time. Option 4 does not specifically address the subject.
Test-Taking Strategy: Focus on the subject, an intervention to alleviate stress. Note the relationship between this subject and the correct option.
Priority Nursing Tip: Raynaud's disease is vasospasm of the arterioles of the upper and lower extremities, which causes constriction of the cutaneous vessels.
Reference: Lewis, S., et al. (2020). *Medical-surgical nursing: Assessment and management of clinical problems* (11th ed., pp. 80–81, 807). Elsevier.

❖ **184.** A client with a history of pulmonary emboli is scheduled for the insertion of an inferior vena cava filter. The nurse checks on the client 1 hour after the primary health care provider has explained the procedure and obtained informed consent from the client. The client is lying in bed, wringing the hands, and states to the nurse, "I'm not sure about this. What if it doesn't work and I'm just as bad off as before?" Which concern for the client would the nurse identify at this time?
1. Anxiety and depression
2. Inability to handle the treatment regimen
3. Lack of knowledge about the surgical procedure
4. Fear about the potential risks and outcomes of surgery

Level of Cognitive Ability: Analyzing
Client Needs: Psychosocial Integrity
Clinical Judgment/Cognitive Skills: Analyze Cues
Integrated Process: Clinical Judgment/Nursing Process/Analysis
Content Area: Adult Health: Cardiovascular
Health Problems: Anxiety
Priority Concepts: Anxiety; Communication

Answer: 4
Rationale: This client has indicated the surgical procedure and its outcome as the object of fear. Anxiety is present when the client cannot identify the source of the uneasy feelings. Presently there are no indications that the client is depressed. A client's inability to handle a treatment regimen would be when the client is not making needed adaptations to deal with daily life. Lack of knowledge would be when there is a lack of appropriate information.
Test-Taking Strategy: Note the subject, the client's concern about the outcome of the surgery. The client is also stating the concerns related to the procedure. Identify the option that addresses surgery, as well as fear. Also note the relationship of the client's statement and the correct option.
Priority Nursing Tip: If a pulmonary embolism is suspected, the nurse would notify the rapid response team; reassure the client and elevate the head of the bed; prepare to administer oxygen; obtain vital signs and check lung sounds; prepare to obtain an arterial blood gas; prepare for the administration of heparin therapy or other therapies; and document the event, the actions taken, and the client's response.
Reference: Ignatavicius, D., et al. (2021). *Medical-surgical nursing: Concepts for interprofessional collaborative care* (10th ed., pp. 588, 591–592). Elsevier.

185. A client diagnosed with acute respiratory failure has an oral endotracheal tube attached to a mechanical ventilator and is about to begin the weaning process. The nurse determines that which item that was previously used to minimize the client's anxiety should now be limited?
1. Radio
2. Television
3. Family visitors
4. Antianxiety medications

Level of Cognitive Ability: Analyzing
Client Needs: Psychosocial Integrity
Clinical Judgment/Cognitive Skills: Generate Solutions
Integrated Process: Clinical Judgment/Nursing Process/Planning
Content Area: Complex Care: Acute Respiratory Failure
Health Problems: Mental Health: Anxiety
Priority Concepts: Anxiety; Gas Exchange

Answer: 4
Rationale: Antianxiety medications and opioid analgesics are used cautiously in the client who is being weaned from a mechanical ventilator. These medications may interfere with the weaning process by suppressing the respiratory drive. The client may exhibit anxiety during the weaning process for a variety of reasons; therefore, distractions such as radio, television, and visitors are still very useful.
Test-Taking Strategy: Focus on the subject, the item that should be limited during weaning from a ventilator. Think about the items that could interfere with the client's strength, endurance, and respiratory drive to maintain independent ventilation. Using this as the guideline, you will realize the only possible choice is the correct option. The side effects of these medications could include sedation, which could interfere with optimal respiratory function.
Priority Nursing Tip: For the client receiving mechanical ventilation, always assess the client first, and then assess the ventilator. Additionally, never set ventilator alarms to the off position.
Reference: Ignatavicius, D., et al. (2021). *Medical-surgical nursing: Concepts for interprofessional collaborative care* (10th ed., pp. 606–607). Elsevier.

❖ **186.** A client scheduled for pulmonary angiography to rule out pulmonary embolism is fearful about the procedure and asks the nurse if the procedure involves significant pain and radiation exposure. Which therapeutic response would the nurse make to the client to provide reassurance?

1. "The procedure is somewhat painful, but there is minimal exposure to radiation."
2. "Discomfort may occur with needle insertion, and there is minimal exposure to radiation."
3. "There is very mild pain throughout the procedure, and the exposure to radiation is negligible."
4. "There is usually no pain, although a moderate amount of radiation must be used to get accurate results."

Level of Cognitive Ability: Applying
Client Needs: Psychosocial Integrity
Clinical Judgment/Cognitive Skills: Take Action
Integrated Process: Clinical Judgment/Nursing Process/Implementation
Content Area: Foundations of Care: Diagnostic Tests
Health Problems: Mental Health: Anxiety
Priority Concepts: Patient Education; Gas Exchange

Answer: 2
Rationale: Pulmonary angiography involves minimal exposure to radiation. The procedure is painless, although the client may feel discomfort with insertion of the needle for the catheter that is used for dye injection. This information supports the fact that the other options are incorrect.
Test-Taking Strategy: Focus on the subject of pulmonary angiography. Eliminate option 4 because of the closed-ended word "no." From the remaining options, recalling that discomfort occurs with needle insertion will direct you to option 2.
Priority Nursing Tip: A pulmonary angiography is an invasive procedure that involves inserting a catheter through the antecubital or femoral vein into the pulmonary artery or one of its branches. It also involves an injection of iodine or radiopaque contrast material; therefore, the nurse needs to assess for an allergy to these substances.
Reference: Pagana, K., Pagana, T., & Pagana, T. N. (2021). *Mosby's Diagnostic and laboratory test reference* (15th ed., pp. 752–753). Elsevier.

187. The nurse is caring for an anxious client who has an open pneumothorax and a sucking chest wound. An occlusive dressing has been applied to the site. Which intervention by the nurse would **best** relieve the client's anxiety?

1. Staying with client
2. Distracting client with television
3. Interpreting the arterial blood gas report
4. Encouraging client to cough and breathe deeply

Level of Cognitive Ability: Applying
Client Needs: Psychosocial Integrity
Clinical Judgment/Cognitive Skills: Take Action
Integrated Process: Clinical Judgment/Nursing Process/Implementation
Content Area: Adult Health: Respiratory
Health Problems: Mental Health: Anxiety
Priority Concepts: Anxiety; Stress and Coping

Answer: 1
Rationale: Staying with the client has a twofold benefit. First, it relieves the anxiety of the dyspneic client. In addition, the nurse must stay with the client to observe respiratory status after the application of the occlusive dressing. It is possible that the dressing could convert the open pneumothorax to a closed (tension) pneumothorax, which would result in a sudden decline in respiratory status and a mediastinal shift. If this occurs, the nurse is present and able to remove the dressing immediately. Option 2 is nontherapeutic. Interpreting the arterial blood gas report and promoting coughing and deep breathing have no immediate benefits for the client who is in distress.
Test-Taking Strategy: Note the strategic word, *best*. Focus on the subject, relieving the anxiety of a client who has an open pneumothorax. Eliminate option 2 first because the client is in distress. From the remaining options, use therapeutic nursing measures to direct you to the correct option.
Priority Nursing Tip: An open pneumothorax occurs when an opening through the chest wall allows the entrance of positive atmospheric air pressure into the pleural space.
Reference: Ignatavicius, D., et al. (2021). *Medical-surgical nursing: Concepts for interprofessional collaborative care* (10th ed., pp. 591–592, 608). Elsevier.

❖ **188.** A client diagnosed with acquired immunodeficiency syndrome (AIDS) shares with the nurse feelings of social isolation. Which strategy would the nurse suggest as the **most** useful way to decrease the client's stated loneliness?
1. Reinstituting contact with client's family, who live in a distant city
2. Contacting a support group for clients with AIDS that is available in the local region
3. Using the internet or the computer to facilitate communication while maintaining isolation
4. Using the television and newspapers to maintain a feeling of being "in touch" with the world

Level of Cognitive Ability: Applying
Client Needs: Psychosocial Integrity
Clinical Judgment/Cognitive Skills: Generate Solutions
Integrated Process: Clinical Judgment/Nursing Process/Planning
Content Area: Adult Health: Immune
Health Problems: Mental Health: Coping
Priority Concepts: Stress and Coping; Immunity

Answer: 2
Rationale: The nurse encourages the client to maintain social contact and support and assists the client with reducing barriers to social contact. This can include educating the client's family about the disease and its transmission, as well as suggesting the use of community resources and support groups. Option 1, although feasible, is less likely to address the client's current feelings of loneliness. Options 3 and 4 will not decrease the client's loneliness.
Test-Taking Strategy: Note the strategic word, *most.* Eliminate options that are comparable or alike in that they relate to keeping socially attached. From the remaining options, note that the wording of option 1 implies that contact has been lost over time, which is not stated in the question.
Priority Nursing Tip: Some of the tests that are used to monitor the progression of human immunodeficiency virus (HIV), which is the virus that leads to AIDS, include complete blood cell count, lymphocyte screen, quantitative immunoglobulin, chemistry panel, anergy panel, hepatitis B surface antigen testing, blood cultures, and chest radiography.
Reference: Ignatavicius, D., et al. (2021). *Medical-surgical nursing: Concepts for interprofessional collaborative care* (10th ed., p. 342). Elsevier.

189. A client was just told by the primary care primary health care provider that the client will have an exercise stress test to evaluate status after recent episodes of severe chest pain. As the nurse enters the examining room, the client states, "Maybe I shouldn't bother going. I wonder if I should just take more medication instead." Which therapeutic response would the nurse make to the client?
1. "Can you tell me more about how you're feeling?"
2. "Don't you really want to control your heart disease?"
3. "Most people tolerate the procedure well without any complications."
4. "Don't worry. Emergency equipment is available if it is needed."

Level of Cognitive Ability: Applying
Client Needs: Psychosocial Integrity
Clinical Judgment/Cognitive Skills: Take Action
Integrated Process: Communication and Documentation
Content Area: Foundations of Care: Diagnostic Tests
Health Problems: Mental Health: Anxiety
Priority Concepts: Anxiety; Communication

Answer: 1
Rationale: Anxiety and fear are often present before stress testing. The nurse needs to explore a client's feelings if concerns are expressed. Option 1 is open-ended and is the only choice that is phrased to engender trust and the sharing of concerns by the client. Eliminate options that are inappropriate statements and limit communication.
Test-Taking Strategy: Use therapeutic communication techniques. Remember to focus on the client's feelings. This will direct you to option 1.
Priority Nursing Tip: A stress test is a noninvasive procedure that studies the heart during activity and detects and evaluates coronary artery disease. Treadmill testing is the most commonly used mode of stress testing.
References: Pagana, K., Pagana, T., & Pagana, T. N. (2021). *Mosby's Diagnostic and laboratory test reference* (15th ed., pp. 214–215). Elsevier; Potter, P., et al. (2021). *Fundamentals of nursing* (10th ed., pp. 333–335). Elsevier.

Client Needs

190. The nurse is giving a client diagnosed with heart failure home care instructions for use after hospital discharge. The client interrupts, saying, "What's the use? I'll never remember all of this, and I'll probably die anyway!" The nurse determines that the client's statement is **most likely** due to which psychosocial concern?

1. Anger about the new medical regimen
2. The teaching strategies used by the nurse
3. Insufficient financial resources to pay for the medications
4. Anxiety about the ability to manage the disease process at home

Level of Cognitive Ability: Analyzing
Client Needs: Psychosocial Integrity
Clinical Judgment/Cognitive Skills: Analyze Cues
Integrated Process: Clinical Judgment/Nursing Process/Analysis
Content Area: Adult Health: Cardiovascular
Health Problems: Mental Health: Coping
Priority Concepts: Anxiety; Stress and Coping

Answer: 4

Rationale: Anxiety and fear often develop after heart failure, and they can further tax the failing heart. The client's statement is made in the middle of receiving self-care instructions. There is no evidence in the question to support option 1, 2, or 3.

Test-Taking Strategy: Note the strategic words, *most likely*. Focus on the subject, a client with heart failure being discharged. Because the client is being prepared for home care, the implication with the question is self-management.

Priority Nursing Tip: Heart failure results in inadequate cardiac output. The diminished cardiac output results in inadequate peripheral tissue perfusion.

Reference: Ignatavicius, D., et al. (2021). *Medical-surgical nursing: Concepts for interprofessional collaborative care* (10th ed., pp. 679–680). Elsevier.

191. Before inserting a peripheral intravenous (IV) catheter into a preoperative client, the nurse notes that the client's muscles are tense and the client is fidgeting with the bed sheet, stating a lack of understanding why the IV is necessary. Which statement would the nurse **first** verbalize to the client?

1. "This will be finished before you know it."
2. "Inserting the IV does not hurt very much."
3. "The IV adds needed fluid into your bloodstream."
4. "The IV catheter is an 18-gauge angiocatheter, which is small."

Level of Cognitive Ability: Applying
Client Needs: Psychosocial Integrity
Clinical Judgment/Cognitive Skills: Take Action
Integrated Process: Clinical Judgment/Nursing Process/Implementation
Content Area: Foundations of Care: Communication
Health Problems: Mental Health: Anxiety
Priority Concepts: Anxiety; Communication

Answer: 3

Rationale: In option 3 the nurse uses simple terms to clearly inform the client about the IV's purpose. Option 1 is an unethical statement for the nurse to make because the information is incorrect. Avoiding the client's feelings in option 2 blocks client communication regarding justifiable fears and feelings related to the IV insertion. Option 4 is an unsuitable statement because the client potentially would not understand the word "angiocatheter."

Test-Taking Strategy: Note the strategic word, *first*. Use therapeutic communication techniques when responding to the client. Nonverbal signals that indicate anxiety should also be noted and addressed using therapeutic communication techniques.

Priority Nursing Tip: Administration of an IV solution or medication provides immediate access to the vascular system. This is a benefit of administering solutions or medications via this route, but it can also present a risk. Therefore, it is critical to ensure that the primary health care provider's prescriptions are checked carefully and the correct solution or medication is administered as prescribed. Always follow the six rights for medication administration.

References: Ignatavicius, D., et al. (2021). *Medical-surgical nursing: Concepts for interprofessional collaborative care* (10th ed., p. 279). Elsevier; Potter, P., et al. (2021). *Fundamentals of nursing* (10th ed., pp. 333–335). Elsevier.

❖ **192.** A client who received an implanted port for intermittent chemotherapy says, "I'm not sure if I can handle having a tube coming out of me. What will my friends think?" Which action would the nurse implement **first**?
1. Show client various central line catheters.
2. Assure client that friends will understand.
3. Explain that implanted ports are subcutaneous and not visible.
4. Notify the primary health care provider of client's concerns.

Level of Cognitive Ability: Applying
Client Needs: Psychosocial Integrity
Clinical Judgment/Cognitive Skills: Take Action
Integrated Process: Clinical Judgment/Nursing Process/Implementation
Content Area: Adult Health: Oncology
Health Problems: Mental Health: Coping
Priority Concepts: Anxiety; Stress and Coping

Answer: 3
Rationale: An implanted port is subcutaneous; it is not visible, and it has no external tubing. Tubing is used when an intravenous line is connected, and the port is accessed for therapy. The remaining options do not correct the client's confusion about the implanted port. Notifying the provider is not indicated. Inquiring about the client's friends is a reasonable response, but it can also provide false hope that the friends will be accepting. In addition, the nurse is likely to cause more anxiety and concern by providing information about the catheter's subcutaneous location. Showing various central line catheters is unlikely to be beneficial because the client will not be using them; in addition, this can heighten client anxiety and concerns.
Test-Taking Strategy: Note the strategic word, *first*. Also note the subject, a client who received an implanted port for intermittent chemotherapy and that the client is concerned. Noting the words *not visible* in option 3 will direct you to this option.
Priority Nursing Tip: Antineoplastic medication causes the rapid destruction of cells, resulting in the release of uric acid. Allopurinol may be prescribed to lower the serum uric acid level.
Reference: Ignatavicius, D., et al. (2021). *Medical-surgical nursing: Concepts for interprofessional collaborative care* (10th ed., pp. 284–285). Elsevier.

193. A postoperative client displays signs of anxiety when the nurse explains that the intravenous (IV) line will need to be discontinued as a result of an infiltration. Which appropriate statement would the nurse make to the client?
1. "This is usually a painless experience. It is nothing to worry about."
2. "I'm sure it will be a real relief for you just as soon as I discontinue this IV for good."
3. "Just relax and take a deep breath. This procedure will not take long, and it will be over soon."
4. "I can see that you're anxious. Removal of the IV shouldn't be painful, but the IV will need to be restarted in another location."

Level of Cognitive Ability: Applying
Client Needs: Psychosocial Integrity
Clinical Judgment/Cognitive Skills: Take Action
Integrated Process: Clinical Judgment/Nursing Process/Implementation
Content Area: Foundations of Care: Communication
Health Problems: Mental Health: Anxiety
Priority Concepts: Anxiety; Communication

Answer: 4
Rationale: The correct option addresses the client's anxiety and honestly informs the client that the IV may need to be restarted. This option uses the therapeutic technique of giving information, and it also acknowledges the client's feelings. Although discontinuing an IV is a painless experience, it is not therapeutic to tell a client not to worry. Option 2 does not acknowledge the client's feelings, and it does not tell the client that an infiltrated IV may need to be restarted. Option 3 does not address the client's feelings.
Test-Taking Strategy: Use therapeutic communication techniques, and recall that an infiltrated IV may need to be restarted. This will direct you to the correct option. In addition, note that the correct option acknowledges the client's feelings.
Priority Nursing Tip: The nurse needs to avoid venipuncture and placing an intravenous line over an area of flexion to prevent infiltration.
Reference: Potter, P., et al. (2021). *Fundamentals of nursing* (10th ed., pp. 333–335, 1006). Elsevier.

❖ **194.** A client has an initial positive result of an enzyme-linked immunosorbent assay (ELISA) test for human immunodeficiency virus (HIV). The client begins to cry and asks the nurse what this means. Which knowledge would the nurse use to provide support to the client?

1. Client is HIV positive, but client's CD4 cell count is high.
2. Client is HIV positive, but the disease has been detected early.
3. There are occasional false-positive readings with this test; results can be verified by repeating it one more time.
4. False-positive results can occur, and more testing is needed before diagnosing client as being HIV positive.

Level of Cognitive Ability: Understanding
Client Needs: Psychosocial Integrity
Clinical Judgment/Cognitive Skills: Generate Solutions
Integrated Process: Clinical Judgment/Nursing Process/Planning
Content Area: Adult Health: Immune
Health Problems: Mental Health: Coping
Priority Concepts: Patient Education; Stress and Coping

Answer: 4
Rationale: If the client tests positive for HIV with the ELISA test, the test is repeated because of the potential for a false-positive result (e.g., from a recent influenza or hepatitis B vaccine) or a false-negative result if drawn too early after infection. If the test is positive a second time, the Western blot (a more specific test) is done to confirm the finding. The client is not diagnosed as HIV positive unless the Western blot is positive. Some laboratories also run the Western blot a second time with a new specimen before making a final determination.
Test-Taking Strategy: Focus on the subject, the procedure for HIV testing and an affirmative diagnosis. Use knowledge about these procedures and recall that, if the client tests positive for HIV with the ELISA test, the test is repeated because of the potential for a false-positive result.
Priority Nursing Tip: Acquired immunodeficiency syndrome (AIDS) is a viral disease caused by HIV.
Reference: Ignatavicius, D., et al. (2021). *Medical-surgical nursing: Concepts for interprofessional collaborative care.* (10th ed., p. 335). Elsevier.

195. When the nurse performs an assessment on a client who is suicidal, which question is the **most appropriate** for the nurse to ask?

1. "Do you have a death wish?"
2. "Do you wish your life was over?"
3. "Do you ever think about ending it all?"
4. "Do you have any thoughts of killing yourself?"

Level of Cognitive Ability: Applying
Client Needs: Psychosocial Integrity
Clinical Judgment/Cognitive Skills: Take Action
Integrated Process: Clinical Judgment/Nursing Process/Assessment
Content Area: Mental Health
Health Problems: Mental Health: Suicide
Priority Concepts: Mood and Affect; Safety

Answer: 4
Rationale: A lethality assessment requires direct communication between the client and the nurse concerning the client's intent. It is important to provide a question that is directly related to lethality. Euphemisms need to be avoided.
Test-Taking Strategy: Note the strategic words, *most appropriate.* Note the relationship between the word *suicidal* in the question and *killing* in the correct option. Although the remaining options infer suicidal intent, the correct option is the most direct.
Priority Nursing Tip: All suicidal behavior is serious regardless of the intent. Suicidal ideation requires constant attention and typically one-on-one observation. The client with a plan must be placed on suicide precautions.
Reference: Varcarolis, E., & Fosbre, C. (2021). *Essentials of psychiatric mental health nursing: A communication approach to evidence-based care* (4th ed., p. 370). Elsevier.

❖ **196.** A client diagnosed with cancer of the bladder is fearful of the potential outcomes of an upcoming cystectomy and urinary diversion. Which statement made to the nurse indicates the client's fear?
1. "I wish I'd never gone to the doctor at all."
2. "I'm so afraid that I won't live through all this."
3. "I'll never feel like myself if I can't go to the bathroom normally."
4. "What if I have no help at home after going through this awful surgery?"

Level of Cognitive Ability: Analyzing
Client Needs: Psychosocial Integrity
Clinical Judgment/Cognitive Skills: Analyze Cues
Integrated Process: Clinical Judgment/Nursing Process/Analysis
Content Area: Adult Health: Oncology
Health Problems: Mental Health: Anxiety
Priority Concepts: Anxiety; Stress and Coping

Answer: 2
Rationale: For fear to be an actual problem, the client must be able to identify the object of fear. In this question, the client is expressing a fear of an uncertain outcome related to cancer and possibly a fear of death. Option 1 is vague and nonspecific. Option 3 reflects a negative self-image. The statement in option 4 reflects potential trouble at home after surgery.
Test-Taking Strategy: Note the subject, client fear related to upcoming cystectomy and urinary diversion surgery. Option 1 is a general statement and should be eliminated first. Options 3 and 4 focus on the client after surgery, but they do not contain statements about an uncertain outcome. In option 2, the client expresses a fear of dying after enduring the ordeal of surgery.
Priority Nursing Tip: The nurse needs to monitor urinary output closely after bladder surgery. The primary health care provider's prescriptions and agency policy regarding bladder irrigation should be followed.
References: Ignatavicius, D., et al. (2021). *Medical-surgical nursing: Concepts for interprofessional collaborative care* (10th ed., pp. 1350–1351). Elsevier; Potter, P., et al. (2021). *Fundamentals of nursing* (10th ed., p. 1068). Elsevier.

197. A client diagnosed with nephrotic syndrome asks the nurse, "Why should I even bother trying to control my diet and the edema? It doesn't really matter what I do if I can never get rid of this kidney problem, anyway!" Which would the nurse identify as the **most appropriate** concern for this client?
1. Anxiety
2. Powerlessness
3. Difficulty coping
4. Negative self-image

Level of Cognitive Ability: Analyzing
Client Needs: Psychosocial Integrity
Clinical Judgment/Cognitive Skills: Analyze Cues
Integrated Process: Clinical Judgment/Nursing Process/Analysis
Content Area: Adult Health: Renal and Urinary
Health Problems: Mental Health: Coping
Priority Concepts: Anxiety; Stress and Coping

Answer: 2
Rationale: Powerlessness is present when the client believes that personal actions will not affect an outcome in any significant way. Because nephrotic syndrome is progressive, the client may feel that personal actions may not affect the disease process. Anxiety is appropriate when the client has a feeling of unease with a vague or undefined source. Difficulty coping occurs when the client has impaired adaptive abilities or behaviors with regard to meeting expected demands or roles. Negative self-image is when there is an alteration in the way that the client perceives their body image.
Test-Taking Strategy: Note the strategic words, *most appropriate*. Focus on the subject, nephrotic syndrome and the client's statement, "It doesn't really matter what I do." This implies that the client feels a lack of control over the situation, and it will direct you to the correct option.
Priority Nursing Tip: The classic manifestations of nephrotic syndrome are massive proteinuria, hypoalbuminemia, and edema.
Reference: Lewis, S., et al. (2020). *Medical-surgical nursing: Assessment and management of clinical problems* (11th ed., pp. 136, 1034–1035). Elsevier.

❖ **198.** A client diagnosed with renal cell carcinoma of the left kidney is scheduled for a nephrectomy. The right kidney appears to be normal at this time. The client is anxious about whether dialysis will ultimately be a necessity. Which information would the nurse **initially** provide to the client?

1. It is very likely that client will need dialysis within 5 to 10 years.
2. One kidney is adequate to meet the needs of the body, as long as it has normal function.
3. There is absolutely no chance of client needing dialysis because of the nature of the surgery.
4. Dialysis could become likely, but it depends on how well client complies with fluid restriction after surgery.

Level of Cognitive Ability: Applying
Client Needs: Psychosocial Integrity
Clinical Judgment/Cognitive Skills: Take Action
Integrated Process: Clinical Judgment/Nursing Process/Implementation
Content Area: Adult Health: Oncology
Health Problems: Mental Health: Anxiety
Priority Concepts: Patient Education; Stress and Coping

Answer: 2

Rationale: Fears about having only one functioning kidney are common among clients who must undergo nephrectomy for renal cancer. These clients need emotional support and reassurance that the remaining kidney will be able to fully meet the body's metabolic needs as long as it has normal function. This information supports that the remaining options are inaccurate.

Test-Taking Strategy: Note the strategic word, *initially*. Focus on the subject, a client who is anxious about an upcoming nephrectomy. Eliminate option 3 because of the words *absolutely no chance*. Knowing that there is no need for fluid restriction with a functioning kidney guides you to eliminate option 4 next. From the remaining options, recalling that an individual can donate a kidney without adverse consequences or the need for dialysis will direct you to option 2.

Priority Nursing Tip: For the client who has undergone a nephrectomy, the nurse needs to monitor specifically for abdominal distention, decreases in urinary output, and alterations in level of consciousness as signs of bleeding; the nurse needs to also check the bed linens under the client for bleeding.

Reference: Lewis, S., et al. (2020). *Medical-surgical nursing: Assessment and management of clinical problems* (11th ed., pp. 1082–1083). Elsevier.

---

199. A charge nurse is supervising a new nurse who is providing care to a client diagnosed with end-stage heart failure. The client is withdrawn and reluctant to talk and shows little interest in participating in hygienic care or activities. Which statement, if made by the new nurse to the client, indicates that the new nurse has a **need for teaching** regarding the use of therapeutic communication techniques?

1. "What are your feelings right now?"
2. "Why don't you feel like getting up for your bath?"
3. "These dreams you mentioned, what are they like?"
4. "Many clients with end-stage heart failure fear death."

Level of Cognitive Ability: Evaluating
Client Needs: Psychosocial Integrity
Clinical Judgment/Cognitive Skills: Evaluate Outcomes
Integrated Process: Clinical Judgment; Nursing Process/Evaluation
Content Area: Foundations of Care: Communication
Health Problems: Adult Health: Cardiovascular: Heart Failure
Priority Concepts: Communication; Leadership

Answer: 2

Rationale: When the nurse asks a "why" question of the client, the nurse is requesting an explanation for feelings and behaviors when the client may not know the reason. Requesting an explanation is a nontherapeutic communication technique. In option 1, the nurse is encouraging the verbalization of emotions or feelings, which is a therapeutic communication technique. In option 3, the nurse is using the therapeutic communication technique of exploring, which involves asking the client to describe something in more detail or to discuss it more fully. In option 4, the nurse is using the therapeutic communication technique of giving information. Identifying the common fear of death among clients with end-stage heart failure may encourage the client to voice concerns.

Test-Taking Strategy: Note the strategic words, *need for teaching*. These words indicate a negative event query and ask you to select an option that is an incorrect statement made by the student. Select the option that is a block to communication. The word *why* in option 2 should guide you to this option.

Priority Nursing Tip: Communication includes verbal and nonverbal expression.

References: Lewis, S., et al. (2020). *Medical-surgical nursing: Assessment and management of clinical problems* (11th ed., p. 742). Elsevier; Potter, P., et al. (2021). *Fundamentals of nursing.* (10th ed., pp. 333–335). Elsevier.

❖ **200.** The nurse is caring for a client diagnosed with acute pulmonary edema. Which psychosocial strategy would the nurse plan to incorporate into the care of the client?
1. Reducing anxiety
2. Increasing fluid volume
3. Decreasing cardiac output
4. Promoting a positive body image

Level of Cognitive Ability: Applying
Client Needs: Psychosocial Integrity
Clinical Judgment/Cognitive Skills: Generate Solutions
Integrated Process: Clinical Judgment/Nursing Process/Planning
Content Area: Adult Health: Cardiovascular
Health Problems: Mental Health: Anxiety
Priority Concepts: Clinical Judgment; Anxiety

Answer: 1
Rationale: Reducing anxiety will help the client during treatment to increase cardiac output and decrease fluid volume. When cardiac output falls as a result of acute pulmonary edema, the sympathetic nervous system is stimulated. Stimulation of the sympathetic nervous system results in the fight-or-flight reaction, which further impairs cardiac function. A disturbed body image is not a common problem among clients with acute pulmonary edema.
Test-Taking Strategy: Focus on the subject, a psychosocial strategy for the client with acute pulmonary edema. Thinking about the physiologic occurrences of this condition will assist you with eliminating the remaining options. In addition, recalling that severe dyspnea occurs will assist with directing you to the correct option.
Priority Nursing Tip: If pulmonary edema occurs, the initial nursing action is to place the client in a high-Fowler's position.
Reference: Lewis, S., et al. (2020). *Medical-surgical nursing: Assessment and management of clinical problems* (11th ed., pp. 532, 1596). Elsevier.

201. A client diagnosed with acute kidney injury is having trouble remembering information and instructions as a result of altered laboratory values. Which actions would the nurse take when communicating with this client? **Select all that apply.**
❑ 1. Give simple, clear directions.
❑ 2. Include the family in discussions related to care.
❑ 3. Explain treatments using understandable language.
❑ 4. Explain the possibility of hemodialysis in simple terms.
❑ 5. Give thorough and complete explanations of treatment options.

Level of Cognitive Ability: Applying
Client Needs: Psychosocial Integrity
Clinical Judgment/Cognitive Skills: Take Action
Integrated Process: Clinical Judgment/Nursing Process/Implementation
Content Area: Foundations of Care: Communication
Health Problems: Mental Health: Anxiety
Priority Concepts: Cognition; Communication

Answer: 1, 2, 3, 4
Rationale: The client with acute kidney injury may have difficulty remembering information and instructions because of anxiety and altered laboratory values. Communications need to be clear, simple, and understandable. The family is included whenever possible. Information about treatment needs to be explained using understandable language. Thorough and complete explanations may be confusing and will not be understandable for the client.
Test-Taking Strategy: Focus on the subject, communicating with the client with acute kidney injury who is experiencing an alteration in cognitive function. Recalling the basic principles of effective communication would lead you to recognize that the correct options are helpful for maintaining effective communication.
Priority Nursing Tip: The signs and symptoms of acute kidney injury are primarily caused by the retention of nitrogenous wastes, the retention of fluids, and the inability of the kidneys to regulate electrolytes.
Reference: Lewis, S., et al. (2020). *Medical-surgical nursing: Assessment and management of clinical problems* (11th ed., p. 1064). Elsevier.

❖ **202.** The rehabilitation nurse witnessed a postoperative client who had a coronary artery bypass graft and the client's spouse arguing after a rehabilitation session. Which would be the **most appropriate** therapeutic statement for the nurse to make to identify the feelings of the client?
  1. "You seem upset."
  2. "Oh, don't let this get you down."
  3. "It will seem better tomorrow. Now smile."
  4. "You shouldn't get upset. It'll affect your heart."

Level of Cognitive Ability: Applying
Client Needs: Psychosocial Integrity
Clinical Judgment/Cognitive Skills: Take Action
Integrated Process: Communication and Documentation
Content Area: Foundations of Care: Communication
Health Problems: Adult Health: Cardiovascular: Coronary Artery Disease
Priority Concepts: Clinical Judgment; Communication

Answer: 1
Rationale: Acknowledging the client's feelings without inserting your own values or judgments is a method of therapeutic communication. Therapeutic communication techniques assist with the flow of communication, and they always focus on the client. Option 1 is an open-ended statement that allows the client to verbalize, which gives the nurse a direction or clarification of the client's true feelings. The remaining options do not encourage verbalization by the client.
Test-Taking Strategy: Note the strategic words, *most appropriate*. Use therapeutic communication techniques. Focusing on the subject of identifying the feelings of the client will direct you to the correct option.
Priority Nursing Tip: After arterial revascularization, the nurse would monitor for a sharp increase in pain because pain is frequently the first indicator of postoperative graft occlusion. If signs of graft occlusion occur, notify the primary health care provider immediately.
References: Ignatavicius, D., et al. (2021). *Medical-surgical nursing: Concepts for interprofessional collaborative care* (10th ed., pp. 771–772). Elsevier; Potter, P., et al. (2021). *Fundamentals of nursing* (10th ed., pp. 333–335). Elsevier.

203. The nurse is monitoring the neurologic status of a client with dementia and assessing the limbic system. Which would the nurse assess to yield the **best** information about this area of functioning?
  1. Judgment
  2. Emotions
  3. Consciousness
  4. Eye movements

Level of Cognitive Ability: Applying
Client Needs: Psychosocial Integrity
Clinical Judgment/Cognitive Skills: Recognize Cues
Integrated Process: Clinical Judgment/Nursing Process/Assessment
Content Area: Health Assessment/Physical Exam: Neurologic
Health Problems: Mental Health: Neurocognitive Impairment
Priority Concepts: Intracranial Regulation; Mood and Affect

Answer: 2
Rationale: Feelings and emotions are part of the role of the limbic system. Eye movements are under the control of cranial nerves III, IV, and VI. The level of consciousness is controlled by the reticular activating system. Insight, judgment, and planning are part of the function of the frontal lobe.
Test-Taking Strategy: Note the strategic word, *best*. Also focus on the subject, assessment of the limbic system. Use knowledge of anatomy and physiology concepts related to the neurologic system to answer correctly. Remember, feelings and emotions are part of the role of the limbic system.
Priority Nursing Tip: Clients with dementia are typically dependent on others. Individuals most at risk for abuse include those who are dependent because of their immobility or altered mental status.
Reference: Lewis, S., et al. (2020). *Medical-surgical nursing: Assessment and management of clinical problems* (11th ed., p. 78). Elsevier.

❖ **204.** A client is admitted to the mental health unit with a diagnosis of panic disorder. The nurse would check the primary health care provider's prescription sheet anticipating that which medication, a benzodiazepine, was prescribed?
1. Doxepin
2. Alprazolam
3. Imipramine
4. Bupropion

Level of Cognitive Ability: Analyzing
Client Needs: Psychosocial Integrity
Clinical Judgment/Cognitive Skills: Generate Solutions
Integrated Process: Clinical Judgment/Nursing Process/Planning
Content Area: Pharmacology: Psychotherapeutics: Barbiturates and Sedative-Hypnotics
Health Problems: Mental Health: Anxiety Disorder
Priority Concepts: Anxiety; Safety

Answer: 2
Rationale: Alprazolam, which is a benzodiazepine antianxiety agent, depresses the central nervous system (CNS) and induces relaxation in clients with panic disorders. The medications mentioned in the remaining options are classified as antidepressants, and they act by stimulating the CNS to elevate mood.
Test-Taking Strategy: Focus on the subject, a benzodiazepine, and use knowledge regarding panic disorders and the classification of the medications identified in the options to answer this question. Eliminate options that are comparable or alike; all are antidepressants.
Priority Nursing Tip: The immediate nursing action for a client with anxiety is to decrease stimuli in the environment and provide a calm and quiet environment.
Reference: Varcarolis, E., & Fosbre, C. (2021). *Essentials of psychiatric mental health nursing: A communication approach to evidence-based care* (4th ed., p. 153). Elsevier.

205. A client diagnosed with empyema is to undergo decortication to remove inflamed tissue, pus, and debris. On the basis of which understanding about this procedure would the nurse offer emotional support to the client?
1. This problem may decrease client's life expectancy.
2. Client is likely to be in excruciating pain after surgery.
3. Client will probably have chronic dyspnea after the surgery.
4. Chest tubes will be in place after surgery, and the healing process is slow.

Level of Cognitive Ability: Understanding
Client Needs: Psychosocial Integrity
Clinical Judgment/Cognitive Skills: Generate Solutions
Integrated Process: Clinical Judgment/Nursing Process/Planning
Content Area: Adult Health: Respiratory
Health Problems: Mental Health: Coping
Priority Concepts: Clinical Judgment; Stress and Coping

Answer: 4
Rationale: The client undergoing decortication to treat empyema needs ongoing support from the nurse. This is especially true because the client will have chest tubes in place after surgery, and these must remain until the former pus-filled space is completely obliterated. This may take some time, and it may be discouraging to the client. Progress is monitored by chest x-ray. This information supports that the remaining options are not accurate.
Test-Taking Strategy: Focus on the subject, a client with empyema who will undergo decortication and the need for emotional support. Recalling that chest tubes are a requirement after this surgery will assist in the selection of the correct option.
Priority Nursing Tip: If the chest tube is pulled out of the chest accidentally, pinch the skin opening together, apply an occlusive sterile dressing, cover the dressing with overlapping pieces of 2-inch tape, and call the primary health care provider immediately.
Reference: Ignatavicius, D., et al. (2021). *Medical-surgical nursing: Concepts for interprofessional collaborative care* (10th ed., pp. 561, 574–575). Elsevier.

❖ **206.** A client who has never been hospitalized before is sharing a hospital room with a roommate. The client is anxious and having trouble initiating a stream of urine. Knowing that there is no pathologic reason for this difficulty, which nursing interventions would be included when assisting the client? **Select all that apply.**
- ❑ 1. Catheterizing client
- ❑ 2. Running tap water in the sink
- ❑ 3. Assisting client to a commode behind a closed curtain
- ❑ 4. Instructing client to pour warm water over the perineum
- ❑ 5. Closing the bathroom door and instructing client to pull the call bell when done

Level of Cognitive Ability: Applying
Client Needs: Psychosocial Integrity
Clinical Judgment/Cognitive Skills: Generate Solutions
Integrated Process: Clinical Judgment/Nursing Process/Planning
Content Area: Skills: Elimination
Health Problems: Mental Health: Anxiety
Priority Concepts: Clinical Judgment; Elimination

Answer: 2, 4, 5
Rationale: A lack of privacy is a key issue that may inhibit the ability of the client to void in the absence of known pathology. Using a commode behind a curtain may inhibit voiding for some individuals, especially with a roommate present. The use of a bathroom is preferable, and this may be supplemented with the use of running water or pouring water over the perineum, as needed. Catheterization is not a nursing intervention and presents a risk of infection. If noninvasive techniques do not work, then the primary health care provider may prescribe that the client be catheterized.
Test-Taking Strategy: Focus on the subject, nursing interventions for a client who is having difficulty voiding. Also, think about the issue related to decreased privacy and its effects on elimination.
Priority Nursing Tip: To aid in initiating the stream of urination, the client needs to be taught to increase ambulation, increase fluid intake unless contraindicated, pour warm water over the perineum, or allow the client to hear running water to promote voiding.
Reference: Potter, P., et al. (2021). *Fundamentals of nursing* (10th ed., p. 1151). Elsevier.

207. The client states to the nurse, "I'm scheduled for outpatient surgery, but I live alone and my only child lives 300 miles away. I'm afraid. What happens if something goes wrong after I go home?" Which statement by the nurse is the **most** therapeutic?
1. "Don't worry about the details. This procedure is done all the time and generally without any problems. You'll be fine!"
2. "They say managed care is no care! Get an alarm system so that if you fall, it will alert someone. If necessary, I'll come."
3. "Your concern is well voiced. I advise you to call your child and insist that your child come home immediately! You can't be too careful."
4. "You seem very concerned about going home without help. Have you discussed your concerns with both your surgeon and your family?"

Level of Cognitive Ability: Applying
Client Needs: Psychosocial Integrity
Clinical Judgment/Cognitive Skills: Take Action
Integrated Process: Clinical Judgment/Nursing Process/Implementation
Content Area: Foundations of Care: Communication
Health Problems: Mental Health: Anxiety Disorder
Priority Concepts: Communication; Stress and Coping

Answer: 4
Rationale: The client has verbalized concerns. In option 4 the nurse uses reflection to direct the client's feelings and concerns. In option 1 the nurse provides false reassurance and then minimizes the client's concerns. In option 2 the nurse is ventilating the nurse's own anger, frustration, and powerlessness. In addition, the nurse is trying to problem-solve for the client but is overly controlling and takes the decision-making out of the client's hands. In option 3, the nurse is projecting the client's own fears, and the problem-solving suggested by the nurse will increase fear and anxiety in the client.
Test-Taking Strategy: Note the strategic word, *most.* Use therapeutic communication techniques. Remember that the priority is to address the client's feelings, and the correct option is the only option that does this.
Priority Nursing Tip: Communication with the client needs to be goal directed and based on the client's concerns.
Reference: Varcarolis, E., & Fosbre, C. (2021). *Essentials of psychiatric mental health nursing: A communication approach to evidence-based care* (4th ed., pp. 93–95). Elsevier.

❖ **208.** During the nursing assessment, the client states, "My surgeon just told me that my cancer has spread, and I have less than 6 months to live." Which nursing response would be the **most** therapeutic?
1. "I am sorry. Would you like to discuss this with me some more?"
2. "I am sorry. There are no easy answers in times like this, are there?"
3. "I hope you'll focus on the fact that your doctor says you have 6 months to live and that you'll think of how you'd like to live."
4. "I know it seems desperate, but there have been a lot of breakthroughs. Something might come along in a month or so to change your status drastically."

Level of Cognitive Ability: Applying
Client Needs: Psychosocial Integrity
Clinical Judgment/Cognitive Skills: Take Action
Integrated Process: Clinical Judgment/Nursing Process/Implementation
Content Area: Adult Health: Oncology
Health Problems: Mental Health: Coping
Priority Concepts: Communication; Stress and Coping

Answer: 1
Rationale: The client has received very distressing news and is most likely still experiencing shock and denial. In option 1 the nurse invites the client to ventilate feelings. Option 2 is social and expresses the nurse's feelings rather than the client's feelings. Option 3 is patronizing and stereotypical. Option 4 provides social communication and false hope.
Test-Taking Strategy: Note the strategic word, *most.* Use therapeutic communication techniques. Note that option 1 provides the opportunity for the client to express feelings. Remember to focus on the client's feelings.
Priority Nursing Tip: The nurse should monitor the client's progression through the stages of grieving. Not all clients will progress in the same manner and may progress from one stage to another in no logical order.
Reference: Potter, P., et al. (2021). *Fundamentals of nursing* (10th ed., pp. 333–335). Elsevier.

209. A client with an endotracheal tube gets easily frustrated when trying to communicate personal needs to the nurse. Which method for communication would the nurse determine may be the **best** for the client?
1. Use a picture or word board.
2. Have the family interpret needs.
3. Devise a system of hand signals.
4. Use a pad of paper and a pencil.

Level of Cognitive Ability: Applying
Client Needs: Psychosocial Integrity
Clinical Judgment/Cognitive Skills: Generate Solutions
Integrated Process: Clinical Judgment/Nursing Process/Planning
Content Area: Foundations of Care: Communication
Health Problems: Mental Health: Coping
Priority Concepts: Clinical Judgment; Communication

Answer: 1
Rationale: The client with an endotracheal tube in place cannot speak, so the nurse devises an alternative communication system with the client. The use of a picture or word board is the simplest method of communication because it requires only pointing at the word or object. The family does not need to bear the burden of communicating the client's needs, and they may not understand the client either. The use of hand signals may not be a reliable method because it may not meet all needs, and it is subject to misinterpretation. A pad of paper and a pencil is an acceptable alternative, but it requires more client effort and time.
Test-Taking Strategy: Note the strategic word, *best.* Options 3 and 4 are not the *best,* and they are therefore eliminated first. Because the family may not necessarily know what the client is trying to communicate, option 2 could cause added frustration for the client.
Priority Nursing Tip: A resuscitation (Ambu) bag must be kept at the bedside of a client with an endotracheal tube or a tracheostomy tube at all times.
Reference: Ignatavicius, D., et al. (2021). *Medical-surgical nursing: Concepts for interprofessional collaborative care* (10th ed., pp. 598, 602). Elsevier.

❖ **210.** The home care nurse visits a client who is receiving total parenteral nutrition, and the client states, "I really miss eating dinner with my family." Which statement from the nurse is the **most** therapeutic?
  1. "What you are feeling is very common."
  2. "Tell me more about your family dinners."
  3. "In a few weeks, you may be allowed to eat."
  4. "You can sit down to dinner even if you do not eat."

Level of Cognitive Ability: Applying
Client Needs: Psychosocial Integrity
Clinical Judgment/Cognitive Skills: Take Action
Integrated Process: Communication and Documentation
Content Area: Skills: Nutrition
Health Problems: Adult Health: Gastrointestinal: Nutrition/Malabsorption Problems
Priority Concepts: Communication; Nutrition

Answer: 2
Rationale: The nurse assists the client with expressing feelings and dealing with the aspects of illness and treatment by clarifying and helping the client to focus on and explore concerns. In option 1 the nurse characterizes and classifies the feelings on the basis of an assumption. Option 3 provides false hope, and option 4 blocks communication by giving advice.
Test-Taking Strategy: Note the strategic word, *most*. Use therapeutic communication techniques. It is important that the nurse validate that the client has concerns and allow them to be discussed. The other options do not allow for the communication exchange about concerns. This will direct you to option 2.
Priority Nursing Tip: The delivery of hypertonic solutions into peripheral veins can cause sclerosis, phlebitis, or swelling, and the nurse needs to monitor for these complications.
Reference: Potter, P., et al. (2021). *Fundamentals of nursing* (10th ed., pp. 333–335, 1122). Elsevier.

211. A client with a diagnosis of depression has been prescribed imipramine. The nurse notifies the primary health care provider if which adverse effect to the medication is noted?
  1. Increased appetite
  2. Increased drowsiness
  3. Reported decrease in anxiety
  4. Increased sense of well-being

Level of Cognitive Ability: Analyzing
Client Needs: Psychosocial Integrity
Clinical Judgment/Cognitive Skills: Take Action
Integrated Process: Clinical Judgment/Nursing Process/Implementation
Content Area: Pharmacology: Psychotherapeutics: Tricyclic Antidepressants
Health Problems: Mental Health: Mood Disorders
Priority Concepts: Collaboration; Safety

Answer: 2
Rationale: Imipramine is a tricyclic antidepressant that is used to treat various forms of depression and anxiety. The client is also often in psychotherapy while prescribed this medication. Adverse effects to report to the primary health care provider include drowsiness, lethargy, and fatigue. Expected effects of the medication include an increased appetite and time spent sleeping, a reduced sense of anxiety, and an improved sense of well-being.
Test-Taking Strategy: Focus on the subject, an adverse effect to imipramine. Recall that this medication is an antidepressant. Options 1, 3, and 4 seem to be reasonable positive responses to this medication.
Priority Nursing Tip: The nurse needs to monitor a depressed client closely for signs of suicidal ideation. If the client presents with increased energy, the nurse needs to monitor the client closely because it could mean that the client now has the energy to perform the suicidal act.
Reference: Varcarolis, E., & Fosbre, C. (2021). *Essentials of psychiatric mental health nursing: A communication approach to evidence-based care* (4th ed., pp. 218–219). Elsevier.

❖ **212.** A client who is to undergo thoracentesis is afraid of not being able to tolerate the procedure. The nurse interprets that the client needs honest support and reassurance that is **best** accomplished with which information?

  1. "I'll be right by your side, but the procedure will be totally painless as long as you don't move."
  2. "The procedure only takes 1 to 2 minutes, so you might try to get through it by mentally counting up to 120."
  3. "The needle hurts when it goes in, and you must remain still. I'll stay with you throughout the entire procedure and help you hold your position."
  4. "The needle is a little bit uncomfortable going in, but this is controlled by rhythmically breathing in and out. I'll be with you to coach your breathing."

Level of Cognitive Ability: Applying
Client Needs: Psychosocial Integrity
Clinical Judgment/Cognitive Skills: Take Action
Integrated Process: Clinical Judgment/Nursing Process/Implementation
Content Area: Foundations of Care: Diagnostic Tests
Health Problems: Mental Health: Coping
Priority Concepts: Caregiving; Communication

Answer: 3
Rationale: The needle insertion for thoracentesis is painful for the client. The nurse tells the client how important it is to remain still during the procedure so that the needle does not injure visceral pleura or lung tissue. The nurse reassures the client during the procedure and helps the client hold the proper position. This information supports that the remaining options are inaccurate statements.
Test-Taking Strategy: Note the strategic word, *best*, and focus on the subject, thoracentesis. Recalling that the client must remain still during the procedure helps you eliminate option 4 first. Knowing that the procedure may be painful for the client and that it takes longer than 1 to 2 minutes helps you eliminate options 1 and 2.
Priority Nursing Tip: The client undergoing thoracentesis needs to be positioned sitting upright with the arms and shoulders supported by a table or lying in bed toward the affected side with the head of the bed elevated.
Reference: Pagana, K., Pagana, T., & Pagana, T. N. (2021). *Mosby's Diagnostic and laboratory test reference* (15th ed., pp. 855, 857–858). Elsevier.

213. A client diagnosed with chronic respiratory failure is dyspneic. The client becomes anxious, which worsens the feelings of dyspnea. The nurse teaches the client which method to **best** interrupt the dyspnea–anxiety–dyspnea cycle?

  1. Guided imagery and limiting fluids
  2. Relaxation and breathing techniques
  3. Biofeedback and coughing techniques
  4. Distraction and increased dietary carbohydrates

Level of Cognitive Ability: Applying
Client Needs: Psychosocial Integrity
Clinical Judgment/Cognitive Skills: Generate Solutions
Integrated Process: Clinical Judgment/Teaching and Learning
Content Area: Adult Health: Respiratory
Health Problems: Mental Health: Anxiety Disorder
Priority Concepts: Client Education; Stress

Answer: 2
Rationale: The anxious client with dyspnea needs to be taught interventions to decrease anxiety, which include relaxation, biofeedback, guided imagery, and distraction. This will stop the escalation of feelings of anxiety and dyspnea. The dyspnea can be further controlled by teaching the client breathing techniques, which include pursed lip and diaphragmatic breathing. Coughing techniques are useful, but breathing techniques are more effective. Limiting fluids will thicken secretions, and increased dietary carbohydrates will increase the production of carbon dioxide by the body.
Test-Taking Strategy: Focus on the subject, relieving anxiety and dyspnea, and note the strategic word, *best*. Limiting fluids and increasing carbohydrates are contraindicated and therefore eliminated. From the remaining options, recall that breathing techniques are more effective than coughing techniques. This will direct you to option 2.
Priority Nursing Tip: Clients with a respiratory disorder need to be positioned with the head of the bed elevated.
Reference: Ignatavicius, D., et al. (2021). *Medical-surgical nursing: Concepts for interprofessional collaborative care* (10th ed., pp. 483, 594). Elsevier.

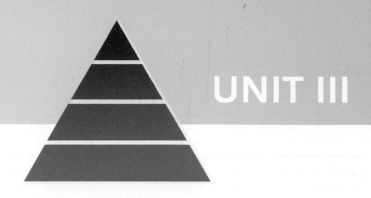

Integrated Processes

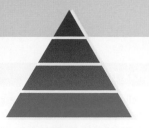

CHAPTER 10

Integrated Processes and the NCLEX-RN® Test Plan

In the new test plan implemented in April 2023, the National Council of State Boards of Nursing (NCSBN) identified a test plan framework based on Client Needs. This framework was selected based on the assessment of the findings in a practice analysis study of newly licensed registered nurses in the United States. This study identified the nursing activities performed by entry-level nurses across all settings for all clients. The NCSBN identified four major categories of Client Needs. These categories—Physiological Integrity, Safe and Effective Care Environment, Health Promotion and Maintenance, and Psychosocial Integrity—are described in Chapter 5.

The 2023 NCLEX-RN® test plan also identifies six processes, titled Integrated Processes, that are a foundation to the practice of nursing. These processes are integrated throughout the four major categories of Client Needs and include Caring, Clinical Judgment, Communication and Documentation, Culture and Spirituality, Nursing Process, and Teaching and Learning (Box 10.1).

Caring

Caring is the essence of nursing, and it is basic to any helping relationship. Caring is central to every encounter that the nurse may have with a client. Through caring, the nurse humanizes the client. Treating the client with respect and dignity is a true expression of caring. In the technological environment of health care, emphasizing the client's individuality counteracts any potential process of depersonalization. Caring is an Integrated Process of the test plan for NCLEX-RN, and the NCSBN describes caring as part of the nurse's role in providing encouragement, hope, support, and compassion. The process of caring is integral to all Client Needs components of the test plan.

For the NCLEX-RN, the process of caring is primary. It is very easy to become involved with looking at a question from a technological viewpoint. However, the process of caring

---

BOX 10.1   Integrated Processes

Caring
Clinical Judgment
Communication and Documentation
Culture and Spirituality
Nursing Process
Teaching and Learning

---

must be addressed when reading a test question and when selecting an option. Always address the client's feelings and provide support. Remember that this examination is all about nursing, and nursing is caring (Box 10.2)!

Clinical Judgment

⚠ Clinical judgment is the observed outcome of critical thinking and decision-making (Dickison, Haerling, & Lasater, 2019).

In recent years, heightened attention has been paid to clinical judgment as a means of teaching, learning, and assessment and testing. The Next Generation NCLEX-RN® (NGN) examination requires candidates to demonstrate a higher level of ability in applying clinical judgment in the delivery of client care. The nurse must be able to make sound clinical judgments when caring for a client and with every interaction or encounter. Therefore, the NCSBN has included Clinical Judgment as an Integrated Process of the Test Plan.

The NCSBN has created a Clinical Judgment Measurement Model (NCJMM) that consists of applying six cognitive skills or processes. These include (1) recognizing cues; (2) analyzing cues; (3) prioritizing hypotheses; (4) generating solutions; (5) taking actions; and (6) evaluating outcomes (Dickison, et al., 2019). Refer to Chapter 1, Table 1.1, which provides a description of these six cognitive skills identified in the NCJMM. Box 10.3 illustrates a sample clinical judgment question.

Communication and Documentation

The process of communication occurs as the nurse interacts either verbally or nonverbally with a client. Therapeutic communication techniques are essential to an effective nurse–client relationship. Communication-type test questions are integrated throughout the NCLEX-RN test plan, and they may address a client situation in any health care setting. The NCSBN describes communication as the verbal and nonverbal interactions that occur in the health care environment.

When answering a question on the NCLEX-RN, notice that the use of therapeutic communication techniques indicates a correct option, and the use of nontherapeutic communication techniques indicates an incorrect option. In addition, some

---

BOX 10.2   Caring

A client who has end-stage cancer is admitted to a hospice care facility from home. Which intervention would the nurse implement to address the client's psychosocial needs?
1. Administer total care for the client.
2. Engage the client in social activities.
3. Allow the client to verbalize feelings.
4. Provide pain medication every 4 hours.

Answer: 3

Focus on the subject, meeting psychosocial needs. The client is experiencing loss from two life-changing experiences: the poor prognosis and the loss of control over the environment, independence, and privacy that accompanies admission to a hospice care facility. To meet the client's psychosocial needs, the nurse would promote a therapeutic relationship and allow the client to verbalize feelings. Options 1 and 4 manage physical needs. Although total care may be necessary, it does not address psychosocial needs. Providing pain medication is indicated as part of effective pain management; however, this can interfere with therapeutic communication if the client is too sedated. Engaging the client in social activities is unlikely to effectively meet the client's psychosocial needs relating to loss; it is more likely to assist in diminishing loneliness and isolation.

---

communication-type questions may focus on psychosocial issues or issues related to client anxiety, fears, or concerns. For communication-type questions, always focus on the client's feelings first. If an option reflects the client's feelings, anxiety, or concerns, select that choice (Box 10.4).

Documentation is a critical component of the nurse's responsibilities. The process of documentation serves many purposes; it provides a comprehensive representation of the client's health status and the care given by all members of the interprofessional team. There are many methods of documentation, but the responsibilities surrounding this practice remain the same. The NCSBN describes documentation as the activities associated with the client's medical record that reflect the highest standards of practice and accountability.

When answering a question on the NCLEX-RN test related to documentation, consider the ethical and legal responsibilities related to documentation and the specific guidelines related to both narrative and computerized documentation systems (see Box 10.4).

Culture and Spirituality

Culture can be described as the knowledge, beliefs, and patterns of behavior, ideas, attitudes, values, and norms that are unique to a particular population or group of people. Spirituality is a broad concept that may have different perspectives for individuals. It can relate to religious beliefs and values and to the soul or human spirit rather than to material and physical things. Spirituality is reflected in how a person lives their life and is shown in their values and beliefs. These values and beliefs can directly affect a person's health choices.

Nurses often care for clients who come from ethnic, cultural, religious, or spiritual backgrounds that are different from their own. The nurse is responsible for providing quality care to all members of society and for providing culturally

---

BOX 10.3   Clinical Judgment

The nurse working on an inpatient oncologic medical unit is performing a physical exam on a 62-year-old client diagnosed with metastatic breast cancer. The nurse collects the following client data:
- Client is having difficulty urinating
- 8/10 Persistent lower back pain with sudden onset
- Lumbar vertebrae tender to palpation
- Hand grips unequal
- Bilateral foot drop
- Diminished sensation to sharp and dull stimuli of bilateral lower extremities
- BP: 98/70 mm Hg
- HR: 98 beats per minute and regular
- Respirations: 18 breaths per minute
- SpO_2: 97% on RA
- Temperature: 98.8° F (37.1° C)

Based on the assessment data, complete the following sentence by choosing from the lists of options provided.

The nurse analyzes the assessment data and recognizes that the client **most likely** has _____[Option 1]_____. The **priority** action to ensure client safety is to _____ [Option 2]_____.

Options for 1	Options for 2
cardiac tamponade	contact the oncologist
spinal cord compression	place the client on strict bed rest
superior vena cava syndrome (SVCS)	perform a straight urinary catheterization
syndrome of inappropriate antidiuretic hormone (SIADH)	administer oral oxycodone as needed for back pain

Answer: The nurse analyzes the assessment data and recognizes that the client **most likely** has spinal cord compression. The **priority** action to ensure client safety is to contact the oncologist.

Focus on the data in the case situation and use knowledge of the complications of cancer to assist in interpreting this client data as clinical manifestations of spinal cord compression. Next, think about the seriousness of the condition to determine the action to take. Also, note the strategic words, *most likely* and *priority*. This requires you to determine which option is of the highest importance as it relates to client safety. Remember that spinal cord compression occurs as a result of a tumor eliciting pressure on the spinal cord and can result in severe, persistent back pain with vertebral tenderness. The condition also results in neurologic symptoms, including motor and sensory deficits, as well as symptoms of autonomic dysfunction, such as alterations with urination or defecation. Treatment is targeted at relieving the spinal cord compression by shrinking the tumor, which is done with radiation therapy, high-dose corticosteroids, or possible surgery. Therefore, the priority nursing action is to contact the oncologist so that further evaluation and management can be initiated as soon as possible.

---

competent care. Awareness of and sensitivity to the unique health and illness beliefs and practices of all populations and those of different backgrounds are essential for the delivery of safe and effective care.

BOX 10.4 Communication and Documentation

Communication

A client with myasthenia gravis is having difficulty with the motor aspects of speech. The client has difficulty forming words, and the voice has a nasal tone. The nurse would plan to use which communication technique when working with this client?

1. Encourage the client to speak quickly.
2. Nod continuously while the client is speaking.
3. Repeat what the client has said to verify the message.
4. Engage the client in lengthy discussions to strengthen their voice.

Answer: *3*

Focus on the **information in the question** and the **subject,** an appropriate communication strategy. The client has speech that is nasal in tone because of cranial nerve involvement in the muscles that govern speech. The nurse should listen attentively and verbally verify what the client has said. Other helpful techniques involve asking questions that require a "yes" or "no" response and developing alternative communication methods (e.g., letter board, picture board, pen and paper, flash cards). Encouraging the client to speak quickly is inappropriate and counterproductive. Continuous nodding may be distracting and is unnecessary. Lengthy discussions will tire the client rather than strengthen the voice.

Documentation

The nurse finds a client lying on the floor. The nurse performs an assessment, assists the client back to bed, and completes an incident report. Which would the nurse document on the incident report?

1. The client fell onto the floor.
2. The client climbed over the side rails.
3. The client was found lying on the floor.
4. The nurse was the only responder to the event.

Answer: *3*

Focus on the **subject,** documenting on an incident report. The incident report contains the client's name, age, and diagnosis and a factual description of the incident; any injuries experienced by those involved; and the outcome of the situation. Option 3 is the only choice that describes the facts as observed by the nurse. The nurse did not witness the events that led up to finding the client on the floor; thus, the nurse cannot comment on how the client got to the floor (options 1 and 2). Option 4 is unsuitable documentation on an incident report because it implies that other staff members failed to respond to the event.

BOX 10.5 Culture and Spirituality

The nurse is performing an educational session on incorporating spiritual assessment in client care. Which statement, if made by one of the participants, indicates a **need for further education** regarding spirituality in health care?

1. "Spirituality has different meanings for different people."
2. "Spirituality can positively influence health and quality of life."
3. "Nurses need to be aware of their own spirituality to address this topic with others."
4. "Spirituality can be a comforting influence; however, there is no scientific evidence of the benefits."

Answer: *4*

Note the **strategic words,** *need for further education.* These words indicate a **negative event query** and the need to select the incorrect statement as the answer. Spirituality is a broad concept that is central to a person's life and their "spirit." The spirit is what defines the person and is at the center of all aspects of a person's life. Spirituality has different meanings for different people. It can positively influence health, quality of life, health promotion behaviors, and disease prevention behaviors. Nurses need to be aware of their own spirituality to accurately assess and address spirituality needs for others. Spirituality can have a comforting influence, and there is research that shows the positive influence it can have on a person's overall well-being.

that address individualized cultural and spiritual needs and goals. This is an essential nursing responsibility to provide culturally competent health care.

When taking the NCLEX-RN examination, be aware of the mention of a specific population or culture in the question. If a specific population or culture is mentioned in the question, then you may need to answer the question based on that population's health care practices and other practices and preferences (Box 10.5).

Nursing Process

The steps of the nursing process provide a systematic and organized method of problem-solving and providing care to clients. As noted by the NCSBN, the nursing process is a scientific and clinical reasoning approach to client care and includes the steps of assessment, analysis, planning, implementation, and evaluation.

Assessment

Assessment is the first step of the nursing process. It involves a systematic method of collecting data about a client to identify existing or potential (at-risk) client health problems and establish a database. The database provides the foundation for the remaining steps of the nursing process; therefore, a thorough and adequate database is essential. Data collection begins with the first contact with the client. During all successive contacts, the nurse continues to collect information that is significant and relevant to the needs of that client.

The NCLEX-RN test plan describes culture and spirituality as the interaction of the nurse and client, which recognizes and considers unique and individual preferences to client care.

Providing individualized and holistic client care that addresses individual beliefs, customs, and practices is a role of the nurse. Cultural awareness is learning about the cultures of clients being cared for; this includes a self-examination of one's own background, and recognizing biases, prejudices, and assumptions about other people. The nurse needs to ask the client about their cultural and spiritual health care practices and preferences so that the nurse can create plans of care

During the assessment process, the nurse collects data about the client from a variety of sources. The client is the primary source of data. Family members and significant others are secondary sources of assessment data, and these sources may supplement or verify the information provided by the client. Data may also be obtained from the client's record through the medical history, laboratory results, and diagnostic reports. Medical records from previous hospital admissions or office or clinic visits may provide additional information about the client. The nurse may also obtain information through consultation with other interprofessional team members who have had contact with the client.

A thorough database is obtained with the use of a health history and a physical assessment. The information collected by the nurse includes both subjective and objective data. Subjective data include the information that the client states. Objective data are the observable, measurable pieces of information about the client, including measurements such as vital signs, laboratory findings, and results of diagnostic tests, as well as information obtained by observing the client. Objective data also include clinical manifestations, such as the signs and symptoms of an illness or health problem.

The process of assessment additionally consists of confirming and verifying client data, communicating information obtained through the assessment process, and documenting assessment findings in a thorough and accurate manner.

On the NCLEX-RN test, remember that assessment is the first step of the nursing process. When answering these types of questions, focus on the data in the question, and select the option that addresses an assessment action. The only exception to selecting an option that addresses an assessment action is if the question presents an emergency situation. In an emergency situation, an intervention may be the priority. In addition, use the skills of prioritizing and the ABCs—airway, breathing, and circulation—to answer the question. However, if the question asks about the procedure for administering cardiopulmonary resuscitation, then follow CAB (circulation [compressions], airway, breathing) guidelines (Box 10.6).

Analysis

Analysis is the second step of the nursing process. During this step, the nurse focuses on the data gathered during the assessment process and identifies existing or potential health care needs, problems, or both. During this process, the nurse summarizes and interprets the assessment data, organizes and validates the data, and determines the need for additional data. Client assessment data are compared with the normal expected findings and behaviors for the client's age, education, and cultural background. The nurse then draws conclusions regarding the client's unique needs and health care problems or risks.

Client health problems are categorized as potential or at-risk problems that require prevention or as existing problems that are being managed or require interventions. The nurse reports the results of the analysis to the appropriate members of the interprofessional team and documents the client's unique health care problems, needs, or both.

On the NCLEX-RN test, questions that address the process of analysis are difficult because they require an understanding of the principles of physiologic responses and an interpretation of the data on the basis of assessment findings or other presented data. Analysis questions require clinical reasoning

---

BOX 10.6   Nursing Process: Assessment

The nurse in a well-baby clinic is collecting data regarding the motor development of a 15-month-old child. Which is the highest level of development that the nurse would expect to observe in this child?
1. The child turns a doorknob.
2. The child unzips a large zipper.
3. The child builds a tower of two blocks.
4. The child puts on simple clothes independently.

Answer: 3

Focus on the subject, the highest level of development for a 15-month-old child. At the age of 15 months, the nurse would expect that the child could build a tower of two blocks. A 24-month-old child would be able to turn a doorknob and unzip a large zipper. At the age of 30 months, the child would be able to put on simple clothes independently.

BOX 10.7   Nursing Process: Analysis

A client is admitted to the cardiac unit and placed on telemetry. The nurse reviews the client's laboratory result for the potassium level. Based on the result and when analyzing the cardiac rhythm, the nurse would expect to note which electrocardiogram (ECG) finding?

Laboratory Results

Test and Results	Reference Range
Potassium 6.3 mEq/L (6.3 mmol/L)	3.5 to 5.0 mEq/L (3.5 to 5.0 mmol/L)

1. A sinus tachycardia with an extra U wave
2. A sinus rhythm with a tall, peaked T wave
3. A sinus rhythm with a depressed ST segment
4. A sinus tachycardia with a prolonged QT interval

Answer: 2

Note the information in the question and focus on the subject, hyperkalemia and the associated ECG finding. A potassium level of more than 5.0 mEq/L (5.0 mmol/L) indicates hyperkalemia, which can be detected on the ECG by the presence of a tall, peaked T wave. A U wave and a depressed ST segment occur with hypokalemia. A prolonged QT interval indicates hypocalcemia.

---

about the data in the question to make a clinical judgment. These questions may address identification of an existing or potential client problem and the communication and documentation of the results of the process of analysis (Box 10.7).

Planning

Planning is the third step of the nursing process. This step involves the functions of setting priorities, determining goals of care, planning actions, collaborating with other interprofessional team members, establishing evaluative criteria, and communicating the plan of care.

Setting priorities assists the nurse with organizing and planning care that solves the most urgent problems. Priorities may change as the client's level of wellness changes. Both existing

BOX 10.8   Nursing Process: Planning

The nurse is planning care for a child admitted to the hospital with an infectious and communicable disease. The nurse would identify which as the **primary** goal?

1. The public health department will be notified.
2. The child will not spread the infection to others.
3. The child will experience only minor complications.
4. The nursing supervisor will be notified about the child's diagnosis.

Answer: 2

Note the **strategic word,** *primary.* The primary goal for a child with an infectious and communicable disease is to prevent the spread of the infection to others. Although the nursing supervisor would be notified of the child's diagnosis and the health department may need to be notified at some point, these are not the primary goals. The child should experience no complications.

BOX 10.9   Nursing Process: Implementation

The nurse in the postpartum unit checks the temperature of a client who delivered a healthy newborn 4 hours ago. The client's temperature is 100.8° F (38.2° C). The nurse provides oral hydration to the client and encourages fluid intake. Four hours later, the nurse rechecks the temperature and notes that it is still 100.8° F (38.2° C). Which action would the nurse take at this time?

1. Document the temperature.
2. Increase the intravenous fluids.
3. Notify the primary health care provider (PHCP).
4. Continue hydration and recheck the temperature in 4 hours.

Answer: 3

Focus on the **information in the question** and note the **subject,** the action the nurse would take at this time. In the postpartum client, a temperature of more than 100.4° F (38° C) at two consecutive readings is considered febrile, and the PHCP should be notified. Options 1, 2, and 4 are inappropriate actions at this time. Although the nurse would document the temperature, this action delays necessary intervention. A PHCP's prescription is needed to increase intravenous fluids. Continuing hydration and rechecking the temperature in 4 hours also delays necessary intervention.

and potential problems need to be considered when establishing priorities. Existing problems are usually more important than potential problems. However, potential problems may, at times, take precedence over existing problems.

After priorities are established, the client and the nurse mutually decide on the expected goals. The expected goals serve as a guide for planning and selecting nursing interventions and determining the criteria for evaluation. Before nursing actions are implemented, mechanisms to determine goal achievement and the effectiveness of nursing interventions are established. Unless criteria have been predetermined, it is difficult to know whether the goal has been achieved or the problem has been resolved.

It is important for the nurse to both identify health or social resources available to the client and collaborate with other interprofessional team members when planning the delivery of care. The nurse needs to communicate the plan of care, review the plan of care with the client, mutually agree with the client on the plan of care, and document the plan of care thoroughly and accurately.

When answering questions on the NCLEX-RN test, remember that this is a nursing exam. In addition, remember that existing problems are usually more important than potential problems, and physiologic needs are usually the priority (Box 10.8).

Implementation

Implementation is the fourth step of the nursing process. Based on clinical judgment, it includes initiating and completing nursing actions that are required to accomplish defined goals. This step is the action phase that involves counseling, teaching, organizing and managing client care, providing care to achieve established goals, assessment, supervising and coordinating the delivery of client care, and communicating and documenting the nursing interventions and client responses.

During implementation, the nurse uses intellectual, interpersonal, and technical skills. Intellectual skills involve clinical reasoning, problem solving, and making clinical judgments. Interpersonal skills involve the ability to communicate, listen, and convey compassion. Technical skills relate to the performance of treatments and procedures and the use of necessary equipment when providing care to the client.

The nurse independently implements actions that include activities that do not require a physician's prescription. The nurse also implements actions collaboratively on the basis of the physician's prescriptions. Collaboration with other interprofessional team members is incorporated into the process of implementation. The implementation step concludes when the nurse's actions are completed and when these actions, including their effects and the client's response, are communicated and documented.

The NCLEX-RN test is an examination about nursing, so focus primarily on nursing actions rather than the medical actions unless the question is asking what prescribed medical action is anticipated. Also, notice that in NGN item types, you will need to use clinical judgment abilities and answer questions anticipating what the physician will prescribe (Box 10.9).

Evaluation

Evaluation is the fifth and final step of the nursing process. The process of evaluation identifies the degree to which the plans for care and interventions have been successful.

Although evaluation is the final step of the nursing process, it is an ongoing and integral component of each step. The process of data collection and assessment is reviewed to determine whether sufficient information was obtained and the information obtained was specific and appropriate. The client's identified existing and potential problems are evaluated for accuracy and completeness on the basis of the client's specific needs. The plan and expected outcomes are examined to determine whether they are realistic, achievable, measurable, and effective. Interventions are examined to determine their effectiveness for achieving the expected outcomes.

Because evaluation is an ongoing process, it is vital to all steps of the nursing process. It is the continuous process of comparing actual outcomes with the expected outcomes of

---

BOX 10.10 Nursing Process: Evaluation

A client has been given a prescription for a course of azithromycin. The nurse determines that the medication is having the intended effect if which is noted?
1. The pain is relieved.
2. The blood pressure is lowered.
3. The joint discomfort is reduced.
4. The signs and symptoms of infection are relieved.

Answer: 4
Focus on the subject, the intended effect of azithromycin. Azithromycin is a macrolide antibiotic that is used to treat infection. It is not prescribed for the treatment of pain, high blood pressure, or joint discomfort.

BOX 10.11 Teaching and Learning

The nurse is preparing a plan regarding home care instructions for the parents of a child with generalized tonic-clonic seizures who is being treated with oral phenytoin. Which instruction would the nurse include in the plan?
1. Monitor the child's intake and output daily.
2. Provide oral hygiene, especially care of the gums.
3. Administer the medication 1 hour before food intake.
4. Check the child's blood pressure before the administration of the medication.

Answer: 2
Focus on the subject, home care instructions regarding phenytoin. Phenytoin is an anticonvulsant medication and causes gum bleeding and hyperplasia; therefore, a soft toothbrush and gum massage should be instituted to diminish this complication and prevent trauma. Intake, output, and blood pressure are not affected by this medication. Directions for administration of this medication include administering it with food to minimize gastrointestinal upset.

---

care, and it provides the means for determining the need to modify the plan of care. Inherent in this step of the nursing process are the communication of evaluation findings and the process of documenting the client's response to treatment, care, and teaching.

Evaluation-type questions on the NCLEX-RN may be written to address a client's response to treatment measures or determine a client's understanding of the prescribed treatment measures (Box 10.10).

Teaching and Learning

Client and family education is a primary nursing responsibility. The NCSBN describes this process as facilitating the acquisition of knowledge, skills, and attitudes that lead to a change in behavior.

The principles related to the teaching and learning process are used when the nurse functions as a teacher. The nurse must remember that the assessment of the client's readiness and motivation to learn is the initial step in the teaching and learning process.

When answering a question on the NCLEX-RN related to the teaching and learning process, use the principles related to teaching and learning theory. If a test question addresses client education, remember that client motivation and readiness to learn are the first priorities (Box 10.11).

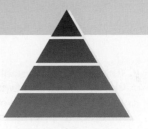
CHAPTER 11

Integrated Processes Practice Questions

Caring

1. A client diagnosed with diabetes mellitus requires the immediate amputation of a leg. The client is very upset and states, "This is the doctor's fault! I did everything that I was told to do!" When considering the grieving process, how would the nurse respond to the client's statement?
   1. Notify the agency's risk management department.
   2. Help the client consider alternatives to treatment.
   3. Allow the client to use anger as a coping mechanism.
   4. Ask the client to list all previous health care providers.

Level of Cognitive Ability: Applying
Client Needs: Psychosocial Integrity
Clinical Judgment/Cognitive Skills: Generate Solutions
Integrated Process: Clinical Judgment; Caring
Content Area: Adult Health: Endocrine
Health Problems: Adult Health: Musculoskeletal: Amputation
Priority Concepts: Caregiving; Stress and Coping

Answer: 3
Rationale: Anger is a stage in the grieving process and an expected response to impending loss. Usually a client directs the anger toward self, God, or another spiritual being, or the caregivers; thus far the client's behavior demonstrates effective coping. Notifying the risk management department is premature, especially because the client has said nothing about legal action. Analyzing alternative treatment options and previous health care providers is likely to interfere with effective coping, and it can delay lifesaving treatment.
Test-Taking Strategy: Focus on the subject, a very upset client. Noting that the client is blaming the doctor and knowledge of the stages of grief associated with loss will direct you to the correct option.
Priority Nursing Tip: A coping mechanism is a method used to decrease anxiety.
References: Ignatavicius, D., et al. (2021). *Medical-surgical nursing: Concepts for interprofessional collaborative care* (10th ed., pp. 1047, 1050). Elsevier; Potter, P., et al. (2021). *Fundamentals of nursing* (10th ed., p. 348). Elsevier.

❖ **2.** The nurse has an established relationship with the family of a client whose death is imminent. Which intervention would the nurse focus on in order to help the family **most effectively** cope with this experience?
1. Limiting time in the client's room to promote privacy
2. Providing education regarding coping mechanisms to use
3. Identifying spiritual measures that work best for dying clients
4. Answering questions clearly and providing resources as requested

Level of Cognitive Ability: Applying
Client Needs: Psychosocial Integrity
Clinical Judgment/Cognitive Skills: Generate Solutions
Integrated Process: Caring
Content Area: Developmental Stages: End-of-Life
Health Problems: Mental Health: Coping
Priority Concepts: Caregiving; Palliative Care

Answer: 4
Rationale: Maintaining effective and open communication among family members affected by death and grief is important to facilitate decision making and effective coping. The nurse maintains and enhances communication and preserves the family's sense of self-direction and control effectively by answering questions clearly and providing information and resources for decision making as requested by the family. Isolating the family from the client by limiting time in the client's room is inappropriate. The nurse should not provide education about coping mechanisms for family members to use because coping mechanisms directed by the nurse are unlikely to be as effective as the methods that the individuals choose for themselves. Identifying spiritual measures that work best for the dying client generalizes and does not reflect individualized care.
Test-Taking Strategy: Note the strategic words, *most effectively*. Focus on therapeutic communication techniques and the role of the nurse in grieving, loss, and crisis, and then choose the most effective intervention. Also note that the correct option uses the words *as requested*.
Priority Nursing Tip: People dealing with crisis usually feel helpless and are unable to control the circumstances; therefore, the nurse must facilitate open communication to determine and then meet the persons' needs.
Reference: Potter, P., et al. (2021). *Fundamentals of nursing* (10th ed., pp. 333–335, 754). Elsevier.

3. A client comes into the emergency department demonstrating manifestations indicative of a severe state of anxiety. What is the **priority** nursing intervention at this time?
1. Remaining with the client
2. Placing the client in a quiet room
3. Teaching the client deep-breathing exercises
4. Encouraging the expression of feelings and concerns

Level of Cognitive Ability: Applying
Client Needs: Psychosocial Integrity
Clinical Judgment/Cognitive Skills: Take Action
Integrated Process: Clinical Judgment; Caring
Content Area: Mental Health
Health Problems: Mental Health: Anxiety Disorder
Priority Concepts: Anxiety; Caregiving

Answer: 1
Rationale: If the client is left alone with severe anxiety, the client may feel abandoned and become overwhelmed. Placing the client in a quiet room is also indicated, but the nurse must stay with the client. It is not possible to teach the client deep-breathing or relaxation exercises until the anxiety decreases. Encouraging the client to discuss concerns and feelings would not take place until the anxiety has decreased.
Test-Taking Strategy: Because the anxiety state is severe, eliminate options 3 and 4. From the remaining choices, consider the strategic word, *priority*, in the question. Focus on the subject, a client in a severe state of anxiety. This will direct you to the correct option.
Priority Nursing Tip: Anxiety occurs as a result of a threat that may be misperceived or misinterpreted or of a threat to identity or self-esteem.
Reference: Varcarolis, E., & Fosbre, C. (2021). *Essentials of psychiatric mental health nursing: A communication approach to evidence-based care* (4th ed., p. 137). Elsevier.

4. When a client is dead on arrival (DOA) to the emergency department, the family states that they do not want an autopsy performed. Which statement would the nurse make in response to the family?
  1. "Autopsies are mandatory for clients who are DOA."
  2. "Federal law requires autopsies for clients who are DOA."
  3. "The medical examiner makes the decision about autopsies."
  4. "I will make sure the medical examiner is aware of your request."

Level of Cognitive Ability: Applying
Client Needs: Safe and Effective Care Environment
Clinical Judgment/Cognitive Skills: Take Action
Integrated Process: Caring
Content Area: Developmental Stages: End of-Life
Health Problems: Mental Health: Grief/Loss
Priority Concepts: Health Care Law; Professional Identity

Answer: 4
Rationale: The nurse needs to notify the medical examiner or the coroner when a family wishes to avoid having an autopsy on a deceased family member. Normally the medical examiner will honor the family request unless there is a state law requiring the autopsy. Depending on the state, it is not mandatory for every client who is DOA to have an autopsy. However, many states require an autopsy in specific circumstances, including sudden death, a suspicious death, and death within 24 hours of admission to the hospital. Autopsy is not a requirement under federal law.
Test-Taking Strategy: Focus on the subject, the laws and issues surrounding autopsy, and use therapeutic communication techniques to answer the question. Eliminate options 1 and 2 because these statements are not accurate. From the remaining choices, option 4 is the most therapeutic and caring response to the family.
Priority Nursing Tip: Special consents are required for performing an autopsy, the use of restraints, receiving blood transfusions, photographing the client, disposal of body parts during surgery, and donating organs after death. It is often times within the client/family's right to deny such a request.
Reference: Potter, P., et al. (2021). *Fundamentals of nursing* (10th ed., pp. 333–335, 755). Elsevier.

5. The nurse is interacting with the family of a client who is unconscious as a result of a head injury. Which approach would the nurse use to help the family cope with their concerns?
  1. Explain equipment and procedures on an ongoing basis.
  2. Discuss displaying their grief only when not in the room with the client.
  3. Discourage them from touching the client in order to minimize stimulation.
  4. Explain that they need their rest so they need to adhere to regular visiting hours.

Level of Cognitive Ability: Applying
Client Needs: Psychosocial Integrity
Clinical Judgment/Cognitive Skills: Take Action
Integrated Process: Caring
Content Area: Adult Health: Neurologic
Health Problems: Adult Health: Neurologic: Head Injury/Trauma
Priority Concepts: Stress and Coping; Family Dynamics

Answer: 1
Rationale: Families often need assistance to cope with the sudden severe illness of a loved one. The nurse should explain all equipment, treatments, and procedures, and should supplement or reinforce the information given by the physician. Displaying grief is a normal process and should not be discouraged. The family should be encouraged to touch and speak to the client and become involved in the client's care in some way if they are comfortable with doing so. The nurse would allow the family to stay with the client whenever possible. This is important for both the client and the family.
Test-Taking Strategy: Use therapeutic communication techniques to answer this question. The correct option provides the family with information that will help them cope with the situation. Each of the incorrect options puts distance between the family and the client.
Priority Nursing Tip: Families of clients who are acutely ill may experience anticipatory grief. Anticipatory grief occurs before the loss and is associated with an acute, chronic, or terminal illness.
Reference: Potter, P., et al. (2021). *Fundamentals of nursing* (10th ed., pp. 333–335). Elsevier.

6. The nurse admits a client who is demonstrating right-sided weakness, aphasia, and urinary incontinence. The client's adult child states, "If this is a stroke, it's the kiss of death." What **initial** response would the nurse make?
  1. "Why would you think like that?"
  2. "You feel your parent is dying?"
  3. "These symptoms are reversible."
  4. "A stroke is not the kiss of death."

Level of Cognitive Ability: Applying
Client Needs: Psychosocial Integrity
Clinical Judgment/Cognitive Skills: Take Action
Integrated Process: Caring
Content Area: Foundations of Care: Communication
Health Problems: Adult Health: Neurologic: Stroke
Priority Concepts: Communication; Stress and Coping

Answer: 2
Rationale: Option 2 allows the client's adult child to verbalize feelings, begin coping, and adapt to what is happening. By restating, the nurse seeks clarification of the adult child's feelings and offers information that potentially helps ease some of the fears and concerns related to the client's condition and prognosis. Option 1 is a disapproving comment that is likely to interfere with communication. Option 3 is potentially misleading and offers false hope. The nurse could reflect back the statement in option 4 to the client's adult child to promote communication. However, as it stands, option 4 is a barrier to communication that contradicts the adult child's feelings.
Test-Taking Strategy: Note the strategic word, *initial*. Use the principles of therapeutic communication to arrive at the option that allows for clarification of the adult child's feelings.
Priority Nursing Tip: A critical factor in the early intervention and treatment of stroke is the accurate identification of stroke manifestations and establishing the onset of manifestations.
References: Ignatavicius, D., et al. (2021). *Medical-surgical nursing: Concepts for interprofessional collaborative care* (10th ed., pp. 903, 905). Elsevier; Potter, P., et al. (2021). *Fundamentals of nursing* (10th ed., pp. 333–335). Elsevier.

7. A birthing client and infant have been diagnosed as being positive for human immunodeficiency virus (HIV). When the client is observed crying, the nurse determines that which intervention will meet the client's **initial** needs?
  1. Discussing how the birthing client was exposed to HIV
  2. Sitting quietly with the birthing client while the client talks and cries
  3. Describing the progressive stages and treatments of HIV
  4. Calling an HIV counselor to make an appointment for the birthing client and infant

Level of Cognitive Ability: Analyzing
Client Needs: Psychosocial Integrity
Clinical Judgment/Cognitive Skills: Generate Solutions
Integrated Process: Clinical Judgment; Caring
Content Area: Pediatrics: Immune
Health Problems: Pediatric-Specific: Immunodeficiency Disease
Priority Concepts: Caregiving; Stress and Coping

Answer: 2
Rationale: This client has just received devastating news and needs to have someone present when beginning to cope with this issue. The nurse needs to sit and actively listen while the birthing client talks and cries. Examining the client and describing the progression and treatment of HIV is not appropriate for this stage of coping. Calling an HIV counselor may be helpful, but it is not what the client needs initially.
Test-Taking Strategy: Note the strategic word, *initial*. Use therapeutic communication techniques, and remember to focus on the client's feelings. This will direct you to the correct option.
Priority Nursing Tip: The nurse must maintain issues of confidentiality surrounding HIV and acquired immunodeficiency syndrome testing while addressing the client's feelings.
Reference: McKinney, E. S., et al. (2022). *Maternal child nursing* (6th ed., pp. 27, 945–946). Elsevier.

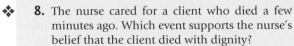

8. The nurse cared for a client who died a few minutes ago. Which event supports the nurse's belief that the client died with dignity?
   1. The family thanks the nurse for facilitating such a peaceful death.
   2. The nurse states that it is difficult to give that kind of care to a dying client.
   3. The physician acknowledges that all of the prescriptions were carried out.
   4. The nurse kept the client's last hours comfortable with increasing doses of pain medication.

Level of Cognitive Ability: Evaluating
Client Needs: Psychosocial Integrity
Clinical Judgment/Cognitive Skills: Evaluate Outcomes
Integrated Process: Clinical Judgment; Caring
Content Area: Developmental Stages: End-of-Life
Health Problems: Mental Health: Grief/Loss
Priority Concepts: Caregiving; Palliative Care

Answer: 1
Rationale: The family response is an external perception, and it is extremely important. Families derive a great deal of comfort from knowing that their loved one received the best care possible. The correct option provides external validation that the client received comprehensive, quality care. Option 2 focuses on the feelings of the nurse, who may be expressing their own anxiety. Option 3 focuses on the provider's prescriptions rather than client care. Option 4 reflects on only one aspect of the care of a dying client.
Test-Taking Strategy: Focus on the subject of whether the client died with dignity. The only choice that addresses this subject is the correct option.
Priority Nursing Tip: Outcomes related to care during illness and the dying experience need to be based on the client's wishes. Pain must be controlled; the dying client needs to be as pain free and comfortable as possible.
References: Lewis, S., et al. (2020). *Medical-surgical nursing: Assessment and management of clinical problems* (11th ed., p. 137). Elsevier; Potter, P., et al. (2021). *Fundamentals of nursing.* (10th ed., p. 755). Elsevier.

9. A client diagnosed with Parkinson's disease is having difficulty adjusting to the disorder. The nurse provides education to the family that focuses on addressing the client's activities of daily living. Which statement indicates that the teaching has been **effective**?
   1. "We need to plan for only a few activities during the day."
   2. "We need to assist with activities of daily living as much as possible."
   3. "We need to cluster activities at the end of the day, to help conserve energy."
   4. "We need to encourage and praise efforts to exercise and perform activities of daily living."

Level of Cognitive Ability: Evaluating
Client Needs: Psychosocial Integrity
Clinical Judgment/Cognitive Skills: Evaluate Outcomes
Integrated Process: Clinical Judgment; Caring
Content Area: Adult Health: Neurologic
Health Problems: Adult Health: Neurologic: Parkinson's Disease
Priority Concepts: Stress and Coping; Functional Ability

Answer: 4
Rationale: The client with Parkinson's disease has a tendency to become withdrawn and depressed, which can be limited by encouraging the client to be an active participant in their own care. The family needs to plan activities intermittently throughout the day to inhibit daytime sleeping and boredom. The family needs to give the client encouragement and praise for their perseverance in these efforts and help only when necessary.
Test-Taking Strategy: Focus on the strategic word, *effective*, and the subject of supporting the client in coping with the effects of Parkinson's disease. Recalling that the client should be an active participant in their own care will direct you to the correct option.
Priority Nursing Tip: The client with Parkinson's disease should exercise in the morning when energy levels are highest.
Reference: Ignatavicius, D., et al. (2021). *Medical-surgical nursing: Concepts for interprofessional collaborative care* (10th ed., pp. 856, 859). Elsevier.

❖ **10.** A community health nurse is caring for a population of people who are unhoused. What is the **most immediate** concern when planning for the potential needs of this group?
1. Finding affordable housing for the group
2. Setting up a 24-hour crisis center and hotline
3. Providing peer support through structured support groups
4. Ensuring that adequate food, shelter, and clothing are available

Level of Cognitive Ability: Analyzing
Client Needs: Physiological Integrity
Clinical Judgment/Cognitive Skills: Prioritize Hypotheses
Integrated Process: Clinical Judgment; Caring
Content Area: Foundations of Care: Community/Public/Population Health
Health Problems: Mental Health: Crisis
Priority Concepts: Caregiving; Health Promotion

Answer: 4
Rationale: The question asks about the situation's most immediate concern. The initial community health concern is always attending to people's basic physiologic needs of food, shelter, and clothing. Finding affordable housing and providing crisis intervention and peer support are meaningful interventions that may be completed at a later time.
Test-Taking Strategy: Note the strategic words, *most immediate*. Use Maslow's Hierarchy of Needs theory to answer the question. The correct option addresses basic physiologic needs. Although the remaining options are also appropriate actions, the correct option is the most immediate concern.
Priority Nursing Tip: Nursing's primary concern is always initially focused on meeting a client's physiologic needs.
Reference: Ignatavicius, D., et al. (2021). *Medical-surgical nursing: Concepts for interprofessional collaborative care* (10th ed., p. 190). Elsevier.

11. A stillborn baby was delivered a few hours ago. After the birth, the family has remained together, holding and touching the baby. The registered nurse is orienting a new nurse and has provided education on how to communicate with the family. Which statement by the new nurse indicates that teaching has been **effective**?
1. "How can I assist you with ways to remember your baby?"
2. "You seem upset. Do you think a tranquilizer would help?"
3. "I feel so bad. I don't understand why this happened either."
4. "I can allow another 15 minutes together for you to grieve."

Level of Cognitive Ability: Evaluating
Client Needs: Psychosocial Integrity
Clinical Judgment/Cognitive Skills: Evaluate Outcomes
Integrated Process: Clinical Judgment; Caring
Content Area: Developmental Stages: End-of-Life
Health Problems: Maternity: Fetal Distress/Demise
Priority Concepts: Caregiving; Communication

Answer: 1
Rationale: Nurses would explore measures that assist the family with creating memories of the infant so that the existence of the child is confirmed and the parents can complete the grieving process. The correct option identifies this measure and also demonstrates a caring and empathetic client-focused response while providing the family with the option to express their needs. Option 2 devalues the parents' feelings and is inappropriate. Option 3 is inappropriate and reflects a lack of knowledge on the nurse's part. Option 4 appears that the nurse is uncaring.
Test-Taking Strategy: Focus on the strategic word, *effective*. Use therapeutic communication techniques to choose the option that demonstrates a caring and empathetic response by the nurse and that meets the psychosocial needs of the grieving client and family.
Priority Nursing Tip: Loss and grief may occur with the birth of a preterm infant, an infant with complications of birth, or an infant with congenital anomalies; it may also occur in a client who is giving up a child for adoption. Beliefs and needs may vary widely across individuals, cultures, and religions.
Reference: McKinney, E. S., et al. (2022). *Maternal child nursing* (6th ed., pp. 27, 520–522). Elsevier.

12. The nurse is caring for a depressed, withdrawn client who was responsible for an automobile accident that recently resulted in the death of a child. What is the nurse's **initial** action?
1. Allow the client to have some time alone to grieve over the loss.
2. Reinforce to the client that the child's death was a result of an accident.
3. Communicate in a manner that acknowledges and respects the client's depressed state.
4. Inform the physician of the client's possible need for medication to cope.

Level of Cognitive Ability: Applying
Client Needs: Psychosocial Integrity
Clinical Judgment/Cognitive Skills: Take Action
Integrated Process: Caring
Content Area: Mental Health
Health Problems: Mental Health: Mood Disorders
Priority Concepts: Communication; Mood and Affect

Answer: 3
Rationale: The nurse's initial intervention is to encourage the client to express feelings, which is facilitated by establishing a nurse–client relationship that is based upon respect. The correct option validates the perception that the client is depressed. This action also allows the nurse to assess the situation. Options 1, 2, and 4 address interventions before assessing the situation and identifying the client's actual needs.
Test-Taking Strategy: Note the strategic word, *initial*, while using therapeutic communication techniques. Select the option that encourages the client to express feelings and maintains communication. Remember to always address the client's feelings.
Priority Nursing Tip: For any client experiencing depression after a traumatic event, the nurse needs to be nonjudgmental and supportive. Encourage the client to express their feelings.
Reference: Varcarolis, E., & Fosbre, C. (2021). *Essentials of psychiatric mental health nursing: A communication approach to evidence-based care* (4th ed., pp. 93–95, 201). Elsevier.

13. The nurse is bathing a client when the client begins to cry. Which action by the nurse is therapeutic at this time?
1. Continue bathing the client and say nothing.
2. Stop the bath, cover the client, and sit with the client.
3. Stop the bath, cover the client, and allow the client private time.
4. Call the physician to report the signs of depression.

Level of Cognitive Ability: Applying
Client Needs: Psychosocial Integrity
Clinical Judgment/Cognitive Skills: Take Action
Integrated Process: Caring
Content Area: Mental Health
Health Problems: Mental Health: Coping
Priority Concepts: Caregiving; Communication

Answer: 2
Rationale: If a client begins to cry, the nurse would stay with the client and let the client know that it is all right to cry. The nurse would ask the client what the client is thinking or feeling at the time. By continuing the bath or by leaving the client, the nurse appears to be ignoring the client's feelings. Crying alone is not necessarily an indication of depression, and calling the physician is a premature action.
Test-Taking Strategy: Focus on the subject, a client who begins to cry. The nurse needs to acknowledge the client's crying and provide emotional support. The correct option is the only one that provides the appropriate care for an emotional client.
Priority Nursing Tip: Used appropriately, silence and listening are therapeutic communication techniques.
Reference: Varcarolis, E., & Fosbre, C. (2021). *Essentials of psychiatric mental health nursing: A communication approach to evidence-based care* (4th ed., pp. 93–95). Elsevier.

14. An older couple was emotionally despondent when their home was severely damaged by flooding. When planning for the couple's **ini-tial** needs, what intervention would the community health nurse implement?
1. Contacting their families
2. Attending to their emotional needs
3. Arranging for the repair of their home
4. Attending to their basic physiologic needs

Level of Cognitive Ability: Analyzing
Client Needs: Physiological Integrity
Clinical Judgment/Cognitive Skills: Prioritize Hypotheses
Integrated Process: Clinical Judgment; Caring
Content Area: Foundations of Care: Community/Public/Population Health
Health Problems: Mental Health: Crisis
Priority Concepts: Clinical Judgment; Caregiving

Answer: 4
Rationale: The question asks about the first thing that the nurse needs to consider when planning for the rescue and relocation of these older residents. The initial concerns of community health are always attending to people's basic needs of food, shelter, and clothing. Contacting family, addressing emotional needs, and arranging for home repairs are needs that may be addressed as needed after physiologic needs are met.
Test-Taking Strategy: Note the strategic word, *initial*. Use Maslow's Hierarchy of Needs theory to answer the question. The correct option addresses basic physiologic needs. Although the remaining options may be appropriate actions at a later time, the correct option is the immediate concern.
Priority Nursing Tip: For any client, the nurse needs to address physiologic needs first; then the nurse would assess safety and psychosocial needs.
Reference: Ignatavicius, D., et al. (2021). *Medical-surgical nursing: Concepts for interprofessional collaborative care* (10th ed., pp. 232–233). Elsevier.

15. The nurse is planning the care of a client newly admitted to the mental health unit for suicidal ideations. To provide a caring, therapeutic environment, which intervention would be included in the nursing care plan?
1. Placing the client in a private room to ensure privacy and confidentiality
2. Interacting with the client demonstrating examples of unconditional positive regard
3. Maintaining a distance of 10 inches to assure client that personal control will be provided
4. Placing the client in charge of a meaningful unit activity, such as the morning chess tournament

Level of Cognitive Ability: Applying
Client Needs: Psychosocial Integrity
Clinical Judgment/Cognitive Skills: Generate Solutions
Integrated Process: Clinical Judgment; Caring
Content Area: Mental Health
Health Problems: Mental Health: Suicide
Priority Concepts: Mood and Affect; Safety

Answer: 2
Rationale: The establishment of a therapeutic relationship with the suicidal client increases feelings of acceptance. Although the suicidal behavior and the client's thinking are undesirable, the use of unconditional positive regard acknowledges the client in a human-to-human context and increases the client's sense of self-worth. The client would not be placed in a private room because this is an unsafe action that may intensify the client's feelings of worthlessness. Distance of 18 inches or less between two individuals constitutes intimate space. The invasion of this space may be misinterpreted by the client and increase the client's tension and feelings of helplessness. Placing the client in charge of the morning chess tournament is a premature intervention that can overwhelm the client and cause the client to fail; this can reinforce the client's feelings of worthlessness.
Test-Taking Strategy: Focus on the subject, providing a therapeutic environment for a client who is suicidal. The correct option is the only choice that addresses a caring and therapeutic environment.
Priority Nursing Tip: Monitor a depressed client closely for signs of suicidal ideation. If the client presents with increased energy, monitor the client closely because it could mean that the client now has the energy to perform the suicide act.
Reference: Varcarolis, E., & Fosbre, C. (2021). *Essentials of psychiatric mental health nursing: A communication approach to evidence-based care* (4th ed., pp. 366, 370). Elsevier.

❖ **16.** Shortly after a client dies, the nurse asks the family about funeral arrangements. When the family refuses to discuss the issue, which intervention by the nurse is appropriate for their stage of grief at this time?
1. Displaying acceptance of the family's issues
2. Providing information about funerals in general
3. Probing for information about funeral arrangements
4. Asking the family if they would like time alone with the client

Level of Cognitive Ability: Applying
Client Needs: Psychosocial Integrity
Clinical Judgment/Cognitive Skills: Generate Solutions
Integrated Process: Caring
Content Area: Developmental Stages: End-of-Life
Health Problems: Mental Health: Grief/Loss
Priority Concepts: Coping; Palliative Care

Answer: 4
Rationale: The family is exhibiting the first stage of grief: denial. By asking the family if they would like time alone with the client, the nurse supports the family's feelings and allows the family to process the death. Option 1 is a suitable intervention for the acceptance or reorganization and restitution stage of grief. Eliminate options 2 and 3 because they are not appropriate at this time since the family has indicated their desire not to discuss funeral arrangements.
Test-Taking Strategy: Focus on the subject of a grieving family. Note the words *at this time* and the stage of grief that the family is demonstrating. This will help you recognize that the family is in denial and direct you to choose the correct option.
Priority Nursing Tip: Grief usually involves moving through a series of stages or tasks to help resolve the grief. Feelings associated with grief include anger, frustration, loneliness, sadness, guilt, regret, and peace.
Reference: Potter, P., et al. (2021). *Fundamentals of nursing* (10th ed., p. 348). Elsevier.

17. A client diagnosed with incurable cancer has a life expectancy of a few weeks. Which response indicates that the client's partner is reacting with an expected coping response?
1. Refusing to visit the client
2. Expressing anger with God
3. Not allowing the death to occur at home
4. Sending the children to live with relatives

Level of Cognitive Ability: Applying
Client Needs: Psychosocial Integrity
Clinical Judgment/Cognitive Skills: Recognize Cues
Integrated Process: Caring
Content Area: Developmental Stages: End-of-Life
Health Problems: Mental Health: Coping
Priority Concepts: Coping; Palliative Care

Answer: 2
Rationale: The expression of anger is a normal response to impending loss, and often the anger is directed internally or at the dying person, God or another spiritual being, or the caregivers. In option 1, the partner is denying the client's situation and needs by refusing to visit. Options 3 and 4 are unilateral decisions made by the partner without considering anyone else's feelings.
Test-Taking Strategy: Focus on the subject, *an expected coping response.* Recalling the stages of grief associated with loss will direct you to the correct option.
Priority Nursing Tip: A coping mechanism is a method used to decrease anxiety. The use of a coping mechanism can be conscious, unconscious, constructive, destructive, task-oriented in relation to direct problem-solving, or defense-oriented and regulating in response to protect oneself.
Reference: Lewis, S., et al. (2020). *Medical-surgical nursing: Assessment and management of clinical problems* (11th ed., p. 136). Elsevier.

Communication and Documentation

 18. The nurse working on the mental health unit is in the orientation (introductory) phase of the therapeutic nurse–client relationship. Which intervention is representative of this phase of the relationship?
1. The nurse and client determine the plan for meetings.
2. The client is encouraged to make use of all services depending on need.
3. The client begins to identify with the nurse, and trust and rapport are maintained.
4. The nurse focuses on facilitating the therapeutic expression of the client's feelings.

Level of Cognitive Ability: Applying
Client Needs: Psychosocial Integrity
Clinical Judgment/Cognitive Skills: Generate Solutions
Integrated Process: Communication and Documentation
Content Area: Mental Health
Health Problems: N/A
Priority Concepts: Communication; Professional Identity

Answer: 1
Rationale: In the orientation (introductory phase) of the therapeutic nurse–client relationship, the client and nurse meet and determine the plan for time, such as how often to meet, the length of the meetings, and when termination is anticipated to occur. Utilizing services, identification with the nurse, and expression of feelings are appropriate for the working phase of the therapeutic nurse–client relationship.
Test-Taking Strategy: Focus on the subject, the orientation (introductory) phase of the therapeutic nurse–client relationship. Recognizing that the correct option contains the only "orienting" actions will assist you in selecting it as the correct option.
Priority Nursing Tip: Acceptance, trust, and boundaries are established in the orientation (introductory) phase of the therapeutic nurse–client relationship.
Reference: Varcarolis, E., & Fosbre, C. (2021). *Essentials of psychiatric mental health nursing: A communication approach to evidence-based care* (4th ed., pp. 108–109). Elsevier.

19. The partner of a client who has an esophageal tube introduced for a second time tells the nurse, "I thought having this tube down the nose the first time would convince anyone to quit drinking." Which response to the statement would the nurse make?
1. "I think you are a good person to stay with your partner."
2. "Alcoholism is a disease that affects the whole family."
3. "Have you discussed this subject at the Al-Anon meetings?"
4. "You sound frustrated dealing with such a drinking problem."

Level of Cognitive Ability: Applying
Client Needs: Psychosocial Integrity
Clinical Judgment/Cognitive Skills: Take Action
Integrated Process: Communication and Documentation
Content Area: Foundations of Care: Communication
Health Problems: Mental Health: Addictions
Priority Concepts: Addiction; Communication

Answer: 4
Rationale: In option 4, the nurse uses the therapeutic communication techniques of clarifying and focusing to assist the client's partner with expressing feelings about the client's chronic illness. Showing approval, stereotyping, and changing the subject are nontherapeutic techniques that block communication.
Test-Taking Strategy: Note the client of the question, the client's partner. Use therapeutic communication techniques. Remembering to always address the client's feelings will direct you to the correct option.
Priority Nursing Tip: Alcohol abuse is an addiction and a relapse in behavior can occur. This can be very frustrating for families to understand and accept.
Reference: Varcarolis, E., & Fosbre, C. (2021). *Essentials of psychiatric mental health nursing: A communication approach to evidence-based care* (4th ed., pp. 57, 93–95). Elsevier.

❖ **20.** The registered nurse is orienting a new nurse on how to care for a client diagnosed with type 2 diabetes mellitus, who was recently hospitalized for hyperglycemic hyperosmolar syndrome (HHS). When preparing for discharge from the hospital, the client expresses anxiety and concerns about the recurrence of HHS. Which response by the new nurse is **best**?
  1. "Do you have concerns about managing your condition?"
  2. "Do you think you might need to go to the nursing home?"
  3. "If you take the correct medications, I doubt this will happen again."
  4. "Don't worry. I'm sure your family will provide all the help you need."

Level of Cognitive Ability: Applying
Client Needs: Psychosocial Integrity
Clinical Judgment/Cognitive Skills: Take Action
Integrated Process: Communication and Documentation
Content Area: Foundations of Care: Communication
Health Problems: Adult Health: Endocrine: Diabetes Mellitus
Priority Concepts: Anxiety; Communication

Answer: 1
Rationale: The nurse needs to provide time and listen to the client's concerns while attempting to clarify the client's feelings as in the correct option. Option 2 is not an appropriate nursing response because it is making suggestions regarding care options without appropriately identifying the client's true concerns. Options 3 and 4 provide inappropriate false hope and disregard the client's concerns.
Test-Taking Strategy: Focus on the **strategic word**, *best*, and use **therapeutic communication techniques** to always address the client's feelings, especially anxiety, to direct you to the correct option.
Priority Nursing Tip: It is inappropriate to tell a client to "not worry" because it is a barrier to effective communication between the client and the nurse.
References: Ignatavicius, D., et al. (2021). *Medical-surgical nursing: Concepts for interprofessional collaborative care* (10th ed., p. 1268). Elsevier; Potter, P., et al. (2021). *Fundamentals of nursing* (10th ed., pp. 333–335). Elsevier.

21. The nurse assesses the client's peripheral intravenous (IV) site and notes that it is cool, pale, and swollen, and the fluid is not infusing. Which condition would the nurse document?
  1. Phlebitis
  2. Infection
  3. Infiltration
  4. Thrombosis

Level of Cognitive Ability: Analyzing
Client Needs: Physiological Integrity
Clinical Judgment/Cognitive Skills: Analyze Cues
Integrated Process: Communication and Documentation
Content Area: Complex Care: Intravenous Therapy
Health Problems: Adult Health: Integumentary: Inflammations/Infections
Priority Concepts: Clinical Judgment; Tissue Integrity

Answer: 3
Rationale: The infusion stops when the pressure in the tissue exceeds the pressure in the tubing. The pallor, coolness, and swelling of the IV site are the result of IV fluid infusing into the subcutaneous tissue. An IV site is infiltrated when it becomes dislodged from the vein and is lying in subcutaneous tissue, so the nurse concludes that the IV is infiltrated. The nurse needs to remove the infiltrated catheter and insert a new IV. All the remaining options are likely to be accompanied by warmth at the site. Eliminate options 1, 2, and 4 that suggest the site appearance as being reddened.
Test-Taking Strategy: Focus on the **subject**, an IV site that is cool, pale, swollen, and not infusing. Use your knowledge regarding the clinical indicators of the complications associated with IV therapy to direct you to the correct option. Eliminate options 1, 2, and 4 that are **comparable or alike** and are characteristic of warmth at the site.
Priority Nursing Tip: Insert an infusion catheter at a distal site to provide the option of proceeding up the extremity if the vein is ruptured or infiltration occurs; for example, if infiltration occurs from the antecubital vein, the lower veins in the same arm usually cannot be used for further puncture sites.
Reference: Ignatavicius, D., et al. (2021). *Medical-surgical nursing: Concepts for interprofessional collaborative care* (10th ed., p. 294). Elsevier.

❖ **22.** The nurse provided education to the unlicensed assistive personnel (UAP) in preparation for communicating with a hearing-impaired client? Which statement(s) by the UAP indicates that teaching has been **effective? Select all that apply.**

☐ 1. "Speak using a normal tone of voice."
☐ 2. "Speak clearly when communicating with the client."
☐ 3. "Speak slowly and directly into the client's impaired ear."
☐ 4. "Face the client directly when carrying on a conversation."
☐ 5. "Be aware of signs that the client does not understand the conversation."

Level of Cognitive Ability: Evaluating
Client Needs: Safe and Effective Care Environment
Clinical Judgment/Cognitive Skills: Evaluate Outcomes
Integrated Process: Clinical Judgment; Communication and Documentation
Content Area: Foundations of Care: Communication
Health Problems: Adult Health: Ear: Hearing Loss
Priority Concepts: Communication; Sensory Perception

Answer: 1, 2, 4, 5
Rationale: When communicating with a hearing-impaired client, the caregiver should speak in a normal tone to the client and should not shout. One should talk directly to the client while facing the client and speak clearly. If the client does not seem to understand what is being said, the caregiver should express the statement differently. Moving closer to the client and toward the better ear may facilitate communication, but one must avoid talking directly into the impaired ear.
Test-Taking Strategy: Focus on the strategic word, *effective*, and the subject, communication techniques for a hearing-impaired client. Knowledge regarding effective therapeutic communication techniques will direct you to the correct options.
Priority Nursing Tip: Hearing impairment occurs with aging; usually high-frequency tones are less perceptible.
References: Ignatavicius, D., et al. (2021). *Medical-surgical nursing: Concepts for interprofessional collaborative care* (10th ed., pp. 958, 964). Elsevier; Potter, P., et al. (2021). *Fundamentals of nursing* (10th ed., pp. 333–335). Elsevier.

23. The nurse creates a plan of care to facilitate effective communication for a client who requests assistance in order to live independently. Which intervention has **highest priority?**

1. Directing the discussions so that teaching needs are met
2. Focusing directly on the client's message regarding needs
3. Reflecting only facts related to the client's expressed concerns
4. Reacting to the client's responses in a matter-of-fact, professional manner

Level of Cognitive Ability: Creating
Client Needs: Psychosocial Integrity
Clinical Judgment/Cognitive Skills: Prioritize Hypotheses
Integrated Process: Clinical Judgment; Communication and Documentation
Content Area: Foundations of Care: Communication
Health Problems: Mental Health: Coping
Priority Concepts: Caregiving; Communication

Answer: 2
Rationale: For effective communication, the nurse uses active listening and assesses verbal and nonverbal communication to receive the client's intended message, thus creating an environment in which the client feels comfortable expressing feelings. An authoritarian approach is directive and not permissive, and it is unlikely to create an environment for the free exchange of thoughts and ideas. Reflecting facts only is a barrier to effective communication because subjective information can also provide a stimulus for effective communication. Reacting in a matter-of-fact manner can be an ineffective strategy for facilitating communication.
Test-Taking Strategy: Note the strategic words, *highest priority*. Eliminate option 3 because of the closed-ended word *only*. Next, use therapeutic communication techniques. This will direct you to the correct option.
Priority Nursing Tip: The nurse needs to use both verbal and nonverbal communication cues to interpret what the client is trying to express.
Reference: Potter, P., et al. (2021). *Fundamentals of nursing* (10th ed., pp. 333–335). Elsevier.

❖ **24.** The nursing student is listening to a lecture on correcting errors in a written narrative on a medical record. Which statement by the nursing student indicates that the teaching has been **effective**?
1. "The correct procedure is to document the correction as a late entry."
2. "The correct procedure is to draw a line through the error and initial and date it."
3. "The correct procedure is to remove the error in a manner approved by the facility."
4. "The correct procedure is to cover the error completely using a permanent marker."

Level of Cognitive Ability: Evaluating
Client Needs: Safe and Effective Care Environment
Clinical Judgment/Cognitive Skills: Evaluate Outcomes
Integrated Process: Clinical Judgment; Communication and Documentation
Content Area: Leadership/Management: Ethical/Legal
Health Problems: N/A
Priority Concepts: Communication; Health Care Law

Answer: 2
Rationale: If the nurse makes a narrative documentation error in the client's record, the agency's policy needs to be followed to correct the error. Agency policy usually includes drawing one line through the error, initialing and dating the line, and then providing the correct information. The nurse uses a late entry to document additional information that was not documented at the time that it occurred. The nurse avoids attempting to remove the error by any means because these actions raise the suspicion of wrongdoing.
Test-Taking Strategy: Focus on the strategic word, *effective*, and the subject, the principles related to a documentation error. The correct option is the only option that represents application of documentation principles because the remaining options either alter the record in some fashion or incorrectly identify the documentation.
Priority Nursing Tip: Principles of documentation must be followed and data recorded accurately, concisely, completely, legibly, and objectively without bias or opinions. Always follow agency protocol for documentation.
Reference: Potter, P., et al. (2021). *Fundamentals of nursing* (10th ed., p. 367). Elsevier.

25. When responding to the call bell, the nurse finds the client lying on the floor beside the bed. After a thorough assessment and appropriate care, the nurse completes an incident report. How would the incident be described in the report?
1. The client fell out of bed and was found on the floor.
2. The client fell while climbing over the bed's side rails.
3. The client was found lying on the floor beside the bed.
4. The client was restless and fell while getting out of bed.

Level of Cognitive Ability: Applying
Client Needs: Safe and Effective Care Environment
Clinical Judgment/Cognitive Skills: Take Action
Integrated Process: Communication and Documentation
Content Area: Leadership/Management: Ethical/Legal
Health Problems: N/A
Priority Concepts: Communication; Health Care Law

Answer: 3
Rationale: The incident report needs to contain the client's name, age, and diagnosis. It also needs to contain a factual description of the incident, any injuries experienced by those involved, and the outcome of the situation. The correct option is the only option that describes the facts as observed by the nurse. All the remaining options are interpretations of the situation and are not factual data as observed by the nurse.
Test-Taking Strategy: Focus on the subject of an incident report and use general documentation guidelines and principles to answer the question. Remembering to focus on factual information when documenting and avoiding the inclusion of interpretations will direct you to option 3.
Priority Nursing Tip: The incident report is used as a means of identifying risk situations and improving client care. The report form should not be copied or placed in the client's record.
Reference: Zerwekh, J., & Zerwekh Garneau, A. (2021). *Nursing today: Transition and trends* (10th ed., pp. 493–494). Elsevier.

❖ **26.** A client diagnosed with angina pectoris appears to be very anxious and states, "So, I had a heart attack, right?" Which response would the nurse make to the client?
1. "No. That is not why you are hospitalized."
2. "No, but there could be some minimal damage to your heart."
3. "No, not this time and we will do our best to prevent a future heart attack."
4. "No, but it's necessary to monitor you and control or eliminate your pain."

Level of Cognitive Ability: Applying
Client Needs: Psychosocial Integrity
Clinical Judgment/Cognitive Skills: Take Action
Integrated Process: Communication and Documentation
Content Area: Foundations of Care: Communication
Health Problems: Adult Health: Cardiovascular: Coronary Artery Disease
Priority Concepts: Communication; Perfusion

Answer: 4
Rationale: Angina pectoris occurs as a result of an inadequate blood supply to the myocardium causing pain; managing the condition will help address the client's pain. The nurse will want to correct the client's misconception regarding a heart attack while addressing the client's concerns. Option 1 does not address the client's concerns. Option 2 is not correct because angina involves interrupted blood supply but does not result in cardiac tissue damage. Neither the nurse nor the physician can guarantee that a heart attack will not occur as option 3 seems to indicate.
Test-Taking Strategy: Use therapeutic communication techniques and focus on the subject, the difference between the pathology of a heart attack and angina. The correct option is the only option that demonstrates correct communication techniques and provides accurate information on the client's condition.
Priority Nursing Tip: By clarifying the client's condition with the client, the nurse will help minimize stress, which is a contributing factor of angina attacks.
References: Ignatavicius, D., et al. (2021). *Medical-surgical nursing: Concepts for interprofessional collaborative care* (10th ed., p. 621). Elsevier; Potter, P., et al. (2021). *Fundamentals of nursing* (10th ed., pp. 333–335). Elsevier.

27. A client diagnosed with delirium anxiously states, "Look at the spiders on the wall." Which response by the nurse addresses the client's concerns therapeutically?
1. "Would you like me to kill the spiders for you?"
2. "While there may be spiders on the wall, they are not going to hurt you."
3. "I know that you are frightened, but I do not see any spiders on the wall."
4. "You are having a hallucination; I'm sure there are no spiders in this room."

Level of Cognitive Ability: Applying
Client Needs: Psychosocial Integrity
Clinical Judgment/Cognitive Skills: Take Action
Integrated Process: Communication and Documentation
Content Area: Mental Health
Health Problems: Mental Health: Neurocognitive Impairment
Priority Concepts: Communication; Psychosis

Answer: 3
Rationale: When hallucinations are present, the nurse needs to reinforce reality with the client while acknowledging the client's feelings as the correct option does. Eliminate options 1, 2, and 4 because they do not reinforce reality but rather support the legitimacy of the hallucination or that reinforces reality but does not address the client's feelings.
Test-Taking Strategy: Use therapeutic communication techniques and focus on the subject, therapeutically responding to a client who is hallucinating. The correct option is the only option that both supports reality and addresses the client's feelings.
Priority Nursing Tip: If the client is hallucinating, ask the client to describe the hallucinations. Avoid reacting to the hallucination as if it were real.
Reference: Varcarolis, E., & Fosbre, C. (2021). *Essentials of psychiatric mental health nursing: A communication approach to evidence-based care* (4th ed., pp. 261–262, 364). Elsevier.

❖ **28.** While in the hospital, a client was diagnosed with coronary artery disease (CAD). Which question by the nurse is likely to elicit the **most** useful response for determining the client's degree of adjustment to the new diagnosis?
1. "Is there anyone to help with housework and shopping?"
2. "How do you feel about making changes to your lifestyle?"
3. "Do you understand the schedule for your new medications?"
4. "Did you make a follow-up appointment with your provider?"

Level of Cognitive Ability: Applying
Client Needs: Health Promotion and Maintenance
Clinical Judgment/Cognitive Skills: Generate Solutions
Integrated Process: Communication and Documentation
Content Area: Foundations of Care: Communication
Health Problems: Adult Health: Cardiovascular: Coronary Artery Disease
Priority Concepts: Communication; Stress and Coping

Answer: 2
Rationale: Exploring feelings assists the nurse with determining the individualized plan of care for the client who is adjusting to a new diagnosis. The correct option is the best question to ask the client because it is likely to elicit the most revealing information about the client's feelings about CAD and the requisite lifestyle changes that can help maintain health and wellness. The remaining choices are aspects of post-hospital care, but they are unlikely to uncover as much information about the client's adjustment to CAD because they are closed-ended questions.
Test-Taking Strategy: Note the strategic word, *most*. Use therapeutic communication techniques. Open-ended questions are needed to explore the client's reactions to or feelings about an identified situation. Closed-ended responses generally elicit a "yes" or "no" response exclusively. All of the incorrect options are closed-ended responses.
Priority Nursing Tip: Increased cholesterol levels, low-density lipoproteins (LDL) levels, and triglyceride levels place the client at risk for CAD.
References: Ignatavicius, D., et al. (2021). *Medical-surgical nursing: Concepts for interprofessional collaborative care* (10th ed., p. 754). Elsevier; Potter, P., et al. (2021). *Fundamentals of nursing* (10th ed., pp. 333–335). Elsevier.

29. A client has been using crutches to ambulate for 1 week and now reports pain, fatigue, and frustration with crutch walking. How would the nurse respond when the client states, "I feel like I will always be crippled"?
1. "Tell me what makes this so bothersome for you."
2. "I know how you feel. I had to use crutches before too."
3. "Why don't you take a couple of days off of work and rest?"
4. "Just remember, you'll be done with the crutches in another month."

Level of Cognitive Ability: Applying
Client Needs: Psychosocial Integrity
Clinical Judgment/Cognitive Skills: Take Action
Integrated Process: Communication and Documentation
Content Area: Foundations of Care: Communication
Health Problems: Adult Health: Musculoskeletal: Skeletal Injury
Priority Concepts: Communication; Stress and Coping

Answer: 1
Rationale: The correct option demonstrates the therapeutic communication technique of clarification and validation and indicates that the nurse is dealing with the client's problem from the client's perspective. Option 2 devalues the client's feelings and thus blocks communication. Option 3 gives advice and is a communication block. Option 4 provides false reassurances because the client may not be done with the crutches in another month. Additionally, it does not focus on the present problem.
Test-Taking Strategy: Use therapeutic communication techniques. The correct option is the only response that encourages communication. The remaining options are comparable or alike because they are blocks to communication.
Priority Nursing Tip: The nurse needs to monitor for compartment syndrome in a client who has a cast. This is a condition in which pressure increases in a confined anatomic space, leading to decreased blood flow, ischemia, and dysfunction of the tissues.
Reference: Potter, P., et al. (2021). *Fundamentals of nursing* (10th ed., pp. 333–335, 798). Elsevier.

❖ **30.** A teenage client is discharged from the hospital after surgery with instructions to use a cane for the next 6 months. What question **best** demonstrates the nurse's ability to use therapeutic communication techniques to **effectively** assess the teenager's feelings about using a cane?

1. "How do you feel about needing a cane to walk?"
2. "Do you have questions about ambulating with a cane?"
3. "Are you worried about what your friends will think about your cane?"
4. "What types of problems do you think you'll have ambulating with a cane?"

Level of Cognitive Ability: Applying
Client Needs: Psychosocial Integrity
Clinical Judgment/Cognitive Skills: Take Action
Integrated Process: Communication and Documentation
Content Area: Developmental Stages: Adolescent
Health Problems: Adult Health: Musculoskeletal: Skeletal Injury
Priority Concepts: Communication; Stress and Coping

Answer: 1
Rationale: The nurse effectively uses therapeutic communication techniques when posing an open-ended question to elicit assessment data about how the teenager feels about using a cane. The remaining options are closed-ended questions. Option 3 makes assumptions about how the teenager feels, and options 2 and 4 focus on the physical aspects of using the cane.
Test-Taking Strategy: Note the strategic words, *best* and *effectively*, in the question. Focus on the subject, the teenager's feelings about the use of the cane. Note the relationship of the subject and the correct option. Also use therapeutic communication techniques and avoid responses that include communication blocks.
Priority Nursing Tip: The nurse would instruct the client using a cane to inspect the rubber tip on the cane regularly for worn places. A worn tip will need to be replaced.
Reference: Potter, P., et al. (2021). *Fundamentals of nursing* (10th ed., pp. 333–335, 797). Elsevier.

31. After the surgical repair of a fractured hip, a client has consistently refused to engage in ambulation as prescribed. Which statement by the nurse will **best** encourage the client's need to ambulate?

1. "What is it about getting out of bed that concerns you?"
2. "If you are afraid of the pain, I can give you medication to help."
3. "If you don't get up and start walking, your recovery will take much longer."
4. "Being dependent on others must be a depressing for an active person like yourself."

Level of Cognitive Ability: Applying
Client Needs: Psychosocial Integrity
Clinical Judgment/Cognitive Skills: Take Action
Integrated Process: Communication and Documentation
Content Area: Foundations of Care: Communication
Health Problems: Adult Health: Musculoskeletal: Skeletal Injury
Priority Concepts: Adherence; Communication

Answer: 1
Rationale: Early ambulation during the postoperative period is very important to a client's health and recovery, but many different factors may be contributing to the client's refusal to ambulate as prescribed. Asking an open-ended question that encourages a discussion about getting out of bed is the best option available to allow the nurse to facilitate the client's plan of care. Pain may be a concern for the client, but again, the nurse is making an unfounded assumption. Although it is true that the recovery might be prolonged by not ambulating and the client may be depressed, these statements make assumptions about the reason the client is refusing to comply with the plan of care.
Test-Taking Strategy: Note the strategic word, *best*. Use the principles of therapeutic communication techniques and your understanding that noncompliance may have many and varied reasons will help direct you to the correct option.
Priority Nursing Tip: Effective communication with the client is a necessary factor in determining the underlying reasons for noncompliance with the plan of care.
References: Lewis, S., et al. (2020). *Medical-surgical nursing: Assessment and management of clinical problems* (11th ed., pp. 1463–1464, 1466); Potter, P., et al. (2021). *Fundamentals of nursing* (10th ed.). Elsevier. pp. 333–335.

❖ **32.** The student nurse is listening to a lecture on caring for clients with thrombophlebitis. Which statement by the student nurse indicates that the teaching has been **effective**?
1. "Elevating the affected leg is indicated."
2. "Keeping the affected leg flat encourages healing."
3. "Engaging in activity as tolerated needs to be encouraged."
4. "Maintaining bathroom privileges is the most important action."

Level of Cognitive Ability: Evaluating
Client Needs: Physiological Integrity
Clinical Judgment/Cognitive Skills: Evaluate Outcomes
Integrated Process: Communication and Documentation
Content Area: Adult Health: Cardiovascular
Health Problems: Adult Health: Cardiovascular: Vascular Disorders
Priority Concepts: Clinical Judgment; Perfusion

Answer: 1
Rationale: The nurse plans to elevate the affected extremity because this facilitates venous return by using gravity to improve blood return to the heart, decreases venous pressure, and helps relieve edema and pain. Option 2 does not facilitate venous return and thus is not indicated for a client with thrombophlebitis. Options 3 and 4 address activity and ambulation and are not the most important or suitable activities for a client with thrombophlebitis.
Test-Taking Strategy: Note the strategic word, *effective,* and focus on the subject, thrombophlebitis, and think about the pathophysiology associated with this condition and how gravity affects venous blood flow and edema. This will direct you to the correct option.
Priority Nursing Tip: Thrombophlebitis is an inflammation of a vein, often accompanied by clot formation that can present serious circulatory problems.
Reference: Ignatavicius, D., et al. (2021). *Medical-surgical nursing: Concepts for interprofessional collaborative care* (10th ed., p. 722). Elsevier.

33. A client who is experiencing paranoid thinking involving food being poisoned is admitted to the mental health unit. Which communication technique would the nurse use to encourage the client to communicate fears?
1. Offering personal opinions about the need to eat
2. Asking open-ended questions and providing for silence
3. Verbalizing reasons why the client may choose not to eat
4. Focusing on self-disclosure of the nurse's own food preferences

Level of Cognitive Ability: Applying
Client Needs: Physiological Integrity
Clinical Judgment/Cognitive Skills: Take Action
Integrated Process: Communication and Documentation
Content Area: Foundations of Care: Communication
Health Problems: Mental Health: Personality Disorders
Priority Concepts: Communication; Psychosis

Answer: 2
Rationale: Open-ended questions and silence are strategies that are used to encourage clients to discuss their feelings in a descriptive manner. Options 1 and 3 are not helpful to the client because they do not encourage the expression of personal feelings. Option 4 is not a client-centered intervention.
Test-Taking Strategy: Use your knowledge of therapeutic communication techniques to identify the usefulness of the techniques suggested in the correct option. The communication techniques identified in the remaining options are nontherapeutic and are blocks to communication.
Priority Nursing Tip: Avoid whispering in the presence of a client who is paranoid because this will intensify feelings of paranoia.
Reference: Varcarolis, E., & Fosbre, C. (2021). *Essentials of psychiatric mental health nursing: A communication approach to evidence-based care* (4th ed., pp. 257–259). Elsevier.

❖ **34.** The nurse is preparing a client for electroconvulsive therapy (ECT). After the client signs the consent form for the procedure, a family member states, "I don't think that this ECT will be helpful, especially since it makes people's memory worse." What form of communication would the nurse implement to address the family member's concern?

1. Ask other family members and the client if they think that ECT makes people worse.
2. Involve the family member in a dialog to ascertain how the family member arrived at this conclusion.
3. Immediately reassure the client and family that ECT will help and that the memory loss is only temporary.
4. Reinforce with the client and the family member that depression causes more memory impairment than ECT.

Level of Cognitive Ability: Applying
Client Needs: Psychosocial Integrity
Clinical Judgment/Cognitive Skills: Generate Solutions
Integrated Process: Communication and Documentation
Content Area: Foundations of Care: Communication
Health Problems: Mental Health: Mood Disorders
Priority Concepts: Communication; Mood and Affect

Answer: 2
Rationale: In option 2, the nurse is looking for data to assist with clarifying information about the procedure with the family, which is necessary in order to deal effectively with their concerns. Option 1 may place family members on the defensive and promote conflict among them. Option 3 does not acknowledge the family member's statement and concerns. Option 4 addresses content clarification but not the assessment process, and it is not the most therapeutic action.
Test-Taking Strategy: Use therapeutic communication techniques and the steps of the nursing process. Remember that assessment is the first step in the nursing process. In the correct option, the nurse gathers more data via the assessment process and addresses the family member's thoughts and feelings.
Priority Nursing Tip: ECT may be prescribed to treat depression. It consists of inducing a seizure by passing an electrical current through the brain via electrodes attached to the temples. ECT is not a permanent cure. It is true that some clients experience temporary memory loss, but it usually centers on the time period around the treatment itself.
Reference: Varcarolis, E., & Fosbre, C. (2021). *Essentials of psychiatric mental health nursing: A communication approach to evidence-based care* (4th ed., pp. 93–95, 221). Elsevier.

Culture and Spirituality

35. The nurse is caring for a postoperative client with spiritual and culturally based eating and food requirements. Which interventions demonstrate the nurse's spiritual and cultural consideration of the client? **Select all that apply.**

☐ 1. Encouraging the client to try new foods only until healing is complete
☐ 2. Suggesting the substitution of similar foods for the culturally appropriate ones
☐ 3. Asking the client to explain the factors that are important to their eating practices
☐ 4. Including the family in discussions regarding the preparation of accepted foods
☐ 5. Discussing the nutritional requirements the client currently has postoperatively

Level of Cognitive Ability: Applying
Client Needs: Safe and Effective Care Environment
Clinical Judgment/Cognitive Skills: Take Action
Integrated Process: Culture and Spirituality
Content Area: Foundations of Care: Diversity, Equity, Inclusion
Health Problems: N/A
Priority Concepts: Clinical Judgment; Culture

Answer: 3, 4, 5
Rationale: Spiritual and cultural consideration reflects attempts to maintain familiar customs to achieve healthy responses. Gaining knowledge of the customs and their importance to the client will be the basis for an understanding that allows for flexibility and compromise when necessary. Including the family in the discussion will assist with the process as will discussing the needs the client has at this particular time to formulate a plan that meets the needs while maintaining cultural customs. Encouraging new foods in place of the usual foods may be viewed as being insensitive and showing a lack of concern. Substitution is not always necessary.
Test-Taking Strategy: Focus on the subject, spiritual and cultural considerations. Eliminate option 1 because of the closed-ended word *only.* Recall that encouraging clients to move away from their usual customs is considered to be a lack of sensitivity and does not indicate cultural competency. Understanding the goals of spiritual and culturally considerate care will direct you to the correct options.
Priority Nursing Tip: Spiritual and cultural consideration is a critical factor in providing quality nursing care and has a direct effect on client recovery and ultimate wellness.
Reference: Jarvis, C. (2020). *Physical examination and health assessment* (8th ed., pp. 19–21). Elsevier.

❖ **36.** The nurse is caring for a client of an unfamiliar ethnic culture. The nurse shows an understanding of the general principles of culturally sensitive interaction when implementing which interventions? **Select all that apply.**

    ❑ **1.** Addressing the client by their full surname in order to display respect

    ❑ **2.** Maintaining eye contact with the client so as to show respect for the client's age

    ❑ **3.** Utilizing the position of authority nurses hold to provide explanation of facility rules

    ❑ **4.** Touching the client only when necessary and only after explaining the need to do so

    ❑ **5.** Avoiding any frequent engagement with the client in conversation of a personal nature

Level of Cognitive Ability: Applying
Client Needs: Safe and Effective Care Environment
Clinical Judgment/Cognitive Skills: Take Action
Integrated Process: Culture and Spirituality
Content Area: Foundations of Care: Diversity, Equity, Inclusion
Health Problems: N/A
Priority Concepts: Clinical Judgment; Culture

Answer: 1, 5
Rationale: Although cultural sensitivities vary, it is generally prudent to show respect for any client of any ethnic background by using their formal name. Personal conversations not required as part of the assessment process need to be avoided, as should a show of authority. Maintaining eye contact is not universally taken to be a positive behavior and so may be limited until it is determined to be acceptable by the client. Physical touching by strangers is not readily accepted in many cultures and should be engaged in cautiously and only when necessary and with permission from the client.
Test-Taking Strategy: Focus on the subject, general principles of cultural sensitivity. Eliminate option 4 because of the closed-ended word *only*. Remember that close and intimate contact generally is avoided to show respect. Understanding the basic principles of culturally sensitive care will direct you to the correct options.
Priority Nursing Tip: Cultural and spiritual practices vary greatly, and the nurse is responsible for acquiring such knowledge to provide culturally sensitive care.
Reference: Potter, P., et al. (2021). *Fundamentals of nursing* (10th ed., p. 517). Elsevier.

37. The nurse is participating in end-of-life care for a client who has recently immigrated to America. Which interventions would the nurse consider in the plan of care for this client? **Select all that apply.**

    ❑ **1.** Respect family requests for use of herbal medicines.

    ❑ **2.** Recognize that the use of healers is a common practice in all non-American cultures.

    ❑ **3.** Have direct conversations with the matriarch of the family only.

    ❑ **4.** Acknowledge that lack of eye contact does not mean disinterest.

    ❑ **5.** Allow someone from the family to stay with the client after death if requested.

Level of Cognitive Ability: Analyzing
Client Needs: Psychosocial Integrity
Clinical Judgment/Cognitive Skills: Generate Solutions
Integrated Process: Clinical Judgment; Culture and Spirituality
Content Area: Foundations of Care: Diversity, Equity, Inclusion
Health Problems: N/A
Priority Concepts: Culture; Palliation

Answer: 1, 4, 5
Rationale: Herbal medicine plays an important role in many cultures in the care of the dying client, and family requests to incorporate its use in care should be acknowledged and discussed with the physician. The nurse must realize that lack of direct eye contact should not be interpreted as a sign of disinterest. If requested, someone from the family should be allowed to stay with the client after death. Use of healers is not a practice of every culture. The nurse needs to assess and determine who the family wishes to be the person as the direct contact for conversations.
Test-Taking Strategy: Focus on the subject, specific knowledge of different cultural groups and religious and spiritual practices. Read each option carefully and eliminate option 2 because of the closed-ended word all, and option 3 because of the word, *only.*
Priority Nursing Tip: An initial step in ensuring culturally competent care is to assess the needs of the client and what the client wishes to be a part of the plan of care.
Reference: Potter, P., et al. (2021). *Fundamentals of nursing* (10th ed., pp. 731, 744). Elsevier.

❖ **38.** The nurse is caring for a client who does not speak English. An interpreter is currently unavailable. The nurse must perform a dressing change. What would the nurse do to enhance communication with this client before changing the dressing?

1. Ask relatives to interpret because an interpreter is unavailable.
2. Speak slowly and allow the client time to interpret what is being said.
3. Use many nonverbal cues and repetition to reinforce what is being said.
4. Use common words in the nurse's language, because the client is likely to be familiar with them.

Level of Cognitive Ability: Applying
Client Needs: Psychosocial Integrity
Clinical Judgment/Cognitive Skills: Take Action
Integrated Process: Culture and Spirituality
Content Area: Foundations of Care: Diversity, Equity, Inclusion
Health Problems: Adult Health: Integumentary: Wounds
Priority Concepts: Communication; Culture

Answer: 2
Rationale: When caring for a client who speaks a language that is different from the nurse's, the nurse ideally can call on a dialect-specific interpreter designated by the health care agency that is the same age and same gender as the client. If an interpreter is unavailable, the nurse should speak slowly and allow the client time to interpret what is being said. The nurse needs to avoid asking relatives to be interpreters to minimize bias and misinterpretation. The nurse needs to avoid using nonverbal facial expressions and body language, because they could be misinterpreted by the client. The nurse should use common words in the client's language if known.
Test-Taking Strategy: Focus on the subject, communication and language barrier. Recalling that family members should not be used as interpreters because of the risk of bias or misinterpretation will assist you in eliminating option 1. Also recalling that nonverbal cues and body language mean different things in different cultures will assist you in eliminating option 3. From the remaining options, read carefully; it is necessary to know that speaking slowly enhances interpretation on the part of the client.
Priority Nursing Tip: Client confidentiality, as well as the delivery of accurate information, may be compromised when a family member or a non–health care provider acts as interpreter.
Reference: Jarvis, C. (2020). *Physical examination and health assessment* (8th ed., pp. 40–41). Elsevier.

39. The nurse is conducting a cultural and spiritual assessment on a newly admitted client. Which factors specifically related to culture and spirituality would the nurse address? **Select all that apply.**

❑ 1. Nutrition
❑ 2. Communication
❑ 3. Insurance coverage
❑ 4. High-risk behaviors
❑ 5. Health care practices
❑ 6. Family roles and organization

Level of Cognitive Ability: Applying
Client Needs: Psychosocial Integrity
Clinical Judgment/Cognitive Skills: Prioritize Hypotheses
Integrated Process: Culture and Spirituality
Content Area: Foundations of Care: Diversity, Equity, Inclusion
Health Problems: N/A
Priority Concepts: Culture; Health Promotion

Answer: 1, 2, 4, 5, 6
Rationale: When performing a cultural and spiritual assessment, the nurse would focus on the following factors: nutrition, communication, high-risk behaviors, health care practices, family roles and organizations, workforce issues, biocultural ecology, overview (e.g., heritage), pregnancy and childbirth practices, death rituals, spirituality preferences, and health care practitioners. Asking the client about insurance coverage is not specifically related to culture or spiritual practices.
Test-Taking Strategy: Focus on the subject, doing a cultural and spiritual assessment. Recognizing that option 3 is the only option that does not specifically relate to values, beliefs, and customs will assist you in eliminating this option.
Priority Nursing Tip: Nurses often care for clients who come from ethnic, cultural, or religious backgrounds that are different from their own. Awareness of and sensitivity to the unique health and illness beliefs and practices of people of different backgrounds are essential for the delivery of safe and effective care.
Reference: Potter, P., et al. (2021). *Fundamentals of nursing* (10th ed., pp. 113–114). Elsevier.

❖ **40.** The nurse is caring for an Orthodox Jewish client of a different sex whose condition is terminal. The nurse is implementing a plan of care and wishes to communicate this plan with the client and family. The nurse would be aware of what end-of-life spiritual and religious practices when planning and communicating with the client and family? **Select all that apply.**

- ❏ 1. Family members might not shake hands with members of a different sex.
- ❏ 2. Religious laws might not be observed during times of severe illness.
- ❏ 3. During the process of dying, visitors and conversation need to be kept to a minimum.
- ❏ 4. Family members might not make direct eye contact with members of a different sex.
- ❏ 5. Clients are usually very quiet and do not express what they are thinking or feeling.

Level of Cognitive Ability: Analyzing
Client Needs: Psychosocial Integrity
Clinical Judgment/Cognitive Skills: Generate Solutions
Integrated Process: Clinical Judgment; Culture and Spirituality
Content Area: Foundations of Care: Diversity, Equity, Inclusion
Health Problems: N/A
Priority Concepts: Caregiving; Culture

Answer: 1, 2, 4
Rationale: The Orthodox Jew strictly follows the laws of Judaism; however, during times of severe illness, Jewish laws are not observed if doing so will endanger the client's health. In the Orthodox Jewish faith, members generally will not shake hands or make direct eye contact with members of a different sex. During times of illness or death, the Orthodox Jewish community, including family and friends, will frequently visit and are considered the nucleus of the Jewish culture. Clients of the Orthodox Jewish faith are generally very verbal about what they are feeling.
Test-Taking Strategy: Note the subject, end-of-life spiritual and religious beliefs of Orthodox Judaism. Think about these religious beliefs to answer correctly. Also, eliminate options 3 and 5 because they are comparable or alike options.
Priority Nursing Tip: According to Jewish law and custom it is very important for the client not to be left alone to die.
References: Giger, J., & Haddad, L. (2021). *Transcultural nursing: Assessment and intervention* (8th ed., pp. 512, 516–517). Elsevier; Lewis, S., et al. (2020). *Medical-surgical nursing: Assessment and management of clinical problems* (11th ed., p. 24). Elsevier.

41. The nurse is caring for a client who reports that they are a practicing Roman Catholic. Which actions by the nurse demonstrates spiritual and cultural sensitivity?

1. Observe fasting rules on Sundays.
2. Inform dietary that meat cannot be served on Fridays.
3. Allow the client to observe communion daily if requested.
4. Discourage anointing by the priest unless the condition becomes terminal.

Level of Cognitive Ability: Applying
Client Needs: Psychosocial Integrity
Clinical Judgment/Cognitive Skills: Take Action
Integrated Process: Culture and Spirituality
Content Area: Foundations of Care: Diversity, Equity, Inclusion
Health Problems: N/A
Priority Concepts: Caregiving; Culture

Answer: 3
Rationale: During response to illness, practicing Roman Catholics may request to be anointed while sick, and this practice should not be discouraged. They may also practice daily Holy Communion. Fasting on Sundays is not a custom. Avoiding meat on Fridays is not a regular custom; it may however be a custom on certain holy days.
Test-Taking Strategy: Focus on the subject, practices of a Roman Catholic client and spiritual and cultural sensitivity. Use knowledge regarding the spiritual practices of the Roman Catholic to answer correctly. Remember that Roman Catholics often practice daily communion and may request to be anointed while sick.
Priority Nursing Tip: It is important to understand the client's religious and spiritual beliefs and how they affect a client's health status. It is also important to have background information regarding holy days and practices for various religions.
Reference: Lewis, S., et al. (2020). *Medical-surgical nursing: Assessment and management of clinical problems* (11th ed., p. 24). Elsevier.

❖ **42.** The nurse is caring for a client who follows a kosher diet. Which foods would the nurse use in meal planning for the client? **Select all that apply.**
- ❑ **1.** Pork
- ❑ **2.** Tuna
- ❑ **3.** Turkey
- ❑ **4.** Chicken
- ❑ **5.** Lobster

Level of Cognitive Ability: Applying
Client Needs: Psychosocial Integrity
Clinical Judgment/Cognitive Skills: Generate Solutions
Integrated Process: Culture and Spirituality
Content Area: Foundations of Care: Diversity, Equity, Inclusion
Health Problems: N/A
Priority Concepts: Culture; Nutrition

Answer: 2, 3, 4
Rationale: Clients who follow a kosher diet avoid meat from carnivores, pork products, and fish without scales or fins, such as shellfish. Tuna, chicken, and turkey are considered kosher and appropriate.
Test-Taking Strategy: Focus on the subject, a kosher diet. Think about what you know about a kosher diet. Clients who follow a kosher diet avoid meat from carnivores, pork products, and fish without scales or fins. This will assist in directing you to the remaining correct options.
Priority Nursing Tip: A kosher diet is a healthy diet because of the strict rules under which foods allowed on the diet are prepared. Foods are prepared so that harmful hormones that transfer from meat and dairy products into our bodies are eliminated.
Reference: Nix, S. (2022). *Williams' Basic nutrition and diet therapy* (16th ed., p. 248). Elsevier; Potter, P., et al. (2021). *Fundamentals of nursing* (10th ed., p. 1110). Elsevier.

43. The nurse is caring for a client who has been admitted for asthma. The nurse is unfamiliar with the cultural and spiritual practices and beliefs of the client's homeland. Which questions are **most appropriate** for the nurse to ask during the admission process? **Select all that apply.**
- ❑ **1.** "What do you believe is causing your illness?"
- ❑ **2.** "Why don't you take some asthma medication?"
- ❑ **3.** "Why do you wear that amulet around your neck?"
- ❑ **4.** "Are there any remedies you have used in the past?"
- ❑ **5.** "Who do you usually see for help when you are sick?"

Level of Cognitive Ability: Applying
Client Needs: Safe and Effective Care Environment
Clinical Judgment/Cognitive Skills: Generate Solutions
Integrated Process: Clinical Judgment; Culture and Spirituality
Content Area: Foundations of Care: Diversity, Equity, Inclusion
Health Problems: Adult Health: Respiratory: Asthma
Priority Concepts: Communication; Culture

Answer: 1, 4, 5
Rationale: Assessment includes cultural and spiritual information. It includes questions regarding clients' health beliefs and practices, their health care providers, and their beliefs regarding the origin of illness. Option 2 may have an accusatory undertone. This type of question will not assist the nurse in developing a rapport. A person's reason for wearing an amulet is not relevant to this situation; this question may be perceived as intrusive.
Test-Taking Strategy: Note the strategic words, *most appropriate*. Focus on the subject, therapeutic communication with a client whose cultural practices are unfamiliar to the nurse. It is also important to keep in mind that the nurse needs to be sensitive to ways in which cultural beliefs and faith impact the client's health care experiences. Think about therapeutic communication techniques, review each option, and then sort the options into therapeutic or nontherapeutic responses to help you eliminate nontherapeutic responses.
Priority Nursing Tip: It is important to ask assessment questions that will assist in gaining information about a client's health care practices. The nurse would avoid gesturing because certain hand or body movements may have adverse connotations in other cultures. The nurse would also evaluate whether questions or instructions have been understood because some clients will nod "yes" but not really comprehend.
Reference: Potter, P., et al. (2021). *Fundamentals of nursing* (10th ed., pp. 113–114, 332). Elsevier.

❖ **44.** The nurse is assessing a client who recently moved to America who presented to the emergency department with complaints of a headache and nausea. The client is accompanied by an adult child. Upon assessment, the nurse notes long, pale red welts on both arms. Which actions would the nurse take **next**? **Select all that apply.**

   ❏ 1. Ask if the client has used any home remedies.

   ❏ 2. Assess cultural health beliefs and practices.

   ❏ 3. Report the presence of welts to social services.

   ❏ 4. Remove the client's adult child from the room immediately.

   ❏ 5. Recognize the redness as a result of a traditional form of healing.

Level of Cognitive Ability: Analyzing
Client Needs: Physiological Integrity
Clinical Judgment/Cognitive Skills: Analyze Cues
Integrated Process: Clinical Judgment; Culture and Spirituality
Content Area: Foundations of Care: Diversity, Equity, Inclusion
Health Problems: N/A
Priority Concepts: Clinical Judgment; Culture

Answer: 1, 2, 5
Rationale: The nurse would ask the client if they are using any home remedies. The nurse would assess cultural health beliefs and practices and understand that "coining or coin rubbing" is a traditional form of healing. The nurse should recognize the redness as a result of coining. The nurse would not report the welts and coining to social services because the practice is not abuse. The client's adult child would not be removed from the room unless the client requests it.
Test-Taking Strategy: Note the strategic word, *next*. Focus on the subject, assessment of a client who presents with long, pale red welts on the arms. Think about the relationship between cultural health beliefs and health care practices. Specific knowledge that coining is a common practice in some cultures is necessary to answer correctly.
Priority Nursing Tip: Coining leaves distinct markings and is often misconstrued as signs of abuse. Coining begins with the use of warm massage oil mixed with essential oils such as peppermint to irritate the skin slightly. The massage relaxes the client in preparation for the next stage in which a coin is repeatedly rubbed against the skin in long flowing movements away from the heart. Blood then rises to the top of the skin. The markings will subside in a few days.
Reference: Giger, J., & Haddad, L. (2021). *Transcultural nursing: Assessment and intervention* (8th ed., p. 393). Elsevier.

45. The hospice nurse is caring for a client of the Muslim faith. Which religious belief would the nurse expect to observe?

   1. The client's bed is positioned toward Mecca.

   2. The client is left alone except for bathing and feeding.

   3. The religious leader is not allowed to visit until the client has died.

   4. Fasting is implemented to promote healing.

Level of Cognitive Ability: Analyzing
Client Needs: Psychosocial Integrity
Clinical Judgment/Cognitive Skills: Recognize Cues
Integrated Process: Clinical Judgment; Culture and Spirituality
Content Area: Foundations of Care: Diversity, Equity, Inclusion
Health Problems: N/A
Priority Concepts: Caregiving; Culture

Answer: 1
Rationale: Mecca is Islam's holiest city. Those of the Muslim faith desire their body to be facing Mecca. It is not common practice to leave the client alone. A family member may wish to remain with the client at all times, if appropriate medically. A religious leader should be made available to the client whenever the client or family requests. Fasting is not a practice.
Test-Taking Strategy: Focus on the subject, religious practices of a Muslim client. It is necessary to have knowledge of these religious practices and beliefs in order to answer correctly.
Priority Nursing Tip: Clients and families of different faiths may deal with and face imminent death differently based on their spiritual beliefs. It is important for the nurse to be familiar with death and dying beliefs and cultural and spiritual practices to provide culturally congruent care.
Reference: Giger, J., & Haddad, L. (2021). *Transcultural nursing: Assessment and intervention* (8th ed., p. 347). Elsevier.

❖ **46.** A biologically born female of the Muslim faith has been stabilized following an assault in the parking lot of a local restaurant. The nurse manager is making assignments for the oncoming shift. Which action by the nurse manager is the **most appropriate** to ensure the client's comfort?

1. Assign the best nurse of the opposite sex to the client.
2. Assign the client a nurse of the same sex for every shift.
3. Allow the client to pick the nurses who will care for them.
4. Remove all of client's clothing each shift to perform a skin assessment.

Level of Cognitive Ability: Applying
Client Needs: Psychosocial Integrity
Clinical Judgment/Cognitive Skills: Take Action
Integrated Process: Culture and Spirituality
Content Area: Foundations of Care: Diversity, Equity, Inclusion
Health Problems: Mental Health: Abuse/Neglect
Priority Concepts: Caregiving; Culture

Answer: 2
Rationale: Information about family and roles will greatly influence the nurse's plan of care. Biologically born female of the Muslim faith can only be cared for by a someone of the same sex. Assigning a nurse of the opposite sex to care for this client would be inappropriate. It would also be inappropriate to place the client in a position to choose a nurse for their care. Unless medically necessary, the client would not need to have a skin assessment every shift. If it is required, a nurse of the same sex must be present to assist in the skin assessment.
Test-Taking Strategy: Focus on the strategic words, *most appropriate.* Note that the client in the question is a biologically born female. Next, think about the cultural beliefs of the Muslim faith and that the subject of the question is that the nurse manager is making an assignment.
Priority Nursing Tip: When assigned to a client, note the client's culture and review any specific beliefs and practices that need to be taken into consideration when planning care.
Reference: Giger, J., & Haddad, L. (2021). *Transcultural nursing: Assessment and intervention* (8th ed., 345–346). Elsevier.

47. The unit manager working on a medical-surgical unit is conducting an in-service session on the provision of spirituality and culturally competent care and factors that contribute to health disparities. Which factors does the manager incorporate into this teaching session? **Select all that apply.**

☐ 1. Age
☐ 2. Genetics
☐ 3. Ethnicity
☐ 4. Education
☐ 5. Past medical history
☐ 6. Health care provider attitudes

Level of Cognitive Ability: Applying
Client Needs: Psychosocial Integrity
Clinical Judgment/Cognitive Skills: Generate Solutions
Integrated Process: Culture and Spirituality
Content Area: Foundations of Care: Diversity, Equity, Inclusion
Health Problems: N/A
Priority Concepts: Culture; Leadership

Answer: 1, 3, 4, 6
Rationale: Many factors contribute to health disparities, including age; ethnicity, race, and culture; education; health care provider attitudes; geographic location; income; occupation; health literacy; and gender. Genetics and past medical history are not factors that influence health disparities.
Test-Taking Strategy: It is necessary to understand the subject of health disparities to answer this question. Recall that disparities relate to a person's position in society, and analyze each of the options and determine whether they would contribute to health disparities.
Priority Nursing Tip: In the provision of spiritual and culturally competent care, the nurse needs to avoid stereotyping and needs to be aware that there are several subcultures within cultures, and there are several dialects within languages.
Reference: Potter, P., et al. (2021). *Fundamentals of nursing* (10th ed., pp. 108–109, 111). Elsevier.

❖ **48.** The nurse is caring for a client of a different culture and is assessing for client perceptions regarding nutrition. Which, in addition to the impact of food on disease and illness, would the nurse consider in order to provide culturally competent care?
1. Educational background and employment history
2. Familial support systems and financial well-being
3. Client perception of body weight and size relative to culture
4. Ability to purchase foods necessary for disease management

Level of Cognitive Ability: Applying
Client Needs: Psychosocial Integrity
Clinical Judgment/Cognitive Skills: Generate Solutions
Integrated Process: Culture and Spirituality
Content Area: Foundations of Care: Diversity, Equity, Inclusion
Health Problems: Adult Health: Gastrointestinal: Nutrition/Malabsorption Problems
Priority Concepts: Clinical Judgment; Culture

Answer: 3
Rationale: When addressing nutrition for clients with diverse cultural backgrounds, the nurse must consider dietary preferences, the impact of food on disease and illness, and client perception of body weight and size relative to culture. For example, some cultures may not consider obesity to be a major health indicator; therefore, teaching regarding weight reduction may be difficult. The other options address social and financial status and are not directly related to cultural considerations with regard to nutrition.
Test-Taking Strategy: Focus on the **subject**, cultural considerations in relation to nutrition. Recognizing that options 1, 2, and 4 are **comparable or alike** and are in some way related to financial status will assist you in eliminating these options. In addition, note the similarity between the question and the option in that both contain the word *culture.*
Priority Nursing Tip: Learn about the cultures of clients with whom you will be working; also, ask clients about their health care practices and preferences.
Reference: Nix, S. (2022). *Williams' Basic nutrition and diet therapy* (16th ed., pp. 236–237). Elsevier; Potter, P., et al. (2021). *Fundamentals of nursing* (10th ed., p. 1111). Elsevier.

49. The nurse is caring for a client in labor who is from the Philippines. The client is 4 cm dilated and 30% effaced. This is a first child. The birthing client is grimacing; pulse, respiratory rate, and blood pressure are elevated. The nurse offers to call the primary health care provider (PHCP) for an epidural prescription. The client declines. The nurse would hypothesize that the client declined the epidural for which reason?
1. Filipino persons decrease their pain through a verbal release.
2. Filipino persons will only accept treatments for pain from their partners and family.
3. Filipino persons are often stoic and view childbirth pain as a normal part of life.
4. Filipino persons believe that pain is a form of spiritual atonement for one's past deeds.

Level of Cognitive Ability: Analyzing
Client Needs: Psychosocial Integrity
Clinical Judgment/Cognitive Skills: Prioritize Hypotheses
Integrated Process: Clinical Judgment; Culture and Spirituality
Content Area: Foundations of Care: Diversity, Equity, Inclusion
Health Problems: Maternity: Discomforts of Pregnancy
Priority Concepts: Communication; Culture

Answer: 4
Rationale: Childbirth experiences differ among different cultures. Filipino persons view pain as part of living an honorable life and view this as an opportunity to reach a fuller spiritual life or to atone for past wrongdoings. The client will not complain of pain despite physiologic indicators. Therefore, the nurse needs to offer and encourage the use of pain medication. The remaining options are not correct information.
Test-Taking Strategy: Focus on the **subject**, the Filipino culture. To plan effective care for clients, the nurse must perform a cultural assessment for each client. To answer correctly it is necessary to know that Filipino persons believe that pain is a form of spiritual atonement.
Priority Nursing Tip: When planning any intervention, the nurse must take a client's culture into consideration.
Reference: Giger, J., & Haddad, L. (2021). *Transcultural nursing: Assessment and intervention* (8th ed., p. 411). Elsevier.

Teaching and Learning

❖ **50.** The nurse is providing discharge teaching for a client diagnosed and treated for tuberculosis (TB). Which statement by the client indicates that teaching has been **effective? Select all that apply.**
- ❏ 1. "All used dishes need to be sterilized."
- ❏ 2. "My close contacts have to be tested for TB."
- ❏ 3. "Soiled tissues need to be disposed of properly."
- ❏ 4. "House isolation is required for at least 8 months."
- ❏ 5. "The mouth needs to always be covered when coughing."

Level of Cognitive Ability: Evaluating
Client Needs: Safe and Effective Care Environment
Clinical Judgment/Cognitive Skills: Evaluate Outcomes
Integrated Process: Clinical Judgment; Teaching and Learning
Content Area: Foundations of Care: Infection Control
Health Problems: Adult Health: Respiratory: Tuberculosis
Priority Concepts: Patient Education; Infection

Answer: 2, 3, 5
Rationale: TB is a communicable disease, and the nurse must teach the client measures to prevent its spread. Any close contacts with the client must be tested and treated if the results of the screening test are positive. Because it is an airborne disease, the client must properly dispose of used tissues and needs to cover the mouth when coughing. There is no evidence to suggest that sterilizing dishes would break the chain of infection with pulmonary TB. It is not necessary for the client to isolate themself in the house. Once the client is treated and results of three sputum cultures are negative, the client will not spread the infection.
Test-Taking Strategy: Focus on the strategic word, *effective,* and the subject, minimizing the spread of TB. Also focusing on the pathophysiology of TB and the associated communicability factors and risks will assist you in answering correctly.
Priority Nursing Tip: Multidrug-resistant strains of TB can result from improper compliance, noncompliance with treatment programs, or development of mutations in tubercle bacillus; the nurse must include the importance of medication compliance when teaching the client with TB.
Reference: Ignatavicius, D., et al. (2021). *Medical-surgical nursing: Concepts for interprofessional collaborative care* (10th ed., pp. 577, 580). Elsevier.

51. A client is receiving intravenous (IV) antibiotic therapy at home via an intermittent IV catheter. In order to facilitate the early detection of IV therapy complications, which intervention would be included in the client's education?
1. Protect the IV site continually.
2. Keep the IV site clean and dry.
3. Report local pain, drainage, or edema.
4. Apply pressure to the IV site if it dislodges.

Level of Cognitive Ability: Applying
Client Needs: Safe and Effective Care Environment
Clinical Judgment/Cognitive Skills: Take Action
Integrated Process: Teaching and Learning
Content Area: Foundations of Care: Fluids and Electrolytes
Health Problems: N/A
Priority Concepts: Patient Education; Safety

Answer: 3
Rationale: The nurse instructs the client to report clinical indicators of an IV site infection, including pain, drainage, and edema because the early detection of infection decreases the risk of septicemia, tissue loss, and devastating complications. The remaining options are reasonable aspects of client teaching for IV therapy at home, but they are not surveillance methods.
Test-Taking Strategy: Focus on the subject, early detection of IV therapy complications. Eliminate options 1, 2, and 4 because these choices describe aspects of IV care to help prevent complications, but they do not contribute to early detection.
Priority Nursing Tip: Any solution administered by the intravenous route directly enters the client's circulatory system. Strict aseptic technique is necessary to prevent infection.
Reference: Ignatavicius, D., et al. (2021). *Medical-surgical nursing: Concepts for interprofessional collaborative care* (10th ed., p. 295). Elsevier.

52. The home care nurse provides instructions about the management of pruritus to a client with hepatitis who developed jaundice. Which statement made by the client suggests to the nurse that the client **needs further teaching?**
1. "I need to wear loose cotton clothing."
2. "A tepid water bath should help stop the itching."
3. "Keeping the house warmer is likely to lessen the itching."
4. "I need to take the prescribed antihistamines as I'm supposed to."

Level of Cognitive Ability: Evaluating
Client Needs: Physiological Integrity
Clinical Judgment/Cognitive Skills: Evaluate Outcomes
Integrated Process: Clinical Judgment; Teaching and Learning
Content Area: Adult Health: Gastrointestinal
Health Problems: Adult Health: Gastrointestinal: Hepatitis
Priority Concepts: Patient Education; Tissue Integrity

Answer: 3
Rationale: Pruritus is caused by the accumulation of bile salts in the skin and results from obstructed biliary excretion. The client would be instructed to keep the house temperature cool to minimize the itching. The client should avoid the use of alkaline soap, and should wear loose, soft, cotton clothing. Antihistamines may relieve the itching, as will tepid water and emollient baths.
Test-Taking Strategy: Note the strategic words, *needs further teaching.* These words indicate a negative event query and ask you to select an option that is an incorrect statement. Recalling that heat causes vasodilation will assist with directing you to the correct option.
Priority Nursing Tip: Jaundice results when the liver is unable to metabolize bilirubin or when edema, fibrosis, and scarring of the hepatic bile ducts interfere with normal bile and bilirubin secretion.
Reference: Lewis, S., et al. (2020). *Medical-surgical nursing: Assessment and management of clinical problems* (11th ed., pp. 596, 972). Elsevier.

53. The nurse has provided home care instructions to a client with prostate cancer who has been hospitalized for a transurethral resection of the prostate (TURP). Which statement by the client indicates the **need for further teaching?**
1. "Prune juice needs to be included in my diet."
2. "I need to avoid strenuous activity for 4 to 6 weeks."
3. "My intake of water needs to be at least six to eight glasses daily."
4. "I can't lift or push objects that weigh more than 30 pounds."

Level of Cognitive Ability: Evaluating
Client Needs: Physiological Integrity
Clinical Judgment/Cognitive Skills: Evaluate Outcomes
Integrated Process: Clinical Judgment; Teaching and Learning
Content Area: Adult Health: Renal and Urinary
Health Problems: Adult Health: Cancer: Prostate
Priority Concepts: Patient Education; Safety

Answer: 4
Rationale: The client needs to be advised to avoid strenuous activity for 4 to 6 weeks and avoid lifting items that weigh more than 20 pounds. Straining during defecation is avoided to prevent bleeding. Prune juice is a satisfactory bowel stimulant. The client needs to consume a daily intake of at least six to eight glasses of nonalcoholic fluids to minimize clot formation.
Test-Taking Strategy: Note the strategic words, *need for further teaching.* These words indicate a negative event query and ask you to select an option that is an incorrect statement. Eliminate options that suggest general postoperative teaching points. Considering the anatomic location of the surgical procedure, it is reasonable to think that constipation needs to be avoided. Also note that lifting items that weigh 30 pounds is excessive.
Priority Nursing Tip: After TURP, monitor for hemorrhage. Postoperative continuous bladder irrigation may be prescribed, which prevents catheter obstruction from clots.
Reference: Ignatavicius, D., et al. (2021). *Medical-surgical nursing: Concepts for interprofessional collaborative care* (10th ed., pp. 1478, 1484). Elsevier.

❖ **54.** A client is being treated for an atrial dysrhythmia with quinidine gluconate. Which statement indicates to the nurse that the client understood the medication instructions about what to do if one dose is missed?
1. "I need to take the next prescribed dose as usual."
2. "I need to take the dose as soon as I realize I've missed it."
3. "I need to call my physician immediately."
4. "I need to take two doses of the medication at the next scheduled time."

Level of Cognitive Ability: Evaluating
Client Needs: Physiological Integrity
Clinical Judgment/Cognitive Skills: Evaluate Outcomes
Integrated Process: Clinical Judgment; Teaching and Learning
Content Area: Pharmacology: Cardiovascular: Antidysrhythmics
Health Problems: Adult Health: Cardiovascular: Dysrhythmias
Priority Concepts: Patient Education; Safety

Answer: 1
Rationale: Quinidine gluconate needs to be taken exactly as prescribed. Because of the action and effects of this medication, the client needs to be instructed to take the medication if remembered within 2 hours of the missed dose, or omit the dose and then resume the normal schedule. There is no need to call the doctor immediately unless more than one dose is missed or if the client experiences cardiac symptoms such as dysrhythmias. It is not safe to take the dose whenever it is remembered or to take an extra dose.
Test-Taking Strategy: Focus on the subject, the principles related to quinidine gluconate administration. Think about the action and effect of the medication. Only the correct option expresses the appropriate measures to take when one medication dose is forgotten.
Priority Nursing Tip: Quinidine gluconate is an antidysrhythmic medication. The client must be instructed to take the medication exactly as prescribed.
Reference: Lilley, L., Rainforth Collins, S., & Snyder J. (2020). *Pharmacology and the nursing process* (9th ed., p. 399). Elsevier.

55. The nurse is educating the client on how to save lives and prevent burn injuries in the event of a fire in the home. Which statement by the client indicates that the teaching has been **effective**?
1. "I need to place escape ladders in the bedrooms."
2. "I need to install a whole-house sprinkler system."
3. "I need to keep fresh batteries in smoke detectors."
4. "I need to mount fire extinguishers in several areas."

Level of Cognitive Ability: Evaluating
Client Needs: Safe and Effective Care Environment
Clinical Judgment/Cognitive Skills: Evaluate Outcomes
Integrated Process: Teaching and Learning
Content Area: Foundations of Care: Safety
Health Problems: Adult Health: Integumentary: Burns
Priority Concepts: Patient Education; Safety

Answer: 3
Rationale: The early detection of smoke using a smoke detector and immediate evacuation from the house have significant and positive effects on mortality rates. This is because the smoke alarm activates before the appearance of open flames, which gives people in the house a chance to evacuate without burn injuries. Option 1 helps people in the house escape from second-story rooms safely, but it does not alert the people to the fire before flames are evident, thus exposing them to the risk of burn injury. Installing a sprinkler system is very expensive, and this is usually not done in private residences. Fire extinguishers are a good idea to have in the kitchen and other areas for small fires, but they are not designed to extinguish large fires.
Test-Taking Strategy: Note the strategic word, *effective*. Focus on the subject, measure to save lives and prevent burn injuries in the event of a fire in the home. This will direct you to the correct option.
Priority Nursing Tip: In the hospital, remember the mnemonic RACE (Rescue the client, Activate the fire alarm, Confine the fire, and Extinguish the fire) to set priorities in the event of a fire.
Reference: Potter, P., et al. (2021). *Fundamentals of nursing* (10th ed., p. 395). Elsevier.

56. A client has had same-day surgery to insert a ventilating tube into the tympanic membrane. Which statement assures the nurse that the client understands the discharge instructions?
1. "I will bathe rather than take a shower for at least a week."
2. "I was told to try and avoid taking medications for pain."
3. "I need to wash my hair quickly; taking 2 minutes or less."
4. "Swimming is allowed only if I keep my head above water."

Level of Cognitive Ability: Evaluating
Client Needs: Physiological Integrity
Clinical Judgment/Cognitive Skills: Evaluate Outcomes
Integrated Process: Teaching and Learning
Content Area: Adult Health: Ear
Health Problems: Adult Health: Ear: Inflammation/Infections/Structural Problems
Priority Concepts: Patient Education; Sensory Perception

Answer: 1
Rationale: After the insertion of tubes into the tympanic membrane, it is important to avoid getting water in the ears. Swimming, showering, and washing the hair are avoided after surgery until the time frame designated for each is identified by the surgeon. The client would take medication as advised for postoperative discomfort.
Test-Taking Strategy: Note the words *understands the discharge instructions*. Eliminate options 3 and 4 because of the word *quickly* and the closed-ended word *only*. From the remaining choices, focusing on the anatomic location of the surgery will direct you to the correct option.
Priority Nursing Tip: Ventilating tubes inserted into the tympanic membranes are tiny, white, spool-shaped tubes. If the tubes fall out, it is not an emergency, but the surgeon needs to be notified.
Reference: Ignatavicius, D., et al. (2021). *Medical-surgical nursing: Concepts for interprofessional collaborative care* (10th ed., p. 963). Elsevier.

57. The nurse has completed diet teaching for a client on a low-sodium diet for the treatment of hypertension. Which statement by the client would indicate to the nurse that there is a **need for further teaching?**
1. "Frozen foods are usually lowest in sodium."
2. "This diet will help lower my blood pressure."
3. "This diet is not a replacement for my antihypertensive medications."
4. "The reason I need to lower my salt intake is to reduce fluid retention."

Level of Cognitive Ability: Evaluating
Client Needs: Physiological Integrity
Clinical Judgment/Cognitive Skills: Evaluate Outcomes
Integrated Process: Teaching and Learning
Content Area: Adult Health: Cardiovascular
Health Problems: Adult Health: Cardiovascular: Hypertension
Priority Concepts: Patient Education; Nutrition

Answer: 1
Rationale: A low-sodium diet is used as an adjunct to antihypertensive medications for the treatment of hypertension. Sodium retains fluid, which leads to hypertension as a result of increased fluid volume. Frozen foods use salt as a preservative, which increases their sodium content. Canned foods are extremely high in sodium. Fresh or frozen foods are best.
Test-Taking Strategy: Note the strategic words, *need for further teaching*. These words indicate a negative event query and ask you to select an option that is an incorrect statement. Eliminate options that are accurate statements related to hypertension. Also, recall that "fresh is best"; fresh foods are lowest in sodium. If fresh is not possible, client should choose frozen, not canned.
Priority Nursing Tip: Emphasize to the client with hypertension that dietary changes are not temporary and must be maintained for life.
Reference: Grodner, M., Escott-Stump, S., & Dorner, S. (2020). *Nutritional foundations and clinical applications* (7th ed., p. 346). Elsevier.

58. The nurse is giving dietary instructions to a client who had a kidney transplant and has been prescribed cyclosporine. Which statement by the client indicates the **need for further teaching?**
1. "Red meats are alright to eat."
2. "Orange juice is a great choice for breakfast."
3. "Grapefruit juice will not interfere with the medication."
4. "Green, leafy vegetables need to be eaten as often as possible."

Level of Cognitive Ability: Evaluating
Client Needs: Physiological Integrity
Clinical Judgment/Cognitive Skills: Evaluate Outcomes
Integrated Process: Teaching and Learning
Content Area: Pharmacology: Immune: Immunosuppressants
Health Problems: Adult Health: Immune: Transplantation
Priority Concepts: Patient Education; Safety

Answer: 3
Rationale: A compound in grapefruit juice inhibits the metabolism of cyclosporine. Thus, drinking grapefruit juice can raise cyclosporine levels by 50% to 100%, greatly increasing the risk of toxicity. The foods in options 1, 2, and 4 are acceptable to consume.
Test-Taking Strategy: Focus on the strategic words, *need for further teaching,* and the subject, the food item to avoid. This creates a negative event query and requires you to select something the client needs to avoid ingesting. Use general medication guidelines to assist in answering the question, and remember that grapefruit juice would not be administered with medications.
Priority Nursing Tip: Cyclosporine is an immunosuppressant medication that can be toxic and cause kidney damage.
Reference: Lilley, L., Rainforth Collins, S., & Snyder J. (2020). *Pharmacology and the nursing process* (9th ed., p. 764). Elsevier.

59. The nurse performs an initial assessment on a pregnant client and determines that the client is at risk for toxoplasmosis. The nurse provides education to the client on how to prevent the disease. Which statement by the client indicates that teaching has been **effective?**
1. "It's alright to eat raw meats."
2. "I need to wash hands only before meals."
3. "I need to avoid exposure to litter boxes used by my cat."
4. "I need to use topical corticosteroid treatments prophylactically."

Level of Cognitive Ability: Evaluating
Client Needs: Safe and Effective Care Environment
Clinical Judgment/Cognitive Skills: Evaluate Outcomes
Integrated Process: Clinical Judgment; Teaching and Learning
Content Area: Foundations of Care: Infection Prevention and Control
Health Problems: Maternity: Infection/Inflammation
Priority Concepts: Patient Education; Infection

Answer: 3
Rationale: Infected house cats transmit toxoplasmosis through the feces. Handling litter boxes can transmit the disease to the pregnant client. Meats that are undercooked can harbor microorganisms that can cause infection. Hands need to be washed frequently throughout the day. The use of topical corticosteroids will not prevent exposure to the disease.
Test-Taking Strategy: Focus on the strategic word, *effective.* Eliminate option 2 because of the closed-ended word *only.* Eliminate option 1 because of the word *raw.* From the remaining choices, focusing on the words *prevent the disease* in the question will direct you to the correct option.
Priority Nursing Tip: Toxoplasmosis is an infection that can be transmitted to the fetus across the placenta. This infection can cause spontaneous abortion in the first trimester.
Reference: McKinney, E. S., et al. (2022). *Maternal child nursing* (6th ed., p. 575). Elsevier.

❖ **60.** A home care nurse is instructing a parent of a child diagnosed with cystic fibrosis (CF) about the appropriate dietary measures. Which diet would the nurse tell the parent that the child needs to consume?
1. Low-calorie, low-fat diet
2. High-calorie, restricted fat
3. Low-calorie, low-protein diet
4. High-calorie, high-protein diet

Level of Cognitive Ability: Applying
Client Needs: Physiological Integrity
Clinical Judgment/Cognitive Skills: Generate Solutions
Integrated Process: Teaching and Learning
Content Area: Foundations of Care: Therapeutic Diets
Health Problems: Pediatric-Specific: Cystic Fibrosis
Priority Concepts: Patient Education; Nutrition

Answer: 4
Rationale: Children with CF are managed with a high-calorie, high-protein diet. Pancreatic enzyme replacement therapy and fat-soluble vitamin supplements are administered. Fat restriction is not necessary.
Test-Taking Strategy: Eliminate options 1 and 2 first because they are comparable or alike, and both restrict fat. From the remaining choices, focus on the subject of nutritional needs of a child with cystic fibrosis (CF) and the pathophysiology related to CF; this will direct you to the correct option.
Priority Nursing Tip: Cystic fibrosis is a progressive and incurable disorder, and respiratory failure is a common cause of death; organ transplantations may be an option to increase survival rates.
Reference: McKinney, E. S., et al. (2022). *Maternal child nursing* (6th ed., p. 1077). Elsevier.

61. The student nurse is listening to an orthopedic lecture on preoperative education and knee surgeries. Which statement by the student nurse indicates that the teaching has been **effective**?
1. "Crutch walking instructions would be scheduled before surgery."
2. "Crutch walking instructions would be given on the first postoperative day."
3. "Crutch walking instructions would be scheduled on the second postoperative day."
4. "Crutch walking instructions would be scheduled at the time of discharge after surgery."

Level of Cognitive Ability: Evaluating
Client Needs: Physiological Integrity
Clinical Judgment/Cognitive Skills: Evaluate Outcomes
Integrated Process: Teaching and Learning
Content Area: Skills: Activity/Mobility
Health Problems: Adult Health: Musculoskeletal: Skeletal Injury
Priority Concepts: Patient Education; Mobility

Answer: 1
Rationale: It is best to assess crutch walking ability and instruct the client with regard to the use of the crutches before surgery because this task can be difficult to learn when the client is in pain and not used to the imbalance that may occur after surgery. None of the remaining options are appropriate times to teach a client about crutch walking.
Test-Taking Strategy: Focus on the strategic word, *effective*, and the subject, the time to schedule crutch walking instructions. Eliminate options 2, 3, and 4 that are comparable or alike in that they address the postoperative period.
Priority Nursing Tip: For the client undergoing knee replacement surgery, the nurse would plan to begin continuous passive motion 24 to 48 hours postoperatively as prescribed to exercise the knee and provide moderate flexion and extension.
Reference: Ignatavicius, D., et al. (2021). *Medical-surgical nursing: Concepts for interprofessional collaborative care* (10th ed., pp. 1012, 1040). Elsevier.

❖ **62.** A client with a short leg plaster cast reports intense itching under the cast. The nurse provides instructions to the client regarding relief measures for the itching. Which statement by the client indicates an understanding of the measures used to relieve the itching?
   1. "I can use the blunt part of a ruler to scratch the area."
   2. "I can trickle small amounts of water down inside the cast."
   3. "I need to obtain assistance when placing an object into the cast for the itching."
   4. "I can use a hair dryer on the cool setting and allow the air to blow into the cast."

Level of Cognitive Ability: Evaluating
Client Needs: Physiological Integrity
Clinical Judgment/Cognitive Skills: Evaluate Outcomes
Integrated Process: Teaching and Learning
Content Area: Foundations of Care: Safety
Health Problems: Adult Health: Musculoskeletal: Skeletal Injury
Priority Concepts: Patient Education; Mobility

Answer: 4
Rationale: Itching is a common complaint of clients with casts. Objects would not be put inside a cast because of the risk of scratching the skin and providing a point of entry for bacteria. A plaster cast can break down when wet. Therefore, the best way to relieve itching is with the forceful injection of air inside the cast.
Test-Taking Strategy: Eliminate options that are comparable or alike and indicate putting objects inside the cast. Next, focus on the subject, proper cast care, to direct you to the correct option.
Priority Nursing Tip: The physician is notified immediately if circulatory impairment occurs in the extremity with a cast.
Reference: Lewis, S., et al. (2020). *Medical-surgical nursing: Assessment and management of clinical problems* (11th ed., p. 1458). Elsevier.

63. Disulfiram has been prescribed for a client, and the nurse provides instructions to the client about the medication. Which statement by the client indicates the **need for further teaching?**
   1. "I must be careful taking cold medicines."
   2. "I will have to check my aftershave lotion."
   3. "I'll be fine as long as I don't drink alcohol."
   4. "I need to be careful with ingredients when I cook."

Level of Cognitive Ability: Evaluating
Client Needs: Physiological Integrity
Clinical Judgment/Cognitive Skills: Evaluate Outcomes
Integrated Process: Teaching and Learning
Content Area: Pharmacology: Psychiatric: Alcohol Deterrents
Health Problems: Mental Health: Addictions
Priority Concepts: Patient Education; Safety

Answer: 3
Rationale: Clients who are taking disulfiram must be taught that substances that contain alcohol can trigger an adverse reaction. Sources of hidden alcohol include foods (soups, sauces, and vinegars), medicine (cold medicine), mouthwashes, and skin preparations (alcohol rubs and aftershave lotions).
Test-Taking Strategy: Note the strategic words, *need for further teaching.* These words indicate a negative event query and ask you to select an option that is an incorrect statement. Remember that disulfiram is used for clients who have alcoholism, and any form of alcohol must be avoided with this medication.
Priority Nursing Tip: Disulfiram is an alcohol deterrent that may be prescribed for alcoholic dependence. The medication sensitizes the client to alcohol, so a disulfiram-alcohol reaction occurs if alcohol is ingested.
Reference: Varcarolis, E., & Fosbre, C. (2021). *Essentials of psychiatric mental health nursing: A communication approach to evidence-based care* (4th ed., pp. 312–313). Elsevier.

❖ **64.** The nurse has provided instructions to a client who is receiving external radiation therapy for a cancerous skin lesion. Which statement by the client indicates a **need for further teaching** regarding self-care related to the radiation therapy?
  1. "I need to eat a high-protein diet."
  2. "I need to avoid exposure to sunlight."
  3. "I need to wash my skin with a mild soap and pat it dry."
  4. "I need to apply pressure on the irritated area to prevent bleeding."

Level of Cognitive Ability: Evaluating
Client Needs: Physiological Integrity
Clinical Judgment/Cognitive Skills: Evaluate Outcomes
Integrated Process: Clinical Judgment; Teaching and Learning
Content Area: Adult Health: Oncology
Health Problems: Adult Health: Cancer: Skin
Priority Concepts: Patient Education; Tissue Integrity

Answer: 4
Rationale: The client receiving external radiation therapy needs to avoid pressure on the irritated area and wear loose-fitting clothing. Specific health care provider instructions would be necessary to obtain if an alteration in skin integrity occurred as a result of the radiation therapy. The remaining options are accurate measures regarding radiation therapy.
Test-Taking Strategy: Note the strategic words, *need for further teaching*. These words indicate a negative event query and ask you to select an option that is an incorrect statement. The word *pressure* in the correct option is an indication that this is an inappropriate measure.
Priority Nursing Tip: The client undergoing external radiation therapy does not emit radiation and does not pose a hazard to anyone else.
Reference: Ignatavicius, D., et al. (2021). *Medical-surgical nursing: Concepts for interprofessional collaborative care* (10th ed., p. 382). Elsevier.

65. During a health assessment the nurse provides instructions to a client regarding the testicular self-examination (TSE). Which statement by the client indicates that the client has a **need for further teaching** regarding TSE?
  1. "I know to report any small lumps."
  2. "I need to examine myself every 2 months."
  3. "I need to examine myself after I take a warm shower."
  4. "I know it's normal to feel something that is cord-like in the back."

Level of Cognitive Ability: Evaluating
Client Needs: Health Promotion and Maintenance
Clinical Judgment/Cognitive Skills: Evaluate Outcomes
Integrated Process: Teaching and Learning
Content Area: Health Assessment/Physical Exam: Testicles
Health Problems: Adult Health: Cancer: Testicular
Priority Concepts: Patient Education; Health Promotion

Answer: 2
Rationale: TSE needs to be performed every month. Small lumps or abnormalities need to be reported. The spermatic cord finding is normal. After a warm bath or shower, the scrotum is relaxed, which makes it easier to perform TSE.
Test-Taking Strategy: Note the strategic words, *need for further teaching*. These words indicate a negative event query and the need to select the incorrect client statement. Remembering that breast self-examination needs to be performed monthly may assist you with recalling that TSE is also performed monthly.
Priority Nursing Tip: Teach the client how to perform TSE; a day of the month is selected, and the examination is performed on the same day each month after a shower or bath when the hands are warm and soapy and the scrotum is warm.
Reference: Potter, P., et al. (2021). *Fundamentals of nursing* (10th ed., p. 575). Elsevier.

66. A client diagnosed with acquired immunodeficiency syndrome (AIDS) is reporting fatigue and asks the nurse about measures to reduce it. The nurse educates the client on ways to conserve energy. Which statement indicates that the teaching was **effective?**
1. "Bathe before eating breakfast."
2. "Sit for as many activities as possible."
3. "Stand in the shower instead of taking a bath."
4. "Group all tasks to be performed early in the morning."

Level of Cognitive Ability: Evaluating
Client Needs: Physiological Integrity
Clinical Judgment/Cognitive Skills: Evaluate Outcomes
Integrated Process: Clinical Judgment; Teaching and Learning
Content Area: Adult Health: Immune
Health Problems: Adult Health: Immune: Immunodeficiency Syndrome
Priority Concepts: Patient Education; Functional Ability

Answer: 2
Rationale: The client is taught to conserve energy by sitting for as many activities as possible, including dressing, shaving, preparing food, and ironing. The client needs to also sit in a shower chair instead of standing while showering. The client needs to prioritize activities such as eating breakfast before bathing, and the client would intersperse each major activity with a period of rest.
Test-Taking Strategy: Focus on the strategic word, *effective,* and the subject of conserving energy. Think about the amount of exertion required by the client to perform each of the activities described in the options. Eliminate options that are obviously taxing for the client. From the remaining choices, recall that bathing may take away energy that could be used for eating and so is not helpful.
Priority Nursing Tip: Acquired immunodeficiency syndrome (AIDS) is a disorder caused by the human immunodeficiency virus (HIV) and characterized by generalized dysfunction of the immune system.
Reference: Ignatavicius, D., et al. (2021). *Medical-surgical nursing: Concepts for interprofessional collaborative care* (10th ed., p. 339). Elsevier.

67. A 10-year-old child has been diagnosed with type 1 diabetes mellitus. What instruction would the nurse provide concerning the monitoring of the child's insulin needs?
1. The child would be taught to self-monitor insulin needs.
2. The parents will need to be available to monitor the child's insulin needs.
3. The child's school teacher will assume responsibility of insulin need monitoring.
4. Friends and family will need to be involved with monitoring the child's insulin needs.

Level of Cognitive Ability: Applying
Client Needs: Physiological Integrity
Clinical Judgment/Cognitive Skills: Generate Solutions
Integrated Process: Teaching and Learning
Content Area: Pediatrics: Metabolic/Endocrine
Health Problems: Pediatric-Specific: Diabetes Mellitus
Priority Concepts: Patient Education; Development

Answer: 1
Rationale: Most children 9 years old or older can understand the principles of monitoring their own insulin requirements. They are usually responsible enough to determine the appropriate intervention needed to maintain their health. Parents, friends, and family cannot always be available. The school teacher should not be expected to take responsibility for health care interventions.
Test-Taking Strategy: Focus on the subject, a 10-year-old child with type 1 diabetes mellitus. Noting the age of the child will indicate that the child is able to take control and responsibility regarding their health care situation. Eliminate options 2, 3, and 4 that are comparable or alike and rely on other individuals to care for the child.
Priority Nursing Tip: The abdomen is the preferred site for infusion set sites and injections. It is easy to see and reach and offers the quickest absorption.
Reference: McKinney, E. S., et al. (2022). *Maternal child nursing* (6th ed., p. 174). Elsevier.

68. The nurse instructs a client diagnosed with oral candidiasis (thrush) about caring for the disorder. Which statement by the client indicates a **need for further teaching?**
  1. "I can eat foods that are liquid or pureed."
  2. "I need to eliminate spicy foods from my diet."
  3. "It's best if I don't drink citrus juices or hot liquids."
  4. "I need to rinse my mouth four times daily with commercial mouthwash."

Level of Cognitive Ability: Evaluating
Client Needs: Physiological Integrity
Clinical Judgment/Cognitive Skills: Evaluate Outcomes
Integrated Process: Teaching and Learning
Content Area: Adult Health: Immune
Health Problems: Adult Health: Integumentary: Inflammation/Infection
Priority Concepts: Patient Education; Infection

Answer: 4
Rationale: Clients with thrush cannot tolerate commercial mouthwashes because the high alcohol concentration in these products can cause pain and discomfort of the lesions. A solution of warm water or mouthwash formulas without alcohol are better tolerated and may promote healing. A change in diet to liquid or pureed food often eases the discomfort of eating. The client needs to avoid spicy foods, citrus juices, and hot liquids.
Test-Taking Strategy: Note the strategic words, *need for further teaching*. These words indicate a negative event query and ask you to select an option that is an incorrect statement. In addition, noting the words *commercial mouthwash* in the correct option will direct you to this option.
Priority Nursing Tip: Candidiasis can be oral or vaginal. Antifungal medications are used to treat this infection. The nurse would encourage increased fluid intake and monitor the client's temperature when the client has an infection and is taking antifungal medication.
Reference: Lewis, S., et al. (2020). *Medical-surgical nursing: Assessment and management of clinical problems* (11th ed., p. 893). Elsevier.

69. The nurse has given instructions about site care to a hemodialysis client who had an implantation of an arteriovenous (AV) fistula in the right arm. Which statement by the client indicates a **need for further teaching?**
  1. "I will need to sleep on my right side."
  2. "It's important that I don't carry heavy objects with the right arm."
  3. "I will perform range-of-motion exercises routinely on my right arm."
  4. "It's important that I report any right arm redness or drainage at the site."

Level of Cognitive Ability: Evaluating
Client Needs: Physiological Integrity
Clinical Judgment/Cognitive Skills: Evaluate Outcomes
Integrated Process: Teaching and Learning
Content Area: Adult Health: Renal and Urinary
Health Problems: Adult Health: Renal and Urinary: Acute Kidney Injury/Chronic Kidney Disease
Priority Concepts: Perfusion; Safety

Answer: 1
Rationale: Routine instructions to the client with an AV fistula, graft, or shunt include avoiding sleeping with the body weight on the extremity with the access site, avoiding carrying heavy objects or compressing the extremity that has the access site, performing routine range-of-motion exercises of the affected extremity, and reporting signs and symptoms of infection.
Test-Taking Strategy: Note the strategic words, *need for further teaching*. These words indicate a negative event query and ask you to select an option that is an incorrect statement. Recalling the importance of maintaining the patency of the AV fistula will direct you to the correct option.
Priority Nursing Tip: Arterial steal syndrome can occur as a result of the presence of an AV fistula. This is a syndrome that can develop after the insertion of an AV fistula when too much blood is diverted to the vein and arterial perfusion to the hand is compromised.
Reference: Ignatavicius, D., et al. (2021). *Medical-surgical nursing: Concepts for interprofessional collaborative care* (10th ed., p. 1399). Elsevier.

❖ **70.** The nurse provides instructions to a client with coronary artery disease about applying a nitroglycerin patch. What statement indicates that the client is using correct technique?
1. "A second patch will be applied if chest pain occurs."
2. "I will apply the patch to a nonhairy area of the body."
3. "I will remove the patch when bathing and reapply it after the bath."
4. "I will remove the patch after gently rubbing the area to activate the medication."

Level of Cognitive Ability: Evaluating
Client Needs: Physiological Integrity
Clinical Judgment/Cognitive Skills: Evaluate Outcomes
Integrated Process: Teaching and Learning
Content Area: Pharmacology: Cardiovascular: Vasodilators
Health Problems: Adult Health: Cardiovascular: Coronary Artery Disease
Priority Concepts: Patient Education; Safety

Answer: 2
Rationale: Topical nitroglycerin is applied to a nonhairy part of the body. It is used on a scheduled basis and is not prescribed specifically for the occurrence of chest pain. The ointment is not rubbed into the skin; it is reapplied only as directed.
Test-Taking Strategy: Focus on the subject, understanding the instructions for applying a nitroglycerin patch. Noting the word *nonhairy* in the correct option will direct you to this choice.
Priority Nursing Tip: Nitroglycerin is a vasodilator and will lower the blood pressure. The nurse needs to wear gloves when applying the topical preparation to a client.
Reference: Ignatavicius, D., et al. (2021). *Medical-surgical nursing: Concepts for interprofessional collaborative care* (10th ed., p. 758). Elsevier.

71. The nurse is giving medication instructions to a client who is receiving furosemide. Which client statement indicates a **need for further teaching**?
1. "I need to change positions slowly."
2. "I need to be careful to not get overheated in warm weather."
3. "I need to talk to my physician about the use of alcohol."
4. "I need to avoid the use of salt substitutes because they contain potassium."

Level of Cognitive Ability: Evaluating
Client Needs: Physiological Integrity
Clinical Judgment/Cognitive Skills: Evaluate Outcomes
Integrated Process: Teaching and Learning
Content Area: Pharmacology: Cardiovascular: Diuretics
Health Problems: Adult Health: Cardiovascular: Heart Failure
Priority Concepts: Patient Education; Safety

Answer: 4
Rationale: Furosemide is a potassium-1osing diuretic, so there is no need to avoid high-potassium products, such as a salt substitute. Orthostatic hypotension is a risk, and the client must use caution when changing positions and with exposure to warm weather. The client needs to discuss the use of alcohol with the physician.
Test-Taking Strategy: Note the strategic words, *need for further teaching.* These words indicate a negative event query and ask you to select an option that is an incorrect statement. Focus on the subject of a client who is receiving furosemide. Recalling that furosemide is a potassium-losing diuretic and that diuretic therapy can induce orthostatic hypotension will direct you to the correct option.
Priority Nursing Tip: The nurse needs to monitor the electrolyte values, specifically the potassium value, when the client is receiving a potassium-losing diuretic.
Reference: Burchum, J., & Rosenthal, L. (2022). *Lehne's Pharmacology for nursing care* (11th ed., pp. 463–464). Elsevier.

72. A client with hypertension has been prescribed a clonidine patch, and the nurse has instructed the client regarding the use of the patch. Which client statement indicates a **need for further teaching**?
1. "I intend to change the patch every 7 days."
2. "I need to trim the patch if an edge becomes loose."
3. "It's important to put the patch on a hairless site on my torso."
4. "It's alright to leave the patch in place during bathing or showering."

Level of Cognitive Ability: Evaluating
Client Needs: Physiological Integrity
Clinical Judgment/Cognitive Skills: Evaluate Outcomes
Integrated Process: Teaching and Learning
Content Area: Adult Health: Cardiovascular
Health Problems: Adult Health: Cardiovascular: Hypertension
Priority Concepts: Patient Education; Safety

Answer: 2
Rationale: The clonidine patch would not be trimmed because it will alter the medication dose. If it becomes slightly loose, it would be covered with an adhesive overlay from the medication package. If it becomes very loose or falls off, it needs to be replaced. It is changed every 7 days and is left in place when bathing or showering. The clonidine patch needs to be applied to a hairless site on the torso or the upper arm. The patch is discarded by folding it in half with the adhesive sides together.
Test-Taking Strategy: Note the strategic words, *need for further teaching.* These words indicate a negative event query and ask you to select an option that is an incorrect statement. Noting the words *trim the patch* will direct you to the correct option because this client's action would alter the medication dose.
Priority Nursing Tip: Clonidine is a centrally acting sympatholytic that is used to treat hypertension. The client is instructed not to discontinue the medication because abrupt withdrawal can cause severe rebound hypertension.
Reference: Skidmore-Roth, L. (2021). *2021 Mosby's Nursing drug reference* (34th ed., p. 306). Elsevier.

73. Cholestyramine is prescribed for a client with coronary artery disease, and the nurse provides instructions to the client about the medication. Which client statement indicates a **need for further teaching**?
1. "I need to take this medication with meals."
2. "I need to mix the medication with juice or applesauce."
3. "I need to increase my fluid intake while taking this medication."
4. "I need to call my primary health care provider immediately if it causes constipation."

Level of Cognitive Ability: Evaluating
Client Needs: Physiological Integrity
Clinical Judgment/Cognitive Skills: Evaluate Outcomes
Integrated Process: Teaching and Learning
Content Area: Pharmacology: Cardiovascular: Antilipemics
Health Problems: Adult Health: Cardiovascular: Coronary Artery Disease
Priority Concepts: Patient Education; Safety

Answer: 4
Rationale: Common side effects of cholestyramine include constipation, nausea, indigestion, and flatulence. Therefore, it is not necessary to contact the primary health care provider immediately if constipation occurs. Cholestyramine must be administered with food to be effective. This medication would not be taken dry, and it can be mixed in water, juice, carbonated beverages, applesauce, or soup. Increasing fluids will minimize the constipating effects of the medication.
Test-Taking Strategy: Note the strategic words, *need for further teaching.* These words indicate a negative event query and ask you to select an option that is an incorrect statement. Select the correct option because of the word *immediately* and because normally measures can be taken to prevent constipation rather than immediately calling the primary health care provider.
Priority Nursing Tip: Cholestyramine is a bile acid sequestrant used to lower the cholesterol level, and client compliance is a problem because of its taste and palatability. Mixing the medication with flavored products or fruit juices can improve the taste.
Reference: Lilley, L., Rainforth Collins, S., & Snyder J. (2020). *Pharmacology and the nursing process* (9th ed., pp. 434–435). Elsevier.

❖ **74.** The nurse is reviewing written medication instructions with a client who is prescribed colestipol hydrochloride as part of the treatment plan for coronary artery disease. Which statement by the client indicates that the teaching has been **effective?**

1. "Vitamin C will help control unintended side effects."
2. "Vitamin B_{12} will help control unintended side effects."
3. "B-complex vitamins will help control unintended side effects."
4. "Fat-soluble vitamins will help control unintended side effects."

Level of Cognitive Ability: Evaluating
Client Needs: Physiological Integrity
Clinical Judgment/Cognitive Skills: Evaluate Outcomes
Integrated Process: Teaching and Learning
Content Area: Pharmacology: Cardiovascular: Antilipemics
Health Problems: Adult Health: Cardiovascular: Coronary Artery Disease
Priority Concepts: Patient Education; Safety

Answer: 4
Rationale: Colestipol hydrochloride, which is a bile-sequestering agent, is used to lower blood cholesterol levels. However, the bile salts (which are rich in cholesterol) interfere with the absorption of the fat-soluble vitamins A, D, E, and K, as well as folic acid. With ongoing therapy, the client is at risk for the deficiency of these vitamins and is counseled to take them as supplements.
Test-Taking Strategy: Focus on the strategic word, *effective*, and the subject, considerations for administration of colestipol hydrochloride and counteracting unintended medication effects. This will help you recall that bile-sequestering agents interfere with the absorption of fat-soluble vitamins and will assist you with eliminating the remaining options. Also, option 4 is the correct option because it is the umbrella option.
Priority Nursing Tip: Bile acid sequestrants bind with acids in the intestines, which prevents reabsorption of cholesterol.
Reference: Burchum, J., & Rosenthal, L. (2022). *Lehne's Pharmacology for nursing care* (11th ed., pp. 579–580). Elsevier.

Nursing Process: Assessment

75. Which data would the nurse expect to obtain during the admission assessment of a child to support the diagnosis of irritable bowel syndrome?

1. Frequent incidents of frothy diarrhea
2. Frequent foul-smelling ribbon stools
3. Profuse, watery diarrhea and nausea and vomiting
4. Diffuse abdominal pain unrelated to meals or activity

Level of Cognitive Ability: Analyzing
Client Needs: Physiological Integrity
Clinical Judgment/Cognitive Skills: Recognize Cues
Integrated Process: Clinical Judgment; Nursing Process/Assessment
Content Area: Pediatrics: Gastrointestinal
Health Problems: N/A
Priority Concepts: Clinical Judgment; Elimination

Answer: 4
Rationale: Irritable bowel syndrome causes diffuse abdominal pain unrelated to meals or activity. Alternating constipation and diarrhea with the presence of undigested food and mucus in the stools may also be noted. Option 1 is a clinical manifestation of lactose intolerance. Option 2 is a clinical manifestation of Hirschsprung's disease. Option 3 is a clinical manifestation of celiac disease.
Test-Taking Strategy: Focus on the subject, manifestations of irritable bowel syndrome. Noting the name of the syndrome will direct you to the correct option because you would expect abdominal pain to occur in clients with this disorder.
Priority Nursing Tip: Stress and emotional factors may contribute to the occurrence of irritable bowel syndrome.
Reference: McKinney, E. S., et al. (2022). *Maternal child nursing* (6th ed., p. 979). Elsevier.

76. The nurse caring for a child diagnosed with rubeola (measles) notes that the primary health care provider (PHCP) has documented the presence of Koplik's spots. On the basis of this documentation, which observation is expected?
1. Pinpoint petechiae noted on both legs
2. Whitish vesicles located across the chest
3. Petechiae spots that are reddish and pinpoint on the soft palate
4. Small, blue-white spots with a red base found on the buccal mucosa

Level of Cognitive Ability: Analyzing
Client Needs: Physiological Integrity
Clinical Judgment/Cognitive Skills: Recognize Cues
Integrated Process: Clinical Judgment; Nursing Process/Assessment
Content Area: Pediatrics: Infectious and Communicable Diseases
Health Problems: Pediatric-Specific: Communicable Diseases
Priority Concepts: Clinical Judgment; Infection

Answer: 4
Rationale: In rubeola (measles), Koplik's spots appear approximately 2 days before the appearance of the rash. These are small, blue-white spots with a red base that are found on the buccal mucosa. The spots last approximately 3 days, after which time they slough off. Based on this information, the remaining options are all incorrect.
Test-Taking Strategy: Eliminate options 1 and 3 that are comparable or alike and address petechiae spots. Focusing on the subject of Koplik's spots will direct you to the correct option.
Priority Nursing Tip: Rubeola (measles) is transmitted via airborne particles, direct contact with infectious droplets, or transplacental contact. The nurse must implement airborne precautions when caring for the hospitalized client with rubeola.
Reference: McKinney, E. S., et al. (2022). *Maternal child nursing* (6th ed., p. 908). Elsevier.

77. Which assessment finding would the nurse expect to note in the child hospitalized with a diagnosis of nephrotic syndrome?
1. Weight loss
2. Constipation
3. Hypotension
4. Abdominal pain

Level of Cognitive Ability: Analyzing
Client Needs: Physiological Integrity
Clinical Judgment/Cognitive Skills: Recognize Cues
Integrated Process: Clinical Judgment; Nursing Process/Assessment
Content Area: Pediatrics: Renal and Urinary
Health Problems: Pediatric-Specific: Nephrotic Syndrome
Priority Concepts: Clinical Judgment; Fluids and Electrolytes

Answer: 4
Rationale: Clinical manifestations associated with nephrotic syndrome include edema, anorexia, fatigue, and abdominal pain from the presence of extra fluid in the peritoneal cavity. Diarrhea caused by the edema of the bowel occurs and may cause decreased absorption of nutrients. Increased weight from fluid build-up and a normal blood pressure are noted.
Test-Taking Strategy: Focus on the subject, the physiology and manifestations associated with nephrotic syndrome. Recalling that edema is a clinical manifestation will direct you to the correct option.
Priority Nursing Tip: The primary objectives of therapeutic management for nephrotic syndrome are to reduce the excretion of urinary protein, maintain protein-free urine, reduce edema, prevent infection, and minimize complications.
Reference: McKinney, E. S., et al. (2022). *Maternal child nursing* (6th ed., p. 1023). Elsevier.

78. A child is admitted to the hospital with a suspected diagnosis of von Willebrand's disease. On assessment of the child, which symptom would **most likely** be noted?
1. Hematuria
2. Presence of hematomas
3. Presence of hemarthrosis
4. Bleeding from the mucous membranes

Level of Cognitive Ability: Analyzing
Client Needs: Physiological Integrity
Clinical Judgment/Cognitive Skills: Recognize Cues
Integrated Process: Clinical Judgment; Nursing Process/Assessment
Content Area: Pediatrics: Hematologic
Health Problems: Pediatric-Specific: Bleeding Disorders
Priority Concepts: Clinical Judgment; Clotting

Answer: 4
Rationale: The primary clinical manifestations of von Willebrand's disease are bruising and mucous membrane bleeding from the nose, mouth, and gastrointestinal tract. Prolonged bleeding after trauma and surgery, including tooth extraction, may be the first evidence of abnormal hemostasis in those with mild disease. In females, menorrhagia and profuse postpartum bleeding may occur. Bleeding associated with von Willebrand's disease may be severe and lead to anemia and shock, but unlike what is seen in clients with hemophilia, deep bleeding into joints and muscles is rare. Options 1, 2, and 3 are characteristic of those signs found in clients with hemophilia.
Test-Taking Strategy: Note the strategic words, *most likely.* Think about the pathophysiology of this disorder and recall that the remaining options are characteristic of hemophilia to assist you with eliminating these options and direct you to the correct option.
Priority Nursing Tip: von Willebrand's disease is a disorder that causes platelets to adhere to damaged endothelium and is characterized by an increased tendency to bleed from mucous membranes.
Reference: McKinney, E. S., et al. (2022). *Maternal child nursing* (6th ed., pp. 1141–1142). Elsevier.

79. A client prescribed dextroamphetamine reports to the nurse difficulty falling asleep at night. The nurse instructs the client on how to minimize sleep disorders. On assessment, which statement by the client indicates that teaching has been **effective?**
1. "I'll take the medication with a bedtime snack."
2. "I'll take the medication upon awaking in the morning."
3. "I'll take the medication two hours before going to bed."
4. "I'll take the medication at least 6 hours before bedtime."

Level of Cognitive Ability: Evaluating
Client Needs: Physiological Integrity
Clinical Judgment/Cognitive Skills: Evaluate Outcomes
Integrated Process: Clinical Judgment; Nursing Process/Assessment
Content Area: Pharmacology: Neurologic: Central Nervous System Stimulants
Health Problems: N/A
Priority Concepts: Patient Education; Safety

Answer: 4
Rationale: Dextroamphetamine is a central nervous system (CNS) stimulant that acts by releasing norepinephrine from the nerve endings. The client needs to take the medication at least 6 hours before going to bed at night to prevent disturbances with sleep. Therefore, the remaining options are incorrect.
Test-Taking Strategy: Focus on the strategic word, *effective,* and the subject, dextroamphetamine and difficulty sleeping. Think about the action and purpose of this medication. Evaluate each of the options in terms of how far removed the scheduled dose is from the client's bedtime. This will direct you to option 4.
Priority Nursing Tip: The client taking a CNS stimulant needs to be instructed to avoid foods containing caffeine to prevent additional stimulation.
Reference: Kizior, R., & Hodgson, B. (2023). *Saunders Nursing drug handbook 2023* (p. 325.). Elsevier.

80. The nurse assessing the level of consciousness of a child with a head injury documents that the child is obtunded. On the basis of this documentation, which observation did the nurse note?
1. The child is unable to think clearly and rapidly.
2. The child is unable to recognize place or person.
3. The child always requires considerable stimulation for arousal.
4. The child has limited interaction with the environment unless aroused.

Level of Cognitive Ability: Analyzing
Client Needs: Physiological Integrity
Clinical Judgment/Cognitive Skills: Recognize Cues
Integrated Process: Clinical Judgment; Nursing Process/Assessment
Content Area: Pediatrics: Neurologic
Health Problems: Pediatric-Specific: Head Injury
Priority Concepts: Cognition; Intracranial Regulation

Answer: 4
Rationale: If the child is obtunded, the child sleeps unless aroused and, when aroused, has limited interaction with the environment. The remaining options describe confusion, disorientation, and stupor.
Test-Taking Strategy: Focus on the subject, that the child is obtunded. Knowledge regarding the standard terms used to identify level of consciousness will direct you to the correct option.
Priority Nursing Tip: Do not place a client with a head injury in a flat or Trendelenburg's position because of the risk of increased intracranial pressure.
Reference: Hockenberry, M., Wilson, D., & Rodgers, C. (2019). *Wong's Nursing care of infants and children* (11th ed., pp. 1113, 1128). Elsevier.

81. The nurse is caring for a client diagnosed with acquired immunodeficiency syndrome (AIDS). Which sign/symptom indicates the presence of an opportunistic respiratory infection?
1. Nausea and vomiting
2. Fever and exertional dyspnea
3. A respiratory rate of 20 breaths/min
4. An arterial blood gas pH of 7.40, reference range 7.35–7.45

Level of Cognitive Ability: Analyzing
Client Needs: Physiological Integrity
Clinical Judgment/Cognitive Skills: Recognize Cues
Integrated Process: Clinical Judgment; Nursing Process/Assessment
Content Area: Adult Health: Immune
Health Problems: Adult Health: Immune: Immunodeficiency Syndrome
Priority Concepts: Immunity; Infection

Answer: 2
Rationale: Fever and exertional dyspnea are signs of *Pneumocystis jiroveci* pneumonia, which is a common, life-threatening opportunistic infection that afflicts those with AIDS. Option 1 is not associated with respiratory infection. Options 3 and 4 are normal findings.
Test-Taking Strategy: Focus on the subject, opportunistic respiratory infection in a client with AIDS. Eliminate options that are comparable or alike and are normal findings. For the remaining options, focusing on the subject, a respiratory infection, will direct you to the correct option.
Priority Nursing Tip: A client with human immunodeficiency virus (HIV) or AIDS is at risk for developing a life-threatening opportunistic infection. Monitor the client closely for signs/symptoms of infection and report these signs immediately if they occur.
Reference: Lewis, S., et al. (2020). *Medical-surgical nursing: Assessment and management of clinical problems* (11th ed., p. 505). Elsevier.

❖ **82.** An adult client seeks treatment in an ambulatory care clinic for reports of a left earache, nausea, and a full feeling in the left ear. The client has an elevated temperature. Which assessment question would the nurse ask **first**?

1. "Do you have a history of a recent brain abscess?"
2. "Do you have a chronic hearing problem in the left ear?"
3. "Do you successfully obtain pain relief with acetaminophen?"
4. "Do you have a history of a recent upper respiratory infection (URI)?"

Level of Cognitive Ability: Analyzing
Client Needs: Physiological Integrity
Clinical Judgment/Cognitive Skills: Recognize Cues
Integrated Process: Clinical Judgment; Nursing Process/Assessment
Content Area: Adult Health: Ear
Health Problems: Adult Health: Ear: Inflammation/Infections/Structural Problems
Priority Concepts: Clinical Judgment; Sensory Perception

Answer: 4
Rationale: Otitis media in the adult is typically one-sided and presents as an acute process with earache; nausea; and possible vomiting, fever, and fullness in the ear. The client may report diminished hearing in that ear during the acute process. The nurse takes a client history first, assessing whether the client has had a recent URI. It is unnecessary to question the client about a brain abscess. The nurse may ask the client if anything relieves the pain, but ear infection pain is usually not relieved until antibiotic therapy is initiated.
Test-Taking Strategy: Focus on the subject, the relationship between an upper respiratory infection and otitis media. Noting the strategic word, *first*, will direct you to the correct option.
Priority Nursing Tip: Infants and children have eustachian tubes that are shorter, wider, and straighter, which makes them more prone to otitis media.
Reference: Ignatavicius, D., et al. (2021). *Medical-surgical nursing: Concepts for interprofessional collaborative care* (10th ed., p. 965). Elsevier.

83. The nurse prepares to administer a continuous intravenous (IV) infusion through a peripheral IV to a dehydrated client. Which **priority** assessment would the nurse obtain before initiating the IV infusion?

1. Daily body weight
2. Serum electrolytes
3. Intake and output records
4. Identifying the client's dominant side

Level of Cognitive Ability: Analyzing
Client Needs: Physiological Integrity
Clinical Judgment/Cognitive Skills: Prioritize Hypotheses
Integrated Process: Clinical Judgment; Nursing Process/Assessment
Content Area: Foundations of Care: Fluids and Electrolytes
Health Problems: Adult Health: Gastrointestinal: Dehydration
Priority Concepts: Clinical Judgment; Fluids and Electrolytes

Answer: 1
Rationale: The nurse obtains the client's baseline body weight as a priority before beginning the IV infusion because body weight is a sensitive and specific indicator of fluid volume status when body weights are compared on a daily basis. This means that as a client receives or accumulates fluid, body weight quickly and proportionately increases and vice versa. The remaining options may also be reasonable assessments to complete before initiating an IV infusion. However, intake, output, and serum electrolytes are potentially affected by more confounding factors; thus, they are less specific and sensitive to fluctuations in body fluid. Determining the client's dominant side assists in deciding a site for inserting the initial IV catheter, but it provides no information about fluid volume status.
Test-Taking Strategy: Focus on the subject, continuous IV infusion through a peripheral IV to a dehydrated client. Note the strategic word, *priority*. Review the options to determine the best method for the nurse to use to evaluate fluid status. Body weight is the best option because it is the most sensitive and specific measurement listed.
Priority Nursing Tip: Clients with respiratory, cardiac, renal, or liver disease; older clients; and very young children are at risk for circulatory overload and may not be able to tolerate an excessive body fluid volume.
References: Lewis, S., et al. (2020). *Medical-surgical nursing: Assessment and management of clinical problems* (11th ed., p. 292). Elsevier; Potter, P., et al. (2021). *Fundamentals of nursing*. (10th ed., p. 1013). Elsevier.

❖ **84.** A client with coronary artery disease is scheduled for an arteriogram using a radiopaque dye. What is the **most important** information the nurse would determine before the procedure to ensure the client's safety?
1. Vital signs
2. Intake and output
3. Height and weight
4. Allergy to iodine or shellfish

Level of Cognitive Ability: Analyzing
Client Needs: Physiological Integrity
Clinical Judgment/Cognitive Skills: Prioritize Hypotheses
Integrated Process: Clinical Judgment; Nursing Process/Assessment
Content Area: Foundations of Care: Diagnostic Tests
Health Problems: Adult Health: Cardiovascular: Coronary Artery Disease
Priority Concepts: Clinical Judgment; Safety

Answer: 4
Rationale: Allergy to iodine or seafood is associated with allergy to the radiopaque dye that is used for medical imaging examinations. Informed consent is necessary because an arteriogram requires the injection of a radiopaque dye into the blood vessel. Although the remaining options are components of the preprocedure assessment, the risks of allergic reaction and possible anaphylaxis are the most critical to the client's safety.
Test-Taking Strategy: Note the strategic words, *most important.* Focusing on the subject of arteriogram using a radiopaque dye will help you recall the risk of anaphylaxis related to the dye; this will direct you to the correct option.
Priority Nursing Tip: If anaphylaxis occurs after the injection of a radiopaque dye, the nurse immediately assesses the client's respiratory status and provides respiratory support and asks another nursing staff member to contact the primary health care provider.
Reference: Pagana, K., Pagana, T., & Pagana, T. N. (2021). *Mosby's Diagnostic and laboratory test reference* (15th ed., p. 113). Elsevier.

85. The nurse is performing a cardiovascular assessment on a client with heart failure. Which item would the nurse assess to obtain the **best** information about the client's left-sided heart function?
1. The status of breath sounds
2. The presence of peripheral edema
3. The presence of hepatojugular reflux
4. The presence of jugular vein distention

Level of Cognitive Ability: Analyzing
Client Needs: Physiological Integrity
Clinical Judgment/Cognitive Skills: Recognize Cues
Integrated Process: Clinical Judgment; Nursing Process/Assessment
Content Area: Health Assessment/Physical Exam: Heart and Peripheral Vascular
Health Problems: Adult Health: Cardiovascular: Heart Failure
Priority Concepts: Gas Exchange; Perfusion

Answer: 1
Rationale: The client with heart failure may present different symptoms depending on whether the right or the left side of the heart is failing. The assessment of breath sounds provides information about left-sided heart function. Peripheral edema, hepatojugular reflux, and jugular vein distention are all signs of right-sided heart function.
Test-Taking Strategy: Focus on the subject, the status of left-sided heart function and the strategic word, *best.* Remember "left" and "lungs." The remaining options reflect right-sided heart failure.
Priority Nursing Tip: Signs of left ventricular failure are evident in the pulmonary system. Signs of right ventricular failure are evident in the systemic circulation.
Reference: Ignatavicius, D., et al. (2021). *Medical-surgical nursing: Concepts for interprofessional collaborative care* (10th ed., p. 671). Elsevier.

❖ **86.** The nurse is obtaining a history from a client who was admitted to the hospital with a thrombotic stroke. What are the **most likely** signs/symptoms the client experienced before the incident occurred? **Select all that apply.**
- ❑ **1.** Temporary aphasia
- ❑ **2.** Throbbing headaches
- ❑ **3.** Transient hemiplegia
- ❑ **4.** Paresthesias on one side of the body
- ❑ **5.** Unexplained loss of consciousness

Level of Cognitive Ability: Analyzing
Client Needs: Physiological Integrity
Clinical Judgment/Cognitive Skills: Recognize Cues
Integrated Process: Clinical Judgment; Nursing Process/Assessment
Content Area: Adult Health: Neurologic
Health Problems: Adult Health: Neurologic: Stroke
Priority Concepts: Clinical Judgment; Intracranial Regulation

Answer: 1, 3, 4
Rationale: Cerebral thrombosis does not occur suddenly. During the few hours or days before a thrombotic stroke, the client may experience a transient loss of speech (aphasia), hemiplegia, or paresthesias on one side of the body. Other signs and symptoms of thrombotic stroke vary, but they may include dizziness, cognitive changes, or seizures. Headache is rare, and a loss of consciousness is not likely to occur.
Test-Taking Strategy: Focus on the subject, symptoms of a thrombotic stroke and the strategic words, *most likely.* Use knowledge about the manifestations of this type of stroke to answer correctly. The remaining options are not associated commonly with this type of stroke and so can be eliminated.
Priority Nursing Tip: A stroke is a syndrome in which the cerebral circulation is interrupted, causing neurologic deficits. Cerebral anoxia lasting longer than 10 minutes causes cerebral infarction with irreversible change.
Reference: Ignatavicius, D., et al. (2021). *Medical-surgical nursing: Concepts for interprofessional collaborative care* (10th ed., p. 900). Elsevier.

87. A client with gastritis in a long-term care facility has had a series of gastrointestinal (GI) diagnostic tests, including an upper and lower GI series and endoscopies. Upon return to the long-term care facility, which **priority** assessment would the nurse focus on?
1. The comfort level
2. Activity tolerance
3. The level of consciousness
4. The hydration and nutrition status

Level of Cognitive Ability: Applying
Client Needs: Physiological Integrity
Clinical Judgment/Cognitive Skills: Prioritize Hypotheses
Integrated Process: Clinical Judgment; Nursing Process/Assessment
Content Area: Foundations of Care: Diagnostic Tests
Health Problems: Adult Health: Gastrointestinal: Gastritis/Gastroenteritis
Priority Concepts: Clinical Judgment; Safety

Answer: 4
Rationale: Many of the diagnostic studies to identify GI disorders require that the GI tract be cleansed (usually with laxatives and enemas) before testing. In addition, the client most often takes nothing by mouth before and during the testing period. Because the studies may be done over a period that exceeds 24 hours, the client may become dehydrated and/or malnourished. Although the remaining options may be components of the assessment, the correct option is the priority.
Test-Taking Strategy: Note the strategic word, *priority.* Use Maslow's Hierarchy of Needs theory to direct you to the correct option. Hydration and nutrition are the priorities.
Priority Nursing Tip: After endoscopic procedures that involve the use of a local throat anesthetic, monitor for the return of a gag reflex before giving the client any oral substance. If the gag reflex has not returned, the client could aspirate.
Reference: Lewis, S., et al. (2020). *Medical-surgical nursing: Assessment and management of clinical problems* (11th ed., p. 841). Elsevier.

❖ **88.** Which aspect would the nurse focus on when assessing a client for the vegetative signs of depression? **Select all that apply.**
- ❑ 1. Weight
- ❑ 2. Appetite
- ❑ 3. Sleep patterns
- ❑ 4. Suicidal ideations
- ❑ 5. Psychomotor activity
- ❑ 6. Rational decision making

Level of Cognitive Ability: Analyzing
Client Needs: Physiological Integrity
Clinical Judgment/Cognitive Skills: Recognize Cues
Integrated Process: Clinical Judgment; Nursing Process/Assessment
Content Area: Mental Health
Health Problems: Mental Health: Mood Disorders
Priority Concepts: Cognition; Mood and Affect

Answer: 1, 2, 3, 5
Rationale: The vegetative signs of depression are changes in physiologic functioning that occur during depression. These include changes in appetite, weight, sleep patterns, and psychomotor activity. The remaining options represent psychologic assessment categories.
Test-Taking Strategy: Focus on the subject, the vegetative signs of depression. Recalling that these are physiologic changes and use of Maslow's Hierarchy of Needs theory will direct you to the correct option.
Priority Nursing Tip: An inappropriate appearance and indications of poor hygiene practices may be signs of depression, manic disorder, dementia, organic brain disease, or another disorder.
Reference: Varcarolis, E., & Fosbre, C. (2021). *Essentials of psychiatric mental health nursing: A communication approach to evidence-based care* (4th ed., p. 208). Elsevier.

89. A client diagnosed with cirrhosis of the liver is receiving oral triamterene daily. Which sign/symptom would indicate to the nurse that the client is experiencing an adverse effect of the medication?
1. Dry skin
2. Excitability
3. Constipation
4. Hyperkalemia

Level of Cognitive Ability: Analyzing
Client Needs: Physiological Integrity
Clinical Judgment/Cognitive Skills: Recognize Cues
Integrated Process: Clinical Judgment; Nursing Process/Assessment
Content Area: Pharmacology: Cardiovascular: Diuretics
Health Problems: Adult Health: Gastrointestinal: Cirrhosis
Priority Concepts: Clinical Judgment; Safety

Answer: 4
Rationale: Triamterene is a potassium-sparing diuretic. Adverse effects include hyperkalemia, dehydration, hyponatremia, and lethargy. Although the concern with most diuretics is hypokalemia, this is a potassium-sparing medication, which means that the concern with the administration of this medication is hyperkalemia. Other effects include nausea, vomiting, cramping, diarrhea, headache, ataxia, drowsiness, confusion, and fever.
Test-Taking Strategy: Focus on the subject, oral triamterene, and think about the classification of the medication. Recalling that this is a potassium-sparing medication will direct you to the correct option.
Priority Nursing Tip: The client with cirrhosis needs to consume foods high in thiamine. Thiamine is present in a variety of foods of plant and animal origin. Pork products are especially rich in this vitamin.
Reference: Burchum, J., & Rosenthal, L. (2022). *Lehne's Pharmacology for nursing care* (11th ed., p. 461). Elsevier.

Integrated Processes

❖ **90.** The nurse is preparing a client in early labor who is experiencing a significant increase in blood pressure for an amniotomy. Which **priority** data would the nurse assess before the procedure?
1. Fetal heart rate
2. Maternal heart rate
3. Fetal scalp sampling
4. Maternal blood pressure

Level of Cognitive Ability: Analyzing
Client Needs: Physiological Integrity
Clinical Judgment/Cognitive Skills: Prioritize Hypotheses
Integrated Process: Clinical Judgment; Nursing Process/Assessment
Content Area: Maternity: Antepartum
Health Problems: Maternity: Gestational Hypertension/Preeclampsia and Eclampsia
Priority Concepts: Reproduction; Safety

Answer: 1
Rationale: Fetal well-being must be confirmed before and after amniotomy. Fetal heart rate needs to be checked by Doppler or with the application of the external fetal monitor. Although maternal vital signs may be assessed, fetal heart rate is the priority. A fetal scalp sampling cannot be done when the membranes are intact.
Test-Taking Strategy: Note the strategic word, *priority*. Eliminate option 3 first, knowing that a fetal scalp sampling cannot be done before an amniotomy. Eliminate options 2 and 4 that are comparable or alike and address maternal vital signs. The correct option addresses fetal well-being.
Priority Nursing Tip: Amniotomy (artificial rupture of the membranes) can be used to induce labor when the condition of the cervix is favorable (ripe) or to augment labor if the progress begins to slow.
Reference: McKinney, E. S., et al. (2022). *Maternal child nursing* (6th ed., pp. 316, 379). Elsevier.

91. The nurse is monitoring a client whose membranes ruptured and is now receiving an oxytocin infusion for the induction of labor. The nurse would suspect water intoxication if which sign or symptom is noted?
1. Fatigue
2. Lethargy
3. Sleepiness
4. Tachycardia

Level of Cognitive Ability: Analyzing
Client Needs: Physiological Integrity
Clinical Judgment/Cognitive Skills: Recognize Cues
Integrated Process: Clinical Judgment; Nursing Process/Assessment
Content Area: Pharmacology: Maternity/Newborn: Uterine Stimulants
Health Problems: N/A
Priority Concepts: Clinical Judgment; Safety

Answer: 4
Rationale: Oxytocin is a uterine stimulant. During an oxytocin infusion, the client is monitored closely for signs of water intoxication, including tachycardia, cardiac dysrhythmias, shortness of breath, nausea, and vomiting. The remaining options are not associated with water intoxication.
Test-Taking Strategy: Focus on the subject of water intoxication. Think about the physiologic response that occurs when fluid overload exists to direct you to the correct option. In addition, eliminate options 1, 2, and 3 that are comparable or alike and are related to energy levels.
Priority Nursing Tip: An oxytocin infusion is discontinued if uterine contraction frequency is less than 2 minutes, the duration is longer than 90 seconds, or fetal distress is noted.
Reference: McKinney, E. S., et al. (2022). *Maternal child nursing* (6th ed., p. 384). Elsevier.

❖ **92.** The nurse reviews the record of a client who is receiving external radiation therapy and notes documentation of a skin finding as moist desquamation. Which finding on assessment of the client would the nurse expect to observe?
   1. A rash
   2. Dermatitis
   3. Reddened skin
   4. Weeping of the skin

Level of Cognitive Ability: Analyzing
Client Needs: Physiological Integrity
Clinical Judgment/Cognitive Skills: Recognize Cues
Integrated Process: Clinical Judgment; Nursing Process/Assessment
Content Area: Adult Health: Integumentary
Health Problems: Adult Health: Integumentary: Inflammations/Infections
Priority Concepts: Clinical Judgment; Tissue Integrity

Answer: 4
Rationale: Moist desquamation occurs when the basal cells of the skin are destroyed. The dermal level is exposed, which results in the leakage of serum. A rash, dermatitis, and reddened skin may occur with external radiation, but these conditions are not described as moist desquamation.
Test-Taking Strategy: Options 1, 2, and 3 are eliminated because they are comparable or alike, and they describe a dry rather than a moist skin alteration. In addition, note the relationship between the word *moist* in the question and *weeping* in the correct option.
Priority Nursing Tip: The nurse needs to teach the client receiving radiation therapy to wash the irradiated area gently each day with warm water alone or mild soap and water. The client needs to use the hand rather than a washcloth to wash the area.
Reference: Lewis, S., et al. (2020). *Medical-surgical nursing: Assessment and management of clinical problems* (11th ed., p. 253). Elsevier.

93. The nurse is performing an assessment on a pregnant client with a history of cardiac disease. Which body area will venous congestion **most** commonly be noted in?
   1. Vulva
   2. Around the eyes
   3. Fingers of the hands
   4. Around the abdomen

Level of Cognitive Ability: Analyzing
Client Needs: Physiological Integrity
Clinical Judgment/Cognitive Skills: Recognize Cues
Integrated Process: Clinical Judgment; Nursing Process/Assessment
Content Area: Health Assessment/Physical Exam: Heart and Peripheral Vascular
Health Problems: Maternity: Cardiac Disease
Priority Concepts: Clinical Judgment; Reproduction

Answer: 1
Rationale: Assessment of the cardiovascular system includes observation for venous congestion that can develop into varicosities. Venous congestion is most commonly noted in the legs, the vulva, or the rectum. Although edema may be noted in the fingers and around the eyes, edema in these areas would not be directly associated with venous congestion. It would be difficult to assess for edema in the abdominal area of a client who is pregnant.
Test-Taking Strategy: Focus on the strategic word, *most*, and note the subject, venous congestion. From the options provided, the only body area in which venous congestion would be noted is the vulva.
Priority Nursing Tip: Varicose veins can occur in the second and the third trimesters of pregnancy. They result from weakening walls of the veins or valves and venous congestion.
Reference: McKinney, E. S., et al. (2022). *Maternal child nursing* (6th ed., pp. 233, 563). Elsevier.

❖ **94.** A client who has been receiving long-term diuretic therapy is admitted to the hospital with a diagnosis of dehydration. The nurse would assess for which sign that correlates with this fluid imbalance?
1. Decreased pulse
2. Bibasilar crackles
3. Increased blood pressure
4. Increased urinary specific gravity

Level of Cognitive Ability: Applying
Client Needs: Physiological Integrity
Clinical Judgment/Cognitive Skills: Recognize Cues
Integrated Process: Clinical Judgment; Nursing Process/Assessment
Content Area: Foundations of Care: Fluids and Electrolytes
Health Problems: Adult Health: Gastrointestinal: Dehydration
Priority Concepts: Clinical Judgment; Fluids and Electrolytes

Answer: 4
Rationale: Assessment findings with fluid volume deficit are increased pulse and respirations, weight loss, poor skin turgor, dry mucous membranes, decreased urine output, concentrated urine with increased specific gravity, increased hematocrit, and altered level of consciousness. The assessment findings in the remaining options are not associated with dehydration.
Test-Taking Strategy: Focus on the subject, a client with dehydration. Think about the pathophysiology associated with dehydration to direct you to the correct option.
Priority Nursing Tip: The nurse needs to monitor for signs of dehydration and electrolyte imbalances in a client receiving diuretic therapy.
Reference: Ignatavicius, D., et al. (2021). *Medical-surgical nursing: Concepts for interprofessional collaborative care* (10th ed., p. 248). Elsevier.

95. A client at 35 weeks' gestation reports a sudden discharge of fluid from the vagina. Based on the data provided, which condition would the nurse suspect?
1. Miscarriage
2. Preterm labor
3. Intrauterine fetal demise
4. Premature rupture of the membranes

Level of Cognitive Ability: Analyzing
Client Needs: Physiological Integrity
Clinical Judgment/Cognitive Skills: Recognize Cues
Integrated Process: Clinical Judgment; Nursing Process/Assessment
Content Area: Maternity: Antepartum
Health Problems: Maternity: Premature Rupture of the Membranes
Priority Concepts: Clinical Judgment; Reproduction

Answer: 4
Rationale: Premature rupture of the membranes is usually manifested by a sudden discharge of fluid from the vagina before 37 weeks of gestation. Miscarriage is typically manifested by vaginal bleeding and abdominal pain. Preterm labor is typically manifested by uterine contractions, cramping, and pressure before 37 weeks' gestation. Intrauterine fetal demise is usually manifested by an absence of fetal movements and heartbeat.
Test-Taking Strategy: Focus on the subject of a client who is at 35 weeks' gestation and reports a sudden discharge of fluid from the vagina. Note that all of the conditions noted in the options may occur during this time; therefore, the answer needs to be determined by looking at the clinical manifestations. Recall that amniotic fluid, rather than blood, would be expelled in premature rupture of the membranes; this will assist in eliminating option 1. From the remaining options, it is necessary to know which signs and symptoms are associated with each disorder in order to answer correctly.
Priority Nursing Tip: Infection can cause premature rupture of the membranes, premature labor, and postpartum endometritis.
Reference: McKinney, E. S., et al. (2022). *Maternal child nursing* (6th ed., pp. 586–587). Elsevier.

❖ **96.** On assessment of the client diagnosed with stage III Lyme disease, the nurse expects to note which clinical manifestation?
   1. Palpitations
   2. A cardiac dysrhythmia
   3. A generalized skin rash
   4. Enlarged and inflamed joints

Level of Cognitive Ability: Analyzing
Client Needs: Physiological Integrity
Clinical Judgment/Cognitive Skills: Recognize Cues
Integrated Process: Clinical Judgment; Nursing Process/Assessment
Content Area: Adult Health: Immune
Health Problems: Adult Health: Immune: Lyme Disease
Priority Concepts: Immunity; Inflammation

Answer: 4
Rationale: Stage III Lyme disease develops within a month to several months after initial infection. It is characterized by arthritic symptoms such as arthralgia and enlarged or inflamed joints, which can persist for several years after the initial infection. A rash occurs during stage I, and cardiac and neurologic dysfunction occur during stage II.
Test-Taking Strategy: Eliminate options that are comparable or alike and are cardiac symptoms. Focusing on the subject of signs and symptoms of stage III Lyme disease will direct you to the correct option.
Priority Nursing Tip: The typical ring-shaped rash of Lyme disease does not occur in all clients. Many clients never develop a rash. Additionally, if a rash does occur, it can arise anywhere on the body, not only at the site of the bite.
Reference: Lewis, S., et al. (2020). *Medical-surgical nursing: Assessment and management of clinical problems* (11th ed., p. 1516). Elsevier.

97. A child experienced a basilar skull fracture that resulted in the presence of Battle's sign. Which would the nurse expect to observe in the child?
   1. Bruising behind the ear
   2. The presence of epistaxis
   3. A bruised periorbital area
   4. An edematous periorbital area

Level of Cognitive Ability: Analyzing
Client Needs: Physiological Integrity
Clinical Judgment/Cognitive Skills: Recognize Cues
Integrated Process: Clinical Judgment; Nursing Process/Assessment
Content Area: Pediatrics: Neurologic
Health Problems: Pediatric-Specific: Head Injury
Priority Concepts: Clinical Judgment; Intracranial Regulation

Answer: 1
Rationale: The most serious type of skull fracture is a basilar skull fracture. Two classic findings associated with this type of skull fracture are Battle's sign and raccoon eyes. Battle's sign is the presence of bruising or ecchymosis behind the ear caused by a leaking of blood into the mastoid sinuses. Raccoon eyes occur as a result of blood leaking into the frontal sinus and causing an edematous and bruised periorbital area.
Test-Taking Strategy: Eliminate options 3 and 4 that are comparable or alike and relate to the periorbital area. Focusing on the subject of the description of Battle's sign will direct you to option 1.
Priority Nursing Tip: Leakage of cerebrospinal fluid (CSF) from the ears or nose may accompany basilar skull fracture. CSF can be distinguished from other body fluids because the drainage will separate into bloody and yellow concentric rings on dressing material, called a halo sign. The CSF fluid also tests positive for glucose.
Reference: McKinney, E. S., et al. (2022). *Maternal child nursing* (6th ed., p. 1301). Elsevier.

❖ **98.** When assessing a child with meningitis, the nurse would note which finding that would indicate the presence of Kernig's sign?
1. Calf pain when the foot is dorsiflexed
2. Pain when the chin is pulled down to the chest
3. The inability of the child to extend the legs fully when lying supine
4. The flexion of the hips when the neck is flexed from a lying position

Level of Cognitive Ability: Analyzing
Client Needs: Physiological Integrity
Clinical Judgment/Cognitive Skills: Recognize Cues
Integrated Process: Clinical Judgment; Nursing Process/Assessment
Content Area: Health Assessment/Physical Exam: Neurologic
Health Problems: Pediatric-Specific: Meningitis
Priority Concepts: Inflammation; Intracranial Regulation

Answer: 3
Rationale: Kernig's sign is the inability of the child to extend the legs fully when lying supine. Brudzinski's sign is flexion of the hips when the neck is flexed from a supine position. Both of these signs are frequently present in clients with bacterial meningitis. Nuchal rigidity is also present with bacterial meningitis, and it occurs when pain prevents the child from touching the chin to the chest. Homans' sign is elicited when pain occurs in the calf region when the foot is dorsiflexed.
Test-Taking Strategy: Focus on the subject, characteristics of Kernig's sign. It is necessary to know that Kernig's sign is the inability of the child to extend the legs fully when lying supine.
Priority Nursing Tip: Meningitis is transmitted by droplet infection. Precautions for this disease include placing the client in a private room or with a cohort client and use of a standard precaution mask.
Reference: McKinney, E. S., et al. (2022). *Maternal child nursing* (6th ed., p. 1313). Elsevier.

99. A home care nurse assesses an older client's functional status and ability to perform activities of daily living (ADLs) since being diagnosed with dementia. What is the focus area of the nurse's assessment?
1. Everyday routines
2. Self-care activities
3. Household management
4. Endurance and flexibility

Level of Cognitive Ability: Applying
Client Needs: Health Promotion and Maintenance
Clinical Judgment/Cognitive Skills: Prioritize Hypotheses
Integrated Process: Nursing Process/Assessment
Content Area: Skills: Activity/Mobility
Health Problems: Mental Health: Neurocognitive Impairment
Priority Concepts: Functional Ability; Health Promotion

Answer: 2
Rationale: To evaluate the client's functional status, the nurse assesses the client's ability to perform self-care or ADLs, including bathing, toileting, ambulating, dressing, and feeding. Everyday routines, household management, and physical condition are not components of functional status.
Test-Taking Strategy: Focus on the subject of the ability to perform ADLs. Recalling that ADLs refer to self-care needs will direct you to the correct option.
Priority Nursing Tip: For the client having a problem with performing ADLs, an occupational therapist would be consulted. An occupational therapist develops adaptive devices that can help the client perform ADLs.
Reference: Touhy, T., & Jett, K. (2022). *Ebersole and Hess' Gerontological nursing & healthy aging* (6th ed., pp. 104–105). Elsevier.

❖ **100.** The nurse is assessing a client diagnosed with Addison's disease for signs of hyperkalemia. Which sign/symptom would the nurse observe with this electrolyte imbalance?
1. Polyuria
2. Cardiac dysrhythmias
3. Dry mucous membranes
4. Prolonged bleeding time

Level of Cognitive Ability: Analyzing
Client Needs: Physiological Integrity
Clinical Judgment/Cognitive Skills: Recognize Cues
Integrated Process: Clinical Judgment; Nursing Process/Assessment
Content Area: Adult Health: Endocrine
Health Problems: Adult Health: Endocrine: Adrenal Disorders
Priority Concepts: Clinical Judgment; Fluids and Electrolytes

Answer: 2
Rationale: The inadequate production of aldosterone in clients with Addison's disease causes the inadequate excretion of potassium and results in hyperkalemia. The clinical manifestations of hyperkalemia are the result of altered nerve transmission. The most harmful consequence of hyperkalemia is its effect on cardiac function. Based on this information, none of the remaining options are manifestations that are associated with Addison's disease or hyperkalemia.
Test-Taking Strategy: Focus on the subject of Addison's disease and hyperkalemia. Think about the effects of potassium on the body and remember that hyperkalemia has a direct effect on cardiac function. This will direct you to the correct option.
Priority Nursing Tip: A low-potassium diet is usually indicated for hyperkalemia, which may be caused by disorders such as impaired renal function, Addison's disease, and potassium-retaining diuretics.
Reference: Ignatavicius, D., et al. (2021). *Medical-surgical nursing: Concepts for interprofessional collaborative care* (10th ed., p. 1239). Elsevier.

101. The nurse performs an Allen's test before blood is drawn from the radial artery for an arterial blood gas (ABG) assessment. This intervention is done to determine the collateral circulatory adequacy of which arterial vessel?
1. Ulnar
2. Carotid
3. Brachial
4. Femoral

Level of Cognitive Ability: Analyzing
Client Needs: Physiological Integrity
Clinical Judgment/Cognitive Skills: Recognize Cues
Integrated Process: Clinical Judgment; Nursing Process/Assessment
Content Area: Foundations of Care: Acid–Base
Health Problems: N/A
Priority Concepts: Acid–Base Balance; Perfusion

Answer: 1
Rationale: Before radial puncture for obtaining an arterial specimen for ABGs, Allen's test is performed to determine adequate ulnar circulation. Failure to assess collateral circulation could result in severe ischemic injury to the hand if damage to the radial artery occurs with arterial puncture. Allen's test does not determine the adequacy of carotid, brachial, or femoral circulation.
Test-Taking Strategy: Note the words *radial artery* in the question. Focus on the subject, arterial blood gas (ABG) assessment drawn from the radial artery, and think about the anatomy of the blood vessels. This will eliminate the remaining options.
Priority Nursing Tip: After obtaining an arterial blood gas specimen, the nurse needs to ensure that pressure is placed over the area of the puncture for at least 5 or 10 minutes and longer if the client is taking an anticoagulant.
Reference: Lewis, S., et al. (2020). *Medical-surgical nursing: Assessment and management of clinical problems* (11th ed., p. 1541). Elsevier.

❖ **102.** A pregnant client diagnosed with diabetes mellitus arrives at the primary health care clinic for a follow-up visit. What **best** assessment would the nurse perform to assess insulin function?
1. Urine for specific gravity
2. For the presence of edema
3. Urine for glucose and ketones
4. Blood pressure, pulse, and respirations

Level of Cognitive Ability: Analyzing
Client Needs: Physiological Integrity
Clinical Judgment/Cognitive Skills: Recognize Cues
Integrated Process: Clinical Judgment; Nursing Process/Assessment
Content Area: Maternity: Antepartum
Health Problems: Maternity: Diabetes
Priority Concepts: Glucose Regulation; Reproduction

Answer: 3
Rationale: In addition to blood glucose testing, the nurse assesses the pregnant client with diabetes mellitus for glucose and ketones in the urine at each prenatal visit because the physiologic changes of pregnancy can drastically alter insulin requirements. It is important to remember, though, that urine testing for glucose may not be beneficial during pregnancy because of the lowered renal threshold for glucose; therefore, the degree of glycosuria does not accurately reflect the blood glucose level. The assessment of urine for specific gravity; the presence of edema; and blood pressure, pulse, and respirations are more related to the client with gestational hypertension.
Test-Taking Strategy: Focus on the *subject* of a pregnant client with diabetes mellitus, and the *strategic word,* *best*. The only option that specifically addresses diabetes mellitus is the correct one.
Priority Nursing Tip: Most oral hypoglycemic agents are not prescribed for use during pregnancy because of their teratogenic effects.
Reference: McKinney, E. S., et al. (2022). *Maternal child nursing* (6th ed., pp. 558–559). Elsevier.

Nursing Process: Analysis

103. A client with acute kidney injury had arterial blood gases drawn. Which disorder would the nurse interpret that the client is experiencing?

LABORATORY RESULTS

Test and Result	Reference Range
pH 7.34	7.35-7.45
PCO_2 37 mm Hg	35-45 mm Hg
PO_2 79 mm Hg	80-100 mm Hg
HCO_3 19 mEq/L	21-28 mEq/L
(19 mmol/L)	(21-28 mmol/L)

1. Metabolic acidosis
2. Metabolic alkalosis
3. Respiratory acidosis
4. Respiratory alkalosis

Level of Cognitive Ability: Analyzing
Client Needs: Physiological Integrity
Clinical Judgment/Cognitive Skills: Analyze Cues
Integrated Process: Clinical Judgment; Nursing Process/Analysis
Content Area: Foundations of Care: Acid–Base
Health Problems: Adult Health: Renal and Urinary: Acute Kidney Injury/Chronic Kidney Disease
Priority Concepts: Acid–Base Balance; Perfusion

Answer: 1
Rationale: Metabolic acidosis occurs when the pH falls to less than 7.35 and the bicarbonate level falls to less than 22 mEq/L (22 mmol/L). With metabolic alkalosis, the pH rises to more than 7.45 and the bicarbonate level rises to more than 27 mEq/L (27 mmol/L). With respiratory acidosis, the pH drops to less than 7.35 and the carbon dioxide level rises to more than 45 mm Hg. With respiratory alkalosis, the pH rises to more than 7.45 and the carbon dioxide level falls to less than 35 mm Hg.
Test-Taking Strategy: Knowing that a pH of 7.34 is acidotic assists you with eliminating options 2 and 4 that are *comparable or alike*. From the remaining choices, focus on the *subject* that involves a metabolic condition that exists when the bicarbonate follows the same up or down pattern as the pH; this will help you to choose the correct option.
Priority Nursing Tip: Causes of metabolic acidosis include diabetes mellitus or diabetic ketoacidosis, excessive ingestion of acetylsalicylic acid (aspirin), a high-fat diet, insufficient metabolism of carbohydrates, malnutrition, renal insufficiency or renal failure, and severe diarrhea.
Reference: Ignatavicius, D., et al. (2021). *Medical-surgical nursing: Concepts for interprofessional collaborative care* (10th ed., pp. 267, 269). Elsevier.

❖ **104.** The nurse caring for a child diagnosed with nephrotic syndrome is analyzing the child's laboratory results. On the basis of this finding, which clinical manifestation would the nurse expect to note in the child?

LABORATORY RESULTS

Test and Result	Reference Range
Sodium 148 mEq/L (148 mmol/L)	135-145 mEq/L (135-145 mmol/L)

1. Lethargy
2. Diaphoresis
3. Cold, wet skin
4. Dry, sticky mucous membranes

Level of Cognitive Ability: Analyzing
Client Needs: Physiological Integrity
Clinical Judgment/Cognitive Skills: Analyze Cues
Integrated Process: Clinical Judgment; Nursing Process/Analysis
Content Area: Pediatrics: Metabolic/Endocrine
Health Problems: Pediatric-Specific: Nephrotic Syndrome
Priority Concepts: Clinical Judgment; Fluids and Electrolytes

Answer: 4
Rationale: Hypernatremia occurs when the sodium level is more than 145 mEq/L (145 mmol/L). Clinical manifestations include intense thirst, oliguria, agitation, restlessness, flushed skin, peripheral and pulmonary edema, dry and sticky mucous membranes, nausea, and vomiting. None of the remaining options are associated with the clinical manifestations of hypernatremia.
Test-Taking Strategy: Focus on the subject of a child with nephrotic syndrome. Note the data in the question and determine that the sodium level is elevated and that the child is experiencing hypernatremia. Eliminate options 2 and 3 that are comparable or alike and relate to the skin. From the remaining choices, recalling that agitation and restlessness (not lethargy) are associated with hypernatremia will direct you to the correct option.
Priority Nursing Tip: Altered cerebral function is a common manifestation of hypernatremia.
Reference: McKinney, E. S., et al. (2022). *Maternal child nursing* (6th ed., pp. 891, 1025). Elsevier.

105. The nurse is caring for an infant admitted to the hospital with a diagnosis of hemolytic disease. Which finding would the nurse expect to note in this infant when reviewing the laboratory results?
1. Decreased bilirubin count
2. Elevated blood glucose level
3. Decreased red blood cell count
4. Decreased white blood cell count

Level of Cognitive Ability: Analyzing
Client Needs: Physiological Integrity
Clinical Judgment/Cognitive Skills: Analyze Cues
Integrated Process: Clinical Judgment; Nursing Process/Analysis
Content Area: Pediatrics: Hematologic
Health Problems: Pediatric-Specific: Anemias
Priority Concepts: Cellular Regulation; Clinical Judgment

Answer: 3
Rationale: The two primary pathophysiologic alterations associated with hemolytic disease are anemia and hyperbilirubinemia. The red blood cell count is decreased because red blood cell production cannot keep pace with red blood cell destruction. Hyperbilirubinemia results from the red blood cell destruction that accompanies this disorder and from the normally decreased ability of the neonate's liver to conjugate and excrete bilirubin efficiently from the body. Hypoglycemia is associated with hypertrophy of the pancreatic islet cells and increased levels of insulin. The white blood cell count is not related to this disorder.
Test-Taking Strategy: Focus on the subject of an infant with hemolytic disease. Noting the word *hemolytic* in the diagnosis will direct you to the correct option.
Priority Nursing Tip: Iron is found predominantly in hemoglobin and acts as a carrier of oxygen from the lungs to the tissues and indirectly aids in the return of carbon dioxide to the lungs.
Reference: Hockenberry, M., Wilson, D., & Rodgers, C. (2019). *Wong's Nursing care of infants and children* (11th ed., pp. 259, 261–262). Elsevier.

❖ **106.** Intravenous immune globulin (IVIG) therapy is prescribed for a child diagnosed with idiopathic thrombocytopenic purpura (ITP). What are the expected results of this medication?

LABORATORY RESULTS

Test and Result	Reference Range
Urinalysis - Glucose positive	Negative
Urinalysis - Specific gravity 1.020	1.003-1.030
Platelets 355,000/mm³ (355 × 10⁹/L)	150,000-400,000/mm³ (150-400 × 10⁹/L)
BUN 22 mg/dL (7.92 mmol/L)	10-20 mg/dL (3.6-7.1 mmol/L)

1. Urine positive for glucose
2. Urine specific gravity of 1.020
3. Platelets of 355,000/mm³ (355 × 10⁹/L)
4. Blood urea nitrogen (BUN) 22 mg/dL (7.92 mmol/L)

Level of Cognitive Ability: Analyzing
Client Needs: Physiological Integrity
Clinical Judgment/Cognitive Skills: Analyze Cues
Integrated Process: Clinical Judgment; Nursing Process/Analysis
Content Area: Pediatrics: Hematologic
Health Problems: Pediatric-Specific: Bleeding Disorders
Priority Concepts: Cellular Regulation; Clinical Judgment

Answer: 3
Rationale: ITP is an immune disorder in which blood clotting is abnormal. ITP can cause excessive bruising and bleeding. An unusually low level of platelets, or thrombocytes, in the blood results in ITP. IVIG is usually effective to rapidly increase the platelet count. It is thought to act by interfering with the attachment of antibody-coded platelets to receptors on the macrophage cells of the reticuloendothelial system. Corticosteroids may be prescribed to enhance vascular stability and decrease the production of antiplatelet antibodies. Based on this information, the remaining options are unrelated to the administration of this medication.
Test-Taking Strategy: Focus on the subject of IVIG therapy for a child with ITP. Note the relationship between the name of the diagnosis *thrombocytopenic purpura* and the word *platelets* in the correct option. This relationship may assist with directing you to the correct option.
Priority Nursing Tip: Manifestations of ITP are first noted in the skin and mucous membranes. Large ecchymotic areas or a petechial rash on the arms, legs, upper chest, and neck may be noted.
Reference: McKinney, E. S., et al. (2022). *Maternal child nursing* (6th ed., pp. 1143–1144). Elsevier.

107. A child was diagnosed with acute poststreptococcal glomerulonephritis and renal insufficiency. Which laboratory result would the nurse expect to note in the child?

LABORATORY RESULTS

Test and Result	Reference Range
Urinalysis – Protein negative	0-trace
Urinalysis – Glucose negative	Negative
WBC 18,000/mm³ (18 × 10⁹/L)	5000-10,000/mm³ (5-10 × 10⁹/L)
Creatinine 2.1 mg/dL (185 mcmol/L)	0.5-1.2 mg/dL (44-106 mcmol/L)

1. Urine negative for protein
2. Urine negative for red blood cells
3. White blood cell count 18,000/mm³ (18 × 10⁹/L)
4. Creatinine level of 2.1 mg/dL (185 mcmol/L)

Level of Cognitive Ability: Analyzing
Client Needs: Physiological Integrity
Clinical Judgment/Cognitive Skills: Analyze Cues
Integrated Process: Clinical Judgment; Nursing Process/Analysis
Content Area: Pediatrics: Renal and Urinary
Health Problems: Pediatric-Specific: Glomerulonephritis
Priority Concepts: Clinical Judgment; Elimination

Answer: 4
Rationale: With poststreptococcal glomerulonephritis, a urinalysis will reveal hematuria with red cell casts. Proteinuria is also present. If renal insufficiency is severe, the BUN and creatinine levels will be elevated. The reference range for BUN is 10–20 mg/dL (3.6–7.1 mmol/L) and creatinine is 0.5–1.2 mg/dL (44–106 mcmol/L). The WBC is usually within normal limits, and mild anemia is common. Platelets would be lower, whereas glucose is not related.
Test-Taking Strategy: Focus on the subject of a child with acute poststreptococcal glomerulonephritis and renal insufficiency. Recalling that the BUN and creatinine levels are laboratory studies that relate to the renal system will direct you to the correct option.
Priority Nursing Tip: In glomerulonephritis, inflammation of the glomeruli results from an antigen-antibody reaction produced by an infection elsewhere in the body. Loss of kidney function develops.
Reference: McKinney, E. S., et al. (2022). *Maternal child nursing* (6th ed., p. 1020). Elsevier.

❖ **108.** A child is admitted to the hospital with a suspected diagnosis of bacterial endocarditis. The child has been experiencing fever, malaise, anorexia, and a headache. Which diagnostic study will confirm the diagnosis?
　1. A blood culture
　2. A sedimentation rate
　3. A white blood cell count
　4. An electrocardiogram (ECG)

Level of Cognitive Ability: Analyzing
Client Needs: Physiological Integrity
Clinical Judgment/Cognitive Skills: Analyze Cues
Integrated Process: Clinical Judgment; Nursing Process/Analysis
Content Area: Pediatrics: Cardiovascular
Health Problems: Pediatric-Specific: Infectious/Communicable Diseases
Priority Concepts: Clinical Judgment; Infection

Answer: 1
Rationale: The diagnosis of bacterial endocarditis is primarily established on the basis of a positive blood culture of the organisms and the visualization of vegetation on echocardiographic studies. Other laboratory tests that may help confirm the diagnosis are an elevated sedimentation rate and the C-reactive protein level. An ECG is not usually helpful for the diagnosis of bacterial endocarditis.
Test-Taking Strategy: Focus on the subject of bacterial endocarditis and its causes. The only test that will confirm the presence of an organism is the blood culture.
Priority Nursing Tip: Instruct the parents of a child who had bacterial endocarditis of the need to inform the dentist and any other health care providers about the condition. Prophylactic antibiotics may be prescribed before dental procedures or any other invasive disorders to prevent the recurrence of endocarditis.
Reference: McKinney, E. S., et al. (2022). *Maternal child nursing* (6th ed., p. 1112). Elsevier.

109. The nurse interprets that which observation is related to the dysfunction of cranial nerve III (oculomotor nerve)?
　1. Mild drowsiness
　2. Unilateral ptosis
　3. Diminished mental acuity
　4. Less frequent spontaneous speech

Level of Cognitive Ability: Analyzing
Client Needs: Physiological Integrity
Clinical Judgment/Cognitive Skills: Analyze Cues
Integrated Process: Clinical Judgment; Nursing Process/Analysis
Content Area: Health Assessment/Physical Exam: Neurologic
Health Problems: N/A
Priority Concepts: Intracranial Regulation; Sensory Perception

Answer: 2
Rationale: Ptosis of the eyelid is caused by pressure on and the dysfunction of cranial nerve III, the oculomotor nerve. The remaining options identify early signs of a deteriorating level of consciousness.
Test-Taking Strategy: Focus on the subject of cranial nerve III dysfunction. Recalling the function of this nerve and that it is the oculomotor nerve will direct you to the correct option.
Priority Nursing Tip: Cranial nerve III, the oculomotor nerve, controls pupillary constriction, upper eyelid elevation, and most eye movement.
Reference: Ignatavicius, D., et al. (2021). *Medical-surgical nursing: Concepts for interprofessional collaborative care* (10th ed., p. 829). Elsevier.

❖ **110.** A client diagnosed with a thrombotic stroke experiences periods of emotional lability. What would the nurse interpret this behavior as indicating?
1. That the client is not adapting well to the disability
2. That the problem is likely to get worse before it gets better
3. That the client is experiencing the usual sequelae of a stroke
4. That the client is experiencing the side effects of prescribed anticoagulants

Level of Cognitive Ability: Analyzing
Client Needs: Psychosocial Integrity
Clinical Judgment/Cognitive Skills: Analyze Cues
Integrated Process: Clinical Judgment; Nursing Process/Analysis
Content Area: Adult Health: Neurologic
Health Problems: Adult Health: Neurologic: Stroke
Priority Concepts: Intracranial Regulation; Mood and Affect

Answer: 3
Rationale: After a thrombotic stroke, the client often experiences periods of emotional lability, which are characterized by sudden bouts of laughing or crying or by irritability, depression, confusion, or being demanding. This is a normal part of the clinical picture of the client with this health problem, although it may be difficult for health care personnel and family members to deal with it. The other options are incorrect.
Test-Taking Strategy: Focus on the subject of emotional lability after thrombotic stroke. Eliminate option 4 first because anticoagulants do not cause emotional lability. From the remaining choices, recalling the emotional changes that accompany a thrombotic stroke will direct you to the correct option.
Priority Nursing Tip: A critical factor in the early intervention and treatment of stroke is the accurate identification of stroke manifestations and establishing the onset of the manifestations. Stroke screening scales may be used to quickly identify stroke manifestations.
Reference: Ignatavicius, D., et al. (2021). *Medical-surgical nursing: Concepts for interprofessional collaborative care* (10th ed., p. 900). Elsevier.

111. The nurse is developing a plan of care for a client in Buck's (extension) traction. The nurse would determine that which is a **priority** client problem?
1. Immobility
2. Risk of infection
3. Altered independence
4. Insufficient sensory stimulation

Level of Cognitive Ability: Analyzing
Client Needs: Physiological Integrity
Clinical Judgment/Cognitive Skills: Prioritize Hypotheses
Integrated Process: Clinical Judgment; Nursing Process/Analysis
Content Area: Skills: Activity/Mobility
Health Problems: Adult Health: Musculoskeletal: Skeletal Injury
Priority Concepts: Clinical Judgment; Mobility

Answer: 1
Rationale: The priority client problem in Buck's traction is immobility. Options 3 and 4 may also be appropriate for the client in traction, but immobility presents the greatest risk for the development of complications. Buck's traction is a skin traction, and there are no pin sites.
Test-Taking Strategy: Focus on the subject, Buck's traction and its possible complications. Eliminate option 2 first because there are no pin sites with Buck's traction. From the remaining choices, focus on the strategic word, *priority*, recalling that the client experiences immobility when in traction. This will direct you to the correct option.
Priority Nursing Tip: Buck's (extension) skin traction is used to alleviate muscle spasms and immobilize a lower limb by maintaining a straight pull on the limb with the use of weights. It is often used in the preoperative period for a client who sustained a hip fracture.
Reference: Ignatavicius, D., et al. (2021). *Medical-surgical nursing: Concepts for interprofessional collaborative care* (10th ed., pp. 1037–1039, 1042). Elsevier.

❖ **112.** A pregnant client diagnosed with mitral valve prolapse is prescribed anticoagulant therapy during pregnancy. The nurse reviews the client's medical record, expecting to note that which medication therapy is prescribed daily?
1. Oral warfarin
2. Intravenous infusion of heparin sodium
3. Subcutaneous administration of terbutaline
4. Subcutaneous administration of heparin sodium

Level of Cognitive Ability: Analyzing
Client Needs: Physiological Integrity
Clinical Judgment/Cognitive Skills: Analyze Cues
Integrated Process: Clinical Judgment; Nursing Process/Analysis
Content Area: Maternity: Antepartum
Health Problems: Maternity: Cardiac Disease
Priority Concepts: Clinical Judgment; Safety

Answer: 4
Rationale: Pregnant women with mitral valve prolapse are frequently given anticoagulant therapy during pregnancy because they are at greater risk for thromboembolic disease during the antenatal, intrapartum, and postpartum periods. Heparin, which does not pass the placental barrier, is a safe anticoagulant therapy during pregnancy, and it would be administered by the subcutaneous route. Warfarin is contraindicated during pregnancy because it passes the placental barrier and causes potential fetal malformations and hemorrhagic disorders. Terbutaline is a medication that is indicated for preterm labor management.
Test-Taking Strategy: Focus on the subject, mitral valve prolapse, anticoagulant therapy, and medication safety during pregnancy. Eliminate options 1 because warfarin is contraindicated in pregnancy. Next, eliminate option 3 because terbutaline is for preterm labor management. From the remaining choices, select option 4 because of the word *subcutaneous*.
Priority Nursing Tip: Bleeding is the primary concern for a client taking an anticoagulant, thrombolytic, or antiplatelet medication.
Reference: McKinney, E. S., et al. (2022). *Maternal child nursing* (6th ed., p. 566). Elsevier.

113. At the last vaginal exam, the client who is in the late first stage of labor was fully effaced, 8 cm dilated, vertex presentation, and station −1. Which observation would indicate that the fetus was in distress?
1. The fetal heart rate slowly drops to 110 beats/min during strong contractions, recovering to 138 beats/min immediately afterward.
2. Fresh meconium is found on the examiner's gloved fingers after a vaginal exam, and the fetal monitor pattern remains essentially unchanged.
3. Fresh, thick meconium is passed with a small gush of liquid, and the fetal monitor shows late decelerations with a variable descending baseline.
4. The vaginal exam continues to reveal some old meconium staining, and the fetal monitor demonstrates a U-shaped pattern of deceleration during contractions, recovering to a baseline of 140 beats/min.

Level of Cognitive Ability: Analyzing
Client Needs: Physiological Integrity
Clinical Judgment/Cognitive Skills: Analyze Cues
Integrated Process: Clinical Judgment; Nursing Process/Analysis
Content Area: Maternity: Intrapartum
Health Problems: Maternity: Fetal Distress/Demise
Priority Concepts: Perfusion; Reproduction

Answer: 3
Rationale: Meconium staining alone is not a sign of fetal distress. Meconium passage is a normal physiologic function that is frequently noted with a fetus of more than 38 weeks' gestation. Fresh meconium, in combination with late decelerations and a variable descending baseline, is an ominous signal of fetal distress caused by fetal hypoxia. It is not unusual for the fetal heart rate to drop to less than the 140- to 160-beats/min range in labor during contractions, and, in a healthy fetus, the fetal heart rate will recover between contractions. Old meconium staining may be the result of a prenatal trauma that is resolved.
Test-Taking Strategy: Note the subject, fetal distress. Eliminate options that indicate a recovering fetal heart rate. From the remaining choices, eliminate option 2 because of the words *fetal monitor pattern remains essentially unchanged*.
Priority Nursing Tip: In the event of fetal distress, prepare the client for emergency cesarean delivery.
Reference: McKinney, E. S., et al. (2022). *Maternal child nursing* (6th ed., pp. 316–317). Elsevier.

❖ **114.** A child diagnosed with seizures is being treated with carbamazepine. The nurse reviews the laboratory report for the results of the drug plasma level (reference range 5-12 mcg/mL [21.16 - 50.80 mcmol/L]) and determines that the plasma level is in a therapeutic range if which result is noted?

1. 1 mcg/mL (4.2 mcmol/L)
2. 10 mcg/mL (42.3 mcmol/L)
3. 18 mcg/mL (76.1 mcmol/L)
4. 20 mcg/mL (84.6 mcmol/L)

Level of Cognitive Ability: Analyzing
Client Needs: Physiological Integrity
Clinical Judgment/Cognitive Skills: Analyze Cues
Integrated Process: Clinical Judgment; Nursing Process/Analysis
Content Area: Pharmacology: Neurologic: Antiseizure
Health Problems: Pediatric-Specific: Seizures
Priority Concepts: Clinical Judgment; Safety

Answer: 2
Rationale: When carbamazepine is administered, plasma levels of the medication need to be monitored periodically to check for the child's absorption of the medication. The amount of the medication prescribed is based on the results of this laboratory test. The therapeutic plasma level of carbamazepine is 5 to 12 mcg/mL (21.16 to 50.80 mcmol/L). Option 1 indicates a low level that possibly necessitates an increased medication dose. Options 3 and 4 identify elevated levels that indicate the need to decrease the medication dose.
Test-Taking Strategy: Focus on the subject, therapeutic plasma level of carbamazepine, to answer the question. Recalling that the therapeutic plasma level is 5 to 12 mcg/mL (21.16 to 50.80 mcmol/L) will direct you to the correct option.
Priority Nursing Tip: Adverse effects of carbamazepine appear as blood dyscrasias, including aplastic anemia, agranulocytosis, thrombocytopenia, and leukopenia; cardiovascular disturbances; thrombophlebitis; dysrhythmias; and dermatologic effects.
References: Kizior, R., & Hodgson, B. (2023). *Saunders Nursing drug handbook 2023* (p. 184). Elsevier; McKinney, E. S., et al. (2022). *Maternal child nursing* (6th ed., p. 1308). Elsevier.

115. The nurse performs an assessment on a client with a history of heart failure who has been taking diuretics on a long-term basis. The nurse reviews the medication record, knowing that which medication, if prescribed for this client, would place the client at risk for hypokalemia?

1. Bumetanide
2. Triamterene
3. Spironolactone
4. Hydrochlorothiazide

Level of Cognitive Ability: Analyzing
Client Needs: Physiological Integrity
Clinical Judgment/Cognitive Skills: Analyze Cues
Integrated Process: Clinical Judgment; Nursing Process/Analysis
Content Area: Pharmacology: Cardiovascular: Diuretics
Health Problems: Adult Health: Cardiovascular: Heart Failure
Priority Concepts: Clinical Judgment; Fluids and Electrolytes

Answer: 1
Rationale: Bumetanide is a loop diuretic. The client on this medication would be at risk for hypokalemia. Triamterene, spironolactone, and hydrochlorothiazide are potassium-sparing diuretics.
Test-Taking Strategy: Focus on the subject of the identification of potassium-losing diuretic. Recalling that bumetanide is a loop diuretic will direct you to option 1. Also note that the remaining options are comparable or alike and are potassium-sparing diuretics.
Priority Nursing Tip: Natriuretic peptides are neuroendocrine peptides that are used to identify the client with heart failure (HF). The brain natriuretic peptide (BNP) is synthesized in the cardiac ventricle muscle. The higher the BNP level, the more severe the HF. If the BNP is elevated, the dyspnea is caused by HF; if it is normal, the dyspnea is caused by a pulmonary problem.
References: Ignatavicius, D., et al. (2021). *Medical-surgical nursing: Concepts for interprofessional collaborative care* (10th ed., pp. 254, 674). Elsevier; Kizior, R., & Hodgson, B. (2023). *Saunders Nursing drug handbook 2023* (p. 162). Elsevier.

❖ **116.** The home care nurse is preparing to visit a client diagnosed with Meniere's disease. The nurse analyzes the physician's prescriptions and expects which diet to be prescribed?
1. A low-fiber diet with decreased fluids
2. A low-sodium diet and fluid restriction
3. A low-fat diet with a restriction of citrus fruits
4. A low-carbohydrate diet and the elimination of red meats

Level of Cognitive Ability: Analyzing
Client Needs: Physiological Integrity
Clinical Judgment/Cognitive Skills: Generate Solutions
Integrated Process: Clinical Judgment; Nursing Process/Analysis
Content Area: Adult Health: Ear
Health Problems: Adult Health: Ear: Meniere's Disease
Priority Concepts: Safety; Sensory Perception

Answer: 2
Rationale: Dietary changes such as salt and fluid restrictions that reduce the amount of endolymphatic fluid are sometimes prescribed for clients with Meniere's disease. None of the remaining options are prescribed for this disorder.
Test-Taking Strategy: Focus on the subject, a client with Meniere's disease. Recalling that salt and fluid restrictions are sometimes necessary to reduce the amount of endolymphatic fluid will assist with directing you to the correct option.
Priority Nursing Tip: A priority nursing intervention in the care of a client with Meniere's syndrome is instituting safety measures because severe vertigo can occur.
Reference: Ignatavicius, D., et al. (2021). *Medical-surgical nursing: Concepts for interprofessional collaborative care* (10th ed., p. 968). Elsevier.

117. The nurse is caring for a client who has been diagnosed with tuberculosis. The client is receiving 600 mg of oral rifampin daily. Which laboratory finding would indicate to the nurse that the client is experiencing an adverse effect?

LABORATORY RESULTS

Test and Result	Reference Range
Sedimentation rate 15 mm/hr	0 - 30 mm/hr
ALT 80 U/L	4 - 36 U/L
Bilirubin 0.3 mg/dL (5.1 mcmol/L)	0.3 - 1.0 mg/dL (5.1 to 17 mcmol/L)
WBC 6000/mm³ (6 × 10⁹/L)	5000 - 10,000/mm³ (5 to 10 × 10⁹/L)

1. A sedimentation rate of 15 mm/hr
2. Alanine aminotransferase (ALT) of 80 U/L
3. A total bilirubin level of 0.3 mg/dL (5.1 mcmol/L)
4. A white blood cell count of 6000 mm³ (6 × 10⁹/L)

Level of Cognitive Ability: Analyzing
Client Needs: Physiological Integrity
Clinical Judgment/Cognitive Skills: Analyze Cues
Integrated Process: Clinical Judgment; Nursing Process/Analysis
Content Area: Pharmacology: Immune: Antimycobacterials
Health Problems: Adult Health: Respiratory: Tuberculosis
Priority Concepts: Clinical Judgment; Safety

Answer: 2
Rationale: Adverse or toxic effects of rifampin include hepatotoxicity, hepatitis, jaundice, blood dyscrasias, Stevens-Johnson syndrome, and antibiotic-related colitis. The nurse monitors for increased liver function, bilirubin, blood urea nitrogen, and uric acid levels because elevations indicate an adverse effect. The reference range for ALT is 4 to 36 U/L. The reference range for total bilirubin level is 0.3 to 1.0 mg/dL (5.1 to 17 mcmol/L). The reference range for sedimentation rate is 0 to 30 mm/hr. The reference range for white blood cell count is 5000 to 10,000/mm³ (5 to 10 × 10⁹/L).
Test-Taking Strategy: Focus on the subject, rifampin and diagnostic results that would indicate a possible adverse effect. Recalling that the medication is metabolized in the liver will assist you with eliminating options because these laboratory studies are not directly related to assessing liver function. From the remaining choices, knowledge of normal laboratory values will direct you to the correct option.
Priority Nursing Tip: A side effect of rifampin, an antituberculosis medication, is red-orange-colored body secretions.
References: Burchum, J., & Rosenthal, L. (2022). *Lehne's Pharmacology for nursing care* (11th ed., pp. 1091–1092, 1097). Elsevier; Pagana, K., Pagana, T., & Pagana, T. N. (2021). *Mosby's Diagnostic and laboratory test reference* (15th ed., p. 17). Elsevier.

❖ **118.** A home care nurse is assessing a client with hypertension who is prescribed prazosin. Which statement by the client would support the **need for further teaching** regarding medication compliance?

1. "If I feel dizzy, I'll skip my dose for a few days."
2. "I can't see the numbers on the label to know how much salt is in the food."
3. "I understand why I have to keep taking the pills even when my blood pressure is normal."
4. "If I have a cold, I shouldn't take any over-the-counter remedies without consulting my doctor."

Level of Cognitive Ability: Analyzing
Client Needs: Physiological Integrity
Clinical Judgment/Cognitive Skills: Analyze Cues
Integrated Process: Clinical Judgment; Nursing Process/Analysis
Content Area: Pharmacology: Cardiovascular: Antihypertensives
Health Problems: Adult Health: Cardiovascular: Hypertension
Priority Concepts: Clinical Judgment; Safety

Answer: 1
Rationale: Prazosin is used to treat hypertension. The side effects of prazosin are dizziness and impotence. The client needs to be instructed to call the physician if these side effects occur. Holding (skipping) medication will cause an abrupt rise in blood pressure. Option 2 indicates difficulty taking care of oneself. The remaining options indicate client understanding regarding the medication.
Test-Taking Strategy: Focus on the subject, prazosin and guidelines for addressing medication compliance. Note the strategic words, *need for further teaching*. These words indicate a negative event query and ask you to select an option that is an incorrect statement. Noting the words, "I'll skip my dose," will direct you to the correct option.
Priority Nursing Tip: Instruct the client taking prazosin to change positions slowly to prevent orthostatic hypotension.
Reference: Burchum, J., & Rosenthal, L. (2022). *Lehne's Pharmacology for nursing care* (11th ed., pp. 172, 181). Elsevier.

119. A client manages peptic ulcer disease (PUD) with excessive amounts of oral antacids. The nurse would assess for which acid-base disorder?

1. Metabolic acidosis
2. Metabolic alkalosis
3. Respiratory acidosis
4. Respiratory alkalosis

Level of Cognitive Ability: Analyzing
Client Needs: Physiological Integrity
Clinical Judgment/Cognitive Skills: Analyze Cues
Integrated Process: Clinical Judgment; Nursing Process/Analysis
Content Area: Pharmacology: Gastrointestinal: Antacids
Health Problems: Adult Health: Gastrointestinal: Peptic Ulcer Disease
Priority Concepts: Acid–Base Balance; Clinical Judgment

Answer: 2
Rationale: Oral antacids can be effective treatment for PUD when administered properly, but when they are taken in excess they can lead to metabolic alkalosis (a pH of more than 7.45 and a bicarbonate ion [HCO_3] level of more than 28 mEq/L [28 mmol/L]). As effective therapy for PUD, antacids bind with the hydrochloric acid (HCl^-) of gastric secretions and halt the corrosive action of the HCl^-. However, antacids are alkaline substances, and excessive administration can exceed the kidney's ability to clear the excess HCO_3, which leads to the accumulation of HCO_3, an increased pH, and metabolic alkalosis. Metabolic acidosis occurs when the pH is low and the HCO_3 is low; respiratory acidosis occurs when the pH is low and the partial pressure of carbon dioxide (Pco_2) is high; and respiratory alkalosis occurs when the pH is high and the Pco_2 is low.
Test-Taking Strategy: Focus on the subject, the use of antacids, and the possible outcome of that behavior. With this in mind, eliminate options 3 and 4 that are comparable and alike because they involve respiratory components. Knowing that the word *antacids* means *working against acids* will help you choose the correct option.
Priority Nursing Tip: To prevent interactions with other medications and the interference with the action of other medications, allow 1 hour between antacid administration and the administration of other medications.
Reference: Ignatavicius, D., et al. (2021). *Medical-surgical nursing: Concepts for interprofessional collaborative care* (10th ed., pp. 271-272). Elsevier.

❖ **120.** The nurse is assessing a 39-year-old Caucasian client with a blood pressure (BP) of 152/92 mm Hg at rest. Laboratory results are available. On which risk factor for coronary artery disease would the nurse place **priority?**

LABORATORY RESULTS

Test and Result	Reference Range
Cholesterol 180 mg/dL (4.5 mmol/L)	<200 mg/dL
Glucose 90 mg/dL (5.14 mmol/L)	70-99 mg/dL (3.9-5.5 mmol/L) Fasting

1. Age
2. Hypertension
3. Hyperlipidemia
4. Glucose intolerance

Level of Cognitive Ability: Analyzing
Client Needs: Health Promotion and Maintenance
Clinical Judgment/Cognitive Skills: Analyze Cues
Integrated Process: Clinical Judgment; Nursing Process/Analysis
Content Area: Health Assessment/Physical Exam: Heart and Peripheral Vascular
Health Problems: Adult Health: Cardiovascular: Coronary Artery Disease
Priority Concepts: Health Promotion; Perfusion

Answer: 2
Rationale: Hypertension, cigarette smoking, and hyperlipidemia are major risk modifiable factors for coronary artery disease. Glucose intolerance, obesity, and response to stress are also contributing factors. An age of more than 40 years is a nonmodifiable risk factor. A cholesterol level of 180 mg/dL (4.5 mmol/L) and a blood glucose level of 90 mg/dL (5.14 mmol/L) are within the reference range. The nurse places priority on major risk factors that need modification.
Test-Taking Strategy: Focus on the subject of risk factors for coronary artery disease, and note the strategic word, *priority.* Note that the only abnormal value is the BP.
Priority Nursing Tip: The goal of treatment for the client with coronary artery disease is to alter the atherosclerotic progression.
Reference: Ignatavicius, D., et al. (2021). *Medical-surgical nursing: Concepts for interprofessional collaborative care* (10th ed., pp. 699–701). Elsevier.

121. What would be the nurse's **priority** for the postprocedure care of a client with renal calculi who has just returned to the unit after a scheduled intravenous pyelogram (IVP)?
1. Maintaining the client on bed rest
2. Ambulating the client in the hallway
3. Encouraging the increased intake of oral fluids
4. Encouraging the client to try to void frequently

Level of Cognitive Ability: Analyzing
Client Needs: Physiological Integrity
Clinical Judgment/Cognitive Skills: Generate Solutions
Integrated Process: Clinical Judgment; Nursing Process/Analysis
Content Area: Foundations of Care: Diagnostic Tests
Health Problems: Adult Health: Renal and Urinary: Calculi
Priority Concepts: Clinical Judgment; Elimination

Answer: 3
Rationale: After IVP, the client needs to take in increased fluids to aid in the clearance of the dye used for the procedure. The client is usually allowed activity as tolerated, without any specific activity guidelines. It is unnecessary to void frequently after the procedure.
Test-Taking Strategy: Note the strategic word, *priority.* Option 4 has no useful purpose and is eliminated first. From the remaining choices, recall that there are no activity guidelines after this procedure. Recalling that fluids are necessary to promote the clearance of the dye from the client's system will direct you to the correct option.
Priority Nursing Tip: An informed consent is required for a diagnostic procedure that is invasive.
Reference: Lewis, S., et al. (2020). *Medical-surgical nursing: Assessment and management of clinical problems* (11th ed., p. 1019). Elsevier.

❖ **122.** A client diagnosed with myasthenia gravis is reporting vomiting, abdominal cramps, and diarrhea. The nurse notes that the client is hypotensive and experiencing facial muscle twitching. Which possible situation does this assessment data support?
1. Myasthenic crisis
2. Cholinergic crisis
3. Systemic infection
4. Reaction to plasmapheresis

Level of Cognitive Ability: Analyzing
Client Needs: Physiological Integrity
Clinical Judgment/Cognitive Skills: Analyze Cues
Integrated Process: Clinical Judgment; Nursing Process/Analysis
Content Area: Adult Health: Neurologic
Health Problems: Adult Health: Neurologic: Myasthenia Gravis
Priority Concepts: Clinical Judgment; Mobility

Answer: 2
Rationale: Signs and symptoms of cholinergic crisis include nausea, vomiting, abdominal cramping, diarrhea, blurred vision, pallor, facial muscle twitching, pupillary miosis, and hypotension. It is caused by overmedication with cholinergic (anticholinesterase) medications, and it is treated by withholding medications. Myasthenic crisis is an exacerbation of myasthenic symptoms caused by undermedication with anticholinesterase medications. There are no data in the question to support the remaining options.
Test-Taking Strategy: Focus on the subject of the client's diagnosis of myasthenia gravis, and the treatment for this disorder. Recalling the effects of cholinergic medications and focusing on the data in the question will direct you to the correct option.
Priority Nursing Tip: In myasthenia gravis, a cholinergic crisis is caused by overmedication with an anticholinesterase medication.
Reference: Lewis, S., et al. (2020). *Medical-surgical nursing: Assessment and management of clinical problems* (11th ed., pp. 1377–1378). Elsevier.

123. The nurse is assigned to care for a child diagnosed with juvenile idiopathic arthritis (JIA). What is the child's **priority** problem?
1. Acute pain
2. Potential difficulty with everyday tasks
3. Impaired mobility causing potential injury
4. Negative view of body because of activity intolerance

Level of Cognitive Ability: Analyzing
Client Needs: Physiological Integrity
Clinical Judgment/Cognitive Skills: Prioritize Hypotheses
Integrated Process: Clinical Judgment; Nursing Process/Analysis
Content Area: Pediatrics: Musculoskeletal
Health Problems: Pediatric-Specific: Juvenile Idiopathic Arthritis
Priority Concepts: Clinical Judgment; Pain

Answer: 1
Rationale: All of the problems identified in the options are appropriate for the child with JIA; however, acute pain must be managed before other problems can be addressed.
Test-Taking Strategy: Note the strategic word, *priority*. Use Maslow's Hierarchy of Needs theory, and remember that physiologic needs receive the highest priority. Option 2 identifies a potential problem rather than an actual problem. Option 3 addresses safety and security needs. Option 4 addresses body image.
Priority Nursing Tip: There are no definitive tests to diagnose JIA.
Reference: McKinney, E. S., et al. (2022). *Maternal child nursing* (6th ed., pp. 1246–1247). Elsevier.

124. A child is admitted to the hospital with a suspected diagnosis of idiopathic thrombocytopenic purpura (ITP), and diagnostic studies are performed. Which diagnostic result is indicative of this disorder?
1. An elevated platelet count
2. Elevated hemoglobin and hematocrit levels
3. Bone marrow aspirate showing increased megakaryocytes
4. Bone marrow aspirate indicating increased immature white blood cells

Level of Cognitive Ability: Analyzing
Client Needs: Physiological Integrity
Clinical Judgment/Cognitive Skills: Analyze Cues
Integrated Process: Clinical Judgment; Nursing Process/Analysis
Content Area: Pediatrics: Hematologic
Health Problems: Hematologic: Bleeding/Clotting Disorders
Priority Concepts: Clinical Judgment; Perfusion

Answer: 3
Rationale: The laboratory manifestations of ITP include the presence of a low platelet count of usually less than 20,000 mm³ (20 × 10⁹/L). Thrombocytopenia is the only laboratory abnormality expected with ITP. If there has been significant blood loss, there is evidence of anemia in the blood cell count. If a bone marrow examination is performed, the results with ITP show a normal or increased number of megakaryocytes, which are the precursors of platelets. Option 4 indicates the bone marrow result that would be found in a client with leukemia.
Test-Taking Strategy: Focus on the subject of ITP and associated diagnostic tests. Think about the pathophysiology of this diagnosis. Recalling that megakaryocytes are the precursors of platelets will assist with directing you to the correct option.
Priority Nursing Tip: For the client with ITP, platelet transfusions may be administered when platelet counts are less than 20,000 cells/mm³ (20 × 10⁹/L).
Reference: McKinney, E. S., et al. (2022). *Maternal child nursing* (6th ed., p. 1142). Elsevier.

125. The parent explains that after meals their infant has been vomiting, and now it is becoming more frequent and forceful. During the assessment, the nurse notes visible peristaltic waves moving from left to right across the infant's abdomen. On the basis of these findings, which condition would the nurse suspect?
1. Colic
2. Intussusception
3. Congenital megacolon
4. Hypertrophic pyloric stenosis

Level of Cognitive Ability: Analyzing
Client Needs: Physiological Integrity
Clinical Judgment/Cognitive Skills: Analyze Cues
Integrated Process: Clinical Judgment; Nursing Process/Analysis
Content Area: Pediatrics: Gastrointestinal
Health Problems: Pediatric-Specific: Developmental GI Defects
Priority Concepts: Clinical Judgment; Safety

Answer: 4
Rationale: In pyloric stenosis, the vomitus contains sour, undigested food but no bile, the infant is constipated, and visible peristaltic waves move from left to right across the abdomen. A movable, palpable, firm, olive-shaped mass in the right upper quadrant may be noted. Crying during the evening hours, appearing to be in pain, but eating well and gaining weight are clinical manifestations of colic. An infant who suddenly becomes pale, cries out, and draws the legs up to the chest is demonstrating physical signs of intussusception. Ribbon-like stool, bile-stained emesis, the absence of peristalsis, and abdominal distention are symptoms of congenital megacolon (Hirschsprung's disease).
Test-Taking Strategy: Focus on the subject of an infant who is vomiting after meals, and it is now becoming more frequent and forceful. Note all the infant's assessment data and the possible diagnoses. Consider each condition presented in the options, and think about the clinical manifestations of each. Recalling the manifestations associated with pyloric stenosis will direct you to the correct option. Also, recalling that stenosis means "narrowing" will direct you to the correct option.
Priority Nursing Tip: In pyloric stenosis, the nurse would monitor for signs of dehydration and electrolyte imbalances.
Reference: McKinney, E. S., et al. (2022). *Maternal child nursing* (6th ed., pp. 988–989). Elsevier.

❖ **126.** The nurse is reviewing the laboratory analysis of cerebrospinal fluid (CSF) obtained during a lumbar puncture from a child who is suspected of having bacterial meningitis. Which result would **most likely** confirm this diagnosis?
1. Clear CSF with low protein and low glucose
2. Cloudy CSF with low protein and low glucose
3. Cloudy CSF with high protein and low glucose
4. Decreased pressure and cloudy CSF with high protein

Level of Cognitive Ability: Analyzing
Client Needs: Physiological Integrity
Clinical Judgment/Cognitive Skills: Analyze Cues
Integrated Process: Clinical Judgment; Nursing Process/Analysis
Content Area: Pediatrics: Neurologic
Health Problems: Pediatric-Specific: Meningitis
Priority Concepts: Clinical Judgment; Infection

Answer: 3
Rationale: A diagnosis of meningitis is made by testing CSF obtained by lumbar puncture. In the case of bacterial meningitis, findings usually include increased pressure and cloudy CSF with high protein and low glucose. Therefore, options 1, 2, and 4 are incorrect.
Test-Taking Strategy: Focus on the subject of the laboratory analysis results of CSF associated with bacterial meningitis. Note the strategic words, *most likely*. Eliminate options 1 and 4 because clear CSF and decreased pressure are not likely to be found with an infectious process such as meningitis. From the remaining choices, recalling that high protein indicates a possible diagnosis of meningitis will direct you to the correct option.
Priority Nursing Tip: Pneumococcal conjugate vaccine is recommended for all children beginning at age 2 months to protect against meningitis.
Reference: McKinney, E. S., et al. (2022). *Maternal child nursing* (6th ed., pp. 1287–1289). Elsevier.

127. A child with profuse diarrhea is admitted to the pediatric unit with a diagnosis of acute gastroenteritis. The nurse monitors the child for signs of hypovolemic shock as a result of fluid and electrolyte losses that have occurred in the child. Which finding would indicate the presence of compensated shock?
1. Bradycardia
2. Hypotension
3. Profuse diarrhea
4. Capillary refill time greater than 3 seconds

Level of Cognitive Ability: Analyzing
Client Needs: Physiological Integrity
Clinical Judgment/Cognitive Skills: Analyze Cues
Integrated Process: Clinical Judgment; Nursing Process/Analysis
Content Area: Complex Care: Shock
Health Problems: Pediatric-Specific: Diarrhea
Priority Concepts: Infection; Perfusion

Answer: 4
Rationale: Shock may be classified as compensated or decompensated. In compensated shock, the child becomes tachycardic in an effort to increase the cardiac output. The blood pressure remains normal. The capillary refill time may be prolonged and more than 3 seconds, and the child may become irritable as a result of increasing hypoxia. The most prevalent cause of hypovolemic shock is fluid and electrolyte losses associated with gastroenteritis. Diarrhea is not a sign of shock; rather, it is a cause of the fluid and electrolyte imbalance.
Test-Taking Strategy: Focus on the subject of compensated shock. Recalling that hypotension is a late sign of shock and indicative of decompensation will assist to eliminate option 2. Recalling that tachycardia rather than bradycardia occurs in shock will assist you with eliminating option 1. From the remaining choices, focusing on the subject of signs of shock will direct you to the correct option.
Priority Nursing Tip: Rotavirus is a cause of serious gastroenteritis and is a nosocomial (hospital-acquired) pathogen that is most severe in children 3 to 24 months old. Children younger than 3 months have some protection because of maternally acquired antibodies.
Reference: McKinney, E. S., et al. (2022). *Maternal child nursing* (6th ed., pp. 766–767, 899). Elsevier.

❖ **128.** A parent whose child is generally alert and participates well in classroom activities is concerned that the teacher now reported that their child has frequent periods during the day when they appear to be staring off into space. The nurse would suspect that the child has which problem?

1. School phobia
2. Absence seizures
3. Behavioral problem
4. Attention-deficit/hyperactivity syndrome

Level of Cognitive Ability: Analyzing
Client Needs: Physiological Integrity
Clinical Judgment/Cognitive Skills: Analyze Cues
Integrated Process: Clinical Judgment; Nursing Process/Analysis
Content Area: Pediatrics: Neurologic
Health Problems: Pediatric-Specific: Seizures
Priority Concepts: Clinical Judgment; Intracranial Regulation

Answer: 2
Rationale: Absence seizures are a type of generalized seizure. They consist of a sudden, brief (usually 5 to 10 seconds) arrest of the child's motor activities accompanied by a blank stare and a loss of awareness. The child's posture is maintained at the end of the seizure, and the child returns to activity that was in process as though nothing has happened. School phobia includes physical symptoms that usually occur at home and that may prevent the child from attending school. Behavior problems would be noted by more overt symptoms than the ones described in this question. A child with attention-deficit/hyperactivity syndrome becomes easily distracted, is fidgety, and has difficulty following directions.
Test-Taking Strategy: Focus on the subject, the child appears to be daydreaming and staring off into space numerous times throughout the day, yet during the remainder of the day, the child is alert and participates in classroom activities. Note the possible diagnoses and the relationship of the information to determine the correct option.
Priority Nursing Tip: Instruct the parents of a child with a seizure disorder to note the time of onset, precipitating events, and behavior before and after the seizure, if one occurs.
Reference: McKinney, E. S., et al. (2022). *Maternal child nursing* (6th ed., p. 1307). Elsevier.

129. A 3-week-old infant is brought to the well-baby clinic for a phenylketonuria (PKU) screening test. The nurse reviews the results of the serum phenylalanine level. What interpretation would the nurse make?

LABORATORY RESULTS

Test and Result	Reference Range
Phenylalanine 1.0 mg/dL (60 mmol/L)	0.8 - 1.8 mg/dL (48 to 109 mmol/L)

1. Report the test as inconclusive.
2. Tell the parent that the test is normal.
3. Prepare to perform another test on client.
4. Notify the pediatrician that the test is moderately elevated.

Level of Cognitive Ability: Analyzing
Client Needs: Physiological Integrity
Clinical Judgment/Cognitive Skills: Analyze Cues
Integrated Process: Clinical Judgment; Nursing Process/Analysis
Content Area: Maternity: Newborn
Health Problems: Pediatric-Specific: Phenylketonuria
Priority Concepts: Clinical Judgment; Health Promotion

Answer: 1
Rationale: The reference range for PKU level is 0.8 to 1.8 mg/dL (48 to 109 mmol/L). With early postpartum discharge, screening is often performed when the infant is less than 2 days old because of the concern that the infant will be lost to follow-up. Infants need to be rescreened by the time that they are 14 days old if the initial screening was done when the infant was 24 to 48 hours old.
Test-Taking Strategy: Focus on the subject, interpretation of the phenylalanine level. Recalling that the reference range is 0.8 to 1.8 mg/dL (48 to 109 mmol/L) will direct you to option 1. Also note that the remaining options are comparable or alike and indicate an other-than-normal finding.
Priority Nursing Tip: All 50 states require routine screening of all newborns for phenylketonuria.
Reference: Hockenberry, M., Wilson, D., & Rodgers, C. (2019). *Wong's Nursing care of infants and children* (11th ed., pp. 63–64). Elsevier.

Nursing Process: Planning

❖ **130.** The nurse is caring for a client who is receiving total parenteral nutrition through a central venous catheter. Which action would the nurse plan to implement to decrease the risk of infection in this client?
1. Track the client's oral temperature.
2. Administer antibiotics intravenously.
3. Evaluate the differential of the leukocytes.
4. Use sterile technique for dressing changes.

Level of Cognitive Ability: Applying
Client Needs: Safe and Effective Care Environment
Clinical Judgment/Cognitive Skills: Generate Solutions
Integrated Process: Nursing Process/Planning
Content Area: Foundations of Care: Infection Control
Health Problems: Adult Health: Gastrointestinal: Nutrition/Malabsorption Problems
Priority Concepts: Infection; Nutrition

Answer: 4
Rationale: Sterile technique is vital during dressing changes of a central venous catheter (CVC). CVCs are large-bore catheters that can serve as a direct-entry point for microorganisms into the heart and circulatory system. Using aseptic technique helps avoid catheter-related infections by preventing the introduction of potential pathogens to the site. Although the remaining options are reasonable nursing interventions for a client with a CVC, none of them prevents infection. Options 1 and 3 are assessment methods, and option 2 is implemented after the confirmation of an existing infection.
Test-Taking Strategy: Focus on the subject of preventing infection. Note the relationship between "infection" in the question and "sterile" in the correct option. In addition, the only option that will prevent infection is the correct option.
Priority Nursing Tip: Use sterile technique when caring for a client receiving total parenteral nutrition (TPN). Because the TPN solution has a high concentration of glucose, it is a medium for bacterial growth.
Reference: Lewis, S., et al. (2020). *Medical-surgical nursing: Assessment and management of clinical problems* (11th ed., pp. 294, 865). Elsevier.

131. The nurse creates a plan of care for a client with a spica cast that covers a lower extremity. Which action would the nurse include in the plan of care to promote bowel elimination?
1. Use a bedside commode.
2. Ambulate to the bathroom.
3. Administer an enema daily.
4. Use a low-profile (fracture) bedpan.

Level of Cognitive Ability: Applying
Client Needs: Physiological Integrity
Clinical Judgment/Cognitive Skills: Generate Solutions
Integrated Process: Nursing Process/Planning
Content Area: Skills: Elimination
Health Problems: Adult Health: Musculoskeletal: Skeletal Injury
Priority Concepts: Elimination; Mobility

Answer: 4
Rationale: A client with a spica cast (body cast) that covers a lower extremity cannot bend at the hips to sit up. A low-profile bedpan or fracture pan is designed for use by clients with body or leg casts and for clients who have difficulty raising the hips to use a standard bedpan; therefore, using a commode or the bathroom is contraindicated. Daily enemas are not a part of routine care.
Test-Taking Strategy: Focus on the subject of spica cast care and the words *covers a lower extremity*. Therefore, choose the measure that promotes elimination for a client who cannot flex the hip.
Priority Nursing Tip: Inform the client and family about keeping the cast clean and dry. The material of a cast can crumble if it becomes wet. This presents a risk of altered skin integrity and subsequent infection.
Reference: Potter, P., et al. (2021). *Fundamentals of nursing* (10th ed., pp. 1210, 1213–1214). Elsevier.

❖ **132.** The nurse is caring for a postpartum client with thromboembolytic disease. Which intervention is **most important** to include when planning care to prevent the complication of pulmonary embolism?
1. Enforce bed rest.
2. Monitor the vital signs frequently.
3. Assess the breath sounds frequently.
4. Administer prescribed anticoagulant therapy.

Level of Cognitive Ability: Analyzing
Client Needs: Physiological Integrity
Clinical Judgment/Cognitive Skills: Generate Solutions
Integrated Process: Clinical Judgment; Nursing Process/Planning
Content Area: Maternity: Postpartum
Health Problems: Adult Health: Hematologic: Bleeding/Clotting Disorders
Priority Concepts: Clotting; Reproduction

Answer: 4
Rationale: The purposes of anticoagulant therapy for the treatment of thromboembolytic disease are to prevent the formation of a clot and to prevent a clot from moving to another area, thus preventing pulmonary embolism. Although the remaining options may be implemented for a client with thromboembolytic disease, the correct option will specifically assist in the prevention of pulmonary embolism.
Test-Taking Strategy: Note the strategic words, *most important.* Focus on the subject of preventing the complication of pulmonary embolism. Recall that anticoagulant therapy is prescribed to treat thromboembolytic disease.
Priority Nursing Tip: Medications containing aspirin would not be given to clients receiving anticoagulant therapy, because aspirin prolongs the clotting time and increases the risk of bleeding.
Reference: McKinney, E. S., et al. (2022). *Maternal child nursing* (6th ed., 613). Elsevier.

133. The physician prescribes an isotonic intravenous solution for a client. The nurse plans for the administration of which solution?
1. 10% dextrose in water
2. 3% sodium chloride
3. 5% dextrose in water
4. 0.45% sodium chloride

Level of Cognitive Ability: Applying
Client Needs: Physiological Integrity
Clinical Judgment/Cognitive Skills: Generate Solutions
Integrated Process: Clinical Judgment; Nursing Process/Planning
Content Area: Foundations of Care: Fluids and Electrolytes
Health Problems: N/A
Priority Concepts: Clinical Judgment; Fluids and Electrolytes

Answer: 3
Rationale: Five percent dextrose in water is an isotonic solution, which means that the osmolality of this solution matches normal body fluids. Other examples of isotonic fluids include 0.9% sodium chloride solution (normal saline) and lactated Ringer's solution. Ten percent dextrose in water and 3% sodium chloride solution are hypertonic solutions, and 0.45% sodium chloride solution is hypotonic.
Test-Taking Strategy: To answer this question accurately, focus on the subject of the tonicity of various intravenous solutions and note the word "isotonic." It is necessary to recall that 5% dextrose in water is an isotonic solution.
Priority Nursing Tip: Isotonic solutions are isotonic to human cells, and thus very little osmosis occurs.
Reference: Lewis, S., et al. (2020). *Medical-surgical nursing: Assessment and management of clinical problems* (11th ed., p. 291). Elsevier.

❖ **134.** The nurse is admitting a client who recently underwent a bilateral adrenalectomy. Which intervention is **essential** for the nurse to include in the client's plan of care?
1. Prevent social isolation.
2. Consider occupational therapy.
3. Discuss changes in body image.
4. Avoid stress-producing situations.

Level of Cognitive Ability: Applying
Client Needs: Physiological Integrity
Clinical Judgment/Cognitive Skills: Generate Solutions
Integrated Process: Clinical Judgment; Nursing Process/Planning
Content Area: Adult Health: Endocrine
Health Problems: Adult Health: Endocrine: Adrenal Disorders
Priority Concepts: Clinical Judgment; Stress

Answer: 4
Rationale: Adrenalectomy can lead to adrenal insufficiency. Adrenal hormones are essential to maintaining homeostasis in response to stressors. None of the remaining options are essential interventions specific to this client's problem.
Test-Taking Strategy: Note the strategic word, *essential.* This indicates the need to prioritize. Remember that, according to Maslow's Hierarchy of Needs theory, physiologic needs come first. The stress reaction involves physiologic processes.
Priority Nursing Tip: Assist a client to identify the source of stress and explore methods to reduce stress.
Reference: Ignatavicius, D., et al. (2021). *Medical-surgical nursing: Concepts for interprofessional collaborative care* (10th ed., pp. 1242, 1245). Elsevier.

135. A perinatal client is admitted to the obstetric unit during an exacerbation of a heart condition. When planning for the nutritional requirements, which dietary intervention would the nurse consult the dietitian about?
1. A low-calorie diet to prevent weight gain
2. A diet low in fluids and fiber to decrease blood volume
3. A diet adequate in fluids and fiber to decrease constipation
4. Unlimited sodium intake to increase circulating blood volume

Level of Cognitive Ability: Applying
Client Needs: Physiological Integrity
Clinical Judgment/Cognitive Skills: Generate Solutions
Integrated Process: Clinical Judgment; Nursing Process/Planning
Content Area: Maternity: Antepartum
Health Problems: Maternity: Cardiac Disease
Priority Concepts: Nutrition; Perfusion

Answer: 3
Rationale: Constipation can cause the client to use Valsalva's maneuver. This maneuver can cause blood to rush to the heart and overload the cardiac system. A low-calorie diet is not recommended during pregnancy. Diets low in fluid and fiber can cause a decrease in blood volume that can deprive the fetus of nutrients; it can also lead to constipation. Therefore, adequate fluid intake and high-fiber foods are important. Sodium needs to be restricted to some degree as prescribed by the physician because this will cause an overload to the circulating blood volume and contribute to cardiac complications.
Test-Taking Strategy: Focus on the subjects, the physiology of the cardiac system, the maternal and fetal needs, and the factors that increase the workload on the heart, to answer the question. Think about what would increase the workload of the heart to direct you to the correct option.
Priority Nursing Tip: Encourage adequate nutrition for the pregnant client with a cardiac condition to prevent anemia. Anemia could worsen the cardiac status.
Reference: McKinney, E. S., et al. (2022). *Maternal child nursing* (6th ed., p. 567). Elsevier.

❖ **136.** The nurse is creating a plan of care for a client with a history of renal calculi, who is prescribed bed rest. Which intervention would the nurse include in the plan to limit renal complications of prolonged immobility?
1. Maintain client in a supine position.
2. Provide a daily fluid intake of 1000 mL.
3. Limit the intake of milk and milk products.
4. Monitor for signs of a low serum calcium level.

Level of Cognitive Ability: Creating
Client Needs: Physiological Integrity
Clinical Judgment/Cognitive Skills: Generate Solutions
Integrated Process: Clinical Judgment; Nursing Process/Planning
Content Area: Skills: Activity/Mobility
Health Problems: Adult Health: Renal and Urinary: Calculi
Priority Concepts: Clinical Judgment; Mobility

Answer: 3
Rationale: The formation of renal and urinary calculi is a complication of immobility. Limiting milk and milk products is the best measure to prevent the formation of calcium stones. A supine position increases urinary stasis; therefore, this position would be limited or avoided. Daily fluid intake should be 2000 mL or more per day, unless contraindicated, but there are no data to indicate that an intake of 2000 mL or more is a contraindication. The nurse would monitor for signs and symptoms of hypercalcemia, such as nausea, vomiting, polydipsia, polyuria, and lethargy.
Test-Taking Strategy: Focus on the subject of the complications of prolonged immobility. Eliminate option 1, which refers to maintaining an immobile client in one position. Eliminate option 2 by noting the amount of fluid suggested. From the remaining choices, recalling the effect of the movement of calcium into the blood from the bones will direct you to the correct option.
Priority Nursing Tip: The client with calcium oxalate stones may be prescribed to follow a diet decreasing the intake of foods high in calcium and avoiding oxalate food sources. This type of diet will help reduce the urinary oxalate content of urine and stone formation. Oxalate food sources include items such as tea, almonds, cashews, chocolate, cocoa, beans, spinach, and rhubarb.
Reference: Ignatavicius, D., et al. (2021). *Medical-surgical nursing: Concepts for interprofessional collaborative care* (10th ed., p. 1345). Elsevier.

137. The nurse determines that a tuberculin skin test is positive. Which diagnostic test would the nurse anticipate will be prescribed to confirm a diagnosis of tuberculosis (TB)?
1. Chest x-ray
2. Sputum culture
3. Complete blood cell count
4. Computed tomography scan of the chest

Level of Cognitive Ability: Applying
Client Needs: Physiological Integrity
Clinical Judgment/Cognitive Skills: Generate Solutions
Integrated Process: Clinical Judgment; Nursing Process/Planning
Content Area: Adult Health: Respiratory
Health Problems: Adult Health: Respiratory: Tuberculosis
Priority Concepts: Clinical Judgment; Infection

Answer: 2
Rationale: Although the findings of the chest x-ray examination are important, it is not possible to make a diagnosis of TB solely on the basis of this examination because other diseases can mimic the appearance of TB. The demonstration of tubercle bacilli bacteriologically is essential for establishing a diagnosis. The microscopic examination of sputum for acid-fast bacilli is usually the first bacteriologic evidence of the presence of tubercle bacilli. Options 3 and 4 will not diagnose TB.
Test-Taking Strategy: Focus on the subject of diagnosing TB. Recalling that the presence of tubercle bacilli indicates TB will direct you to the correct option.
Priority Nursing Tip: Tuberculosis has an insidious onset, and many clients are not aware that the symptoms are associated to TB until the disease is well advanced.
Reference: Ignatavicius, D., et al. (2021). *Medical-surgical nursing: Concepts for interprofessional collaborative care* (10th ed., p.578). Elsevier.

❖ **138.** The home care nurse is creating a plan of care for a client diagnosed with Meniere's disease. Which nursing intervention would the nurse include to assist the client with controlling vertigo?
1. Instruct the client to cut down on cigarette smoking.
2. Encourage the client to increase the daily fluid intake.
3. Encourage the client to avoid sudden head movements.
4. Instruct the client to increase the amount of sodium in the diet.

Level of Cognitive Ability: Creating
Client Needs: Physiological Integrity
Clinical Judgment/Cognitive Skills: Generate Solutions
Integrated Process: Clinical Judgment; Nursing Process/Planning
Content Area: Adult Health: Ear
Health Problems: Adult Health: Ear: Meniere's Disease
Priority Concepts: Patient Education; Sensory Perception

Answer: 3
Rationale: Meniere's disease refers to dilation of the endolymphatic system by overproduction or decreased resorption of endolymphatic fluid. The nurse instructs the client to make slow head movements to prevent worsening of the vertigo. Clients are advised to stop smoking because of its vasoconstrictive effects. Dietary changes such as salt and fluid restrictions that reduce the amount of endolymphatic fluid are sometimes prescribed.
Test-Taking Strategy: Identify the subject of the question, controlling vertigo. Note the relationship between the words *vertigo* and the correct option, which recommends the avoidance of sudden head movements. Noting the words *cut down* in option 1 will assist you with eliminating this option. Recalling that salt and fluid restrictions are sometimes prescribed will also assist you with eliminating options.
Priority Nursing Tip: Instruct the client experiencing an episode of vertigo to avoid watching television because flickering of lights may exacerbate symptoms.
Reference: Ignatavicius, D., et al. (2021). *Medical-surgical nursing: Concepts for interprofessional collaborative care* (10th ed., p. 968). Elsevier.

139. A client is admitted to a mental health unit with a diagnosis of anorexia nervosa. When planning care for this client, which **primary** intervention would health promotion focus on?
1. Providing a supportive environment
2. Examining intrapsychic conflicts and past issues
3. Emphasizing social interaction with clients who are withdrawn
4. Helping the client identify and examine dysfunctional thoughts and beliefs

Level of Cognitive Ability: Applying
Client Needs: Psychosocial Integrity
Clinical Judgment/Cognitive Skills: Prioritize Hypotheses
Integrated Process: Clinical Judgment; Nursing Process/Planning
Content Area: Mental Health
Health Problems: Mental Health: Eating Disorders
Priority Concepts: Clinical Judgment; Nutrition

Answer: 4
Rationale: Health promotion focuses on helping clients identify and examine dysfunctional thoughts, as well as identifying and examining the values and beliefs that maintain these thoughts. Providing a supportive environment is important, but it is not as primary as option 4 for this client. Examining intrapsychic conflicts and past issues is not directly related to the client's problem. Emphasizing social interaction is not appropriate at this time.
Test-Taking Strategy: Note the strategic word, *primary*. Focus on the subject of health promotion in a client diagnosed with anorexia nervosa. The correct option is the only choice that is specifically client centered. This option also focuses on assessment, which is the first step of the nursing process.
Priority Nursing Tip: Explain treatments and procedures to a client in a quiet and simple manner. Always allow the client the opportunity to express fears.
Reference: Varcarolis, E., & Fosbre, C. (2021). *Essentials of psychiatric mental health nursing: A communication approach to evidence-based care* (4th ed., p. 186). Elsevier.

❖ **140.** The nurse is preparing discharge plans for a hospitalized client who attempted suicide. Which intervention would the nurse include in the plan as an **immediate** resource?
1. Scheduling weekly follow-up appointments
2. Establishing a contact with a specific crisis resource person
3. Encouraging family and friends to be with the client at all times
4. Providing phone numbers for the physician and psychiatrist

Level of Cognitive Ability: Applying
Client Needs: Psychosocial Integrity
Clinical Judgment/Cognitive Skills: Generate Solutions
Integrated Process: Clinical Judgment; Nursing Process/Planning
Content Area: Mental Health
Health Problems: Mental Health: Suicide
Priority Concepts: Mood and Affect; Safety

Answer: 2
Rationale: Crisis times may occur between appointments. Establishing a specific contact with a crisis resource person provides the client with a direct connection for communication and immediate crisis intervention. Providing phone numbers will not ensure available and immediate crisis intervention. Family and friends cannot always be present.
Test-Taking Strategy: Focus on the subject, the availability of immediate resources for the client who attempted suicide, and the strategic word, *immediate.* Eliminate option 3 first because this is unrealistic. Next, eliminate options 1 and 4 because these will not necessarily provide immediate resources.
Priority Nursing Tip: Discharge planning and follow-up care are important for the continued well-being of the client with a mental health disorder. Aftercare case managers are used to facilitate the client's adaptation back into the community and provide early referral if the treatment plan is unsuccessful.
Reference: Varcarolis, E., & Fosbre, C. (2021). *Essentials of psychiatric mental health nursing: A communication approach to evidence-based care* (4th ed., p. 373). Elsevier.

141. The nurse is creating a plan of care for a newborn diagnosed with bilateral club feet. Which information would the nurse plan to include in the parent's education?
1. The regimen of manipulation and casting is effective in all cases of bilateral club feet.
2. Genetic testing is wise for future pregnancies because other children born to this couple may also be affected.
3. If casting is needed, it will begin at birth and continue for 12 weeks, at which time the condition will be reevaluated.
4. Surgery performed immediately after birth has been found to be the most effective for achieving a complete recovery.

Level of Cognitive Ability: Creating
Client Needs: Physiological Integrity
Clinical Judgment/Cognitive Skills: Generate Solutions
Integrated Process: Clinical Judgment; Nursing Process/Planning
Content Area: Pediatrics: Musculoskeletal
Health Problems: Pediatric-Specific: Clubfoot
Priority Concepts: Patient Education; Mobility

Answer: 3
Rationale: For the infant with clubfoot, casting would begin at birth and continue for at least 12 weeks or until maximum correction is achieved. At this time, corrective shoes may provide support to maintain alignment, or surgery can be performed. Surgery is usually delayed until the child is 4 to 12 months old. Options 1 and 4 are inaccurate. Option 2 does not specifically address the subject of the question.
Test-Taking Strategy: Focus on the subject, parent instructions for the child with bilateral club feet. Eliminate option 1 because of the closed-ended word "all." Eliminate option 2 because it does not specifically address the subject of the question, and relates to the future. Eliminate option 4 because of the word *immediately.*
Priority Nursing Tip: The nurse needs to monitor the child with a cast or brace for signs of neurovascular impairment. If signs occur, the physician is notified immediately.
Reference: McKinney, E. S., et al. (2022). *Maternal child nursing* (6th ed., p. 1243). Elsevier.

❖ **142.** Which items would the nurse plan to provide to optimally maintain the integrity of a set of arterial blood gas measurements?
1. A syringe that contains a preservative
2. A heparinized syringe and a bag of ice
3. A heparinized syringe and a preservative
4. A syringe that contains a preservative and a bag of ice

Level of Cognitive Ability: Applying
Client Needs: Physiological Integrity
Clinical Judgment/Cognitive Skills: Generate Solutions
Integrated Process: Nursing Process/Planning
Content Area: Foundations of Care: Acid–Base
Health Problems: N/A
Priority Concepts: Clinical Judgment; Acid–Base Balance

Answer: 2
Rationale: The arterial blood gas sample is obtained using a heparinized syringe. The sample of blood is placed on ice and sent to the laboratory immediately. A preservative is not used.
Test-Taking Strategy: Focus on the subject of arterial blood gas measurements; specific knowledge regarding this procedure is needed to answer this question. Remember that an arterial blood gas sample is obtained using a heparinized syringe, is placed on ice, and is sent to the laboratory immediately.
Priority Nursing Tip: Assist with the specimen draw for an arterial blood gas by preparing a heparinized syringe (if one is not already pre-packaged); otherwise, the blood may clot.
References: Lewis, S., et al. (2020). *Medical-surgical nursing: Assessment and management of clinical problems* (11th ed., p. 470). Elsevier; Pagana, K., Pagana, T., & Pagana, T. N. (2021). *Mosby's Diagnostic and laboratory test reference* (15th ed., p. 109). Elsevier.

143. A client is experiencing diabetes insipidus as a result of cranial surgery. Which anticipated therapy would the nurse plan to implement?
1. Fluid restriction
2. Administering diuretics
3. Increased sodium intake
4. Intravenous (IV) replacement of fluid losses

Level of Cognitive Ability: Analyzing
Client Needs: Physiological Integrity
Clinical Judgment/Cognitive Skills: Generate Solutions
Integrated Process: Clinical Judgment; Nursing Process/Planning
Content Area: Adult Health: Neurologic
Health Problems: Adult Health: Endocrine: Pituitary Disorders
Priority Concepts: Clinical Judgment; Fluids and Electrolytes

Answer: 4
Rationale: The client with diabetes insipidus excretes large amounts of extremely dilute urine. This usually occurs as a result of decreased synthesis or the release of antidiuretic hormone in clients with conditions such as head injury, surgery near the hypothalamus, or increased intracranial pressure. Corrective measures include allowing ample oral fluid intake, administering IV fluid as needed to replace sensible and insensible losses, and administering vasopressin. Diuretics are not administered. Sodium is not administered because the serum sodium level is usually high, as is the serum osmolality.
Test-Taking Strategy: Focus on the subject, diabetes insipidus as a result of cranial surgery, and recall that a large fluid loss is the problem in this client. This will assist you with eliminating options 1 and 2. From the remaining choices, recalling that the serum sodium level is already elevated in clients with this disorder or knowing that fluid replacement is the most direct form of therapy for fluid loss will direct you to the correct option.
Priority Nursing Tip: For the client with diabetes insipidus, monitor electrolyte values and monitor for signs of dehydration, and maintain an adequate intake of fluids.
Reference: Ignatavicius, D., et al. (2021). *Medical-surgical nursing: Concepts for interprofessional collaborative care* (10th ed., pp. 1235–1236). Elsevier.

❖ **144.** The nurse is caring for a client diagnosed with dementia. Which nutritional goal would the nurse plan for with this client?
1. Client will be free of hallucinations.
2. Client will feed self with cueing within 24 hours.
3. Client will be able to prepare simple foods by discharge.
4. Client will identify favorite foods by the time of discharge.

Level of Cognitive Ability: Applying
Client Needs: Physiological Integrity
Clinical Judgment/Cognitive Skills: Generate Solutions
Integrated Process: Nursing Process/Planning
Content Area: Mental Health
Health Problems: Mental Health: Neurocognitive Impairment
Priority Concepts: Cognition; Nutrition

Answer: 2
Rationale: The correct option identifies a goal that is directly related to the client's ability to care for self. None of the remaining options are related to the client's self-care needs.
Test-Taking Strategy: Focus on the **subject**, needs of a client with dementia. The correct option is the only option that addresses a physiologic need. In addition, on the basis of **Maslow's Hierarchy of Needs theory**, physiologic needs take precedence. This will direct you to the correct option.
Priority Nursing Tip: In dementia, long-term and short-term memory loss occurs, with impairment in judgment, abstract thinking, problem-solving, and behavior.
Reference: Varcarolis, E., & Fosbre, C. (2021). *Essentials of psychiatric mental health nursing: A communication approach to evidence-based care* (4th ed., pp. 290, 295). Elsevier.

145. The nurse is preparing to care for an infant diagnosed with pertussis. Which **priority** problem would the nurse address when planning care?
1. Infection
2. Fluid overload
3. Impaired sleep patterns
4. Inability to expectorate secretions

Level of Cognitive Ability: Analyzing
Client Needs: Physiological Integrity
Clinical Judgment/Cognitive Skills: Prioritize Hypotheses
Integrated Process: Clinical Judgment; Nursing Process/Planning
Content Area: Pediatrics: Throat/Respiratory
Health Problems: Pediatric-Specific: Communicable Diseases
Priority Concepts: Clinical Judgment; Gas Exchange

Answer: 4
Rationale: The priority problem for the child with pertussis relates to adequate air exchange. Because of the copious, thick secretions that occur with pertussis and the small airways of an infant, air exchange is critical. Infection is an important consideration, but airway is the priority. A deficient fluid volume is more likely to occur in this infant because of the thick secretions and vomiting. Sleep patterns may be disturbed because of the coughing, but this is not the critical issue.
Test-Taking Strategy: Use the ABCs—airway, breathing, and circulation—and note the strategic word, *priority.* Airway is always the priority. This will direct you to the correct option.
Priority Nursing Tip: For the client with a respiratory problem, reduce environmental factors that cause coughing spasms, such as dust, smoke, and sudden changes in temperature.
Reference: McKinney, E. S., et al. (2022). *Maternal child nursing* (6th ed., pp. 921–922). Elsevier.

❖ **146.** The nurse is planning care for an infant who has a diagnosis of hypertrophic pyloric stenosis and is scheduled for surgery. Which intervention would the nurse include to meet the infant's preoperative needs?
1. Administer enemas until returns are clear.
2. Provide the parent privacy to breast-feed/chest-feed every 2 hours.
3. Monitor the intravenous (IV) infusion, intake, output, and weight.
4. Provide small, frequent feedings of glucose, water, and electrolytes.

Level of Cognitive Ability: Analyzing
Client Needs: Physiological Integrity
Clinical Judgment/Cognitive Skills: Generate Solutions
Integrated Process: Clinical Judgment; Nursing Process/Planning
Content Area: Pediatrics: Gastrointestinal
Health Problems: Pediatric-Specific: Developmental GI Defects
Priority Concepts: Clinical Judgment; Safety

Answer: 3
Rationale: Preoperatively, important nursing responsibilities for the child with hypertrophic pyloric stenosis include monitoring the IV infusion, intake, output, and weight and obtaining urine specific gravity measurements. Additionally, weighing the infant's diapers provides information regarding output. Enemas until clear would further compromise the fluid volume status. Preoperatively, the infant receives nothing by mouth unless otherwise prescribed by the physician.
Test-Taking Strategy: Focus on the subject of preoperative care of a child with pyloric stenosis. Eliminate options 2 and 4 based on the fact that the infant needs to receive nothing by mouth during the preoperative period. Eliminate option 1 knowing that enemas would further compromise the fluid balance status.
Priority Nursing Tip: When preparing the infant with hypertrophic pyloric stenosis for surgery, monitor intake and output, the number and character of stools, and patency of the nasogastric tube used for stomach decompression.
Reference: McKinney, E. S., et al. (2022). *Maternal child nursing* (6th ed., pp. 989–990). Elsevier.

147. A client who was a victim of a gunshot incident states, "I feel like I am losing my mind. I keep hearing the gunshots and seeing my friend lying on the ground." Which strategy would the nurse include when **initially** formulating a therapeutic relationship?
1. Teaching the client, a variety of relaxation techniques
2. Asking the psychiatrist to prescribe appropriate medication
3. Encouraging the client to talk about the incident and feelings related to it
4. Encouraging the client to think about just how lucky they are to still be alive

Level of Cognitive Ability: Analyzing
Client Needs: Psychosocial Integrity
Clinical Judgment/Cognitive Skills: Generate Solutions
Integrated Process: Clinical Judgment; Nursing Process/Planning
Content Area: Mental Health
Health Problems: Mental Health: Post-Traumatic Stress Disorder
Priority Concepts: Clinical Judgment; Communication

Answer: 3
Rationale: When developing a therapeutic relationship, the nurse must acknowledge and validate the client's feelings. Although teaching the client relaxation techniques may be helpful at some point, it is not related to the subject of the question. Options 2 and 4 are nontherapeutic techniques, and they do not promote a therapeutic relationship.
Test-Taking Strategy: Focus on the subject, initiating a therapeutic relationship with a gunshot victim, and note the strategic word, *initially*. Eliminate options that do not encourage further discussion about the client's feelings. Teaching the client how to relax may be helpful at some point, but not at the beginning of the therapeutic relationship. Remember to address the client's feelings.
Priority Nursing Tip: The nurse would always encourage the client to express thoughts and feelings as they address identified areas of concern.
Reference: Varcarolis, E., & Fosbre, C. (2021). *Essentials of psychiatric mental health nursing: A communication approach to evidence-based care* (4th ed., pp. 93–95, 382.). Elsevier.

❖ **148.** The nurse is caring for a hospitalized child with a diagnosis of rheumatic fever who has developed carditis. The parent asks the nurse to explain the meaning of carditis. On which description of this complication of rheumatic fever would the nurse plan to base a response?
1. Involuntary movements affecting the legs, arms, and face
2. Inflammation of all parts of the heart, primarily the mitral valve
3. Tender, painful joints, especially in the elbows, knees, ankles, and wrists
4. Red skin lesions that start as flat or slightly raised macules, usually over the trunk, and that spread peripherally

Level of Cognitive Ability: Applying
Client Needs: Physiological Integrity
Clinical Judgment/Cognitive Skills: Generate Solutions
Integrated Process: Clinical Judgment; Nursing Process/Planning
Content Area: Pediatrics: Cardiovascular
Health Problems: Pediatric-Specific: Rheumatic Fever
Priority Concepts: Patient Education; Inflammation

Answer: 2
Rationale: Carditis is the inflammation of all parts of the heart, primarily the mitral valve, and it is a complication of rheumatic fever. Option 1 describes chorea. Option 3 describes polyarthritis. Option 4 describes erythema marginatum.
Test-Taking Strategy: Focus on the *subject* of the complications of rheumatic fever-induced carditis. Note the relationship between the word *carditis* in the question and *heart* in the correct option.
Priority Nursing Tip: Initiate seizure precautions if a child with rheumatic fever is experiencing chorea.
Reference: McKinney, E. S., et al. (2022). *Maternal child nursing* (6th ed., p. 1116). Elsevier.

149. The nurse preparing to admit a 7-month-old infant with febrile seizures would anticipate the need for which equipment when planning care for this infant?
1. Restraints at the bedside
2. A code cart at the bedside
3. Suction equipment and an airway at the bedside
4. A padded tongue blade taped to the head of the bed

Level of Cognitive Ability: Applying
Client Needs: Physiological Integrity
Clinical Judgment/Cognitive Skills: Generate Solutions
Integrated Process: Clinical Judgment; Nursing Process/Planning
Content Area: Pediatrics: Neurologic
Health Problems: Pediatric-Specific: Seizures
Priority Concepts: Intracranial Regulation; Safety

Answer: 3
Rationale: Suctioning may be required during a seizure to remove secretions that obstruct the airway. An airway would also be readily available for use after the seizure subsides if needed. During a seizure, the infant needs to be placed in a side-lying position but would not be restrained. It is not necessary to place a code cart at the bedside, but a cart needs to be readily available on the nursing unit. A padded tongue blade would never be used; in fact, nothing would ever be placed in the mouth during a seizure.
Test-Taking Strategy: Use the ABCs—airway, breathing, and circulation—to answer the question. Option 3 is the only choice that specifically relates to the airway.
Priority Nursing Tip: If a child experiences a seizure, lower the child to the floor and protect the child's head from injury.
Reference: McKinney, E. S., et al. (2022). *Maternal child nursing* (6th ed., p. 1309). Elsevier.

❖ **150.** A 10-month-old infant is hospitalized for respiratory syncytial virus (RSV). On the basis of the developmental stage of the infant, what intervention would the nurse include in the plan of care?

1. Restrain the infant with a total body restraint to prevent any tubes from being dislodged.
2. Follow the home feeding schedule, and allow the infant to be held only when the parents visit.
3. Wash hands, wear a mask when caring for the infant, and keep the infant as quiet as possible.
4. Provide a consistent routine, and touch, rock, and cuddle the infant throughout the hospitalization.

Level of Cognitive Ability: Applying
Client Needs: Physiological Integrity
Clinical Judgment/Cognitive Skills: Generate Solutions
Integrated Process: Clinical Judgment; Nursing Process/Planning
Content Area: Developmental Stages: Infant
Health Problems: Pediatric-Specific: Bronchitis/Bronchiolitis/Respiratory Syncytial Virus
Priority Concepts: Development; Health Promotion

Answer: 4
Rationale: A 10-month-old infant is in the trust versus mistrust stage of psychosocial development, according to Erik Erikson, and the sensorimotor period of cognitive development, according to Jean Piaget. Hospitalization may have an adverse effect. A consistent routine accompanied by touching, rocking, and cuddling will help the child develop trust and provide sensory stimulation. Total body restraint is unnecessary and an incorrect action. Touching and holding the infant only when the parents visit will not provide adequate stimulation and interpersonal contact for the infant. RSV is not airborne (a mask is not required, unless mandated by institution protocol), and it is usually transmitted by the hands.
Test-Taking Strategy: Focus on the subject, a 10-month-old infant who is hospitalized with RSV and appropriate interventions based on the child's developmental state. Note the age and diagnosis of the infant to answer correctly. Also, eliminate options 1 and 2 because of the closed-ended words *total* and *only*, respectively.
Priority Nursing Tip: According to Erikson's theory of psychosocial development, each psychosocial crisis must be resolved for the child or adult to progress emotionally. Unsuccessful resolution can leave the person emotionally disabled.
Reference: McKinney, E. S., et al. (2022). *Maternal child nursing* (6th ed., pp. 67, 1056). Elsevier.

151. A child with a diagnosis of Reye's syndrome is being admitted to the hospital. The nurse creates a plan of care for the child that includes which **priority** nursing action?

1. Monitoring for hearing loss
2. Monitoring intake and output (I&O)
3. Repositioning the child every 2 hours
4. Providing a quiet environment with dimmed lighting

Level of Cognitive Ability: Creating
Client Needs: Physiological Integrity
Clinical Judgment/Cognitive Skills: Prioritize Hypotheses
Integrated Process: Clinical Judgment; Nursing Process/Planning
Content Area: Pediatrics: Neurologic
Health Problems: Pediatric-Specific: Reye's Syndrome
Priority Concepts: Intracranial Regulation; Safety

Answer: 4
Rationale: Cerebral edema is a progressive part of the disease process of Reye's syndrome. A priority component of care for a child with Reye's syndrome is maintaining effective cerebral perfusion and controlling intracranial pressure. Decreasing stimuli in the environment would decrease the stress on the cerebral tissue, as well as neuron responses. Hearing loss does not occur in clients with this disorder. Although monitoring I&O may be a component of the plan, it is not the priority nursing action. Changing the body position every 2 hours would not affect the cerebral edema and intracranial pressure directly. The child needs to be in a head-elevated position to decrease the progression of cerebral edema and promote the drainage of cerebrospinal fluid.
Test-Taking Strategy: Note the strategic word, *priority*. Recalling that increased intracranial pressure is a concern for the child with Reye's syndrome will direct you to the correct option.
Priority Nursing Tip: The nurse needs to assess the neurologic status of a child with Reye's syndrome. Signs of neurologic deterioration need to be reported immediately.
Reference: McKinney, E. S., et al. (2022). *Maternal child nursing* (6th ed., pp. 917, 1290). Elsevier.

❖ **152.** A nursing student is preparing to conduct a clinical conference regarding cerebral palsy. Which characteristic related to this disorder would the student plan to include in the discussion?
1. Cerebral palsy is an infectious disease of the central nervous system.
2. Cerebral palsy is an inflammation of the brain as a result of a viral illness.
3. Cerebral palsy is a chronic disability characterized by difficulty with muscle control.
4. Cerebral palsy is a congenital condition that results in moderate to severe retardation.

Level of Cognitive Ability: Applying
Client Needs: Physiological Integrity
Clinical Judgment/Cognitive Skills: Generate Solutions
Integrated Process: Nursing Process/Planning
Content Area: Pediatrics: Musculoskeletal
Health Problems: Pediatric-Specific: Cerebral Palsy
Priority Concepts: Functional Ability; Mobility

Answer: 3
Rationale: Cerebral palsy is a chronic disability that is characterized by difficulty with controlling the muscles because of an abnormality in the extrapyramidal or pyramidal motor system. Meningitis is an infectious process of the central nervous system. Encephalitis is an inflammation of the brain that occurs as a result of viral illness or central nervous system infections. Down syndrome is an example of a congenital condition that results in moderate to severe retardation.
Test-Taking Strategy: Eliminate options 1 and 2 that are comparable or alike and focus on cause of the disorder. Next, note the relationship between "palsy" in the question and "muscle" in the correct option.
Priority Nursing Tip: Provide the parents of a child with cerebral palsy with information about the disorder, treatment plan, and support services, including support groups.
Reference: McKinney, E. S., et al. (2022). *Maternal child nursing* (6th ed., pp. 1297–1299). Elsevier.

153. A nursing student is asked to conduct a clinical conference about autism. Which characteristic associated with autism would the student plan to include?
1. Normal social play that ceases by age 5
2. Lack of social interaction and awareness
3. The consistent imitation of others' actions
4. Normal verbal but abnormal nonverbal communication

Level of Cognitive Ability: Applying
Client Needs: Psychosocial Integrity
Clinical Judgment/Cognitive Skills: Generate Solutions
Integrated Process: Nursing Process/Planning
Content Area: Pediatrics: Neurologic
Health Problems: Pediatric-Specific: Autism Spectrum Disorders
Priority Concepts: Functional Ability; Mood and Affect

Answer: 2
Rationale: Autism is a severe developmental disorder that begins in infancy or toddlerhood. A primary characteristic is a lack of social interaction and awareness. Social behaviors in children with autism include a lack of or abnormal imitations of others' actions and a lack of or abnormal social play. Additional characteristics include a lack of or impaired verbal communication and marked abnormal nonverbal communication.
Test-Taking Strategy: Focus on the subject, characteristics of autism. It is necessary to recall that the primary characteristic is a lack of social interaction and awareness.
Priority Nursing Tip: For the child with autism, determine the child's routines, habits, and preferences and maintain consistency as much as possible. Provide support to parents.
Reference: McKinney, E. S., et al. (2022). *Maternal child nursing* (6th ed., pp. 1360–1362). Elsevier.

❖ **154.** Which interventions are appropriate to include in the plan of care for a child after a tonsillectomy? **Select all that apply.**
- ❑ **1.** Offer clear, cool liquids when awake.
- ❑ **2.** Administer pain medication as prescribed.
- ❑ **3.** Monitor for bleeding from the surgical site.
- ❑ **4.** Suction every 15 minutes and PRN as necessary.
- ❑ **5.** Initially eliminate milk or milk products from the diet.

Level of Cognitive Ability: Applying
Client Needs: Physiological Integrity
Clinical Judgment/Cognitive Skills: Generate Solutions
Integrated Process: Clinical Judgment; Nursing Process/Planning
Content Area: Pediatrics: Throat/Respiratory
Health Problems: Pediatric-Specific: Tonsillitis and Adenoiditis
Priority Concepts: Clinical Judgment; Safety

Answer: 1, 2, 3, 5
Rationale: After tonsillectomy, clear, cool liquids are encouraged. Options 2 and 3 are important interventions after any type of surgery. Suction equipment needs to be available, but suctioning is not performed unless there is an airway obstruction. Milk and milk products are avoided initially because they coat the throat; this causes the child to clear the throat, thereby increasing the risk of bleeding.
Test-Taking Strategy: Focus on the subject of post-tonsillectomy interventions. Think about the location and complications of this procedure to answer correctly.
Priority Nursing Tip: After tonsillectomy, suction equipment needs to be available, but suctioning is not done unless there is airway obstruction because it will disrupt the integrity of the surgical site and cause bleeding.
Reference: McKinney, E. S., et al. (2022). *Maternal child nursing* (6th ed., pp. 1047–1048). Elsevier.

155. The school nurse is preparing to perform health screening for scoliosis on children aged 9 through 14. Which instruction would the nurse plan to provide to each child?
1. Lie flat and lift the legs straight up.
2. Lie on the right side and then roll to the left side while the arms are held overhead.
3. Walk 10 feet forward and then 10 feet backward with the arms held overhead at both sides.
4. Stand with weight equally on both feet with the legs straight, and the arms hanging loosely at both sides.

Level of Cognitive Ability: Applying
Client Needs: Health Promotion and Maintenance
Clinical Judgment/Cognitive Skills: Generate Solutions
Integrated Process: Clinical Judgment; Nursing Process/Planning
Content Area: Health Assessment/Physical Exam: Musculoskeletal
Health Problems: Pediatric-Specific: Scoliosis
Priority Concepts: Health Promotion; Mobility

Answer: 4
Rationale: To perform this screening test, the child would be asked to disrobe or wear underpants only so that the chest, back, and hips can be clearly seen. The child is asked to stand with weight equally on both feet with the legs straight and the arms hanging loosely at both sides. The nurse assesses the child's posture, spinal column, shoulder height, and leg lengths. Lying down positions and walking forward and backward are incorrect assessment techniques.
Test-Taking Strategy: Focus on the subject, plan of care for scoliosis screening procedure. Recall the anatomic location of this disorder and then visualize the screening procedure and the preparation required to adequately assess for this disorder.
Priority Nursing Tip: A complication after surgical treatment of scoliosis is superior mesenteric artery syndrome. This disorder is caused by mechanical changes in the position of the child's abdominal contents that occurs during surgery.
Reference: McKinney, E. S., et al. (2022). *Maternal child nursing* (6th ed., pp. 1231–1232). Elsevier.

❖ **156.** The nurse is creating a plan of care for a child diagnosed with leukemia who is beginning chemotherapy. Which intervention would the nurse include?
  1. Monitor rectal temperatures every 4 hours.
  2. Monitor the mouth and perianal area each shift for signs of breakdown.
  3. Encourage the child to consume fresh fruits and vegetables to maintain nutritional status.
  4. Provide meticulous mouth care several times daily using an alcohol-based mouthwash and a toothbrush.

Level of Cognitive Ability: Creating
Client Needs: Physiological Integrity
Clinical Judgment/Cognitive Skills: Generate Solutions
Integrated Process: Clinical Judgment; Nursing Process/Planning
Content Area: Pediatrics: Oncologic
Health Problems: Pediatric-Specific: Cancers
Priority Concepts: Cellular Regulation; Infection

Answer: 2
Rationale: When the child is receiving chemotherapy, the nurse would assess the mouth and perianal area each shift for ulcers, erythema, or breakdown. The nurse needs to avoid taking rectal temperatures. Oral temperatures are also avoided if mouth ulcers are present. Axillary or temporal temperatures would be taken to prevent alterations in skin integrity. Bland, nonirritating foods and liquids would be provided to the child. Fresh fruits and vegetables need to be avoided because they can harbor organisms. Chemotherapy can cause neutropenia, and the child would be maintained on a low-bacteria diet if the white blood cell count is low. Meticulous mouth care needs to be performed, but the nurse would avoid alcohol-based mouthwashes and should use a soft-bristled toothbrush.
Test-Taking Strategy: Focus on the subject, interventions for the child receiving chemotherapy. Think about the adverse effects that can occur with chemotherapy to assist in answering correctly. Remember that life-threatening neutropenia and thrombocytopenia can occur.
Priority Nursing Tip: Chemotherapy can cause life-threatening neutropenia and thrombocytopenia.
Reference: McKinney, E. S., et al. (2022). *Maternal child nursing* (6th ed., pp. 1153–1154). Elsevier.

157. The nurse is preparing to admit a client from the postanesthesia care unit who has had microvascular decompression of the trigeminal nerve. Which **essential** equipment would the nurse ask the assistive personnel to make sure is at the bedside when the client arrives?
  1. Flashlight and pulse oximeter
  2. Cardiac monitor and suction equipment
  3. Padded bed rails and suction equipment
  4. Blood pressure cuff and cardiac monitor

Level of Cognitive Ability: Applying
Client Needs: Physiological Integrity
Clinical Judgment/Cognitive Skills: Generate Solutions
Integrated Process: Clinical Judgment; Nursing Process/Planning
Content Area: Adult Health: Neurologic
Health Problems: Adult Health: Neurologic: Trigeminal Neuralgia
Priority Concepts: Clinical Judgment; Intracranial Regulation

Answer: 1
Rationale: The postoperative care of the client having microvascular decompression of the trigeminal nerve is the same as for the client undergoing craniotomy. This client requires hourly neurologic assessment as well as monitoring of the cardiovascular and respiratory statuses. Therefore, a flashlight and pulse oximetry are essential items. Cardiac monitoring and padded bed rails are not required, unless there is a special need based on a client history of cardiac disease or seizures, respectively. Suctioning is performed cautiously and only when necessary, after craniotomy to avoid increasing the intracranial pressure.
Test-Taking Strategy: Note the strategic word, *essential,* on the subject of required assessments and the essential equipment for a client who just had microvascular decompression of the trigeminal nerve. The client is not necessarily at risk for seizures postoperatively, so option 3 is eliminated first. Eliminate options 2 and 4 because no data in the question indicate that the client had a history of a cardiac problem. In addition, knowing that the procedure is performed via craniotomy enables you to recall that suctioning is done cautiously and only when necessary and also that neurologic assessment is needed, so a flashlight would be required to perform a neurologic assessment.
Priority Nursing Tip: After surgery for microvascular decompression of the trigeminal nerve, the client's pain is compared with the preoperative pain level.
Reference: Ball, J., et al. (2019). *Seidel's Guide to physical examination: An interprofessional approach* (9th ed., pp. 575–576). Elsevier; Ignatavicius, D., et al. (2021). *Medical-surgical nursing: Concepts for interprofessional collaborative care* (10th ed., pp. 175, 924–925). Elsevier.

❖ **158.** The nurse is receiving a client from the emergency department who has a diagnosis of Guillain-Barré syndrome. The client's chief sign/symptom is an ascending paralysis that has reached the level of the waist. Which items would the nurse plan to have available for emergency use?

1. Nebulizer and pulse oximeter
2. Blood pressure cuff and flashlight
3. Flashlight and incentive spirometer
4. Cardiac monitor and intubation tray

Level of Cognitive Ability: Applying
Client Needs: Physiological Integrity
Clinical Judgment/Cognitive Skills: Generate Solutions
Integrated Process: Clinical Judgment; Nursing Process/Planning
Content Area: Adult Health: Neurologic
Health Problems: Adult Health: Neurologic: Guillain-Barré Syndrome
Priority Concepts: Gas Exchange; Mobility

Answer: 4
Rationale: The client with Guillain-Barré syndrome is at risk for respiratory failure as a result of ascending paralysis. An intubation tray needs to be available for emergency use. Another complication of this syndrome is cardiac dysrhythmias, which necessitates the need for cardiac monitoring. Although some of the items in the remaining options may be kept at the bedside (e.g., pulse oximeter, blood pressure cuff, flashlight), they are not necessarily needed for emergency use in this situation.
Test-Taking Strategy: Focus on the **subject**, equipment needed for possible emergency use in a client with Guillain-Barré syndrome who is experiencing ascending paralysis. These words tell you that the correct answer will be an option that contains equipment that is not routinely used to provide care. With this in mind, eliminate options 2 and 3 based on the fact that a flashlight is needed for routine neurologic assessment. From the remaining choices, recalling the complications of this syndrome will direct you to the correct option.
Priority Nursing Tip: Monitor respiratory and cardiac status closely and prepare to initiate respiratory support for the client with Guillain-Barré syndrome.
Reference: Lewis, S., et al. (2020). *Medical-surgical nursing: Assessment and management of clinical problems* (11th ed., pp. 1424–1425). Elsevier.

159. The nurse is informed that a newborn infant whose birth parent is Rh negative will be admitted to the nursery. When planning care for the infant's arrival, which action would the nurse take?

1. Obtain the newborn infant's blood type and direct Coombs' results from the laboratory.
2. Obtain the necessary equipment from the blood bank needed for an exchange transfusion.
3. Call the maintenance department and ask for a phototherapy unit to be brought to the nursery.
4. Obtain a vial of vitamin K from the pharmacy and prepare to administer an injection to prevent isoimmunization.

Level of Cognitive Ability: Applying
Client Needs: Physiological Integrity
Clinical Judgment/Cognitive Skills: Generate Solutions
Integrated Process: Clinical Judgment; Nursing Process/Planning
Content Area: Maternity: Newborn
Health Problems: Newborn: Erythroblastosis Fetalis
Priority Concepts: Clinical Judgment; Perfusion

Answer: 1
Rationale: To further plan for the newborn infant's care, the infant's blood type and direct Coombs' results must be known. Umbilical cord blood is taken at the time of delivery to determine blood type, Rh factor, and antibody titer (direct Coombs' test) of the newborn infant. The nurse would obtain these results from the laboratory. Options 2 and 3 are inappropriate at this time, and additional data are needed to determine whether these actions are needed. Option 4 is incorrect because vitamin K is given to prevent hemorrhagic disease of the newborn infant.
Test-Taking Strategy: Focus on the **subject,** the birth parent being Rh negative. Note the relationship between the **subject** of the question and the correct option. In addition, note that the correct option is the only option that addresses assessment.
Priority Nursing Tip: For the infant with erythroblastosis fetalis, the newborn's blood is replaced with Rh-negative blood to stop the destruction of the newborn's red blood cells; the Rh-negative blood is replaced with the newborn's own blood gradually.
Reference: McKinney, E. S., et al. (2022). *Maternal child nursing* (6th ed., pp. 552, 649). Elsevier.

❖ **160.** The nurse is preparing to assist in the administration of a chemotherapeutic agent via intraperitoneal (IP) therapy for the treatment of ovarian cancer. In which position would the nurse plan to place the client before administering this therapy?
1. Supine
2. Semi-Fowler's
3. Trendelenburg's
4. Dorsal recumbent

Level of Cognitive Ability: Applying
Client Needs: Physiological Integrity
Clinical Judgment/Cognitive Skills: Generate Solutions
Integrated Process: Clinical Judgment; Nursing Process/Planning
Content Area: Adult Health: Oncology
Health Problems: Adult Health: Cancer: Cervical/Uterine/Ovarian
Priority Concepts: Clinical Judgment; Safety

Answer: 2
Rationale: IP therapy is the administration of chemotherapeutic agents into the peritoneal cavity. This therapy is used for intra-abdominal malignancies such as ovarian and gastrointestinal tumors that have moved into the peritoneum after surgery. The client would be placed in a semi-Fowler's position for this infusion because the client may experience nausea and vomiting caused by increasing pressure on the internal organs. Additionally, this treatment may also place pressure on the diaphragm. The positions indicated in the rest of the options would increase pressure in the peritoneal cavity.
Test-Taking Strategy: Focus on the subject, care of the client receiving IP therapy. Recalling that this therapy can increase intra-abdominal pressure and cause nausea and vomiting will assist you in eliminating the incorrect options.
Priority Nursing Tip: Malignancies of the abdomen may be treated with the instillation of chemotherapeutic agents into the peritoneal cavity or with external radiation.
Reference: Ignatavicius, D., et al. (2021). *Medical-surgical nursing: Concepts for interprofessional collaborative care* (10th ed., p. 302). Elsevier.

161. The nurse plans care for a client with alcohol abuse disorder based on which support system?
1. Fresh Start, an option for families of addicts
2. Families Anonymous, an option for those addicted to nicotine
3. Al-Anon, an option for parents of children who abuse substances
4. Alcoholics Anonymous, a major self-help organization for the treatment of alcohol abuse

Level of Cognitive Ability: Applying
Client Needs: Safe and Effective Care Environment
Clinical Judgment/Cognitive Skills: Generate Solutions
Integrated Process: Nursing Process/Planning
Content Area: Mental Health
Health Problems: Mental Health: Addictions
Priority Concepts: Addiction; Health Promotion

Answer: 4
Rationale: Alcoholics Anonymous is a major self-help organization for the treatment of alcoholism. Option 1 is a group for families of alcoholics. Option 2 is for nicotine addicts. Option 3 is for the parents of children who abuse substances.
Test-Taking Strategy: Focus on the subject, resources for a client who is personally dealing with alcohol abuse. Note the relationship of this subject and the correct option.
Priority Nursing Tip: As part of the assessment of a client who abuses alcohol, the nurse would ask about the type of alcohol used, how much is consumed, and for how many years.
Reference: Varcarolis, E., & Fosbre, C. (2021). *Essentials of psychiatric mental health nursing: A communication approach to evidence-based care* (4th ed., p. 325). Elsevier.

❖ **162.** A client hospitalized after a stroke is prepared for discharge. The primary health care provider (PHCP) has prescribed range-of-motion (ROM) exercises for the client's right side. Which intervention would the home care nurse include when planning for the client's care?

1. Implements ROM exercises to the point of pain for client
2. Considers the use of active, passive, or active-assisted exercises in the home
3. Encourages dependence on the home care nurse to complete the exercise program
4. Develops a schedule involving ROM exercises every 3 hours during daylight hours

Level of Cognitive Ability: Applying
Client Needs: Physiological Integrity
Clinical Judgment/Cognitive Skills: Generate Solutions
Integrated Process: Clinical Judgment; Nursing Process/Planning
Content Area: Skills: Activity/Mobility
Health Problems: Adult Health: Neurologic: Stroke
Priority Concepts: Clinical Judgment; Mobility

Answer: 2

Rationale: The home care nurse must consider all forms of ROM for the client. Even if the client has right hemiplegia, the client can assist with some of their own rehabilitative care. In addition, the goal of home care nursing is for the client to assume as much self-care and independence as possible. The nurse needs to teach so that the client becomes self-reliant. Options 1 and 4 are incorrect from a physiologic standpoint.

Test-Taking Strategy: Focus on the subject, appropriate implementation of ROM exercise. Eliminate options 1 and 4 because the suggested actions may be harmful to the client. From the remaining choices, recalling that dependency is not in the best interest of a client's sense of health promotion will help you eliminate option 3. In addition, note that the correct option is the umbrella option.

Priority Nursing Tip: The nurse would assist the client who had a stroke establish a balanced exercise and rest program.

References: Ignatavicius, D., et al. (2021). *Medical-surgical nursing: Concepts for interprofessional collaborative care* (10th ed., pp. 977–978). Elsevier; Potter, P., et al. (2021). *Fundamentals of nursing* (10th ed., pp. 828–829). Elsevier.

Nursing Process: Implementation

163. A client diagnosed with heart failure is receiving furosemide and digoxin daily. When the nurse enters the room to administer the morning doses, the client reports anorexia, nausea, and yellow vision. Which intervention would the nurse implement **first**?

1. Administer the medications.
2. Contact the physician.
3. Check the morning serum digoxin level.
4. Check the morning serum potassium level.

Level of Cognitive Ability: Analyzing
Client Needs: Physiological Integrity
Clinical Judgment/Cognitive Skills: Take Action
Integrated Process: Clinical Judgment; Nursing Process/Implementation
Content Area: Pharmacology: Cardiovascular: Cardiac Glycosides
Health Problems: Adult Health: Cardiovascular: Heart Failure
Priority Concepts: Clinical Judgment; Safety

Answer: 3

Rationale: The nurse would check the result of the digoxin level that was drawn because the client's symptoms are compatible with digoxin toxicity. A low potassium level may contribute to digoxin toxicity, so checking the serum potassium level may give useful additional information, but the digoxin level needs to be checked first. The medications would be withheld until both levels are known. If the digoxin level is elevated or the potassium level is not within the normal range, then the physician needs to be notified. If the morning digoxin level is within the therapeutic range, then the client's complaints are unrelated to the digoxin.

Test-Taking Strategy: Note the strategic word, *first*. This will assist you with determining that the nurse's action is to further investigate the cause of the client's complaints. Recalling the manifestations of digoxin toxicity and noting the relationship of the name of the medication to option 3 will direct you to this option.

Priority Nursing Tip: The nurse must count the apical heart rate for 1 full minute in a client who is receiving digoxin. If the rate is less than 60 beats/min, the medication is withheld and further investigation is done, because this finding could indicate digoxin toxicity.

Reference: Burchum, J., & Rosenthal, L. (2022). *Lehne's Pharmacology for nursing care* (11th ed., pp. 530, 538–539). Elsevier.

❖ **164.** The nurse is checking the fundus of a postpartum client and notes that the uterus is soft and spongy. Which nursing action is appropriate **initially?**
1. Encourage the client to ambulate.
2. Notify the primary health care provider.
3. Massage the fundus gently until it is firm.
4. Document fundal position, consistency, and height.

Level of Cognitive Ability: Applying
Client Needs: Physiological Integrity
Clinical Judgment/Cognitive Skills: Take Action
Integrated Process: Clinical Judgment; Nursing Process/Implementation
Content Area: Maternity: Postpartum
Health Problems: Maternity: Postpartum Uterine Problems
Priority Concepts: Clinical Judgment; Reproduction

Answer: **3**
Rationale: If the fundus is boggy (soft), it needs to be massaged gently until it is firm and the client is observed for increased bleeding or clots. Option 1 is an inappropriate action at this time. The nurse would document the fundal position, consistency, and height; the need to perform fundal massage; and the client's response to the intervention. The primary health care provider will need to be notified if uterine massage is not helpful.
Test-Taking Strategy: Note the strategic word, *initially.* Focus on the data in the question and note the relationship of these data (soft and spongy) and the data in the correct option (massage the fundus gently until it is firm).
Priority Nursing Tip: The nurse needs to gently massage the fundus of a client experiencing uterine atony and take care not to overmassage.
Reference: McKinney, E. S., et al. (2022). *Maternal child nursing* (6th ed., pp. 605–606). Elsevier.

165. A primipara is being evaluated in the clinic during the second trimester of pregnancy. The nurse checks the fetal heart rate (FHR) and notes that it is 190 beats/min. What is the appropriate **initial** nursing action?
1. Document the finding.
2. Tell the client that the FHR is fast.
3. Consult with the primary health care provider (PHCP).
4. Recheck the FHR with the client in the standing position.

Level of Cognitive Ability: Applying
Client Needs: Physiological Integrity
Clinical Judgment/Cognitive Skills: Take Action
Integrated Process: Clinical Judgment; Nursing Process/Implementation
Content Area: Maternity: Antepartum
Health Problems: Maternity: Fetal Distress/Demise
Priority Concepts: Clinical Judgment; Perfusion

Answer: **3**
Rationale: The FHR should be between 110 and 160 beats/min. In this situation, the FHR is elevated from the normal range, and the nurse needs to consult with the primary health care provider. The FHR would be documented, but option 3 is the appropriate action. The nurse would not tell the client that the FHR is fast at this point in time. Option 4 is an inappropriate action.
Test-Taking Strategy: Focus on the subject, FHR of 190 beats/min, as well the strategic word, *initial.* Recalling that the normal FHR is between 110 and 160 beats/min will direct you to the correct option.
Priority Nursing Tip: The normal FHR is 160 to 170 beats/min in the first trimester, but slows with fetal growth to 110 to 160 beats/min near or at term. The primary health care provider must be notified if the FHR is outside these parameters.
Reference: McKinney, E. S., et al. (2022). *Maternal child nursing* (6th ed., pp. 311, 448). Elsevier.

❖ **166.** A client tells the clinic nurse that their skin is very dry and irritated. Which product would the nurse suggest that the client apply to the dry skin?
  1. Myoflex
  2. Aspercreme
  3. Topical emollient
  4. Acetic acid solution

Level of Cognitive Ability: Applying
Client Needs: Health Promotion and Maintenance
Clinical Judgment/Cognitive Skills: Take Action
Integrated Process: Nursing Process/Implementation
Content Area: Adult Health: Integumentary
Health Problems: Adult Health: Integumentary: Inflammations/Infections
Priority Concepts: Patient Education; Tissue Integrity

Answer: **3**
Rationale: A topical emollient is used for dry, cracked, and irritated skin. Aspercreme and Myoflex are used to treat muscular aches. Acetic acid solution is used for irrigating, cleansing, and packing wounds infected with *Pseudomonas aeruginosa*.
Test-Taking Strategy: Focus on the subject, treatment for dry and irritated skin. Note the relationship of the subject and the word *emollient* in the correct option.
Priority Nursing Tip: To sustain the hydrating effect, it is best to apply cream or ointment emollients (moisturizers) after bathing.
Reference: Lewis, S., et al. (2020). *Medical-surgical nursing: Assessment and management of clinical problems* (11th ed., p. 425). Elsevier.

167. A client with a history of hypertension has been prescribed triamterene. The nurse provides information to the client about the medication and instructs the client to avoid consuming which fruit?
  1. Pears
  2. Apples
  3. Bananas
  4. Cranberries

Level of Cognitive Ability: Applying
Client Needs: Health Promotion and Maintenance
Clinical Judgment/Cognitive Skills: Take Action
Integrated Process: Nursing Process/Implementation
Content Area: Adult Health: Cardiovascular
Health Problems: Adult Health: Cardiovascular: Hypertension
Priority Concepts: Patient Education; Nutrition

Answer: **3**
Rationale: Triamterene is a potassium-sparing diuretic, and the client needs to avoid foods that are high in potassium. Fruits that are naturally higher in potassium include avocados, bananas, oranges, mangoes, cantaloupe, strawberries, nectarines, papayas, and dried prunes.
Test-Taking Strategy: Focus on the subject, the fruit that the client needs to avoid. Note that this is a negative event query asking you to choose the fruit the client should not eat. Recall that triamterene is a potassium-sparing diuretic and the intake of potassium presents dietary concerns related to the medication.
Priority Nursing Tip: Normal potassium levels range from 3.5 to 5.0 mEq/L (3.5 to 5.0 mmol/L). A potassium level outside of these parameters needs to be reported.
Reference: Lilley, L., Rainforth Collins, S., & Snyder J. (2020). *Pharmacology and the nursing process* (9th ed., pp. 449, 453). Elsevier.

❖ **168.** A client in the late, active, first stage of labor has just reported a gush of vaginal fluid. The nurse observes a fetal monitor pattern of variable decelerations during contractions followed by a brief acceleration. After that, there is a return to baseline until the next contraction, when the pattern is repeated. On the basis of these data, what is the nurse's **initial** intervention?

1. Take the client's vital signs.
2. Perform a Leopold's maneuver.
3. Perform a manual sterile vaginal exam.
4. Test the vaginal fluid with a Nitrazine strip.

Level of Cognitive Ability: Applying
Client Needs: Physiological Integrity
Clinical Judgment/Cognitive Skills: Take Action
Integrated Process: Clinical Judgment; Nursing Process/Implementation
Content Area: Maternity: Intrapartum
Health Problems: Maternity: Fetal Distress/Demise
Priority Concepts: Perfusion; Reproduction

Answer: 3
Rationale: Variable deceleration with brief acceleration after a gush of amniotic fluid is a common clinical manifestation of cord compression caused by occult or frank prolapse of the umbilical cord. A manual vaginal exam can detect the presence of the cord in the vagina, which confirms the problem. On the basis of the data in the question, none of the remaining options are initial actions.
Test-Taking Strategy: Note the **strategic word**, *initial*. Focusing on the **data in the question** and determining the significance of the data will direct you to the correct option.
Priority Nursing Tip: Compression of the cord between the fetal head and the forceps used during delivery can cause a drop in the fetal heart rate (FHR). The FHR and pattern are checked, reported, and recorded before and after forceps are applied.
Reference: McKinney, E. S., et al. (2022). *Maternal child nursing* (6th ed., pp. 349, 598–599). Elsevier.

169. The nurse prepares to administer an enteral feeding to a client through a nasogastric tube (NGT). Which is the **priority** intervention for the nurse to complete before administering the feeding?

1. Determining tube placement
2. Auscultating the bowel sounds
3. Measuring the intake and output
4. Establishing the client's baseline weight

Level of Cognitive Ability: Applying
Client Needs: Physiological Integrity
Clinical Judgment/Cognitive Skills: Take Action
Integrated Process: Clinical Judgment; Nursing Process/Implementation
Content Area: Skills: Tube Care
Health Problems: Adult Health: Gastrointestinal: Nutrition/Malabsorption Problems
Priority Concepts: Clinical Judgment; Safety

Answer: 1
Rationale: The nurse avoids instilling any substance into a client's NGT before verifying tube placement because NGTs can migrate out of the stomach. If the NGT is not in the correct location, subsequent infusions or feedings through the tube can lead to serious complications such as aspiration. None of the remaining options are priorities before administering an enteral feeding.
Test-Taking Strategy: Note the **strategic word**, *priority*. Use the **ABCs—airway, breathing, and circulation**—to answer the question. The correct option relates to the risk of aspiration.
Priority Nursing Tip: After insertion of an NGT, an abdominal x-ray study needs to be done to confirm placement of the tube. If the tube is incorrectly placed, the client is at risk for aspiration.
Reference: Potter, P., et al. (2021). *Fundamentals of nursing* (10th ed., pp. 1134–1135). Elsevier.

❖ **170.** The nurse is asked to assist another health care team member with providing care for a client. On entering the client's room, the nurse notes that the client is placed in this position (**refer to the figure**). The nurse maintains the client's position knowing that this client is **most likely** being treated for which condition?

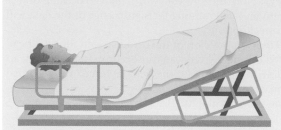

(Figure from Black, J., & Hawks, J. [2009]. *Medical-surgical nursing: Clinical management for positive outcomes.* 8th ed. Saunders.)

1. Shock
2. A head injury
3. Respiratory insufficiency
4. Increased intracranial pressure

Level of Cognitive Ability: Analyzing
Client Needs: Physiological Integrity
Clinical Judgment/Cognitive Skills: Take Action
Integrated Process: Clinical Judgment; Nursing Process/Implementation
Content Area: Complex Care: Shock
Health Problems: Adult Health: Cardiovascular: Shock
Priority Concepts: Clinical Judgment; Perfusion

Answer: 1
Rationale: A client in shock is placed in a modified Trendelenburg's position that includes elevating the legs, leaving the trunk flat, and elevating the head and shoulders slightly. This position promotes increased venous return from the lower extremities without compressing the abdominal organs against the diaphragm. The Trendelenburg's position is no longer recommended for hypotensive clients because the client is predisposed to aspiration and worsens gas exchange. The remaining options identify conditions in which the head of the client's bed would be elevated.
Test-Taking Strategy: Note the strategic words, *most likely.* Focus on the subject of the position identified in the figure. Eliminate options 2 and 4 that are comparable or alike, and both relate to a neurologic condition. From the remaining choices, eliminate option 3, recalling that the head of the bed is elevated for respiratory conditions.
Priority Nursing Tip: Shock results from the loss of circulatory fluid volume, which is usually caused by hemorrhage. Shock can also be caused by sepsis or hypovolemia (dehydration).
Reference: Ignatavicius, D., et al. (2021). *Medical-surgical nursing: Concepts for interprofessional collaborative care* (10th ed., p. 739). Elsevier.

---

171. The nurse needs to administer 7.5 mg of a medication intramuscularly. The medication label reads "10 mg/mL." How much medication would the nurse administer in mL? **Fill in the blank.**

_____ mL

Level of Cognitive Ability: Applying
Client Needs: Physiological Integrity
Clinical Judgment/Cognitive Skills: Generate Solutions
Integrated Process: Clinical Judgment; Nursing Process/Implementation
Content Area: Skills: Dosage Calculations
Health Problems: N/A
Priority Concepts: Clinical Judgment; Safety

Answer: 0.75
Rationale: Use the following formula to calculate the medication dose:

$$\frac{\text{Desired}}{\text{Available}} \times \text{Volume} = \text{mL per dose}$$

$$\frac{7.5 \text{ mg}}{10 \text{ mg}} \times 1 \text{ mL} = 0.75 \text{ mL}$$

Test-Taking Strategy: Focus on the subject, mL of medication per dose. Use the formula to determine the correct dosage, and use a calculator to verify your answer.
Priority Nursing Tip: After performing a medication calculation problem, ensure that the answer or the amount of medication to be administered makes sense and is not an excessive or extremely small dose.
Reference: Potter, P., et al. (2021). *Fundamentals of nursing* (10th ed., pp. 599–601). Elsevier.

❖ **172.** A client diagnosed with obsessive-compulsive rituals often misses the unit's morning activities because of a bed-making ritual. What nursing action would be therapeutic?
1. Verbalize tactful, mild disapproval of the behavior.
2. Discuss the social implications of the behavior with the client.
3. Help the client to make the bed so that the task can be finished quicker.
4. Offer reflective feedback, such as, "I see that you have made your bed several times."

Level of Cognitive Ability: Applying
Client Needs: Psychosocial Integrity
Clinical Judgment/Cognitive Skills: Take Action
Integrated Process: Nursing Process/Implementation
Content Area: Mental Health
Health Problems: Mental Health: Obsessive-Compulsive Disorder
Priority Concepts: Clinical Judgment; Anxiety

Answer: 4
Rationale: Reflective feedback acknowledges the client's behavior. Verbalizing disapproval and discussing social implications would increase the client's anxiety and reinforce the need to perform the ritual. The client is usually aware of the implications of the behavior. Helping with the ritual is nontherapeutic and also reinforces the behavior.
Test-Taking Strategy: Focus on the subject, a client with obsessive-compulsive rituals. Recalling that the purpose of the ritual is to relieve anxiety would assist you with eliminating options 1 and 2 that would increase the client's anxiety. Eliminate option 3 because there is no therapeutic value in participating in the ritual.
Priority Nursing Tip: If a client is experiencing anxiety, assist the client to perform relaxation techniques.
Reference: Varcarolis, E., & Fosbre, C. (2021). *Essentials of psychiatric mental health nursing: A communication approach to evidence-based care* (4th ed., pp. 93–95, 144). Elsevier.

173. A client who has undergone internal fixation after fracturing a left hip has developed a reddened left heel. What equipment would the nurse use to manage this problem?
1. Trapeze
2. Bed cradle
3. Draw sheet
4. Alternating pressure mattress

Level of Cognitive Ability: Applying
Client Needs: Physiological Integrity
Clinical Judgment/Cognitive Skills: Take Action
Integrated Process: Nursing Process/Implementation
Content Area: Skills: Activity/Mobility
Health Problems: Adult Health: Musculoskeletal: Skeletal Injury
Priority Concepts: Clinical Judgment; Tissue Integrity

Answer: 4
Rationale: The reddened heel results from the pressure of the foot against the mattress. An alternating pressure mattress is effective at minimizing pressure points. The bed cradle will keep the linens off of the client's lower extremities but will not assist with the management of a reddened heel. A draw sheet and trapeze are of general use for this client, but they are not specific for dealing with the reddened heel.
Test-Taking Strategy: Note the subject, a reddened left heel after internal fixation surgery. Think about the item in each option and how it may assist in managing the problem, a reddened heel. The items in options 1, 2, and 3 will have no helpful effect. The correct option addresses the problem stated in the question.
Priority Nursing Tip: The nurse needs to perform frequent skin assessments on the immobile client.
Reference: Potter, P., et al. (2021). *Fundamentals of nursing* (10th ed., pp. 1256–1257). Elsevier.

❖ **174.** The nurse is caring for an infant after a pylo-romyotomy is performed to treat hypertrophic pyloric stenosis. In which position would the nurse place the infant after surgery?
1. Flat on the operative side
2. Flat on the unoperative side
3. Prone with the head of the bed elevated
4. Supine with the head of the bed elevated

Level of Cognitive Ability: Applying
Client Needs: Physiological Integrity
Clinical Judgment/Cognitive Skills: Take Action
Integrated Process: Clinical Judgment; Nursing Process/Implementation
Content Area: Pediatrics: Gastrointestinal
Health Problems: Pediatric-Specific: Developmental GI Defects
Priority Concepts: Clinical Judgment; Safety

Answer: **3**
Rationale: After pyloromyotomy, the head of the bed is elevated, and the infant is placed prone to reduce the risk of aspiration. Based on this information, the remaining options are incorrect positions after this type of surgery. The surgeon's prescriptions for positioning would always be followed.
Test-Taking Strategy: Focus on the subject, proper positioning after pyloromyotomy. Consider the anatomic location of the surgical procedure and the risks associated with the procedure to answer the question. Visualize each of the positions identified in the options. Keeping in mind that aspiration is a major concern will direct you to the correct option.
Priority Nursing Tip: After pyloromyotomy to treat hypertrophic pyloric stenosis, small frequent feedings are introduced as prescribed. This is followed by a gradual increase in the amount and interval between feedings until a full feeding schedule had been reinstated.
Reference: McKinney, E. S., et al. (2022). *Maternal child nursing* (6th ed., pp. 875–876, 990). Elsevier.

175. A parent of a child with mumps calls the health care clinic to tell the nurse that the child has been lethargic and vomiting. What instruction would the nurse give to the parent?
1. To continue to monitor the child
2. That lethargy and vomiting are normal manifestations of mumps
3. That, as long as there is no fever, there is nothing to be concerned about
4. To bring the child to the clinic to be seen by the physician

Level of Cognitive Ability: Applying
Client Needs: Physiological Integrity
Clinical Judgment/Cognitive Skills: Take Action
Integrated Process: Clinical Judgment; Nursing Process/Implementation
Content Area: Pediatrics: Infectious and Communicable Diseases
Health Problems: Pediatric-Specific: Communicable Diseases
Priority Concepts: Clinical Judgment; Infection

Answer: **4**
Rationale: Mumps generally affects the salivary glands, but it can also affect multiple organs. The most common complication is septic meningitis, with the virus being identified in the cerebrospinal fluid. Common signs include nuchal rigidity, lethargy, and vomiting. The child needs to be seen by the physician.
Test-Taking Strategy: Focus on the subject, a child with mumps who has been lethargic and vomiting. Recalling that meningitis is a complication of mumps will direct you to the correct option.
Priority Nursing Tip: Inform the parents of a child with mumps that bed rest would be encouraged until the parotid swelling subsides.
Reference: McKinney, E. S., et al. (2022). *Maternal child nursing* (6th ed., p. 918). Elsevier.

❖ **176.** The nurse is reviewing the physician's prescriptions for a child who was admitted to the hospital with vaso-occlusive pain crisis resulting from sickle cell anemia. Which prescription would the nurse question?
1. Bed rest
2. Intravenous fluids
3. Supplemental oxygen
4. Meperidine hydrochloride

Level of Cognitive Ability: Applying
Client Needs: Safe and Effective Care Environment
Clinical Judgment/Cognitive Skills: Take Action
Integrated Process: Clinical Judgment; Nursing Process/Implementation
Content Area: Pediatrics: Hematologic
Health Problems: Pediatric-Specific: Sickle Cell
Priority Concepts: Collaboration; Safety

Answer: 4
Rationale: Meperidine hydrochloride is contraindicated for ongoing pain management because of the increased risk of seizures associated with the use of the medication. The management of vaso-occlusive pain generally includes the use of strong opioid analgesics such as morphine sulfate or hydromorphone. These medications are usually most effective when given as a continuous infusion or at regular intervals around the clock. The remaining options are appropriate prescriptions for treating vaso-occlusive pain crisis.
Test-Taking Strategy: Focus on the subject, the prescription to question for treatment of vaso-occlusive pain crisis. Remember that meperidine hydrochloride is associated with an increased risk of seizures.
Priority Nursing Tip: The priority of care for a child with vaso-occlusive pain crisis from sickle cell anemia is to provide hydration and relieve pain.
Reference: McKinney, E. S., et al. (2022). *Maternal child nursing* (6th ed., pp. 1131, 1133). Elsevier.

177. The nurse is caring for an infant diagnosed with laryngomalacia (congenital laryngeal stridor). In which position would the nurse place the infant to decrease the incidence of stridor?
1. Prone
2. Supine
3. Supine with the neck flexed
4. Prone with the neck hyperextended

Level of Cognitive Ability: Applying
Client Needs: Physiological Integrity
Clinical Judgment/Cognitive Skills: Take Action
Integrated Process: Clinical Judgment; Nursing Process/Implementation
Content Area: Pediatrics: Throat/Respiratory
Health Problems: Newborn: Disorders of Prenatal Development
Priority Concepts: Gas Exchange; Safety

Answer: 4
Rationale: The prone position with the neck hyperextended improves the child's breathing. Based on that information, none of the remaining options are appropriate positions.
Test-Taking Strategy: Focus on the subject, positioning a child diagnosed with laryngomalacia in order to minimize stridor. Visualize each of the positions identified in the options and how they may or may not improve breathing to assist with directing you to the correct option.
Priority Nursing Tip: A child experiencing respiratory difficulty is never left unattended.
Reference: McKinney, E. S., et al. (2022). *Maternal child nursing* (6th ed., p. 1048). Elsevier.

❖ **178.** The nurse prepares to admit a newborn with spina bifida, myelomeningocele. Which nursing action is **most important** for the care for this infant?
1. Monitoring the temperature
2. Monitoring the blood pressure
3. Inspecting the anterior fontanel for bulging
4. Monitoring the specific gravity of the urine

Level of Cognitive Ability: Applying
Client Needs: Physiological Integrity
Clinical Judgment/Cognitive Skills: Prioritize Hypotheses
Integrated Process: Clinical Judgment; Nursing Process/Implementation
Content Area: Maternity: Newborn
Health Problems: Pediatric-Specific: Neural Tube Defects
Priority Concepts: Intracranial Regulation; Tissue Integrity

Answer: 3
Rationale: Increased intracranial pressure is a complication that is associated with spina bifida. A sign of increased intracranial pressure in the newborn infant with spina bifida is a bulging anterior fontanel. The newborn infant is at risk for infection before the surgical procedure and the closure of the gibbus, and monitoring the temperature is an important intervention; however, assessing the anterior fontanel for bulging is most important. A normal saline dressing is placed over the affected site to maintain the moisture of the sac and its contents. This prevents tearing or breakdown of skin integrity at the site. Blood pressure is difficult to assess during the newborn period, and it is not the best indicator of infection or a potential complication. Urine concentration is not well developed during the newborn stage of development.
Test-Taking Strategy: Focus on the strategic words, *most important.* Eliminate options 2 and 4 because blood pressure and specific gravity are common assessments, but they are not as reliable indications of changes in the status of a newborn as they would be for an older child. From the remaining choices, focusing on the strategic words will direct you to the correct option.
Priority Nursing Tip: In myelomeningocele, the sac (defect) is covered by a thin membrane and is prone to leakage or rupture.
Reference: McKinney, E. S., et al. (2022). *Maternal child nursing* (6th ed., pp. 1294, 1296). Elsevier.

179. During the assessment, the nurse notes that the child's genitals are swollen. The nurse suspects that the child is being sexually abused. Which **priority** action would the nurse take?
1. Document the child's physical findings.
2. Report the case because abuse is suspected.
3. Refer the family to appropriate support groups.
4. Assist the family with identifying resources and support systems.

Level of Cognitive Ability: Applying
Client Needs: Psychosocial Integrity
Clinical Judgment/Cognitive Skills: Take Action
Integrated Process: Clinical Judgment; Nursing Process/Implementation
Content Area: Leadership/Management: Ethical/Legal
Health Problems: Mental Health: Abusive Behaviors
Priority Concepts: Health Care Law; Interpersonal Violence

Answer: 2
Rationale: The primary legal responsibility of the nurse when child abuse is suspected is to report the case. All 50 states require health care professionals to report all cases of suspected abuse. Although documenting the assessment findings, assisting the family, and referring the family to appropriate resources and support groups is important, the primary legal responsibility is to report the case. Although the remaining options are appropriate, reporting the findings has priority.
Test-Taking Strategy: Note the strategic word, *priority.* Focus on the subject, the possible sexual abuse of a child. Recall that abuse is a crime. Keeping this in mind will direct you to the correct option.
Priority Nursing Tip: The nurse needs to document information related to suspected child abuse in an objective manner.
Reference: McKinney, E. S., et al. (2022). *Maternal child nursing* (6th ed., p. 709). Elsevier. p. 1339; Potter, P., et al. (2021). *Fundamentals of nursing* (10th ed., p. 709). Elsevier.

❖ **180.** The nurse is planning care for an infant with a diagnosis of an encephalocele located in the occipital area. Which item would the nurse use to assist with positioning the child to avoid pressure on the encephalocele?

1. Sandbags
2. Sheepskin
3. Feather pillows
4. Foam half donut

Level of Cognitive Ability: Applying
Client Needs: Physiological Integrity
Clinical Judgment/Cognitive Skills: Take Action
Integrated Process: Clinical Judgment; Nursing Process/Implementation
Content Area: Pediatrics: Neurologic
Health Problems: Pediatric-Specific: Neural Tube Defects
Priority Concepts: Safety; Tissue Integrity

Answer: 4
Rationale: The infant is positioned to avoid pressure on the lesion. If the encephalocele is in the occipital area, a foam half donut may be useful for positioning to prevent this pressure. A sandbag, sheepskin, or feather pillow will not protect the encephalocele from pressure.
Test-Taking Strategy: Eliminate options 1, 2, and 3 that are comparable or alike in that they would require the head to remain flat and therefore would not protect the lesion.
Priority Nursing Tip: The nurse needs to monitor the infant with encephalocele closely for signs of neurologic deterioration.
Reference: Hockenberry, M., Wilson, D., & Rodgers, C. (2019). *Wong's Nursing care of infants and children* (11th ed., pp. 1310, 1318). Elsevier.

181. The nurse caring for a child who has sustained a head injury notes that the physician has documented decorticate posturing. During the assessment, the nurse notes the extension of the upper extremities and the internal rotation of the upper arms and wrists and that the lower extremities are extended, with some internal rotation noted at the knees and feet. On the basis of these findings, what is the **initial** nursing action?

1. Notify the physician of the change in posturing.
2. Document that the original positioning is unchanged.
3. Attempt to assess the flexibility of the child's lower extremities.
4. Plan to continue to monitor the child for posturing every 2 hours.

Level of Cognitive Ability: Analyzing
Client Needs: Physiological Integrity
Clinical Judgment/Cognitive Skills: Take Action
Integrated Process: Clinical Judgment; Nursing Process/Implementation
Content Area: Complex Care: Emergency Situations/ Management
Health Problems: Pediatric-Specific: Head Injury
Priority Concepts: Clinical Judgment; Intracranial Regulation

Answer: 1
Rationale: Decorticate (flexion) posturing refers to the flexion of the upper extremities and the extension of the lower extremities. Plantar flexion of the feet may also be observed. Decerebrate (extension) posturing involves the extension of the upper extremities with the internal rotation of the upper arms and wrists. The lower extremities will extend with some internal rotation noted at the knees and feet. The progression from decorticate to decerebrate posturing usually indicates deteriorating neurologic function and warrants physician notification. Although documentation is appropriate, it is not the initial action in this situation. The other options are not appropriate.
Test-Taking Strategy: Focus on the subject, decerebrate and decorticate positioning. Also note the strategic word, *initial*. Recalling that progression from decorticate to decerebrate posturing usually indicates deteriorating neurologic function will direct you to the correct option.
Priority Nursing Tip: Decorticate (flexion) posturing is seen with severe dysfunction of the cerebral cortex. Decerebrate (extension) posturing is a sign of dysfunction at the level of the midbrain.
Reference: McKinney, E. S., et al. (2022). *Maternal child nursing* (6th ed., pp. 1292–1293). Elsevier.

❖ **182.** The parent of the child with a diagnosis of hepatitis B calls the health care clinic to report that the jaundice seems to be worsening. Which response would the nurse make to the mother?
1. "It sounds as if the hepatitis may be worsening."
2. "It is necessary to isolate the child from others in the home."
3. "The jaundice may appear to get worse before it begins to resolve."
4. "You need to bring the child to the health care clinic to see the physician."

Level of Cognitive Ability: Applying
Client Needs: Physiological Integrity
Clinical Judgment/Cognitive Skills: Take Action
Integrated Process: Clinical Judgment; Nursing Process/Implementation
Content Area: Pediatrics: Gastrointestinal
Health Problems: Pediatric-Specific: Hepatitis
Priority Concepts: Clinical Judgment; Infection

Answer: 3
Rationale: The parents would be instructed that jaundice may appear to get worse before it resolves. The parents of a child with hepatitis would also be taught the danger signs that could indicate a worsening of the child's condition, specifically changes in neurologic status, bleeding, and fluid retention. Based on this information, the statements in the remaining options are incorrect.
Test-Taking Strategy: Focus on the subject, the physiology associated with hepatitis to answer this question. Remember that jaundice worsens before it resolves. This will direct you to the correct option.
Priority Nursing Tip: Proper hand washing and standard precautions can help prevent the spread of viral hepatitis.
Reference: Murray, S., et al. (2019). *Foundations of maternal-newborn and women's health nursing* (7th ed., p. 528). Elsevier.

183. The nurse is preparing to suction a tracheotomy on an infant. The nurse prepares the equipment for the procedure and would turn the suction to which setting?
1. 60 mm Hg
2. 90 mm Hg
3. 110 mm Hg
4. 120 mm Hg

Level of Cognitive Ability: Applying
Client Needs: Physiological Integrity
Clinical Judgment/Cognitive Skills: Take Action
Integrated Process: Clinical Judgment; Nursing Process/Implementation
Content Area: Skills: Tube Care
Health Problems: N/A
Priority Concepts: Gas Exchange; Safety

Answer: 2
Rationale: The suctioning procedure for pediatric clients varies from that used for adults. Suctioning in infants and children requires the use of a smaller suction catheter and lower suction settings as compared with those used for adults. Suction settings for a neonate are usually 60 to 80 mm Hg; for an infant, 80 to 100 mm Hg; and, for larger children, 100 to 120 mm Hg. The physician prescription and agency procedures are always followed.
Test-Taking Strategy: Focus on the subject of the suctioning of an infant's tracheotomy. Recalling the procedure that is used for an adult will assist with directing you to the correct option.
Priority Nursing Tip: The nurse would always hyperoxygenate the infant before performing respiratory suctioning.
Reference: McKinney, E. S., et al. (2022). *Maternal child nursing* (6th ed., pp. 846–847). Elsevier.

❖ **184.** A client begins to experience seizure activity while in bed. The nurse would provide which intervention to prevent aspiration?
1. Raise the head of the bed.
2. Loosen restrictive clothing.
3. Remove the pillow and raise the padded side rails.
4. Position client on the side with the head flexed forward.

Level of Cognitive Ability: Applying
Client Needs: Physiological Integrity
Clinical Judgment/Cognitive Skills: Take Action
Integrated Process: Clinical Judgment; Nursing Process/Implementation
Content Area: Adult Health: Neurologic
Health Problems: Adult Health: Neurologic: Seizure Disorder/Epilepsy
Priority Concepts: Intracranial Regulation; Safety

Answer: 4
Rationale: Positioning the client on one side with the head flexed forward allows the tongue to fall forward and facilitates the drainage of secretions, which could help prevent aspiration. The nurse would not raise the head of the client's bed. The nurse would remove restrictive clothing and the pillow and raise the padded side rails, if present, but these actions would not decrease the risk of aspiration; rather, they are general safety measures to use during seizure activity.
Test-Taking Strategy: Focus on the subject of preventing aspiration. Focus on the ABCs—airway, breathing, and circulation—and then visualize the effect that each remaining option would have on airway and aspiration to direct you to the correct option.
Priority Nursing Tip: Never place anything into the mouth of a client experiencing a seizure.
Reference: Ignatavicius, D., et al. (2021). *Medical-surgical nursing: Concepts for interprofessional collaborative care* (10th ed., p. 865). Elsevier.

185. A client who has experienced a stroke has episodes of coughing while swallowing liquids. The client has developed a temperature of 101° F (38.3° C) and an oxygen saturation of 91% (down from 98% previously), is slightly confused, and has noticeable dyspnea. Which action would the nurse take?
1. Notify the physician.
2. Administer an acetaminophen suppository.
3. Encourage the client to cough and deep breathe.
4. Administer a bronchodilator prescribed on an as-needed basis.

Level of Cognitive Ability: Analyzing
Client Needs: Physiological Integrity
Clinical Judgment/Cognitive Skills: Take Action
Integrated Process: Clinical Judgment; Nursing Process/Implementation
Content Area: Adult Health: Neurologic
Health Problems: Adult Health: Neurologic: Stroke
Priority Concepts: Clinical Judgment; Gas Exchange

Answer: 1
Rationale: The client is exhibiting clinical signs and symptoms of aspiration, which include fever, dyspnea, decreased arterial oxygen levels, and confusion. Other symptoms that occur with this complication are difficulty with managing saliva or coughing or choking while eating. Because the client has developed a complication that requires medical intervention, the most appropriate action is to contact the physician. The remaining options are not related to the management of aspiration.
Test-Taking Strategy: Focus on the subject, a client who has experienced a stroke and episodes of coughing while swallowing liquids, as well as the client's specific sign/symptoms. This will indicate that aspiration has most likely occurred. Eliminate options 2, 3, and 4 as they do not assist with alleviating this life-threatening condition.
Priority Nursing Tip: During the acute phase of a stroke, monitor the client for signs of increased intracranial pressure because the client is most at risk during the first 72 hours after the stroke.
Reference: Ignatavicius, D., et al. (2021). *Medical-surgical nursing: Concepts for interprofessional collaborative care* (10th ed., pp. 902, 907). Elsevier.

❖ **186.** Which action would the nurse implement as part of care for a client with suspected multiple myeloma after a bone biopsy?
1. Monitor the vital signs once per day.
2. Keep the area in a dependent position.
3. Administer intramuscular opioid analgesics.
4. Monitor the site for swelling, bleeding, or hematoma formation.

Level of Cognitive Ability: Applying
Client Needs: Physiological Integrity
Clinical Judgment/Cognitive Skills: Take Action
Integrated Process: Clinical Judgment; Nursing Process/Implementation
Content Area: Foundations of Care: Diagnostic Tests
Health Problems: Adult Health: Cancer: Multiple Myeloma
Priority Concepts: Clinical Judgment; Safety

Answer: 4
Rationale: Nursing care after bone biopsy includes monitoring the site for swelling, bleeding, or hematoma formation. The vital signs are monitored every 4 hours for 24 hours. The biopsy site is elevated for 24 hours to reduce edema. A dependent position will increase the risk for bleeding. The client usually requires mild analgesics; more severe pain usually indicates that complications are arising.
Test-Taking Strategy: Focus on the subject, care of the client after bone biopsy. Begin to answer this question by recalling that after this procedure the client must have periodic assessments. With this in mind, eliminate option 1 because the time frame is too infrequent. Knowing that the procedure is done under local anesthesia helps you eliminate option 3 next. From the remaining choices, recall the principles related to circulation and positioning to direct you to the correct option.
Priority Nursing Tip: Inform the client that mild to moderate discomfort is normal after a bone biopsy.
Reference: Heuther, S., McCance, K., & Brashers, V. (2020). *Understanding pathophysiology* (7th ed., p. 533). Elsevier; Pagana, K., Pagana, T., & Pagana, T. N. (2021). *Mosby's Diagnostic and laboratory test reference* (15th ed., p. 166). Elsevier.

187. The nurse is caring for a client with rheumatoid arthritis who is scheduled for an arthrogram involving the use of a contrast medium. Which action by the nurse is the **priority?**
1. Determining the presence of client allergies
2. Asking if the client has any last-minute questions
3. Telling the client to try to void before leaving the unit
4. Emphasizing to the client the importance of remaining still during the procedure

Level of Cognitive Ability: Applying
Client Needs: Physiological Integrity
Clinical Judgment/Cognitive Skills: Take Action
Integrated Process: Clinical Judgment; Nursing Process/Implementation
Content Area: Foundations of Care: Diagnostic Tests
Health Problems: Adult Health: Musculoskeletal: Rheumatoid Arthritis and Osteoarthritis
Priority Concepts: Clinical Judgment; Safety

Answer: 1
Rationale: Because of the risk of allergy to contrast medium, the nurse places the highest priority on assessing whether the client has an allergy to iodine or shellfish. The nurse also reinforces information about the test and reminds the client about the need to remain still during the procedure. It is helpful to have the client void before the procedure for comfort.
Test-Taking Strategy: Note the strategic word, *priority.* Recalling the risk associated with the administration of contrast medium will direct you to the correct option.
Priority Nursing Tip: The priority nursing action before any procedure involving the injection of a contrast medium is to assess the client for any allergies.
Reference: Ignatavicius, D., et al. (2021). *Medical-surgical nursing: Concepts for interprofessional collaborative care* (10th ed., p. 157). Elsevier.

❖ **188.** The nurse responds to a call bell and finds a client lying on the floor after a fall. The nurse suspects that the client's arm may be broken. Which **immediate** action would the nurse take?
1. Immobilize the arm.
2. Take a set of vital signs.
3. Call the radiology department.
4. Ask the client to describe what happened.

Level of Cognitive Ability: Applying
Client Needs: Physiological Integrity
Clinical Judgment/Cognitive Skills: Take Action
Integrated Process: Clinical Judgment; Nursing Process/Implementation
Content Area: Adult Health: Musculoskeletal
Health Problems: Adult Health: Musculoskeletal: Skeletal Injury
Priority Concepts: Clinical Judgment; Mobility

Answer: 1
Rationale: When a fracture is suspected, it is imperative that the area be splinted before the client is moved. Emergency help needs to be called for if the client is external to a hospital, and a physician is called if the client is hospitalized. Vital signs would be taken, but this is not the immediate action. The physician rather than the nurse prescribes an x-ray examination. The nurse would remain with the client and provide realistic reassurance. Although the details of the fall are important, such a discussion is not an immediate need.
Test-Taking Strategy: Note the strategic word, *immediate.* Eliminate option 3 because the physician will prescribe radiology films. Option 4 is eliminated next because such a discussion is not a priority. From the remaining choices, noting that a fracture is suspected will direct you to the correct option.
Priority Nursing Tip: If a fracture is suspected, immobilize the extremity by splinting, including the joints above and below the fracture site. Monitor circulatory status closely after splinting the extremity.
Reference: Ignatavicius, D., et al. (2021). *Medical-surgical nursing: Concepts for interprofessional collaborative care* (10th ed., p. 1035). Elsevier.

189. The nurse is caring for a hospitalized 14-year-old adolescent client who is placed in Crutchfield traction. The adolescent is having difficulty adjusting to the length of the hospital confinement. Which nursing action would be appropriate to meet the adolescent's needs?
1. Allow the adolescent to play loud music in the hospital room.
2. Let the adolescent wear their own clothing when friends visit.
3. Allow the adolescent to have their hair dyed if the parent agrees.
4. Allow the adolescent to keep the shades closed and the room darkened.

Level of Cognitive Ability: Applying
Client Needs: Psychosocial Integrity
Clinical Judgment/Cognitive Skills: Take Action
Integrated Process: Clinical Judgment; Nursing Process/Implementation
Content Area: Developmental Stages: Adolescent
Health Problems: Mental Health: Coping
Priority Concepts: Clinical Judgment; Development

Answer: 2
Rationale: An adolescent needs to identify with peers and has a strong need to belong to a group. The adolescent should be allowed to wear their own clothes to feel a sense of belonging to the group. The adolescent likes to dress like the group and to wear similar hairstyles. Loud music may disturb others in the hospital. Because Crutchfield traction involves the use of skeletal pins, hair dye is not appropriate. The adolescent's request for a darkened room is indicative of a possible problem with depression that may require further evaluation and intervention.
Test-Taking Strategy: Focus on the subject, a 14-year-old having difficulty adjusting to the length of the hospital confinement. Specific knowledge of Crutchfield traction and its limitations, as well as of growth and development concepts, will direct you to the correct option.
Priority Nursing Tip: Hospitalized adolescents become upset if friends go on with their lives, excluding them. For the hospitalized adolescent, separation from friends is a source of anxiety.
Reference: McKinney, E. S., et al. (2022). *Maternal child nursing* (6th ed., p. 791). Elsevier.

❖ **190.** The nurse prepares for a client in leg traction to be admitted to the nursing unit. The nurse asks the assistive personnel to obtain which **essential** item that will be needed to assist the client to move in bed while in leg traction?

1. A foot board
2. Extra pillows
3. A bed trapeze
4. An electric bed

Level of Cognitive Ability: Applying
Client Needs: Physiological Integrity
Clinical Judgment/Cognitive Skills: Take Action
Integrated Process: Clinical Judgment; Nursing Process/Implementation
Content Area: Skills: Activity/Mobility
Health Problems: Adult Health: Musculoskeletal: Skeletal Injury
Priority Concepts: Clinical Judgment; Mobility

Answer: 3
Rationale: A trapeze is essential to allow the client to lift straight up while being moved so that the amount of pull exerted on the limb in traction is not altered. A foot board and extra pillows do not facilitate moving. Either an electric bed or a manual bed can be used for traction, but this does not specifically assist the client with moving in bed.
Test-Taking Strategy: Note the strategic word, *essential*. Attempt to visualize the items identified in the options, and focus on the subject of helping the client in leg traction to move in bed. This will direct you to the correct option.
Priority Nursing Tip: For the client in traction, ensure that pulleys in the traction device are not obstructed and ropes in the pulleys move freely.
References: Lewis, S., et al. (2020). *Medical-surgical nursing: Assessment and management of clinical problems* (11th ed., p. 1458). Elsevier; Potter, P., et al. (2021). *Fundamentals of nursing* (10th ed., p. 844). Elsevier.

191. A pregnant client is receiving rehabilitative services for alcohol abuse. How would the nurse provide supportive care? **Select all that apply.**

1. Assist the client in identifying supportive strategies.
2. Initiate the possibility of placing the baby up for adoption.
3. Stress the need for Alcoholics Anonymous (AA) meetings.
4. Encourage the client to continue counseling after the birth.
5. Encourage the client to participate in their rehabilitation care.
6. Minimize communication with codependent family members.

Level of Cognitive Ability: Analyzing
Client Needs: Health Promotion and Maintenance
Clinical Judgment/Cognitive Skills: Take Action
Integrated Process: Clinical Judgment; Nursing Process/Implementation
Content Area: Maternity: Antepartum
Health Problems: Mental Health: Addictions
Priority Concepts: Addiction; Reproduction

Answer: 1, 3, 4, 5
Rationale: The nurse provides supportive care by encouraging the client to participate in care and to identify coping strategies. Counseling needs to continue after the infant is born. Communication with family members is important but not when they are supporting the addiction. It is not appropriate to suggest adoption.
Test-Taking Strategy: Focus on the subject, supportive care to a pregnant client for alcohol abuse. Only the correct options provide the client with an active role in care. The incorrect options create barriers for long-term success in dealing with the problem.
Priority Nursing Tip: Fetal alcohol syndrome is caused by maternal alcohol use during pregnancy.
Reference: Varcarolis, E., & Fosbre, C. (2021). *Essentials of psychiatric mental health nursing: A communication approach to evidence-based care* (4th ed., pp. 308–309, 323). Elsevier.

❖ **192.** A client in the second trimester of pregnancy is being assessed at the primary health care clinic. The nurse notes that the fetal heart rate (FHR) is 100 beats/min. Which nursing action would be appropriate **initially**?
1. Document the findings as normal.
2. Notify the physician of the finding.
3. Inform client that the assessment is normal and everything is fine.
4. Instruct client to return to the clinic in 8 hours for reevaluation of the FHR.

Level of Cognitive Ability: Applying
Client Needs: Physiologic Integrity
Clinical Judgment/Cognitive Skills: Take Action
Integrated Process: Clinical Judgment; Nursing Process/Implementation
Content Area: Maternity: Antepartum
Health Problems: Maternity: Fetal Distress/Demise
Priority Concepts: Perfusion; Reproduction

Answer: 2
Rationale: The FHR should be between 110 and 160 beats/min during pregnancy. An FHR of 100 beats/min would require that the physician be notified and the client be further evaluated. Although the nurse would document the findings, the most appropriate nursing action is to notify the physician. Based on this information, eliminate the options that suggest inaccurate nursing actions.
Test-Taking Strategy: Note the strategic word, *initially*. Eliminate options 1 and 3 that are comparable or alike and inaccurate so that they can be eliminated first. From the remaining choices, focus on the subject of FHR recalling that the normal range for the FHR is between 110 and 160 beats/min; this will direct you to the correct option.
Priority Nursing Tip: The FHR is usually about twice the maternal heart rate. However, an FHR outside the parameters of 110 and 160 beats/min during pregnancy warrants physician notification.
Reference: McKinney, E. S., et al. (2022). *Maternal child nursing* (6th ed., p. 448). Elsevier.

193. A client admitted to the hospital with a diagnosis of a leaking cerebral aneurysm is scheduled for surgery. Which intervention would the nurse implement during the preoperative period?
1. Place the client on bed rest.
2. Allow the client to ambulate only in the room.
3. Obtain a bedside commode for the client's use.
4. Encourage the client to be up at least twice per day.

Level of Cognitive Ability: Applying
Client Needs: Physiological Integrity
Clinical Judgment/Cognitive Skills: Take Action
Integrated Process: Clinical Judgment; Nursing Process/Implementation
Content Area: Adult Health: Neurologic
Health Problems: Adult Health: Neurologic: Aneurysm
Priority Concepts: Clinical Judgment; Intracranial Regulation

Answer: 1
Rationale: The client is placed on aneurysm precautions, and the client's activity is kept to a minimum to prevent Valsalva's maneuver. Clients often hold their breath and strain while pulling up to get out of bed. This exertion may cause a rise in blood pressure, which increases bleeding. Clients who have bleeding aneurysms in any vessel will have activity curtailed. Therefore, the rest of the options are incorrect actions.
Test-Taking Strategy: Focus on the subject, the client's diagnosis of a leaking cerebral aneurysm, and the words *preoperative period*. Eliminate options 2, 3, and 4 that are comparable or alike in that they all involve out-of-bed activity and are incorrect.
Priority Nursing Tip: The primary concern for a client with a cerebral aneurysm is rupture.
Reference: Lewis, S., et al. (2020). *Medical-surgical nursing: Assessment and management of clinical problems* (11th ed., p. 812). Elsevier.

❖ **194.** Which is the **most important** laboratory result for the nurse to present to the physician on a client who is receiving total parenteral nutrition (TPN)?
1. White blood cell count
2. Serum electrolyte levels
3. Arterial blood gas levels
4. Hemoglobin and hematocrit levels

Level of Cognitive Ability: Analyzing
Client Needs: Physiological Integrity
Clinical Judgment/Cognitive Skills: Prioritize Hypotheses
Integrated Process: Clinical Judgment; Nursing Process/Implementation
Content Area: Skills: Nutrition
Health Problems: Adult Health: Gastrointestinal: Nutrition/Malabsorption Problems
Priority Concepts: Clinical Judgment; Nutrition

Answer: 2
Rationale: Total parenteral nutrition solutions contain amino acids and dextrose in solution with electrolytes, trace elements, and other agents added. The provider uses the electrolyte values (including sodium, potassium, and chloride) and the glucose level to determine the effectiveness of the solution, makes changes to the solution as necessary, and decreases the client's risk of a fluid and electrolyte imbalance. It is important to monitor the serum glucose because parenteral nutrition is usually composed of 10% or more dextrose in water. The remaining options can be suitable tests for a client who is receiving total parenteral nutrition, but these results cover a narrower range of information than serum electrolytes.
Test-Taking Strategy: Note the strategic words, *most important*, to choose the laboratory test that provides better information than the other options. Thinking about the purpose of TPN and its components will direct you to option 2.
Priority Nursing Tip: Assess the client who is to receive total parenteral nutrition for a history of glucose intolerance. If the client receives the solution too rapidly, does not receive enough insulin, or contracts an infection, hyperglycemia can occur.
Reference: Lewis, S., et al. (2020). *Medical-surgical nursing: Assessment and management of clinical problems* (11th ed., p. 864). Elsevier.

Nursing Process: Evaluation

195. The nurse is evaluating the effects of care for the client with nephrotic syndrome. Which finding demonstrates the least amount of improvement over 2 days of care?

LABORATORY RESULTS

Test and Result	Reference Range
Albumin 1.9 g/dL (19 g/L)	3.5 - 5 g/dL (35 to 50 g/L)

1. Initial weight 208 pounds, down to 203 pounds
2. Blood pressure 160/90 mm Hg, down to 130/78 mm Hg
3. Serum albumin 1.9 g/dL (19 g/L), up to 2.0 g/dL (20 g/L)
4. Daily intake and output record of 2100 mL intake and 1900 mL output and 2000 mL intake and 2900 mL output

Level of Cognitive Ability: Evaluating
Client Needs: Physiological Integrity
Clinical Judgment/Cognitive Skills: Evaluate Outcomes
Integrated Process: Clinical Judgment; Nursing Process/Evaluation
Content Area: Adult Health: Renal and Urinary
Health Problems: Adult Health: Renal and Urinary: Urinary Tract Inflammation/Infection/Trauma
Priority Concepts: Clinical Judgment; Safety

Answer: 3
Rationale: The goal of therapy in nephrotic syndrome is to heal the leaking glomerular membrane. This would then control edema by stopping the loss of protein in the urine. Fluid balance and albumin levels are monitored to determine the effectiveness of therapy. The least amount of improvement is in the serum albumin level because the normal albumin level is 3.5 to 5 g/dL (35 to 50 g/L). Option 1 represents a loss of fluid that slightly exceeds 2 L and represents a significant improvement. Option 2 shows improvement because both systolic and diastolic blood pressures are lower. Option 4 represents an increased fluid loss, which indicates improvement.
Test-Taking Strategy: Focus on the subject, the information that identifies the least amount of improvement. Option 1 illustrates the greatest improvement and is eliminated first. Option 4 is also a significant improvement and is eliminated next. From the remaining choices, noting that the blood pressure has decreased significantly will direct you to the correct option.
Priority Nursing Tip: For the client with nephrotic syndrome, bed rest is important if severe edema is present.
Reference: Ignatavicius, D., et al. (2021). *Medical-surgical nursing: Concepts for interprofessional collaborative care* (10th ed., p. 1362). Elsevier.

❖ **196.** A client is being discharged after the application of a plaster leg cast. The nurse determines that the client understands the proper care of the cast when the client states the need to engage in which action?
1. Avoid getting the cast wet.
2. Cover the casted leg with warm blankets.
3. Use the fingertips to lift and move the leg.
4. Use a padded coat hanger end to scratch under the cast.

Level of Cognitive Ability: Evaluating
Client Needs: Physiological Integrity
Clinical Judgment/Cognitive Skills: Evaluate Outcomes
Integrated Process: Nursing Process/Evaluation
Content Area: Adult Health: Musculoskeletal
Health Problems: Adult Health: Musculoskeletal: Skeletal Injury
Priority Concepts: Patient Education; Mobility

Answer: 1
Rationale: A plaster cast must remain dry to keep its strength. Air needs to circulate freely around the cast to help it dry. Additionally, the cast also gives off heat as it dries. The cast needs to be handled using the palms of the hands rather than the fingertips until it is fully dry. The client would never scratch under the cast. A cool hair dryer may be used to relieve an itch.
Test-Taking Strategy: Focus on the subject, cast care. Option 4 is dangerous to skin integrity and is eliminated first. Recalling that the cast needs to dry eliminates option 2. Knowing that a wet cast can be dented with the fingertips causing pressure underneath helps you eliminate option 3. Remember that plaster casts, when they have dried after application, should not become wet.
Priority Nursing Tip: The client with a plaster cast needs to be taught to keep the cast clean and dry.
Reference: Lewis, S., et al. (2020). *Medical-surgical nursing: Assessment and management of clinical problems* (11th ed., p. 1458). Elsevier.

197. The client recovering from an acute kidney injury demonstrates an understanding of the therapeutic dietary regimen when indicating a need to limit which dietary factor?
1. Fats
2. Vitamins
3. Potassium
4. Carbohydrates

Level of Cognitive Ability: Evaluating
Client Needs: Physiological Integrity
Clinical Judgment/Cognitive Skills: Evaluate Outcomes
Integrated Process: Nursing Process/Evaluation
Content Area: Adult Health: Renal and Urinary
Health Problems: Adult Health: Renal and Urinary: Acute Kidney Injury and Chronic Kidney Disease
Priority Concepts: Patient Education; Nutrition

Answer: 3
Rationale: Most of the excretion of potassium and the control of potassium balance are normal functions of the kidneys. In the client with renal failure, potassium intake must be restricted as much as possible (30 to 50 mEq/day). The primary mechanism of potassium removal with acute kidney injury is dialysis. None of the remaining options are normally restricted in the client with acute kidney injury unless a secondary health problem warrants the need to do so.
Test-Taking Strategy: Focusing on the subject, a client recovering from acute kidney injury, will assist you with answering this question. Recalling that potassium balance and excretion are controlled by the kidney will direct you to the correct option.
Priority Nursing Tip: Foods that are low in potassium include green beans, applesauce, cabbage, lettuce, peppers, grapes, blueberries, cooked summer squash or turnip greens, pineapple, or raspberries.
Reference: Ignatavicius, D., et al. (2021). *Medical-surgical nursing: Concepts for interprofessional collaborative care* (10th ed., p. 1381). Elsevier.

❖ **198.** The nurse teaches the client with a history of anxiety and command hallucinations to harm self or others appropriate management techniques. Which client statement indicates that the client understands these techniques?
1. "I can go to group and talk about my feelings to hurt myself or others."
2. "If I take my prescribed medication as I'm supposed to, I won't be as anxious."
3. "I can call my counselor so that I can talk about my feelings and not hurt anyone."
4. "If I get enough sleep and eat well, I won't be as likely to get anxious and hear things."

Level of Cognitive Ability: Evaluating
Client Needs: Psychosocial Integrity
Clinical Judgment/Cognitive Skills: Evaluate Outcomes
Integrated Process: Nursing Process/Evaluation
Content Area: Mental Health
Health Problems: Mental Health: Anxiety Disorder
Priority Concepts: Anxiety; Psychosis

Answer: 3
Rationale: There may be an increased risk for impulsive or aggressive behavior if a client is receiving command hallucinations to harm self or others. The client would be asked if they have intentions to hurt self or others. Talking about auditory hallucinations can interfere with the subvocal muscular activity that is associated with a hallucination. The remaining options are general interventions, but they are not specific to anxiety and hallucinations.
Test-Taking Strategy: Focus on the subject, anxiety and hallucinations. The incorrect options are all interventions that a client can do to aid general wellness. The correct option is specific to the subject and indicates self-responsible commitment and control over the client's own behavior.
Priority Nursing Tip: Monitor the client experiencing command hallucinations for signs of increasing fear, anxiety, or agitation.
Reference: Varcarolis, E., & Fosbre, C. (2021). *Essentials of psychiatric mental health nursing: A communication approach to evidence-based care* (4th ed., pp. 255, 264). Elsevier.

199. A perinatal client has been instructed about the prevention of genital tract infections. Which statement by the client indicates an understanding of these preventive measures?
1. "I can douche anytime I want."
2. "I can wear my tight-fitting jeans."
3. "I should avoid the use of condoms."
4. "I should wear underwear with a cotton panel liner."

Level of Cognitive Ability: Evaluating
Client Needs: Health Promotion and Maintenance
Clinical Judgment/Cognitive Skills: Evaluate Outcomes
Integrated Process: Nursing Process/Evaluation
Content Area: Maternity: Antepartum
Health Problems: Maternity: Infections/Inflammations
Priority Concepts: Infection; Sexuality

Answer: 4
Rationale: Wearing items with a cotton panel liner allows for air movement in and around the genital area. Douching is to be avoided. Wearing tight clothes irritates the genital area and does not allow for air circulation. Condoms need to be used to minimize the spread of genital tract infections.
Test-Taking Strategy: Focus on the subject, the client's understanding of preventing genital tract infections. Options 1, 2, and 3 are all incorrect statements regarding prevention of infections.
Priority Nursing Tip: Instruct the client with a genital tract infection to avoid the use of perfumed toilet paper, sanitary napkins, and feminine hygiene sprays. These items will irritate the genital area.
Reference: Lowdermilk, D., et al. (2020). *Maternity & women's health care* (12th ed., p.277). Elsevier.

❖ **200.** The nurse has given the client with coronary artery disease information about the use of sublingual nitroglycerin tablets prescribed for as-needed use if chest pain occurs. Which client statement helps assure the nurse that the client understands how to self-administer the medication?
1. "I will keep the nitroglycerin in a shirt pocket close to my body."
2. "I won't take the medication until the chest pain actually begins and intensifies."
3. "If I get a headache when I first start taking the nitroglycerin, then I will take an aspirin."
4. "I will discard unused nitroglycerin tablets 3 to 6 months after the bottle is opened, and obtain a new prescription."

Level of Cognitive Ability: Evaluating
Client Needs: Physiological Integrity
Clinical Judgment/Cognitive Skills: Evaluate Outcomes
Integrated Process: Nursing Process/Evaluation
Content Area: Pharmacology: Cardiovascular: Vasodilators
Health Problems: Adult Health: Cardiovascular: Coronary Artery Disease
Priority Concepts: Patient Education; Safety

Answer: 4
Rationale: Nitroglycerin may be self-administered sublingually 5 to 10 minutes before an activity that triggers chest pain; waiting for the pain to intensify is incorrect because the client could be experiencing myocardial infarction. Tablets need to be discarded 3 to 6 months after opening the bottle (per expiration date), and a new bottle of pills would be obtained from the pharmacy. Nitroglycerin is unstable and is affected by heat and cold, so it would not be kept close to the body (warmth) in a shirt pocket; rather, it would be kept in a jacket pocket or a purse. Headache often occurs with early use and diminishes in time. Acetaminophen may be used to treat headache.
Test-Taking Strategy: Focus on the subject, self-administration of nitroglycerin. Recalling that nitroglycerin loses its potency in 3 to 6 months will direct you to the correct option.
Priority Nursing Tip: The nurse needs to teach a client taking nitroglycerin to store the medication in a dark, tightly closed bottle. Additionally, the client needs to be informed that tablets will not relieve chest pain if they have expired.
Reference: Ignatavicius, D., et al. (2021). *Medical-surgical nursing: Concepts for interprofessional collaborative care* (10th ed., p. 774). Elsevier.

201. A client who had a laryngectomy for laryngeal cancer has started oral intake. The nurse determines that the first stage of dietary advancement has been tolerated when the client ingests which type of diet without aspirating or choking?
1. Bland
2. Full liquids
3. Clear liquids
4. Semisolid foods

Level of Cognitive Ability: Evaluating
Client Needs: Physiological Integrity
Clinical Judgment/Cognitive Skills: Evaluate Outcomes
Integrated Process: Clinical Judgment; Nursing Process/Evaluation
Content Area: Foundations of Care: Therapeutic Diets
Health Problems: Adult Health: Cancer: Laryngeal and Lung
Priority Concepts: Nutrition; Safety

Answer: 4
Rationale: Oral intake after laryngectomy is started with semisolid foods. When the client can manage this type of food, liquids may be introduced. A bland diet is not appropriate. The client may not be able to tolerate the texture of some of the solid foods that would be included in a bland diet. Thin liquids are not given until the risk of aspiration is negligible.
Test-Taking Strategy: Focus on the subject, swallowing and aspiration concerns related to a postoperative laryngectomy. Eliminate options 2 and 3 by recalling that a client with swallowing difficulty will not be able to manage liquids. From the remaining choices, recall that a bland diet provides no control over the consistency or texture of the food.
Priority Nursing Tip: After laryngectomy (radical neck dissection), place the client in a semi-Fowler's to Fowler's position to maintain a patent airway and minimize edema.
References: Ignatavicius, D., et al. (2021). *Medical-surgical nursing: Concepts for interprofessional collaborative care* (10th ed., pp. 527–528). Elsevier; Potter, P., et al. (2021). *Fundamentals of nursing* (10th ed., p. 1122). Elsevier.

❖ **202.** An older client is a victim of elder abuse. The client and family have been attending counseling sessions for the past month. Which statement, made by the abusive family member, would indicate an understanding of more positive coping skills?

1. "I will be more careful to make sure that my parent's needs are 100% met."
2. "I am so sorry and embarrassed that the abusive event occurred. It won't happen again."
3. "I feel better equipped to care for my parent now that I know where to turn if I need assistance."
4. "Now that my parent is going to move into my home with me, I will have to stop drinking alcohol."

Level of Cognitive Ability: Evaluating
Client Needs: Psychosocial Integrity
Clinical Judgment/Cognitive Skills: Evaluate Outcomes
Integrated Process: Nursing Process/Evaluation
Content Area: Mental Health
Health Problems: Mental Health: Abuse/Neglect
Priority Concepts: Coping; Interpersonal Violence

Answer: 3
Rationale: Elder abuse is sometimes caused by family members who are being expected to care for their aging parents. This care can cause the family to become overextended, frustrated, or financially depleted. Knowing where to turn in the community for assistance with caring for an aging family member can bring much-needed relief. Using these alternatives is a positive coping skill for many families. The rest of the options are statements of good faith or promises, which may or may not be kept in the future.
Test-Taking Strategy: Focus on the subject, positive coping skills. The correct option is the only choice that identifies a means of coping with the issues and that outlines a definitive plan for how to handle the pressure associated with the parent's care.
Priority Nursing Tip: When working with caregivers, assess the need for respite care or the need for other support systems.
Reference: Varcarolis, E., & Fosbre, C. (2021). *Essentials of psychiatric mental health nursing: A communication approach to evidence-based care* (4th ed., pp. 350–352). Elsevier.

203. A 24-hour-old term infant whose birthing parent has diabetes had a confirmed episode of hypoglycemia when 1 hour old. Which observation by the nurse would indicate the **need for follow-up?**

LABORATORY RESULTS

Test and Result	Reference Range
Glucose 40 mg/dL (2.28 mmol/L)	70-99 mg/dL (3.9-5.5 mmol/L) Fasting

1. Weight loss of 4 ounces and dry, peeling skin
2. Blood glucose level of 40 mg/dL (2.28 mmol/L) before the last feeding
3. Breast/chest-feeding for 20 minutes or more, with strong sucking
4. High-pitched cry, drinking 10 to 15 mL of formula per feeding

Level of Cognitive Ability: Evaluating
Client Needs: Physiological Integrity
Clinical Judgment/Cognitive Skills: Evaluate Outcomes
Integrated Process: Clinical Judgment; Nursing Process/Evaluation
Content Area: Maternity: Newborn
Health Problems: Newborn: Newborn of a Diabetic Birthing Parent
Priority Concepts: Clinical Judgment; Glucose Regulation

Answer: 4
Rationale: Hypoglycemia causes central nervous system symptoms (high-pitched cry), and it is also exhibited by a lack of strength for eating enough for growth. At 24 hours old, a term infant needs to be able to consume at least 1 ounce of formula per feeding. A high-pitched cry is indicative of neurologic involvement. Weight loss over the first few days of life and dry, peeling skin are normal findings for term infants. Blood glucose levels are acceptable at 40 mg/dL (2.28 mmol/L) during the first few days of life. Breast/chest-feeding for 20 minutes with a strong suck is an excellent finding.
Test-Taking Strategy: Note the strategic words, *need for follow-up.* These words indicate a negative event query and ask you to select an option that is an abnormal finding. Eliminate options 1, 2, and 3 that are comparable or alike and are normal findings. The words *high-pitched cry* will direct you to the correct option.
Priority Nursing Tip: In the newborn, a low blood glucose level is prevented through early feedings.
Reference: Lowdermilk, D., et al. (2020). *Maternity & women's health care* (12th ed., p. 510). Elsevier.

❖ **204.** A home care nurse visits a child with a diagnosis of celiac disease. Which finding **best** indicates that a gluten-free diet is being maintained and has been **effective?**
1. The child is free of diarrhea.
2. The child is free of bloody stools.
3. The child tolerates dietary wheat and rye.
4. A balanced fluid and electrolyte status is noted on the laboratory results.

Level of Cognitive Ability: Evaluating
Client Needs: Physiological Integrity
Clinical Judgment/Cognitive Skills: Evaluate Outcomes
Integrated Process: Clinical Judgment; Nursing Process/Evaluation
Content Area: Pediatrics: Gastrointestinal
Health Problems: Pediatric-Specific: Nutrition Problems
Priority Concepts: Clinical Judgment; Elimination

Answer: 1
Rationale: Watery diarrhea is a frequent clinical manifestation of celiac disease. The absence of diarrhea indicates effective treatment. Bloody stools are not associated with this disease. The grains of wheat and rye contain gluten and are not allowed. A balance of fluids and electrolytes does not necessarily demonstrate the improved status of celiac disease.
Test-Taking Strategy: Note the strategic words, *best* and *effective*. Focus on the subject, a child with celiac disease. Recalling that watery diarrhea is a manifestation of celiac disease will direct you to the correct option.
Priority Nursing Tip: The nurse needs to instruct the parents of a child with celiac disease about lifelong elimination of gluten sources.
Reference: McKinney, E. S., et al. (2022). *Maternal child nursing* (6th ed., p. 997). Elsevier.

205. A client in labor is receiving oxytocin by intravenous infusion. The nurse monitors the client, knowing that which finding indicates an adequate contraction pattern?
1. One contraction per minute, with resultant cervical dilation
2. Four contractions every 5 minutes, with resultant cervical dilation
3. One contraction every 10 minutes, without resultant cervical dilation
4. Three to five contractions in a 10-minute period, with resultant cervical dilation

Level of Cognitive Ability: Evaluating
Client Needs: Physiological Integrity
Clinical Judgment/Cognitive Skills: Evaluate Outcomes
Integrated Process: Clinical Judgment; Nursing Process/Evaluation
Content Area: Pharmacology: Maternity/Newborn: Uterine Stimulants
Health Problems: N/A
Priority Concepts: Clinical Judgment; Reproduction

Answer: 4
Rationale: The preferred oxytocin dosage is the minimal amount necessary to maintain an adequate contraction pattern characterized by three to five contractions in a 10-minute period, with resultant cervical dilation. If contractions are more frequent than every 2 minutes, contraction quality may be decreased.
Test-Taking Strategy: Focus on the subject of an adequate contraction pattern in a client receiving oxytocin. Recall that an adequate contraction pattern is characterized by three to five contractions in a 10-minute period, with resultant cervical dilation; this will assist you with eliminating the incorrect options.
Priority Nursing Tip: A client in labor who is receiving oxytocin would not be left unattended.
Reference: McKinney, E. S., et al. (2022). *Maternal child nursing* (6th ed., pp. 382, 385). Elsevier.

❖ **206.** A home care nurse is assigned to visit a preschooler who has a diagnosis of scarlet fever and is on bed rest. What data obtained by the nurse would indicate that the child is coping with the illness and bed rest?

1. The child insists that their parent stay in the room.
2. The child is coloring and drawing pictures in a notebook.
3. The parent keeps providing new activities for the child to do.
4. The child sucks their thumb whenever they does not get what they asked for.

Level of Cognitive Ability: Evaluating
Client Needs: Health Promotion and Maintenance
Clinical Judgment/Cognitive Skills: Evaluate Outcomes
Integrated Process: Clinical Judgment; Nursing Process/Evaluation
Content Area: Developmental Stages: Preschool
Health Problems: Pediatric-Specific: Communicable Diseases
Priority Concepts: Coping; Development

Answer: 2
Rationale: According to Jean Piaget, for the preschooler, play is the best way for children to understand and adjust to life's experiences. They are able to use pencils and crayons, and they can draw stick figures and other rudimentary things. A child with scarlet fever needs quiet play, and drawing will provide that. Based on this information, none of the remaining options address positive coping mechanisms.
Test-Taking Strategy: Note the subject of the coping behavior of a preschooler with scarlet fever. Think about the developmental level of a preschooler. Look at the data obtained by the nurse to determine if the child is coping with the disease and bed rest. The correct option is a positive coping mechanism for preschoolers. None of the remaining options address positive coping mechanisms.
Priority Nursing Tip: Scarlet fever is transmitted via direct contact with an infected person or droplet spread, or indirectly by contact with infected articles, ingestion of contaminated milk, or other foods.
Reference: McKinney, E. S., et al. (2022). *Maternal child nursing* (6th ed., pp. 67, 922–924). Elsevier.

207. A client with gastritis has just taken a dose of trimethobenzamide. When the client states relief of which sign/symptom, it is appropriate for the nurse to determine that the medication has been **effective?**

1. Nausea
2. Heartburn
3. Constipation
4. Abdominal pain

Level of Cognitive Ability: Evaluating
Client Needs: Physiological Integrity
Clinical Judgment/Cognitive Skills: Evaluate Outcomes
Integrated Process: Clinical Judgment; Nursing Process/Evaluation
Content Area: Pharmacology: Gastrointestinal: Antiemetics
Health Problems: Adult Health: Gastrointestinal: Gastritis/Gastroenteritis
Priority Concepts: Clinical Judgment; Safety

Answer: 1
Rationale: Trimethobenzamide is an antiemetic agent that is used for the treatment of nausea and vomiting. The medication is not used to treat heartburn, constipation, or abdominal pain.
Test-Taking Strategy: Note the strategic word, *effective.* Focus on the subject, the intended effect of trimethobenzamide. Recalling that trimethobenzamide is an antiemetic will direct you to option 1.
Priority Nursing Tip: Antinausea medications cause drowsiness; therefore, safety is a concern when they are administered.
Reference: Skidmore-Roth, L. (2021). *2021 Mosby's Nursing drug reference* (34th ed., p. 1271). Elsevier.

❖ **208.** The nurse is providing instructions to the parent of a child with a diagnosis of strabismus of the left eye. Which statement by the parent indicates an understanding of the procedure for patching?

1. "I will place the patch on both eyes."
2. "I will place the patch on the left eye."
3. "I will place the patch on the right eye."
4. "I will alternate the patch from the right eye to the left eye every hour."

Level of Cognitive Ability: Evaluating
Client Needs: Physiological Integrity
Clinical Judgment/Cognitive Skills: Evaluate Outcomes
Integrated Process: Clinical Judgment; Nursing Process/Evaluation
Content Area: Pediatrics: Eye/Ear
Health Problems: Pediatric-Specific: Eye Focus and Alignment Disorders
Priority Concepts: Patient Education; Sensory Perception

Answer: 3
Rationale: Patching may be used for the treatment of strabismus to strengthen the weak eye. With this treatment, the good eye is patched; this encourages the child to use the weaker eye. The treatment is most successful when it is performed during the preschool years. The schedule for patching is individualized and prescribed by the ophthalmologist.
Test-Taking Strategy: Focus on the subject, patching the eye related to the treatment of strabismus. Remembering that this condition involves a lazy eye will direct you to the correct option. It makes sense to patch the unaffected eye to strengthen the muscles in the affected eye.
Priority Nursing Tip: Strabismus is also known as "squint" or "lazy eye."
Reference: McKinney, E. S., et al. (2022). *Maternal child nursing* (6th ed., pp. 1369–1370). Elsevier.

209. The nurse is assessing a client with gestational hypertension who was admitted to the hospital 48 hours ago. Which current assessment data would indicate that the condition has not yet resolved?

1. Increased urinary output
2. Presence of trace urinary protein
3. Client complaints of blurred vision
4. Blood pressure reading at prenatal baseline

Level of Cognitive Ability: Evaluating
Client Needs: Physiological Integrity
Clinical Judgment/Cognitive Skills: Evaluate Outcomes
Integrated Process: Clinical Judgment; Nursing Process/Evaluation
Content Area: Maternity: Antepartum
Health Problems: Maternity: Gestational Hypertension/Preeclampsia and Eclampsia
Priority Concepts: Perfusion; Reproduction

Answer: 3
Rationale: Client complaints of headache or blurred vision indicate a worsening of the condition and warrant immediate further evaluation. The remaining options are all signs that the gestational hypertension is being resolved.
Test-Taking Strategy: Note the words, *not yet resolved*. This asks you to select an option that is an abnormal finding. Focus on the subject, to identify a symptom of gestational hypertension that still exists. Eliminate options that are normal findings (options 1 and 4). From the remaining choices, note that option 2 contains the word *trace* and is the most normal finding of options 2 and 3.
Priority Nursing Tip: Signs of preeclampsia are hypertension and proteinuria.
Reference: McKinney, E. S., et al. (2022). *Maternal child nursing* (6th ed., pp. 542–543). Elsevier.

❖ **210.** A client has begun medication therapy with betaxolol. The nurse determines that the client is experiencing the intended effect of therapy if which observation is noted?

1. Edema present at 3+
2. Weight loss of 5 pounds within 2 days
3. Pulse rate increased from 58 to 74 beats/min
4. Blood pressure decreased from 142/94 mm Hg to 128/82 mm Hg

Level of Cognitive Ability: Evaluating
Client Needs: Physiological Integrity
Clinical Judgment/Cognitive Skills: Evaluate Outcomes
Integrated Process: Clinical Judgment; Nursing Process/Evaluation
Content Area: Pharmacology: Cardiovascular: Beta Blockers
Health Problems: Adult Health: Cardiovascular: Hypertension
Priority Concepts: Clinical Judgment; Perfusion

Answer: 4
Rationale: Betaxolol is a beta-adrenergic blocking agent used to lower blood pressure, relieve angina, or eliminate dysrhythmias. Side/adverse effects include bradycardia and symptoms of heart failure, such as weight gain and increased edema.
Test-Taking Strategy: Focus on the subject, the intended effect of the betaxolol. Remember that beta-adrenergic blocking agent medication names end with the suffix *-lol*. Recalling the action of the medication will direct you to the correct option.
Priority Nursing Tip: Beta-adrenergic blocking agents are used with caution in clients with diabetes mellitus because they may mask the symptoms of hypoglycemia.
Reference: Lewis, S., et al. (2020). *Medical-surgical nursing: Assessment and management of clinical problems* (11th ed., p. 687). Elsevier.

211. The nurse has taught a client with asthma who is prescribed a xanthine bronchodilator about beverages to avoid. The nurse determines that the client understands the information if the client chooses which beverage from the dietary menu?

1. Cola
2. Coffee
3. Chocolate milk
4. Cranberry juice

Level of Cognitive Ability: Evaluating
Client Needs: Physiological Integrity
Clinical Judgment/Cognitive Skills: Evaluate Outcomes
Integrated Process: Nursing Process/Evaluation
Content Area: Pharmacology: Respiratory: Restrictive Airway Disease Agents
Health Problems: Adult Health: Respiratory: Asthma
Priority Concepts: Patient Education; Safety

Answer: 4
Rationale: Cola, coffee, and chocolate contain xanthine and needs to be avoided by the client who is taking a xanthine bronchodilator. This could lead to an increased incidence of cardiovascular and central nervous system side effects that can occur with the use of these types of bronchodilators.
Test-Taking Strategy: Focus on the subject, an acceptable beverage to consume. Note that options 1, 2, and 3 are comparable or alike in that they all contain some form of stimulant; therefore, these options can be eliminated.
Priority Nursing Tip: Theophylline, a bronchodilator, increases the risk of digoxin toxicity and decreases the effects of lithium and phenytoin.
Reference: Lilley, L., Rainforth Collins, S., & Snyder J. (2020). *Pharmacology and the nursing process* (9th ed., p. 581). Elsevier.

❖ **212.** A client is prescribed glipizide once daily. What intended effect of this medication would the nurse observe for?
1. Weight loss
2. Resolution of infection
3. Decreased blood glucose
4. Decreased blood pressure

Level of Cognitive Ability: Evaluating
Client Needs: Physiological Integrity
Clinical Judgment/Cognitive Skills: Evaluate Outcomes
Integrated Process: Clinical Judgment; Nursing Process/Evaluation
Content Area: Pharmacology: Endocrine: Oral Hypoglycemics
Health Problems: Adult Health: Endocrine: Diabetes Mellitus
Priority Concepts: Clinical Judgment; Glucose Regulation

Answer: 3
Rationale: Glipizide is an oral hypoglycemic agent that is taken in the morning. It is not used to enhance weight loss, treat infection, or decrease blood pressure.
Test-Taking Strategy: Focus on the **subject**, the intended effect of glipizide. Recalling that this medication is an oral hypoglycemic will direct you to the correct option.
Priority Nursing Tip: Clients prescribed hypoglycemic agents require education regarding the possible side and adverse effects, including signs of hypoglycemia.
Reference: Lilley, L., Rainforth Collins, S., & Snyder J. (2020). *Pharmacology and the nursing process* (9th ed., p. 502). Elsevier.

213. A client regularly takes nonsteroidal antiinflammatory drugs (NSAIDs) and misoprostol has been added to the medication regimen. The nurse would monitor the client for the relief of which sign/symptom?
1. Diarrhea
2. Bleeding
3. Infection
4. Epigastric pain

Level of Cognitive Ability: Evaluating
Client Needs: Physiological Integrity
Clinical Judgment/Cognitive Skills: Evaluate Outcomes
Integrated Process: Clinical Judgment; Nursing Process/Evaluation
Content Area: Pharmacology: Gastrointestinal: Gastric Protectants
Health Problems: Adult Health: Gastrointestinal: Gastritis/Gastroenteritis
Priority Concepts: Clinical Judgment; Pain

Answer: 4
Rationale: The client who regularly takes NSAIDs is prone to gastric mucosal injury, which gives the client epigastric pain as a symptom. Misoprostol is administered to prevent this occurrence. Diarrhea can be a side effect of the medication, but its relief is not an intended effect. Bleeding and infection are unrelated to the question.
Test-Taking Strategy: Focus on the **subject**, the relief of a sign/symptom in a client taking both NSAIDs and misoprostol. This tells you that the misoprostol is being given to treat or prevent the occurrence of a specific sign/symptom. Recalling that NSAIDs can cause gastric mucosal injury will direct you to the correct option.
Priority Nursing Tip: NSAIDs are contraindicated in clients with hypersensitivity or liver or renal disease.
Reference: Lilley, L., Rainforth Collins, S., & Snyder J. (2020). *Pharmacology and the nursing process* (9th ed., pp. 680–681). Elsevier.

❖ **214.** A client has received a dose of an as-needed medication loperamide. The nurse evaluates the client after administration to determine if the client has relief of which sign/symptom?
1. Diarrhea
2. Tarry stools
3. Constipation
4. Abdominal pain

Level of Cognitive Ability: Evaluating
Client Needs: Physiological Integrity
Clinical Judgment/Cognitive Skills: Evaluate Outcomes
Integrated Process: Clinical Judgment; Nursing Process/Evaluation
Content Area: Pharmacology: Gastrointestinal: Antidiarrheals
Health Problems: Adult Health: Gastrointestinal: Nutrition/Malabsorption Problems
Priority Concepts: Clinical Judgment; Elimination

Answer: 1
Rationale: Loperamide is an antidiarrheal agent, and it is commonly administered after loose stools. It is used for the management of acute diarrhea and also for chronic diarrhea, such as with inflammatory bowel disease. It can also be used to reduce the volume of drainage from an ileostomy. It is not intended to treat any of the other options.
Test-Taking Strategy: Focus on the subject, the intended effect of loperamide. Recalling that this medication is an antidiarrheal agent will direct you to the correct option.
Priority Nursing Tip: Goals for a client with diarrhea are to identify and treat the underlying cause, treat dehydration, replace fluids and electrolytes, relieve abdominal discomfort and cramping, and reduce the passage of stool.
Reference: Lilley, L., Rainforth Collins, S., & Snyder J. (2020). *Pharmacology and the nursing process* (9th ed., pp. 798–799). Elsevier.

215. The nurse has provided discharge instructions to the parent of a child who has undergone heart surgery. Which statement by the parent would indicate the **need for further teaching?**
1. "My child can return to school for full days one week after discharge."
2. "I will allow my child to play inside but omit outside play at this time."
3. "I need to have my child avoid crowds and people for 2 weeks after discharge."
4. "I need to call the surgeon if my child develops faster or harder breathing than normal."

Level of Cognitive Ability: Evaluating
Client Needs: Safe and Effective Care Environment
Clinical Judgment/Cognitive Skills: Evaluate Outcomes
Integrated Process: Clinical Judgment; Nursing Process/Evaluation
Content Area: Pediatrics: Cardiovascular
Health Problems: Pediatric-Specific: Congenital Cardiac Defects
Priority Concepts: Patient Education; Safety

Answer: 1
Rationale: The child may return to school the third week after hospital discharge, but they should go to school for half days for the first week. Outside play needs to be omitted for several weeks, with inside play allowed as tolerated. The child needs to avoid crowds of people for 2 weeks after discharge, including crowds at day care centers and churches. If any difficulty with breathing occurs, the parent needs to notify the surgeon.
Test-Taking Strategy: Note the strategic words, *need for further teaching*. This indicates a negative event query and asks you to select an option that is an incorrect statement. Recalling the principles related to the prevention of infection and the complications of surgery will direct you to the correct option.
Priority Nursing Tip: After cardiac surgery, the parents would be instructed to keep the child away from crowds for 2 weeks after discharge to decrease the risk of contracting an infection.
Reference: McKinney, E. S., et al. (2022). *Maternal child nursing* (6th ed., p. 1111). Elsevier.

❖ **216.** A client has been taking nadolol for the past month. Which finding would indicate a therapeutic effect of the medication?
1. The client is afebrile.
2. The client has clear breath sounds.
3. The client reports no episodes of headache.
4. The client has a blood pressure of 118/72 mm Hg.

Level of Cognitive Ability: Evaluating
Client Needs: Physiological Integrity
Clinical Judgment/Cognitive Skills: Evaluate Outcomes
Integrated Process: Clinical Judgment; Nursing Process/Evaluation
Content Area: Pharmacology: Cardiovascular: Beta Blockers
Health Problems: Adult Health: Cardiovascular: Hypertension
Priority Concepts: Clinical Judgment; Perfusion

Answer: 4
Rationale: Nadolol is a beta-adrenergic blocking agent that is used to treat hypertension. Therefore, a blood pressure within the normal range would indicate an effective response to the medication. Based on this information the remaining options are unrelated to the action of this medication.
Test-Taking Strategy: Focus on the subject, the therapeutic effect of nadolol. Remember that an evaluation-type question addresses a client's response to a treatment measure. In addition, recalling that medication names that end with -lol are beta-blocking agents will direct you to the correct option.
Priority Nursing Tip: Beta blockers may be prescribed to treat angina, dysrhythmias, hypertension, migraine headaches, and glaucoma and prevent myocardial infarction.
Reference: Lewis, S., et al. (2020). *Medical-surgical nursing: Assessment and management of clinical problems* (11th ed., p. 687). Elsevier.

217. The nurse is assigned to care for a client diagnosed with acquired immunodeficiency syndrome (AIDS) who is receiving amphotericin B for a fungal respiratory infection. When evaluating the effects of the medication, which would indicate an adverse effect?
1. Hypokalemia
2. Hypernatremia
3. Hypochloremia
4. Hypercalcemia

Level of Cognitive Ability: Evaluating
Client Needs: Physiological Integrity
Clinical Judgment/Cognitive Skills: Evaluate Outcomes
Integrated Process: Clinical Judgment; Nursing Process/Evaluation
Content Area: Pharmacology: Immune: Antifungals
Health Problems: Adult Health: Immune: Immunodeficiency Syndrome
Priority Concepts: Clinical Judgment; Safety

Answer: 1
Rationale: Clients receiving amphotericin B may develop hypokalemia, which can be severe and lead to extreme muscle weakness and electrocardiogram changes. Distal renal tubular acidosis commonly occurs, and this contributes to the development of hypokalemia. High potassium levels do not occur. The medication does not cause sodium, chloride, or calcium levels to fluctuate.
Test-Taking Strategy: Focus on the subject, an adverse effect of amphotericin B, and recall that it is an antifungal medication. It is necessary to recall that hypokalemia is an adverse effect of this medication. This will direct you to the correct option.
Priority Nursing Tip: Amphotericin B is nephrotoxic and the nurse needs to monitor the client closely for signs of nephrotoxicity such as decreased urine output and elevated blood urea nitrogen levels or creatinine levels.
Reference: Lilley, L., Rainforth Collins, S., & Snyder J. (2020). *Pharmacology and the nursing process* (9th ed., p. 659). Elsevier.

❖ **218.** A client is seen in the health care clinic, and a diagnosis of conjunctivitis is made. The nurse provides instructions to the client regarding the care of the disorder while at home. Which statement by the client indicates the **need for further teaching?**
1. "I can use an ophthalmic analgesic ointment at night if I have eye discomfort."
2. "I do not need to be concerned about spreading this infection to others in my family."
3. "I need to apply warm compresses before instilling antibiotic drops if purulent discharge is present in my eye."
4. "I need to perform saline eye irrigation before instilling the antibiotic drops into my eye if purulent discharge is present."

Level of Cognitive Ability: Evaluating
Client Needs: Safe and Effective Care Environment
Clinical Judgment/Cognitive Skills: Evaluate Outcomes
Integrated Process: Clinical Judgment; Nursing Process/Evaluation
Content Area: Adult Health: Eye
Health Problems: Adult Health: Eye: Inflammation/Infection/Trauma
Priority Concepts: Patient Education; Infection

Answer: 2
Rationale: Conjunctivitis is highly contagious. Antibiotic drops are usually administered four times a day. Ophthalmic analgesic ointment or drops may be instilled, especially at bedtime because discomfort becomes more noticeable when the eyelids are closed. When purulent discharge is present, saline eye irrigations or applications of warm compresses to the eye may be necessary before instilling the medication.
Test-Taking Strategy: Note the strategic words, *need for further teaching.* This indicates a negative event query and asks you to select an incorrect statement. Knowing that this disorder is considered highly contagious will direct you to the correct option.
Priority Nursing Tip: Instruct the client with conjunctivitis about the importance of infection control measures such as good hand washing and not sharing towels and washcloths.
Reference: Heuther, S., McCance, K., & Brashers, V. (2020). *Understanding pathophysiology* (7th ed., pp. 341–342). Elsevier.

219. The nurse reviews the nursing care plan of a hospitalized preschool child who is immobilized as a result of skeletal traction. The nurse notes concerns related to the child's development because of immobilization and hospitalization. Which evaluative statement indicates a positive outcome for the child?
1. The fracture heals without complications.
2. The caregivers verbalize safe and effective home care.
3. The child maintains normal joint and muscle integrity.
4. The child displays age-appropriate developmental behaviors.

Level of Cognitive Ability: Evaluating
Client Needs: Health Promotion and Maintenance
Clinical Judgment/Cognitive Skills: Evaluate Outcomes
Integrated Process: Clinical Judgment; Nursing Process/Evaluation
Content Area: Pediatrics: Musculoskeletal
Health Problems: Pediatric-Specific: Fractures
Priority Concepts: Development; Health Promotion

Answer: 4
Rationale: Regression and inappropriate developmental behaviors may be displayed in response to immobilization and hospitalization. With individualized care planning, a positive outcome of age-appropriate behavior can be achieved. The remaining options are appropriate evaluative statements for an immobilized child, but they do not directly address the child's development.
Test-Taking Strategy: Focus on the subject, concerns regarding growth and development. Recalling that issues with development involve an individual not performing age-appropriate tasks will direct you to the correct option. All options are evaluative statements, but only the correct option addresses development.
Priority Nursing Tip: For the hospitalized child who is immobilized, focus on the child's ability and needs. Accept regression in the child but encourage independence.
Reference: McKinney, E. S., et al. (2022). *Maternal child nursing* (6th ed., pp. 792–793, 1220). Elsevier.

❖ **220.** The nurse has been encouraging the intake of oral fluids for a client in labor to improve hydration. Which indicates a successful outcome of this action?

LABORATORY RESULTS

Test and Result	Reference Range
Urine Specific Gravity 1.020	1.003-1.030

1. Ketones in the urine
2. A urine specific gravity of 1.020
3. A blood pressure of 150/90 mm Hg
4. The continued leaking of amniotic fluid during labor

Level of Cognitive Ability: Evaluating
Client Needs: Physiological Integrity
Clinical Judgment/Cognitive Skills: Evaluate Outcomes
Integrated Process: Clinical Judgment; Nursing Process/Evaluation
Content Area: Maternity: Intrapartum
Health Problems: N/A
Priority Concepts: Fluids and Electrolytes; Reproduction

Answer: 2
Rationale: Urine specific gravity (reference range 1.003–1.030) measures the concentration of the urine. During the first stage of labor, the renal system has a tendency to concentrate urine. Labor and birth require hydration and caloric intake to replenish energy expenditure and promote efficient uterine function. An elevated blood pressure and ketones in the urine are not expected outcomes related to labor and hydration. After the membranes have ruptured, it is expected that amniotic fluid may continue to leak.
Test-Taking Strategy: Focus on the subject, a successful outcome related to oral intake. Recalling the relationship of oral intake to urine concentration will direct you to the correct option.
Priority Nursing Tip: The client in labor is at risk for hypovolemia because of the dehydrating effects of labor. However, if the laboring client is receiving intravenous fluids, the risk of hypervolemia is present.
Reference: McKinney, E. S., et al. (2022). *Maternal child nursing* (6th ed., pp. 318, 1010). Elsevier.

221. A goal for a postpartum client states, "The client will remain free of infection during their hospital stay." Which assessment data would support that the goal has been met?
1. Normal appetite
2. Absence of fever
3. Minimal vaginal bleeding
4. Moderate breast tenderness

Level of Cognitive Ability: Evaluating
Client Needs: Physiological Integrity
Clinical Judgment/Cognitive Skills: Evaluate Outcomes
Integrated Process: Clinical Judgment; Nursing Process/Evaluation
Content Area: Maternity: Postpartum
Health Problems: Maternity: Infections/Inflammations
Priority Concepts: Infection; Reproduction

Answer: 2
Rationale: Fever is the first indication of an infection. Therefore, the absence of a fever indicates that an infection is not present. The remaining options are not associated with a postpartum infection.
Test-Taking Strategy: Focus on the subject, the physical indications of an infection. The question is asking for a means of evaluating the effectiveness of a goal that relates to infection. Options 1, 3, and 4 are not related to postpartum infection.
Priority Nursing Tip: In the postpartum client, a temperature up to 100.4° F (38° C) is normal because of the dehydrating effects of labor.
Reference: McKinney, E. S., et al. (2022). *Maternal child nursing* (6th ed., p. 406). Elsevier.

❖ **222.** The nurse is monitoring the nutritional status of a client who is receiving enteral nutrition. Which would the nurse monitor as the **best** clinical indicator of the client's nutritional status?
1. Daily weight
2. Calorie count
3. Skinfold measurement
4. Serum prealbumin level

Level of Cognitive Ability: Evaluating
Client Needs: Physiological Integrity
Clinical Judgment/Cognitive Skills: Evaluate Outcomes
Integrated Process: Clinical Judgment; Nursing Process/Evaluation
Content Area: Skills: Nutrition
Health Problems: Adult Health: Gastrointestinal: Nutrition/Malabsorption Problems
Priority Concepts: Clinical Judgment; Nutrition

Answer: 4
Rationale: A serum prealbumin level is the most important parameter for determining the effectiveness of a client's nutritional management and nutritional status. Because prealbumin is a major plasma protein with a short half-life, it is sensitive to changes in protein synthesis and catabolism, and it is thus the best clinical indicator of nutritional status. It is a better nutritional index than a daily weight because body weight can be skewed quickly by changes in total body fluid. It is also a better index than anthropomorphic measurements because nutritional status is not necessarily related to skinfold thickness. The calorie count reports the total calories provided to the client without data regarding the client's use of the calories and nutrients.
Test-Taking Strategy: Note the strategic word, *best.* This tells you that the correct option is a better indicator of nutritional status than the remaining options. Remember that the prealbumin is a major plasma protein and is sensitive to changes in protein synthesis and catabolism.
Priority Nursing Tip: Enteral nutrition provides liquefied foods into the gastrointestinal tract via a tube.
Reference: Lewis, S., et al. (2020). *Medical-surgical nursing: Assessment and management of clinical problems* (11th ed., pp. 854, 862–863). Elsevier.

---

223. An adult client with hyperkalemia is prescribed sodium polystyrene sulfonate. Knowing that the reference range is 3.5 to 5.0 mEq/L (3.5 to 5.0 mmol/L), which serum potassium level is a clinical indicator of **effective** therapy?

1. 4.9 mEq/L (4.9 mmol/L)
2. 5.4 mEq/L (5.4 mmol/L)
3. 5.8 mEq/L (5.8 mmol/L)
4. 6.2 mEq/L (6.2 mmol/L)

Level of Cognitive Ability: Evaluating
Client Needs: Physiological Integrity
Clinical Judgment/Cognitive Skills: Evaluate Outcomes
Integrated Process: Clinical Judgment; Nursing Process/Evaluation
Content Area: Pharmacology: Fluid and Electrolyte Balance: Electrolytes
Health Problems: N/A
Priority Concepts: Clinical Judgment; Fluids and Electrolytes

Answer: 1
Rationale: The reference range for serum potassium level for an adult is 3.5 to 5.0 mEq/L (3.5 to 5.0 mmol/L). Option 1 is the only option that reflects a value within this range. The remaining options identify hyperkalemic levels.
Test-Taking Strategy: Note the strategic word, *effective.* Without knowing the mechanism of action of sodium polystyrene sulfonate, compare each value with normal serum potassium levels. Note that only one value is within normal limits and that effective therapy is very likely to achieve normal results.
Priority Nursing Tip: Electrocardiographic changes in hyperkalemia include tall-peaked T waves, flat P waves, widened QRS complexes, and prolonged PR intervals.
Reference: Lewis, S., et al. (2020). *Medical-surgical nursing: Assessment and management of clinical problems* (11th ed., pp. 279, 1063). Elsevier.

❖ **224.** The nurse assesses a client after abdominal surgery who has a nasogastric (NG) tube in place that is connected to suction. Which observation by the nurse indicates **most** reliably that the tube is functioning properly?
1. The suction gauge reads low intermittent suction.
2. The client indicates that pain is a 3 on a scale of 0 to 10.
3. The distal end of the NG tube is pinned to the client's gown.
4. The client denies nausea and has 250 mL of fluid in the suction collection container.

Level of Cognitive Ability: Evaluating
Client Needs: Physiological Integrity
Clinical Judgment/Cognitive Skills: Evaluate Outcomes
Integrated Process: Nursing Process/Evaluation
Content Area: Skills: Tube Care
Health Problems: Adult Health: Gastrointestinal: Nutrition/Malabsorption Problems
Priority Concepts: Clinical Judgment; Safety

Answer: 4
Rationale: An NG tube connected to suction is used postoperatively to decompress and rest the bowel. The gastrointestinal tract lacks peristaltic activity as a result of manipulation during surgery. The client should not experience symptoms of ileus (nausea and vomiting) if the tube is functioning properly. Although the nurse makes pertinent observations of the tube to ensure that it is secure and properly connected to suction, the client is assessed for the effect. A pain indicator of 3 is an expected finding in a postoperative client.
Test-Taking Strategy: Note the strategic word, *most.* Focus on the subject that the NG tube is functioning properly. Recalling the purpose of an NG tube in a postoperative client will direct you to the correct option.
Priority Nursing Tip: To determine the true or actual amount of NG drainage during a nursing shift, subtract the amount of irrigating solution used during the shift from the amount of drainage in the collection device.
Reference: Lewis, S., et al. (2020). *Medical-surgical nursing: Assessment and management of clinical problems* (11th ed., p. 342). Elsevier.

225. The nurse is caring for a client who has returned from the postanesthesia care unit after prostatectomy. The client has a three-way indwelling urinary catheter with an infusion of continuous bladder irrigation (CBI). Which color description of the urinary drainage would lead the nurse to determine that the flow rate is adequate?
1. Dark cherry
2. Clear as water
3. Pale yellow or slightly pink
4. Concentrated yellow with small clots

Level of Cognitive Ability: Evaluating
Client Needs: Physiological Integrity
Clinical Judgment/Cognitive Skills: Evaluate Outcomes
Integrated Process: Clinical Judgment; Nursing Process/Evaluation
Content Area: Adult Health: Renal and Urinary
Health Problems: Adult Health: Renal and Urinary: Urinary Tract Inflammation/Infection/Trauma
Priority Concepts: Clinical Judgment; Elimination

Answer: 3
Rationale: The infusion of bladder irrigant is not at a preset rate; rather, it is increased or decreased to maintain urine that is a clear, pale yellow color or has just a slight pink tinge. The infusion rate would be increased if the drainage is cherry colored or if clots are seen. Alternatively, the rate can be slowed down slightly if the returns are as clear as water.
Test-Taking Strategy: Note the subject, an indication of an adequate flow rate of CBI. With this in mind, eliminate option 4 because clots are not expected. Eliminate options 1 and 2 that reflect inadequate or excessive irrigation flow, respectively.
Priority Nursing Tip: If the client is receiving an infusion of CBI, use only sterile bladder irrigation solution or the prescribed solution to prevent water intoxication.
Reference: Lewis, S., et al. (2020). *Medical-surgical nursing: Assessment and management of clinical problems* (11th ed., p. 1261). Elsevier.

❖ **226.** The nurse caring for a client with Graves' disease is concerned about the client's calorie intake because of the resulting hypercatabolic state of the disorder. Which situation indicates a successful outcome for this concern?

1. The client verbalizes the need to avoid snacking between meals.
2. The client discusses the relationship between mealtime and the blood glucose level.
3. The client maintains a normal weight or gradually gains weight if it is below normal.
4. The client demonstrates knowledge regarding the need to consume a diet that is high in fat and low in protein.

Level of Cognitive Ability: Evaluating
Client Needs: Physiological Integrity
Clinical Judgment/Cognitive Skills: Evaluate Outcomes
Integrated Process: Clinical Judgment; Nursing Process/Evaluation
Content Area: Adult Health: Endocrine
Health Problems: Adult Health: Endocrine: Thyroid Disorders
Priority Concepts: Hormonal Regulation; Nutrition

Answer: **3**
Rationale: Graves' disease causes a state of chronic nutritional and caloric deficiency caused by the metabolic effects of excessive T3 and T4. Clinical manifestations are weight loss and increased appetite. Therefore, it is a nutritional goal that the client will not lose additional weight and they will gradually return to the ideal body weight, if necessary. To accomplish this, the client must be encouraged to eat frequent high-calorie, high-protein, and high-carbohydrate meals and snacks.
Test-Taking Strategy: Focus on the subject, the client's need to manage their own hypercatabolic state. Eliminate options 1 and 4 as they would not be beneficial for a client in a hypercatabolic state. Option 2 can be eliminated because discussing the fluctuation in the blood glucose level will not be helpful for a client who is hypermetabolic.
Priority Nursing Tip: Provide a high-calorie diet to a client with Graves' disease because of the increased metabolic effects that is characteristic of the disorder.
Reference: Lewis, S., et al. (2020). *Medical-surgical nursing: Assessment and management of clinical problems* (11th ed., p. 1163). Elsevier.

227. The nurse is reviewing the results of a client's phenytoin level that was drawn that morning. The nurse is preparing to discharge once the level is therapeutic. Which result indicates that this goal has been met?

LABORATORY RESULTS

Test and Result	Reference Range
Phenytoin 15 mcg/mL (59.5 mcmol/L)	10 - 20 mcg/mL (40 to 79 mcmol/L)

1. 3 mcg/mL (11.9 mcmol/L)
2. 8 mcg/mL (31.7 mcmol/L)
3. 15 mcg/mL (59.5 mcmol/L)
4. 24 mcg/mL (95.2 mcmol/L)

Level of Cognitive Ability: Evaluating
Client Needs: Physiological Integrity
Clinical Judgment/Cognitive Skills: Evaluate Outcomes
Integrated Process: Clinical Judgment; Nursing Process/Evaluation
Content Area: Pharmacology: Neurologic: Antiseizure
Health Problems: Adult Health: Neurologic: Seizure Disorder/Epilepsy
Priority Concepts: Clinical Judgment; Safety

Answer: **3**
Rationale: The therapeutic range for serum phenytoin levels is 10 to 20 mcg/mL (40 to 79 mcmol/L) in clients with normal serum albumin levels and renal function. A level below this range indicates that the client is not receiving sufficient medication and is at risk for seizure activity. In this case, the medication dose would be adjusted upward. A level above the therapeutic range indicates that the client is entering the toxic range and is at risk for toxic side effects of the medication. In this case, the dose would be adjusted downward.
Test-Taking Strategy: Focus on the subject, the therapeutic drug serum level. Recalling that this level for phenytoin is to 10 to 20 mcg/mL (40 to 79 mcmol/L) will direct you to the correct option.
Priority Nursing Tip: The client prescribed the anticonvulsant phenytoin needs to be informed of the need for monitoring therapeutic serum drug levels to assess for toxicity.
Reference: Kizior, R., & Hodgson, B. (2023). *Saunders Nursing drug handbook 2023* (p. 925). Elsevier.

❖ **228.** The nurse instructs a parent regarding the appropriate actions to take when the toddler has a temper tantrum. Which statement by the parent indicates a successful outcome of the teaching?

1. "I will ignore the tantrums as long as there is no physical danger."
2. "I will give frequent reminders that only bad children have tantrums."
3. "I will send my child to a room alone for 10 minutes after every tantrum."
4. "I will reward my child with candy at the end of each day without a tantrum."

Level of Cognitive Ability: Evaluating
Client Needs: Health Promotion and Maintenance
Clinical Judgment/Cognitive Skills: Evaluate Outcomes
Integrated Process: Nursing Process/Evaluation
Content Area: Developmental Stages: Toddler
Health Problems: N/A
Priority Concepts: Patient Education; Development

Answer: 1
Rationale: Ignoring a negative attention-seeking behavior is considered the best way to extinguish it, provided that the child is safe from injury. Option 2 is untrue and negative. Option 3 gives attention to the tantrum and also exceeds the recommended time of 1 minute per year of age for a time-out. Providing candy for rewards is unhealthy and unlikely to be effective at the end of the day.
Test-Taking Strategy: Focus on the subject, toddler tantrum management. Recalling that ignoring a tantrum is the best way to extinguish it will direct you to the correct option.
Priority Nursing Tip: Anticipate temper tantrums from a toddler. Ensure a safe environment if the toddler displays physical acting-out behaviors.
Reference: McKinney, E. S., et al. (2022). *Maternal child nursing* (6th ed., p. 127). Elsevier.

229. The nurse is caring for a client who is placed in seclusion because of violent behavior. Which client statement indicates to the nurse that the seclusion is no longer necessary?

1. "I am in control of myself now."
2. "I need to use the restroom right away."
3. "I'd like to go back to my room and be alone for a while."
4. "I can't breathe in here. It feels like the walls are closing in on me."

Level of Cognitive Ability: Evaluating
Client Needs: Psychosocial Integrity
Clinical Judgment/Cognitive Skills: Evaluate Outcomes
Integrated Process: Clinical Judgment; Nursing Process/Evaluation
Content Area: Mental Health
Health Problems: Mental Health: Violence
Priority Concepts: Clinical Judgment; Safety

Answer: 1
Rationale: Option 1 indicates that the client may be safely removed from seclusion. The client in seclusion must be assessed at regular intervals (usually every 15 to 30 minutes) for physical needs, safety, and comfort. Option 2 indicates a physical need that could be met with a urinal, bedpan, or commode; it does not indicate that the client has calmed down enough to leave the seclusion room. Option 3 could be an attempt to manipulate the nurse; it gives no indication that the client will control themself when alone in the room. Option 4 could be handled by supportive communication or an as-needed medication, if indicated; it does not necessitate discontinuing seclusion.
Test-Taking Strategy: Focus on the subject, removing a client from seclusion. Recalling the purpose and the use of seclusion will direct you to the correct option.
Priority Nursing Tip: Within 1 hour of the initiation of restraints or seclusion of a client with a mental health disorder, the psychiatrist must make a face-to-face assessment and evaluation of the client. Agency and state policies and procedures regarding the use of restraints and seclusion are always followed.
Reference: Varcarolis, E., & Fosbre, C. (2021). *Essentials of psychiatric mental health nursing: A communication approach to evidence-based care* (4th ed., pp. 383–385). Elsevier.

❖ **230.** The nurse has created a plan of care to include interventions focused on reassuming self-care for a client who is in traction. The nurse evaluates the plan of care and determines that which observation indicates a successful outcome?
1. The client denies a need for assistance with care.
2. The client allows the family to perform the care.
3. The client assists in self-care as much as possible.
4. The client allows the nurse to complete the care on a daily basis.

Level of Cognitive Ability: Evaluating
Client Needs: Physiological Integrity
Clinical Judgment/Cognitive Skills: Evaluate Outcomes
Integrated Process: Clinical Judgment; Nursing Process/Evaluation
Content Area: Adult Health: Musculoskeletal
Health Problems: Adult Health: Musculoskeletal: Skeletal Injury
Priority Concepts: Clinical Judgment; Health Promotion

Answer: 3
Rationale: A successful outcome for reassuming self-care is for the client to do as much of the self-care as possible. The nurse would promote independence in the client and allow the client to perform as much self-care as is optimal considering the client's condition. The nurse would determine that the outcome is unsuccessful if the client refuses care or allows others to perform the care.
Test-Taking Strategy: Focus on the subject, reassuming of self-care. Option 1 can be eliminated first because the client is denying a need for assistance. Eliminate options 2 and 4 that are comparable or alike in that they indicate relying on others to perform care.
Priority Nursing Tip: To maintain self-esteem and client dignity, the nurse would encourage and maintain client independence in the performance of activities of daily living as much as possible.
Reference: Ignatavicius, D., et al. (2021). *Medical-surgical nursing: Concepts for interprofessional collaborative care* (10th ed., pp. 1039–1040). Elsevier.

231. The nurse is monitoring a biologically born male client with a spinal cord injury who is experiencing spinal shock. Which findings indicate that the spinal shock is resolving? **Select all that apply.**
❑ 1. Flaccidity
❑ 2. Presence of a gag reflex
❑ 3. Positive Babinski's reflex
❑ 4. Development of hyperreflexia
❑ 5. Return of the bulbocavernosus reflex
❑ 6. Return of reflex emptying of the bladder

Level of Cognitive Ability: Evaluating
Client Needs: Physiological Integrity
Clinical Judgment/Cognitive Skills: Evaluate Outcomes
Integrated Process: Clinical Judgment; Nursing Process/Evaluation
Content Area: Adult Health: Neurologic
Health Problems: Adult Health: Neurologic: Spinal Cord Injury
Priority Concepts: Intracranial Regulation; Mobility

Answer: 3, 4, 5, 6
Rationale: Spinal shock is associated with acute injury to the spinal cord with temporary suppression of reflexes controlled by segments below the level of injury. It may last for 1 to 6 weeks. Indications that spinal shock is resolving include return of reflexes, development of hyperreflexia rather than flaccidity, and return of reflex emptying of the bladder. The return of the bulbocavernosus reflex in biologically born male clients is also an early indicator of recovery from spinal shock. Babinski's reflex (dorsiflexion of the great toe with fanning of the other toes when the sole of the foot is stroked) is an early returning reflex. The gag reflex is not lost in spinal shock; therefore, its presence is not an indication of resolving spinal shock.
Test-Taking Strategy: Focus on the subject, indications that spinal shock is resolving. As you read each option, recall that spinal shock is associated with acute injury to the spinal cord with temporary suppression of reflexes controlled by segments below the level of injury. This will assist in eliminating flaccidity and the presence of a gag reflex as signs that spinal shock is resolving.
Priority Nursing Tip: For clients with spinal cord injuries above the level of T6, autonomic dysreflexia may occur as a result of autonomic nervous system overstimulation. The clinical manifestations include severe hypertension, throbbing headaches, diaphoresis, nasal stuffiness, flushing above the level of the injury, and bradycardia.
Reference: Heuther, S., McCance, K., & Brashers, V. (2020). *Understanding pathophysiology* (7th ed., pp. 376, 389–390). Elsevier.

❖ **232.** The nurse is monitoring a client on mechanical ventilation via an oral endotracheal tube. Which of the following would be indicative of possible causes of the high-pressure alarm sounding? **Select all that apply.**

❑ 1. A kink in the tube
❑ 2. The client fighting the ventilator
❑ 3. Increased secretions in the airway
❑ 4. A cuff leak in the endotracheal tube
❑ 5. The client biting on the endotracheal tube
❑ 6. The ventilator tubing disconnecting from the endotracheal tube

Level of Cognitive Ability: Evaluating
Client Needs: Physiological Integrity
Clinical Judgment/Cognitive Skills: Recognize Cues
Integrated Process: Clinical Judgment; Nursing Process/Evaluation
Content Area: Complex Care: Mechanical Ventilation
Health Problems: Adult Health: Respiratory: Artificial Airways
Priority Concepts: Clinical Judgment; Gas Exchange

Answer: 1, 2, 3, 5

Rationale: The high-pressure alarm sounds when the peak inspiratory pressure reaches the set alarm limit. Causes include obstruction of the endotracheal tube because of the client lying on the tube or water or a kink in the tubing; the client being anxious or fighting the ventilator; an increased amount of secretions in the airways or a mucous plug; the client coughing, gagging, or biting on the oral endotracheal tube; decreased airway size related to wheezing or bronchospasm; pneumothorax; and displacement of the artificial airway and the endotracheal tube slipping into the right main stem bronchus. The low-pressure alarm sounds when there is a leak or disconnection in the ventilator circuit or a leak in the client's artificial airway cuff.

Test-Taking Strategy: Focus on the subject, the triggers of the high-pressure alarm. Recalling that the high-pressure alarm sounds when the peak inspiratory pressure reaches the set alarm limit assists in eliminating options 4 and 6. In addition, remember that "L" in "low" can be associated with "L" in "leak" for low-pressure alarms.

Priority Nursing Tip: The nurse never shuts the alarms on a ventilator to the off position.

Reference: Ignatavicius, D., et al. (2021). *Medical-surgical nursing: Concepts for interprofessional collaborative care* (10th ed., p. 603). Elsevier.

233. The clinic nurse is observing a student perform a complete physical assessment on a client. During the respiratory assessment, the clinic nurse determines that the student is performing which physical assessment technique correctly? **Refer to figure.**

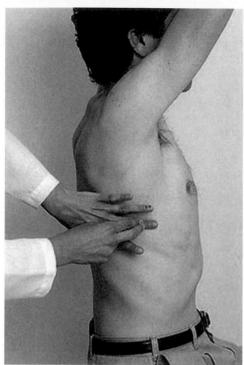

(From Wilson, S. F., & Giddens, J. F. [2013]. *Health assessment for nursing practice* [5th ed.] Mosby.)

1. Palpation
2. Inspection
3. Percussion
4. Auscultation

Level of Cognitive Ability: Evaluating
Client Needs: Health Promotion and Maintenance
Clinical Judgment/Cognitive Skills: Evaluate Outcomes
Integrated Process: Clinical Judgment; Nursing Process/Evaluation
Content Area: Health Assessment/Physical Exam: General Assessment Techniques
Health Problems: N/A
Priority Concepts: Gas Exchange; Health Promotion

Answer: 3
Rationale: To perform percussion, the nurse places the middle finger of the nondominant hand against the body's surface. The tip of the middle finger of the dominant hand strikes the top of the middle finger of the nondominant hand. Palpation is performed using the sense of touch. Inspection is the process of observation. Auscultation involves listening to the sounds produced by the body.
Test-Taking Strategy: Focus on the **subject**, identifying assessment techniques. Recalling the definition of each technique listed in the options will direct you to the correct option. Remember that inspection is observing, palpation uses the sense of touch, and auscultating is listening.
Priority Nursing Tip: When auscultating breath sounds, instruct the client to breathe through the mouth. Monitor the client for dizziness and provide a rest period if dizziness occurs.
Reference: Jarvis, C. (2020). *Physical examination and health assessment* (8th ed., pp. 113–114). Elsevier.

❖ **234.** The nurse is reviewing a plan of care prepared by a nursing student for an infant being admitted to the hospital with a diagnosis of congestive heart failure. Which intervention would the nurse recognize as needing revision?
1. Elevate the head of the bed.
2. Provide oxygen during stressful periods.
3. Limit the time that the infant is allowed to bottle-feed.
4. Wake the infant for feedings to ensure adequate nutrition.

Level of Cognitive Ability: Evaluating
Client Needs: Physiological Integrity
Clinical Judgment/Cognitive Skills: Evaluate Outcomes
Integrated Process: Clinical Judgment; Nursing Process/Evaluation
Content Area: Pediatrics: Cardiovascular
Health Problems: Pediatric-Specific: Congestive Heart Failure
Priority Concepts: Development; Perfusion

Answer: 4
Rationale: Awaking the child is not therapeutic in this situation. Measures that will decrease the workload on the heart include limiting the time that the infant is allowed to bottle-feed or breast-/chest-feed, elevating the head of the bed, allowing for uninterrupted rest periods, and providing oxygen during stressful periods.
Test-Taking Strategy: Focus on the subject, the intervention that needs revision. This asks you to select an incorrect measure. Review each option carefully, and recall that the goal for an infant with congestive heart failure is to decrease the workload on the heart. The correct option is the only one that will not ensure this goal.
Priority Nursing Tip: An early sign of congestive heart failure in an infant is tachycardia, especially during rest or with slight exertion.
Reference: Hockenberry, M., Wilson, D., & Rodgers, C. (2019). *Wong's Nursing care of infants and children* (11th ed., pp. 967, 975). Elsevier.

235. The nurse has provided self-care activity instructions to a client after the insertion of an internal cardioverter-defibrillator (ICD). The nurse determines that there is a **need for further teaching** if the client makes which statement?
1. "I need to avoid doing anything where there would be rough contact with the ICD insertion site."
2. "I can perform activities and operate heavy equipment such as my lawn mower or tractor as I need to."
3. "I need to try to avoid doing strenuous things that would make my heart rate go up to or above the rate cut-off on the ICD."
4. "I need to keep away from electromagnetic sources such as transformers, large electrical generators, and metal detectors, as well as running motors."

Level of Cognitive Ability: Evaluating
Client Needs: Safe and Effective Care Environment
Clinical Judgment/Cognitive Skills: Evaluate Outcomes
Integrated Process: Clinical Judgment; Nursing Process/Evaluation
Content Area: Adult Health: Cardiovascular
Health Problems: Adult Health: Cardiovascular: Dysrhythmias
Priority Concepts: Patient Education; Perfusion

Answer: 2
Rationale: Postdischarge instructions typically include avoiding the following: tight clothing or belts over the ICD insertion site; rough contact with the ICD insertion site; electromagnetic fields, such as those surrounding electrical transformers; radio, television, and radar transmitters; metal detectors; and the running motors of cars or boats. Clients must also alert health care providers or dentists to the presence of the device because certain procedures such as diathermy, electrocautery, and magnetic resonance imaging may need to be avoided to prevent device malfunction. Clients need to follow the specific advice of the cardiologist regarding activities that are potentially hazardous to the self or others, such as operating heavy equipment.
Test-Taking Strategy: Note the strategic words, *need for further teaching,* and that this indicates a negative event query. Options 1 and 3 can be eliminated because they are comparable or alike to standard post–pacemaker insertion instructions. From the remaining choices, noting the words *heavy equipment* will direct you to the correct option.
Priority Nursing Tip: The nurse who is caring for the client after insertion of an ICD needs to assess the device settings. Care is similar to that implemented after insertion of a permanent pacemaker.
Reference: Lewis, S., et al. (2020). *Medical-surgical nursing: Assessment and management of clinical problems* (11th ed., p. 771). Elsevier.

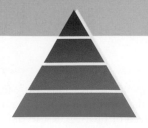

References

American Academy of Pediatrics. (2023). *Car seats: Information for families*. Retrieved from https://www.healthychildren.org/English/safety-prevention/on-thego/Pages/Car-Safety-Seats-Information-for-Families.aspx.

American Heart Association. (2020). *Highlights of the 2020 American Heart Association Guidelines for CPR and ECC* (p. 11). Hghlghts_2020_ECC_Guidelines_English.pdf.

Ard, K., & Makadon, H. (2016). *Improving the health care of lesbian, gay, bisexual and transgender (LGBT) people: Understanding and eliminating health disparities*. https://www.lgbthealtheducation.org/wp-content/uploads/Improving-the-Health-of-LGBT-People.pdf.

Ball, J., et al. (2019). *Seidel's Guide to physical examination: An interprofessional approach* (9th ed.). Elsevier.

Bandura, A. (1997). *Self-efficacy: The exercise of control*. New York: W.H. Freeman and Company.

Bandura, A. (1977). *Social learning theory*. Upper Saddle River, NJ: Pearson Prentice Hall.

Burchum, J., & Rosenthal, L. (2019). *Lehne's Pharmacology for nursing care* (10th ed). Elsevier.

Burchum, J., & Rosenthal, L. (2022). *Lehne's Pharmacology for nursing care* (11th ed.). Elsevier.

Centers for Disease Control and Prevention (CDC). (2020). *Coronavirus (COVID-19)*. Retrieved from https://www.cdc.gov/coronavirus/2019-ncov/index.html.

Centers for Disease Control and Prevention (CDC). (2019). *Isolation precautions*. Retrieved from https://www.cdc.gov/infectioncontrol/guidelines/isolation/index.html.

Centers for Disease Control and Prevention (CDC). (2021). *2020 National and State Healthcare-Associated Infections Progress Report*. Retrieved from https://www.cdc.gov/hai/data/archive/2020-HAI-progress-report.html.

Centers for Disease Control and Prevention (CDC). (2022). *When and how to wash hands*. Retrieved from https://www.cdc.gov/features/handwashing/index.html.

Dickison, P., Haerling, K. A., & Lasater, K. (2019). Integrating the National Council of State Boards of Nursing Clinical Judgment Model into nursing educational frameworks. *Journal of Nursing Education, 58*(2), 72–78.

Dorlands's Illustrated Medical Dictionary (33rd ed.) (2020). Elsevier.

Federal Emergency Management Agency (n.d.). *Official website of the United States Government*. http://fema.gov/.

Foster, K., et al. (2021). *Mental health in nursing: Theory and practice for clinical settings* (5th ed.). Elsevier.

Gahart, B., Nazareno, A., & Ortega, M. (2021). *Gahart's 2021 Intravenous medications: A handbook for nurses and health professionals* (37th ed.). Elsevier.

Giger, J., & Haddad, L. (2021). *Transcultural nursing: Assessment and intervention* (8th ed.). Elsevier.

Grodner, M., Escott-Stump, S., & Dorner, S. (2020). *Nutritional foundations and clinical applications* (7th ed.). Elsevier.

Henry, J., & Kaiser Family Foundation. (2017). *Key facts about the uninsured population*. Retrieved from https://www.kff.org/uninsured/fact-sheet/key-facts-about-the-uninsured-population/.

Heuther, S., McCance, K., & Brashers, V. (2020). *Understanding pathophysiology* (7th ed.). Elsevier.

Hockenberry, M., Wilson, D., & Rodgers, C. (2019). *Wong's Nursing care of infants and children* (11th ed.). Elsevier.

iPledge. (2021). *What is the iPLEDGE® REMS (Risk Evaluation and Mitigation Strategy)?*. Retrieved from https://www.ipledgeprogram.com.

Ignatavicius, D., et al. (2021). *Medical-surgical nursing: Concepts for interprofessional collaborative care* (10th ed.). Elsevier.

International Association for the Study of Pain, (n.d.). *IASP's 50th Anniversary: Working together for pain relief throughout the world*. Retrieved from https://www.iasp-pain.org.

Issues in Science and Technology. (n.d.). *Correctional health is community health*. Retrieved from https://issues.org/correctional-health-is-community-health/.

Jarvis, C. (2020). *Physical examination and health assessment* (8th ed.). Elsevier.

Kizior, R., & Hodgson, B. (2022). *Saunders Nursing drug handbook 2022*. Elsevier.

Kizior, R., & Hodgson, B. (2023). *Saunders Nursing drug handbook 2023*. Elsevier.

Lewis, S., et al. (2020). *Medical-surgical nursing: Assessment and management of clinical problems* (11th ed.). Elsevier.

Lewis, S., et al. (2023). *Medical-surgical nursing: Assessment and management of clinical problems* (12th ed.). Elsevier.

Lilley, L., Rainforth Collins, S., & Snyder, J. (2020). *Pharmacology and the nursing process* (9th ed.). Elsevier.

Lowdermilk, D., et al. (2020). *Maternity & women's health care* (12th ed.). Elsevier.

McKinney, E. S., et al. (2022). *Maternal child nursing* (6th ed.). Elsevier.

MD+Calc. (2005-2023). *Parkland Formula for burns*. https://www.mdcalc.com/parkland-formula-for-burns.

Murray, S., et al. (2019). *Foundations of maternal-newborn and women's health nursing* (7th ed.). Elsevier.

National Center for Complementary and Integrative Health. (2023). *Herbs at a glance*. Retrieved from https://nccih.nih.gov/health/herbsataglance.

National Council of State Boards of Nursing. (2023). *Next Generation NCLEX® NCLEX-RN® test plan*. National Council of State Boards of Nursing. Retrieved from http://www.ncsbn.org.

National Council of State Boards of Nursing. (2021). *Next Generation NCLEX News* at https://www.ncsbn.org/NGN_Summer21_Eng.pdf.

National Council of State Boards of Nursing. (2021). *Braving new pathways: Leading the way for regulatory transformation*. 2021 NCSBN Annual Meeting.

National Council of State Boards of Nursing. (2021). *Next Generation NCLEX News*. Retrieved from https://www.ncsbn.org/NGN_Summer21_Eng.pdf

National Domestic Violence Hotline. https://www.thehotline.org. 1-800-799-SAFE (7233).

Nix, S. (2022). *Williams' Basic nutrition and diet therapy* (16th ed.). Elsevier.

Pagana, K., Pagana, T., & Pagana, T. N. (2021). *Mosby's Diagnostic and laboratory test reference* (15th ed.). Elsevier.

Petersen, E., Betts, J., & Muntean, W. (2020). *Next Generation NCLEX® (NGN) Webinar*. Chicago: NCSBN.

Potter, P., et al. (2021). *Fundamentals of nursing* (10th ed.). Elsevier.

Potter, P., et al. (2023). *Fundamentals of nursing* (11th ed.). Elsevier.

ProEdit. (2019). *Understanding Bloom's (and Anderson and Krathwohl's) Taxonomy*. Retrieved from https://proedit.com/understanding-blooms-and-anderson-and-krathwohls-taxonomy/.

Skidmore-Roth, L. (2021). *2021 Mosby's Nursing drug reference* (34th ed.). Elsevier.

Skidmore-Roth, L. (2022). *2022 Mosby's Nursing drug reference* (35th ed.). Elsevier.

Sleep Foundation. (2023). *Better sleep for a better you*. Retrieved from https://sleepfoundation.org.

StopBullying.gov (n.d.). *Prevention: Learn how to identify bullying and stand up to it safely*. Retrieved from http://www.stopbullying.gov.

Sweet, V., & Foley, P. (2020). *Sheehy's Emergency nursing: Principles and practice* (7th ed.). Elsevier.

Touhy, T., & Jett, K. (2022). *Ebersole and Hess' Gerontological nursing & healthy aging* (6th ed.). Elsevier.

Traditional Chinese Medicine World Foundation (n.d.). *TCM healing modalities*. https://www.tcmworld.org/what-is-tcm/healing-modalities/.

United Ostomy Associations of America (n.d.). Retrieved from https://www.uoaa.org.

Urden, L., Stacy, K., & Lough, M. (2022). *Critical care nursing: Diagnosis and management* (9th ed.). Elsevier.

Urden, L., Stacy, K., & Lough, M. (2020). *Priorities in critical care nursing* (8th ed.). Elsevier.

U.S. Department of Health and Human Resources (n.d.). *Child welfare information Gateway*. Retrieved from https://www.childwelfare.gov.

Varcarolis, E., & Fosbre, C. (2021). *Essentials of psychiatric mental health nursing: A communication approach to evidence-based care* (4th ed.). Elsevier.

WebMD. (2005-2023). *Senna tablet laxatives: Uses, side effects, and more*. Retrieved from http://www.webmd.com/drugs/2/drug-1557/senna-oral/details.

Zerwekh, J., & Zerwekh Garneau, A. (2021). *Nursing today: Transition and trends* (10th ed.). Elsevier.